ABDOMINAL-PELVIC MRI

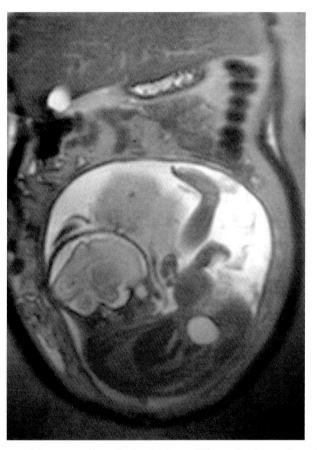

He who sees things grow from the beginning will have the finest view of them.
—*Aristotle*

ABDOMINAL-PELVIC MRI

Richard C. Semelka, M.D.

Director, Magnetic Resonance Services
Professor and Vice Chairman,
Department of Radiology
University of North Carolina at Chapel Hill

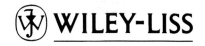

A JOHN WILEY & SONS, INC., PUBLICATION

Cover Concept: Sharon Casey
Cover Illustration: Diane Armao (redrawn after Erich Lepier)

This book is printed on acid-free paper. ⊗

For ordering and customer service information please call 1-800-CALL-WILEY.

Library of Congress Cataloging-in-Publication Data:

Semelka, Richard C.
    Abdomino-pelvic MR / Richard C. Semelka.
       p. ; cm.
    Includes bibliographical references and index.
    ISBN 0-471-41476-X (cloth : alk. paper)
      1. Abdomen—Magnetic resonance imaging.   2. Pelvis—Magnetic resonance imaging.
    3. Abdomen—Magnetic resonance imaging—Atlases.   4. Pelvis—Magnetic resonance imaging—Atlases.   I. Title.
      [DNLM: 1. Abdomen—pathology.   2. Digestive System Diseases—diagnosis.
    3. Magnetic Resonance Imaging.   4. Pelvis—pathology.   WI 900 S471a 2002]
    RC944.S46   2002
    617.5′507548—dc21   2001026773

Printed in the United States of America.

10 9 8 7 6 5 4 3 2

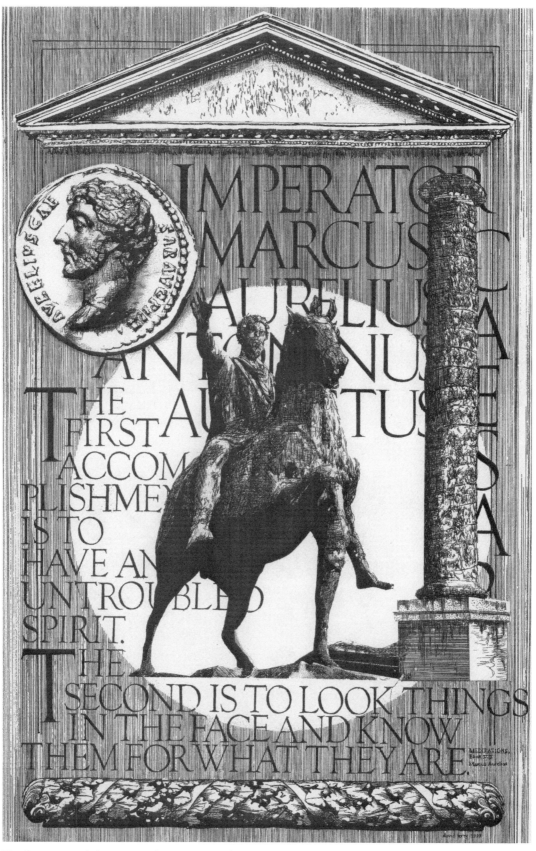

The first accomplishment is to have an untroubled spirit. The second is to look things in the face and know them for what they are.

—*Marcus Aurelius*

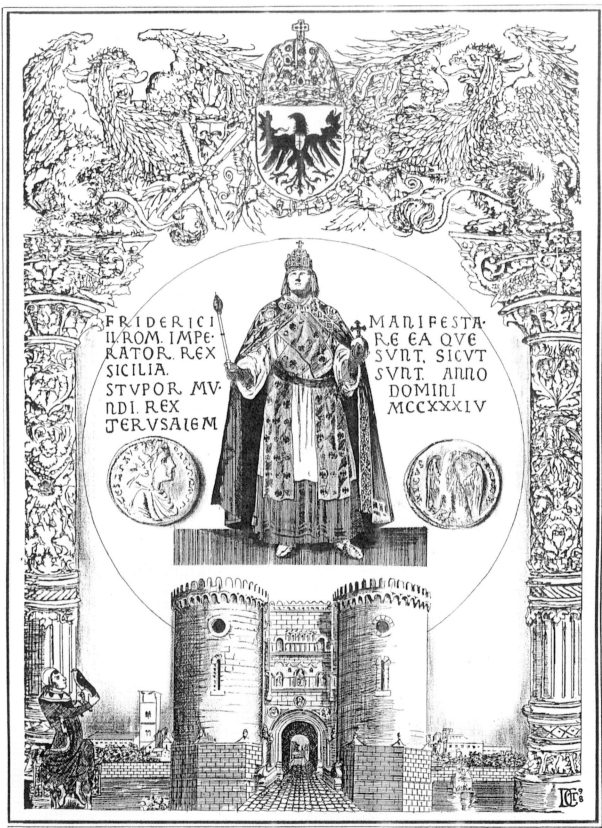

FRIDERICI
II.ROM. IMPE-
RATOR. REX
SICILIA.
STVPOR MV-
NDI. REX
JERVSAIEM

MANIFESTA-
RE EA QVE
SVNT. SICVT
SVNT. ANNO
DOMINI
MCCXXXIV

Manifestare ea qve svnt, sicvt svnt (To show things that are as they are).
—*Frederick II*

CONTENTS

PREFACE

The purpose of this book is to provide a clear and balanced text and atlas comprehensively describing disorders of the abdomen and pelvis imaged by MRI. Modern diagnostic MRI is based upon the fundamental principles of high image quality and reproducibility, conspicuity of disease, and comprehensive imaging information. These objectives are consistently met using short duration sequences in various planes with contrast administration. In MRI, the process of seeing and discriminating between diseases is largely via pattern recognition in the context of imaging sequences. This pattern recognition approach is emphasized throughout the text. Although this book is richly illustrated, showing T1, T2, early and late post gadolinium contrast appearances, emphasis is placed on an understanding of the morphological characteristics and pathologic criteria necessary to assess and diagnose disease. In this regard, pathologic descriptions and fundamental MR appearances on T1- and T2-weighted and contrast enhanced images are enduring, whereas particular imaging sequences become outmoded and change with time. Therefore, clinical-pathologic correlation is stressed and incorporated into the discussion of many disorders. New modifications of MR sequences are described but not emphasized.

The sweeping changes that have occurred in medicine over the past several years have added great pressure to the subspecialty fields, including radiology. While government and patients demand continued use of highly technologic diagnostic tests, reduced examination time and cost containment are held at a premium. In this book, we stress the importance of achieving reproducible, consistently sound image quality. We encourage the development and dissemination of imaging protocols in order to increase their standardization and use in body MR. This effort may result in earlier diagnosis and earlier appropriate patient management which would translate into health care savings.

In conclusion, much like a painting, MRI is a visual document. It creates a picture and tells a story that is unique for each patient. This book is dedicated to all those patients whose stories lie within, and their physicians, devoted to their care.

ACKNOWLEDGMENTS

The authors would like to acknowledge Hedvig Hricak, M.D., Ph.D., Susan M. Ascher, M.D., Caroline Reinhold, M.D., Charles B. Higgins, M.D., Alexander R. Margulis, M.D., Joseph K. T. Lee, M.D., Milton Lautatzis, M.D., Donald G. Mitchell, M.D., J. Patrick Shoenut, B.Sc., Howard M. Greenberg, M.D., and our referring physicians for their support.

RICHARD C. SEMELKA, M.D.

CONTRIBUTORS

DIANE ARMAO, M.D., Research Associate, Departments of Radiology and Pathology, University of North Carolina, Chapel Hill, North Carolina

SUSAN M. ASCHER, M.D., Professor, Department of Radiology, Director, Division of Abdominal Imaging, Georgetown University Hospital, Washington, DC

TILL R. BADER, M.D., Clinical Research Fellow in Magnetic Resonance Imaging, University of North Carolina, Chapel Hill, North Carolina. Associate Professor, Department of Radiology, University of Vienna, Vienna, Austria

N. CEM BALCI, M.D., Department of Radiology, Florence Nightingale Hospital, Istanbul, Turkey

DEBORAH A. BAUMGARTEN, M.D., Assistant Professor Emory University Hospital, The Emory Clinic and Grady Memorial Hospital, Atlanta, Georgia

KIMBERLY L. BEAVERS, M.D., Clinical Instructor, Department of Medicine, Division of Digestive Diseases, University of North Carolina, Chapel Hill, North Carolina

LARISSA BRAGA, M.D., Clinical Research Fellow in Magnetic Resonance Imaging, University of North Carolina, Chapel Hill, North Carolina. Post-Graduation Program, University of Sao Paulo, Brazil. Supported by CAPES, Brasilia, Brazil

ELIZABETH DENNY BROWN, M.D., Greensboro Radiology, P.A., Greensboro, North Carolina

HECTOR COOPER, M.D., Abdominal Imaging Fellow, Department of Radiology, University of North Carolina, Chapel Hill, North Carolina

LARA B. EISENBERG, M.D., Director of CT and Body MRI Services, Suburban Hospital, Bethesda, Maryland

NIKOLAOS L. KELEKIS, M.D., Assistant Professor of Radiology, General Regional Hospital of Larissa, University of Thessalia, Larissa, Greece

RAHEL A. KUBIK-HUCH, PD DR. MED., Institute of Diagnostic Radiology, University Hospital Zurich, Zurich, Switzerland

HANI B. MARCOS, M.D., Imaging Sciences Program, Diagnostic Radiology Department, Clinical Center, National Institutes of Health, Bethesda, Maryland

DIEGO R. MARTIN, M.D., PH.D., F.R.C.P. (C), Head of Abdominal Imaging, Director MR Imaging, Associate Professor, Department of Radiology, Robert C. Byrd Health Sciences Center, Morgantown, West Virginia

SVEN CLAUDE ANDRÉ MICHEL M.D., Institute of Diagnostic Radiology, University Hospital Zurich, Zurich, Switzerland

TOMOFUMI MOTOHARA, M.D., Research Fellow, Abdominal Magnetic Resonance Imaging Section, Department of Radiology, University of North Carolina, Chapel Hill, North Carolina. Instructor, Department of Radiology, Shimane Medical University, Izumo, Japan.

LARISSA L. NAGASE, M.D., Clinical Research Fellow in Magnetic Resonance Imaging, Department of Radiology, University of North Carolina, Chapel Hill, North Carolina

TARA C. NOONE, M.D., Assistant Professor, Director of Magnetic Resonance Imaging, Department of Radiology, Medical University of South Carolina, Charleston, South Carolina

ERIC K. OUTWATER, M.D., Professor of Radiology, University of Arizona, Tucson, Arizona

MONICA S. PEDRO, M.D., Clinical Research Fellow in Magnetic Resonance Imaging, University of North Carolina, Chapel Hill, North Carolina

CAROLINE REINHOLD, M.D., Associate Professor of Radiology, Gastroenterology & Gynecology, Director, MRI, Director, Fellowship Program, Department of Radiology, Montreal General Hospital, Montreal, PQ, Canada

RICHARD C. SEMELKA, M.D., Professor of Radiology, Director, Magnetic Resonance Services, Vice Chair of Research, Department of Radiology, University of North Carolina, Chapel Hill, North Carolina

EVAN S. SIEGELMAN, M.D., Associate Professor of Radiology, Section Chief: Body MRI, Department of Radiology, University of Pennsylvania Medical Center, Philadelphia, Pennsylvania

SHAMBHAVI VENKATARAMAN, M.B.B.S., M.R.C.P. (UK), Clinical Research Fellow in Magnetic Resonance Imaging, Department of Radiology, University of North Carolina, Chapel Hill, North Carolina

KATHY P. WILBER, R.T., Research Associate, Department of Radiology, University of North Carolina, Chapel Hill, North Carolina

ABDOMINAL-PELVIC MRI

CHAPTER 1

DIAGNOSTIC APPROACH TO PROTOCOLING AND INTERPRETING MR STUDIES OF THE ABDOMEN AND PELVIS

RICHARD C. SEMELKA, M.D., KATHY P. WILBER, R.T., AND LARISSA BRAGA, M.D.

High image quality, reproducibility of image quality, and good conspicuity of disease require the use of sequences that are robust and reliable and avoid artifacts [1–5]. Maximizing these principles to achieve high-quality diagnostic MR images usually requires the use of fast scanning techniques, with the overall intention of generating images with consistent image quality that demonstrate consistent display of disease processes. The important goal of shorter examination time may also be achieved with the same principles that maximize diagnostic quality. With the decrease of imaging times for individual sequences, a variety of sequences may be employed to take advantage of the major strength of MRI, which is comprehensive information on disease processes.

Respiration and bowel peristalsis are the major artifacts that have lessened the reproducibility of MRI. Breathing-independent sequences and breath-hold sequences form the foundation of high-quality MRI studies of the abdomen. Breathing artifact is less problematic in the pelvis, and high-spatial and contrast-resolution imaging have been the mainstay for maximizing image quality for pelvis studies.

Disease conspicuity depends on the principle of maximizing the difference in signal intensities between diseased tissues and the background tissue. For disease processes situated within or adjacent to fat, this is readily performed by manipulating the signal intensity of fat, which can range from low to high in signal intensity on both T1-weighted and T2-weighted images. For example, diseases that are low in signal intensity on T1-weighted images, such as peritoneal fluid or retroperitoneal fibrosis, are most conspicuous on T1-weighted sequences in which fat is high in signal intensity (i.e., sequences without fat suppression). Conversely, diseases that are high in signal intensity, such as subacute blood or proteinaceous fluid, are more conspicuous if fat is rendered low in signal intensity with the use of fat suppression techniques. On T2-weighted images, diseases that are low in signal intensity, such as fibrous tissue, are most conspicuous on sequences in which background fat is high in signal intensity, such as echo-train spin-echo sequences. Diseases that are moderate to high in signal intensity, such as lymphadenopathy or ascites, are most conspicuous on sequences in which fat signal intensity is low, such as fat-suppressed sequences.

Gadolinium chelate enhancement may be routinely useful because it provides at least two further imaging properties that facilitate detection and characterization of disease, specifically the pattern of blood delivery (i.e., capillary enhancement) and the size and/or rapidity of drainage of the interstitial space (i.e., interstitial enhancement) [6]. Capillary-phase image acquisition is achieved by using a short-duration sequence initiated immediately after gadolinium injection. Spoiled gradient-echo (SGE) sequence, performed as multisection acquisition, is an ideal sequence to use for capillary phase imaging. The majority of focal mass lesions are best evaluated in the capillary phase of enhancement, particularly lesions that do not distort the margins of the organs in which they are located (e.g., focal liver, spleen, or pancreatic lesions). Images acquired 1.5–10 min after contrast administration are in the interstitial phase of enhancement with the optimal window being 2–5 min postcontrast. Diseases that are superficial, spreading, or inflammatory in nature are generally well shown on interstitial phase images. The concomittant use of fat suppression serves to increase the conspicuity of disease processes characterized by increased enhancement on interstitial phase images including peritoneal metastases, cholangiocarcinoma, ascending cholangitis, inflammatory bowel disease, and abscesses [7, 8].

The great majority of diseases can be characterized by defining their appearance on T1, T2, and early and late postgadolinium images. Throughout this text the combination of these four parameters for the evaluation of abdomino-pelvic disease will be stressed.

T1-WEIGHTED SEQUENCES

T1-weighted sequences are routinely useful for investigating diseases of the abdomen, and they supplement T2-weighted images for investigating disease of the pelvis. The primary information that precontrast T1-weighted images provide includes 1) information on abnormally increased fluid content or fibrous tissue content that appears low in signal intensity on T1-weighted images and 2) information on the presence of subacute blood or concentrated protein, which are both high in signal intensity. T1-weighted sequences obtained without fat suppression also demonstrate the presence of fat as high-signal intensity tissue. The routine use of an additional fat attenuating technique permits reliable characterization of fatty lesions.

Spoiled Gradient-Echo (SGE) Sequences

SGE sequences are the most important and versatile sequences for studying abdominal disease. They provide true T1-weighted imaging and, with the use of phased-array multicoil imaging, may be used to replace longer duration sequences such as the T1-weighted spin-echo (SE) sequence. Image parameters for SGE are (1) relatively long repetition time (TR) (approximately 150 ms) to maximize signal-to-noise ratio and the number of sections that can be acquired in one multisection acquisition and (2) the shortest in-phase echo time (TE)

(approximately 6.0 ms at 1.0 T and 4.2–4.5 ms at 1.5 T) to maximize signal-to-noise ratio and the number of sections per acquisition [2]. For routine T1-weighted images, in-phase TE may be preferable to the shorter out-of-phase echo times (4.0 ms at 1.0 T and 2.2–2.4 ms at 1.5 T), to avoid both phase-cancellation artifact around the borders of organs and fat-water phase cancellation in tissues containing both fat and water protons. Flip angle should be approximately 70–90° to maximize T1-weighted information. With the use of the body coil, the signal-to-noise ratio of SGE sequences is usually suboptimal with section thickness less than 8 mm, whereas with the phased-array multicoil, section thickness of 5 mm results in diagnostically adequate images. On new MRI machines more than 22 sections may be acquired in a 20-s breath-hold.

An important feature of the multisection acquisition of SGE is that the central phase encoding steps (which determine the bulk signal in the image) are acquired over 6 s for both the entire data set and each individual section. Thereby the data acquisition is sufficiently short for the entire data set to isolate a distinct phase of enhancement (e.g., hepatic arterial dominant phase) while at the same time the data acquisition of each individual section is sufficiently long to compensate for slight variations in patient cardiac output, peak lesion enhancement, and injection technique.

In addition to its use as precontrast T1-weighted images, SGE should be routinely used for capillary-phase image acquisition after gadolinium administration for investigation of the liver, spleen, pancreas, and kidneys. SGE may also be modified as a single-shot technique using the minimum TR to achieve breathing-independent images for noncooperative patients.

SGE sequences can be performed as three-dimensional (3D) acquisition, which can be used both for volumetric imaging of organs such as the liver and for pre- and postgadolinium administration. Gadolinium-enhanced 3D gradient-echo sequences also are the most clinically effective techniques for MR angiography (MRA) of the body (see Chapter 10, *Retroperitoneum and Body Wall*).

Fat-Suppressed SGE Sequences

Fat-suppressed (FS) SGE sequences are routinely used as precontrast images for evaluating the pancreas and for the detection of subacute blood. Image parameters are similar to those for standard SGE; however, it is advantageous to employ a lower out-of-phase echo time (2.2–2.5 ms at 1.5 T), which benefits from additional fat-attenuating effects and also increases signal-to-noise ratio and the number of sections per acquisition. On state-of-the-art MRI machines fat-suppressed SGE may acquire 22 sections in a 20-s breath-hold with reproducible uniform fat suppression.

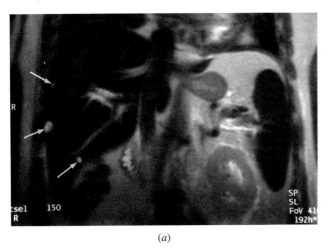

(a)

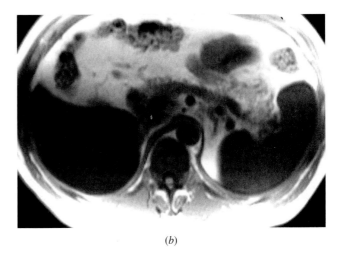

(b)

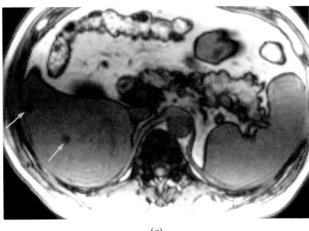

(c)

FIG. 1.1 Iron effects. Coronal T2-weighted single-shot echo train spin echo (a), TE = 4 ms in-phase (b), and TE = 2 ms out-of-phase (c) sequences. Iron in the reticuloendothelial system from transfusional siderosis results in low signal of the liver and spleen on T2-weighted images (a). The liver and spleen are low signal on the longer TE in-phase sequence (b) and increase in signal on the shorter TE out-of-phase (c) sequence because of decreasing susceptibility effects on the shorter TE sequence. Note the excellent conspicuity of small liver cysts on the T2-weighted image (arrows, a). The high fluid content of cysts in a background of iron-deposited liver renders them very high in signal. On T1-weighted images, the low signal of cysts results in no signal difference from liver on the TE = 4 ms in-phase sequence because of the concurrent low signal of liver. On the TE = 2 ms sequence, liver becomes higher in signal and the cysts are visible (arrows, c).

Fat-suppressed SGE images are used to acquire interstitial-phase gadolinium-enhanced images. The complementary roles of gadolinium enhancement, which generally increases the signal intensity of disease tissue, and fat suppression, which diminishes the competing high signal intensity of background fat, are particularly effective at maximizing conspicuity of diseased tissue. The principle of maximizing signal difference between diseased tissue and background tissue is achieved in the majority of MRI examinations with this approach.

If fat-suppressed SGE sequences cannot be performed on an MRI system, then fat-suppressed SE sequences can be substituted, with little loss of diagnostic information.

Out-of-Phase SGE Sequences

Out-of-phase (opposed-phase) SGE images are useful for demonstrating diseased tissue in which fat and water protons are present within the same voxel. A TE of 2 ms is advisable at 1.5 T, and 4 ms is advisable at 1.0 T. A TE of 6 ms is also out of phase at 1.5 T, but the shorter TE of 2 ms is preferable because more sections can be acquired per sequence acquisition, signal is higher, the

sequence is more T1 weighted, there is lesser problems with magnetic susceptibility, and in combination with a T2-weighted sequence, it is easier to distinguish fat and iron in the liver. At TE = 6 ms both fat and iron in the liver result in signal loss relative to the TE = 4 in-phase sequence, whereas on TE = 2 out-of-phase sequences fat is darker and iron is brighter relative to TE = 4, facilitating their distinction (fig. 1.1). The most common indications for an out-of-phase sequence are the detection of the presence of fat within the liver and the detection of lipid within adrenal masses to characterize them as adenomas. Another useful feature is that the generation of a phase-cancellation artifact around high-signal intensity masses, located in water-based tissues, confirms that these lesions are fatty. Examples of this include angiomyolipomas of the kidney and ovarian dermoids. In addition to out-of-phase effects, the different TE, for the out-of-phase sequence compared to the in-phase sequence, provides information on magnetic susceptibility effects, which increase with increase in TE. This can be used to distinguish iron-containing structures (e.g., surgical clips, gamna gandy bodies in the spleen) from nonmagnetic signal void structures (e.g., calcium). To illustrate this point, the signal void susceptibility artifact from surgical clips increase in size, from a shorter TE (e.g., 2 ms) out-of-phase sequence to a longer TE (e.g., 4 ms) in-phase sequence, whereas the signal void from calcium remains unchanged.

Magnetization-Prepared Rapid-Acquisition Gradient-Echo (MP-RAGE) Sequences

MP-RAGE sequences include turbo fast low-angle shot (turboFLASH). These techniques are generally performed as a single shot with image acquisition duration of 1–2 s, which renders them relatively breathing independent. Magnetization preparation is currently performed with a 180° inversion pulse to achieve T1-weighted information. The inversion pulse may be either slice or non-slice selective. Slice-selective means that only the tissue section that is being imaged experiences the inverting pulse, whereas non-slice-selective means that all the tissue in the bore of the magnet experience the inverting pulse. The advantage of a slice-selective inversion pulse is that no time delay is required between acquisition of single sections in multiple single-section acquisition. A stack of single-section images can be acquired in a rapid fashion. This is important for dynamic gadolinium-enhanced studies. A non-slice-selective inversion pulse results in slightly better image quality, particularly because flowing blood is signal void (fig. 1.2).

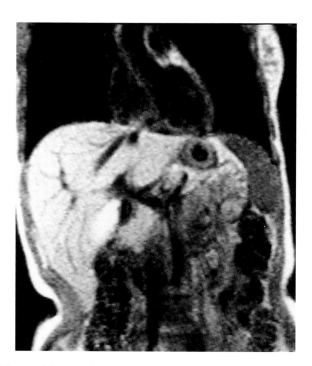

F I G. 1.2 Non-slice-selective 180° magnetization prepared gradient echo. A coronal image through the liver demonstrates good T1 weighting, evidenced by a moderately high-signal intensity liver and moderately low-signal intensity spleen. The infracardiac portion of the left lobe is artifact free. Blood vessels in the liver and the cardiac chambers are seen signal void.

Approximately 3 s of tissue relaxation are required between acquisition of individual sections, which limits the usefulness of this sequence for dynamic gadolinium-enhanced acquisitions. Current versions of MP-RAGE are limited because of low signal-to-noise, ratio varying signal intensity and contrast between sections, unpredictable bounce-point boundary artifacts due to signal-nulling effects caused by the inverting 180° pulse, and unpredictable nulling of tissue enhanced with gadolinium. Research is ongoing to alleviate these problems with MP-RAGE so that it may assume a more important clinical role. Routine use of a high-quality MP-RAGE sequence would further increase the reproducibility of MR image quality by obviating the need for breath-holding, particularly in patients unable to suspend respiration.

T2-WEIGHTED SEQUENCES

The predominant information provided by T2-weighted sequences are 1) the presence of increased fluid in diseased tissue, which results in high signal intensity, 2) the presence of chronic fibrotic tissue, which results in low signal intensity, and 3) the presence of iron deposition, which results in very low signal intensity.

Echo-Train Spin-Echo Sequences

Echo-train spin-echo sequences are termed fast spin-echo, turbo spin-echo, or rapid acquisition with relaxation enhancement (RARE) sequences. The principle of echo-train spin-echo sequences is to summate multiple echoes within the same repetition time interval to decrease examination time, increase spatial resolution, or both. Echo-train spin-echo has achieved widespread use because of these advantages. Conventional T2 spin-echo sequences are lengthy and suffer from patient motion and increased examination time, factors that are lessened with echo-train spin-echo. The major disadvantage of echo-train sequences is that T2 differences between tissues are minimized. This generally is not problematic in the pelvis because of the substantial differences in the T2 values between diseased and normal tissue. In the liver, however, the T2 difference between diseased and background liver may be small, and the T2-averaging effects of summated multiple echoes blur this T2 difference. These effects are most commonly observed with hepatocellular carcinoma. Fortunately, diseases with T2 values similar to those of liver generally have longer T1 values than liver, so that lesions poorly visualized on echo-train spin-echo are generally apparent on SGE or immediate postgadolinium SGE images as low-signal lesions.

Echo-train spin-echo, and T2-weighted sequences in general, are important for evaluating the liver and pelvis.

T2-weighted sequences are often useful for the pancreas, in demonstrating the pancreatic and common bile ducts, evaluating cystic masses and pseudocysts, and detecting islet cell tumors. Breathing-independent single-shot T2-weighted sequences are useful for investigation of bowel and peritoneum. Use of the single-shot technique for many applications of a T2 sequence is recommended, because the image quality is consistent. Although the detection of lesions with subtle T2 difference from background organ/tissue is compromised (e.g., hepatocellular carcinoma), the major application that we employ for T2-weighted sequences is to provide information on fluid content of disease processes for disease characterization. This information is reliably provided by single-shot echo-train spin-echo.

Fat is high in signal intensity on echo-train spin-echo sequences in comparison to conventional spin-echo sequences, in which fat is intermediate in signal intensity. The MR imaging determination of recurrent malignant disease versus fibrosis for pelvic malignancies illustrates this difference. Recurrent malignant disease in the pelvis (e.g., cervical, endometrial, bladder, or rectal cancer) generally appears high in signal intensity on conventional spin-echo sequences because of the higher signal intensity of the diseased tissue relative to the moderately low-signal intensity fat. In contrast, fat is high in signal intensity on echo-train spin-echo images, and recurrent disease will commonly appear relatively lower in signal intensity. The fact that abnormal tissue is not high in signal intensity on T2-weighted images relative to fat cannot be relied upon to exclude recurrence. Caution must therefore be exercised not to misinterpret recurrent disease as fibrotic tissue, by making the assumption that recurrence is higher in signal intensity than background fat. Fat may also be problematic in the liver because fatty liver will be high in signal intensity on echo-train spin-echo sequences, thereby diminishing contrast with the majority of liver lesions, which are generally high in signal intensity on T2-weighted images. It may be essential to use fat suppression on T2-weighted echo-train spin-echo sequences for liver imaging.

Echo-train spin-echo sequences, acquired as contiguous thin two-dimensional (2D) sections or as a thick 3D volume slab, form the basis for MR cholangiography (see Chapter 3, *Gallbladder and Biliary System*) and MR urography (see Chapter 9, *Kidneys*).

Single-Shot Echo-Train Spin-Echo Sequence

Single-shot echo-train spin-echo sequence [e.g., half-Fourier snapshot turbo spin-echo (HASTE) or single shot fast spin echo (SSFSE)] is a breathing-independent T2-weighted sequence that has had a substantial impact on

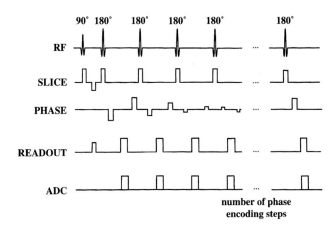

FIG. 1.3 Single-shot echo train spin echo timing diagram.

abdominal imaging [3]. Typical imaging parameters include a 400-ms image acquisition time in which K space is filled in one data acquisition using half-Fourier reconstruction (fig. 1.3). Shorter effective echo time (e.g., 60 ms) is recommended for bowel-peritoneal disease, and longer effective echo time (e.g., 100 ms and greater) is recommended for liver-biliary disease. Other parameters are a repetition time that is infinite and echo train length of 104 or longer. A stack of sections should be acquired in single-section mode in one breath-hold to avoid slice misregistration. Most recently, 3D versions of this technique have been implemented. Motion artifacts from respiration and bowel peristalsis are obviated; chemical-shift artifact is negligible; and susceptibility artifact from air in bowel, lungs, and other locations is minimized, such that bowel wall is clearly demonstrated. Similarly, susceptibility artifact from metallic devices such as surgical clips or hip prostheses is minimal (fig. 1.4). All of these effects render single-shot echo-train spin-echo an attractive sequence for evaluating abdomino-pelvic disease. In patients with implanted metallic devices and extensive surgical clips, single-shot echo-train spin-echo is the sequence least affected by metal susceptibility artifact.

Fat-Suppression (FS) Single-Shot Echo-Train Spin-Echo Sequence

This technique may be useful for investigating focal liver disease to attenuate the high signal intensity of fatty infiltration, if present. Fatty liver is high in signal intensity on echo-train spin-echo sequences, in particular single-shot versions, which lessens the conspicuity of high-signal intensity liver lesions. Diminishing fat signal intensity with fat suppression accentuates the high signal intensity of focal liver lesions (fig. 1.5). FS single-shot echo-train spin-echo is also useful for evaluating the biliary tree. Fat suppression appears to diminish the image quality

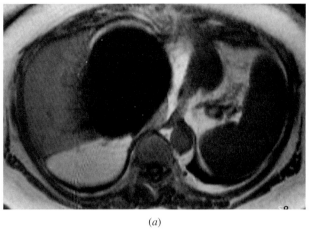

(a)

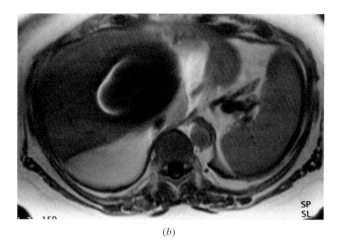

(b)

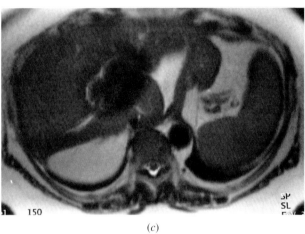

(c)

FIG. 1.4 Metallic susceptibility artifact. SGE (*a*), T1 spin echo (T1-SE) (*b*), and single-shot echo-train spin-echo (SS-ETSE) (*c*) images. Severe susceptibility artifact is present on the gradient echo image (*a*), with the result that the images of the liver are not interpretable. T1-SE (*b*) is relatively resistant to image degradation by susceptibility artifact; however, substantial artifact still renders much of the liver uninterpretable. The SS-ETSE image (*c*) is the least sensitive MR sequence and less sensitive than CT imaging for artifacts generated by metallic devices. Only a small portion of the liver is not interpretable with SS-ETSE (*c*).

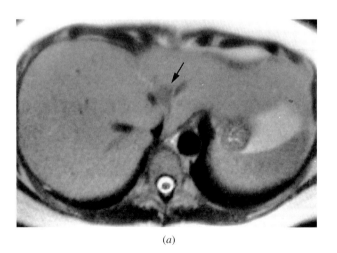

(a)

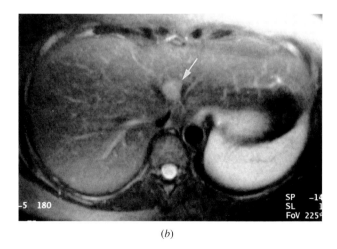

(b)

FIG. 1.5 Focal liver lesion in a fatty liver. Single-shot echo train spin echo (SS-ETSE) (*a*) and fat suppressed (FS)-SS-ETSE (*b*) image. The liver appears high in signal intensity on the SS-ETSE image (*a*) due to the presence of fatty liver. A focal liver lesion (focal nodular hyperplasia) is identified, which is mildly lower in signal intensity than liver parenchyma. On the FS-SS-ETSE image (*b*), the liver has decreased in signal intensity and the liver lesion (arrow, *b*) now appears moderately high in signal intensity relative to liver. Good liver-spleen contrast is also apparent on the fat-suppressed image (*b*), with no liver-spleen contrast on the nonsuppressed sequence (*a*).

of bowel because of susceptibility artifact from air-bowel wall interface and is not recommended for bowel studies.

Turbo Short Tau Inversion Recovery (TurboSTIR) Sequence

TurboSTIR is a short-duration T2-type sequence that can be performed in a breath-hold [4]. Five sections may be acquired in a 20-s breath-hold. Lesion conspicuity is high for focal liver lesions, but image quality generally is fair. As the sequence is fundamentally different from single-shot echo-train spin-echo, it may be useful to combine both short-duration sequences for the liver in place of longer, breathing averaged echo-train spin-echo (fig. 1.6).

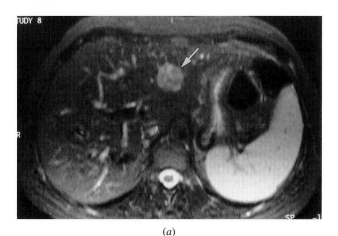

(a)

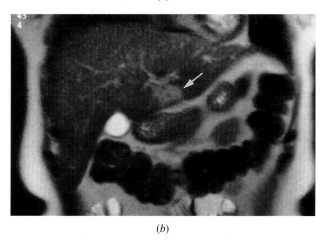

(b)

FIG. 1.6 Echo-train STIR (*a*) and SS-ETSE (*b*). Transverse echo train STIR (*a*) and coronal SSETSE (*b*) images in a patient with colon cancer liver metastases. A moderately high-signal intensity metastasis is present in the left lobe of the liver on the echo train STIR (arrow, *a*). Background fat is nulled. The liver metastasis is also shown on the coronal SSETSE image (arrow, *b*). Background fat is high in signal intensity. Variations in the signal intensity of the background fat provide differing contrast relationships.

GADOLINIUM-ENHANCED T1-WEIGHTED SEQUENCES

Gadolinium contrast agent is most effective when it is administered as a rapid bolus and imaging is performed with a T1-weighted SGE sequence obtained in a dynamic serial fashion. A minimum of two postcontrast sequences is needed, one acquired in the hepatic arterial dominant phase, within 30 s of contrast administration, and the second in the hepatic venous or interstitial phase at approximately 2–5 min. For liver imaging an intermediate-timed third pass, termed portal venous or early hepatic venous, at 1 min postcontrast, is useful as well [6]. Little additional information is provided if more than four sequences are acquired. Features of these phases of enhancement are as follows.

Hepatic Arterial Dominant (Capillary) Phase

The hepatic arterial dominant (capillary) phase is the single most important data set when using a nonspecific extracellular gadolinium chelate [6]. This technique is essential for imaging the liver, spleen, and pancreas, and it provides useful information on the kidneys, adrenals, vessels, bladder, and uterus. The timing for this phase of enhancement is the only timing for postcontrast sequences that is crucial. It is essential to capture the "first pass" or capillary bed enhancement of tissues during this phase. Demonstration of gadolinium in hepatic arteries and portal veins and absence of gadolinium in hepatic veins are reliable landmarks (fig. 1.7). At this

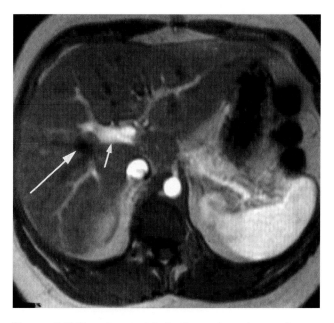

FIG. 1.7 Hepatic arterial dominant-phase image demonstrates gadolinium in portal veins (short arrow) and lack of contrast in hepatic veins (long arrow).

phase of enhancement, although contrast is present in portal veins, the majority of the gadolinium present in the liver has been delivered by hepatic arteries. The absolute volume of hepatic artery-delivered gadolinium is greater in this phase of enhancement than the data acquired when gadolinium is only present in hepatic arteries; therefore, more hepatic arterial enhancement information is available. This is important because most focal liver lesions, especially metastases and hepatocellular carcinoma, are fed primarily by hepatic arteries. Imaging slightly earlier than this, when only hepatic arteries are opacified (hepatic arteries-only phase) may approach the diagnostic utility of the hepatic arterial dominant phase if the injection rate of contrast is very fast (e.g., 5 ml/s) and data is acquired late in the hepatic arteries-only phase (within 1 or 2 s of gadolinium appearing in the portal veins). It is very difficult to achieve these objectives in the hepatic arteries-only phase, and it is also difficult to judge whether image acquisition is too early in this phase, when the liver is essentially unenhanced. Appropriate timing, as judged by vessel enhancement, is also important for the evaluation of surrounding organs. Too little pancreatic enhancement is consistent with pancreatic fibrosis or chronic pancreatitis, and too little enhancement of renal cortex may imply ischemic nephropathy or acute cortical necrosis. This can be reliably judged on hepatic arterial dominant phase images because of the fixed landmarks of contrast in portal veins and absence in hepatic veins. In the hepatic arteries-only phase minimal enhancement of pancreas or renal cortex may reflect too-early image acquisition rather than disease process. Because this immediate postgadolinium phase of enhancement is also used to diagnose adequate perfusion of these organs, it is oxymoronic to use enhancement of these organs as the determination of the appropriateness of the phase of image acquisition timing. Although enhancement of pancreas or renal cortex is used as ancillary information for assessment of timing, it is not the major determinant, because the extent of enhancement of these organs is also evaluated at this phase. In the liver, imaging too early in the hepatic arteries-only phase diminishes the ability to recognize the distinctive patterns of lesion enhancement for different lesion types because the absolute volume of hepatic artery-delivered contrast may be too small and may cause lesions to be mischaracterized (fig. 1.8).

On hepatic arterial dominant phase T1-weighted SGE images, various types of liver lesions have distinctive enhancement patterns: cysts show lack of enhancement, hemangiomas show peripheral nodules of enhancement in a discontinuous ring, nonhemorrhagic adenomas and focal nodular hyperplasia show intense uniform enhancement, metastases show ring enhancement, and hepatocellular carcinomas show diffuse heterogeneous enhancement. The ability to use this information to characterize lesions as small as 1 cm may be

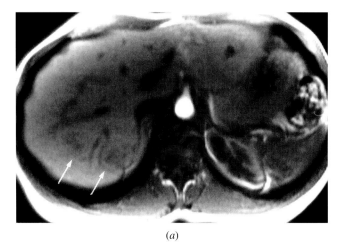

(a)

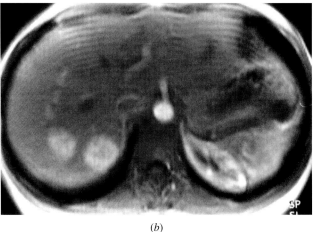

(b)

FIG. 1.8 Hepatic arteries-only (a) and hepatic arterial dominant (b) phase images in a patient with focal nodular hyperplasias. Image acquisition in the hepatic arteries-only phase results in too little enhancement of liver lesions such that the focal nodular hyperplasia tumors appear to have diffuse mild heterogenerous enhancement with negligible enhancement (arrows, a) simulating hepatocellular carcinoma. Repeat examination with data acquisition in the hepatic arterial dominant phase demonstrates intense lesion enhancement with negligible enhancement of the small central scars, diagnostic for focal nodular hyperplasia. Data acquisition in the hepatic arterial dominant phase provides diagnostic information on the enhancement features of liver tumors.

unique to MRI. Appearances of less common liver lesions on immediate postgadolinium images have also been reported, many of which show overlap with the above-described patterns of common liver lesions. To a somewhat lesser extent, appreciation of the capillary phase enhancement of lesions in the pancreas, spleen, and kidneys provides information on lesion characterization that will be described in the respective chapters of these organ systems. Clinical history is often important, despite the high diagnostic accuracy of current MRI imaging protocols. In addition, many different histologic types of liver lesions when they measure less than 1 cm demonstrate virtually identical uniform enhancement, for example, hemangiomas, adenomas, focal nodular hyperplasia, metastases, and hepatocellular carcinoma. Ancillary information to assist in characterization of lesions is crucial, including T2-weighted images that demonstrate lesion fluid content (e.g., high for hemangioma and often high for hypervascular metastases and relatively low for adenoma, focal nodular hyperplasia, and hepatocellular carcinoma), appearance of other concomitant large lesions, and clinical history (e.g., history of known primary tumor that can result in hypervascular metastases, such as gastrointestinal leiomyosarcoma).

Various enhancement patterns of liver and other organ parenchyma are also demonstrated on hepatic arterial dominant phase images. One of the most common perfusion abnormalities observed in the liver is transient increased segmental enhancement in liver segments with compromised portal venous flow due to compression or thrombosis. Other hepatic diseases that demonstrate perfusional abnormalities on immediate postgadolinium images include Budd-Chiari syndrome, with different enhancement patterns for acute, subacute, and chronic disease and severe acute hepatitis with hepatocellular injury. Perfusional abnormalities of the kidneys are also relatively common and are clearly shown on early- and late-phase gadolinium-enhanced images.

Examination for liver metastases may be the most common indication for liver MR examination. Liver metastases have been classified as hypovascular (typical examples are colon cancer and transitional cell carcinoma) or hypervascular (typical examples are islet cell tumors, renal cell carcinoma, and breast cancer). A third category of vascularity has not been described well in the past, and this is near-isovascular with liver. Near-isovascular refers to lesion enhancement that is very comparable to that of liver on early and late postgadolinium images. Near isovascularity is most readily appreciated when lesions are poorly seen on postgadolinium images but well seen on precontrast images (fig. 1.9). Liver metastases from primaries of colon, thyroid, and endometrium may show this type of enhancement pattern. The most common setting is postchemotherapy, although this may also be observed in untreated patients. Fortunately many of these tumors are moderately low signal intensity on T1-weighted images, rendering them readily apparent, and on occasion they may also be moderately high signal intensity on T2-weighted images. Rarely, they may also be near isointense on T1-weighted and T2-weighted images and therefore can escape detection. The rarity of this occurrence illustrates one of the great strengths of MRI over sonography and computed tomography: the greater the number of distinctly different data sets that are acquired, the less likely it is for disease to escape detection. MRI has more acquisitions of different types of data than ultrasound or CT.

Chemotherapy-treated liver metastases deserve special mention in that chemotherapy is routinely given to

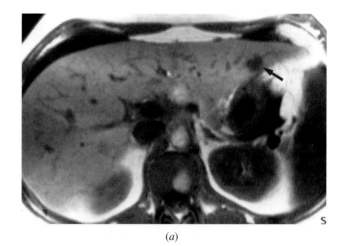

(a)

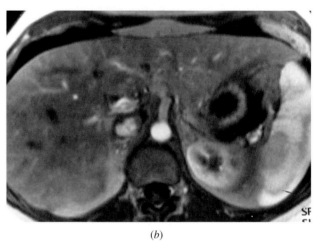

(b)

FIG. 1.9 Near-isovascular liver metastases. SGE (*a*) and hepatic arterial dominant phase gadolinium-enhanced SGE (*b*) images. In this patient with liver metastases, who is at 9 months after initiation of chemotherapy, liver metastases are clearly shown on noncontrast T1-weighted images (arrow, *a*) but poorly seen after gadolinium administration. This enhancement pattern, termed near isovascular, is most commonly observed in liver metastases in a subacute phase of response to chemotherapy.

the majority of patients with liver metastases and it alters the imaging features of metastases. Chemotherapy induces change in the signal intensity and imaging features of metastases such that they may resemble cysts, hemangiomas, or scar tissue [6]. As mentioned above, they may also become near isovascular on postgadolinium images.

Portal Venous Phase or Early Hepatic Venous Phase

This phase is acquired at 45–60 s postinitiation of gadolinium injection. In this phase hepatic parenchyma is maximally enhanced, so hypovascular lesions (cysts, hypovascular metastases, and scar tissue) are best shown as regions of lesser enhancement. Patency or thrombosis of hepatic vessels are also best shown in this phase.

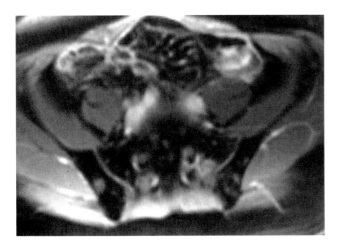

FIG. 1.10 Bone metastases. Two-minute gadolinium-enhanced T1-weighted fat-suppressed SGE image demonstrates multiple rounded enhancing bone metastases that are clearly defined in a background of suppressed fatty marrow.

Hepatic Venous (Interstitial) Phase

Hepatic venous phase or interstitial phase is acquired 90 s–5 min after initiation of contrast injection. Late enhancement features of focal liver lesions are shown that aid in lesion characterization, such as persistent lack of enhancement of cysts, coalescence and centripetal progression of enhancing nodules in hemangiomas, homogeneous fading of enhancement of adenomas and focal nodular hyperplasia to near isointensity with liver, late enhancement of central scar in some focal nodular hyperplasias, peripheral or heterogeneous washout of contrast in liver metastases, washout to hypointensity with liver in small liver metastases and hepatocellular carcinoma, heterogeneous washout of hepatocellular carcinoma, and delayed capsule enhancement in hepatocellular carcinoma (less commonly, adenoma). Enhancement of peritoneal metastases, inflammatory disease, bone metastases (fig. 1.10), and circumferential, superficial spreading cholangiocarcinoma is also well shown at this time frame. Concomitant use of fat suppression is essential for optimized demonstration of these findings. Additional documentation of vascular thrombosis is also provided on these images.

MULTIPLE IMAGING VARIABLES

On MR images it is common that multiple imaging properties are present concurrently. The contributions of these various properties must be separately determined so that appropriate diagnosis is made. Common potentially competing imaging characteristics include T2 and fat suppression effects, T1 out-of-phase and magnetic susceptibility effects, and gadolinium washout and fat suppression effects, T2 and fat suppression effects can

usually be separated by employing both nonsuppressed and fat-suppressed T2-weighted sequences. Low signal due to fat suppression effects can be correctly ascertained by the demonstration of higher signal intensity of the structure on non-fat-suppressed T2 sequences relative to the T2 fat-suppressed sequences. Out-of-phase and magnetic susceptibility signal loss can be separated by observing that susceptibility effects increase with increasing TE on gradient echo sequences and are generally also observed as low signal on T2-weighted sequences, whereas out-of-phase lipid signal effects cycle with in- and out-of-phase echo times. Distinction between gadolinium washout and fat suppression effects on the 2-min postgadolinium T1-weighted fat-suppressed SGE sequence must also be established. In problem cases, there is the observation of low signal of a structure on later postgadolinium fat-suppressed sequences that appeared high signal on early postgadolinium nonsuppressed sequences. The question arises whether this reflects a fat suppression effect rather than a gadolinium washout effect. In the liver this can usually be distinguished by the observation that a lesion that is fatty is low signal on a 2-min postgadolinium fat-suppressed sequence but isointense or hyperintense on both the immediate and the 1-min nonsuppressed portal venous phase SGE sequences. Generally, if a liver lesion washes out at 2 min, it has most often already shown evidence of washout by 1 min on the portal venous phase non-fat-suppressed SGE images. Further information supportive of a fat effect is evidence that the lesion appears fatty on any of the other sequences employed in the imaging protocol (e.g., out-of-phase or noncontrast fat-suppressed sequences). Figure 1.11 illustrates many of these combined imaging properties in one situation.

SIGNAL INTENSITY OF VESSELS

Inhomogeneous signal intensity of vessels is a disgnostic problem not infrequently encountered on MR images. In general, we have found that image acquisition between 1 and 2 min postgadolinium using SGE results in consistently high signal of patent arteries and veins. Unfortunately, data acquisition often falls beyond this range, particularly in the setting of acquiring images of the pelvis after images of the abdomen. If patency of vessels is a particular diagnostic concern then we employ sequences that consistently show high signal in patent vessels, often by combining intrinsic inflow effects and gadolinium effects. Sequences we employ include gadolinium-enhanced slice-selective 180° MP-RAGE (particularly useful for noncooperative patients), gadolinium-enhanced water excitation SGE, and gradient echo sequences with gradient echo refocusing (±gadolinium) (e.g., true FISP, GRASS). Acquisition of

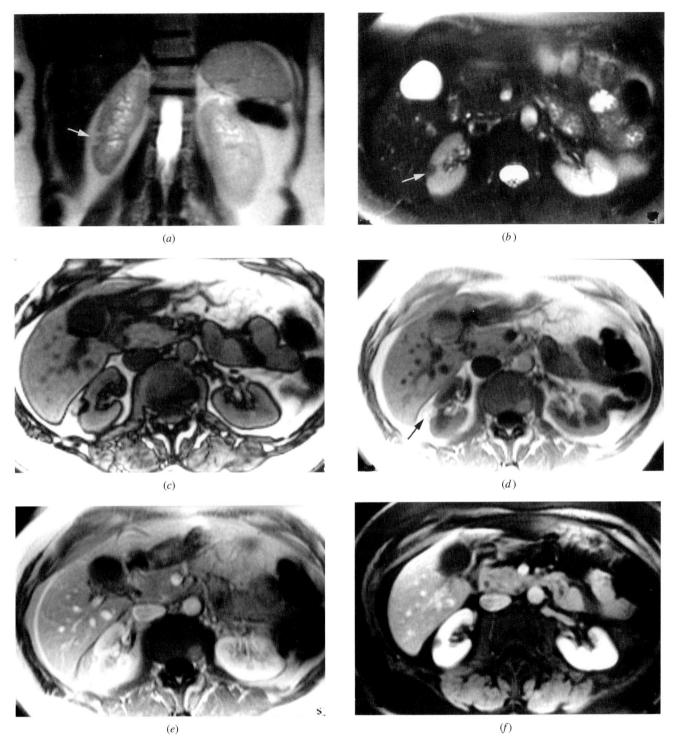

(a)

(b)

(c)

(d)

(e)

(f)

F IG . 1.11 Fat effects, gadolinium effects, and their distinction. Coronal T2-weighted single-shot echo train spin echo (*a*), T2-weighted fat-suppressed single-shot echo train spin echo (*b*), T1-weighted out-of-phase SGE (*c*), T1-weighted in-phase SGE (*d*), 1 min postgadolinium SGE (*e*), and 1.5 min gadolinium-enhanced fat-suppressed SGE (*f*) images. It is always useful to compare noncontrast nonsuppressed (*a*) and fat-suppressed (*b*) sequences to ascertain whether high-signal structures observed on nonsuppressed sequences represent fat or lower-signal structures observed on fat-suppressed sequences represent fat and not low fluid content solid masses. Comparing out-of-phase (*c*) to in-phase (*d*) sequences also permits characterization of fatty tumors. In this patient, a right renal angiomyolipoma is present, which on the basis of the fat-suppressed T2-weighted sequence alone (arrow, *b*) may be considered a possible renal cancer or hemorrhagic cyst because of its low signal. Comparison with the non-fat-suppressed sequence (*a*) reveals that the tumor is high signal intensity in the absence of suppression (arrow, *a*), showing that it represents fat. Another approach is to show that the high-signal mass on the in-phase image (arrow, *d*) develops a phase cancellation black ring interface with renal parenchyma on the out-of-phase image (*c*). By noting that the mass is fatty, high signal on early postgadolinium images (arrow, *d*) can be recognized as a fat effect and not enhancement, and loss of signal on the 1.5 min gadolinium-enhanced fat-suppressed image is not misinterpreted as washout but correctly observed as a fat suppression effect.

additional planes are also useful, for example, coronal plane of the liver postgadolinium and sagittal plane of the pelvis postgadolinium.

IMAGING STRATEGIES

High diagnostic accuracy can be achieved by describing the T1-, T2-, capillary, and interstitial phase gadolinium-enhanced T1-weighted sequence appearance of various disease processes. In practice, it is also important to recognize which technique is the most consistent in demonstrating various lesions to target these lesions in an imaging protocol. Table 1.1 lists the MR sequences on which certain disease processes are consistently shown. A major strength of MRI is the variety of types of information that the modality is able to generate. As a result, MRI is able to provide comprehensive information on organ systems and disease entities. The use of a diverse group of sequences, acquired in multiple planes, minimizes the likelihood of not detecting disease or misclassifying disease. This is a reflection of the fact that the more different information that is acquired, the less likely it is that disease will escape detection. Attention to length of examination is critical because longer examinations result in fewer patients who can be examined and a decrease in patient cooperation. Ideally, many of the different sequences employed should be of short duration and breath-hold or breathing independent. An

attempt should be made to achieve this goal in protocol design. Another consideration is reproducibility of examination protocols. Efficient operation of an MRI system requires the use of set protocols, which serves to speed up examinations, render exams reproducible, and increase utilization by familiarity with a standard approach. A useful approach is to have sufficient redundancy in sequences that if one or two sequences are unsatisfactory there still is enough information for the study to be diagnostic, while at the same time not to have so much redundancy that study times are long and patient cooperation diminishes toward the latter part of the study. MRI techniques are in continuous evolution, and when new sequences are developed it is important to replace older sequences with newer sequences rather than simply adding new sequences onto an existing protocol. Speed of data acquisition, image quality, disease display, and consistency of image quality are all important considerations when evaluating new sequences. For example, we anticipate that in the near future the image quality of 3D T1-weighted gradient echo imaging will improve to the point that it is comparable to 2D imaging. At that time we will replace all 2D SGE sequences in our protocols with 3D imaging. The rationale to utilize 3D imaging includes thinner section data acquisition, lesser problems with motion and phase artifact, and the ability to use the same data set to generate an MRA exam [9, 10].

The protocoling of MRI studies that investigate the abdomen and pelvis in the same setting may be rendered

Table 1.1 MR Imaging Sequences That Show Consistent Display of Various Disease Processes

Sequences	Disease Process	Appearance
T1	Fluid	↓↓
T1 Out of phase	Adrenal adenoma Fatty liver	↓
T1 Fat suppressed	Normal pancreas Subacute hematoma Endometriosis (subacute blood)	↑
T2	Fluid	↑↑
T2	Iron (including hemosiderin)	↓↓
T2	Uterine cervix, prostate	Zonal anatomy, cancer
Capillary phase Gad	Focal lesions liver, spleen, pancreas	Distinctive patterns
Capillary phase Gad	Inflammatory disease	↑
Capillary phase Gad	Arterial compromise	↓
Capillary phase Gad	Portal vein compromise	↑

Interstitial phase
  Gad
	Inflammatory disease, peritoneal
	   metastases, bone metastases,
	   lymphadenopathy
		↑

most efficient by acquiring a complete study of the upper abdomen initially, using precontrast SGE, T2-weighted FS-echo-train spin-echo, and serial postgadolinium SGE and FS-SGE images, and then acquiring the pelvis study, including postgadolinium FS-SGE followed by T2-weighted sequences (fig. 1-12). Comprehensive examination of all organs and tissues in the abdomen and pelvis can be achieved with this approach, which permits detection of a full range of disease, including unsuspected disease (fig. 1.13). This strategy minimizes table motion and repositioning of the phased-array coil, which are time-consuming procedures. Although it is not generally desired to acquire T2-weighted images after gadolinium we have not appreciated that T2-weighted images of the pelvis obtained after gadolinium degrade the T2 effects. The presence of concentrated low-signal intensity gadolinium in the bladder on T2-weighted im-

ages may in fact be beneficial by increasing conspicuity of bladder involvement from malignant pelvic diseases. The liver is the organ that benefits the most from immediate postgadolinium imaging, and imaging protocols should be designed in a fashion to image the liver immediately after gadolinium administration. If, however, liver metastases are unlikely and the pelvis is the major focus of investigation, studies can be structured to acquire immediate postgadolinium images of the pelvis (e.g., for the evaluation of bladder tumors).

Patient set up can be performed as follows: the phased-array coil is initially placed over the upper abdomen, and image acquisition is centered over the liver. After precontrast sequences, with the patient positioned in the bore of the magnet, gadolinium is injected as a forceful hand bolus injection over 5 s, followed by injection of a normal saline flush over 3 s. Image

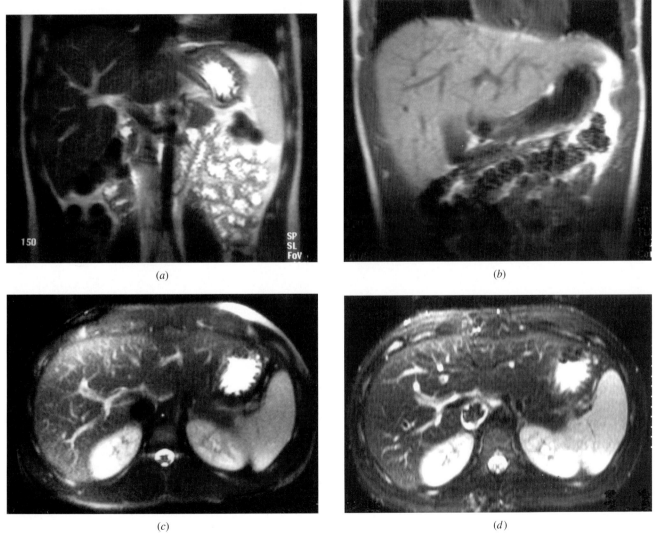

(a)

(b)

(c)

(d)

FIG. 1.12 Liver and pelvis protocol. Coronal T2-weighted single-shot echo train spin echo (a), coronal T1-weighted SGE (b), T2-weighted fat-suppressed single-shot echo train spin echo (c), T2-weighted breath hold STIR (d).

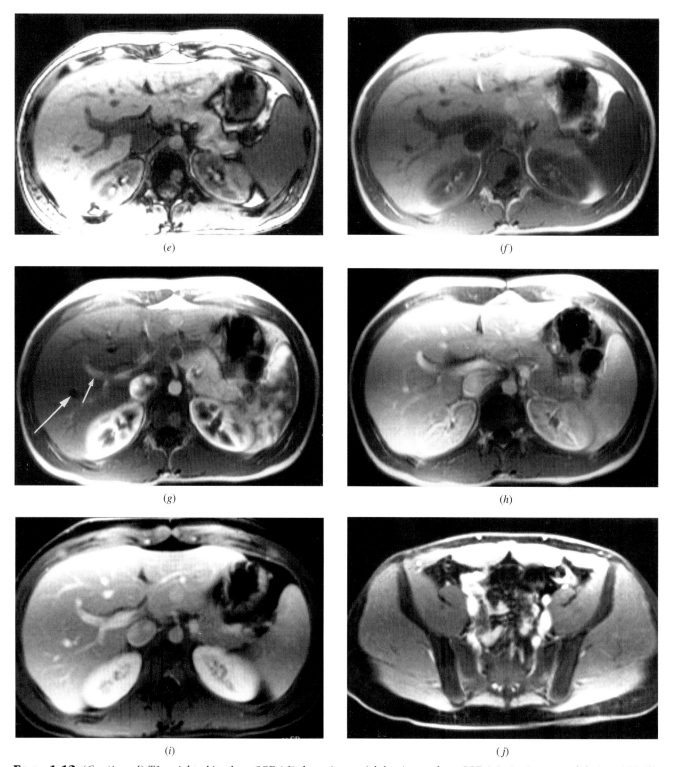

FIG. 1.12 (*Continued*) T1-weighted in-phase SGE (*f*), hepatic arterial dominant phase SGE (*g*), 1 min postgadolinium SGE (*h*), 1.5 min postgadolinium fat-suppressed SGE (*i*), transverse (*j*) and sagittal (*k*) 4 min postgadolinium fat-suppressed SGE, and transverse (*l*) and sagittal (*m*) T2-weighted single-shot echo train spin echo images. Pre- and postgadolinium multiplanar T1- and T2-weighted images of the abdomen (*a–i*) and postgadolinium images of the pelvis (*j–m*).

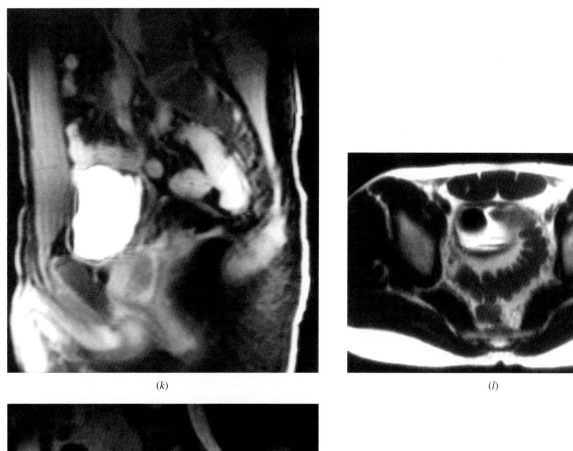

(k)

(l)

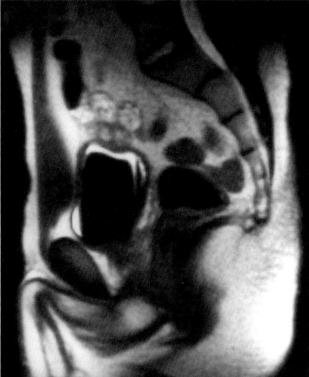

(m)

F I G . 1.12 (*Continued*) A combination of breath hold (*b, d, e-k*) and breathing-independent (*a, c, l, m*) sequences are used to ensure consistent image quality in cooperative patients resulting in a short study duration, typically 30-40 min. On the hepatic arterial dominant phase image, note the presence of gadolinium in portal veins (short arrow, *g*) and not hepatic veins (long arrow, *g*).

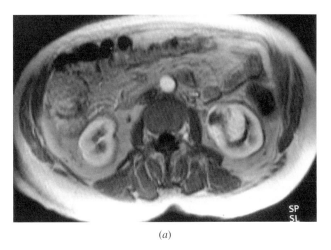

(a)

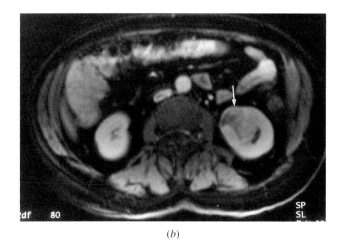

(b)

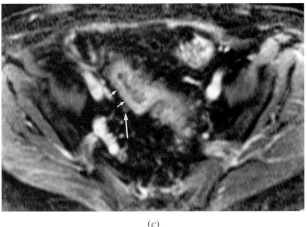

(c)

FIG. 1.13 Concurrent renal cell cancer and colon cancer. Immediate postgadolinium SGE (*a*), 90 s postgadolinium fat-suppressed SGE (*b*), and 3 min postgadolinium fat-suppressed SGE (*c*). Selected images from a liver pelvis protocol in a patient evaluated for colon cancer demonstrate an incidental left renal tumor that enhances intensely on immediate postgadolinium images (*a*) and washes out (arrow, *b*) on the fat-suppressed image, diagnostic for renal cell cancer. Thickening of the sigmoid colon representing cancer (small arrows, *c*) is appreciated on images acquired of the pelvis. A small regional involved lymph node (long arrow, *c*) is well shown on the gadolinium-enhanced fat-suppressed image.

acquisition is initiated immediately after the normal saline flush with the SGE sequence. Another approach, using a power injector, is to administer contrast at 2 ml/s and to initiate the scan 17 s after the start of contrast injection. Other researchers have also recommended using a timing bolus to increase the reproducibility of data acquisition in a correct phase of enhancement [10]. After the postgadolinium sequences of the upper abdomen, the phased-array coil is then shifted over the pelvis and the table is repositioned for image acquisition centered on the pelvis. Initial pelvic images should be T1-weighted images to utilize the presence of gadolinium before too much washout has occurred (e.g., within 10 min). We employ T1-weighted fat-suppressed SGE in the transverse and sagittal plane. T2-weighted images then follow. If small-volume disease is suspected (e.g., prostate cancer, small cervical cancer) then we use breathing-averaged high-resolution (512 matrix) T2-weighted echo-train spin echo. If the pelvic images are more of a survey for disease (e.g., intra-abdominal abscess) then we employ single-shot T2-weighted echo-train spin echo. This approach sacrifices precontrast SGE images of the pelvis. The major disadvantage of this is that hemorrhagic pelvic lesions may not be demonstrated, but in practice this mainly decreases the abil-

ity to detect endometriosis. When investigation of endometriosis is required, precontrast FS-SGE images are obtained and a dedicated pelvis protocol is performed. On the most recent MR systems, remote table motion, performed at the imaging console, and the ability to use either two phased-array torso coils overlying the abdomen and pelvis or one extended-coverage torso coil covering the abdomen and pelvis, are available. This permits time-efficient imaging of the abdomen and pelvis such that precontrast imaging of the pelvis can be performed as well, if needed.

In patients with malignant disease, it is also useful to screen for pulmonary metastases. The 3D GE sequence is effective in this capacity as artifact from cardiac motion is minimized, and rapid consistant image quality of the lungs can be obtained [11]. We acquire thorough images between the imaging of the abdomen and the pelvis.

Tables 1.2–1.26 show the current protocols that are useful for the investigation of abdominopelvic disease when imaging at 1.5 T using a phased-array multicoil.

The sequence protocols are designed for a Siemens system. Vendor-specific variations in imaging parameters should be employed as needed. Variations in TR/TE/flip angle for SGE sequences should generally be avoided. Imaging parameters of echo-train spin-echo sequences

Table 1.2 Liver

Sequence	Plane	TR	TE	FOV	Thickness/Gap	Flip	Matrix
Localizer							
SS-ETSE	Coronal	∞	90	350–400	8–10 mm/20%	150°	192 × 256
T1 SGE	Coronal	140	4.1	350–400	8–10 mm/20%	80°	128 × 256
SS-ETSE fat suppressed	Transverse	∞	90	350–400	8–10 mm/20%	150°	192 × 256
ET-STIR	Transverse	5110	76	350–400	8–10 mm/20%	160°	99 × 256
T1 SGE out-of-phase	Transverse	140	2.2	350–400	8–10 mm/20%	80°	128 × 256
T1 SGE	Transverse	140	4.1	350–400	8–10 mm/20%	80°	128 × 256
T1 SGE 1, 45 s post-Gd	Transverse	140	4.1	350–400	8–10 mm/20%	80°	128 × 256
T1 SGE fat suppressed 90 s post-Gd	Transverse	145	4.1	350–400	8–10 mm/20%	80°	144 × 256

SGE = spoiled gradient echo; SS-ETSE = single-shot echo-train spin echo; ET-STIR = echo-train short inversion time inversion recovery

Table 1.3 Liver and Pancreas

Sequence	Plane	TR	TE	FOV	Thickness/Gap	Flip	Matrix
Localizer							
SS-ETSE (liver-pancreas)	Coronal	∞	90	350–400	8 mm/20%	150°	192 × 256
SS-ETSE (liver-pancreas)	Transverse	∞	90	350–400	8 mm/20%	150°	192 × 256
SS-ETSE fat suppressed	Transverse	∞	90	350–400	8–10 mm/20%	150°	192 × 256
T1 SGE fat suppressed; (pancreas)	Transverse	145	4.1	350–400	6–8 mm/20%	80°	144 × 256
T1 SGE out-of-phase (liver)	Transverse	140	2.2	350–400	8–10 mm/20%	80°	128 × 256
T1 SGE (liver-pancreas)	Transverse	140	4.1	350–400	8–10 mm/20%	80°	128 × 256
T1 SGE (liver-pancreas) 1, 45 s post-Gd	Transverse	140	4.1	350–400	8–10 mm/20%	80°	128 × 256
T1 SGE fat suppressed 90 s (liver)	Transverse	145	4.1	350–400	8–10 mm/20%	80°	144 × 256

SGE = spoiled gradient echo; SS-ETSE = single-shot echo-train spin echo

Table 1.4 Liver and Kidney

Sequence	Plane	TR	TE	FOV	Thickness/Gap	Flip	Matrix
Localizer							
SS-ETSE (liver-kidney)	Coronal	∞	90	450	8–10 mm/20%	150°	128 × 256
SS-ETSE (liver-kidney)	Transverse	∞	90	450	8–10 mm/20%	150°	128 × 256
T1 SGE fat suppressed (kidney)	Transverse	145	4.1	350	8–10 mm/20%	80°	144 × 256
T1 SGE (liver + kidney)	Transverse	140	4.1	350–400	8–10 mm/20%	80°	128 × 256
T1 SGE (liver + kidney) 1, 45 s post-Gd	Transverse	140	4.1	350–400	8–10 mm/20%	80°	128 × 256
T1 SGE fat suppressed (kidney) 90 s	Transverse	145	4.1	350–400	8–10 mm/20%	80°	144 × 256
T1 SGE fat suppressed (kidney)	Sagittal	145	4.1	350	8–10 mm/20%	80°	144 × 256

SGE = spoiled gradient echo; SS-ETSE = single-shot echo-train spin echo

Table 1.5 Liver and Pelvis

Sequence	Plane	TR	TE	FOV	Thickness/ Gap	Flip	Matrix
Localizer							
SS-ETSE (liver)	Coronal	∞	90	350–400	8–10 mm/20%	150°	192 × 256
T1 SGE (liver)	Coronal	140	4.5	350–400	8–10 mm/20%	80°	128 × 256
SS-ETSE fat suppressed (liver)	Transverse	∞	90	350–400	8–10 mm/20%	150°	192 × 256
ET-STIR	Transverse	5110	76	350–400	8–10 mm/20%	160°	99 × 256
T1 SGE out of phase (liver)	Transverse	140	2.2	350–400	8–10 mm/20%	80°	128 × 256
T1 SGE (liver)	Transverse	140	4.5	300–400	8–10 mm/20%	80°	128 × 256
T1 SGE (liver) 1, 45 s post-Gd	Transverse	140	4.5	350–400	8–10 mm/20%	80°	128 × 256
T1 SGE fat suppressed 90 s post-Gd (liver + mid abd)	Transverse	145	4.1	350–400	8–10 mm/20%	80°	144 × 256
T1 SGE fat suppressed (pelvis)	Transverse	145	4.1	350–400	8 mm/20%	80°	144 × 256
T1 SGE fat suppressed (pelvis)	Sagittal	145	4.1	350–400	8 mm/20%	80°	144 × 256
SS-ETSE (pelvis)	Transverse	∞	90	350–400	8–10 mm/20%	150°	192 × 256
SS-ETSE (pelvis)	Sagittal	∞	90	350–400	8–10 mm/20%	150°	192 × 256

SGE = spoiled gradient echo; SS-ETSE = single-shot echo-train spin echo; ET-STIR = echo-train short inversion time inversion recovery
Note: For rectal cancer substitute T2 high-resolution ETSE for the postcontrast pelvic SS-ETSE.

Table 1.6 Abdomen (Agitated Noncooperative)

Sequence	Plane	TR	TE	FOV	Thickness/ Gap	Flip	Matrix
Localizer							
SS-ETSE	Coronal	∞	90	400	8 mm/20%	150°	192 × 256
SS-ETSE	Transverse	∞	90	350	8 mm/20%	150°	192 × 256
SS-ETSE fat suppressed	Transverse	∞	90	350	8 mm/20%	150°	192 × 256
MP-RAGE non-slice selective	Coronal	11	4.2	400	8–10 mm/20%	15°	128 × 256
MP-RAGE non-slice selective	Transverse	11	4.2	350	8–10 mm/20%	15°	128 × 256
MP-RAGE slice selective 9 s post-Gd	Transverse	11	4.2	350	8–10 mm/20%	15°	128 × 256
MP-RAGE slice selective post-Gd	Coronal	11	4.2	400	8–10 mm/20%	15°	128 × 256

SS-ETSE = single-shot echo-train spin echo; MP-RAGE = magnetization prepared-rapid acquisition gradient echo

Table 1.7 Abdomen (Sedated)

Sequence	Plane	TR	TE	FOV	Thickness/Gap	Flip	Matrix
Localizer							
SS-ETSE	Coronal	∞	90	400	8 mm/20%	150°	192 × 256
MP-RAGE non-slice selective	Coronal	11	4.2	400	8–10 mm/20%	15°	128 × 256
T2 ETSE fat suppressed	Transverse	4300	120	350–400	6–10 mm/20%	180°	140 × 256
T1 SE fat suppressed	Transverse	500	15	350–400	8–10 mm/20%	90°	144 × 256
MP-RAGE slice selective 9 s post-Gd	Transverse	11	4.2	350	8–10 mm/20%	15°	128 × 256
MP-RAGE slice selective post-Gd	Coronal	11	4.2	400	8–10 mm/20%	15°	128 × 256
T1 SE fat suppressed post-Gd	Transverse	500	15	350–400	8–10 mm/20%	90°	144 × 256

ETSE = echo-train spin echo; T1 SE = T1 spin echo; MP-RAGE = magnetization prepared-rapid acquisition gradient echo

Table 1.8 Bowel

Sequence	Plane	TR	TE	FOV	Thickness/Gap	Flip	Matrix
Localizer							
T1 SGE (abdomen)	Coronal	140	4.5	400	8–10 mm/20%	80°	128 × 256
SS-ETSE (abdomen)	Coronal	∞	90	400	8 mm/20%	150°	192 × 256
SS-ETSE (abdomen)	Transverse	∞	90	350	8 mm/20%	150°	192 × 256
T1 SGE (abdomen)	Transverse	140	4.5	350	8–10 mm/20%	80°	128 × 256
T1 SGE fat suppressed (1 and 45 s post-Gd)(Abd)	Transverse	145	4.1	350	8–10 mm/20%	80°	144 × 256
T1 SGE fat suppressed (pelvis)	Coronal	145	4.1	350	8–10 mm/20%	80°	144 × 256
T1 SGE fat suppressed (pelvis)	Sagittal	145	4.1	350	8–10 mm/20%	80°	144 × 256
SS-ETSE	Coronal	∞	90	400	8 mm/20%	150°	192 × 256
SS-ETSE	Transverse	∞	90	350	8 mm/20%	150°	192 × 256
SS-ETSE	Sagittal	∞	90	350	8 mm/20%	150°	192 × 256

SGE = spoiled gradient echo; SS-ETSE = single-shot echo-train spin echo
Note: For rectal cancer, use T2 high-resolution echo-train sagittal + transverse.

Table 1.9 Pancreas

Sequence	Plane	TR	TE	FOV	Thickness/Gap	Flip	Matrix
Localizer							
SS-ETSE (liver-pancreas)	Coronal	∞	90	350–400	8 mm/20%	150°	192 × 256
SS-ETSE (liver-pancreas)	Transverse	∞	90	350–400	8 mm/20%	150°	192 × 256
SS-ETSE fat suppressed	Transverse	∞	90	350–400	8–10 mm/20%	150°	192 × 256
T1 SGE fat suppressed (pancreas)	Transverse	145	4.1	350–400	6–8 mm/20%	80°	144 × 256
T1 SGE (liver-pancreas)	Transverse	140	4.5	350–400	8–10 mm/20%	80°	128 × 256
T1 SGE (liver-pancreas) 1, 45 s post-Gd	Transverse	140	4.5	350–400	8–10 mm/20%	80°	128 × 256
T1 SGE fat suppressed 90 s (pancreas)	Transverse	145	4.5	350–400	8–10 mm/20%	80°	144 × 256

SGE = spoiled gradient echo; SS-ETSE = single-shot echo-train spin echo

Table 1.10 MR Cholangiogram

Sequence	Plane	TR	TE	FOV	Thickness/Gap	Flip	Matrix
Localizer							
SS-ETSE	Oblique (coronal to sagittal 23°)	∞	95	300	4 mm/0%	150°	240 × 256
Optional							
TSE	Coronal	2800	1100	300	70 mm/0%	150°	240 × 256
TSE	Coronal	2800	1100	300	50 mm/0%	150°	240 × 256
TSE	Coronal	2800	1100	300	30 mm/0%	150°	240 × 256

SS-ETSE = single-shot echo-train spin echo

Table 1.11 Adrenal

Sequence	Plane	TR	TE	FOV	Thickness/Gap	Flip	Matrix
Localizer							
SS-ETSE	Coronal	∞	90	400	8 mm/20%	150°	192 × 256
T1 SGE (diaphragm to aortic bifurcation)	Coronal	140	4.5	350–400	8–10 mm/20%	80°	128 × 256
SS-ETSE fat suppressed (diaphragm to aortic bifurcation)	Transverse	∞	90	350–400	8–10 mm/ 20%	150°	192 × 256
T1 SGE fat suppressed	Transverse	145	4.1	350–400	6 mm/20%	80°	144 × 256
T1 SGE out of phase	Transverse	140	2.2	350–400	8 mm/20%	80°	128 × 256
T1 SGE	Transverse	140	4.5	350–400	8 mm/20%	80°	128 × 256
T1 SGE (1, 45 s post-Gd)	Transverse	140	4.5	350–400	8 mm/20%	80°	128 × 256
T1 SGE fat suppressed (90 s post-Gd)	Transverse	145	4.1	350–400	7 mm/20%	80°	144 × 256

SGE = spoiled gradient echo; SS-ETSE = single-shot echo-train spin echo

Table 1.12a Kidney

Sequence	Plane	TR	TE	FOV	Thickness/Gap	Flip	Matrix
Localizer							
T1 SGE fat suppressed	Transverse	145	4.1	350–400	8–10 mm/20%	80°	144 × 256
T1 SGE	Transverse	140	4.5	350–400	8–10 mm/20%	80°	128 × 256
T1 SGE (1 s post-Gd)	Transverse	140	4.5	350–400	8–10 mm/20%	80°	128 × 256
T1 SGE fat suppressed (45 and 90 s post-Gd)	Transverse	145	4.1	350–400	8–10 mm/20%	80°	144 × 256
T1 SGE fat suppressed (3 min post-Gd)	Sagittal or coronal	140	4.5	350–400	8–10 mm/20%	80°	128 × 256

SGE = spoiled gradient echo; SS-ETSE = single-shot echo-train spin echo
Notes: *If possible, cover liver as well as kidneys on 1-s post-Gd FLASH.
*Renal artery studies require an MRA study, and this can be performed in place of the 1-s post-Gd T1 SGE.

Table 1.12b Renal Artery MRA (Substitute the Following for Postcontrast Sequences in Routine Kidney Protocol)

Sequence	Plane	TR	TE	FOV	Thickness/Gap	Flip	Matrix
Turbo MRA-3D GE (3–6 s post-Gd)	Coronal	4.0	1.6	300–450	2–3 mm/32 partitions 1Aq/3 meas	30°	180 × 256
T1 SGE fat suppressed (90 s post-Gd)	Transverse	145	4.1	350–400	8–10 mm/20%	80°	144 × 256
T1 SGE fat suppressed	Coronal	145	4.1	350–400	8–10 mm/20%	80°	144 × 256

Table 1.13 Male: Screening Abdomen and Pelvis

Sequence	Plane	TR	TE	FOV	Thickness	Flip	Matrix
Localizer							
T1 SGE (liver)	Coronal	140	4.5	350–400	8–10 mm/20%	80°	128 × 256
SS-ETSE (liver)	Coronal	∞	90	350–400	8–10 mm/20%	150°	128 × 256
T1 SGE (liver)	Transverse	140	2.5	350–400	8–10 mm/20%	80°	128 × 256
T1 SGE (liver)	Transverse	140	4.5	350–400	8–10 mm/20%	80°	128 × 256
T1 SGE (1, 45 s post-Gd) (liver)	Transverse	140	4.5	350–400	8–10 mm/20%	80°	128 × 256
T1 SGE fat suppressed (liver-mid abdomen)	Transverse	145	4.1	350–400	10 mm/20%	80°	144 × 256
T1 SGE fat suppressed (pelvis)	Transverse	145	4.1	350–400	10 mm/20%	80°	144 × 256
T1 SGE fat suppressed (pelvis)	Sagittal	145	4.1	350–400	10 mm/20%	80°	144 × 256
SS-ETSE (pelvis)	Sagittal	∞	90	350–400	8–10 mm/20%	150°	128 × 256
SS-ETSE (pelvis)	Transverse	∞	90	350–400	8–10 mm/20%	150°	128 × 256

SGE = spoiled gradient echo; SS-ETSE = single-shot echo-train spin echo
Note: For rectal cancer substitute T2 high-resolution ETSE sagittal and transverse for the SS-ETSE sagittal and transverse pelvis.

Table 1.14 Prostate

Sequence	Plane	TR	TE	FOV	Thickness/Gap	Flip	Matrix
Localizer							
T1 SGE (mid-abdomen)	Transverse	140	4.5	350–400	8–10 mm/20%	90°	144 × 256
T1 SGE (pelvis)	Transverse	140	4.5	350–400	7 mm/20%	90°	144 × 256
T1 SGE fat suppressed (pelvis)	Transverse	145	4.1	350	8–10 mm/20%	80°	128 × 256
T2-high-resolution ETSE (pelvis)	Transverse	5000	132	350–400	5 mm/20%	180°	270 × 512
T2-high-resolution ETSE (pelvis)	Sagittal	5000	132	350–400	5 mm/20%	180°	270 × 512
T1 SGE fat suppressed (10 s post-Gd) (pelvis)	Transverse	145	4.1	350–400	10 mm/20%	80°	128 × 256
T1 SGE fat suppressed (pelvis)	Sagittal	145	4.1	350–400	10 mm/20%	80°	128 × 256
T1 SGE fat suppressed post-Gd (mid-abdomen)	Transverse	145	4.1	350	8–10 mm/20%	80°	128 × 256

SGE = spoiled gradient echo; ETSE = T2-echo train spin echo

Table 1.15   Female: Screening Abdomen and Pelvis

Sequence	Plane	TR	TE	FOV	Thickness/Gap	Flip	Matrix
Localizer							
T1 SGE (liver)	Coronal	140	4.5	350–400	8–10 mm/20%	80°	128 × 256
SS-ETSE (liver)	Coronal	∞	90	350–400	8 mm/20%	150°	192 × 256
T1 SGE (liver)	Transverse	140	4.5	350–400	8–10 mm/20%	80°	128 × 256
T1 SGE (1, 45 s post-Gd) (liver)	Transverse	140	4.5	350–400	8–10 mm/20%	80°	128 × 256
T1 SGE fat suppressed post-Gd (liver)	Transverse	145	4.1	350–400	10 mm/20%	80°	128 × 256
T1 SGE fat suppressed post-Gd (pelvis)	Transverse	145	4.1	350–400	8 mm/20%	80°	128 × 256
T2 high-resolution ETSE (pelvis)	Sagittal	5000	132	350	7 mm/20%	180°	270 × 512
T2 high-resolution ETSE (pelvis)	Transverse	5000	132	350	6 mm/20%	180°	270 × 512

SGE = spoiled gradient echo; ETSE = echo train spin echo
Note: For the short version, substitute SS-ETSE for T2 echo train spin echo.

Table 1.16   Uterus (Benign Disease)

Sequence	Plane	TR	TE	FOV	Thickness/Gap	Flip	Matrix
Localizer							
SS-ETSE (pelvis)	Coronal	∞	90	350–400	8–10 mm/20%	150°	128 × 256
T2 high-resolution ETSE (pelvis)	Transverse	5000	132	250	5 mm/20%	180°	270 × 512
T2 high-resolution ETSE (pelvis)	Sagittal	5000	132	250	5 mm/20%	180°	270 × 512
T1 SGE (pelvis)	Transverse	140	4.5	350–400	8 mm/20%	80°	128 × 256
T1 SGE (pelvis)	Sagittal	140	4.5	350–400	7 mm/20%	80°	128 × 256
T1 SGE fat suppressed (pelvis)	Transverse	145	4.1	350	7 mm/20%	80°	128 × 256

SS-ETSE = single-shot echo-train spin echo; SGE = spoiled gradient echo; T2-ETSE = T2-echo-train spin echo
Note: Long-axis and short-axis views of the uterus should be considered for some congenital uterine anomalies.

Table 1.17   Endometrial/Cervical Cancer

Sequence	Plane	TR	TE	FOV	Thickness/Gap	Flip	Matrix
Localizer							
SS-ETSE (liver)	Coronal	∞	90	350–400	8 mm/20%	150°	192 × 256
T1 SGE (liver)	Transverse	140	4.5	350–400	8–10 mm/20%	80°	128 × 256
T1 SGE (1, 45 s post-Gd) (liver)	Transverse	140	4.5	350–400	8–10 mm/20%	80°	128 × 256
T1 SGE fat suppressed post-Gd (liver-midabdomen)	Transverse	145	4.1	350–400	10 mm/20%	80°	128 × 256
T1 SGE fat suppressed post-Gd (pelvis)	Transverse	145	4.1	350–400	8 mm/20%	80°	128 × 256
T1 SGE fat suppressed post-Gd (pelvis)	Sagittal	145	4.1	350–400	8 mm/20%	80°	128 × 256
T2 high-resolution ETSE (pelvis)	Transverse	5000	132	350	6 mm/20%	180°	270 × 512
T2 high-resolution ETSE (pelvis)	Sagittal	5000	132	350	7 mm/20%	180°	270 × 512

SS-ETSE = single-shot echo train spin echo; SGE = spoiled gradient echo; ETSE = echo-train spin echo

Table 1.18 Endometriosis

Sequence	Plane	TR	TE	FOV	Thickness/Gap	Flip	Matrix
Localizer							
SS-ETSE (pelvis)	Coronal	∞	90	350–400	8–10 mm/20%	150°	128 × 256
T2 high-resolution ETSE (pelvis)	Transverse	5000	132	350–400	5 mm/20%	180°	270 × 512
T2 high-resolution ETSE (pelvis)	Sagittal	5000	132	350–400	5 mm/20%	180°	270 × 512
T1 SGE (pelvis)	Transverse	140	4.5	350–400	8 mm/20%	80°	128 × 256
T1 SGE fat-suppressed (pelvis)	Transverse	145	4.1	350–400	7 mm/20%	80°	128 × 256
T1 SGE fat-suppressed (pelvis)	Sagittal	145	4.1	350	8 mm/20%	80°	128 × 256

SGE = spoiled gradient echo; ETSE = echo-train spin echo

Table 1.19 Ovarian Cancer

Sequence	Plane	TR	TE	FOV	Thickness/Gap	Flip	Matrix
Localizer							
SS-ETSE (liver)	Coronal	∞	90	350–400	8 mm/20%	150°	128 × 256
T1 SGE (liver)	Coronal	140	4.5	400	8 mm/20%	80°	128 × 256
SS-ETSE fat suppressed (liver)	Transverse	∞	90	350	8 mm/20%	150°	128 × 256
ET-STIR	Transverse	5110	76	350–400	8–10 mm/20%	160°	99 × 256
T1 SGE	Transverse	140	4.5	350–400	8–10 mm/20%	80°	128 × 256
T1 SGE (liver) 1, 45 s post-Gd	Transverse	140	4.5	350	8–10 mm/20%	80°	128 × 256
T1 SGE fat suppressed (upper abd)	Transverse	145	4.1	400	8–10 mm/20%	80°	128 × 256
T1 SGE fat suppressed (upper abd)	Coronal	145	4.1	350	8–10 mm/20%	80°	128 × 256
T1 SGE fat suppressed (lower abd/pelvis)	Transverse	145	4.1	350	8 mm/20%	80°	128 × 256
T1 SGE fat suppressed (lower abd/pelvis)	Sagittal	145	4.1	350	8 mm/20%	80°	128 × 256
SS-ETSE (pelvis)	Coronal	∞	90	350–400	8 mm/20%	150°	128 × 256
T2 high-resolution ETSE (pelvis)	Transverse	5000	132	350	7–8 mm/20%	180°	270 × 512

SS-ETSE = single-shot echo-train spin echo; SGE = spoiled gradient echo; ETSE = echo-train spin echo
Note: T2 ETSE sagittal should be added to the pelvis if this is initial presentation.

Table 1.20 Pelvis (with Gadolinium)

Sequence	Plane	TR	TE	FOV	Thickness/Gap	Flip	Matrix
SS-ETSE	Coronal	4.4	90	400	8 mm/20%	150°	192 × 256
T2 high-resolution ETSE	Transverse	5000	132	350–400	5 mm/20%	180°	270 × 512
T2 high-resolution ETSE	Sagittal	5000	132	350–400	5 mm/20%	180°	270 × 512
SGE	Transverse	140	4.1	350–400	8 mm/20%	80°	128 × 256
SGE fat suppressed	Transverse	145	4.1	350	8 mm/20%	80°	128 × 256
SGE (10 s. post-Gd)	Transverse	140	4.1	350	8 mm/20%	80°	128 × 256
SGE fat suppressed post-Gd	Transverse	140	4.1	350	8 mm/20%	80°	128 × 256
SGE fat suppressed post-Gd	Transverse	145	4.1	350–400	8 mm/20%	80°	128 × 256

SS-ETSE = single-shot echo-train spin echo; ETSE = echo-train spin echo; SGE = spoiled gradient echo

Table 1.21   Abdomen Pelvis--Agitated Noncooperative

Sequence	Plane	TR	TE	FOV	Thickness/Gap	Flip	Matrix
Localizer							
SS-ETSE (abdomen)	Coronal	∞	90	350	8 mm/20%	150°	192 × 256
SS-ETSE (abdomen)	Transverse	∞	90	350	8 mm/20%	150°	192 × 256
SS-ETSE fat suppressed (abdomen)	Transverse	∞	90	350	8 mm/20%	150°	192 × 256
SGE fat suppressed (abdomen)	Transverse	145	4.1	350–400	8–10 mm/20%	80°	96 × 256
SGE fat suppressed (abdomen)	Transverse	145	4.1	350–400	8–10 mm/20%	80°	96 × 256
MP-RAGE non-slice selective (abdomen)	Coronal	11	4.2	400	8–10 mm/20%	15°	128 × 256
MP-RAGE non-slice selective (abdomen)	Transverse	11	4.2	350	8–10 mm/20%	15°	128 × 256
MP-RAGE non-slice selective (9 s post-gd) (abdomen)	Transverse	11	4.2	350	8–10 mm/20%	15°	128 × 256
MP-RAGE non-slice selective (abdomen)	Coronal	11	4.2	400	8–10 mm/20%	15°	128 × 256
SGE fat suppressed (pelvis)	Transverse	145	4.1	350–400	8–10 mm/20%	80°	96 × 256
SGE fat suppressed (pelvis)	Sagittal	145	4.1	350–400	8–10 mm/20%	80°	96 × 256
SS-ETSE (pelvis)	Transverse	∞	90	350–400	8–10 mm/20%	150°	192 × 256
SS-ETSE (pelvis)	Sagittal	∞	90	350	8–10 mm/20%	150°	192 × 256

MP-RAGE = magnetization prepared rapid acquisition gradient echo; SS-ETSE = single-shot echo-train spin echo; SGE = spoiled gradient echo

Table 1.22   Abdomen and Pelvis—Sedated Patient

Sequence	Plane	TR	TE	FOV	Thickness/Gap	Flip	Matrix
Localizer							
SS-ETSE (abdomen)	Coronal	∞	90	400	8 mm/20%	150°	192 × 256
MP-RAGE non-slice selective (abdomen)	Coronal	11	4.2	400	8 mm/20%	15°	192 × 256
T2 Turbo SE fat suppressed (abdomen)	Transverse	4500	22/90	350	8 mm/20%	180°	140 × 256
T1 SE fat suppressed (abdomen)	Transverse	500	15	350–400	8–10 mm/20%	90°	128 × 256
MP-RAGE slice selective post-Gd (abdomen)	Transverse	11	4.2	350	8 mm/20%	15°	128 × 256
MP-RAGE slice selective post-Gd (abdomen)	Coronal	11	4.2	400	8 mm/20%	15°	128 × 256
T1 SE fat suppressed (abdomen)	Transverse	500	15	350–400	8–10 mm/20%	90°	128 × 256
T1 SE fat suppressed (pelvis)	Transverse	500	15	350–400	8–10 mm/20%	90°	128 × 256
SS-ETSE (pelvis)	Transverse	∞	90	350	8 mm/20%	150°	192 × 256
SS-ETSE (pelvis)	Sagittal	∞	90	350	8 mm/20%	150°	192 × 256

MP-RAGE = magnetization prepared rapid acquisition gradient echo; SS-ETSE = single-shot echo train spin echo; SGE = spoiled gradient echo
Optional: T2 TSE transverse if pelvic disease is strongly suspected.

Table 1.23 Abdominal Aorta

Sequence	Plane	TR	TE	FOV	Thickness/Gap	Flip	Matrix
Localizer							
T1 SGE (diaphragm to bifurcation of femoral arteries)	Transverse	140	4.5	350–400	8–10 mm/20%	80°	128 × 256
SS-ETSE black blood	Coronal	800	43	400	8 mm/20%	150°	192 × 256
SS-ETSE black blood	Transverse	800	43	350	8 mm/20%	150°	192 × 256
Turbo MRA-3D GE (diaphragm to bifurcation of femoral arteries) (3–6 s post-Gd)	Coronal	4.0	1.6	300–450	2 mm/48 partitions 1 Aql/3 meas	30°	180 × 256
T1 SGE fat suppressed (diaphragm to bifurcation of femoral arteries)	Transverse	145	4.1	350–400	8 mm/20%	80°	128 × 256
T1 SGE fat suppressed (diaphragm to bifurcation of femoral arteries)	Coronal	145	4.1	350–400	8 mm/20%	80°	128 × 256

SGE = spoiled gradient echo; SS-ETSE = single-shot echo-train spin echo

Table 1.24 General MRA Including Dissection of Abdominal Aorta

Sequence	Plane	TR	TE	FOV	Thickness/Gap	Flip	Matrix
Localizer							
SGE	Transverse	140	4.1	320–400	8–10 mm/20%	80°	128 × 256
SS-ETSE (black blood)	Coronal	800	43	350	8 mm/20%	150°	192 × 256
SS-ETSE (black blood)	Transverse	800	43	350	8 mm/20%	150°	192 × 256
Turbo MRA-3D GE (diaphragm to bifurcation of femoral arteries) (3–6 s post-Gd)	Coronal	4.0	1.6	300–450	2 mm/48 partitions	30°	180 × 256
SGE fat suppressed (post-Gd)	Coronal	145	4.1	320–400	6–8 mm/20%	80°	128 × 256
SGE fat suppressed (post-Gd)	Transverse	145	4.1	320–400	6–8 mm/20%	80°	128 × 256

SS-ETSE = single-shot echo train spin echo; SGE = spoiled gradient echo
An optional water excitation SGE may be added postcontrast.
Note: Area of interest from the diaphragm to bifurcation of the abdominal aorta 3D-MRA run 2 passes sequentially; for venous assessment may run 3 passes.
Plane for 3D-MRA: abdominal aorta-coronal celiac and SMA-sagittal

Table 1.25 Chest/Abdomen/Pelvis

Sequence	Plane	TR	TE	FOV	Thickness/ Gap	Flip	Matrix
Localizer							
SS-ETSE (liver)	Coronal	4.4	90	350–400	8 mm/20%	150°	192 × 256
SGE (liver) out of phase	Transverse	140	2.2	350–400	8–10 mm/20%	80°	128 × 256
SGE (liver)	Coronal	140	4.1	350–400	8–10 mm/20%	80°	128 × 256
SGE (liver)	Transverse	140	4.1	350–400	8–10 mm/20%	80°	128 × 256
SGE (liver) 1, 45 s post-Gd	Transverse	140	4.1	350–400	8–10 mm/20%	80°	128 × 256
SGE fat suppressed 90 s post-Gd (liver + mid abd)	Transverse	145	4.1	350–400	8–10 mm/20%	80°	128 × 256
3D GE (chest)	Transverse	4.6	1.8	400	8 mm/14 partitions	15°	200 × 512
3D GE (chest)	Coronal	4.6	1.8	400	8 mm/14 partitions	15°	200 × 512
SS-ETSE (black blood) (chest)	Coronal	800	43	350–400	8–10 mm/20%	150°	128 × 256
SS-ETSE (black blood) (chest)	Transverse	800	43	350–400	8–10 mm/20%	150°	128 × 256
SGE fat suppressed (pelvis)	Transverse	145	4.1	350–400	8 mm/20%	80°	128 × 256
SGE fat suppressed (pelvis)	Sagittal	145	4.1	400	8 mm/20%	80°	128 × 256
SS-ETSE (pelvis)	Transverse	4.4	90	350–400	6–8 mm/20%	150°	192 × 256
SS-ETSE (pelvis)	Sagittal	4.4	90	350–400	6–8 mm/20%	150°	192 × 256

SS-ETSE = single-shot echo train spin echo; SGE = spoiled gradient echo; 3D GE = 3D gradient echo

Table 1.26 Chest

Sequence	Plane	TR	TE	FOV	Thickness/ Gap	Flip	Matrix
Localizer							
SS-ETSE (black blood)	Coronal	800	43	350–400	8–10 mm/20%	150°	128 × 256
SS-ETSE (black blood)	Transverse	800	43	350–400	8–10 mm/20%	150°	128 × 256
3D GE	Coronal	4.6	1.8	400	8 mm/14 partitions	15°	200 × 512
3D GE	Transverse	4.6	1.8	400	8 mm/14 partitions	15°	200 × 512
3D GE post-Gd	Transverse	4.6	1.8	400	8 mm/14 partitions	15°	200 × 512
3D GE post-Gd	Coronal	4.6	1.8	400	8 mm/14 partitions	15°	200 × 512
SGE fat suppressed post-Gd	Transverse	145	4.1	350–400	8 mm/20%	80°	128 × 256

SS-ETSE = single-shot echo train spin echo; SGE = spoiled gradient echo; 3D GE = 3D gradient echo are more flexible, with minor changes resulting in no substantial loss of diagnostic information. With the use of phased-array multicoils both slice thickness and FOV can be substantially modified for many protocols (e.g., slice thickness of 5 mm for the pancreas, adrenals, and pelvis, and FOV of 200 mm for the pelvis).

SERIAL MRI EXAMINATION

MRI is currently considered the most expensive imaging modality, which has hampered its appropriate utilization. The expense of MRI studies can be dramatically reduced by decreasing study time and the number of sequences employed. This may be done most reasonably in the setting of follow-up examinations. Depending on the amount of information needed, a follow-up study that employs coronal single-shot echo-train spin echo, transverse precontrast SGE, immediate and 45-s postgadolinium SGE, and 2-min postgadolinium fat-suppressed SGE provides relatively comprehensive information in a 10-min study time [5]. Even more curtailed examination can be performed if only change in size is examined for. An adrenal mass or lymphadenopathy may be adequately followed by precontrast SGE alone,

or, in the case of an adrenal adenoma, in combination with out-of-phase SGE.

NONCOOPERATIVE PATIENTS

It is crucial to recognize that separate protocols are required for noncooperative patients. In general, noncooperative patients fall into two categories: (1) those who cannot suspend respiration but breathe in a regular fashion and (2) those who cannot suspend respiration and cannot breathe in a regular fashion. The most common patient population that fits into the first group are sedated pediatric patients. Agitated patients are the most commonly encountered population who fit into the second group. Imaging strategies differ for each.

In sedated patients, substitution of breath-hold images (e.g., SGE) can be made readily with breathing-averaged spin echo images, the image quality of which is improved by using fat suppression. With sedation, breathing is in a more regular pattern than that observed for all other patients. Additionally, breathing-independent T2-weighted single-shot echo-train spin-echo is useful, as is T1-weighted MP-RAGE, if dynamic gadolinium-enhanced images are required (fig. 1.14).

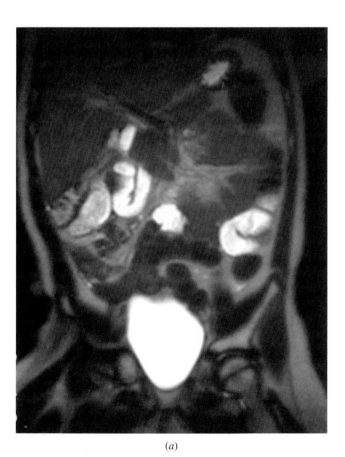
(a)

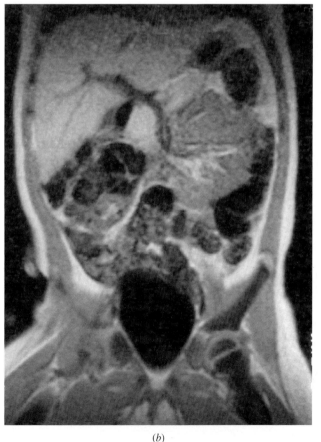
(b)

FIG. 1.14 Sedated patient protocol, abdomen and pelvis. Coronal T2-weighted single-shot echo train spin echo (*a*), coronal T1-weighted single-shot non-slice-selective 180° magnetization prepared gradient echo (*b*).

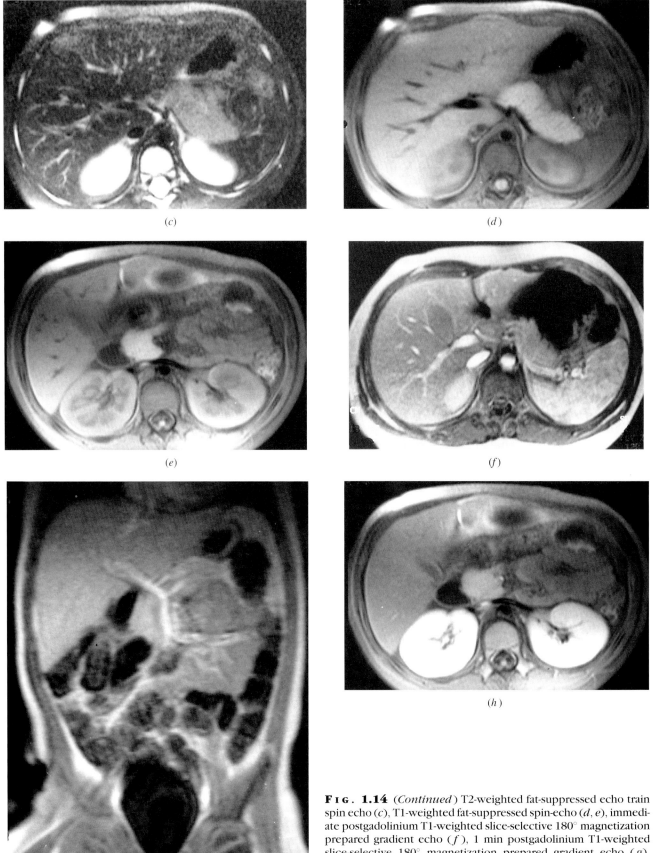

(c)

(d)

(e)

(f)

(g)

(h)

FIG. 1.14 (*Continued*) T2-weighted fat-suppressed echo train spin echo (*c*), T1-weighted fat-suppressed spin-echo (*d*, *e*), immediate postgadolinium T1-weighted slice-selective 180° magnetization prepared gradient echo (*f*), 1 min postgadolinium T1-weighted slice-selective 180° magnetization prepared gradient echo (*g*), 1.5 min gadolinium-enhanced T1-weighted fat-suppressed spin echo (*h*).

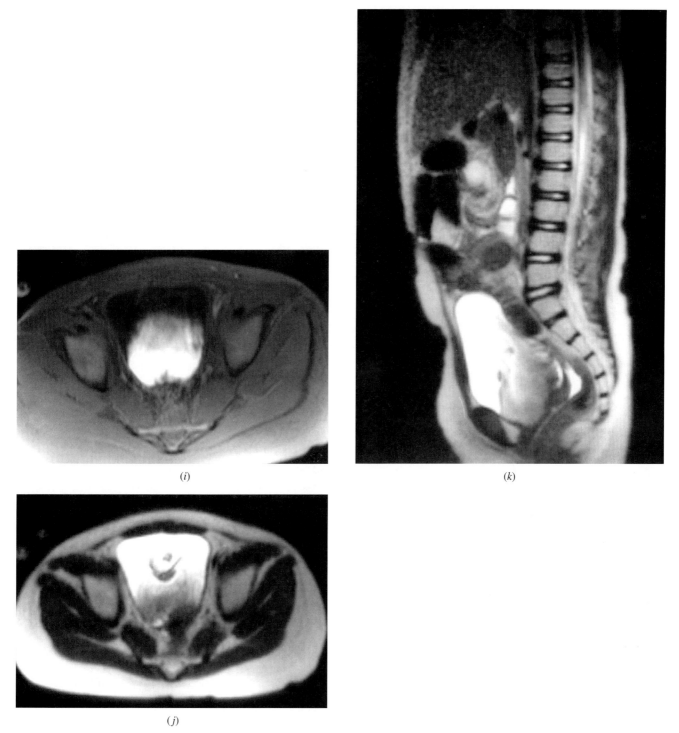

FIG. 1.14 (*Continued*) 5 min gadolinium-enhanced T1-weighted fat-suppressed spin echo (*i*), and transverse (*j*) and coronal (*k*) T2-weighted single-shot echo train spin echo images. Images of the abdomen are acquired first, pre- and postgadolinium (*a–b*), followed by imaging of the pelvis (*i–k*). In sedated patients, a combination of longer-duration, breathing-averaged sequences (*c–e, h, i*) and breathing-independent single-shot techniques (*a, b, f, g, j, k*) are used. In this patient, the T2-weighted images of the pelvis were acquired using single-shot technique. If there was a high index of suspicion of pelvic disease, breathing-averaged sequences could have been performed. Note the excellent demonstration of the pancreas on the noncontrast breathing-averaged fat-suppressed T1-weighted spin echo images (*d, e*).

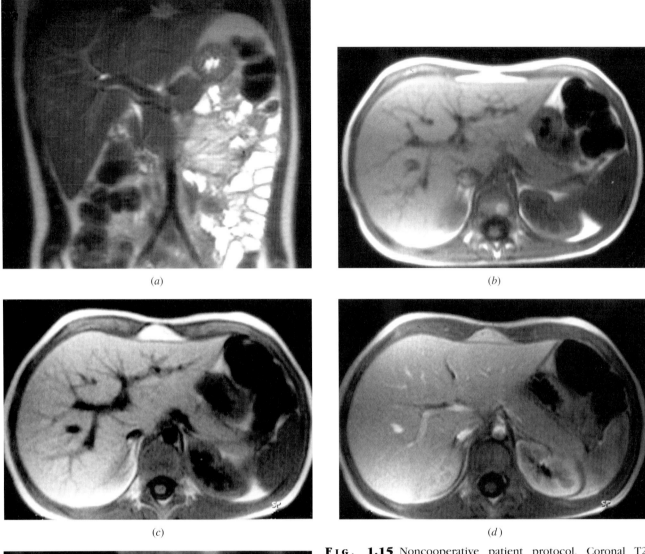

(a)

(b)

(c)

(d)

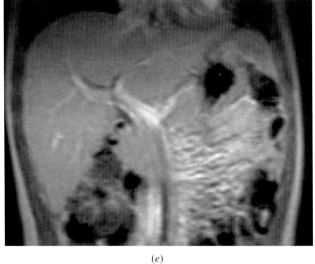

(e)

FIG. 1.15 Noncooperative patient protocol. Coronal T2-weighted single-shot echo train spin echo (*a*), reduced matrix (96 × 128) shortened TR (100 ms) SGE (*b*), non-slice-selective 180° magnetization prepared gradient echo (*c*), immediate post-gadolinium slice-selective 180° magnetization prepared gradient echo (*d*), and coronal 1 min postgadolinium slice-selective 180° magnetization prepared gradient echo (*e*) images. An imaging protocol for a patient who cannot suspend respiration or breathe in a regular fashion includes breathing-independent sequences (*a, c–e*). Attempt should be made, as in this patient, to reduce matrix size, field of view and TR time on the SGE sequence to render it a 10-s breath hold. In this patient, this reduced parameter SGE sequence (*b*) resulted in acceptable image quality for this acquisition but was not reproducible. The study was switched to perform only breathing-independent sequences (*c–e*). Note the comparison between SGE (*b*) and non-slice-selective 180° magnetization prepared gradient echo (*c*). The former sequence has mirror artifacts from the aorta (arrow, *b*); the latter sequence has very good signal void in vessels, no mirror artifacts, and strong T1 weighting, as evidenced by excellent liver-spleen contrast. Drawbacks of non-slice-selective 180° magnetization prepared gradient echo include low signal to noise, lengthy total imaging time, and variable image quality outside the liver.

In patients who are agitated, only single-shot techniques should be used, including breathing-independent T2-weighted single-shot echo train spin echo and T1-weighted MP-RAGE pre- and postgadolinium administration (fig. 1.15).

REFERENCES

1. Brown MA, Semelka RC: *MRI: basic principles and applications.* 2nd ed. New York: Wiley-Liss, 1999.
2. Semelka RC, Willms AB, Brown MA, Brown ED, Finn JP: Comparison of breath-hold T1-weighted MR sequences for imaging of the liver. *J Magn Reson Imaging* 4: 759–765, 1994.
3. Semelka RC, Kelekis NL, Thomasson D, Brown MA, Laub GA: HASTE MR imaging: Description of technique and preliminary results in the abdomen. *J Magn Reson Imaging* 6: 698–699, 1996.
4. Gaa J, Hutabu H, Jenkins RL, Finn JP, Edelman RR: Liver masses: replacement of conventional T2-weighted spin echo MR imaging with breath-hold MR imaging. *Radiology* 200: 459–464, 1996.
5. Semelka RC, Balci NC, Op de Beeck B, Reinhold C: Evaluation of a 10-minute comprehensive MR imaging examination of the upper abdomen. *Radiology* 211: 189–195, 1999.
6. Semelka RC, Helmberger T: Contrast agents for MR imaging of the liver: State-of-the-art. *Radiology* 218: 27–38, 2001.
7. Low RN, Semelka RC, Worawattanakul S, Alzate GD: Extrahepatic abdominal imaging in patients with malignancy: comparison of MR imaging and helical CT in 164 patients. *J Magn Reson Imaging* 12: 269–277, 2001.
8. Low RN, Semelka RC, Worawwattanakul S, Alzate GD, Sigeti JS: Extrahepatic abdominal imaging in patients with malignancy: comparison of MR imaging and helical CT, with subsequent surgical correlation. *Radiology* 210: 625–632, 1999.
9. Rofsky NM, Lee VS, Laub G, Pollack MA, Krinsky GA, Thomasson D, Ambrosino MM, Weinreb JC: Abdominal MR imaging with a volumetric interpolated breath-hold examination. *Radiology* 212: 876–884, 1999.
10. Lee VS, Lavelle MT, Rofsky NM, Laub G, Thomasson DM, Krinsky GA, Weinreb JC: Hepatic MR imaging with a dynamic contrast-enhanced isotropic volumetric interpolated breath-hold examination: feasibility, reproducibility, and technical quality. *Radiology* 215: 365–372, 2001.
11. Semelka RC, Balci NC, Wilber KP, Fisher LL, Brown MA, Gomez-Caminero A, Molina PL. Breath-hole 3D gradient-echo MR imaging of the lung parenchyma: evaluation of reproducibility of image quality in normals and preliminary observations in patients with disease. JMRI 11: 195–200, 2000.

CHAPTER 2

LIVER

RICHARD C. SEMELKA, M.D., LARISSA BRAGA, M.D., DIANE ARMAO, M.D., DIEGO R. MARTIN, M.D., PH.D., F.R.C.P., TILL BADER, M.D., KIMBERLY L. BEAVERS, M.D., SHAMBHAVI VENKATARAMAN, M.B.B.S., M.R.C.P., AND MONICA S. PEDRO, M.D.

Early civilizations considered the liver as the seat of the soul. The liver's unique regenerative power is embodied in Greek mythology in the tale of Prometheus. Zeus punished Prometheus, in part for stealing fire for mankind. Prometheus was taken to the Caucasus, where he was bound.

> To a high-piercing, headlong rock
> In adamantine chain that none can break . . .
> An eagle red with blood
> Shall come, a guest unbidden to your banquet.
> All day long he will tear to rags your body.
> Feasting in fury on the blackened liver.
>   Edith Hamilton MYTHOLOGY

Because of its remarkable capacity for regeneration, the liver can restore approximately three-quarters of its own mass within six months.

NORMAL ANATOMY

The liver is the most massive of the viscera and commands the right upper quadrant of the abdomen.

The current classification system of liver segmental anatomy, as refined by Couinaud [1], describes the liver as divided into eight independent functioning units or segments, each of which is served by its own vascular pedicle (arterial, portal venous, and lymphatic) and biliary drainage. This improved understanding of the intrahepatic architecture has fueled technical progress in liver surgery and transplantation. Vessels are clearly discernible with MRI, which makes this technique ideally suited to the study of the functional segmental anatomy of the liver (fig. 2.1).

With respect to the imaging features of liver, there are three fissures that help define functional right and left hepatic lobes and the major hepatic segments. The interlobar fissure, located on the inferior liver margin, is oriented along a line passing through the gallbladder fossa inferiorly and the middle hepatic vein superiorly [2]. Although well defined in some patients, the interlobar fissure is usually difficult to identify. The left intersegmental fissure (fissure for the ligamentum teres) forms a well-defined sagittally oriented cleft in the caudal aspect of the left hepatic lobe, serving to divide the lobe into medial and lateral segments. The ligamentum teres, or obliterated vestige of the left umbilical vein, normally ensconced in a small amount of fat, runs through this fissure after entering it via the free margin of the falciform ligament. The third fissure, or fissure for the ligamentum venosum, is oriented in a coronal or oblique plane

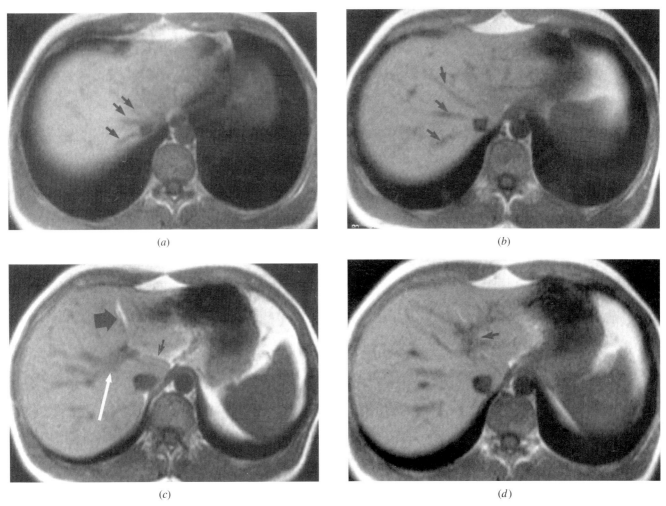

(a)   (b)

(c)   (d)

F I G . 2.1 Normal anatomy. Transverse SGE (*a, b, c, d*) images. The vascular anatomy of the liver includes the hepatic venous system—superior, middle, and inferior hepatic veins (arrows, *a, b*); portal venous system—right portal vein (long white arrow, *c*) and left portal vein (arrow, *d*). Note the caudate lobe, the fissure for the ligamentum venosum (small black arrow, *c*), and the fissure for the ligamentum teres (Large black arrow, *c*).

between the posterior aspect of the left lateral hepatic segment and the anterior aspect of the caudate lobe [2]. This fissure forms a continuum with the intersegmental fissure. The fissure for the ligamentum venosum cuts deeply anterior to the caudate lobe and contains the two layers of the lesser omentum.

The porta hepatis is a deep transverse fissure situated between the medial segment anteriorly and the caudate process posteriorly. At the porta hepatis, the portal vein, hepatic artery, and hepatic nerve plexus enter the liver and the right and left hepatic ducts and lymphatic vessels emerge from it. The caudate lobe stands at the watershed between right and left portobiliary arterial territories. Because the caudate lobe drains directly into the inferior vena cava, it may escape injury from venous outflow obstruction [3]. Whereas branches of the hepatic artery, portal vein, and tributaries of the bile ducts travel together serving segments of the liver, hepatic veins run independently and are intersegmental (fig. 2.2). The close relationship of the hepatic artery,

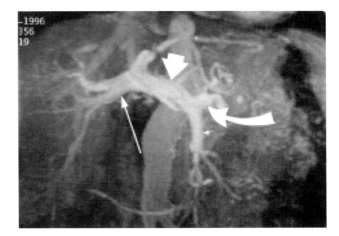

F I G . 2.2 Portal venous system. Anteroposterior projection from 3D MIP reconstruction of a set of coronal gadolinium-enhanced 2-mm 3D MRA source images. Superior mesenteric vein (small arrow), splenic vein (curved arrow), main portal vein (large arrow), and intrahepatic portal veins (long arrow) are well defined on this gadolinium-enhanced 3D MRA source image.

portal vein, and bile ducts on a macroscopic level is mirrored on a microscopic level by the presence of portal triads comprising hepatic arterioles, portal venules, and interlobular bile ducts.

MRI TECHNIQUE

The current standard MRI examination of the liver includes a T1-weighted sequence, a T2-weighted sequence, and a contrast-enhanced sequence (fig. 2.3). The most comprehensive contrast administration approach is the use of gadolinium chelate, as a rapid bolus injection with serial imaging using a spoiled gradient-echo (SGE) sequence. A variety of sequences exist that generate T1- and T2-weighted images. Field strength and gradient factors of the MRI machine generally dictate the type of sequences employed. At lower field strength (<1 T) spin-echo sequences are generally used because of gradient strength and signal-to-noise ratio limitations. At high field strength ($\geq$1 T) gradient-echo sequences are generally used for T1-weighted sequences, and echo-train sequences are used for T2-weighted sequences. See Chapter 1 for a more complete description of standard liver imaging protocols. The vast majority of liver diseases can be characterized by the combined information provided by T1, T2, and early (hepatic arterial dominant) and late (hepatic venous) SGE images (figs. 2.4–2.6). Table 2.1 describes the appearance of common focal liver lesions using this approach [4].

LIVER CONTRAST AGENTS

Intravenously administered contrast agents have been used in clinical magnetic resonance imaging of the liver since 1988. The need for more accurate detection and characterization of the full spectrum of liver pathology has been the major impetus for continued development in intravenous contrast agents [5]. The first category of contrast agents to be used in clinical practice was that of nonspecific extracellular gadolinium chelates. Since then, other classes of contrast agents have been developed for liver MR studies. There are two histologically and functionally distinct populations of cells in the liver. Liver epithelial cells, or hepatocytes, carry out the major metabolic activities. Hepatocyte function is assisted by another major class of cells, the reticuloendothelial system, which possess storage, phagocytic, and mechanically supportive functions. In recent years, hepatocyte-selective contrast agents and reticuloendothelial system (RES)-specific contrast agents have targeted these cell populations and added a new dimension to hepatic MR imaging. Clinically available liver contrast agents can be categorized as:

1. Nonspecific extracellular contrast: **Gadolinium chelates**
2. Hepatocyte-selective: **Mn-DPDP (mangafodipir trisodium)**
3. Agents with combined early nonspecific extracellular and late hepatocyte-selective properties: **Gd-EOB-DTPA (gadolinium ethoxybenzyl diethylenetriaminepentaacetic acid) and Gd-BOPTA (gadolinium benzyloxypropionictetraacetate)** [6–8]
4. RES-specific: **superparamagnetic iron oxide particles (SPIO)** [9–11]
5. Agents with combined early blood pool and late RES-specific properties: **ultrasmall paramagnetic iron oxide particles)** [12].

Nonspecific extracellular gadolinium chelates are the standard contrast agents to image liver and other organs and tissues in patients evaluated with MR imaging for a diverse range of indications. These paramagnetic contrast agents provide important information about tumor perfusion, which is a key factor in the assessment of liver masses [13–15]. Gadolinium chelates are optimally used when administered as a rapid bolus and imaging is performed with a T1-weighted spoiled GRE sequence that is repeated in a dynamic serial fashion. This is best achieved at high field strength [5]. The elimination is 100% renal [5]. The most important phase of enhancement may be termed the hepatic arterial dominant phase, with contrast present in hepatic arteries and portal veins and before contrast appears in hepatic veins. The hepatic arterial phase has contrast present only in the hepatic arteries (see figs. 2.5 and 2.6). See Chapter 1 for a more complete description.

Hepatocyte-selective contrast agents undergo uptake by hepatocytes and are eliminated through the renal and biliary system [5]. This category of contrast agents—Mn-DPDP, Gd-EOB-DTPA, and Gd-BOPTA—are all T1-relaxation-enhancing agents that are taken up by and result in an increase in the signal intensity of normal liver tissue and hepatocyte-containing tumors. Gd-EOB-DTPA and Gd-BOPTA exhibit early per fusisnal information as well. These contrast agents are not taken up by non-hepatocyte-containing masses (e.g., hemangioma, metastases) on late, >10 min, post contrast images; therefore, they leave signal unchanged in these entities on T1-weighted images. Non-hepatocyte-containing masses are rendered more conspicuous by the increase in signal of background liver tissue. Advantages of T1-relaxation agents include the following. (1) Use with SGE (as 2D or 3D sequences with or without fat suppression) results in robust, reproducible image quality with complete liver coverage in one breath hold. (2) They do not result in artifacts, such as susceptibility artifact, that can mask small lesions. The only hepatocyte-selective contrast agent that is at present licensed for use in the

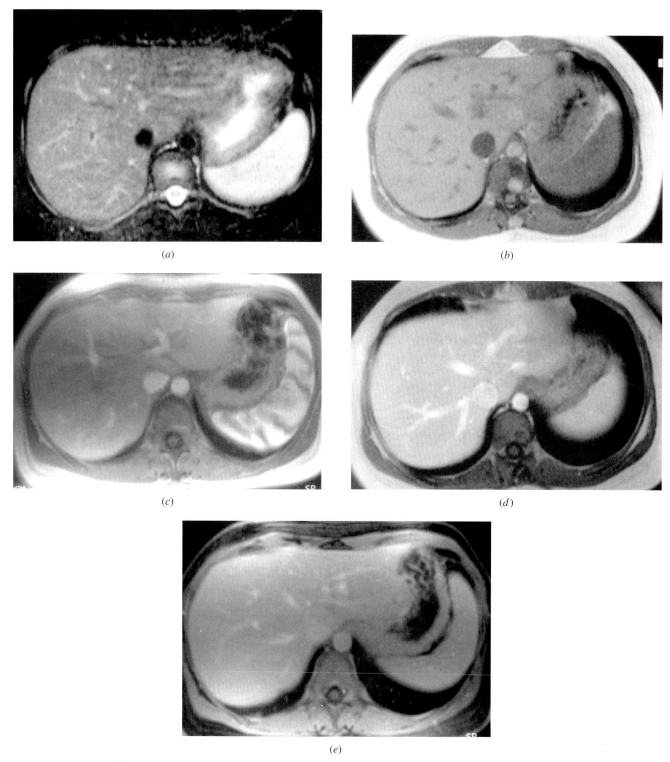

F I G . 2.3 Normal liver and sequences. Transverse T2-weighted fat-suppressed SS-ETSE (*a*), SGE (*b*), immediate postgadolinium (*c*), 45-s postgadolinium SGE (*d*), and 90-s postgadolinium fat-suppressed SGE (*e*) images. Liver is lower in signal than normal, non-iron-deposited spleen on the T2- (*a*) and higher in signal intensity than spleen on the T1-weighted (*b*) images. A liver imaging protocol should include noncontrast T2- (*a*) and T1-weighted (*b*) sequences, hepatic arterial dominant phase (*c*), early hepatic venous phase (*d*), and fat-suppressed hepatic venous phase (*e*) sequences.

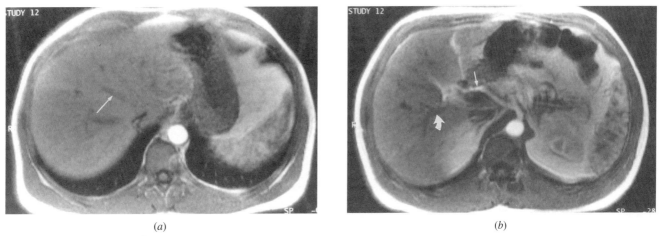

F I G . 2.4 Hepatic arterial-phase qadolinium-enhanced SGE images. Transverse hepatic arterial phase images from the level of the hepatic veins (*a*) and portal vein (*b*). The hepatic artery (thin arrow, *b*) is enhanced. Hepatic veins (arrow, *a*) and portal vein (curved arrow, *b*) are not enhanced. Some enhancement is appreciated in the splenic parenchyma and superior aspect of the left kidney, showing that these images were acquired in approximately the middle of the hepatic arterial enhancement phase.

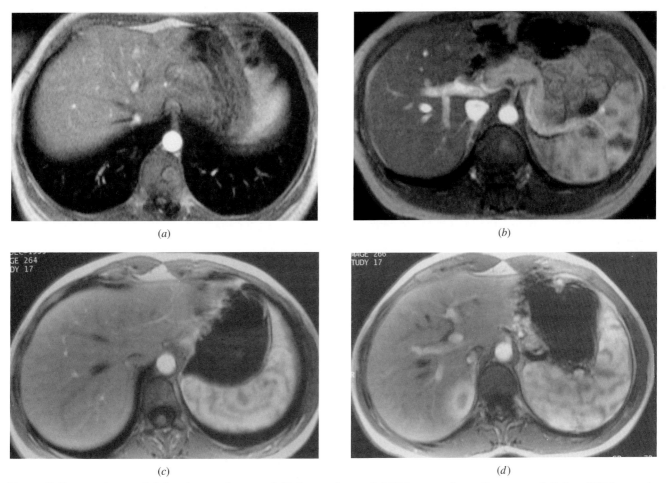

F I G . 2.5 Hepatic arterial dominant-phase gadolinium-enhanced SGE images. Immediate postgadolinium SGE images in 2 patients [(*a*, *b*) and (*c*, *d*), respectively]. Images acquired from the higher tomographic sections (*a*, *c*) demonstrate absence of gadolinium in hepatic veins, and images acquired from the more inferior tomographic sections (*b*, *d*) demonstrate presence of gadolinium in hepatic arteries and portal veins.

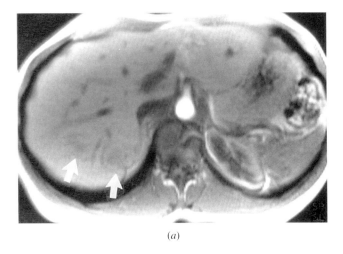

(a)

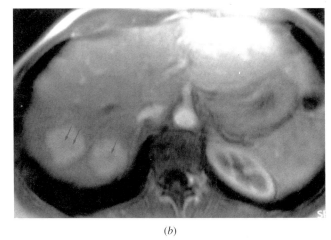

(b)

F I G . 2.6 Hepatic arterial dominant versus hepatic arterial phase. Hepatic arterial (*a*), hepatic arterial dominant postgadolinium (*b*), and Mn-DPDP-enhanced SGE (*c*) images. Two lobular lesions are seen in the right hepatic lobe and demonstrate moderate high signal after manganese administration (*c*). Hepatic arterial phase (*a*) shows faint heterogeneous enhancement that may suggest a hepatocellular carcinoma. The intense blush on hepatic arterial dominant phase (*b*), with a central scar (arrows, *b*) is, however, characteristic for a FNH. Note that on hepatic arterial phase the lesions are not as evident (arrows, a) as in hepatic arterial dominant phase (*b*). Note that uptake of Mn-DPDP by the lesions is consistant with FNHs (*c*).

(c)

United States is Mn-DPDP. This agent is administered as a slow (1 min) intravenous infusion, and the maximal imaging window is between 15 min and 4 h [5]. Dynamic images are not required, and it is not necessary that the MR machine have high field strength. At this stage of clinical use, this agent appears to be safe and well tolerated. At present, the best clinical use for Mn-DPDP is to improve detection of the number and extension of focal liver metastases from colon cancer in patients in whom hepatic resection is being contemplated [5]. In a recent report with 21 patients, no adverse reaction was observed or reported subsequently [16]. The combined use of conventional gadolinium chelates and Mn-DPDP has been described. This approach combines the perfusional information of gadolinium with the hepatocyte uptake information of Mn-DPDP (fig. 2.7) [16]. In selected cases, the combination of gadolinium chelates and liver-specific contrast agents may provide additional information [16, 17].

 Gd-EOB-DTPA (fig. 2.8) and Gd-BOPTA are combined extracellular/hepatocyte agents that can be used to acquire early perfusional information similar to standard gadolinium chelates and late (>15 min) hepatocyte enhancement [18]. The early perfusional informa-

tion is very important for lesion characterization with the additional benefit of improved detection, particularly for hypervascular lesions. The late images may be used for lesion detection with some additional information to distinguish hepatocyte-containing from non-hepatocyte-containing tumors. Although hepatocyte-specific agents permit distinction between hepatocyte-containing tumors (e.g., adenoma, focal nodular hyperplasia, hepatocellular carcinoma) and non-hepatocyte containing tumors (e.g., hemangioma, metastases), it is generally more important to distinguish between benign and malignant tumors. Early perfusional information generally achieves this goal.

 Iron oxide particle agents are selectively taken up by RES in the liver, spleen, and bone marrow. This class of contrast agent is also termed superparamagnetic iron oxide, and the first of these agents licensed for use in the United States are the ferumoxides. RES cell-specific contrast agents are T2-relaxation-enhancing agents that lower the signal intensity of normal RES cell-containing liver tissue on T2-weighted images and do not alter the signal intensity of mass lesions that do not contain RES cells (e.g., metastases). Blood pool effects may be observed with hemangiomas, which can result

Table 2.1 Liver Lesion Pattern Recognition

	T1	T2	Early Gd	Late Gd	Other Features
Cyst	↓↓	↑↑	◯	◯	well defined
Hamartoma	↓↓	↑↑	thin rim	thin rim	<1 cm
Hemangioma	↓↓	↑↑	peripheral nodules	nodules coalesce, retain contrast	<1.5-cm lesion may enhance homogeneously
FNH	↓−φ	φ−↑	homogeneous intense, negligible scar enhancement	homogeneous washout, late scar enhancement	central scar liver is commonly fatty
Adenoma	↓−↑	φ−↑	homogeneous intense	homogeneous washout	uniform signal loss on out-of-phase T1, hemorrhage not uncommon
Metastases	↓	↑	ring	progressive with heterogeneous washout	<1.5-cm lesion may enhance homogeneously
HCC	↓−↑	φ−↑	diffuse heterogeneous	heterogeneous late capsule enhance washout	<1.5-cm lesion may enhance homogeneously
Bacterial abscess	↓↓	↑−↑↑	perilesional enhancement, capsule enhances	perilesional enhancement fades capsule remains enhanced	resemble metastases but no progressive lesion enhancement
Lymphoma secondary	↓	↑	ring	progressive mild enhancement	resemble mestastases
Lymphoma primary	↓	↑	diffuse heterogeneous	progressive with heterogeneous washout	resemble HCC
Regenerative nodule	↓−φ	↓−φ	negligible	negligible	lesions generally <1.5 cm and homogeneous
Mildly dysplastic nodule	↓−↑	—	minimal	minimal	lesions generally <1.5 cm and homogeneous
Severely dysplastic nodules	↓−↑	—	homogeneous intense	fade to isointense with liver	lesions generally <1.5 cm, homogeneous, and no capsule

↓↓ moderately decreased signal intensity
↓ mildly decreased signal intensity
φ isointense
↑ mildly increased etc
↑↑ moderately to mildly etc.
◯ no enhancement

in T1 shortening on T1-weighted sequences. This results in an increase in detection and in the conspicuity of liver tumors that are moderately high in signal intensity on T2-weighted images (fig. 2.9). The patient group in which this role for ferumoxides may be the most applicable is patients with liver metastases from colon cancer who are considered to be candidates for hepatic resection [5]. Studies have shown that ferumoxide-enhanced T2-weighted MR imaging has performance comparable to that of CT during arterial portography for the demonstration of liver metastases [5]. A cautionary note with this agent is that susceptibility artifact may potentially interfere with detection of subcentimeter lesions such as metastases. A number of sequences have been employed to improve image quality, including gradient echo sequences with a longer TE (≥6ms), single-shot or breath hold echo-train spin echo, and breathing-averaged proton density echo-train spin echo. Combined use of superparamagnetic iron oxide and conventional gadolinium chelates has been de-

scribed. This approach combines the perfusional information of gadolinium with the RES information of superparamagnetic iron oxide. It may be expected that their combined use would be more effective for detection and characterizing focal lesions than either contrast agent alone [17]. The long infusion period (30 min) is an inconvenient aspect of this agent, which necessitates two imaging sessions for nonenhanced and enhanced images. Attractive features of the agent include the long imaging window (1–4 h), no need for precise dynamic image acquisition related to contrast material administration, and acceptable image quality with machines of various field strength [5]. Although serious adverse events are rare, approximately 3% of patients will experience severe back pain while the contrast agent is being administered. This back pain appears to be a side effect of particulate agents in general and develops in patients in whom the contrast agent is administered too rapidly [5]. This agent can also be administered as a small-volume rapid bolus, which is greatly advantageous

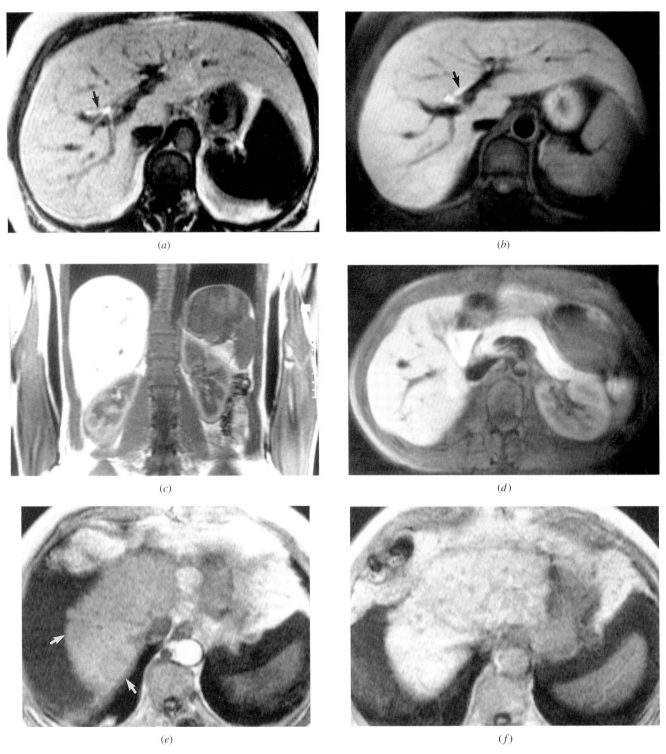

(a)   (b)

(c)   (d)

(e)   (f)

FIG. 2.7 Mn-DPDP-enhancement. Mn-DPDP-enhanced SGE (*a*) and Mn-DPDP-enhanced T1-weighted fat-suppressed SE (*b*) images in a normal patient. Normal liver homogeneously enhances with Mn-DPDP because of its T1-shortening effect. Excretion of Mn-DPDP in the biliary system is shown as high-signal intensity fluid in biliary ducts (arrow, *a*, *b*).

Coronal Mn-DPDP-enhanced SGE (*c*) and transverse Mn-DPDP-enhanced T1-weighted fat-suppressed spin-echo (*d*) images in a second patient. Note the increased signal intensity of normal liver tissue after administration of Mn-DPDP.

SGE (*e*) and 30-min post-Mn-DPDP SGE (*f*) images in a third patient. Subtle low-signal intensity mass lesions are apparent on the precontrast image (arrows, *e*). After Mn-DPDP enhancement (*f*) the HCCs enhance slightly more intensely than background liver, rendering the tumors minimally hyperintense. A pseudocapsule is appreciated around the more posterior tumor on both the precontrast and postcontrast images.

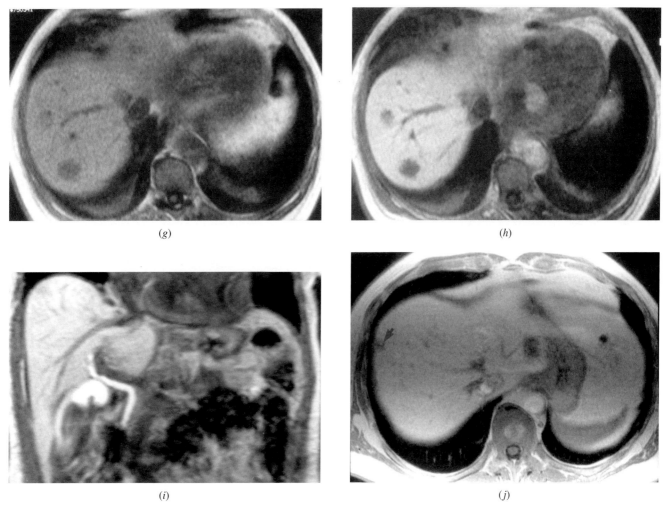

(g)   (h)

(i)   (j)

FIG. 2.7 (*Continued*) Transverse noncontrast SGE (*g*), 10-min post-Mn-DPDP-enhanced SGE (*h*) and coronal 10-min Mn-DPDP-enhanced SGE (*i*) images in a fourth patient who has liver metastases. The liver increases in signal from pre- (*g*) to post-Mn (*h*) images, increasing the conspicuity of the metastases. Note the excretion of Mn-DPDP into the biliary system (*i*).

Mn-DPDP-enhanced 512 resolution SGE image (*j*) in a fifth patient who has a liver metastasis (arrow, *j*). The liver detail is greater than usual, reflecting the use of 512 matrix.

over the larger particulate agent superparamagnetic iron oxide.

Ultrasmall paramagnetic iron oxide particles have blood pool effects that may be helpful in detecting or characterizing vascular lesions such as hemangiomas [12] and provide bright vessel enhancement in the vascular phase, which can be used for MR angiography [5].

Other newer tissue-specific contrast agents are under development such as those targeted to cell membrane antigens [19]. The application and role of new contrast agents will ultimately depend on how they compare with nonspecific extracellular gadolinium chelates. Recent studies have compared contrast agents in an attempt to define clinical uses [7, 18–20]. Defined clinical roles are under development for these new agents. It is

likely that the majority of these agents cannot replace extracellular gadolinium entirely because of its broad applicability.

NORMAL VARIATIONS

A number of normal variations in liver size and shape occur. Common variations include horizontal elongation of the lateral segment of the left lobe, hypoplasia of the left lobe, and vertical elongation of the right lobe, termed the Riedel lobe. The Riedel lobe is fairly common and is characterized by a downward tonguelike projection of the right lobe. This anatomical variation is more frequent in women [21]. Correct identification of a Riedel lobe is

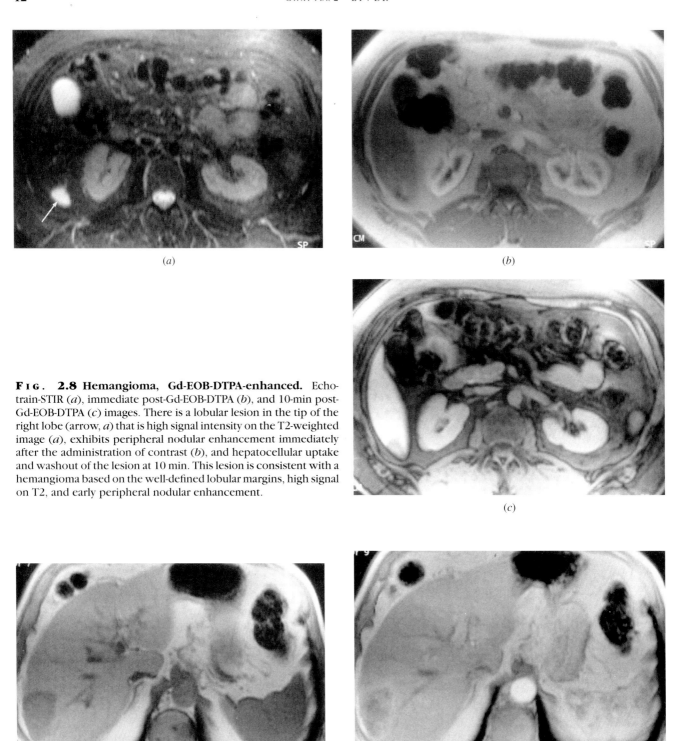

(a)

(b)

(c)

FIG. 2.8 Hemangioma, Gd-EOB-DTPA-enhanced. Echo-train-STIR (*a*), immediate post-Gd-EOB-DTPA (*b*), and 10-min post-Gd-EOB-DTPA (*c*) images. There is a lobular lesion in the tip of the right lobe (arrow, *a*) that is high signal intensity on the T2-weighted image (*a*), exhibits peripheral nodular enhancement immediately after the administration of contrast (*b*), and hepatocellular uptake and washout of the lesion at 10 min. This lesion is consistent with a hemangioma based on the well-defined lobular margins, high signal on T2, and early peripheral nodular enhancement.

(a)

(b)

FIG. 2.9 Gadolinium and iron oxide. Noncontrast SGE (*a*), immediate postgadolinium SGE (*b*), iron oxide-enhanced SGE (*c*), and iron oxide-enhanced T2 fat-suppressed (*d*) images in a patient with colon carcinoma imaged with a Gd study performed 19 days before an iron oxide study. A 3-cm metastasis is seen in the right hepatic lobe, which is moderately low signal on the noncontrast SGE image (*a*), and demonstrates a peripheral ring enhancement on the immediate postgadolinium SGE image (*b*) consistent with metastasis. On the iron oxide-enhanced SGE image (*c*), a lowered signal intensity in the liver and spleen is noted, diminishing the conspicuity of the metastasis. On the iron oxide-enhanced T2-weighted image (*d*), the signal intensity of the liver and spleen are markedly lower, increasing the conspicuity of the metastasis.

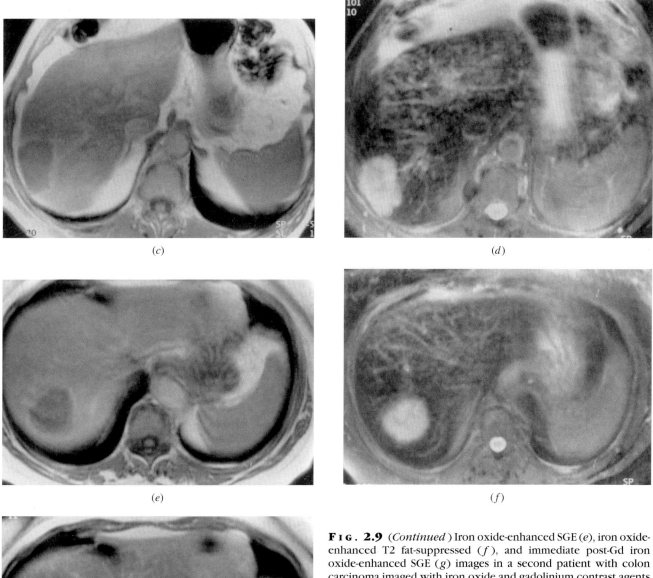

(c)

(d)

(e)

(f)

(g)

F I G . 2.9 (*Continued*) Iron oxide-enhanced SGE (*e*), iron oxide-enhanced T2 fat-suppressed (*f*), and immediate post-Gd iron oxide-enhanced SGE (*g*) images in a second patient with colon carcinoma imaged with iron oxide and gadolinium contrast agents with iron oxide imaged first in a combined protocol. A lesion is present in the right hepatic lobe, which is low signal intensity on the iron oxide-enhanced SGE image (*e*) and high signal intensity on the iron oxide-enhanced T2-weighted image (*f*). The lesion enhances with a peripheral rim pattern consistent with a metastasis on the immediate post-Gd iron oxide-enhanced SGE image (*g*). Lesion conspicuity is high on the post-Gd iron oxide-enhanced image because of the lowered signal intensity of the background liver parenchyma and intense early enhancement of the neoplasm. (Reproduced with permission from Semelka RC, Lee JKT, Worawattanakul S, Noone TC, Patt RH, Asher SM. Sequential use of ferumoxide particles and gadolinium chelate for the evaluation of focal liver lesions on MRI. *J Magn Reson Imaging* 8: 670–674, 1998.)

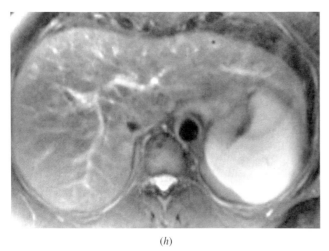
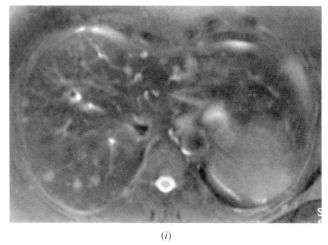

(h)   *(i)*

F I G . 2.9 *(Continued)* Nonenhanced (*h*) and iron oxide particulate-enhanced (*i*) T2-weighted fat-suppressed ETSE images in a third patient, who has liver metastases. After contrast administration (*i*), a greater number of <1-cm metastases are identified in the liver.

necessary to avoid confusion with hepatomegaly. Transverse and coronal images are effective at demonstrating this variant, and coronal images are useful for excluding an exophytic mass lesion such as hepatic adenoma or metastasis (fig. 2.10).

An elongated lateral segment may wrap around the anterior aspect of the upper abdomen and extend laterally to the spleen. This variation is also more common in women. A clear distinction between liver and spleen may be made with T2-weighted images in which normal spleen is high in signal intensity and distinct from the lower-signal intensity liver (fig. 2.11).

Hypoplasia of the left lobe does not generally result in diagnostic difficulties, although it may simulate a left hepatectomy, which clinical history readily establishes.

Diaphragmatic insertions are not an uncommon finding along the lateral aspect of the liver. They tend to be multiple and closely related to overlying ribs, having wedge-shaped margins with the capsular surface of the liver (fig. 2.12). Insertions are low in signal on T1- and T2-weighted images. These features help to distinguish diaphragmatic insertions from peripheral mass lesions.

PARTIAL HEPATECTOMY

Partial hepatectomy is a common procedure. Imaging findings after partial hepatectomy vary depending on the remoteness of the resection. Magnetic susceptibility artifact, related to surgical clips, is often present along the resection margin of the liver. Hyperplasia of the remaining liver may be appreciated as early as 3 months after surgery. Within 1 year, general enlargement of the remaning liver occurs. After right hepatectomy, hypertrophy of the medial segment may create the appearance of a pseudo-right lobe (fig. 2.13).

DISEASE OF THE HEPATIC PARENCHYMA

Mass Lesions

Benign Masses

Solitary (nonparasitic) Cysts. Hepatic cysts are common lesions and are usually divided into unilocular (95%) or multilocular varieties. Although the pathogenesis of these cysts is not clear, developmental and acquired causes are postulated. Acquired cysts are thought to represent retention cysts of bile ductule derivation [22]. Pathologically, the lining of the cyst shows a single layer of cuboidal to columnar epithelial cells. Lining epithelium rests on an underlying fibrous stroma. On imaging, cysts are homogeneous, well-defined lesions that possess a sharp margin with the liver. Although slight variations are common, cysts are usually oval-shaped (figs. 2.14–2.16) [23]. Occasionally, cysts are so closely grouped that they resemble a multicystic mass. Cysts are low in signal intensity on T1-weighted images and high in signal intensity on T2-weighted images, and thus retain signal intensity on longer echo time (e.g., >120 ms) T2-weighted images. Because cysts do not enhance with gadolinium on MR images, delayed postgadolinium images (up to 5 min) may be useful to ensure that lesions are cysts and not poorly vascularized metastases that show gradual enhancement [24]. An advantage of MRI over computed tomography (CT) imaging in the characterization of cysts is that on gadolinium-enhanced MR images cysts are nearly signal void, whereas cysts on contrast-enhanced CT images are a light gray in attenuation. Single-shot breathing-independent T2-weighted sequences (e.g., SS-ETSE) are especially effective at showing small (≤5 mm) cysts. MRI is particularly valuable when lesions are small and the patient has a known primary malignancy.

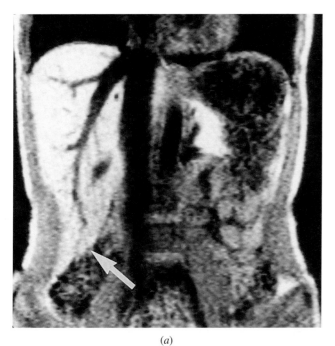

(a)

FIG. 2.10 Riedel lobe. Coronal snap-shot magnetization-prepared gradient-echo image (*a*) demonstrates elongation of the inferior aspect of the right lobe of the liver (arrow, *a*) consistent with Riedel lobe.

Coronal T2-weighted SS-ETSE (*b*) and SGE (*c*) images in a second patient exhibit a Riedel lobe with bulbous inferior aspect.

Coronal T2-weighted SS-ETSE (*d*) and SGE (*e*) images in a third patient that demonstrates hypertrophy of the Riedel lobe, with a convex medial border.

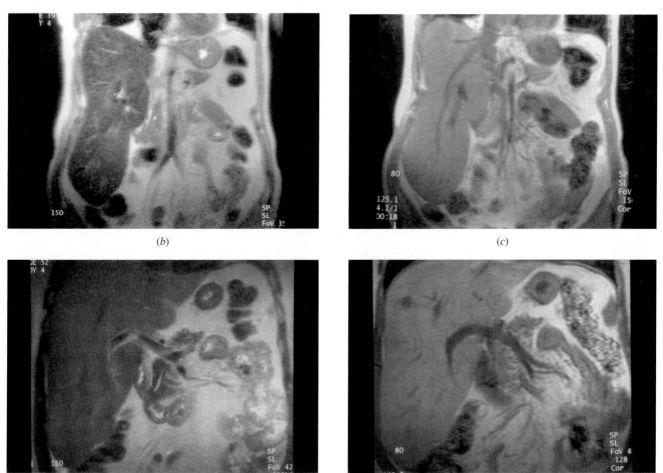

(b)

(c)

(d)

(e)

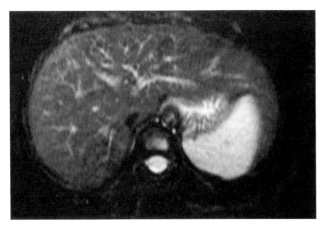

FIG. 2.11 Elongated lateral segment of the left lobe. T2-weighted fat-suppressed ETSE image demonstrates an elongated lateral segment that extends lateral to the spleen. Clear distinction is made between lower-signal intensity liver and moderately high-signal intensity spleen on T2-weighted images.

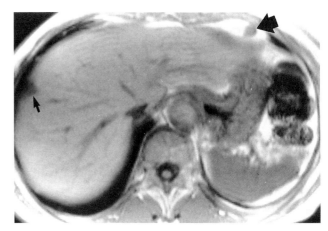

FIG. 2.12 Diaphragmatic insertion. SGE image demonstrates a wedge-shaped defect along the lateral superior margin of the liver (arrow). Diaphragmatic insertions are usually multiple but may be single as in this case. Incidental note is made of a subdiaphragmatic lymph node (large arrow).

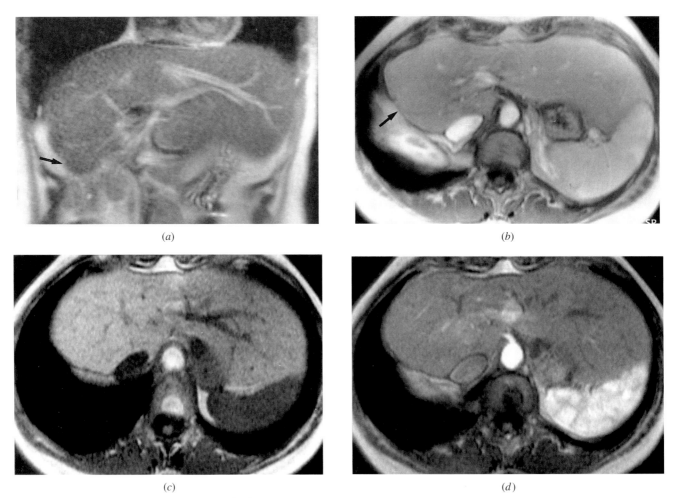

(a)

(b)

(c)

(d)

FIG. 2.13 Liver regeneration after right hepatectomy. Coronal T2-weighted SS-ETSE (*a*) and immediate postgadolinium SGE (*b*) images. The lateral segment of the left lobe is enlarged and rounded in contour (*a, b*). Hypertrophy of the medial segment results in an appearance of a pseudo-right lobe (arrow, *a*). A relatively sharp resection margin is noted (arrow, *b*) with no abnormal tissue apparent.

Transverse SGE (*c*) and immediate postgadolinium SGE (*d*) images in a second patient with hypertrophy of the left liver lobe after right lobectomy. Note that the lateral segment of the left lobe is enlarged but there is a clear distinction between the liver and the spleen.

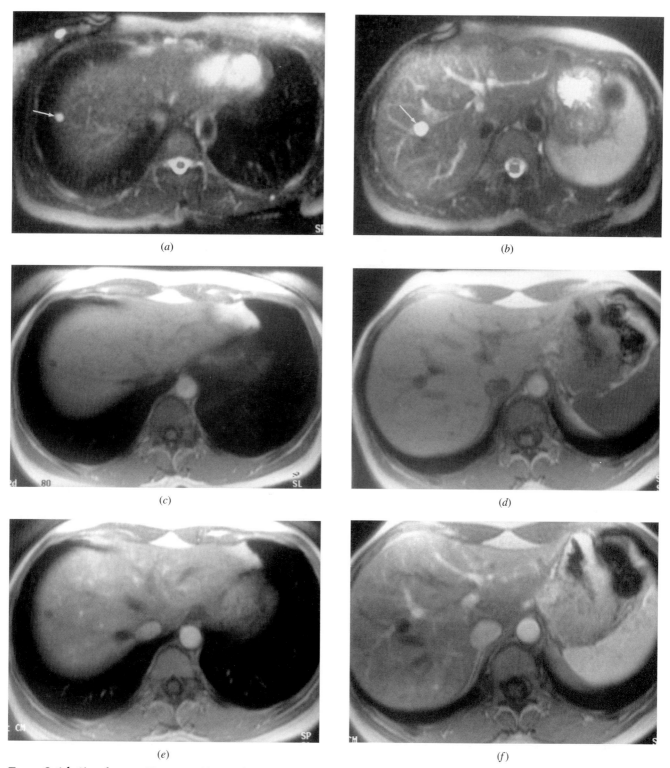

F I G . 2.14 Simple cyst. Transverse T2-weighted fat-suppressed SS-ETSE (*a*, *b*), SGE (*c*, *d*), immediate postgadolinium (*e*, *f*) and 90-s postgadolinium fat-suppressed SGE (*g*, *b*) images. There are two homogeneous, well-defined lesions (arrow, *a*, *b*) that are high signal on T2 (*a*, *b*) and low signal on T1-weighted images (*c*, *d*) that do not enhance after administration of gadolinium on early (*e*, *f*) and late (*g*, *b*) postcontrast images, consistent with simple liver cysts.

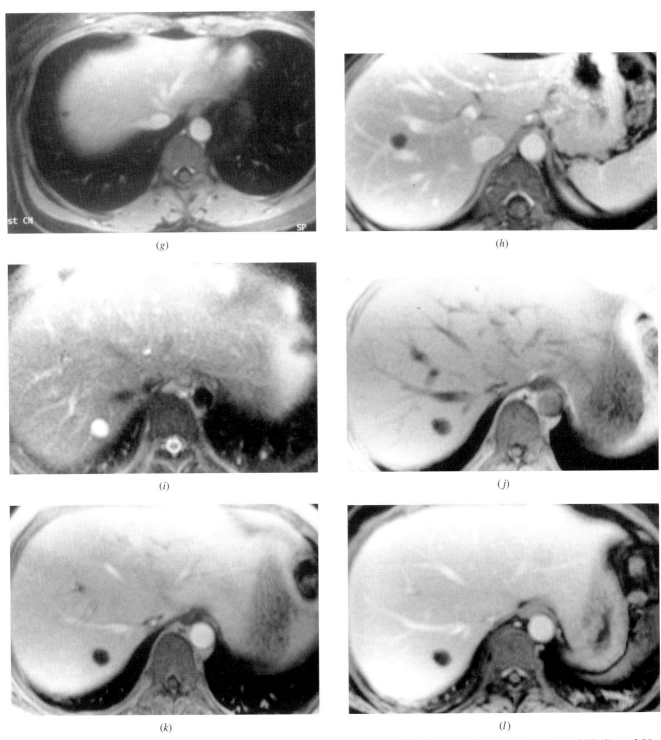

FIG. 2.14 (*Continued*) Transverse T2-weighted fat-suppressed SS-ETSE (*i*), SGE (*j*), immediate postgadolinium SGE (*k*), and 90-s postgadolinium fat-suppressed SGE (*l*) images in a second patient. A small lesion is present, which demonstrates increased signal on T2- (*i*) and decreased signal on T1-weighted (*j*) images, and shows no enhancement after gadolinium administration on early (*k*) and late (*l*) postcontrast images.

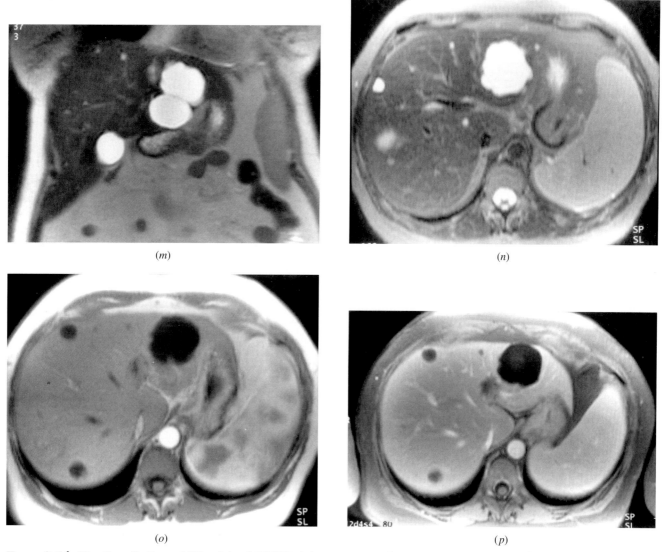

(m)   *(n)*

(o)   *(p)*

Fɪɢ. 2.14 (*Continued*) Coronal T2-weighted SS-ETSE (*m*), transverse echo-train-STIR (*n*), immediate postgadolinium SGE (*o*), and 90-s postgadolinium fat-suppressed SGE (*p*) images in a third patient. Multiple homogeneous simple cysts of different sizes are scattered throughout the hepatic parenchyma.

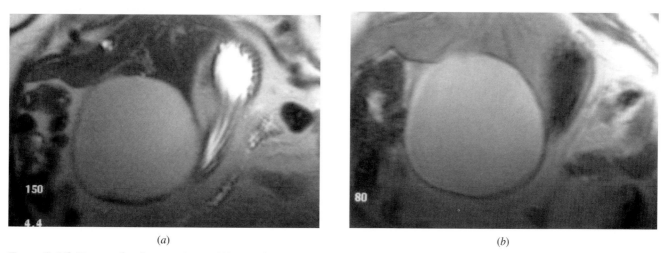

(a)   *(b)*

Fɪɢ. 2.15 Hemorrhagic cyst. Coronal T2-weighted SS-ETSE (*a*), Coronal SGE (*b*), transverse immediate postgadolinium SGE (*c*), and 90-s postgadolinium fat-suppressed SGE (*d*) images.

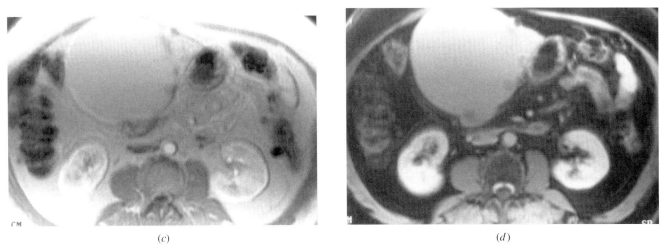

(c)   *(d)*

FIG. 2.15 *(Continued)* A large cystic mass with thickened and irregular wall arises from the lateral segment and demonstrates increased signal on T2- (*a*) and T1-weighted (*b*) images and no enhancement on early (*c*) and late (*d*) postcontrast images. A blood-filled cyst was proven by histopathology.

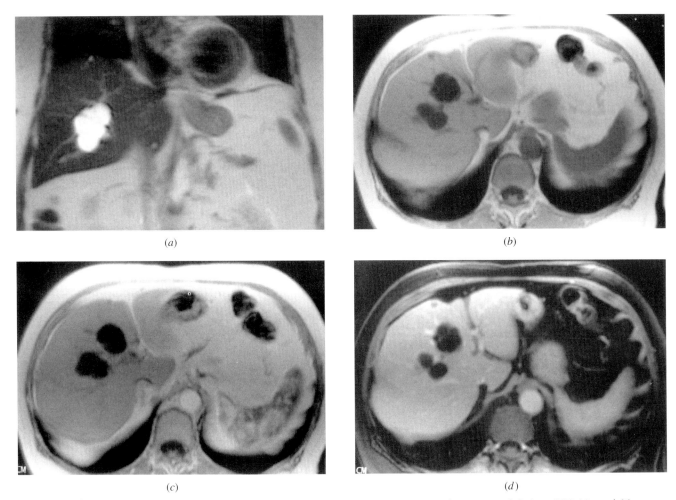

(a)   *(b)*

(c)   *(d)*

FIG. 2.16 Multi-septated cysts. Coronal T2-weighted SS-ETSE (*a*), SGE (*b*), immediate postgadolinium SGE (*c*), and 90-s postgadolinium fat-suppressed SGE (*d*) images. Multiple cystic lesions with internal septations are present in the right hepatic lobe.

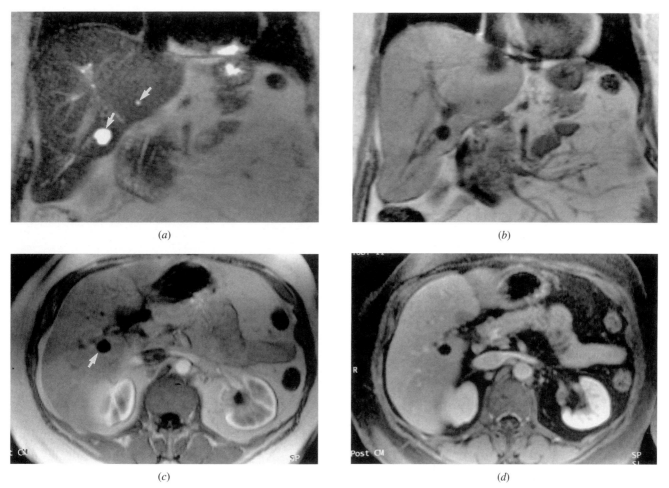

FIG. 2.17 Liver cysts. Coronal T2-weighted SS-ETSE (*a*), coronal SGE (*b*), immediate postgadolinium SGE (*c*), and 90-s postgadolinium fat-suppressed SGE (*d*) images. Two cysts, 2 mm and 10 mm, are present on coronal images (arrows, *a*). Cysts measuring <5 mm are most clearly shown on T2-weighted SS-ETSE images. Cysts are high signal intensity on T2-weighted images (*a*) and low signal intensity on T1-weighted images (*b*). The 10-mm cyst is signal void on early (arrow, *c*) and later (*d*) postgadolinium images.

The vast majority of liver cysts are simple in type. Therefore, the majority are low in signal intensity on T1-weighted images, high in signal intensity on T2-weighted images, and nearly signal void on postgadolinium images (fig. 2.17).

Ciliated Hepatic Foregut Cysts. Foregut cysts are an uncommon type of solitary unilocular cyst. These congenital lesions are believed to arise from the embryonic foregut and to differentiate toward bronchial tissue in the liver. Pathologically, the cyst wall consists of four layers: pseudostratified ciliated columnar epithelium with mucous cells, subepithelial connective tissue, abundant smooth muscle, and an outermost fibrous capsule. These cysts are most frequently located at the anterosuperior margin of the liver but may be situated elsewhere, superficially along the external surface of the liver, typically at intersegmental locations. Foregut cysts range from hypo- to hyperintense on T1-weighted images, are hyperintense on T2-weighted images, and do not enhance with gadolinium [25, 26]. The presence of mucin in these cysts results in high signal intensity on T1-weighted images, with the extent of increase in signal intensity dependent on the concentration of mucin. These cysts characteristically bulge the liver contour and possess a perceptible enhancing cyst wall on postgadolinium images (figs. 2.18 and 2.19). The presence of a cystic lesion with an enhancing wall and extension beyond the contour of the liver may also be observed in some forms of metastatic disease such as hepatic metastasis from ovarian malignancies. For this reason, a diagnosis of foregut cyst on imaging studies should only be made in the absence of peritoneal disease and a clinical history of malignancy.

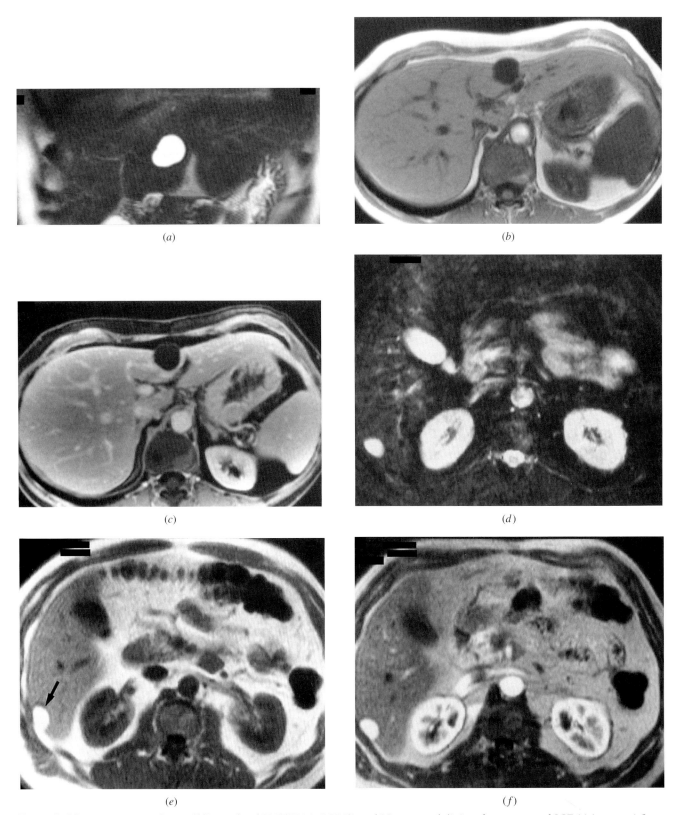

(a)

(b)

(c)

(d)

(e)

(f)

F I G . 2.18 Foregut cyst. Coronal T2-weighted SS-ETSE (*a*), SGE (*b*) and 90-s postgadolinium fat-suppressed SGE (*c*) images. A 3-cm cystic lesion is noted superiorly on the border between medial and lateral segments. The lesion extends beyond the contour of the liver and has a thin perceptible wall, features that are characteristic of foregut cysts.

T2-weighted fat-suppressed SS-ETSE (*d*), SGE (*e*), and immediate postgadolinium SGE (*f*) images in a second patient demonstrate a 1.5-cm lesion along the lateral inferior aspect of the right lobe of the liver (arrow, *e*). The lesion is sharply demarcated and is high in signal intensity on the T2- (*d*) and T1-weighted (*e*) images and does not change in shape or appearance after gadolinium administration (*f*). The lesion extends beyond the contour of the liver. The high concentration of mucin in the cyst accounts for the high signal intensity on the T1-weighted (*e*) images.

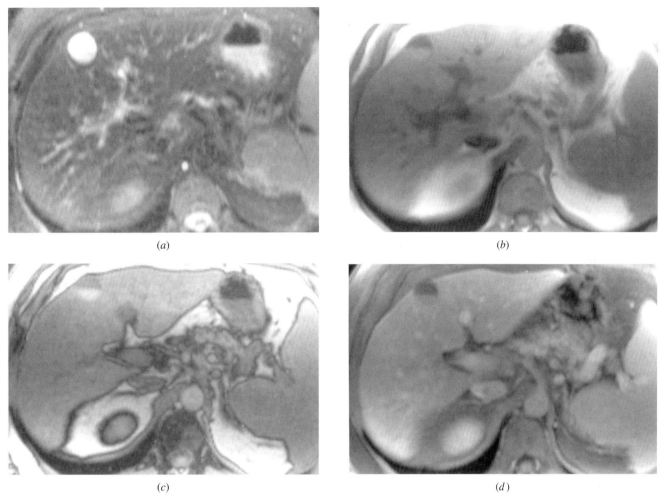

(a)

(b)

(c)

(d)

F I G . 2.19 Foregut cyst with layering. Echo train-STIR (*a*), SGE (*b*), out-of-phase SGE (*c*), and 90-s postgadolinium fat-suppressed SGE (*d*) images. A cystic lesion is identified in *segment 4* that distorts the anterior liver contour. The lesion is high signal on T2- (*a*) and demonstrates layering with high signal intensity on the T1-weighted image (*b*), which does not lose signal on out-of-phase SGE (*c*), consistent with proteinaceous material (mucin) observed in these cysts.

Autosomal Dominant Polycystic Kidney Disease. In autosomal dominant polycystic kidney disease, the liver is the most common extrarenal organ in which cysts occur. Although these cysts vary in number and size, they tend to be multiple and smaller than the renal cysts, measuring less than 2 cm (figs. 2.20 and 2.21). They generally do not distort hepatic architecture or undergo hemorrhage. Extensive hepatic replacement with large cysts has been described [27].

Biliary Hamartoma. Biliary hamartomas are benign biliary malformations, which are currently considered as part of the spectrum of fibropolycystic diseases of the liver due to ductal plate malformation [28]. This entity is common and estimated to be present in approximately 3% of patients. Histopathologically biliary hamartomas consist of a collection of small, sometimes dilated, irregular and branching bile ducts embedded in a fibrous stroma. A few of the ducts may contain inspissated bile. In general, biliary hamartomas contain no or few vascular channels. Tumors may be solitary (fig. 2.22) or multiple, and multiple tumors can be extensive (fig. 2.23). On MR images, tumors are small (usually <1 cm) and well defined. The high fluid content renders these lesions low signal on T1, high signal on T2, and negligible enhancement on early and late postgadolinium images. Although this appearance resembles simple cysts, biliary hamartomas demonstrate a thin rim of enhancement on early and late postcontrast images [28]. The major potential diagnostic error is to misclassify these lesions as metastases due to the presence of ring enhancement. The thin enhancing rim of biliary hamartomas, visualized on imaging, may be correlated histopathologically with the presence of compressed hepatic parenchyma bordering the lesion [28]. In contrast, the pattern of ring enhancement displayed by metastases relates histopathologically with

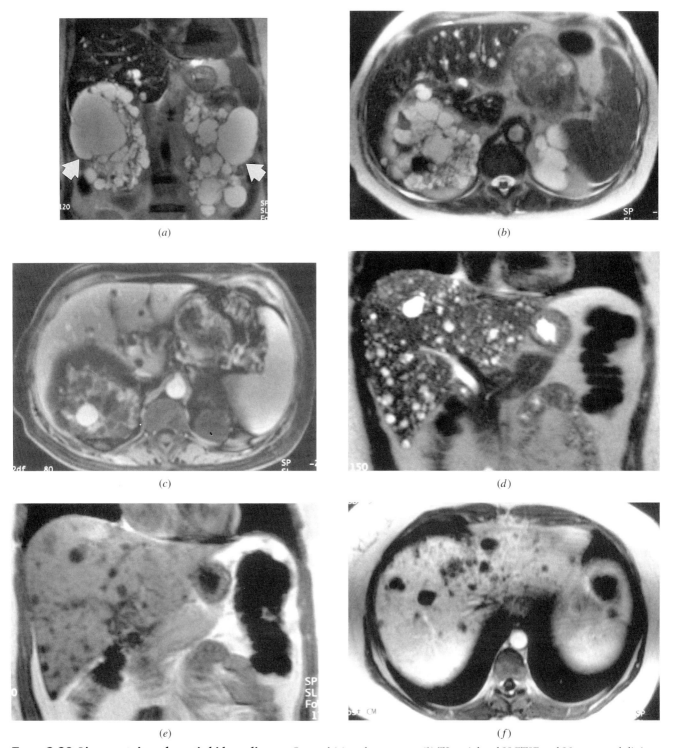

(a)

(b)

(c)

(d)

(e)

(f)

F I G . 2.20 Liver cysts in polycystic kidney disease. Coronal (*a*) and transverse (*b*) T2-weighted SS-ETSE and 90-s postgadolinium fat-suppressed SGE (*c*) images. The kidneys are massively enlarged and contain multiple cysts of varying size with no definable renal parenchyma (arrows, *a*). Multiple <1-cm cysts are present and scattered throughout the liver that are high in signal intensity on T2-weighted images (*a*, *b*) and do not enhance after gadolinium administration (*c*).

Coronal T2-weighted SS-ETSE (*d*), SGE (*e*), transverse 1-min postgadolinium SGE (*f*) images in a second patient show cysts scattered throughout the liver parenchyma with no evidence of hemorrhage or distortion of hepatic architecture.

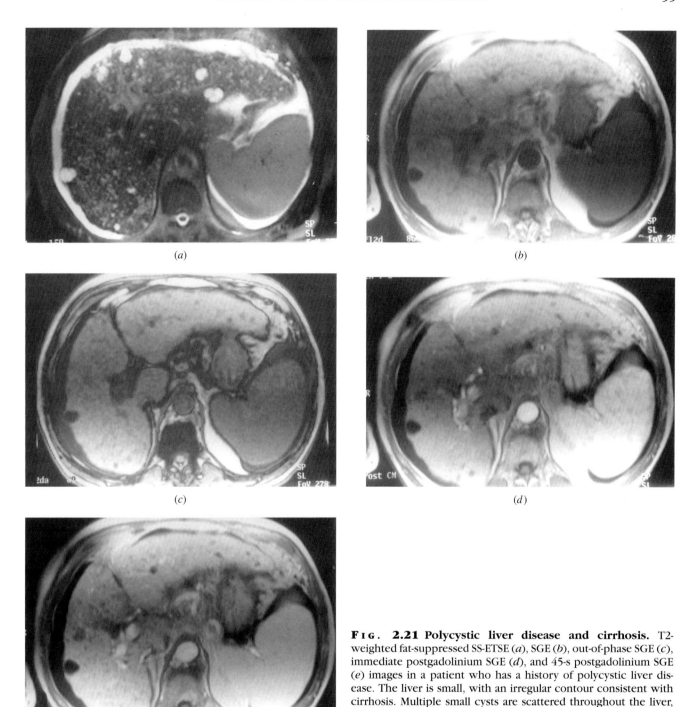

(a)

(b)

(c)

(d)

(e)

FIG. 2.21 Polycystic liver disease and cirrhosis. T2-weighted fat-suppressed SS-ETSE (*a*), SGE (*b*), out-of-phase SGE (*c*), immediate postgadolinium SGE (*d*), and 45-s postgadolinium SGE (*e*) images in a patient who has a history of polycystic liver disease. The liver is small, with an irregular contour consistent with cirrhosis. Multiple small cysts are scattered throughout the liver, compatible with liver cysts seen in autosomal dominant polycystic kidney disease.

the outer, most vascularized portion of the tumor. Peritumoral enhancement is also observed in some metastases as described below [29]. MR imaging further corroborates the different histologic profiles of the two processes through the observation that enhancement in biliary hamartoma does not progress centrally, whereas enhancement in metastases most often progresses centrally (fig. 2.24).

Extramedullary Hematopoiesis. Focal intrahepatic extramedullary hematopoiesis (EH) is an unusual condition that may appear as focal hepatic masses in the setting of hereditary disorders of hematopoiesis or in long-standing hematologic malignancies. EH is a compensatory phenomenon that occurs when erythrocyte production is diminished or destruction is accelerated [30]. EH is usually microscopic and commonly involves

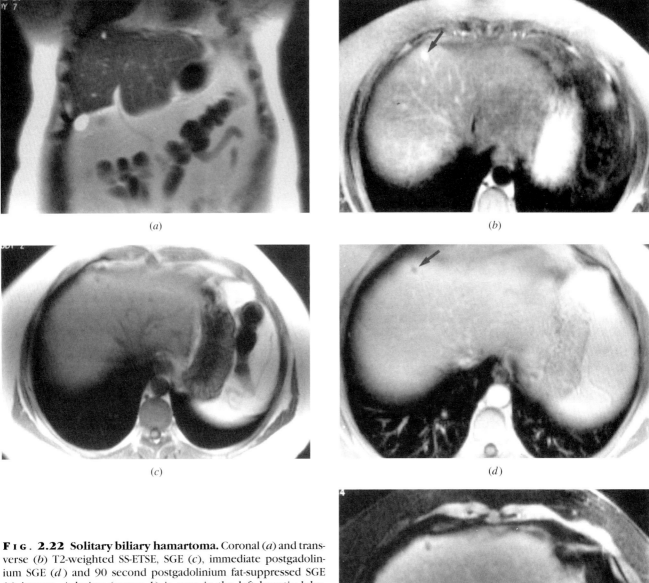

(a)

(b)

(c)

(d)

(e)

F I G . 2.22 Solitary biliary hamartoma. Coronal (*a*) and transverse (*b*) T2-weighted SS-ETSE, SGE (*c*), immediate postgadolinium SGE (*d*) and 90 second postgadolinium fat-suppressed SGE (*e*) images. A lesion (arrow, *b*) is seen in the left hepatic lobe, near the dome, which is well-defined, and high signal on the T2- (*a, b*) and low signal on the T1-weighted (*c*) images. On the immediate postgadolinium image (*d*), the lesion does not enhance with gadolinium, but a thin perilesional rim of enhancement is appreciated (arrow, *d*). (Reproduced with permission from Semelka RC, Hussain SM, Marcos HB, Woosley JT. Biliary hamartomas: Solitary and multiple lesions shown on current MR techniques including gadolinium enhancement. *J Magn Reson Imaging* 10: 196–201, 1999.)

the liver, spleen, and lymph nodes. Rarely, the involvement may be macroscopic [30]. The focal hepatic disease can manifest as solitary or multiple lesions [31], and the masses tend to be homogeneous and moderately high in signal intensity on T2-weighted images and to enhance in a diffuse homogeneous fashion on immediate postgadolinium images (fig. 2.25). A histopathological specimen is required for definitive diagnosis.

Angiomyolipomas. Angiomyolipomas of the liver are uncommon benign mesenchymal tumors. Histologically, the tumor is composed of mature fat, blood vessels, and smooth muscle. Some tumors may contain foci of extramedullary hematopoiesis (angiomyomyelolipomas). Some patients have tuberous sclerosis [32]; although the association is less strong than with renal angiomyolipomas. Angiomyolipomas are well-defined,

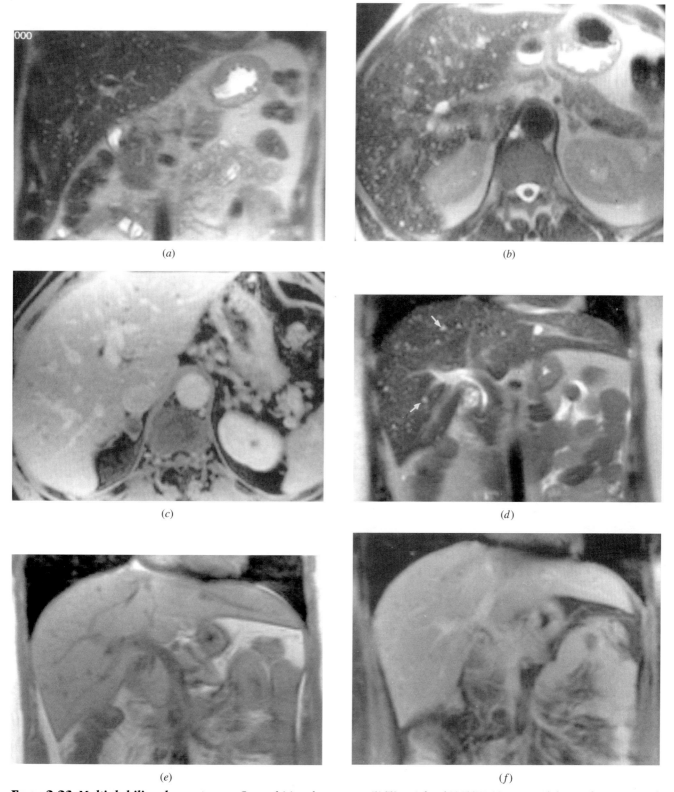

F I G . 2.23 Multiple biliary hamartomas. Coronal (*a*) and transverse (*b*) T2-weighted SS-ETSE, 90-s postgadolinium fat-suppressed SGE (*c*), coronal T2-weighted SS-ETSE (*d*), coronal SGE (*e*), coronal (*f*), and transverse (*g*) 2-min postgadolinium fat-suppressed SGE images in two different patients. In both patients there are multiple well defined lesions, <1 cm, scattered throughout the liver. They are high signal intensity on T2- (arrows, *d*) and low signal intensity on noncontrast T1-weighted (*e*) images and demonstrate thin perilesional rim enhancement on postgadolinium images. These lesions represent biliary hamartomas.

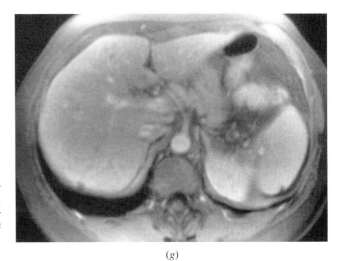

(g)

Fig. 2.23 (*Continued*) (Images *d* and *e* reproduced with permission from Semelka RC, Hussain SM, Marcos HB, Woosley JT. Biliary hamartomas: Solitary and multiple lesions shown on current MR techniques including gadolinium enhancement. *J Magn Reson Imaging* 10: 196–201, 1999.)

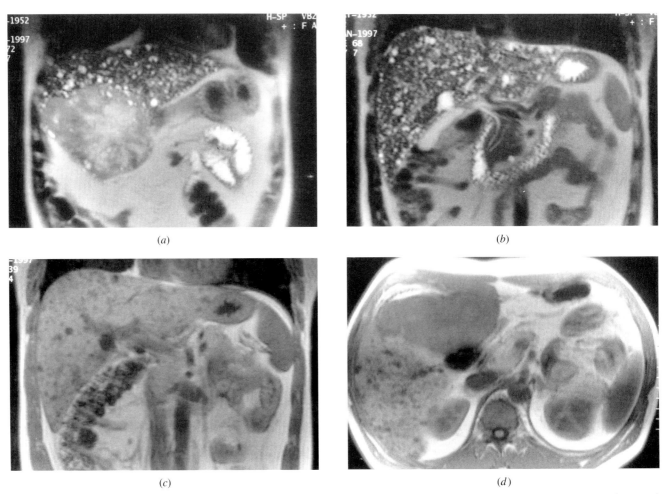

(a)

(b)

(c)

(d)

Fig. 2.24 Multiple biliary hamartomas and colon cancer metastases. Coronal T2-weighted SS-ETSE (*a, b*), coronal (*c*), and transverse (*d*) SGE, immediate postgadolinium SGE (*e, f*), and 90-s postgadolinium fat-suppressed SGE (*g, h*) images in a patient who has a history of colon cancer.

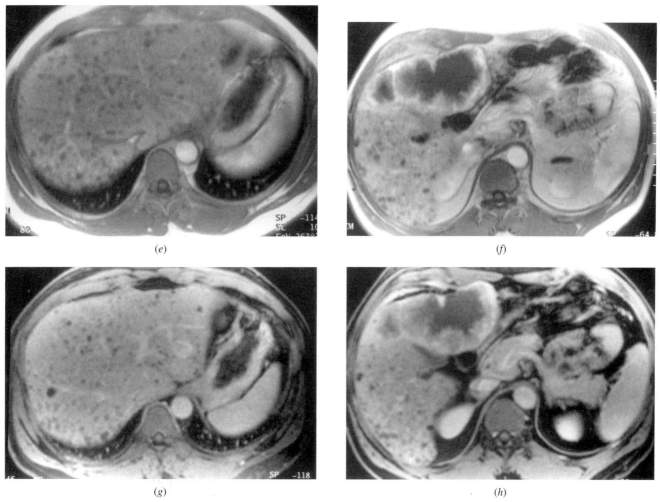

(e)   (f)

(g)   (h)

F I G . 2.24 (*Continued*) There is a large mass in *segments 4/5* that demonstrates heterogeneous and moderately high signal on T2 (*a*), moderately low signal on T1 (*d*), and ring enhancement postcontrast (*f, h*) consistent with a metastasis. The liver is riddled with many small well-defined lesions, measuring <1 cm, that demonstrate thin ring enhancement after contrast administration, consistent with biliary hamartomas. Note that the metastasis progress in enhancement from early (*f*) to late (*h*) images, whereas biliary hamartomas show identical ring enhancement on early and late images with no progressive enhancement.

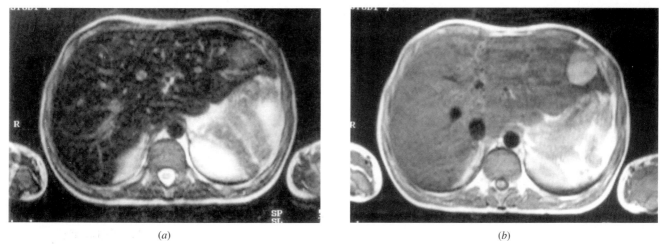

(a)   (b)

F I G . 2.25 Extramedullary Hematopoiesis. T2-weighted SS-ETSE (*a*), T1-weighted spin-echo (*b*) and 1-min postgadolinium SGE (*c*) images.

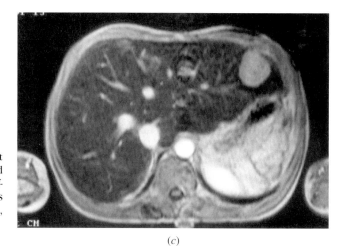

FIG. 2.25 (*Continued*) A rounded lesion is present in the left lobe that demonstrates slight increase in signal on T2- (*a*) and T1- weighted (*b*) images and mild homogeneous enhancement after administration of gadolinium (*c*). Extramedullary hematopoiesis was present at histopathology. (Courtesy of N. Cem Balci M.D., Florence Nightingale Hospital, Istanbul).

(*c*)

sharply marginated masses, frequently have a high fat content, and therefore are high in signal intensity on T1-weighted images and low in signal intensity on fat-suppressed images. Angiomyolipomas may also have a low fat content and appear moderately low in signal intensity on T1-weighted images, appear moderately high in signal intensity on T2-weighted images, and enhance in a diffuse heterogeneous fashion on immediate postgadolinium SGE images (figs. 2.26 and 2.27) [33]. A similar enhancement pattern is observed in well-differentiated hepatocellular carcinoma, and this enhancement reflects the appearance of well-defined tumors of hepatic origin. The pattern of enhancement of angiomyolipomas tends to be much more orderly than well-differentiated hepatocellular carcinomas.

Lipomas. Hepatic lipomas are rarer than angiomyolipomas. On imaging, tumors are commonly multiple and appear as fatty tumors that are high in signal intensity on T1-weighted sequences and low in signal intensity with fat-suppressed techniques (fig. 2.28) [34]. These lesions show negligible enhancement on postgadolinium images.

Hemangiomas. Hemangiomas are the most common benign hepatic neoplasm, with an autopsy incidence between 0.4 and 20% [35, 36]. Hemangiomas are more frequent in women. They not uncommonly coexist with focal nodular hyperplasia (FNH) lesions, particularly in the setting of the multiple FNH syndrome [37]. Hemangiomas are usually multiple (fig. 2.29), rarely

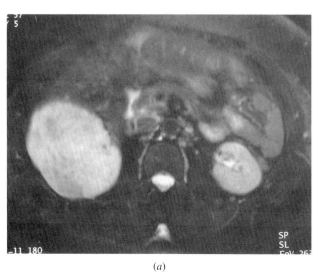

(*a*)

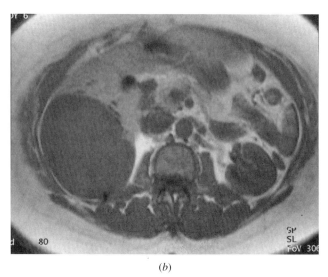

(*b*)

FIG. 2.26 Angiomyolipoma with minimal fat. T2-weighted fat-suppressed ETSE (*a*), SGE (*b*), immediate postgadolinium SGE (*c*), and 90-s postgadolinium SGE (*d*) images. The angiomyolipoma is moderately hyperintense with slight heterogeneity on the T2-weighted image (*a*) and moderately hypointense on the T1-weighted image (*b*) and enhances intensely in a diffuse heterogeneous fashion on the immediate postgadolinium SGE image (*c*).

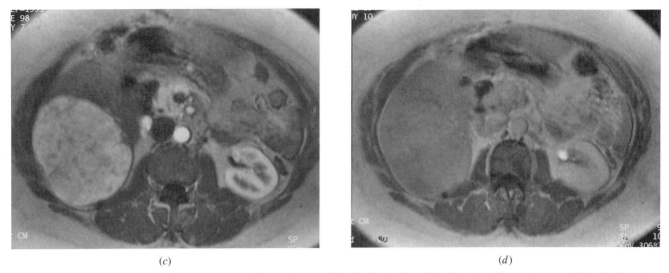

(c)   (d)

F I G . 2.26 (*Continued*) On the 90-s postgadolinium image (*d*), the lesion has faded in signal intensity to slightly higher than background liver. This angiomyolipoma is unusual in that it contains minimal fat. The diffuse heterogeneous enhancement is typical of tumors of hepatic origin.

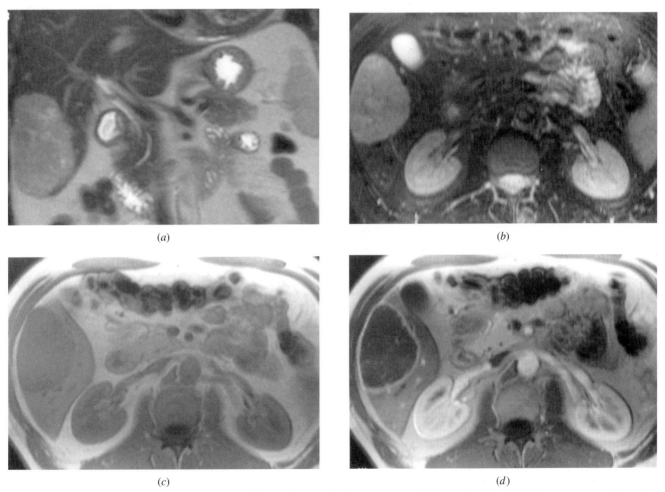

(a)   (b)

(c)   (d)

F I G . 2.27 Angiomyolipoma with minimal fat and vascular tissue. Coronal T2-weighted SS-ETSE (*a*), transverse echo train-STIR (*b*), SGE (*c*), immediate postgadolinium SGE (*d*), and 90-s postgadolinium fat-suppressed SGE (*e*) images.

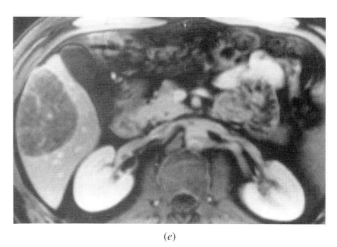

(e)

FIG. 2.27 (*Continued*) There is a well-circumscribed lesion in the right hepatic lobe that demonstrates moderately high signal intensity on T2 (*a, b*), low signal intensity on T1 (*c*), and capsular enhancement on immediate postgadolinium (*d*) images that fades by 90 s (*e*). On the early (*d*) and late (*e*) images there is a fine regular network of vessels apparent within the lesion. Angiomyolipoma with minimal fat was present at histopathology. Blood vessels are well organized throughout the tumor, unlike the irregular pattern observed in HCC. There is also a paucity of vascular tissue in this tumor.

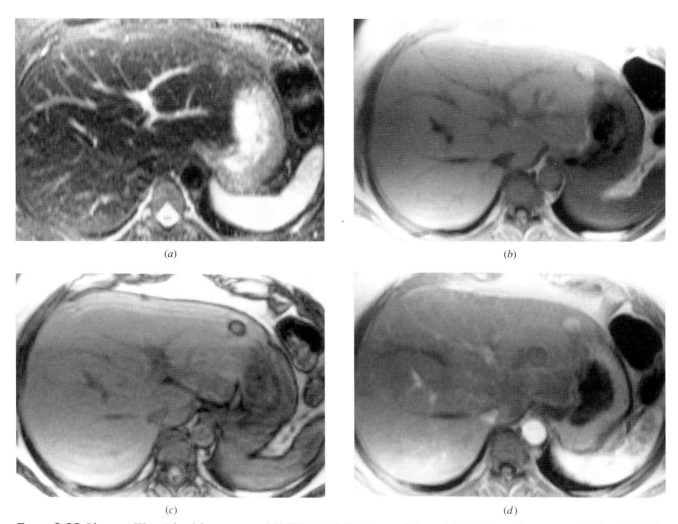

(a)   (b)

(c)   (d)

FIG. 2.28 Lipoma. T2-weighted fat suppressed SS-ETSE (*a*), SGE (*b*), out-of-phase SGE (*c*), immediate postgadolinium SGE (*d*), and 90-s postgadolinium fat-suppressed SGE (*e*) images. A 2.5-cm lipoma is present in the left lobe that demonstrates the same signal as fat on all imaging sequences. Note the development of a phase cancellation artifact on the out-of-phase image (*c*), which shows that the high-signal lesion is fatty.

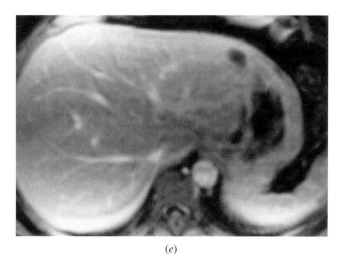

(e)

FIG. 2.28 (*Continued*) Care should be exercised not to attribute the high signal of fat as enhancement in fatty lesions on gadolinium-enhanced nonsuppressed images (*d*) or attribute the effect of fat suppression as washout on later fat-suppressed images (*e*).

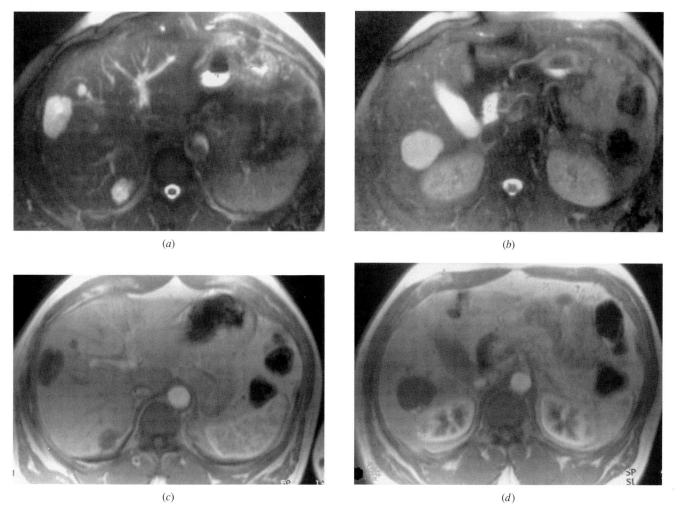

(a)   (b)

(c)   (d)

FIG. 2.29 Multiple Hemangiomas. T2-weighted fat-suppressed SS-ETSE (*a, b*), immediate postgadolinium SGE (*c, d*) and 90-s postgadolinium fat-suppressed SGE (*e, f*) images. Multiple hemangiomas are appreciated throughout the liver.

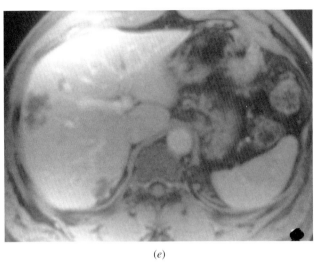

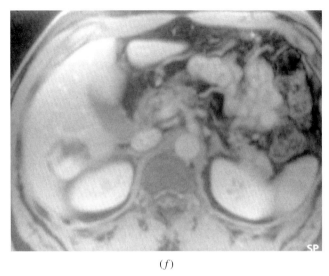

(e)   *(f)*

F I G . 2.29 *(Continued)* All of these lesions show increased T2 signal intensity (*a*, *b*), peripheral nodular enhancement after contrast administration (*c*, *d*), and enlargement and coalescence of nodules on delayed postcontrast images (*e*, *f*), consistent with hemangiomas.

produce symptoms, and are usually detected incidentally. The great majority of these benign vascular lesions are cavernous hemangiomas, but in rare instances they may represent capillary telangiectasias. Pathologically, hemangiomas are characterized grossly as well-circumscribed, spongelike blood-filled mesenchymal tumors. Microscopically, hemangiomas reveal numerous large vascular channels lined by a single layer of flat endothelial cells separated by slender fibrous septa. Foci of thrombosis, extensive fibrosis, and calcification may be present. On imaging, cavernous hemangiomas are composed primarily of large vascular lakes and channels. Some of the vascular channels undergo thrombosis and fibrous organization [38]. Hemangiomas have long T1 and T2 values, so they are low in signal intensity on T1-weighted images and high in signal intensity on T2-weighted images, maintaining signal intensity on longer echo times (e.g., >120 ms) [39, 40]. Hemangiomas have well-defined round or lobular borders [39, 40]. Small lesions typically appear round, whereas larger lesions have either a round or lobular margin. T2 measurements are less than those of cysts. Hemangiomas typically enhance in a peripheral nodular fashion on dynamic serial gadolinium-enhanced MR images with slow progressive complete or nearly complete fill-in of the entire lesion by 10 min [41–43]. This enhancement pattern is characterized by enlargement and coalescence of enhancing nodules. Serial gadolinium-enhanced SGE images have been shown to be effective in distinguishing benign from malignant hepatic masses [44, 45].

The MRI appearances of small (<1.5 cm), medium (1.5–5.0 cm), and large (15.0 cm) hemangiomas have been reported in a multi-institutional study [46]. Among the 154 hemangiomas in 66 patients, 81 lesions were small, 56 medium, and 17 large. Hemangiomas were multiple in 68% of patients. All lesions were high in signal intensity on T2-weighted images. Three types of enhancement patterns were observed: (1) uniform high signal intensity immediately after contrast (Type 1), (2) peripheral nodular enhancement with centripetal progression to uniform high signal intensity (Type 2), and (3) peripheral nodular enhancement with centripetal progression and a persistent central scar (Type 3). Type 1 enhancement was observed only in small tumors. Type 2 and Type 3 enhancements were observed in all size categories. Type 3 enhancement was observed in 16 of 17 large tumors. A variation in the Type 2 or 3 enhancement pattern consists of enhancement that spreads at a fairly rapid rate with complete enhancement at 1–2 min [46]. Similar findings also have been described in an Asian patient population [47].

Hemangiomas vary in the rate and completeness of tumor enhancement. Rapidity of enhancement has been determined on 90-s images as slow (approximately 25% of tumor enhancement at the maximum transverse diameter), medium (approximately 50% enhancement), and fast (approximately 75% enhancement) [46, 48]. Tumors at all sizes may enhance very slowly to very quickly and enhance minimally to complete enhancement, with the exception that >5-cm tumors almost invariably demonstrate lack of central enhancement. Slow enhancement of hemangiomas permits distinction from most tumors. The only other neoplasm that may show comparable slow enhancement is chemotherapy-treated metastases (as described below).

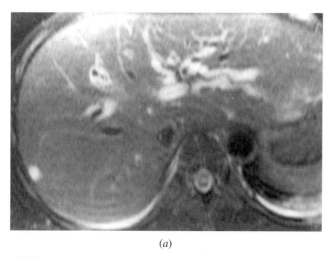

(a)

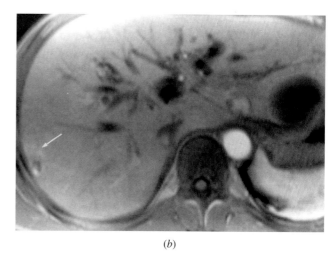

(b)

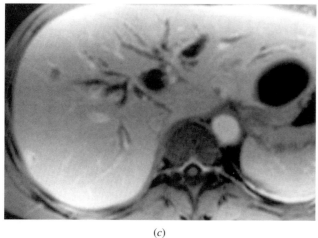

(c)

FIG. 2.30 Hemangioma with perilesional enhancement. T2-weighted SS-ETSE (*a*), immediate postgadolinium SGE (*b*), and 90-s postgadolinium fat-suppressed SGE (*c*) images. This patient, who has an inflammatory pseudotumor arising in the common hepatic duct that causes dilatation of the biliary tree, also demonstrates a round, well-defined lesion, which is hyperintense on T2 (*a*) and shows peripheral nodular enhancement on the immediate postcontrast image (*b*) with nearly complete fill-in of the lesion on the delayed image (*c*). Note the transient ill-defined increased perilesional enhancement (arrow, *b*) on the immediate postcontrast image (*b*) that reflects high flow in vessels related to the hemangioma.

Fast-enhancing hemangiomas show enhancement patterns that can resemble other tumors, with metastases being the most difficult to distinguish. Fast-enhancing hemangiomas can also demonstrate perilesional high signal on T2 and perilesional increased enhancement that likely reflects high flow in efferent veins (fig. 2.30). These findings are rare in hemangiomas and are more commonly observed in metastases, especially colon cancer metastases. A recent study correlated the temporal parenchyma enhancement surrounding hepatic cavernous hemangiomas with the rapidity of intratumoral contrast material enhancement and tumor volume. Thirty-two of the 167 hemangiomas (19%) had temporal peritumoral enhancement, and this was more common in hemangiomas with rapid enhancement (41%). However, there was no statistically significant relationship between peritumoral enhancement and tumor volume. The mean diameter of hemangioma with peritumoral enhancement was not significantly different from that of hemangioma without peritumoral enhancement [49].

Small hemangiomas most commonly demonstrate Type 2 enhancement. The peripheral nodules of enhancement are typically very small (fig. 2.31). Type 1 en-

hancement is the next most common pattern (fig. 2.32), whereas type 3 enhancement is uncommonly observed (fig. 2.33). Small hemangiomas are difficult to distinguish from other types of liver lesions, specifically liver metastases, and MRI follow-up is generally required.

The great majority of medium-sized hemangiomas exhibit Type 2 enhancement (figs. 2.34 and 2.35) and represent the classic hemangiomas. Type 3 enhancement is the next most common enhancement pattern (figs. 2.36 and 2.37), whereas type 1 enhancement is exceedingly rare. Lesions larger than 1.5 cm with Type 1 enhancement either represent well-differentiated tumors of hepatocellular origin or hypervascular liver metastases.

Giant hemangiomas most frequently have a central scar [46, 50], and virtually all giant hemangiomas have Type 3 enhancement (fig. 2.38). Absence of a central scar should raise the concern that the mass may represent another lesion. Large hemangiomas frequently have mildly complex signal intensity on T2-weighted images with the frequent presence of low signal strands (fig. 2.39), which reflects the internal network of fibrous stroma that is observed histologically. In rare instances, large hemangiomas may compress adjacent portal veins resulting in

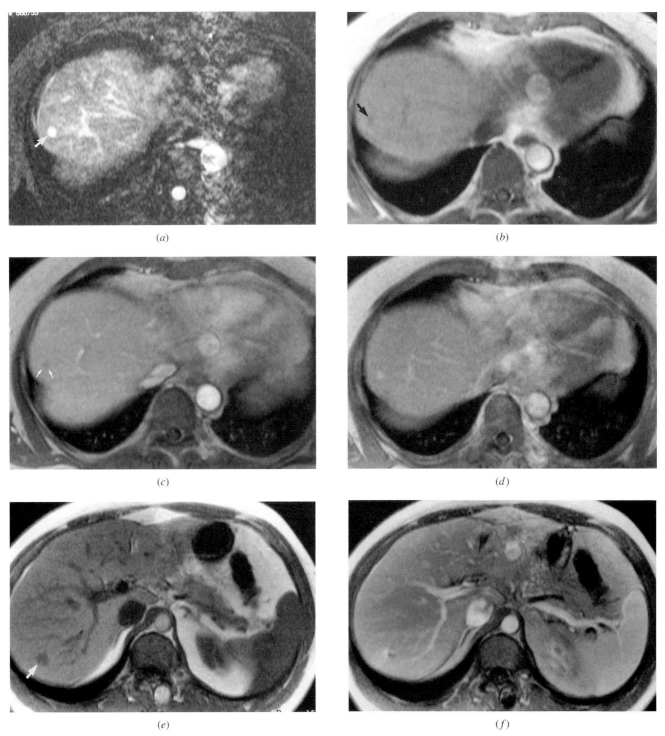

(a)

(b)

(c)

(d)

(e)

(f)

F ɪ ɢ . 2.31 Small hemangiomas, Type 2 enhancement. T2-weighted fat-suppressed ETSE (*a*), SGE (*b*), and immediate (*c*) and 5-min (*d*) postgadolinium SGE images. A 1-cm hemangioma is present in the right lobe that is high in signal intensity on the T2 images (arrow, *a*) and mildly low in signal intensity on the T1 images (arrow, *b*), demonstrates peripheral nodular enhancement (arrows, *c*) on the early postcontrast image (*c*), and is uniformly homogeneous and moderately high in signal intensity on the delayed image (*d*).

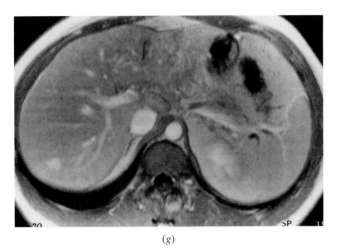

(g)

FIG. 2.31 (*Continued*) SGE (*e*), and immediate (*f*) and 90-s (*g*) postgadolinium SGE images in a second patient demonstrate a 1-cm lesion that is moderately hypointense on the T1-weighted image (arrow, *e*), develops peripheral nodular enhancement on the immediate postgadolinium image (*f*), and is uniform and moderately high in signal intensity on the 90-s postgadolinium image (*g*).

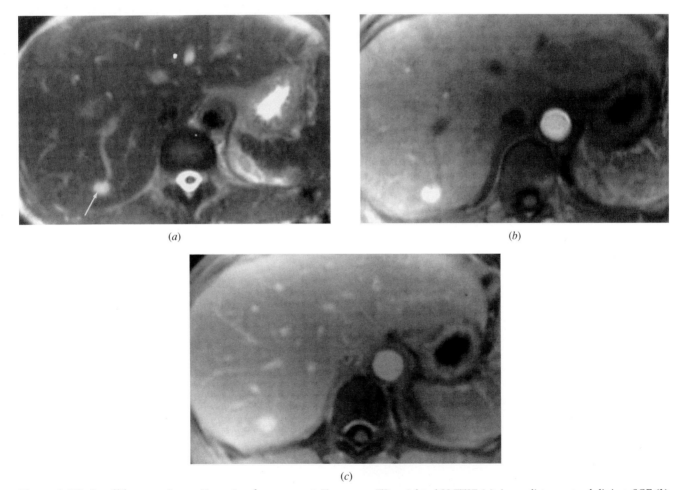

(a)   (b)

(c)

FIG. 2.32 Small hemangioma, Type 1 enhancement. Transverse T2-weighted SS-ETSE (*a*), immediate postgadolinium SGE (*b*) and 90-s postgadolinium fat-suppressed SGE (*c*) images. A lesion (arrow, *a*) is present in the right hepatic lobe that shows low signal on T1 (not shown), high signal on T2 (*a*), and intense uniform enhancement immediately after gadolinium administration (*b*) that persists at 90 s (*c*). These findings represent a hemangioma type 1.

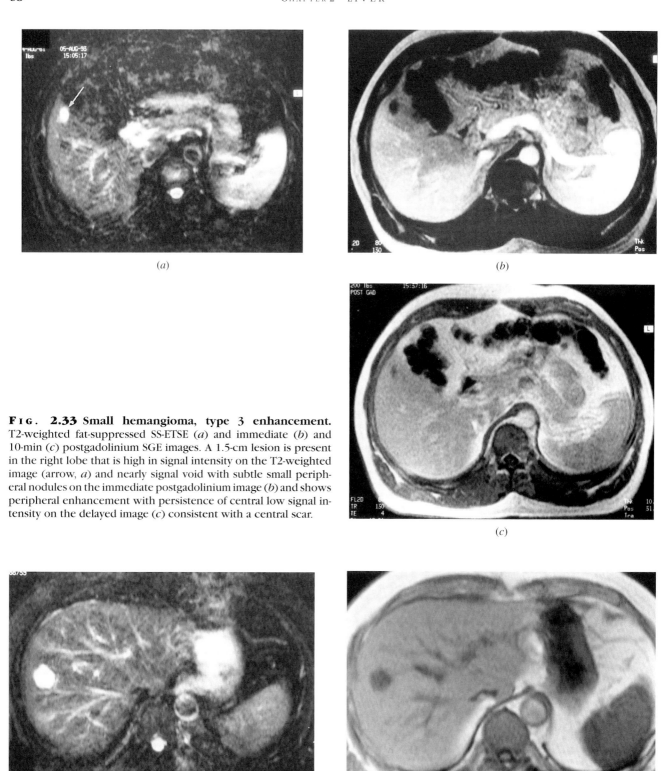

FIG. 2.33 Small hemangioma, type 3 enhancement.
T2-weighted fat-suppressed SS-ETSE (*a*) and immediate (*b*) and
10-min (*c*) postgadolinium SGE images. A 1.5-cm lesion is present
in the right lobe that is high in signal intensity on the T2-weighted
image (arrow, *a*) and nearly signal void with subtle small peripheral nodules on the immediate postgadolinium image (*b*) and shows
peripheral enhancement with persistence of central low signal intensity on the delayed image (*c*) consistent with a central scar.

(*a*) (*b*) (*c*) (*a*) (*b*)

FIG. 2.34 Medium-sized hemangioma, type 2 enhancement. Transverse T2-weighted fat-suppressed ETSE (*a*), SGE (*b*) immediate (*c*) and 5-min (*d*) postgadolinium SGE images demonstrate a well-defined, round lesion that is high signal on T2-weighted
(*a*) and moderately low signal on T1-weighted (*b*) images and enhances in a peripheral nodular fashion (*c*) with complete filling of
the entire lesion on the late image (*d*), consistent with hemangioma.

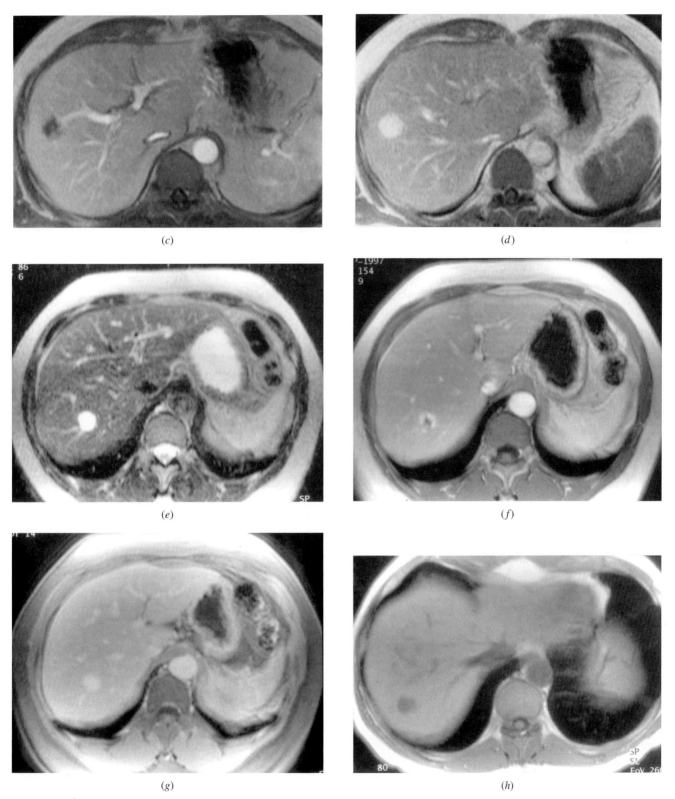

(c)

(d)

(e)

(f)

(g)

(h)

FIG. 2.34 (*Continued*) T2-weighted SS-ETSE (*e*), immediate postgadolinium SGE (*f*), and 90-s postgadolinium fat-suppressed SGE (*g*) images in a second patient. A 2.1-cm hemangioma is high in signal intensity on the T2 (*e*), enhances in a peripheral nodular fashion on the immediate postgadolinium image (*f*), and is uniformly high in signal intensity on the late postgadolinium image (*g*).

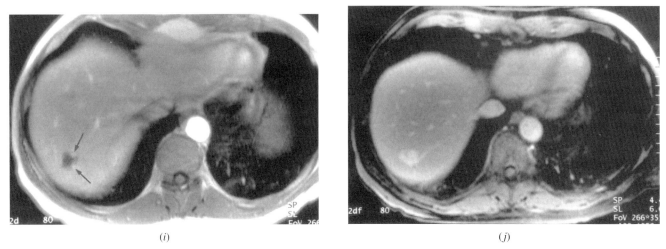

(i)   *(j)*

F I G . 2.34 (*Continued*) SGE (*h*), immediate postgadolinium SGE (*i*), and 90-s postgadolinium fat-suppressed SGE (*j*) images in a third patient. There is a 2-cm hemangioma in the right lobe that exhibits peripheral nodular enhancement (arrows, *i*) in a discontinuous ring on immediate postgadolinium image (*i*) with complete lesion enhancement by 90 s (*j*).

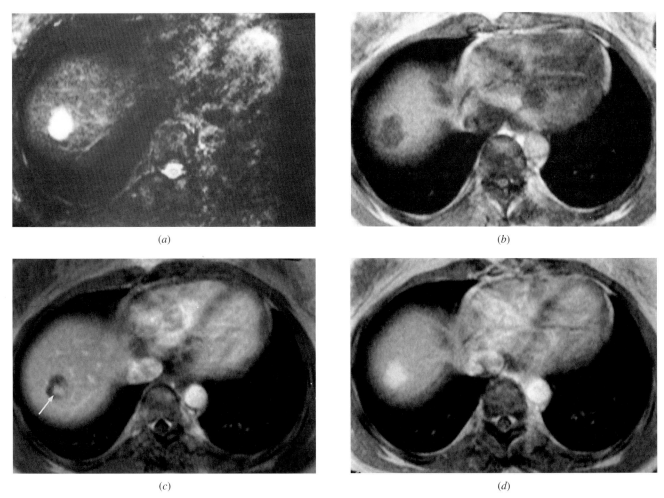

(a)   *(b)*

(c)   *(d)*

F I G . 2.35 Medium-sized hemangiomas, type 2 enhancement with central nodular enhancement. T2-weighted fat-suppressed ETSE (*a*), SGE (*b*) and 45-s (*c*) and 10-min (*d*) postgadolinium SGE images. A 2.5-cm hemangioma is present that demonstrates high signal on T2- (*a*), moderately low signal on T1-weighted (*b*) images, and nodular progressive enhancement (*c, d*). In this patient, the early postcontrast image demonstrates one predominant enhancing nodule that is almost central in location (arrow, *c*).

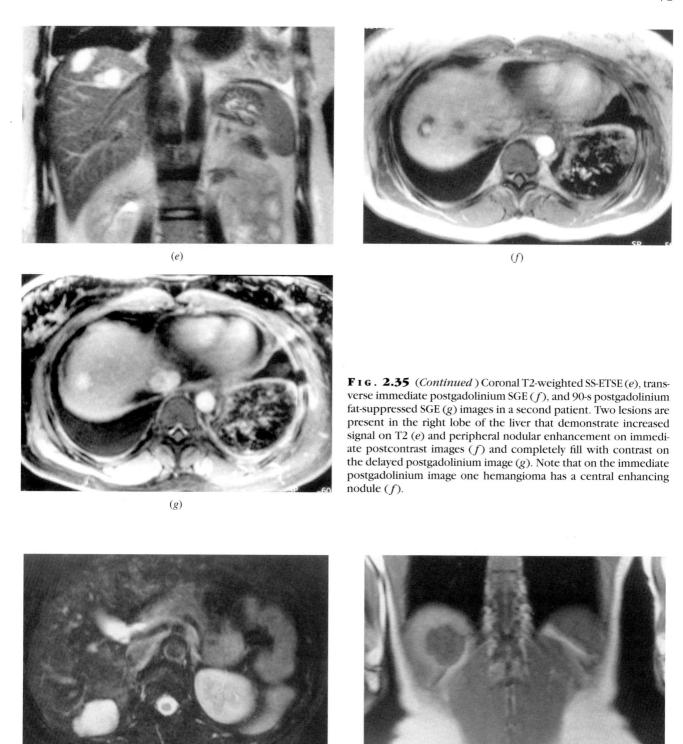

(e)

(f)

(g)

Fig. 2.35 (*Continued*) Coronal T2-weighted SS-ETSE (*e*), transverse immediate postgadolinium SGE (*f*), and 90-s postgadolinium fat-suppressed SGE (*g*) images in a second patient. Two lesions are present in the right lobe of the liver that demonstrate increased signal on T2 (*e*) and peripheral nodular enhancement on immediate postcontrast images (*f*) and completely fill with contrast on the delayed postgadolinium image (*g*). Note that on the immediate postgadolinium image one hemangioma has a central enhancing nodule (*f*).

(a)

(b)

Fig. 2.36 Medium-sized hemangioma, Type 3 enhancement. T2-weighted fat-suppressed ETSE (*a*), coronal SGE (*b*), immediate postgadolinium (*c*), 90-s (*d*) and 10-minute transverse (*e*) and coronal (*f*) SGE images. The hemangioma is high in signal intensity on the T2 (*a*) and moderately low in signal intensity on the T1 (*b*) and demonstrates peripheral nodular enhancement (*c*) that progresses centripetally (*d*). Persistent central low signal intensity is present on the delayed images (*e*, *f*) consistent with a central scar.

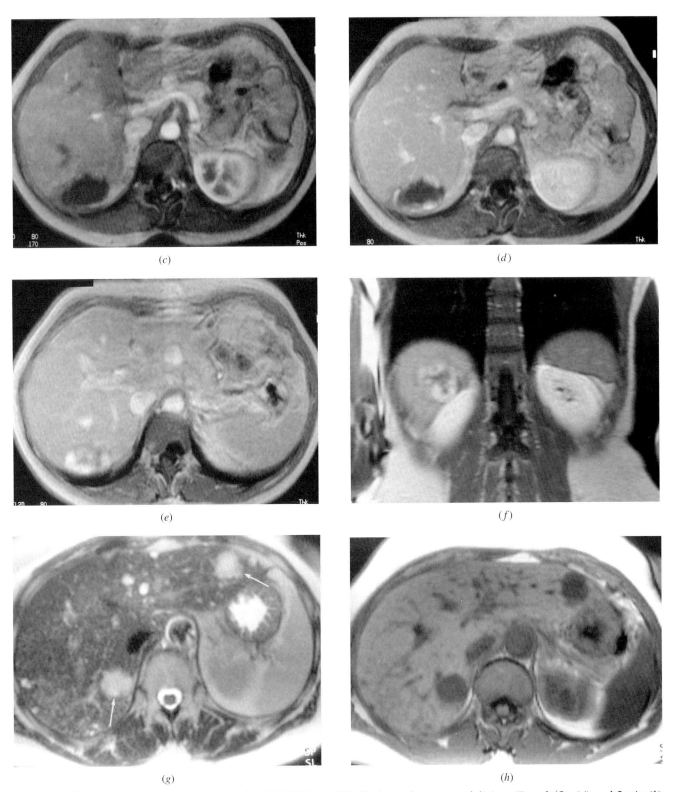

F I G . 2.36 (*Continued*) Transverse T2-weighted SS-ETSE (*g*), SGE (*h*), immediate postgadolinium (*i*) and 45-s (*j*) and 5-min (*k*) postgadolinium SGE images in a second patient. There are two lobular lesions that appear high signal on T2 (arrows, *g*) and decreased signal on T1-weighted (*h*) images. The first one is situated in the left lobe, demonstrates peripheral nodular enhancement after administration of gadolinium and gradually fills in completely on delayed images (*k*) consistent with a type 2 hemangioma.

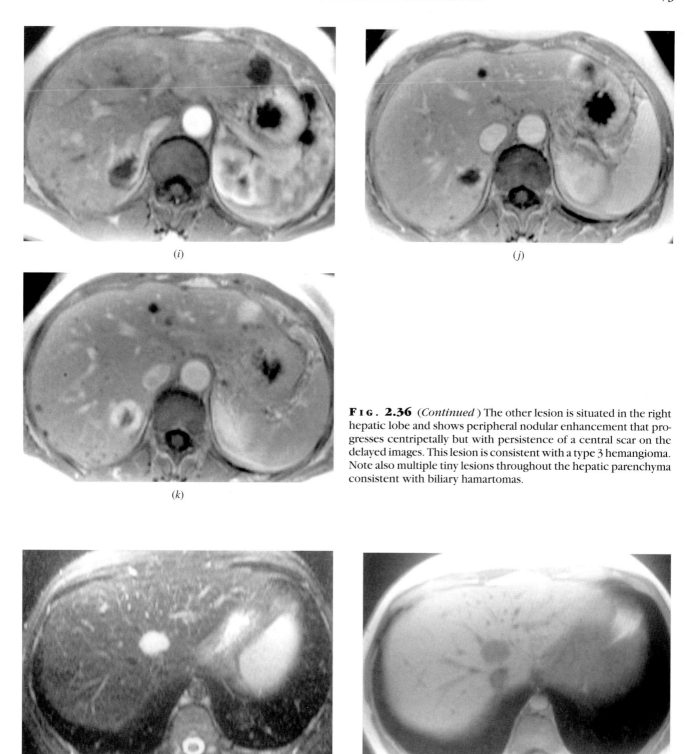

(i)

(j)

(k)

FIG. 2.36 (*Continued*) The other lesion is situated in the right hepatic lobe and shows peripheral nodular enhancement that progresses centripetally but with persistence of a central scar on the delayed images. This lesion is consistent with a type 3 hemangioma. Note also multiple tiny lesions throughout the hepatic parenchyma consistent with biliary hamartomas.

(a)

(b)

FIG. 2.37 Hypovascular medium sized hemangioma, type 3 enhancement. Echo-train STIR (*a*), SGE (*b*), immediate postgadolinium SGE (*c, d*), and 90-s postgadolinium fat-suppressed SGE (*e*) images. There is a lobular lesion that demonstrates high signal intensity on T2 (*a*) and low signal intensity on T1 (*b*), small peripheral nodules of enhancement after contrast administration (*c*), and lack of progression of enhancement on delayed images (*e*). This is consistent with a hemangioma type 3 enhancement.

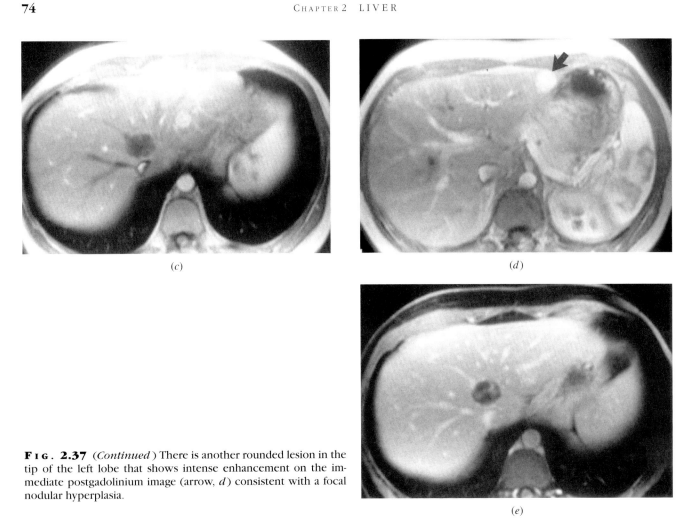

(c)

(d)

(e)

FIG. 2.37 (*Continued*) There is another rounded lesion in the tip of the left lobe that shows intense enhancement on the immediate postgadolinium image (arrow, *d*) consistent with a focal nodular hyperplasia.

(a)

(b)

FIG. 2.38 Giant hemangioma. SGE (*a*), immediate postgadolinium (*b*) and 90-s (*c*) and 10-min (*d*) postgadolinium SGE images. A hemangioma is present in the left lobe that is moderately low in signal intensity on T1 (*a*), demonstrates peripheral nodular enhancement in a discontinuous ring on the immediate postcontrast image (*b*),

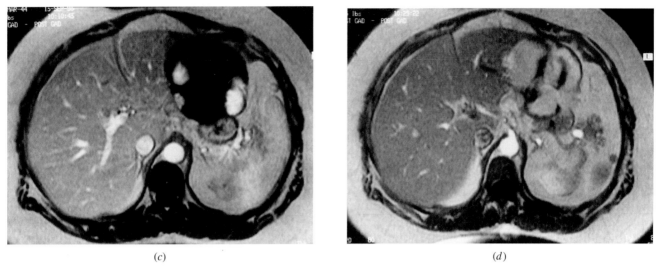

(c)

(d)

F I G. 2.38 (*Continued*) and gradually enhances in a centripetal fashion (*c*) with persistent low signal intensity centrally at 10 min (*d*), consistent with a central scar.

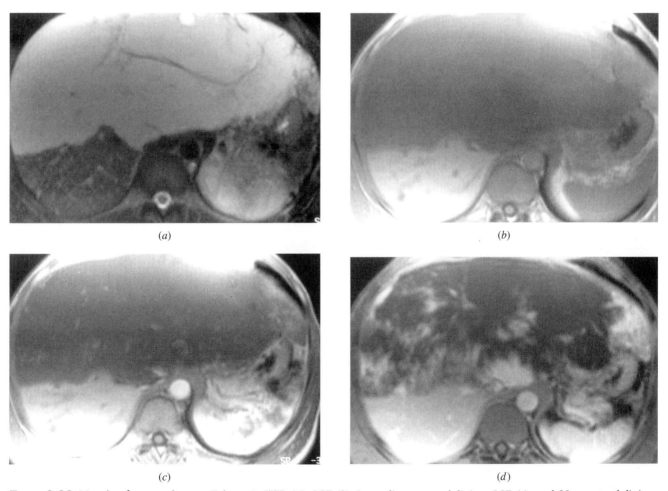

(a)

(b)

(c)

(d)

F I G. 2.39 Massive hemangiomas. Echo-train-STIR (*a*), SGE (*b*), immediate postgadolinium SGE (*c*), and 90-s postgadolinium fat-suppressed SGE (*d*) images. A massive tumor replaces the majority of the liver with sparing of *segments 6* and 7 in the right hepatic lobe. After administration of gadolinium, this lesion demonstrates discontinuous peripheral nodular enhancement with enlargement and coalescence of the nodules. The appearance is consistent with a massive hemangioma.

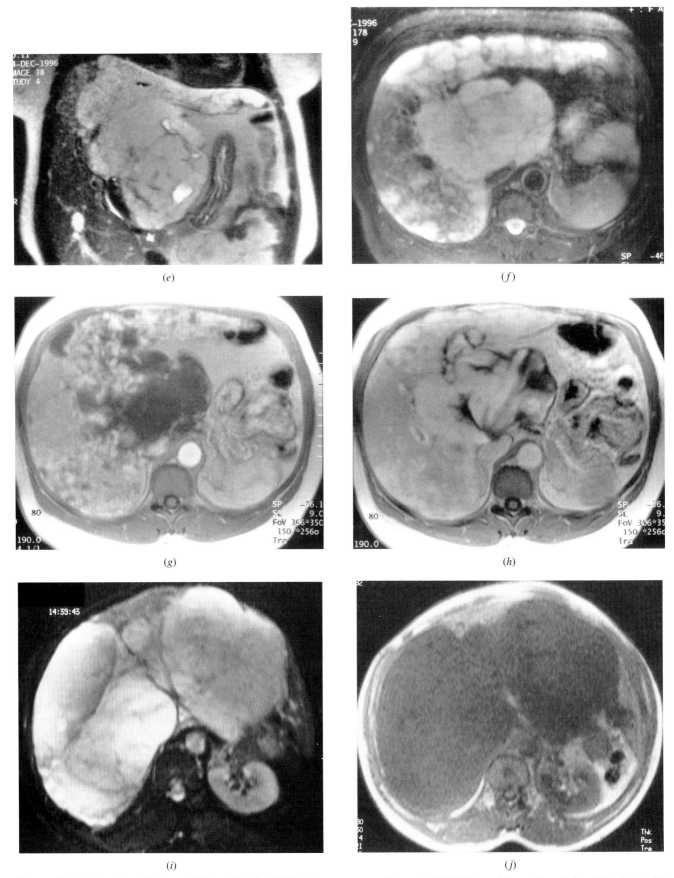

(e)

(f)

(g)

(h)

(i)

(j)

F I G . 2.39 (*Continued*) Coronal T2-weighted SS-ETSE (*e*), transverse echo-train STIR (*f*), and immediate (*g*) and 5-minute (*h*) postgadolinium SGE images in a second patient.

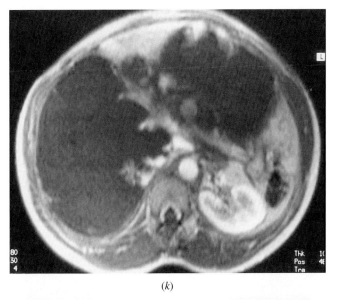

(k)

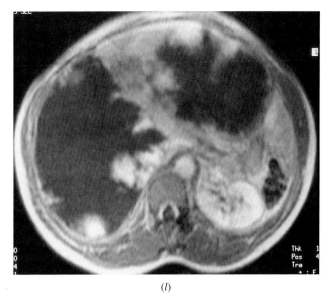

(l)

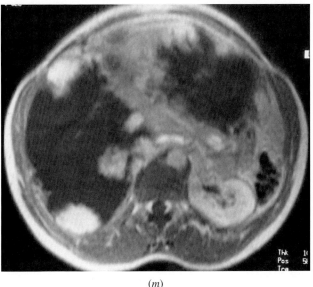

(m)

FIG. 2.39 (*Continued*) A massive lobulated lesion is present, which is high signal (*e, f*), contains multiple low-signal strands on T2, and demonstrates discontinuous nodular enhancement (*g*) with centripetal progression (*h*) after the administration of gadolinium. Regions of hypointense central scar persist on the delayed images (*h*).

T2-weighted fat-suppressed ETSE (*i*), SGE (*j*), immediate postgadolinium (*k*), 90-s (*l*), and 5-min (*m*) postgadolinium SGE images in a second patient. The liver is largely replaced with massive hemangiomas. They are high in signal intensity with multiple low-signal intensity linear strands on T2 (*i*), moderately low-signal intensity on T1 (*j*) and demonstrate peripheral nodular enhancement (*k*) that progresses centrally (*l, m*). Large central unenhanced regions persist on the 5-min image (*m*). Low-signal intensity linear strands are common on T2-weighted images in giant hemangiomas and represent bands of collagenous tissue. This patient underwent liver transplantation because of the extensive hepatic replacement by hemangiomas.

transient segmental increased enhancement on immediate postgadolinium images secondary to autoregulatory increased hepatic arterial supply (fig. 2.40). On rare occasions, large hemangiomas may also hemorrhage.

The most distinctive imaging feature of hemangiomas is the demonstration of a discontinuous ring of nodules immediately after gadolinium administration [44, 46, 51]. Nodular enhancement is most frequently eccentric in location and may originate from the superior or inferior aspect of the hemangioma, simulating central enhancement on transverse images (fig. 2.41). True, central enhancement may rarely occur. The appearance of central enhancement is rare for all histologic types of tumors, and occurs by early filling of a large central lake by a narrow feeding vessel.

Hemangiomas may fade in signal intensity over time, but they will fade in a homogeneous fashion with no evidence of peripheral or heterogeneous washout [44, 46].

Hemangiomas may fade in signal to isointensity with liver but will not fade to hypointensity. Small hemangiomas with Type 1 enhancement may be indistinguishable from hypervascular malignant liver lesions such as hepatocellular carcinomas or leiomyosarcoma. Small hemangiomas are high in signal intensity on T2-weighted images, whereas small hepatocellular carcinomas are often near isointensity. Small hypervascular metastases may appear identical in appearance to small hemangiomas on all sequences. Usually, however, a large lesion is also present that will exhibit the enhancement features of either a hemangioma or a metastasis, so that the histology of the small lesions may be inferred.

Chemotherapy-treated liver metastases, when chemotherapy treatment has been initiated between 2- to 12-months prior to imaging, may resemble the appearance of hemangiomas (see below) [52]. A less

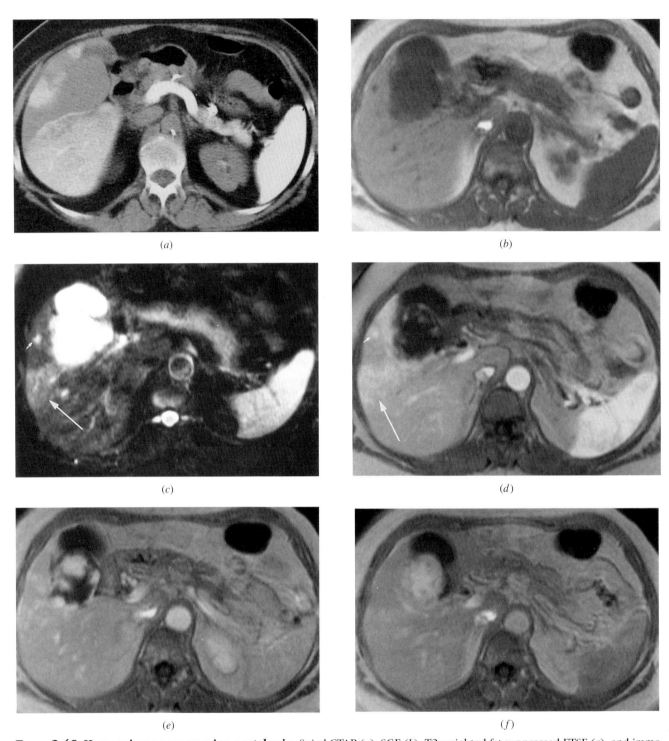

(a)   *(b)*

(c)   *(d)*

(e)   *(f)*

F I G . 2.40 Hemangioma compressing portal vein. Spiral CTAP (*a*), SGE (*b*), T2-weighted fat-suppressed ETSE (*c*), and immediate (*d*), 90-s (*e*), and 10-min (*f*) postgadolinium SGE images. A 6-cm lesion is present in the anterior segment of the right lobe
that causes distal wedge-shaped diminished portal venous perfusion on the CTAP image (*a*), findings that were considered consistent
with a malignant tumor. The tumor is moderately low in signal intensity on the T1-weighted image (*b*), high in signal intensity on
the T2-weighted image (*c*) and has peripheral nodular enhancement on the immediate postgadolinium image (*d*) that progresses in a
centripetal fashion (*e*) to hyperintensity at 10 min (*f*) with small, central low-signal intensity foci consistent with a central scar. The
perfusion defect observed on the CTAP image is noted to be wedge-shaped and minimally hyperintense on the T2-weighted image
(long arrow, *c*) and enhances in a transient fashion greater than adjacent liver on the immediate postgadolinium image (long arrow,
d), findings consistent with portal vein compression. Additional note is made of a 6-mm hemangioma lateral to the large hemangioma
(small arrow, *c*), which enhances homogeneously after gadolinium administration (small arrow, *d*) in a type 1 pattern of enhancement.

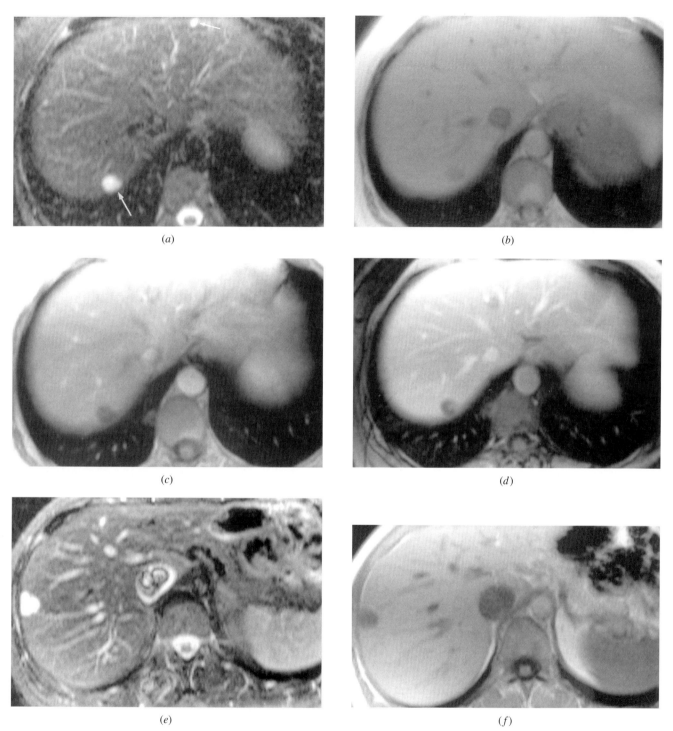

F I G . 2.41 Hemangioma with central filling. Transverse T2-weighted fat suppressed SS-ETSE (*a*), SGE (*b*), immediate post-gadolinium SGE (*c*), and 90-s postgadolinium fat-suppressed SGE (*d*) images. There are two lesions (arrows, *a*) located in the right and left hepatic lobe. The lesion in the right lobe is increased signal on T2 (*a*) and decreased signal on T1 (*b*), and shows peripheral and central nodules on early (*c*) and late (*d*) postcontrast images. On the delayed image, there is a prominant central enhanced nodule. The small left lobe lesion is hyperintense on the T2-weighted image and is barely perceptible on any of the other sequences. This is not uncommon with <1-cm hemangiomas with type 1 enhancement, in which enhancement may be minimally greater and comparable in intensity to background liver on immediate postgadolinium images, and lesions fade to isointensity by 1-2 min. Note a phase encoding mirror artifact from the IVC that should not be mistaken for a lesion. The artifact is equidistant to the IVC from a second artifact posterior to the IVC that assists in making the correct observation.

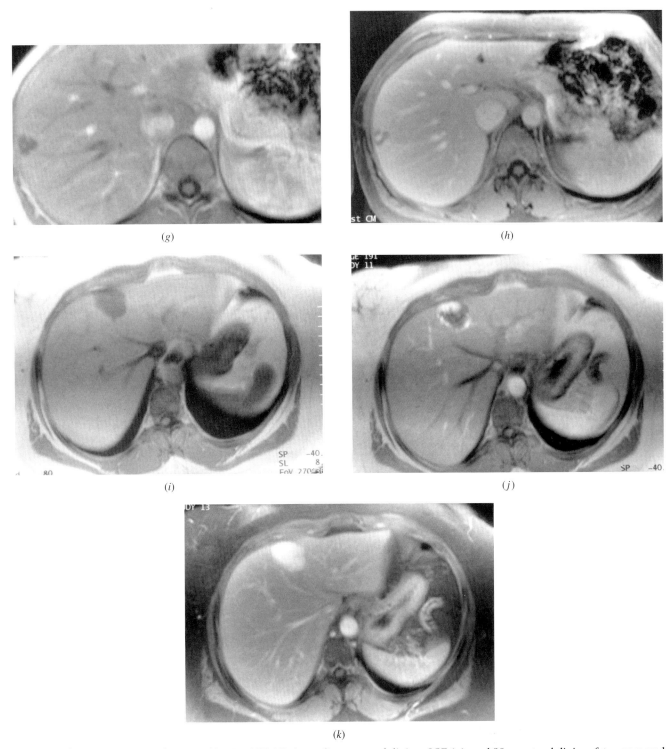

(g)

(h)

(i)

(j)

(k)

F i g . 2.41 (*Continued*) Echo-train STIR (*e*), SGE (*f*), immediate postgadolinium SGE (*g*), and 90-s postgadolinium fat-suppressed SGE (*h*) images in a second patient. A lobulated lesion is seen along the lateral edge of the right hepatic lobe and demonstrates peripheral and central nodular filling enhancement, which progresses on interstitial phase (*h*) images.

SGE (*i*), immediate postgadolinium SGE (*j*), and 90-s postgadolinium fat-suppressed SGE (*k*) images in a third patient. There is a mildly lobular lesion in the left lobe that demonstrates low signal on the T1-weighted image (*i*), enhances in a peripheral nodular pattern on the immediate postgadolinium image (*j*), and fills in completely on the delayed image (*k*), consistent with hemangioma.

aggressive enhancement pattern that develops in chemotherapy-treated liver metastasis may be reflective of underlying histologic changes associated with a salutary response to chemotherapy, that is, an antiangiogenic effect with altered vascularity. Angiosarcomas may resemble hemangiomas; however, central hemorrhage and less orderly nodular progressive enhancement are features consistent with angiosarcoma [53]. Clinical history is important because patients with hypervascular malignant liver lesions usually have a known primary tumor [54] and history of chemotherapy can be established.

Advantages of MRI over CT imaging in the evaluation of hemangiomas include (1) the greater ability to image the entire liver in the same phase of contrast enhancement, which is particularly useful when multiple lesions are present, (2) greater lesion enhancement on contrast-enhanced images such that lesions are comparatively brighter than background liver (fig. 2.42), (3) superior detection of small hemangiomas and (4) effective lesion detection and characterization with T2-weighted images, for which CT does not have an analogous technique.

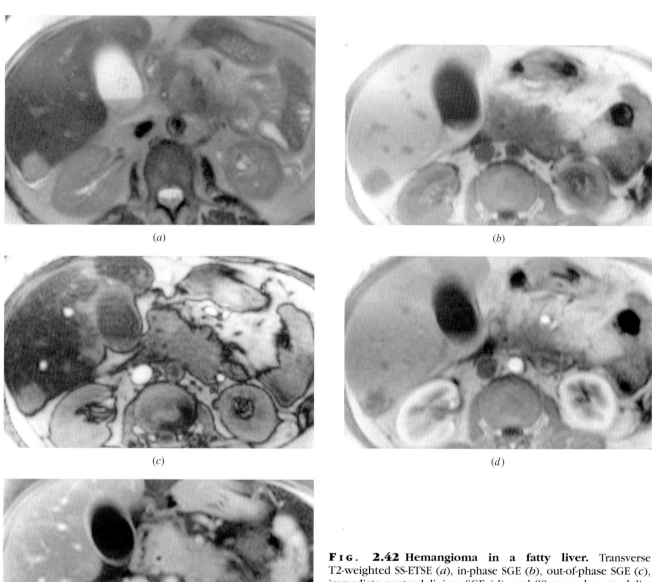

(a)

(b)

(c)

(d)

(e)

F I G . 2.42 Hemangioma in a fatty liver. Transverse T2-weighted SS-ETSE (*a*), in-phase SGE (*b*), out-of-phase SGE (*c*), immediate postgadolinium SGE (*d*), and 90 second postgadolinium fat-suppressed SGE (*e*) images. A lobulated lesion is present in the right hepatic lobe, which shows peripheral nodular enhancement on early postgadolinium images (*d*) and gradually fills with contrast (*e*). Note the presence of a central scar on the delayed image. The liver is diffusely fatty infiltrated (*c*), which renders the lesion relatively high signal on the out-of-phase sequence (*c*).

Reports have shown that hemangiomas may be reliably distinguished from metastases on T2-weighted images based on the smooth lobular margins and the higher calculated T2 values of hemangiomas (mean of 140 ms) [55]. Although this may be true in the majority of patients, cumulative experience from many centers has shown that T2-weighted images alone may not allow characterization of small tumors or allow reliable distinction between hemangiomas and hypervascular malignant tumors (such as leiomyosarcoma and islet-cell tumors). For this reason, long-TE T2-weighted sequences for hemangiomas are not performed at our institution because some diagnostically difficult lesions, such as hypervascular metastases, may also show long T2 values. The routine combination of T2-weighted information with serial gadolinium-enhanced SGE is useful to increase observer confidence for establishing the correct diagnosis and also to maximize evaluation of other hepatic and extrahepatic diseases (fig. 2.43).

An unusual benign tumor that resembles a hemangioma is the littoral cell angioma (fig. 2.44).

Liver Cell Adenomas. Liver cell adenomas are benign epithelial neoplasms. Approximately 90% of liver cell adenomas occur in young women [56, 57]. These lesions are associated with the use of oral contraceptive steroids. Other much less frequent associations include the use of anabolic steroids and disorders associated with abnormal carbohydrate metabolism, such as familial diabetes mellitus, galactosemia, and glycogen storage disease type Ia [37]. With the increased use of MR in patients, it is clear that the majority of liver cell adenomas are small, and if patients are withdrawn from birth control pill use, the tumors will involute spontaneously. Patients may present with acute abdominal pain related to hemorrhage into the tumor. Rarely, rupture into the peritoneal cavity may occur that requires emergency intervention [58].

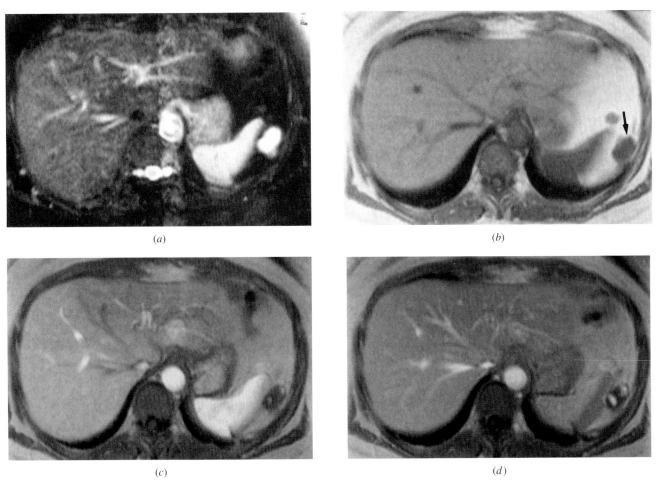

(a)   *(b)*

(c)   *(d)*

F I G . 2.43 Exophytic Hemangioma. T2-weighted fat-suppressed ETSE (*a*), SGE (*b*), and immediate (*c*), 90-s (*d*), and 10-min (*e*) postgadolinium SGE images. A pedunculated 2.5-cm mass (arrow, *b*) arises from the tip of the lateral segment of the liver.

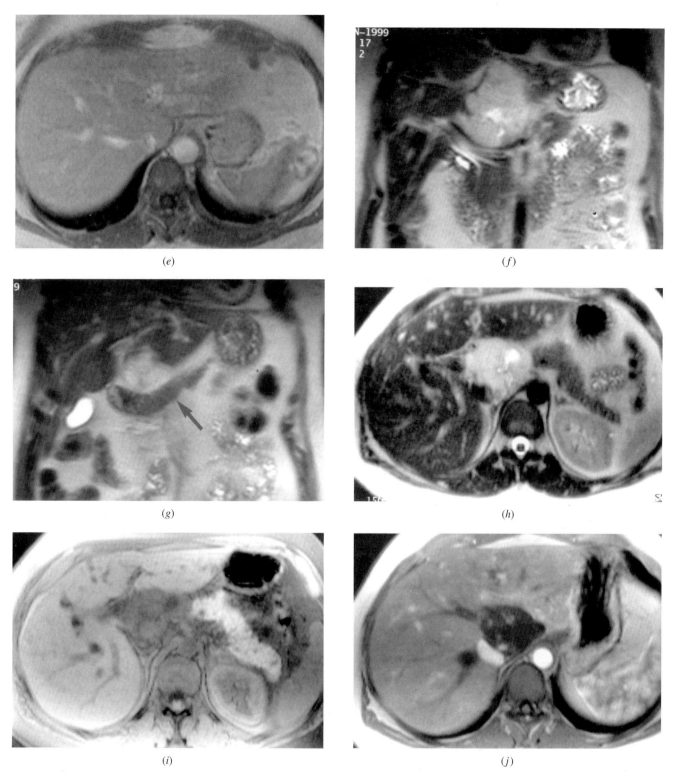

(e)

(f)

(g)

(h)

(i)

(j)

F I G . 2.43 (*Continued*) The mass is high in signal intensity on the T2 (*a*) and moderately low in signal intensity on the T1-weighted image (*b*), enhances in a peripheral nodular fashion on the immediate postgadolinium SGE image (*c*) with centripetal progression on the 90-s postgadolinium SGE image (*d*), and progresses to hyperintensity with small, low-signal intensity foci on the 10-min postgadolinium SGE image (*e*). Despite the thin stalk of the hemangioma, it exhibits circumlesional peripheral nodular enhancement, comparable to standard intraparenchymal hemangiomas.

Coronal (*f, g*) and transverse (*h*) T2-weighted SS-ETSE, T1-weighted fat-suppressed SGE (*i*), immediate postgadolinium SGE (*j*), and 90-s postgadolinium fat-suppressed SGE (*k*) images in a second patient. There is a large mass arising from *segment 1* of the liver, with extension into the porta hepatis, that demonstrates high signal on T2 (*f, g, h*) and low signal on T1 (*i*).

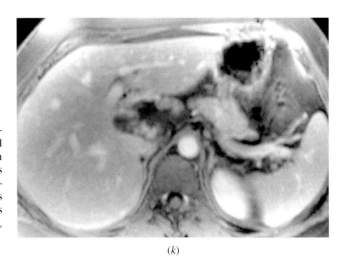

(k)

FIG. 2.43 (*Continued*) Immediately after gadolinium administration (*j*), multiple peripheral enhancing nodules are identified that enlarge and coalesce on later images (*k*), consistent with an exophytic hemangioma. On an outside CT examination this was thought to arise from the pancreas. The coronal T2-weighted image (*g*) demonstrates inferior displacement of an intact pancreas (arrow, *g*). Additionally, the pancreas distal to the mass exhibits normal high signal on the T1-weighted fat-suppressed image (*i*), which essentially excludes a pancreatic parenchymal mass.

Pathologically, liver cell adenomas are most commonly solitary tumors characterized as a bulging mass with dilated blood vessels traversing the surface. Liver cell adenomas are partially or completely enclosed by a pseudocapsule derived from compressed and collapsed hepatic parenchyma [59]. Sectioning reveals a spherical, well-demarcated, richly vascular lesion, frequently with areas of hemorrhage or necrosis. Focal scar formation is indicative of remote infarction. The histologic hallmark consists of clusters of benign hepatocytes arranged in slender plates of two- to three-cell thickness. These plates are separated by slitlike sinusoids and numerous thin-walled veins. Bile ducts are absent. Malignant transformation is rare.

On imaging, adenomas may contain substantial fat. Occasionally, the presence of central fibrosis may cause

diagnostic confusion with FNH [37]. On MRI, the appearance of adenomas typically varies in signal intensity from mildly hypointense to moderately hyperintense on T1-weighted images, and they are generally mildly hyperintense on T2-weighted images (fig. 2.45). The degree of high signal intensity on T1-weighted images reflects the quantity of fat. Tumors may decrease in signal intensity on out-of-phase or fat-suppressed images because of their fat content (fig. 2.46) [60]. Homogeneous drop in signal intensity on out-of-phase images is a relatively common feature of fat-containing adenomas and is rarely observed in hepatocellular carcinoma, and then only in <2-cm tumors. Adenomas may be nearly isointense with liver on all imaging sequences, reflecting similarity to liver parenchyma. Tumors may also have mixed high signal intensity on T1- and T2-weighted

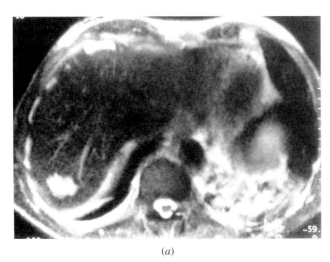

(a)

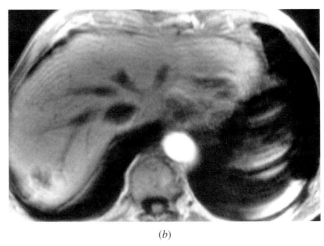

(b)

FIG. 2.44 **Littoral cell angioma of the liver.** T2-weighted SS-ETSE (*a*) and immediate postgadolinium SGE (*b*) images. There is a lobular lesion in the right hepatic lobe that is high signal on T2 (*a*) and low signal on T1 (not shown) and has peripheral nodular enhancement after administration of contrast (*b*). Littoral cell angioma of the liver was present at histopathology. Note that the lesion has a similar appearance to a hemangioma, although the peripheral nodules are not as well defined.

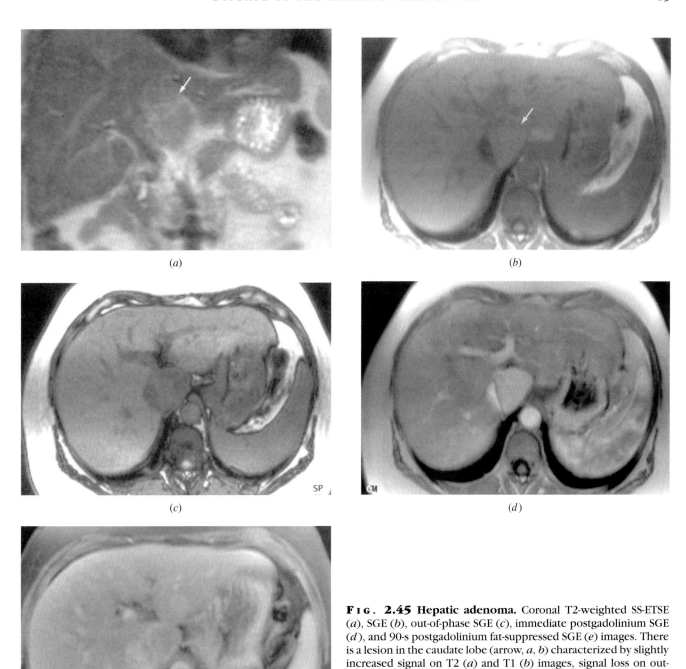

FIG. 2.45 Hepatic adenoma. Coronal T2-weighted SS-ETSE (*a*), SGE (*b*), out-of-phase SGE (*c*), immediate postgadolinium SGE (*d*), and 90-s postgadolinium fat-suppressed SGE (*e*) images. There is a lesion in the caudate lobe (arrow, *a*, *b*) characterized by slightly increased signal on T2 (*a*) and T1 (*b*) images, signal loss on out-of-phase images (*c*), diffuse homogeneous enhancement immediately after administration of gadolinium (*d*), and fading to near-isointensity on delayed gadolinium-enhanced images (*e*). Loss of signal on the out-of-phase image (*c*) is characteristic of hepatic adenoma. Late capsular enhancement (*e*), as observed in this case, may be occasionally observed in hepatic adenomas.

images due to the presence of hemorrhage [60, 61] (fig. 2.47). Rarely, the arrangement of vessels and stroma in adenomas may result in an intense marbled pattern of enhancement that may be difficult to distinguish from hepatocellular carcinoma. Characteristically, tumors have a transient blush immediately after gadolinium chelate administration that fades by 1 min.

Because adenomas contain hepatocytes, hepatocyte-specific contrast agents (e.g., Mn-DPDP) will be taken up by these tumors [16, 62].

Liver adenomatosis is an uncommon condition first described in 1985 by Flejou et al. [63]. As a separate clinical entity, liver adenomatosis may be distinguished from liver cell adenoma by the presence of numerous

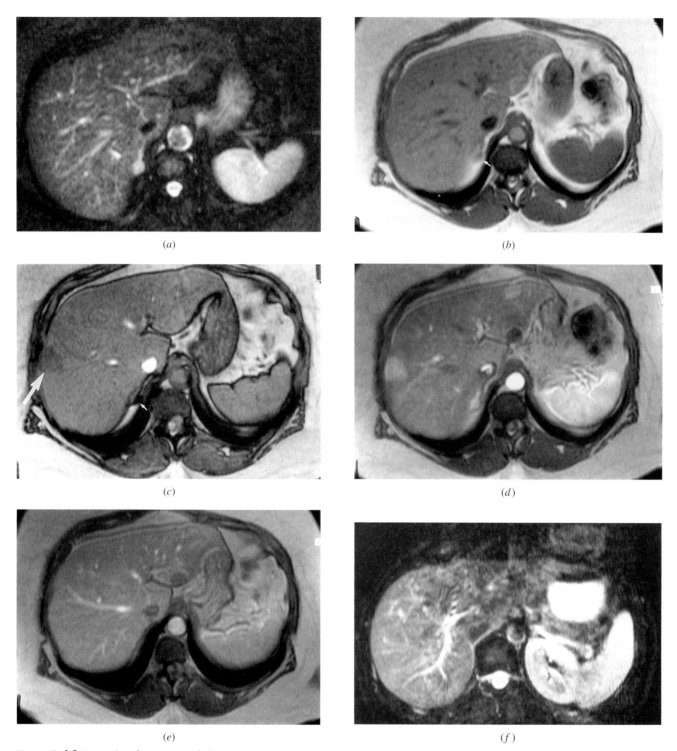

(a)

(b)

(c)

(d)

(e)

(f)

F I G . 2.46 Hepatic adenoma with fat. T2-weighted fat-suppressed ETSE (*a*), SGE (*b*), out-of-phase SGE (*c*), and immediate (*d*) and 90-s (*e*) postgadolinium SGE images. No focal liver lesions are apparent on the T2 (*a*) or T1-weighted (*b*) images. On the out-of-phase image (*c*) the adenoma is shown as a low signal mass (arrow) due to signal dropout caused by the presence of fat within the tumor. The adenoma enhances with a characteristic uniform hepatic arterial dominant phase blush (*d*), which rapidly washes out, rendering the tumor isointense with liver by 90 s (*e*). Incidental note is made of a right adrenal mass (small arrow, *b, c*) that drops in signal intensity from in-phase (*b*) to out-of-phase (*c*) images, which is diagnostic for adrenal adenoma.

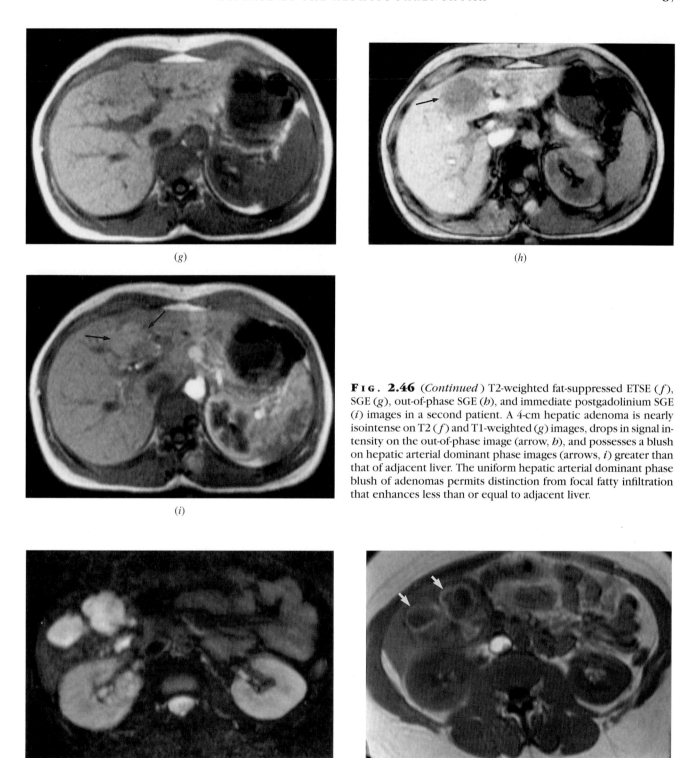

(g)

(h)

(i)

F I G . 2.46 (*Continued*) T2-weighted fat-suppressed ETSE (*f*), SGE (*g*), out-of-phase SGE (*h*), and immediate postgadolinium SGE (*i*) images in a second patient. A 4-cm hepatic adenoma is nearly isointense on T2 (*f*) and T1-weighted (*g*) images, drops in signal intensity on the out-of-phase image (arrow, *h*), and possesses a blush on hepatic arterial dominant phase images (arrows, *i*) greater than that of adjacent liver. The uniform hepatic arterial dominant phase blush of adenomas permits distinction from focal fatty infiltration that enhances less than or equal to adjacent liver.

(a)

(b)

F I G . 2.47 Hepatic adenoma complicated by hemorrhage. T2-weighted fat-suppressed ETSE (*a*), SGE (*b*), and immediate postgadolinium SGE (*c*) images. An 8-cm mass arises from the inferior aspect of the right lobe of the liver. Regions within the mass possess high signal intensity on the T2-weighted image (*a*) and high signal intensity peripheral rims on the T1-weighted image (arrows, *b*) consistent with blood. Heterogeneous enhancement of the nonhemorrhagic portions of the mass is identified on the immediate postgadolinium image (*c*). The patient discontinued birth control pills and on the 3-month follow-up study the mass had decreased in size to 3.5 cm and was heterogeneously high in signal intensity on the T2-weighted ETSE fat-suppressed (*d*) and T1-weighted (*e*) images, consistent with subacute blood.

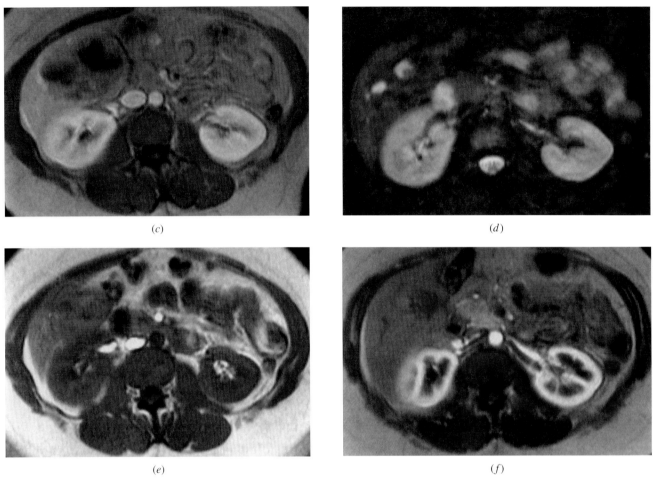

(c)

(d)

(e)

(f)

FIG. 2.47 (*Continued*) The peripheral, viable portion of the tumor enhances greater than background liver on the immediate postgadolinium SGE image (*f*).

adenomas (>10), lack of correlation with steroid medication, equal involvement in men and women, abnormal liver function tests, and a higher incidence of hemorrhage and malignant transformation (fig. 2.48) [64].

Focal Nodular Hyperplasia. Focal Nodular Hyperplasia (FNH) is an uncommon lesion defined by a localized region of hyperplasia within otherwise normal liver. Although the lesion may occur in all age groups and both sexes, FNH predominantly is found in women during the third to fifth decades of life [65]. In contrast to liver cell adenoma, FNH does not appear to have a clear-cut association with oral contraceptive use. Generally, FNH is a solitary lesion [65]. Multicentric lesions may be encountered as part of the multiple FNH syndrome including other lesions such as liver hemangioma, meningioma, astrocytoma, telangiectasias of the brain, berry aneurysm, dysplastic systemic arteries, and portal vein atresia [66]. On imaging, background fatty liver may be more common in FNH than that observed with other focal liver lesions, except metastases. A collar of higher-concentration perilesional fatty infiltration may rarely be present [67], which differs from the perilesional fatty sparing of metastasis. FNH does not exhibit malignant potential, and hemorrhage is exceedingly rare, encountered only in large lesions [37, 57].

The most common appearance on noncontrast MR images is slight hypointensity on T1-weighted images and slight hyperintensity on T2-weighted images, although tumors may be nearly isointense on both of these sequences. Unlike adenomas, FNH rarely has higher signal intensity than liver on T1-weighted images. High signal intensity on T2-weighted images of the central scar is a characteristic feature of FNH but is observed in only 10–49% of patients [65, 68–71]. The central scar has a typical appearance of a relatively small size with sharp angular margins. The hyperintense appearance of the central scar on T2-weighted images may correlate with the presence of vascular channels, bile ducts, fibrosis, chronic inflammation, and edema noted histopathologically.

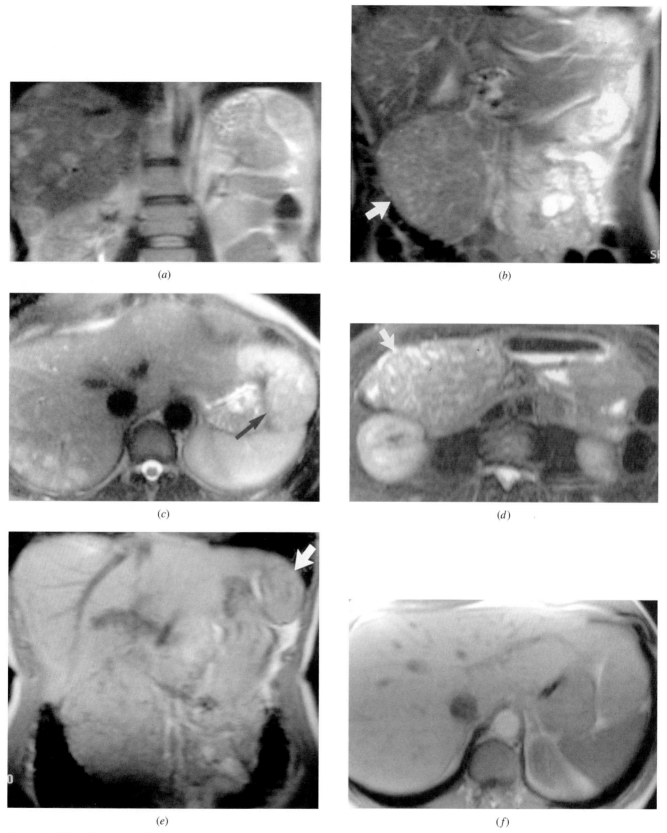

(a)

(b)

(c)

(d)

(e)

(f)

F I G . 2.48 Adenomatosis. Coronal (*a*, *b*) and transverse (*c*, *d*) T2-weighted SS-ETSE, coronal (*e*) and transverse (*f*, *g*) SGE, out-of-phase SGE (*h*, *i*), immediate postgadolinium SGE (*j*, *k*), and 90-s postgadolinium fat-suppressed SGE (*l*, *m*) images. Multiple small lesions are scattered throughout the hepatic parenchyma, predominantly in the right lobe, that demonstrate slight high signal on T2-weighted images (*a*, *c*), near isointensity on T1-weighted images (*f*), and mildly intense homogeneous enhancement immediately after administration of contrast (*j*, *k*) and become isointense with the liver by 90 s (*l*, *m*).

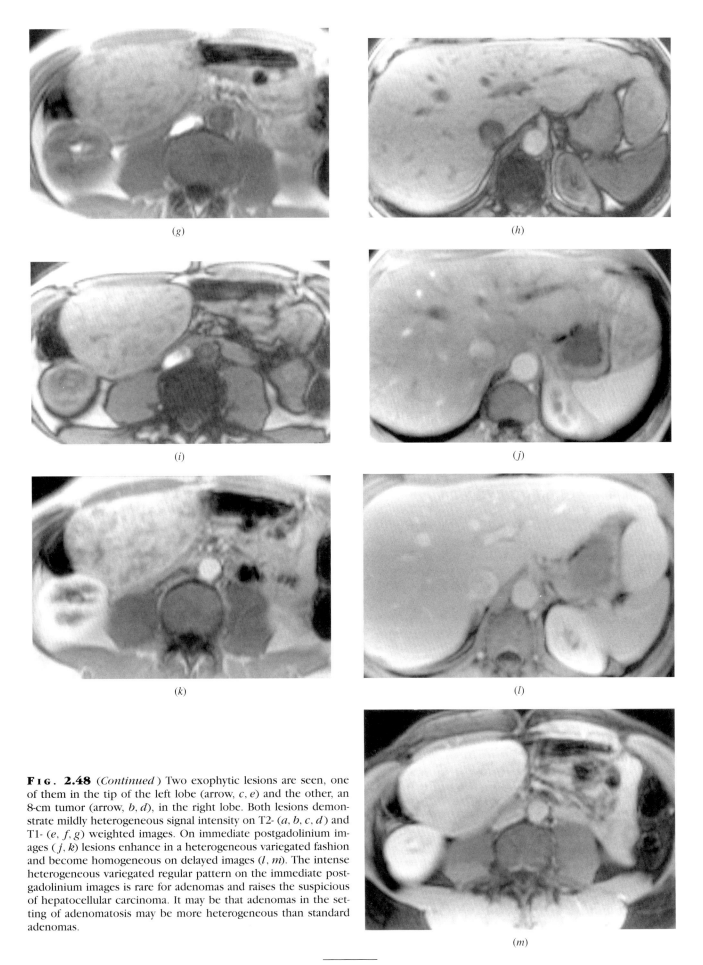

(g)

(h)

(i)

(j)

(k)

(l)

(m)

F I G . 2.48 (*Continued*) Two exophytic lesions are seen, one of them in the tip of the left lobe (arrow, *c, e*) and the other, an 8-cm tumor (arrow, *b, d*), in the right lobe. Both lesions demonstrate mildly heterogeneous signal intensity on T2- (*a, b, c, d*) and T1- (*e, f, g*) weighted images. On immediate postgadolinium images (*j, k*) lesions enhance in a heterogeneous variegated fashion and become homogeneous on delayed images (*l, m*). The intense heterogeneous variegated regular pattern on the immediate postgadolinium images is rare for adenomas and raises the suspicious of hepatocellular carcinoma. It may be that adenomas in the setting of adenomatosis may be more heterogeneous than standard adenomas.

Although the patho-etiology of FNH is incompletely understood, it has been proposed that the lesion is developmental in origin, consisting of a hyperplastic response of hepatic parenchyma to a preexisting arterial malformation [72]. From a pathologic perspective, FNH is characterized grossly as a sharply circumscribed, but uncapsulated, rounded or lobulated mass. The cut surface reveals a central stellate scar, often containing large, malformed blood vessels. This feature is detected in approximately one-half of cases by MRI techniques [69, 73]. It is postulated that the spiderlike branches of the anomalous vessels provide excellent blood supply to the component nodules; hence, these tumors are usually homogeneous (with internal necrosis and hemorrhage being rare events) [74]. Microscopically, fibrous septa radiating from the central scar contain vascular channels, exuberant bile duct proliferation, and intense inflammation. Parenchyma between the septa show benign hepatocytes.

Two subtypes of FNH have been described: (1) the solid type, which is most common and is characterized by the presence of a central fibrous scar containing enlarged malformed arteries that may be inconspicuous or absent in lesions smaller than 1 cm, and (2) the telangiectatic type, which is characterized by the presence of centrally located multiple dilated blood filled spaces. This subtype is enriched with more abundant and smaller arteries than the solid type. The telangiectatic type of FNH is more commonly associated with the multiple FNH sydrome [37].

FNH enhances with a dramatic uniform blush on immediate postgadolinium images and fades rapidly to near isointensity (typically at 1 min after contrast)

(fig. 2.49) [73]. When observed, the central scar is low in signal intensity on immediate post-gadolinium images and gradually enhances to hyperintensity over time (figs. 2.50 and 2.51). This enhancement pattern is that of scar tissue independent of location. There is a tendency for larger FNHs to have central scars that show only partial enhancement on delayed images, which may reflect more mature, less vascularized scar tissue. FNH may also occur as exophytic lesions and the attachment to liver may be a thin stalk. Even exophytic tumors possess the characteristic imaging appearance (fig. 2.52).

As diffuse fatty liver is common in patients with FNH, the tumor may be mildly hypointense on in-phase T1-weighted images and hyperintense on out-of-phase images (fig. 2.53). Unlike the situation with adenomas, we have not observed signal drop of FNH on out-of-phase images, reflecting the lesser occurrence and lesser volume of fat that may be present in FNH. Fatty infiltration of FNH is rare and only sporadically mentioned in the literature. In previous reports describing the presence of fat in FNH, fatty infiltration of the lesion was interpreted as an extension of the patient's underlying disease, that is, hepatic steatosis. In theory, intralesional steatosis in FNH may be encountered in several types of hepatic injury associated with steatosis, including alcoholic toxicity, obesity, diabetes, and malnutrition [65].

Lesions that are isointense on all precontrast images may be appreciated only on the immediate postgadolinium SGE image as a mass that transiently enhances in a uniform homogeneous fashion. This is a common apperance for small, <1.5-cm FNHs. The central scar is often not apparent in the small FNHs as well.

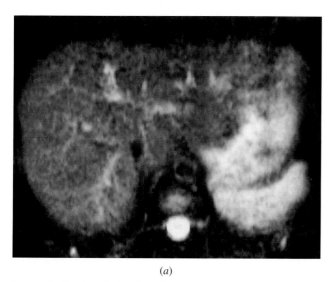

(a)

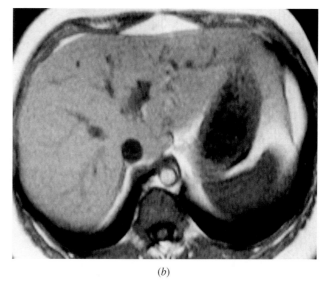

(b)

F I G . 2.49 Small focal nodular hyperplasia. T2-weighted fat-suppressed ETSE (*a*), SGE (*b*), out-of-phase SGE (*c*), and immediate (*d*) and 90-s (*e*) postgadolinium SGE images. A 1.5-cm focal nodular hyperplasia is present in the lateral segment that is isointense on T2 (*a*) and out-of-phase (*c*) images and near isointense on T1 (*b*).

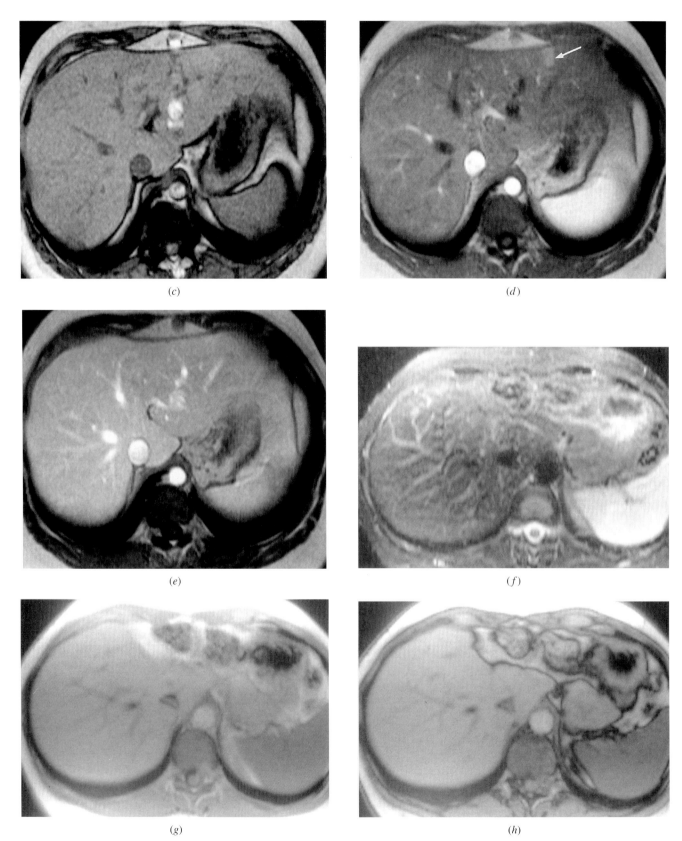

(c)

(d)

(e)

(f)

(g)

(h)

FIG. 2.49 (*Continued*) The tumor is only visualized on the immediate postgadolinium SGE image by the presence of a hepatic arterial dominant blush (arrow, *d*). The tumor fades by 90 s to isointensity with background liver (*e*).

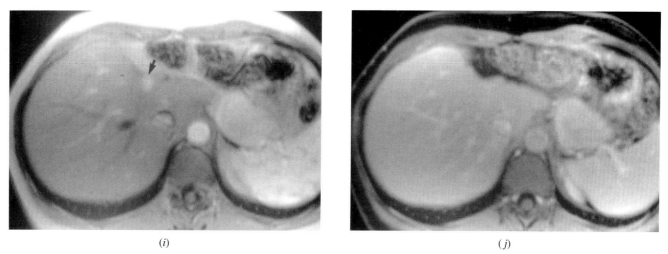

(i)   (j)

F I G . 2.49 (*Continued*) Echo-train STIR (*f*), SGE (*g*), out-of-phase SGE (*h*), immediate postgadolinium (*i*), and 90-s postgadolinium fat-suppressed SGE (*j*) images in a second patient who has a history of left hepatectomy for focal nodular hyperplasia. There is a small lesion in *segment 8*, which is isointense on all imaging sequences except for the transient tumor blush (arrow, *i*) on the immediate postgadolinium image. The appearance of the 1-cm FNH in these two patients is typical for these tumors when they are small in size, in that they may be only visible on hepatic arterial dominant phase images. A central scar is often not visualized in small FNHs.

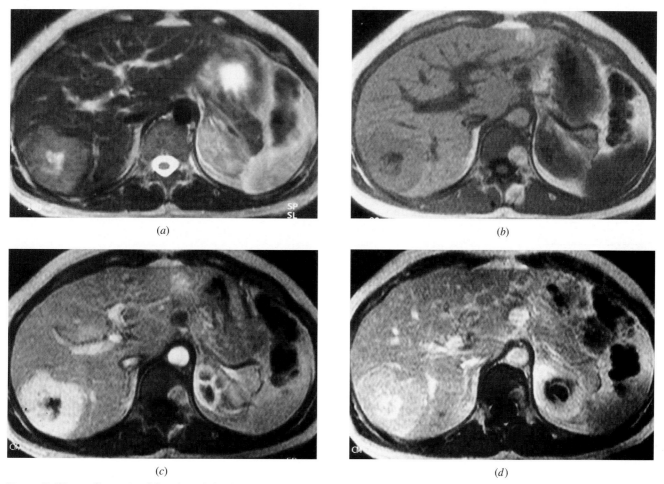

(a)   (b)

(c)   (d)

F I G . 2.50 Medium-sized focal nodular hyperplasia. T2-weighted ETSE (*a*), SGE (*b*), immediate postgadolinium (*c*), and 5-min postgadolinium SGE (*d*) images. A 5.5-cm mass is present in the right lobe of the liver.

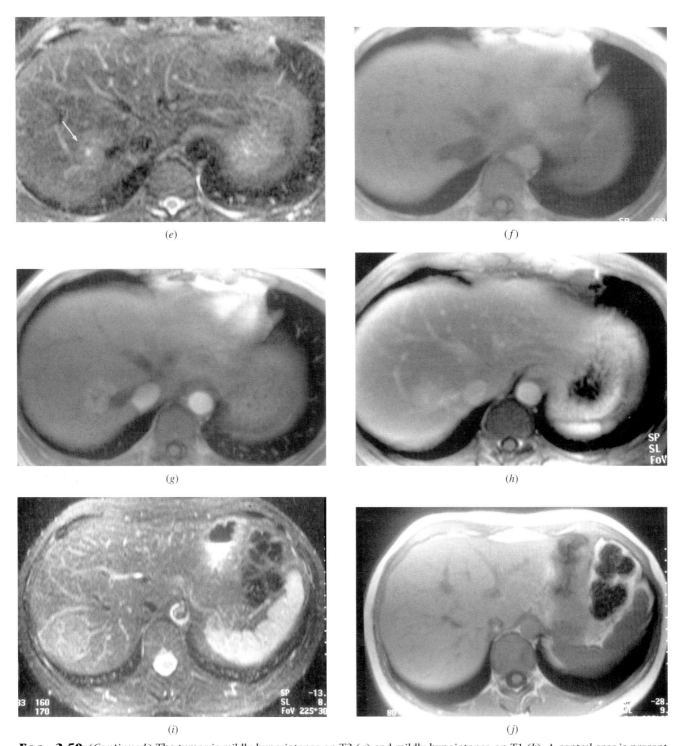

(e)

(f)

(g)

(h)

(i)

(j)

FIG. 2.50 (*Continued*) The tumor is mildly hyperintense on T2 (*a*) and mildly hypointense on T1 (*b*). A central scar is present that is low in signal intensity on T1 (*b*) and high in signal intensity on T2 (*a*). On the immediate postgadolinium image (*c*), the tumor enhances with a uniform capillary blush, whereas the central scar remains low in signal intensity. On the late postgadolinium image (*d*), the tumor fades to near isointensity with background liver whereas the central scar shows delayed enhancement. This lesion is a classic focal nodular hyperplasia. (Courtesy of Susan M. Ascher, MD, Department of Radiology, Georgetown University Medical Center.)

Echo-train STIR (*e*), SGE (*f*), immediate postgadolinium SGE (*g*), and 90-s postgadolinium SGE (*h*) images in a second patient. There is a lesion in the right hepatic lobe (arrow, *e*) that demonstrates minimally high signal on the T2-weighted image (*e*) and isointensity on the T1-weighted image (*f*), enhances with a uniform blush on the immediate postgadolinium image (*g*), and fades to near isointensity on the delayed image (*h*). Note the small central scar that is high signal intensity on T2 (*e*) and low signal intensity on T1 (*f*) and immediate postgadolinium (*g*) images and enhances to hyperintensity over time (*h*).

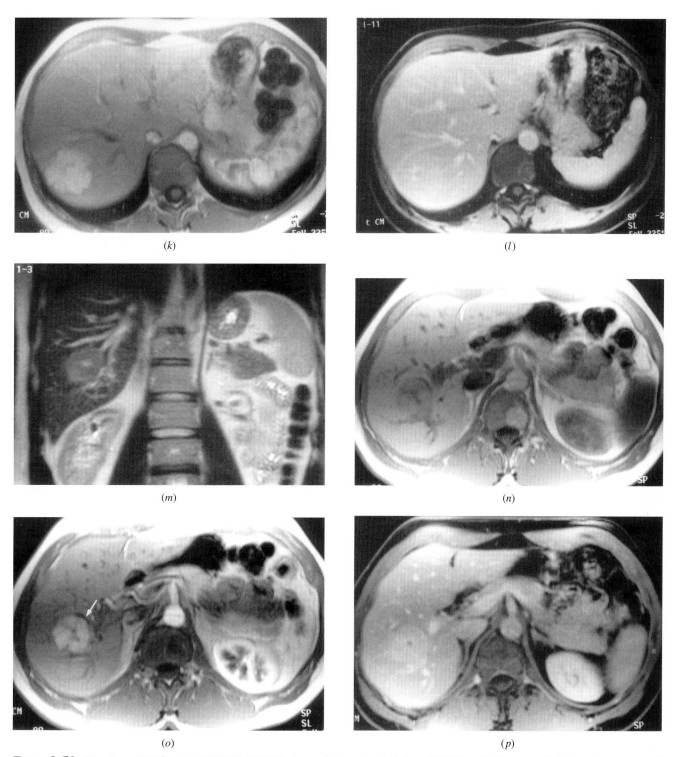

F I G . 2.50 (*Continued*) Echo-train STIR (*i*), SGE (*j*), immediate postgadolinium SGE (*k*), and 90-s postgadolinium fat-suppressed SGE (*l*) images in a third patient. There is a lobular lesion in the right hepatic lobe that has minimally increased signal on T2 (*i*), near isointensity on T1 (*j*), demonstrates intense uniform enhancement on the immediate postgadolinium image (*k*), and fades to near isointensity on late image (*l*). There is a small central scar best seen as a low-signal linear structure on the immediate postcontrast image (*k*).

Coronal T2-weighted SS-ETSE (*m*), SGE (*n*), immediate postgadolinium SGE (*o*) and 90-s postgadolinium fat-suppressed SGE (*p*) images in a fourth patient. The 3.5-cm FNH has a partial pseudocapsule (arrow, *o*). The pseudocapsule and central scar show partial enhancement on the delayed image (*p*). The lesion otherwise has a typical MRI appearance for a FNH.

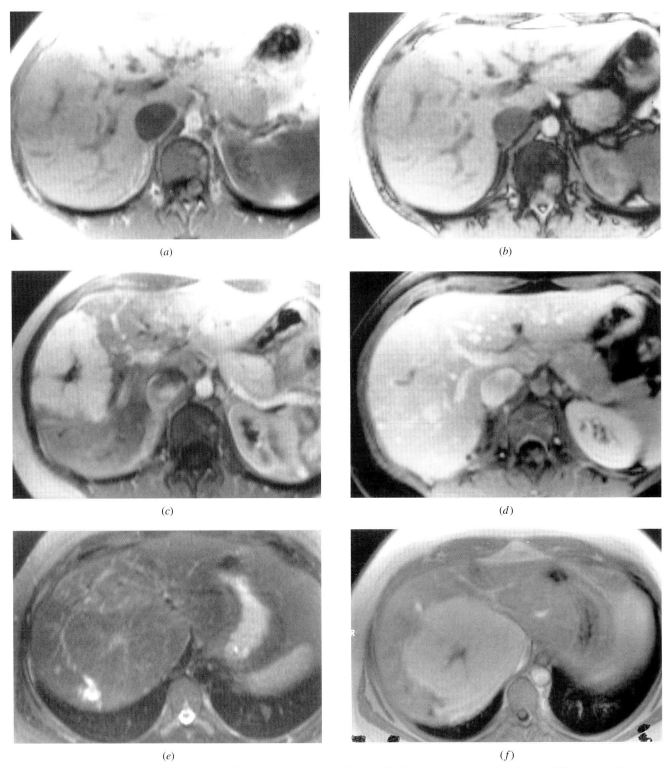

(a)

(b)

(c)

(d)

(e)

(f)

FIG. 2.51 Large focal nodular hyperplasia. SGE (*a*), out-of-phase SGE (*b*), immediate postgadolinium SGE (*c*), and 90-s post-gadolinium SGE (*d*) images. A large lesion is seen in the right hepatic lobe which is mildly hypointense on T1 (*a*) and does not drop in signal on out-of-phase (*b*), and shows homogeneous enhancement with lack of enhancement of the central scar on immediate postgadolinium images. The central scar shows partial enhancement on the late postcontrast image (*d*). The central scar in FNH is commonly small in size with angular margins. FNH almost never drop in signal on out-of-phase images, unlike adenomas, which commonly do.

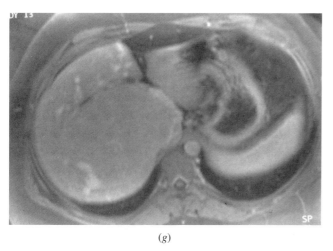

(*g*)

FIG. 2.51 (*Continued*) Echo-train STIR (*e*), immediate post-gadolinium SGE (*f*), and 90-s postgadolinium fat-suppressed SGE (*g*) images in a second patient. There is a large mass that has a small central scar with angular margins. The tumor has comparable signal to surrounding liver on T2 (*e*). Intense homogeneous enhancement of the lesion, with negligible enhancement of the small central scar, is apparent on the immediate postgadolinium images (*f*). The FNH fades to isointensity on the interstitial phase image (*g*). Note that the central scar is slightly hyperintense on T2 (*e*), and hypointense on the immediate postgadolinium T1 (*f*), and enhances to hyperintensity over time (*g*).

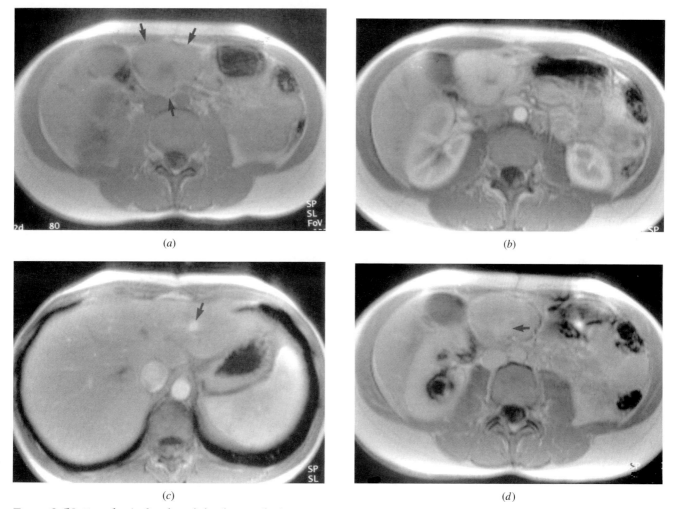

(*a*)   (*b*)

(*c*)   (*d*)

FIG. 2.52 Exophytic focal nodular hyperplasia. SGE (*a*), immediate (*b, c*) and 3-min (*d*) postgadolinium SGE, and sagittal 3.5-min postgadolinium fat-suppressed SGE (*e*) images. There is a lobular mass with a central scar in the anterior upper abdomen, which abuts the left hepatic lobe. This lesion is isointense on T1 (arrows, *a*) and demonstrates a transient blush on the immediate postgadolinium image with lack of enhancement of the central scar (*b*). Note early filling of the left hepatic vein (arrow, *c*), which drains the tumor, confirming its hepatic origin.

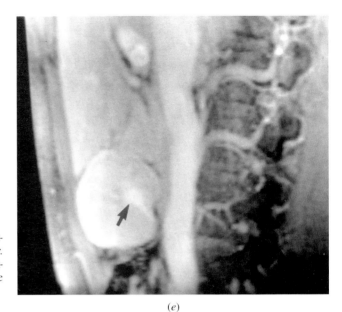

FIG. 2.52 (*Continued*) Transverse (*d*) and sagittal (*e*) late post-contrast images demonstrate late enhancement of the central scar. Despite its completely exophytic origin to the liver, the tumor exhibits the classic imaging features of FNH, which establishes the diagnosis.

(*e*)

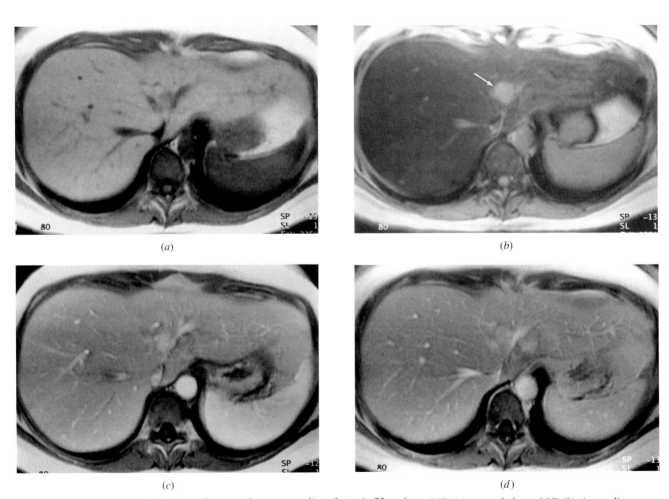

(*a*)

(*b*)

(*c*)

(*d*)

FIG. 2.53 Focal nodular hyperplasia with surrounding fatty infiltration. SGE (*a*), out-of-phase SGE (*b*), immediate post-gadolinium SGE (*c*), and 90-s postgadolinium SGE (*d*) images. A 2-cm focal nodular hyperplasia is present in the medial segment that is hypointense on the in-phase (*a*) and hyperintense on the out-of-phase (arrow, *b*) images because of signal dropout of the fatty liver. The tumor enhances with a uniform blush on the immediate postgadolinium image (*c*) and fades in signal intensity by 90 s (*d*).

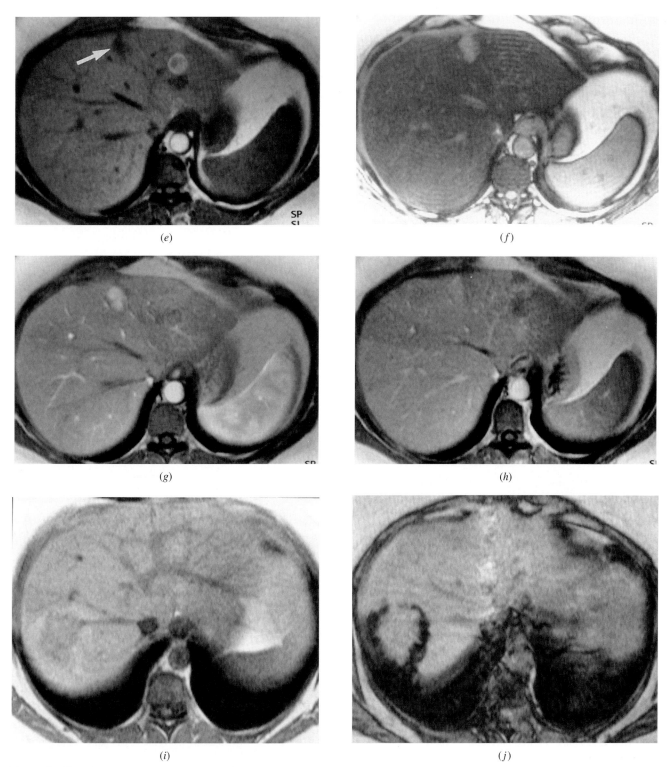

(e)

(f)

(g)

(h)

(i)

(j)

FIG. 2.53 (*Continued*) SGE (*e*), out-of-phase SGE (*f*), and immediate (*g*) and 90-s (*h*) postgadolinium SGE images in a second patient, who has diffuse fatty infiltration of the liver and a 2-cm focal nodular hyperplasia in the medial segment (arrow, *e*). The identical imaging findings are present as those shown in the prior patient.

A 4-cm focal nodular hyperplasia in a third patient demonstrates a collar of condensed fatty infiltration. The perilesional fat is moderately high in signal intensity on the in-phase SGE image (*i*) and drops to nearly signal void on the out-of-phase SGE image (*j*).

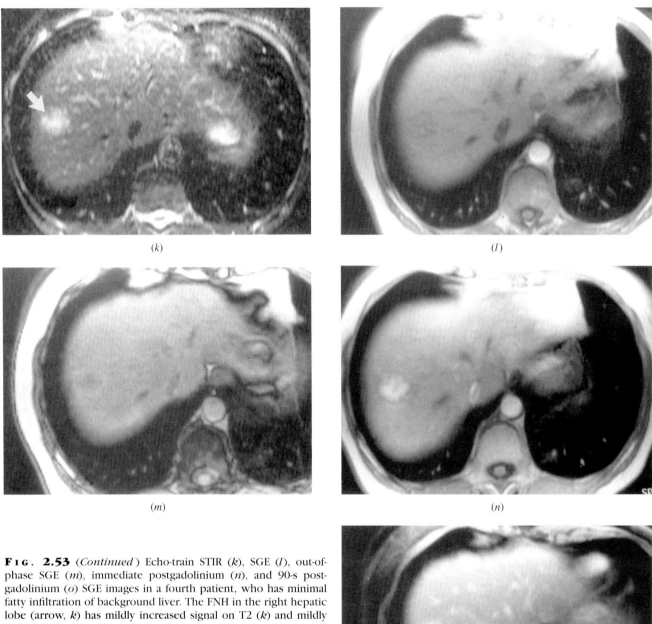

(k)   *(l)*

(m)   *(n)*

FIG. 2.53 (*Continued*) Echo-train STIR (*k*), SGE (*l*), out-of-phase SGE (*m*), immediate postgadolinium (*n*), and 90-s postgadolinium (*o*) SGE images in a fourth patient, who has minimal fatty infiltration of background liver. The FNH in the right hepatic lobe (arrow, *k*) has mildly increased signal on T2 (*k*) and mildly low signal on T1 (*l*) and becomes near isointense on the out-of-phase image (*m*), reflecting slight drop in signal of background liver. Note that the pseudocapsule appears slightly hyperintense on out of phase. This lesion exhibits a central scar more evident, as a low signal linear structure, on immediate postcontrast image (*n*). The lesion remains hyperintense on the 90 second fat-suppressed image, which may reflect signal loss in background liver more than retention of contrast in the lesion.

These cases illustrate that fatty infiltration of background liver is not uncommon in the setting of focal nodular hyperplasia.

(o)

The distinction between FNH and liver cell adenomas may be based on the following features. A central scar that shows delayed enhancement is typical for FNH, whereas pseudocapsule, internal hemorrhage, focal necrosis, and intralesional fat are features more commonly noted in liver cell adenomas [60]. Both lesions have an early transient tumor blush on gadolinium enhanced images [41, 73], and both may take up Mn-DPDP (fig. 2.54) [62, 75].

On Gd-EOB-DTPA enhanced images, FNH will show an early capillary blush and late hepatocellular uptake. An atypical feature of FNH is lack of the capillary blush

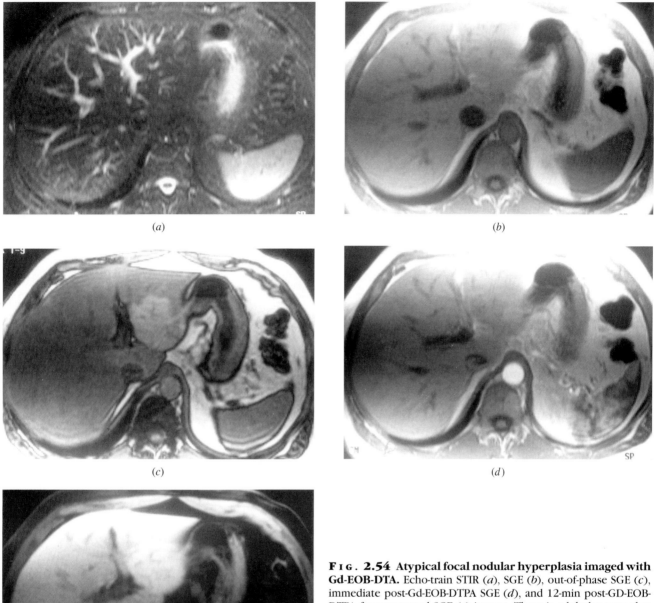

(a)

(b)

(c)

(d)

(e)

FIG. 2.54 Atypical focal nodular hyperplasia imaged with Gd-EOB-DTA. Echo-train STIR (*a*), SGE (*b*), out-of-phase SGE (*c*), immediate post-Gd-EOB-DTPA SGE (*d*), and 12-min post-GD-EOB-DTPA fat-suppressed SGE (*e*) images. There is a lobular mass that is isointense on T2 (*a*) and T1 (*b*) images and is well shown on the out-of-phase image (*c*) as a high-signal mass because of signal drop of surrounding fatty liver. Atypical for FNH is negligible enhancement immediately after gadolinium administration (*d*). Note the high signal of the mass on the late fat-suppressed (*e*) image that reflects both signal loss in the fatty liver and Gd-EOB-DTPA uptake in the hepatocytes of the FNH.

(fig. 2.54). A uniform capillary blush and uptake of Mn-DPDP must be cautiously interpreted because they are features of well-differentiated tumors of hepatocellular origin, including well-differentiated or early hepatocellular carcinoma.

Malignant Masses

Liver Metastases. Metastases are the most common malignant tumors of the liver in western contries.

Pathologically, liver metastases usually appear as solitary or multiple nodules, with rare appearances including confluent masses or small, infiltrative lesions mimicking cirrhosis. Tumors may be complicated by central necrosis or cystic change.

Optimal hepatic imaging evaluation involves both detection and characterization of focal lesions [41, 75–77]. Detection involves identification of the presence of lesions and the segmental extent of liver involvement

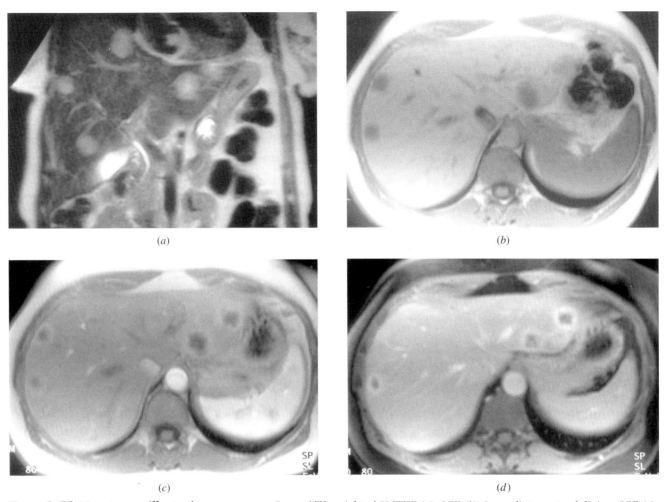

(a)   *(b)*

(c)   *(d)*

F I G . 2.55 Metastases—illustrating sequences. Coronal T2-weighted SS-ETSE (*a*), SGE (*b*), immediate postgadolinium SGE (*c*), and 90-s postgadolinium fat-suppressed SGE (*d, e*) images in a patient with metastases from cloacogenic carcinoma. An MR study of the liver should include coronal (*a*) in addition to transverse plane images, T2 (*a*), T1 (*b*), immediate postgadolinium (*c*) and interstitial-phase (*d*) fat-suppressed images. Multiple metastases are present throughout the liver. Well-defined ring enhancement is appreciated on immediate postgadolinium images (*c*). Attention to lung bases must be made to evaluate for lung metastases (arrow, *e*).

[76]. Demonstration that malignant disease has limited hepatic involvement may have a substantial impact on patient management. Survival of patients with colorectal metastases may be improved by partial hepatectomy, if metastases are localized to three or fewer segments [78, 79]. MRI is superior to CT imaging in the evaluation of the liver [41, 54, 80–83]. The current challenge is whether the superior performance of MRI translates into a beneficial effect on patient management, disease outcome, and health care costs. New MR sequences, phased-array surface coils, and tissue-specific MR contrast agents suggest that MRI may further exceed the diagnostic ability of CT imaging.

An imaging protocol including T1-weighted SGE, T2-weighted, and serial gadolinium-enhanced SGE images acquired with whole liver coverage per acquisition achieves good lesion detection (T2-weighted and imme-

diate postgadolinium SGE images) and characterization (T2-weighted and serial postgadolinium SGE images) (fig. 2.55). The use of fat suppression on T2-weighted sequences is advisable because it facilitates detection of subcapsular lesions [84]. Fat suppression is especially important to apply on echo-train spin-echo sequences, because fat liver results in a bright liver on nonsuppressed T2-weighted echo-train sequences that can obscure liver metastases. In addition to histologic features of the metastases themselves, histologic changes often occur in the uninvolved portion of liver near the tumor. Patchy fatty infiltration of liver may also be noted.

On out-of-phase SGE images, liver metastases may appear high in signal intensity because of signal drop of background liver parenchyma (fig. 2.56). On occasion, this may facilitate lesion detection, particularly if lesions are intrinsically high in signal intensity (fig. 2.57). More

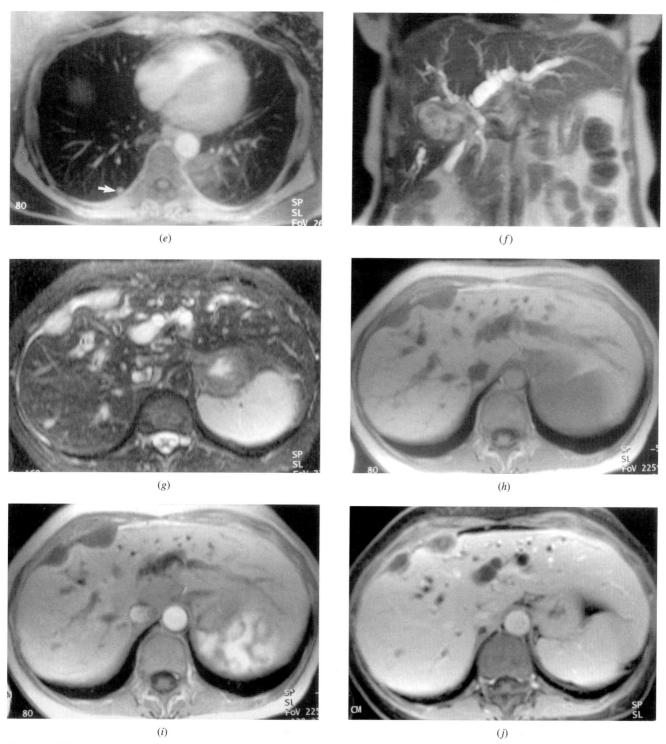

F I G . 2.55 (*Continued*) Coronal T2-weighted SS-ETSE (*f*) and transverse echo-train STIR (*g*), SGE (*h*), immediate postgadolinium SGE (*i*), and interstitial-phase gadolinium-enhanced SGE (*j*) images in a second patient with capsule-based metastases who has colon cancer. Two capsule-based metastases are present that demonstrate scalloping of the liver margin. A large metastasis in *segment 5* is also present which obstructs the common hepatic duct (*f*).

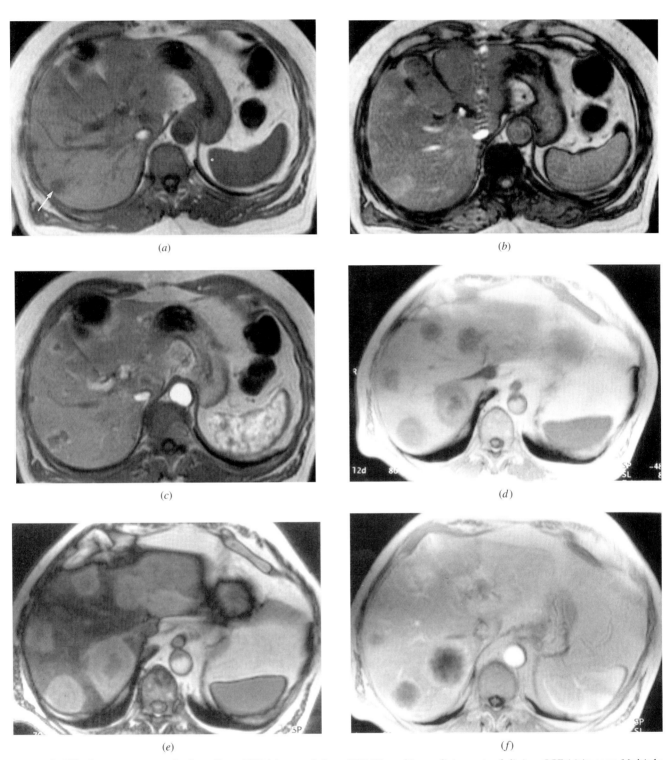

(a)

(b)

(c)

(d)

(e)

(f)

F I G . 2.56 Liver metastases in fatty liver. SGE (*a*), out-of-phase SGE (*b*), and immediate postgadolinium SGE (*c*) images. Multiple low-signal intensity metastases are present in the liver on the in-phase T1-weighted image (arrow, *a*). On the out-of-phase T1-weighted image (*b*), the liver diminishes in signal intensity, rendering the metastases mildly high in signal intensity relative to liver. Immediate postgadolinium SGE image (*c*) shows that the lesions enhance in a peripheral ring fashion, consistent with metastases.

SGE (*d*), out-of-phase SGE (*e*), and immediate postgadolinium SGE (*f*) images in a second patient with colon cancer liver metastases. Fatty liver may arise as a response to the presence of liver metastases or also as a response to the chemotherapy directed at the metastases.

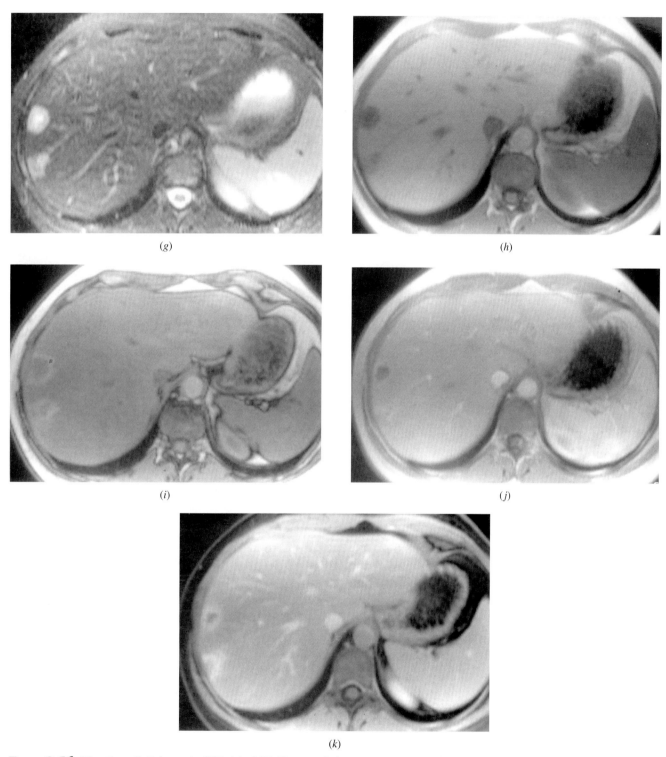

(g)

(h)

(i)

(j)

(k)

F ɪ ɢ . 2.56 (*Continued*) Echo train-STIR (*g*), SGE (*h*), out-of-phase SGE (*i*), immediate postgadolinium SGE (*j*), and 90-s post-gadolinium fat-suppressed (*k*) images in a third patient, who has breast cancer. There are two lesions in the right hepatic lobe that demonstrate high signal on T2 (*g*), low signal on T1 (*h*), and ring enhancement aftering contrast administration (*j*, *k*) consistent with metastases. Note that the liver drops moderately in signal on the out-of-phase image (*i*) and a bright rim is present around the lesions consistent with compressed liver parenchyma, which is unable to accumulate intracytoplasmic lipid.

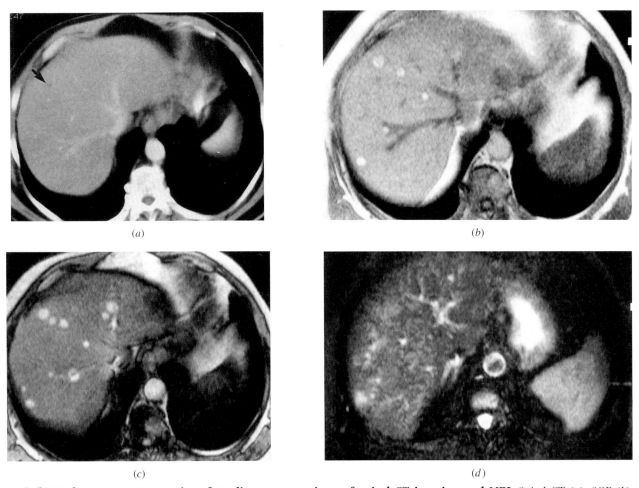

(a)

(b)

(c)

(d)

FIG. 2.57 Melanoma metastases in a fatty liver—comparison of spiral CT imaging and MRI. Spiral CT (*a*), SGE (*b*), out-of-phase SGE (*c*), and T2-weighted fat-suppressed ETSE (*d*) images. A solitary melanoma metastasis is apparent on the spiral CT image (arrow, *a*). Multiple mildly hyperintense metastases smaller than 1 cm are identified on the SGE image (*b*), and these high-signal intensity lesions become more conspicuous on the out-of-phase image (*c*). Lesions are apparent on the T2-weighted images (*d*), but are not as clearly shown as on the out-of-phase images (*c*). The presence of fatty infiltration of the liver has resulted in a signal drop on out-of-phase images (*c*), which has increased the conspicuity of the high T1-weighted signal intensity liver metastases.

often, however, lesions are rendered less conspicuous because the lowered signal of the liver reduces the contrast with low-signal focal liver lesions. Pathologically, in the setting of liver metastasis, surrounding parenchyma may show compression or atrophy of hepatocyte cords, scattered foci of chronic inflammation replacing lost hepatocytes, and the absence of fatty change. On out-of-phase images this zone of compressed liver parenchyma bordering on the metastasis appears as a moderately bright rim. This finding is relatively common in the setting of colon cancer metastases with background fatty liver and may occasionally be seen in other lesions including hemangiomas.

The acquisition of at least one sequence in the coronal plane may be of value in evaluating the superior and inferior margins of the liver, particularly the infracardiac portion of the left lobe [85]. Short duration techniques

such as SGE, SS-ETSE, or both are useful for this purpose (fig. 2.58). A study that compared nonspiral dynamic contrast-enhanced CT imaging and MRI employing T2-weighted fat-suppressed spin-echo, SGE, and dynamic serial postgadolinium SGE images in 73 patients with clinically suspected liver disease demonstrated greater lesion detection and characterization by MRI (fig. 2.59) [41]. Lesion detection was greatest with T2 fat suppression (T2-FS) (272 lesions) and contrast-enhanced SGE (244 lesions) images, which was statistically greater than with CT (220 lesions) and SGE (219 lesions) images ($P < 0.03$) [41]. Lesion characterization was greatest with contrast-enhanced SGE images (236 lesions) ($P < 0.01$), followed by CT (199 lesions), SGE (164 lesions), and T2-FS (144 lesions) images. A follow-up study compared these MRI sequences to dynamic nonspiral contrast-enhanced CT images in 20 patients with

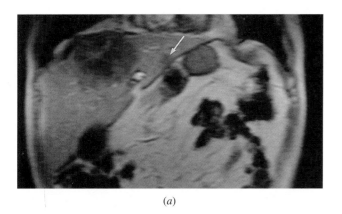

(a)

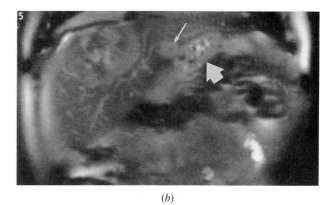

(b)

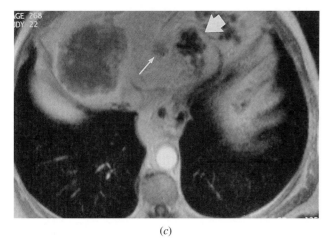

(c)

FIG. 2.58 Liver metastases, coronal images. Coronal magnetization-prepared gradient echo (a), coronal T2-weighted SS-ETSE (b), and 45-s postgadolinium SGE (c) images. A 6-cm colon cancer metastasis is present in the medial segment that is heterogeneous and low in signal intensity on the T1-weighted image (a) and heterogeneous and mildly hyperintense on the T2-weighted image (b). A 1-cm capsule-based metastasis is identified in the lateral segment (arrows, a, b) that has signal intensity features similar to those of the larger metastasis. Close proximity to the stomach (large arrow, b) is appreciated. The transverse postgadolinium image (c) demonstrates ring enhancement around the large heterogeneously low signal intensity metastasis. Ring enhancement is also appreciated around the small lesion (arrow, c). This lesion could easily be mistaken for a partial volume artifact with the nearby stomach (large arrow, c) on transverse sections. At least one coronal acquisition is recommended to minimize potential errors of ascribing lesions on the superior and inferior edges of the liver as partial volume effects.

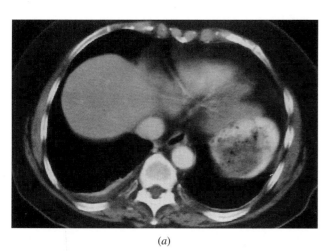

(a)

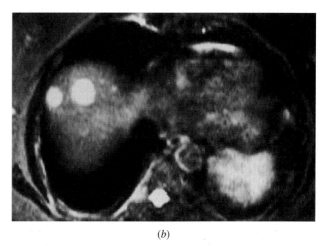

(b)

FIG. 2.59 Liver metastases, dynamic contrast-enhanced CT imaging versus MRI. Dynamic contrast-enhanced CT (a), T2-weighted fat-suppressed SS-ETSE (b), and immediate postgadolinium SGE (c, d) images. Few lesions are apparent on the dynamic contrast-enhanced CT image, including no lesions at the dome of the liver (a). At this tomographic level two well-defined high signal intensity masses are identified on the T2-weighted image (b). These lesions are distinguished from hemangiomas by the demonstration of uniform ring enhancement on the immediate postgadolinium image (arrow, c). On the immediate postgadolinium image from a more inferior tomographic section (d), multiple ring enhancing (long arrows, d) and uniform enhancing (short arrows, d) metastases are identified.

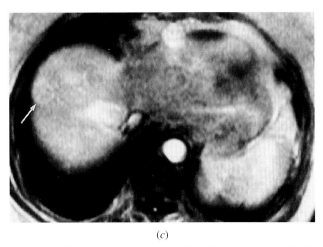

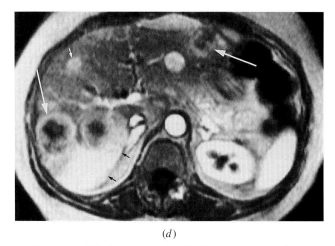

(c)   *(d)*

F I G . 2.59 (*Continued*) Intense ill-defined perilesional enhancement is present (black arrows, *d*), which is commonly observed with colon cancer liver metastases.

solitary hepatic metastases detected by CT imaging and demonstrated that MRI detected more than one lesion in 6 of 20 (30%) patients [80].

Characterization of focal liver lesions as benign or malignant is important because patients with known primary malignancies commonly have small hepatic lesions that are benign cysts or hemangiomas. A previous report described the detection of small (<15 mm) lesions in 254 of 1/454 patients who underwent CT examination [86]. The majority of patients (82%) with liver lesions in this study had a known primary tumor, yet lesions in 51% of these patients were benign. Another report described a large series of cancer patients in whom 41.8% of detected focal liver lesions were benign [87].

We reported on a consecutive population of women with newly diagnosed breast cancer and suspected liver metastases who were referred to MRI [88]. A total of 11 of 34 (32%) had benign lesions only. Twenty-one (62%) patients had malignant lesions, two of whom had coexistent benign lesions. Patients with malignant disease may have a variety of lesions, many of which may be benign, multiple, and scattered throughout the liver. Therefore, the whole organ coverage per acquisition of SGE permits optimal evaluation of the entire liver in distinct phases of enhancement using serial image acquisition after gadolinium administration. In the presence of multiple liver lesions, the distinction of benign and malignant lesions is of critical importance and is performed well by MRI (fig. 2.60).

Comparison between spiral CT arterial portography (CTAP) and current MRI techniques for diagnostic accuracy, cost, and effect on patient management has been studied using a population of 26 patients referred for hepatic surgery with suspected malignant liver lesions [89]. Regarding lesion detection, CTAP and MRI, respectively, showed 185 and 176 true-positive malig-

nant lesions, 15 and 0 false-positive malignant lesions, 0 and 18 true-negative malignant lesions, and 13 and 22 false-negative malignant lesions. Regarding segmental involvement, CTAP and MRI, respectively, showed 107 and 105 true-positive segments, 11 and 0 false-positive segments, 80 and 91 true-negative segments, and 4 and 6 false-negative segments. A statistically significant difference in specificity of segmental involvement was observed between MRI (1.0 ± 0) and CTAP (0.88 ± 0.05) ($P < 0.03$). Total procedural charges were $3499 for CTAP and $1224 for MRI. Findings at MR imaging altered patient treatment in seven patients, whereas findings at CTAP did not impact on patient treatment in any of the cases; this result was statistically significant ($P = 0.015$). The results of this study demonstrated that state-of-the-art MRI has higher diagnostic accuracy and greater effect on patient management than spiral CTAP and is 64% less expensive. A follow-up study comparing spiral CTAP and MRI in 20 surgically staged patients showed a trend that MR was superior for lesion detection and segmental involvement [53]. CTAP and MR images demonstrated, respectively, 54 and 60 true-positive lesions, 6 and 1 false-positive lesions, 15 and 22 true-negative (i.e., benign) lesions, and 8 and 2 false-negative lesions. CTAP and MR images demonstrated, respectively, 57 and 62 true-positive segmental involvements, 6 and 1 false-positive segmental involvements, 89 and 95 true-negative segmental involvements, and 8 and 2 false-negative segmental involvements [53]. A major problem with CTAP is the frequent occurrence of perfusion defects that can resemble a focal mass or can mask the presence of metastases on CTAP images. Perfusion defects are rarely problematic on MR images (figs. 2.61 and 2.62).

We reported a comparison between MRI using T2-weighted fat-suppressed echo-train spin-echo and immediate postgadolinium SGE with single-phase spiral CT

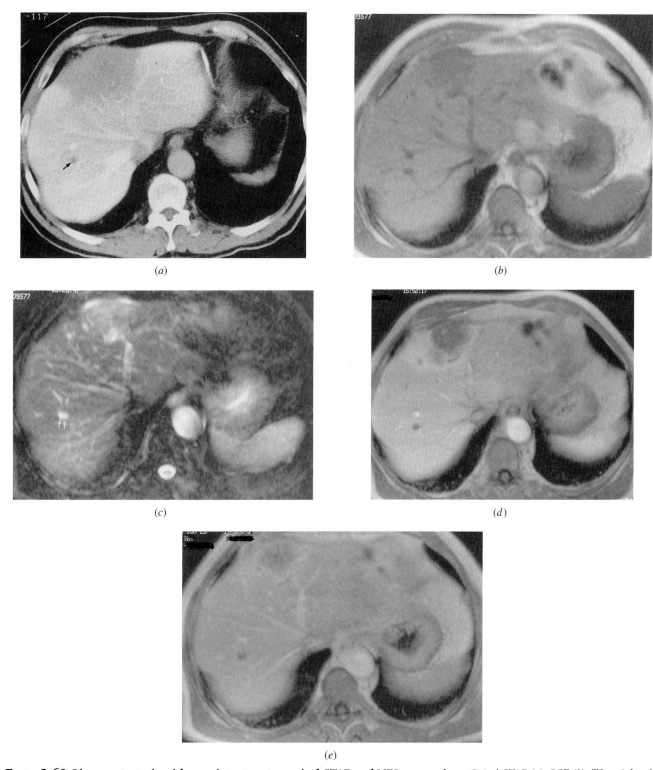

(a)   *(b)*

(c)   *(d)*

(e)

F I G . 2.60 Liver metastasis with coexistent cysts—spiral CTAP and MRI comparison. Spiral CTAP (*a*), SGE (*b*), T2-weighted fat-suppressed ETSE (*c*), and immediate (*d*), and 5-min postgadolinium SGE (*e*) images. The CTAP image (*a*) demonstrates a large perfusional defect in the medial segment related to a colon cancer metastasis. A 6-mm lesion in the anterior segment (arrow, *a*) was interpreted as one of several similar-appearing small lesions consistent with metastases scattered throughout the remainder of the liver. The MR images demonstrate a 4-cm mass in the medial segment with the imaging features of a colon cancer metastasis, including transient ill-defined perilesional enhancement on the immediate postgadolinium image (*d*). The lesion in the anterior segment represents two 3-mm juxtaposed cysts (arrows, *c*) that are small, sharply marginated, low in signal intensity on the T1-weighted image (*b*), and high in signal intensity on the T2-weighted image (*c*). Lack of enhancement on early (*d*) and later (*e*) postgadolinium-enhanced images are diagnostic for cysts. The remaining small liver lesions scattered throughout the liver were all shown to be cysts on MR images. The patient was operated on based on the MRI findings of a solitary liver metastases and multiple coexistent cysts. Intraoperative sonography-guided aspiration demonstrated that these small lesions were cysts. MRI was more diagnostically accurate than CTAP and had a greater effect on patient management.

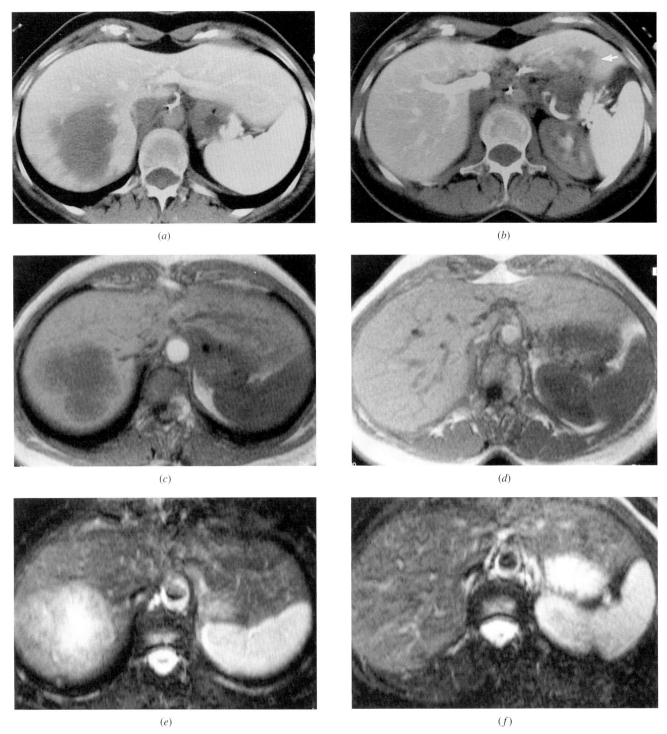

(a)

(b)

(c)

(d)

(e)

(f)

FIG. 2.61 Liver metastases—spiral CT arterial portography versus MRI. Spiral CTAP (*a, b*), SGE (*c, d*), T2-weighted fat-suppressed SS-ETSE (*e, f*), and immediate postgadolinium SGE (*g, h*) images from superior (*a, c, e, g*) and more inferior (*b, d, f, h*) tomographic sections. A large metastasis is present in the right lobe of the liver shown on all imaging techniques (*a, c, e, g*). A second metastasis was suspected on the CTAP image (arrow, *b*) in the lateral segment. No lesion was identified in this location on any MRI sequence. CTAP findings would have precluded surgery. However, the decision to operate was based on MRI findings. No liver metastasis was identified in the lateral segment by surgical palpation or interoperative sonography. The patient is disease free for more than 5 years since right hepatectomy. MRI was more accurate and had a greater impact on patient management and outcome than CTAP.

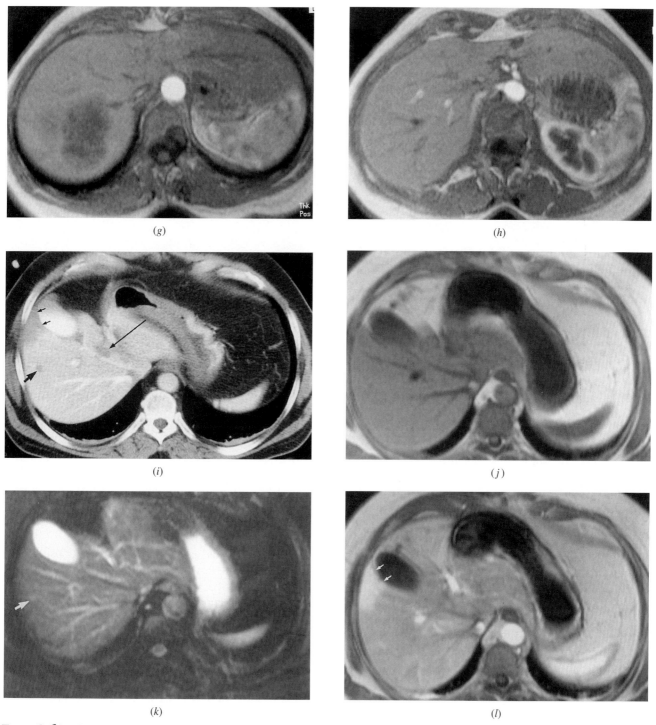

FIG. 2.61 (*Continued*) Spiral CTAP (*i*), SGE (*j*), T2-weighted fat-suppressed SS-ETSE (*k*), and immediate postgadolinium SGE (*l*) images in a second patient with liver metastases from colon cancer. Spiral CTAP and MR images demonstrate an 8-mm metastasis in the anterior segment of the right lobe (arrow, *i*, *k*) and a perfusional abnormality related to a metastasis in the anterior segment of the right lobe (short arrows, *i*, *l*). A focal defect interpreted as metastasis on the CTAP image (long arrow, *i*) is apparent in the medial segment, but is not identified on any of the MR images (*j–l*). No metastasis in this location was identified at surgery and intraoperative sonography.

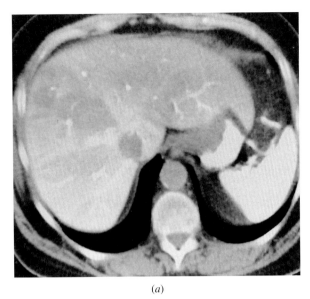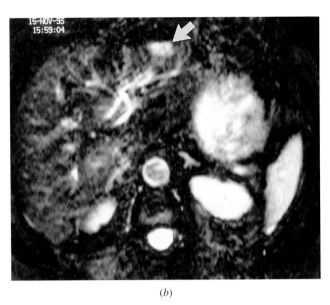

(a)   (b)

F I G . 2.62 Liver metastases—perfusional defect. Spiral CTAP (*a*) and T2-weighted fat-suppressed SS-ETSE (*b*) images. Multiple large perfusional defects are present on the CTAP image (*a*) with the entire left lobe exhibiting diminished perfusion. A 1.5-cm liver metastasis is present on the T2-weighted image (arrow, *b*), which was masked by the perfusion defect on the CTAP image.

for the detection and characterization of hepatic lesions in 89 patients [89]. Regarding true-positive lesion detection, 295 and 519 lesions were detected on spiral CT and MR images, respectively, which was significantly different on a patient-by-patient basis ($P<0.001$). More lesions were detected on MR than on spiral CT in 44 of 89 patients (49.4%), and 11 of these 44 patients had lesions shown on MRI that were not apparent on CT images. No patients had true-positive lesions shown on spiral CT that were not shown on MRI. Regarding lesion characterization, 129 and 486 lesions were characterized on spiral CT and MRI images, respectively, which was significantly different on a patient-by-patient basis ($P < 0.001$). More lesions were characterized on MR than CT images in 68 (76.4%) patients. Regarding effect on patient management, findings on MRI provided information that altered patient compared to findings on spiral CT in 57 patients.

A follow-up study comparing dual-phase spiral CT and the above-described sequences in 22 patients showed that MR and dual-phase spiral CT detected 53 and 63 lesions, and characterized 39 and 62 lesions, respectively [90].

Metastases vary substantially in appearance on T1- and T2-weighted images. Borders are usually ill-defined but may be sharp. Lesion shape is frequently irregular but may be regular, round or oval. Metastases generally are moderately low in signal intensity on T1-weighted images and modestly high in signal intensity on T2-weighted images. Some metastases, particularly vascular metastases from islet cell tumors, leiomyosarcoma, pheochromocytoma, renal cell carcinoma, necrotic metastases, or cystic metastases from

ovarian cancer, may be high in signal intensity on T2-weighted images, rendering distinction from hemangiomas difficult [39, 54, 91, 92].

Metastases do not have the classical enhancement patterns of benign lesions (i.e., no enhancement as seen with cysts, peripheral nodular enhancement as seen with hemangiomas, or, in metastases >2 cm, transient immediate postgadolinium homogeneous blush as seen with FNH or adenomas) [41, 44, 45, 54, 73, 74]. Transient tumor blush, however, is commonly observed in small (<2 cm) hypervascular metastases.

Homogeneous enhancement may be observed in large metastases; however, these lesions often possess a radial spoke-wheel appearance with thin radial strands of lesser enhancement. Clinical history of a primary hypervascular tumor is usually present facilitating correct diagnosis. In some cases, liver cell adenoma, FNH and metastasis may present as large focal lesions showing homogeneous enhancement. However, benign primary tumors of the liver, such as adenomas and FNH almost invariably show only mild hyperintensity on T2-weighted images. This is not the case in hypervascular metastases, which exhibit moderate to high signal. The most common enhancement feature of metastases is a peripheral ring of enhancement on immediate postgadolinium SGE images [54, 91]. Central progression of contrast enhancement is common. Irregular or peripheral contrast washout is also observed [44, 54, 93] and is common in hypervascular metastases.

Certain histologic types of metastases may display distinctive morphology or patterns of enhancement (figs. 2.63–2.65). When tumors exceed 3 cm in diameter,

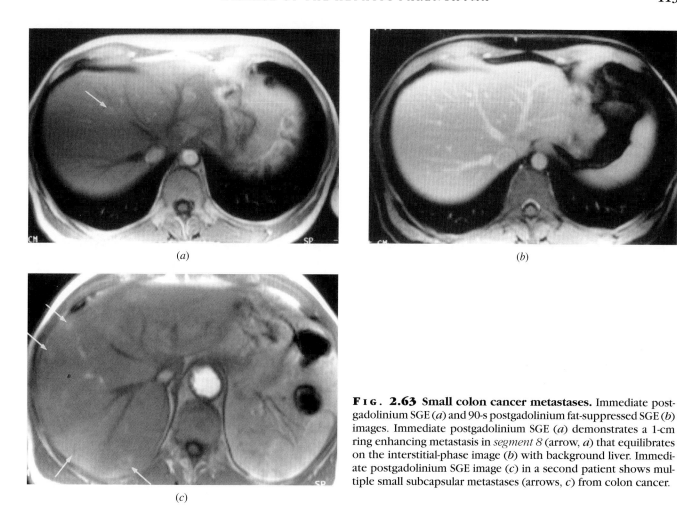

(a)

(b)

(c)

F I G . 2.63 Small colon cancer metastases. Immediate postgadolinium SGE (*a*) and 90-s postgadolinium fat-suppressed SGE (*b*) images. Immediate postgadolinium SGE (*a*) demonstrates a 1-cm ring enhancing metastasis in *segment 8* (arrow, *a*) that equilibrates on the interstitial-phase image (*b*) with background liver. Immediate postgadolinium SGE image (*c*) in a second patient shows multiple small subcapsular metastases (arrows, *c*) from colon cancer.

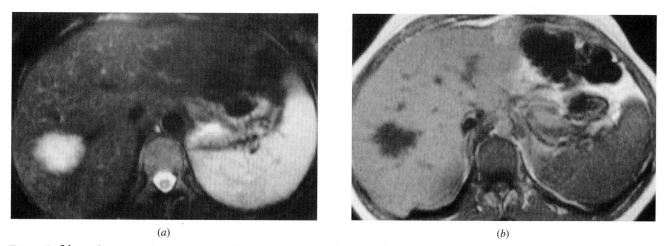

(a)

(b)

F I G . 2.64 Medium-sized colon cancer liver metastases. T2-weighted fat-suppressed ETSE (*a*), SGE (*b*), and immediate postgadolinium SGE (*c*) images. An irregularly marginated mass is present in the right lobe that is moderately high in signal intensity on the T2-weighted image (*a*) and moderately low in signal intensity on the T1-weighted image (*b*) and demonstrates intact ring enhancement on the immediate postgadolinium image (*c*) with an irregular inner margin to the ring. A faint region of ill-defined transient increased enhancement is present on the immediate postgadolinium image (*c*).

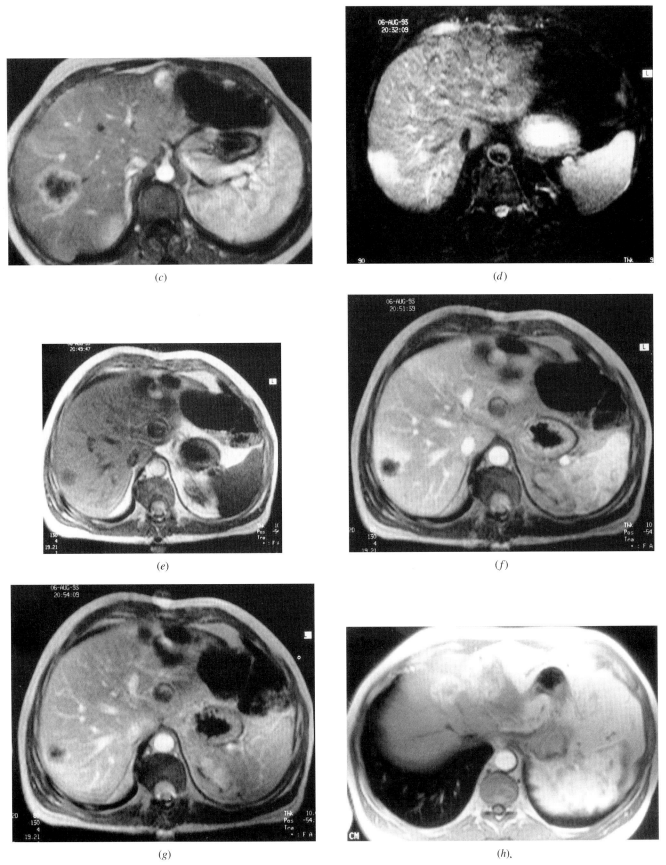

(c)

(d)

(e)

(f)

(g)

(h).

F I G . 2.64 (*Continued*) T2-weighted fat-suppressed SS-ETSE (*d*), SGE (*e*), and immediate (*f*) and 90-s postgadolinium SGE (*g*) images in a second patient.

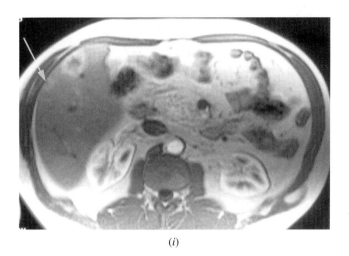

(*i*)

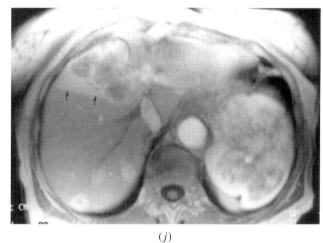

(*j*)

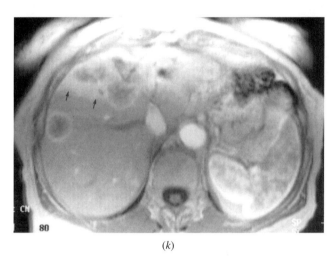

(*k*)

FIG. 2.64 (*Continued*) A 2-cm liver metastasis is present in the right lobe of the liver that is moderately high in signal intensity on the T2-weighted image (*d*), and moderately low in signal intensity on the T1-weighted image (*e*), and demonstrates ring enhancement on the immediate postgadolinium image (*f*) with ill-defined perilesional enhancement. Ill-defined perilesional enhancement resolves at 90 s after gadolinium (*g*).

Immediate postgadolinium SGE images (*h, i*) in a third patient demonstrate irregular ring-enhancing lesions consistent with metastases. Even metastases <1 cm exhibit ring enhancement (arrow, *i*).

Immediate postgadolinium SGE images (*j, k*) in a fourth patient with colon cancer demonstrate multiple metastatic foci, several small rounded masses, and one large cauliflower-shaped lesion, all with ring enhancement. Note ill-defined perilesional enhancement (arrows, *j, k*) around the cauliflower-shaped metastasis, characteristic for colon cancer metastases.

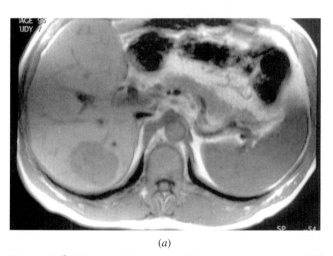

(*a*)

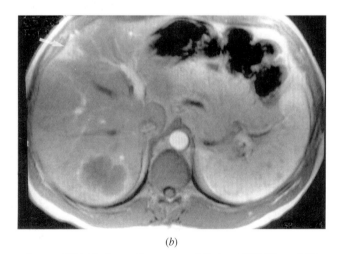

(*b*)

FIG. 2.65 **Large colon cancer liver metastases—cauliflower shape.** SGE (*a*), immediate postgadolinium SGE (*b*), and 90-s postgadolinium fat-suppressed SGE (*c*) images demonstrate a colon cancer metastasis with a cauliflower shape. A small peripheral metastasis with intense wedge-shaped perilesional enhancement (arrow, *b*) is present.

Coronal T2-weighted SS-ETSE (*d*), transverse immediate postgadolinium SGE (*e*), and 90-s postgadolinium fat-suppressed SGE (*f*) images in a second patient demonstrate a large, centrally located metastasis that has a cauliflower shape. Note that the central location of the metastases has resulted in bile duct obstruction (*d*).

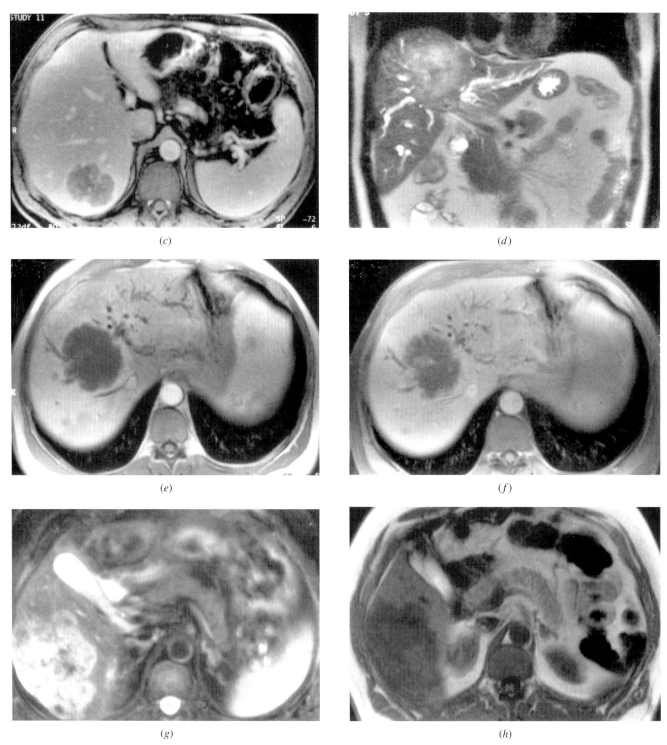

F I G . 2.65 (*Continued*) T2-weighted fat-suppressed SS-ETSE (*g*), SGE (*h*). immediate postgadolinium SGE (*i*), and 45-s postgadolinium SGE (*j*) images in a third patient demonstrates a large cauliflower-shaped metastasis that has ring enhancement with peripheral areas of contrast with arcs of peripheral enhancement that extend into the lesion.

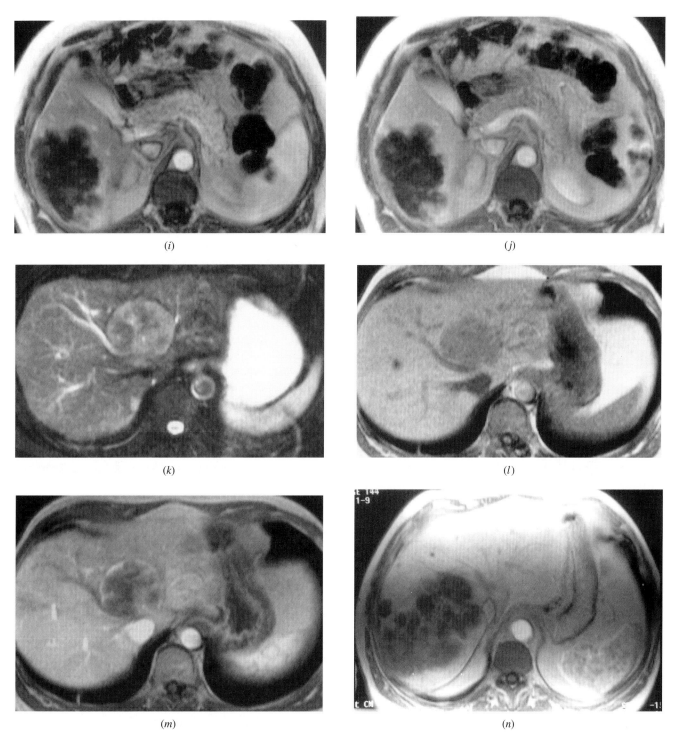

(i)

(j)

(k)

(l)

(m)

(n)

FIG. 2.65 (*Continued*) T2-weighted fat-suppressed SS-ETSE (*k*), SGE (*l*), and immediate postgadolinium SGE (*m*) images in a fourth patient. This lesion possesses the typical imaging features of a colon cancer metastasis. The metastasis is heterogeneous and moderately hyperintense on T2 (*k*) and mildly hypointense on T1 (*l*) images and has ring enhancement with peripheral arcs of contrast on the immediate postgadolinium image (*m*).

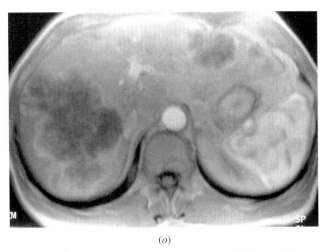
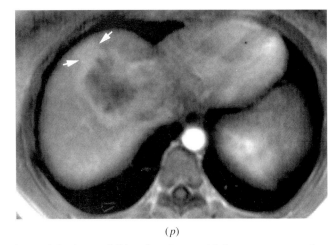

(o)   (p)

FIG. 2.65 (*Continued*) Immediate postgadolinium SGE images (*n, o, p*) in three additional patients with large metastases that exhibit the characteristic cauliflower shape of colon cancer metastases. Ill-defined perilesional enhancement (arrows, *p*) is observed in the third patient.

metastases from colorectal cancer typically develop a cauliflower-type appearance. Large solitary metastases are most commonly observed in colon carcinoma. This imaging observation may in part reflect the fact that colon cancer is the most commonly encountered liver metastasis, although minimal involvement of the liver with metastatic disease explains why colon cancer is one of the few malignancies amenable to curative surgical resection of liver metastases.

Ill-defined increased perilesional and subsegmental enhancement is common with both colorectal cancer and pancreatic ductal adenocarcinoma metastases but uncommon with other metastases. Perilesional enhancement is rare in hypervascular tumors such as islet cell tumors or renal cell carcinomas, implying that increased hepatic arterial supply is not the cause of perilesional enhancement. Perilesional enhancement with colon cancer is more typically ill-defined circumferential, whereas with pancreatic ductal adenocarcinoma it is often more sharply demarcated wedge-shaped enhancement. A recent publication reported that microscopic examination of liver tissue surrounding metastases showed variable degrees of hepatic parenchyma compression, desmoplastic reaction, inflammatory infiltrates, and neovascularization [94]. This histopathological zone, surrounding the metastasis, was termed the tumor border. Tumors with more extensive perilesional enhancement had thicker tumor borders [94]. The area of perilesional enhancement observed on imaging (fig. 2.66) was, however, broader than the tumor border noted on histopathologic inspection, suggesting the possibility that vascular changes extended beyond the outer confines of compressed liver tissue. Hypothetically, hepatocellular damage induced by the presence of nearby tumor or secretion of tumor metabolites into the vincinty adjacent to tumor may have incited an inflammatory response and neovascularization, contributing to the perilesional enhancement seen on MR images.

Metastases from squamous cell lung cancer are generally characterized as well-defined rounded masses that have a high-signal intensity rim and low-signal intensity center on T2-weighted images and show intense enhancement of the outer rim on early postgadolinium images (fig. 2.67). Squamous cell carcinomas from other sites of origin also tend to be rounded and have uniform ring enhancement on immediate postgadolinium SGE images (see fig. 2.67).

Poorly differentiated adenocarcinomas frequently demonstrate numerous metastases smaller than 2 cm scattered throughout the entire liver. These metastases are typically high in signal intensity on T2-weighted images and show peripheral ring enhancement on immediate postgadolinium images (fig. 2.68). These metastases range from hypovascular to very hypervascular. Small cell and other aggressive nonsquamous cell lung cancers have similar imaging findings (figs. 2.68 and 2.69).

Metastases may undergo hemorrhage resulting in varying high-and low-signal intensity lesions on T1- and T2-weighted images. Coagulative necrosis may produce central low signal intensity on T2-weighted images surrounded by **higher-signal intensity viable tumor** [95]. This appearance may be observed with colorectal metastases.

Melanoma metastases may represent a mixture of high- and low-signal intensity lesions on T1- and T2-weighted images because of the paramagnetic property of melanin (fig. 2.70) [95]. Melanoma metastases must be highly pigmented, well-differentiated lesions to produce this paramagnetic effect. Amelanocitic malignant melanomas or poorly differentiated tumors will not produce the paramagnetic effect and will appear mildly hypointense on T1 and mildly hyperintense on T2.

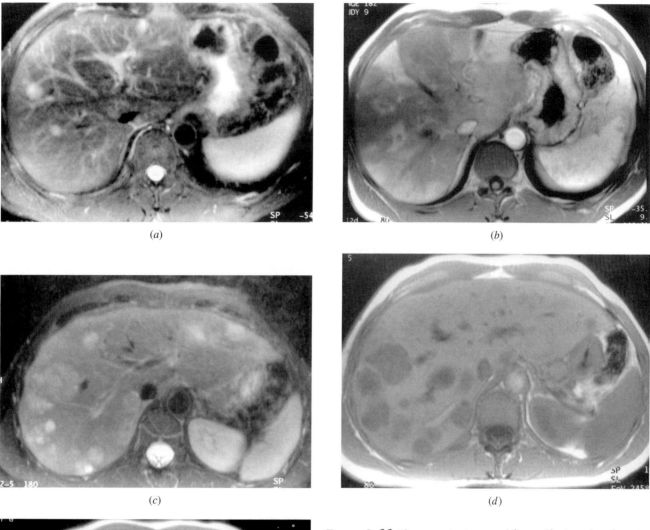

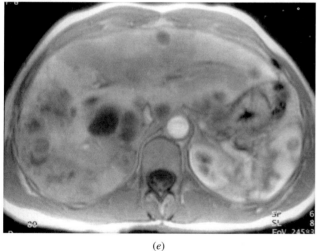

F I G . 2.66 Liver metastases with perilesional enhancement. Echo-train STIR (*a*) and immediate postgadolinium SGE (*b*) images. Multiple metastases from pancreatic ductal adenocarcinoma are seen throughout the hepatic parenchyma. The >1-cm metastases demonstrate moderately high signal on T2 (*a*). Many more lesions are identified on the immediate postgadolinium images (*b*) with several associated with peripheral wedge-shaped perilesional enhancement. Wedge-shaped perilesional enhancement is somewhat characteristic for pancreatic cancer liver metastases, unlike colon cancer metastases that typically possess ill-defined circumferential perilesional enhancement.

Echo-train STIR (*c*), SGE (*d*), and immediate postgadolinium SGE (*e*) images in a second patient with gastric adenocarcinoma. Note the perilesional enhancement after administration of contrast (*e*). These lesions resemble colon cancer metastases with perilesional enhancement, however cauliflower shape is unusual in gastric cancer liver metastases.

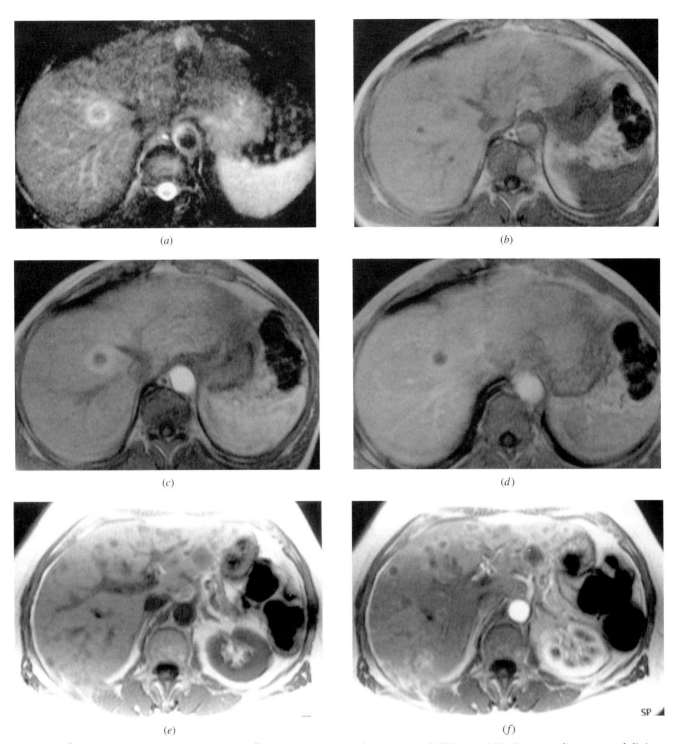

(a)

(b)

(c)

(d)

(e)

(f)

F I G . 2.67 Liver metastases, squamous cell type. T2-weighted fat-suppressed ETSE (*a*), SGE (*b*), immediate postgadolinium SGE (*c*), and 90-s postgadolinium SGE (*d*) images. A well-defined 2-cm metastasis is present in the anterior segment of the right lobe that appears as a moderately high-signal intensity ring with central isointensity on T2 (*a*) and mildly low in signal intensity on T1 (*b*) images, has a uniform ring enhancement on the immediate postgadolinium SGE image (*c*), and fades over time with negligible central enhancement (*d*). The enhancing ring on the immediate postgadolinium image (*c*) corresponds to the high signal intensity rim on the T2-weighted image (*a*). This is a typical appearance for liver metastases from squamous cell lung cancer.

SGE (*e*), immediate postgadolinium SGE (*f*), and 90-s postgadolinium fat-suppressed SGE (*g*) images in a second patient with squamous cell lung cancer. There are multiple rounded lesions scattered throughout the liver that demonstrate low signal on T1-weighted images (*e*) and ring enhancement immediately after gadolinium administration (*f*), consistent with metastases.

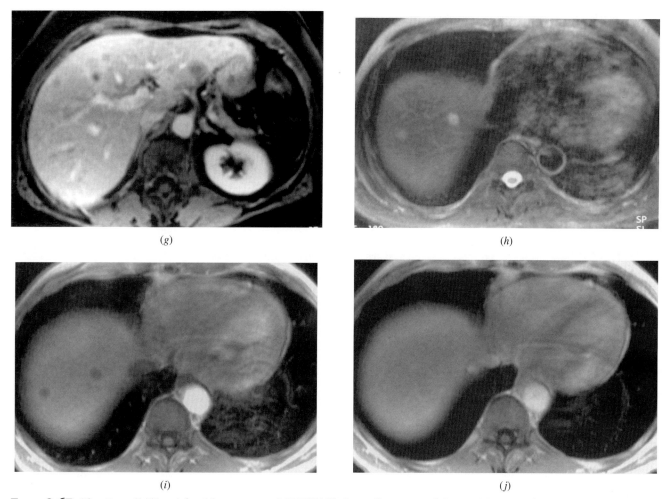

(g)

(h)

(i)

(j)

FIG. 2.67 (*Continued*) T2-weighted fat-suppressed SS-ETSE (*h*), immediate postgadolinium SGE (*i*), and 90-s postgadolinium SGE (*j*) images in a third patient, who has liver metastases from esophageal squamous cell cancer. The metastases are round, well defined, and high in signal on the T2-weighted image (*h*) enhance with uniform rings on the immediate postgadolinium SGE image (*i*), and become isointense with liver at 90 s (*j*).

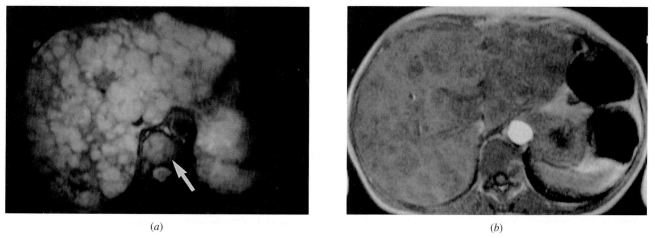

(a)

(b)

FIG. 2.68 Liver metastases, poorly differentiated small cell cell type. T2-weighted fat-suppressed ETSE (*a*), SGE (*b*), and immediate postgadolinium SGE (*c*) images. The liver is extensively replaced by numerous metastatic lesions smaller than 2 cm.

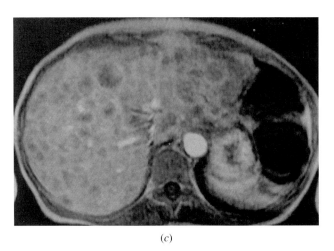

FIG. 2.68 (*Continued*) Lesions are high in signal intensity on T2 (*a*) mildly low in signal intensity on T1 (*b*) and demonstrate intact ring enhancement on the immediate postgadolinium images (*c*). High signal intensity is also apparent in the bone marrow on the T2 image (arrow, *a*), which represents bone metastases. Poorly differentiated or anaplastic malignancies not uncommonly result in this pattern of liver metastases. This patient has small cell lung cancer.

(*c*)

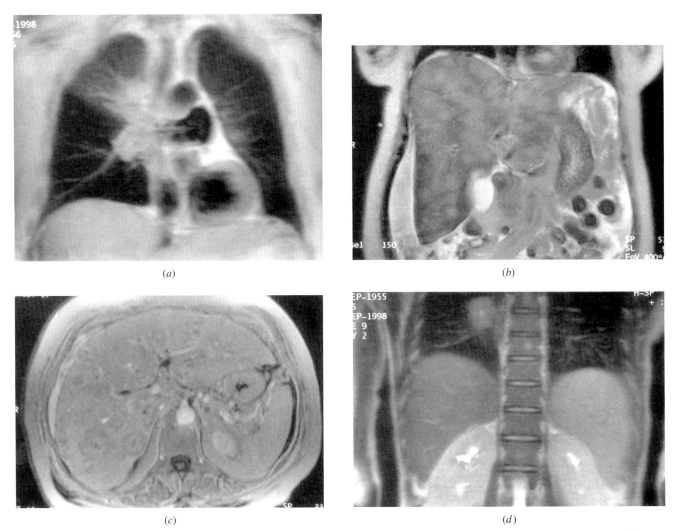

(*a*)   (*b*)

(*c*)   (*d*)

FIG. 2.69 Metastases from lung cancer. Coronal T2-weighted SS-ETSE (*a, b*) and transverse immediate postgadolinium magnetization-prepared gradient-echo (*c*) images. Multiple lesions are scattered throughout the liver, which appear high signal on T2-weighted images (*b*) and show ring enhancement on immediate postgadolinium images (*c*). Note the right hilar mass associated with an alveolar infiltrate due to postobstructive pneumonia.

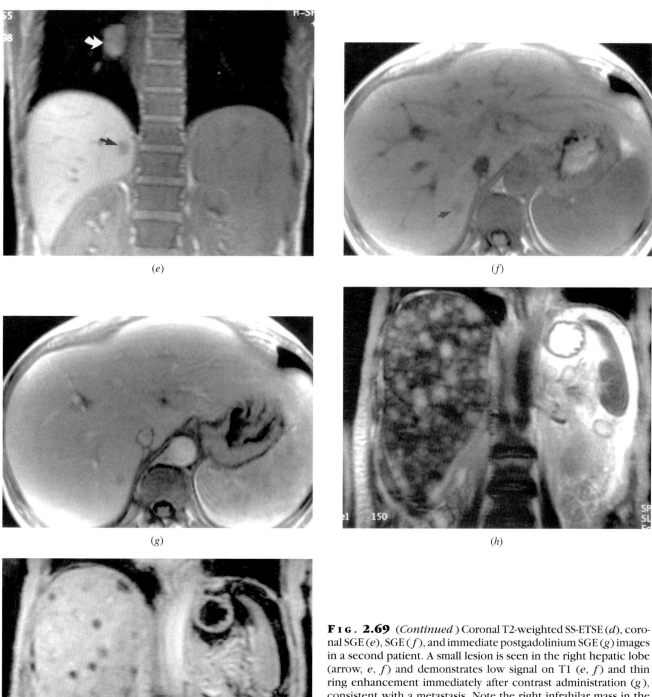

(e)

(f)

(g)

(h)

(i)

F I G . 2.69 (*Continued*) Coronal T2-weighted SS-ETSE (*d*), coronal SGE (*e*), SGE (*f*), and immediate postgadolinium SGE (*g*) images in a second patient. A small lesion is seen in the right hepatic lobe (arrow, *e*, *f*) and demonstrates low signal on T1 (*e*, *f*) and thin ring enhancement immediately after contrast administration (*g*), consistent with a metastasis. Note the right infrahilar mass in the lung (curved arrow, *e*).

Coronal T2-weighted SS-ETSE (*h*) and coronal immediate postgadolinium magnetization-prepared gradient-echo (*i*) images in a third patient. There are numerous metastases scattered throughout the liver, which exhibit high signal on T2 (*h*) and ring enhancement after gadolinium administration (*i*), consistent with metastases from non-small cell carcinoma.

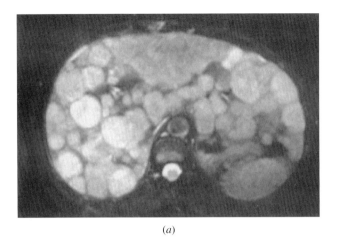

(a)

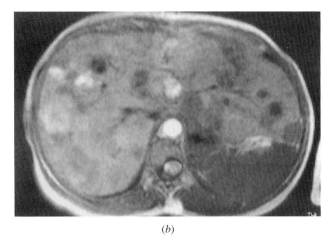

(b)

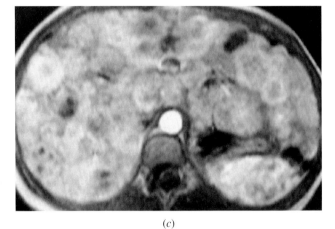

(c)

F I G . 2.70 Melanoma metastasis. T2-weighted fat-suppressed ETSE (*a*), SGE (*b*), and immediate postgadolinium SGE (*c*) images. Melanoma metastases are a mixed population of low- to high-signal intensity lesions on T2- (*a*) and T1- (*b*) weighted images. This reflects the paramagnetic properties of melanin. Intense ring enhancement is present on the immediate postgadolinium image (*c*), demonstrating the hypervascularity of these metastases.

Metastases from mucin-producing tumors such as ovarian cancer or mucinous cystadenocarcinoma of the pancreas may result in liver metastases that are high in signal intensity on T1-weighted images because of the protein content (fig. 2.71).

Metastases that are active in protein synthesis, such as in the production of enzymes or hormones (e.g., carcinoid tumors) may also be high in signal intensity on T1-weighted images because of the presence of a high concentration of protein (fig. 2.72).

Capsule-based metastases frequently occur in the setting of tumors that metastasize by intraperitoneal spread (fig. 2.73). Ovarian cancer most commonly results in capsule-based metastases (fig. 2.74), followed by colon cancer (fig. 2.75). However, a variety of malignancies can produce capsule-based metastases (see fig. 2.75).

■ HYPOVASCULAR METASTASES

Primary tumors that commonly result in hypovascular metastases include colorectal carcinoma (fig. 2.76) and

transitional cell carcinoma. Lymphoma and hepatocellular carcinomas are other malignant lesions that are occasionally hypovascular. Presumably, malignant hypovascular metastases possess a diminished blood supply, usually as a result of pronounced fibrosis, necrosis, or confluent dense cellularity (fig. 2.77).

Lesions are usually low in signal on T1- and T2-weighted images, signal features that are comparable to those of muscle or fibrous tissue. They are hypointense relative to liver on T1-weighted images and are often nearly isointense on T2-weighted images [96]. These tumors are usually most conspicuous on portal-phase gadolinium-enhanced SGE images [96]. However, because of the high sensitivity of MR to gadolinium, hepatic arterial dominant phase images are usually the best images to demonstrate hypovascular metastases with a frequently discernible peripheral ring of enhancement (fig. 2.78). Hypovascular metastases may contain a large volume of extracellular fluid and mimic the appearance of benign cysts (fig. 2.79) (i.e., high signal intensity on T2-weighted images and nearly signal void immediately after gadolinium administration). This is particularly true for cystic subcapsular metastases, that are most commonly observed with ovarian cancer. Delayed

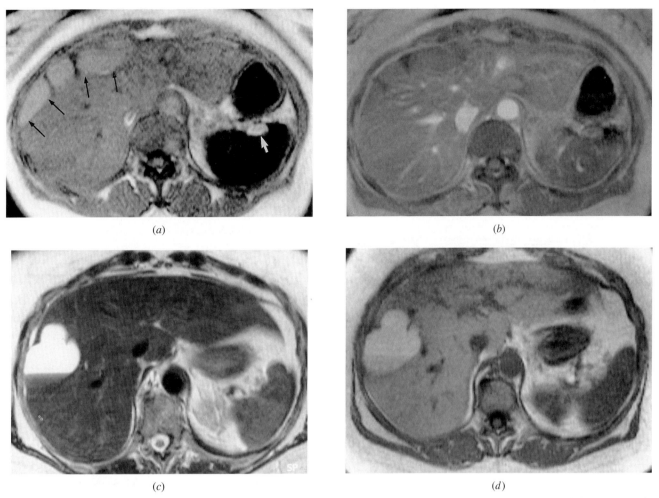

(a)   *(b)*

(c)   *(d)*

F I G . 2.71 High T1 signal mucin-producing liver metastases, ovarian cancer. SGE (*a*) and 90-s postgadolinium SGE (*b*) images. A large capsule-based metastasis is present along the lateral margin of the liver (black arrows, *a*), and a smaller subcapsular metastasis is present in the spleen (white arrow, *a*). The metastases are high in signal intensity because of high mucin content. Enhancement of cyst walls is present on postgadolinium images (*b*). The spleen is nearly signal void on these T1-weighted images because of transfusional hemosiderosis.

T2-weighted ETSE (*c*) and SGE (*d*) images in a second patient demonstrate a cystic ovarian metastasis located superficially in the right lobe of the liver. On the T2-weighted images (*c*), low-signal intensity material layers in the dependent portion of the metastasis. The high mucin content of the cystic metastasis renders it high in signal intensity on the T1-weighted image (*d*).

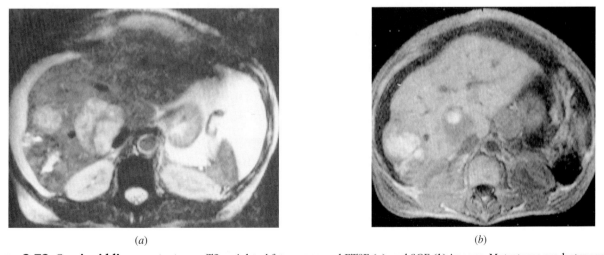

(a)   *(b)*

F I G . 2.72 Carcinoid liver metastases. T2-weighted fat-suppressed ETSE (*a*) and SGE (*b*) images. Metastases are heterogeneous with mixed high-signal intensity on T2 (*a*) and T1 (*b*) images. The high signal intensity on the T1-weighted image (*b*) reflects a high protein concentration due to protein synthesis from hormone production. The high signal on T1 is an uncommon appearance for carcinoid metastases.

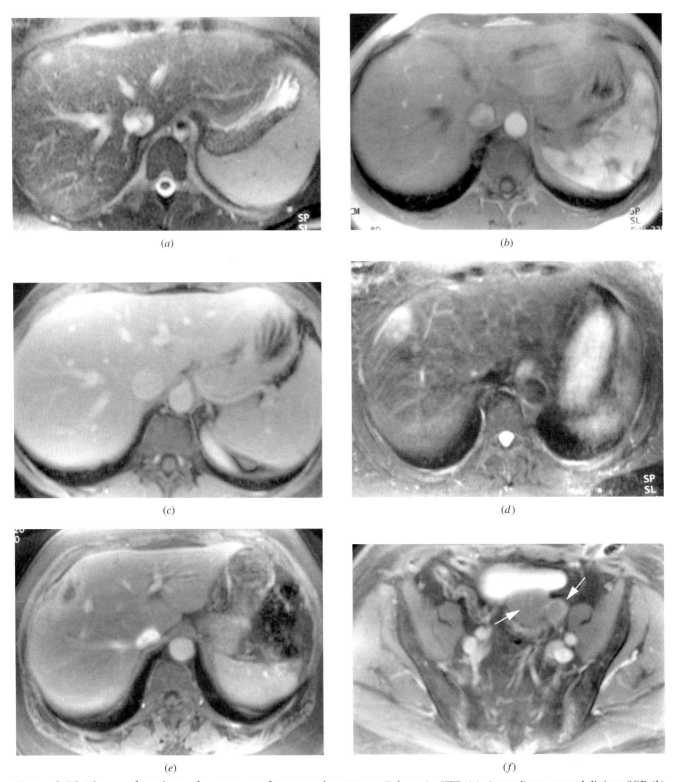

(a)

(b)

(c)

(d)

(e)

(f)

FIG. 2.73 Liver and peritoneal metastases from ovarian tumor. Echo-train STIR (*a*), immediate postgadolinium SGE (*b*) and 90 second postgadolinium fat-suppressed SGE (*c*) images in one patient; and echo-train STIR (*d*), and 90-s postgadolinium fat-suppressed SGE (*e*, *f*) images in a second patient, both of whom have ovarian cancer and peritoneal metastases. Both patients demonstrate liver metastases characterized by high signal on T2-weighted images (*a*, *d*) and ring enhancement on early (*b*) and late (*c*, *e*) postgadolinium images. Note the presence of recurrent pelvic tumor (arrows, *f*) in the second patient.

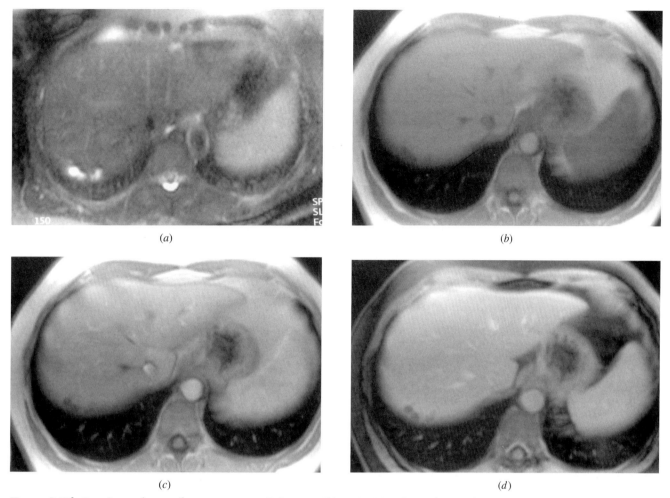

F I G . 2.74 Ovarian subcapsular metastases. Echo-train STIR (*a*), SGE (*b*), and immediate (*c*) and 90-s postgadolinium fat-suppressed SGE (*d*) images. There is a cluster of small lesions in a subcapsular location along the dome of the liver, which demonstrate high signal on T2 (*a*), low signal on T1 (*b*), and faint ring enhancement on early (*c*) and late (*d*) postgadolinium images consistent with capsule-based metastatic implants. This is the most common pattern of involvement of the liver with ovarian cancer and represents part of the generalized process of intraperitoneal seeding and spread.

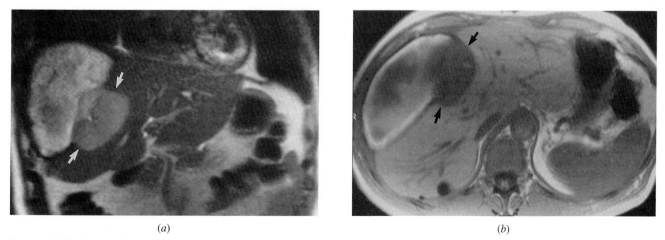

F I G . 2.75 Capsule-based liver metastases. Coronal T2-weighted SS-ETSE (*a*), transverse SGE (*b*), and immediate postgadolinium SGE (*c*) images. A large capsule-based metastasis is present along the lateral margin of the liver with a solid tumor component (arrows, *a, b*) from synovial sarcoma. Hemorrhage is heterogeneous on the T2-weighted image (*a*). On the noncontrast T1-weighted image (*b*), a peripheral rim of high signal intensity is present from recent hemorrhage. On the immediate postgadolinium image (*c*), the solid tumor component enhances uniformly.

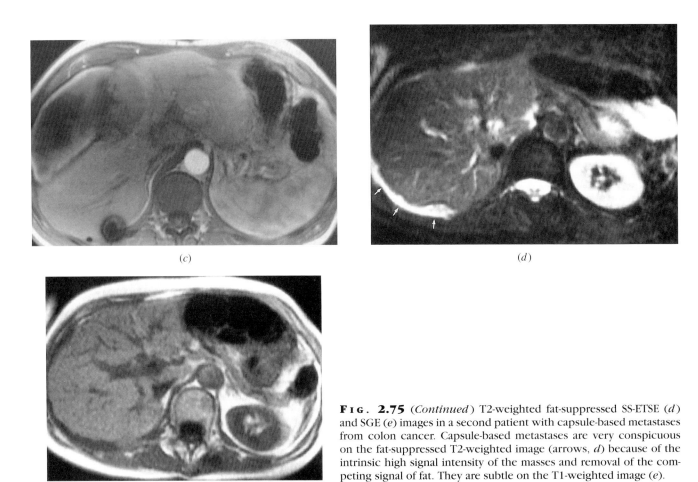

(c)

(d)

(e)

FIG. 2.75 (*Continued*) T2-weighted fat-suppressed SS-ETSE (*d*) and SGE (*e*) images in a second patient with capsule-based metastases from colon cancer. Capsule-based metastases are very conspicuous on the fat-suppressed T2-weighted image (arrows, *d*) because of the intrinsic high signal intensity of the masses and removal of the competing signal of fat. They are subtle on the T1-weighted image (*e*).

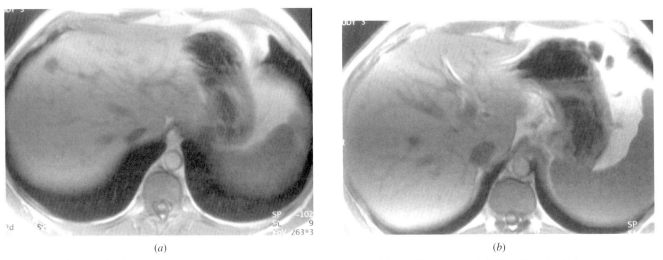

(a)

(b)

FIG. 2.76 Low fluid content colon cancer metastases. SGE (*a*, *b*) and immediate postgadolinium SGE (*c*, *d*) images.

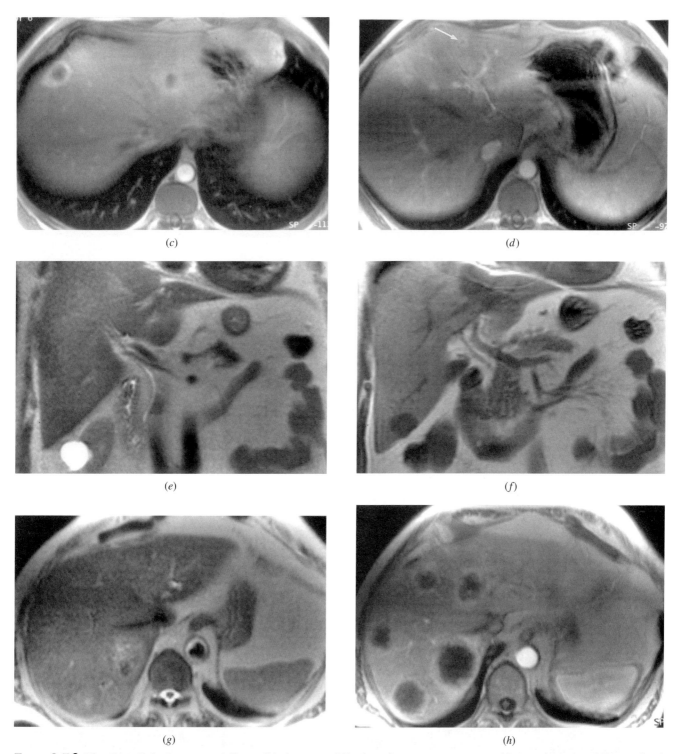

(c)

(d)

(e)

(f)

(g)

(h)

F I G . 2.76 (*Continued*) Lesions, especially small lesions, are difficult to discern on noncontrast T2 (not shown) and T1-weighted images (*a, b*). On immediate postgadolinium images (*c, d*), lesions are rendered conspicuous because of ring enhancement. Lesions <1 cm in size may be detected and characterized with this technique.

Coronal T2-weighted SS-ETSE (*e*), coronal SGE (*f*), transverse T2-weighted SS-ETSE (*g*), and transverse immediate postgadolinium SGE (*h*) images in a second patient. There are multiple metastases in the liver that are near isointense on T2 (*e, g*), hypointense on T1-weighted images (*f*), and demonstrate ring enhancement on postgadolinium images (*h*). These liver metastases are poorly seen on T2 (*e, g*), well seen on T1 (*f*), and very well shown on immediate postgadolinium images (*h*).

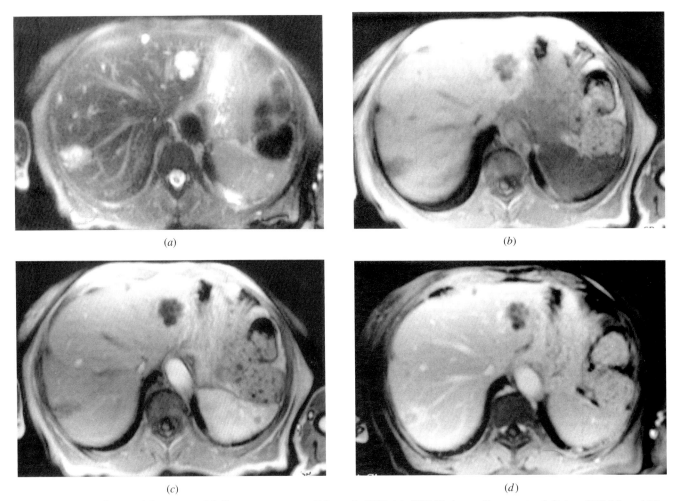

(a)

(b)

(c)

(d)

F I G . 2.77 Endometrial cancer with liver metastases. Echo-train STIR (*a*), SGE (*b*), immediate postgadolinium SGE (*c*), and 90-s postgadolinium fat-suppressed SGE (*d*) images in a patient who has endometrial cancer. There are multiple lesions that demonstrate high signal on T2 (*a*) and low signal on T1-weighted images (*b*) and exhibit ring enhancement on immediate postgadolinium images (*c*), which persists on interstitial-phase images (*d*).

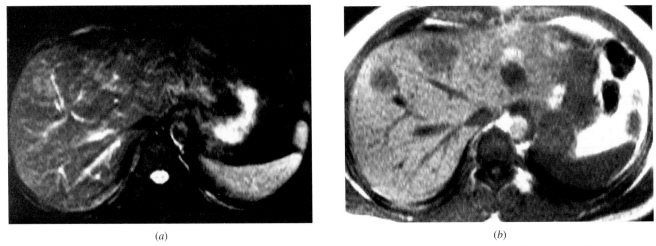

(a)

(b)

F I G . 2.78 Hypovascular liver metastases with low fluid content. T2-weighted fat-suppressed ETSE (*a*), SGE (*b*), and immediate postgadolinium SGE (*c*) images. Hypovascular liver metastases with low fluid content are usually low in signal intensity on T2- and T1-weighted images, which renders them isointense to minimally hyperintense signal intensity relative to liver on T2-weighted images (*a*) and low in signal relative to liver on T1-weighted images (*b*). Hypovascular liver metastases with low fluid content possess imaging features comparable to those of fibrous tissue. Despite their hypovascularity, these metastases exhibit faint peripheral rim enhancement on the immediate postgadolinium SGE image (*c*). (Reproduced with permission from Semelka RC, Shoenut JP, Greenberg HM, Micflikier AB. The liver. In: Semelka RC, Shoenut JP, eds. *MRI of the Abdomen with CT Correlation.* New York: Raven, p. 13–41, 1993.)

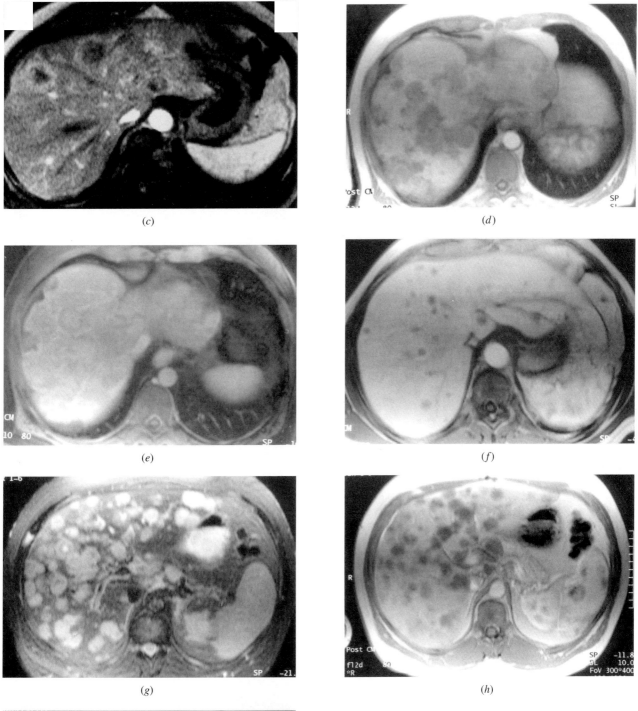

(c)

(d)

(e)

(f)

(g)

(h)

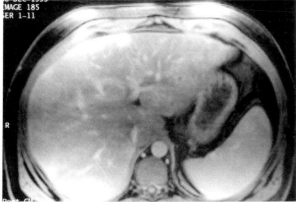

(i)

FIG. 2.78 (*Continued*) Immediate postgadolinium SGE (*d*) and 90-s postgadolinium fat-suppressed SGE (*e*) images in a second patient, who has a history of bladder carcinoma. On the immediate postgadolinium image (*d*), the lesions exhibit negligible enhancement, and on the interstitial-phase image (*e*) they become heterogeneously isointense with liver.

Immediate postgadolinium SGE (*f*) image in a third patient. Multiple hypointense lesions with faint ring enhancement are seen in the hepatic parenchyma consistent with metastases.

Echo-train STIR (*g*), immediate postgadolinium SGE (*h*), and 90-s postgadolinium fat-suppressed SGE (*i*) images. Extensive metastases are scattered throughout the liver that appear moderately high signal on T2 (*g*) and moderately low signal on T1 (not shown), show ring enhancement on immediate postgadolinium images (*h*), and enhance to near isointensity on late images (*i*).

131

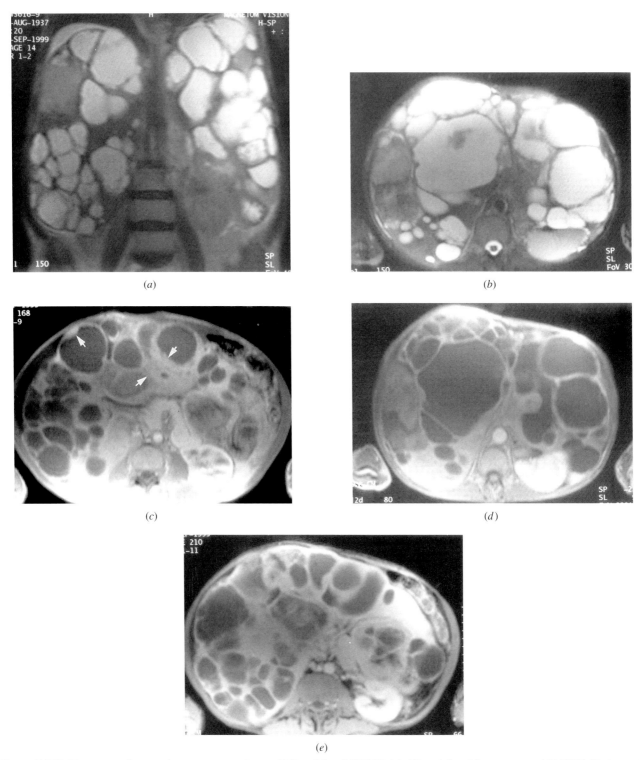

(a)

(b)

(c)

(d)

(e)

FIG. 2.79 Hypovascular cystic metastases. Coronal T2-weighted SS-ETSE (*a*), T2-weighted fat-suppressed SS-ETSE (*b*), immediate postgadolinium SGE (*c*), and 90-s postgadolinium fat-suppressed SGE (*d, e*) images. The liver is massively expanded with multiple cysts of varying sizes that replace the parenchyma. Some of these cysts have relatively uniform walls, some contain debris, and some cystic lesions have mural nodules (arrows, *c*) and intervening tumor stroma. On interstitial phase images (*d, e*) some progressive enhancement of tumor stroma is appreciated. The metastases are from epithelioid stromal tumor.

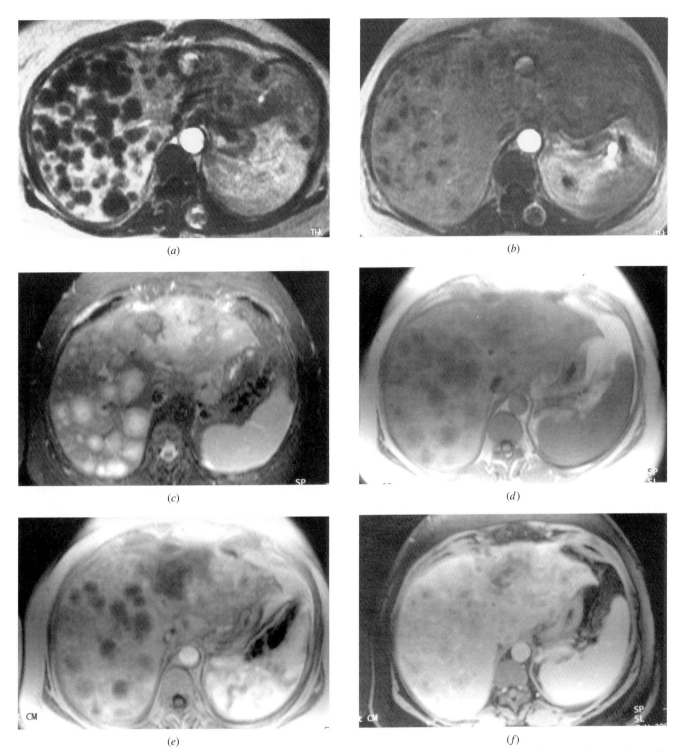

(a)

(b)

(c)

(d)

(e)

(f)

F I G . 2.80 Hypovascular liver metastases with high fluid content from adenocarcinoma of unknown primary. Immediate (*a*) and 10-min (*b*) postgadolinium SGE images. Hypovascular liver metastases with a high fluid content are low in signal intensity on T1 (not shown) and high in signal intensity on T2 (not shown) images. On immediate postgadolinium images (*a*) they may appear well defined and nearly signal void, mimicking the appearance of cysts. On delayed postgadolinium images (*b*) these lesions will partially enhance and decrease in size, permitting correct characterization. (Reproduced with permission from Semelka RC, Shoenut JP, Greenberg HM, Micflikier AB. The liver. In: Semelka RC, Shoenut JP, eds. *MRI of the Abdomen with CT Correlation*. New York: Raven, p. 13–41, 1993.)

Echo-train STIR (*c*), SGE (*d*), immediate postgadolinium SGE (*e*), and 90-s postgadolinium fat-suppressed SGE (*f*) images in a second patient with adenocarcinoma of unknown primary. There are multiple metastases scattered throughout the liver that exhibit high signal on T2 (*c*), low signal on T1-weighted images (*d*), and ring enhancement on immediate postgadolinium images (*e*) with progressive enhancement of the lesions on delayed images (*f*).

As these cases illustrate, patients with adenocarcinoma of unknown primary often have extensive liver metastases that also may be of relatively low vascularity.

postgadolinium images demonstrate indistinct lesions borders and a decrease in lesion size due to peripheral enhancement (fig. 2.80). This feature distinguishes hypovascular metastases from true cysts because the latter lesions remain sharply circumscribed with no change in size on late postcontrast images.

HYPERVASCULAR METASTASES

The malignancies that most commonly result in hypervascular liver metastases include renal cell carcinoma, carcinoid, islet cell tumor, leiomyosarcoma, and malignant melanoma [54]. Other malignancies that occasionally result in hypervascular liver metastases include colon carcinoma, pancreatic ductal carcinoma, and lung cancer. Although breast carcinoma results in metastases of increased vascularity, it rarely matches the hypervascularity of the previously cited tumors. A variety of appearances are observed for breast cancer liver metastases. Breast cancer liver metastases have a greater range of MR findings than other common types of liver metastases. These patterns include ring, miliary, and confluent segmental (figs. 2.81–2.83).

Hypervascular metastases are generally high in signal intensity on T2-weighted images and possess an intense peripheral ring of enhancement immediately after gadolinium administration (figs. 2.84–2.87) [44, 54, 91]. In many of these lesions, contrast will progress in a centripetal fashion [54].

Dynamic serial gadolinium-enhanced MR images are particularly important for lesion detection and characterization in patients with known vascular primary tumors (fig. 2.88). Vascular metastases from gastrinomas enhance with a uniform peripheral ring pattern on immediate postgadolinium images (fig. 2.89) and have a particular propensity to fade peripherally on more delayed images [97]. Hypervascular metastases from renal cell cancer, bowel cancer, carcinoid (fig. 2.90), or nongastrinoma islet cell tumors tend to be irregular in size and shape and to enhance with a thick, irregular rim that may gradually fill in. Enhancement of hypervascular metastases is better shown on MR than on CT images because of the higher sensitivity of MRI for gadolinium chelates, the more compact bolus of contrast delivered to the hepatic parenchyma, and the better temporal resolution for dynamic image acquisition (fig. 2.91).

Features that are more consistently observed with malignant lesions versus hemangiomas are, in the former, (1) early intense peripheral ring, (2) uniformity of the thickness of the ring, (3) jagged or serrated internal margin of the ring rather than a lobular margin, and (4) peripheral washout of the ring with persistent central enhancement (fig. 2.92) [44, 45, 54, 91, 93]. Features that are more consistent with hemangiomas include (1) dis-

continuous nodular ring of enhancement on immediate post-gadolinium images, (2) progressively increased intensity of enhancement between immediate and 90 second post gadolinium images and (3) round or lobular internal margin of enhancement.

Small (<1.5 cm) hypervascular metastases often enhance in an intense homogeneous fashion, fade to near isointensity by 1 minute and may only be demonstrated on hepatic arterial dominant phase images [54]. Some small hemangiomas may enhance as rapidly; however, hemangiomas tend to retain contrast and remain high in signal intensity for a more prolonged period. Small hemangioma may fade in signal, by as early as 2 minutes, to isointensity with liver. This feature is also observed in small hypervascular metastases. However, unlike metastases, small hemangiomas will not fade to a signal lower than liver. Often at least one lesion greater than 2 cm in diameter is present that possesses the typical enhancement features of a metastasis or hemangioma, allowing inference of the nature of the smaller lesions. The hepatic arterial dominant phase of enhancement is the most important phase of image acquisition both for detection and characterization.

SECONDARY INFECTION OF LIVER METASTASES

Secondary infection of metastases may occur in the liver and is most commonly observer with colon cancer metastases. It is postulated that the high content of intraluminal bacteria within the colon may be conducive to embolization of coliform bacteria with tumor cells. Experimental data suggests that certain anaerobic bacteria grow selectively in tumor nodules but not in the normal tissues of a tumor-bearing host [98]. Secondary infection of liver metastases after chemoembolization of these lesions has been reported [99]. Infected metastases may simulate both the clinical and imaging features of liver abscesses.

Infected metastases tend to have thickened, irregular walls and heterogeneous intermediate signal intensity on T2-weighted images and show some progressive central enhancement on delayed images (fig. 2.93). Abscesses tend to have thinner walls and higher signal intensity on T2-weighted images and do not demonstrate progressive lesion enhancement over time, even in abscesses with thick walls and internal septations. Both types of lesions will show transient, ill-defined perilesional enhancement reflecting an inflammatory hyperemic response in the liver.

Lymphoma. Secondary involvement of the liver by Hodgkin and non-Hodgkin lymphoma is common in

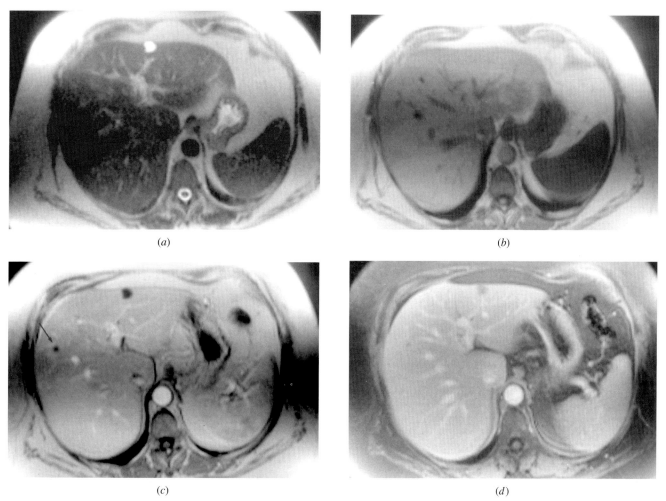

(a)   (b)

(c)   (d)

F I G . 2.81 Breast cancer liver metastases—ring enhancement. T2-weighted SS-ETSE (*a*), SGE (*b*), immediate postgadolinium SGE (*c*), and 90-s postgadolinium fat-suppressed SGE (*d*) images. There is a small lesion in the right lobe that is almost imperceptible on T2 (*a*) and T1 (*b*) images. The metastasis exhibits ring enhancement (arrow, *c*) on immediate postgadolinium images that render it conspicuous. The metastasis fades on the interstitial-phase image (*d*). This lesion was not seen on spiral CT. Note also a ciliated hepatic foregut cyst between *segments 4* and *2* anteriorly.

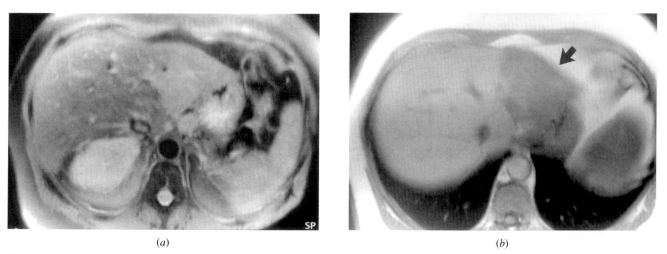

(a)   (b)

F I G . 2.82 Breast cancer liver metastases—confluent pattern. T2-weighted fat-suppressed SS-ETSE (*a*), SGE (*b*), and immediate postgadolinium SGE (*c*) images.

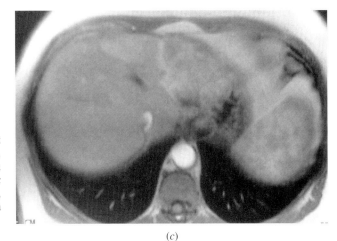

(c)

F I G . 2.82 (*Continued*) There is a mass (arrow, *b*) in the left hepatic lobe that demonstrates slightly increased signal on T2 (*a*), decreased signal on T1 (*b*), and heterogeneous enhancement on immediate postgadolinium images (*c*), consistent with metastatic disease. The confluent involvement of a segment, as in this case, is characteristic of breast cancer but represents an uncommon pattern.

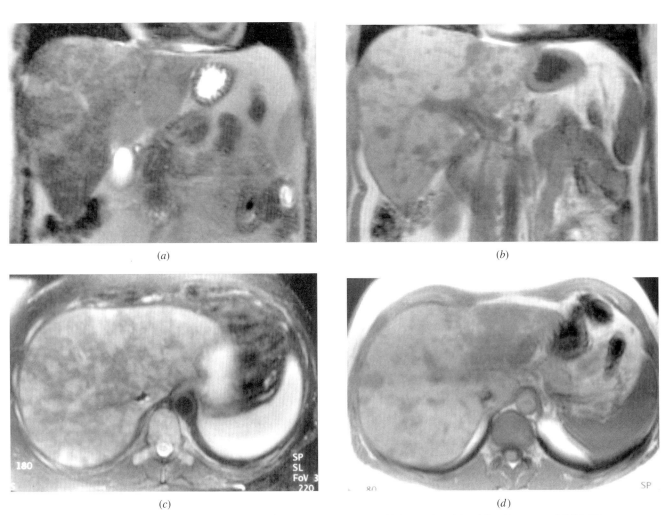

(a)   (b)

(c)   (d)

F I G . 2.83 Breast cancer liver metastases—miliary pattern. Coronal T2-weighted SS-ETSE (*a*), coronal SGE (*b*), transverse T2-weighted fat-suppressed ETSE (*c*), SGE (*d*), and immediate postgadolinium SGE (*e*) images. There are numerous lesions scattered throughout the hepatic parenchyma that demonstrate moderate signal on T2 (*a, c*), moderately low signal on T1 (*b, d*), and ring enhancement on immediate postgadolinium images (*e*), consistent with metastases.

T2-weighted fat-suppressed SS-ETSE (*f*), SGE (*g*), immediate postgadolinium fat-suppressed SGE (*h*), and 90-s postgadolinium SGE (*i*) images in a second patient. Extensive liver metastases, <5 mm in size, are present throughout the liver with a miliary pattern of involvement.

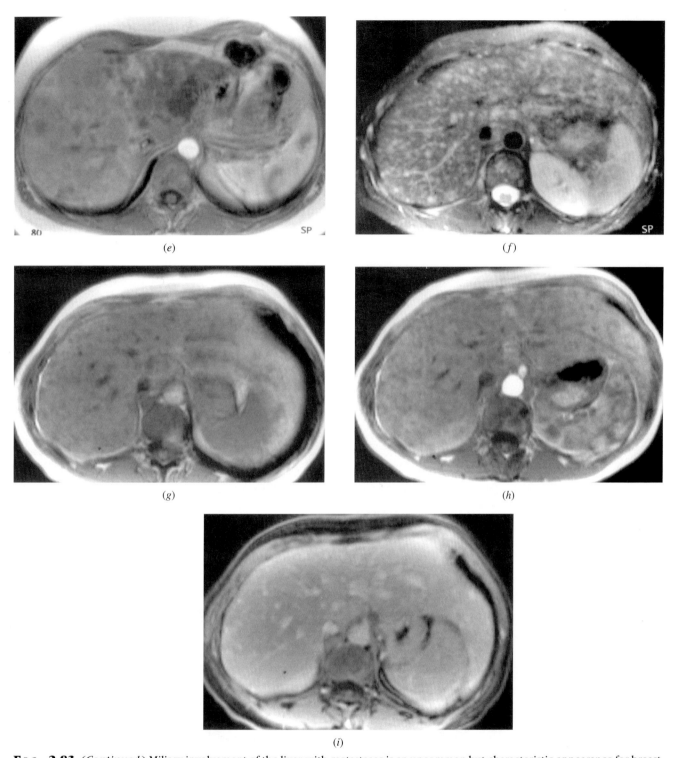

F I G. 2.83 (*Continued*) Miliary involvement of the liver with metastases is an uncommon but characteristic appearance for breast cancer liver metastases. Note in both cases that coexistent bone metastases are present in vertebral bodies that are high-signal small foci on fat-suppressed T2 and exhibit uniform enhancement on interstitial-phase fat-suppressed SGE images. If liver metastases respond to chemotherapy with this pattern of involvement, the liver develops extensive fibrosis with an appearance that resembles cirrhosis.

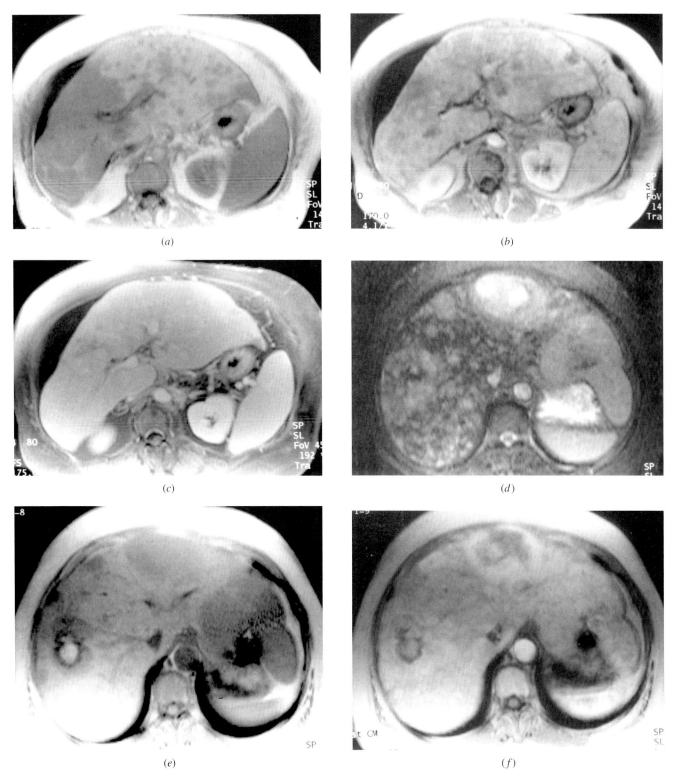

(a)

(b)

(c)

(d)

(e)

(f)

FIG. 2.84 Hypervascular liver metastases from adenocarcinoma of unknown primary. SGE (*a*), immediate postgadolinium SGE (*b*), and 90-s postgadolinium fat-suppressed SGE (*c*) images. There are numerous lesions scattered throughout the hepatic parenchyma, which are low signal on T1-weighted image (*a*), exhibit ring enhancement immediately after gadolinium administration (*b*), and enhance to near isointensity with liver on interstitial-phase images (*c*).

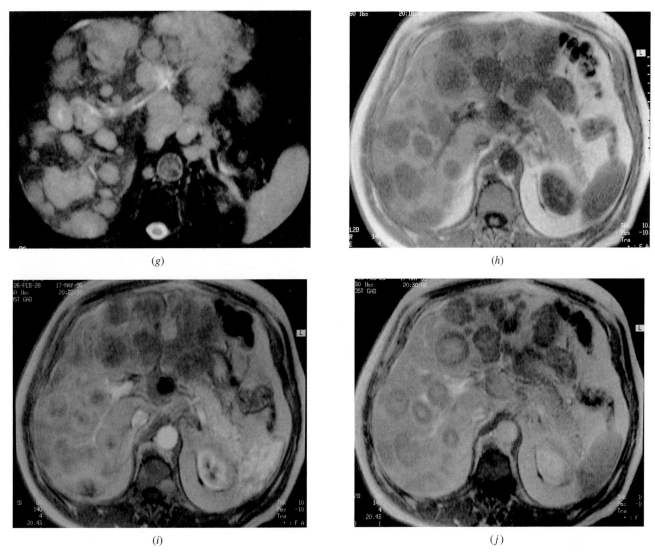

(g)

(h)

(i)

(j)

F I G . 2.84 (*Continued*) Echo-train STIR (*d*), SGE (*e*), and immediate postgadolinium SGE (*f*) images in a second patient. There are numerous metastases in the liver. One lesion has mildly increased high signal on T2 (*d*) and high signal on the T1-weighted image (*e*) consistent with hemorrhage. Note that many of the <1-cm metastases exhibits intense uniform enhancement (*f*).

T2-weighted fat-suppressed ETSE (*g*), SGE (*h*), immediate postgadolinium SGE (*i*), and 2-min postgadolinium SGE (*j*) images. The liver contains numerous metastases scattered throughout all segments that are moderately high signal intensity on T2 (*g*), well defined and moderately low in signal intensity on T1 (*h*), and have prominent thick uniform rings of enhancement on immediate postgadolinium images (*i*). Peripheral washout with centripetal progression of enhancement is noted on the delayed postcontrast image (*j*). Peripheral washout is common in hypervascular tumors that possess uniform intense rings of enhancement on immediate postgadolinium images.

stage IV disease [100]. On imaging, non-Hodgkin lymphoma more frequently results in focal hepatic lesions than Hodgkin disease. Lesions are typically low in signal intensity on T1-weighted images but vary in signal intensity from low to moderately high on T2-weighted images. Enhancement on immediate postgadolinium images tends to parallel the signal intensity on T2-weighted images; lesions that are low in signal intensity on T2-weighted images tend to enhance minimally (fig. 2.94), whereas lesions that are high in signal intensity tend to enhance in a substantial fashion (fig. 2.95) [101]. As with liver metastases, enhancement on immediate post-

gadolinium images usually is predominantly peripheral. Lesions of malignant lymphoma may possess transient, ill-defined perilesional enhancement on immediate postgadolinium images independent of the degree of enhancement of the lesions themselves (fig. 2.96). Rarely tumors may directly invade vessels producing an angiotropic pattern of involvement (fig. 2.97). Histopathologically, secondary involvement of the liver by malignant lymphoma is heralded by tumor deposits within the portal tracts. A clinical correlate with this microscopic appearance may be reflected on MR imaging with the appearance of periportal tumor tracking. This particular

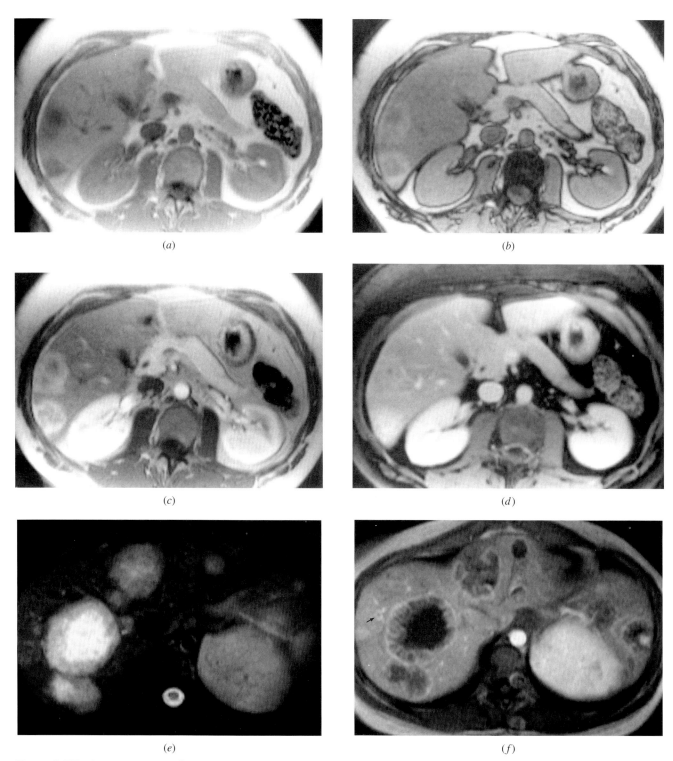

(a)

(b)

(c)

(d)

(e)

(f)

F I G . 2.85 Liver metastases from ovarian cancer. SGE (*a*), out-of-phase SGE (*b*), immediate postgadolinium SGE (*c*), and 90-s postgadolinium fat-suppressed SGE (*d*) images. There are two lesions in the right hepatic lobe that exhibit low signal on T1 (*a*) and intense ring enhancement on immediate postgadolinium images (*c*), consistent with metastases. Enhancement of lesions diminishes substantially in the interstitial phase (*d*). Note that the liver drops in signal on the out-of-phase image (*b*) because of the presence of fatty liver and the lesions develop a high signal peripheral rim of compressed nonfatty liver and/or other tumor border.

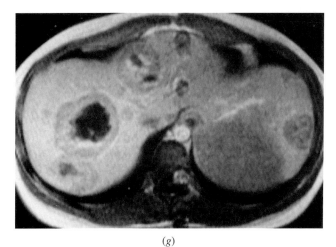

(g)

FIG. 2.85 (*Continued*) T2-weighted fat-suppressed ETSE (*e*), immediate SGE (*f*), and 10-min postgadolinium SGE (*g*) images in a second patient with ovarian cancer. Multiple varying sized metastases are scattered throughout the liver. The largest metastasis is high in signal intensity centrally on the T2-weighted image (*e*) because of central necrosis. Metastases are better shown on the immediate postgadolinium image and appear as multiple hypervascular lesions with ring enhancement. Ring enhancement is appreciated in metastases as small as 6 mm (arrow, *f*). Peripheral washout of metastases is apparent on the 10-min postgadolinium image (*g*).

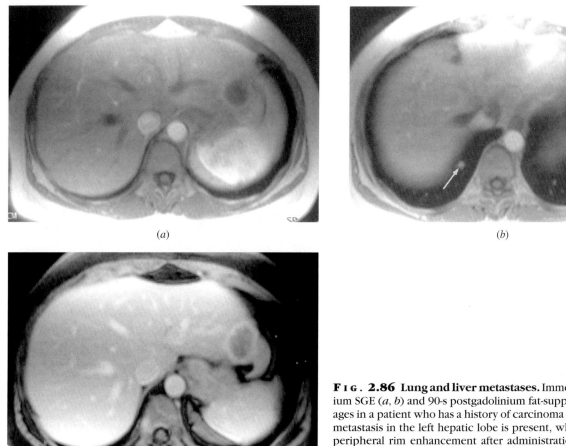

(a)

(b)

(c)

FIG. 2.86 Lung and liver metastases. Immediate postgadolinium SGE (*a, b*) and 90-s postgadolinium fat-suppressed SGE (*c*) images in a patient who has a history of carcinoma of the sphenoid. A metastasis in the left hepatic lobe is present, which demonstrates peripheral rim enhancement after administration of contrast (*a*) that persists on the late image (*c*), consistent with a metastasis. Note that lung metastases are also present (arrows, *b*).

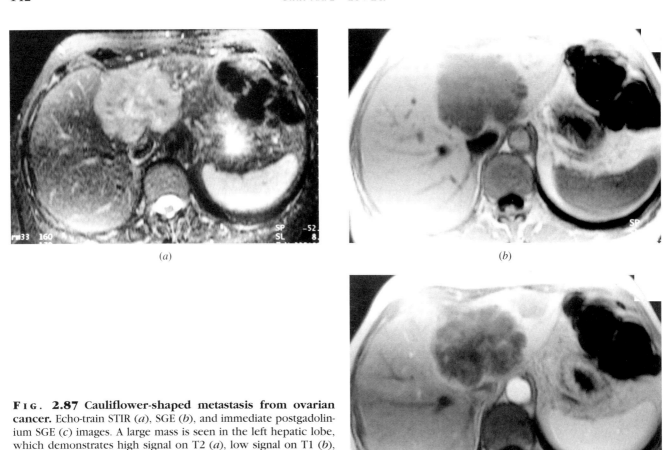

(a)

(b)

(c)

FIG. 2.87 Cauliflower-shaped metastasis from ovarian cancer. Echo-train STIR (*a*), SGE (*b*), and immediate postgadolinium SGE (*c*) images. A large mass is seen in the left hepatic lobe, which demonstrates high signal on T2 (*a*), low signal on T1 (*b*), and ring enhancement on immediate postgadolinium images (*c*). Note that the lesion resembles a colon cancer metastasis because of its cauliflower shape.

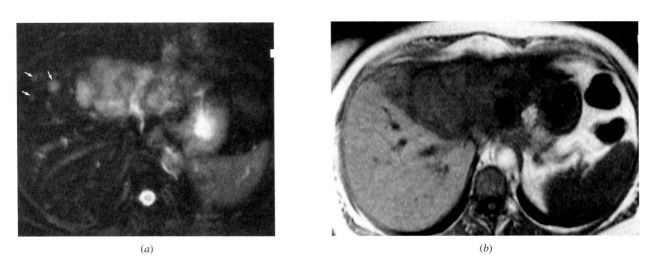

(a)   (b)

FIG. 2.88 Hypervascular liver metastases. T2-weighted fat-suppressed ETSE (*a*), SGE (*b*), immediate postgadolinium SGE (*c*), and 90-s postgadolinium SGE (*d*) images. A 7-cm metastasis is identified in the left lobe of the liver (*a–d*). Several metastases smaller than 1 cm are present in the medial and anterior segments. These small metastases are moderately high in signal intensity on T2 (arrows, *a*) and not visible on T1 (*b*), enhance intensely on immediate postgadolinium images (arrows, *c*), and washout to lower signal intensity than liver on 90-s postgadolinium images (*d*). On the immediate postgadolinium image (*c*) the smallest lesions enhance homogeneously, whereas the 1-cm metastasis has ring enhancement.

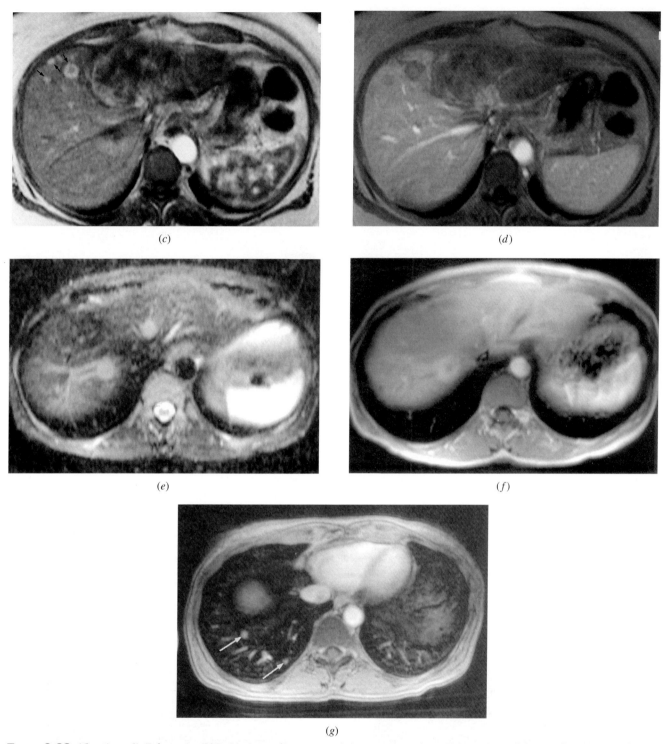

FIG. 2.88 (*Continued*) Echo-train STIR (*e*), immediate postgadolinium SGE (*f*), and 90-s postgadolinium fat-suppressed SGE (*g*) images in a second patient, who has a history of thyroid cancer. Two lesions are seen in the liver that are high signal on T2 (*e*) and enhance intensely on immediate postgadolinium images (*f*) consistent with hypervascular metastases. Note also the presence of lung metastases (arrows, *g*).

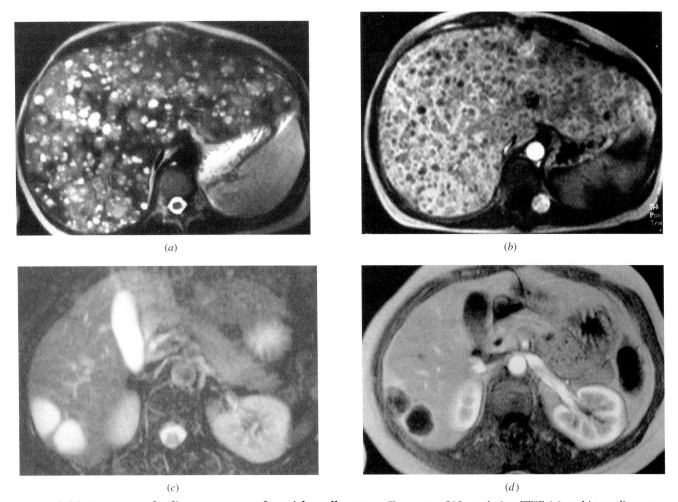

(a)

(b)

(c)

(d)

F I G . 2.89 Hypervascular liver metastases from islet cell tumors. Transverse 512 resolution ETSE (*a*) and immediate post-gadolinium SGE (*b*) images in a patient with gastrinoma. Numerous metastases smaller than 1 cm are scattered throughout all segments, many of which are well defined and high in signal intensity on the T2-weighted image (*a*). The immediate postgadolinium image (*b*) demonstrates that the metastases have intact ring enhancement.

T2-weighted fat-suppressed ETSE (*c*) and immediate postgadolinium SGE (*d*) images in a second patient who has an untyped islet cell tumor. The metastases are well-defined round masses that are high in signal intensity on the T2-weighted image (*c*) and have calculated T2 values of 160 ms. On the immediate postgadolinium image (*d*), the lesions possess intact rings of enhancement that are a feature of metastases and not of hemangiomas. Prior outside MRI performed with conventional spin-echo techniques and original outside interpretation of percutaneous biopsy specimen suggested the diagnosis of hemangiomas. On the gadolinium-enhanced images, hypervascular cystic liver metastases and a 2-cm islet cell tumor in the head of the pancreas were shown. The histology specimen was reexamined, and the diagnosis of islet cell tumor was confirmed.

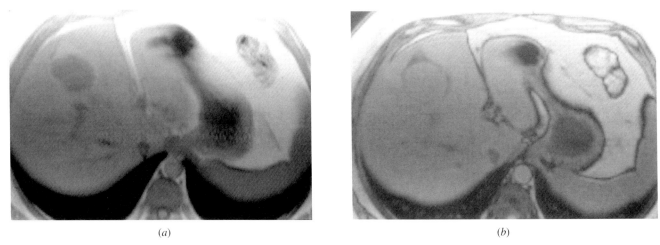

(a)

(b)

F I G . 2.90 Hypervascular liver metastases from carcinoid tumor. SGE (*a*), out-of-phase SGE (*b*), and immediate postgadolinium SGE (*c*) images.

144

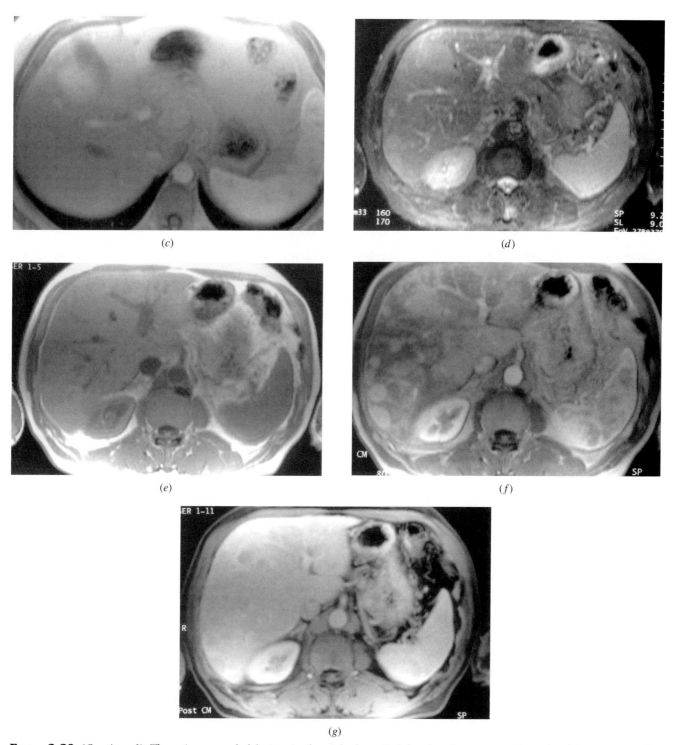

(c)

(d)

(e)

(f)

(g)

FIG. 2.90 (*Continued*) There is a rounded lesion in the right hepatic lobe that demonstrates low signal intensity on the T1-weighted image (*a*), does not drop signal on the out-of-phase image (*b*), and shows intense and homogeneous enhancement after gadolinium administration (*c*), consistent with a hypervascular metastasis. Carcinoid tumor was present at histopathology.

Echo-train STIR (*d*), SGE (*e*), immediate postgadolinium SGE (*f*), and 90-s postgadolinium fat-suppressed SGE (*g*) images. Numerous metastases are scattered throughout the hepatic parenchyma that demonstrate near-isointense signal on T2- (*d*) and T1- (*e*) weighted images and intense enhancement on immediate postgadolinium images (*f*) that washout on later images (*g*), consistent with hypervascular metastases metastases. The difference in lesion conspicuity between immediate postgadolinium images and other sequences, including noncontrast T2- and T1-weighted images and late postgadolinium images, is particularly impressive in the setting of hypervascular malignant disease.

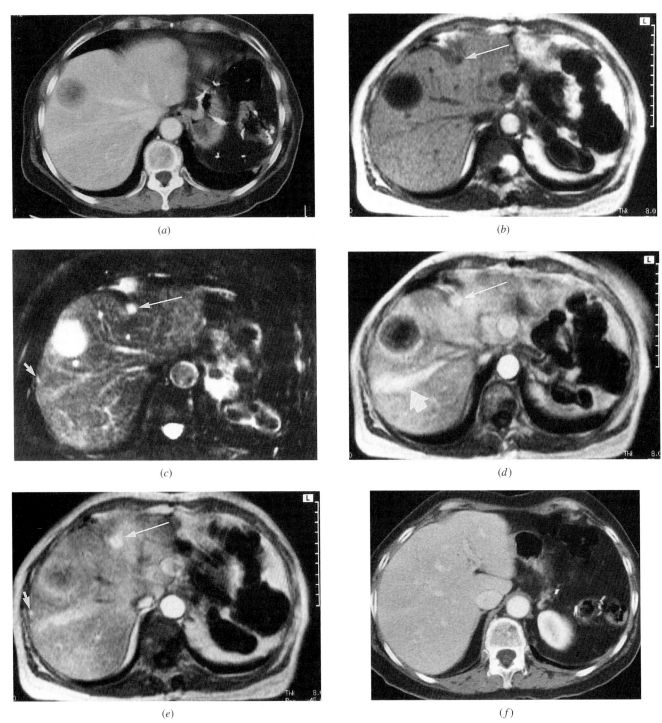

(a) *(b)* *(c)* *(d)* *(e)* *(f)*

FIG. 2.91 Hypervascular liver metastases from small bowel leiomyosarcoma. Dynamic contrast-enhanced CT (*a*), SGE (*b*), T2-weighted fat-suppressed SE (*c*), and immediate postgadolinium SGE (*d, e*) images. A 4-cm metastasis was appreciated on the CT imaging study (*a*). The SGE image (*b*) demonstrated a second 8-mm lesion in the lateral segment (arrow, *b*). The T2-weighted fat-suppressed SE image (*c*) demonstrated the lesion in the lateral segment (long arrow, *c*) and 5-mm subcapsular lesion in the anterior segment (short arrow, *c*). Immediate postgadolinium SGE images (*d, e*) demonstrate ring enhancement around the 4-cm metastases and uniform enhancement of the 8-mm metastases in the lateral segment (long arrow, *d, e*) and of the 5-mm subcapsular metastases (short arrow, *e*). Wedge-shaped transient increased enhancement is present in the posterior segment (large arrow, *d*), which is also faintly apparent on the CT image (*a*). Dynamic contrast-enhanced CT (*f*), SGE (*g*), T2-weighted fat-suppressed SE (*h*), and immediate (*i*) and 45-s (*j*) postgadolinium SGE images from the midhepatic level in the same patient. A 7-mm metastasis is present in the right lobe of the liver that is not visualized on the CT (*f*) or noncontrast T1-weighted (*g*) or T2-weighted (*h*) images but is well shown as a uniform enhancing lesion (arrow, *i*) on the immediate postgadolinium SGE image (*i*).

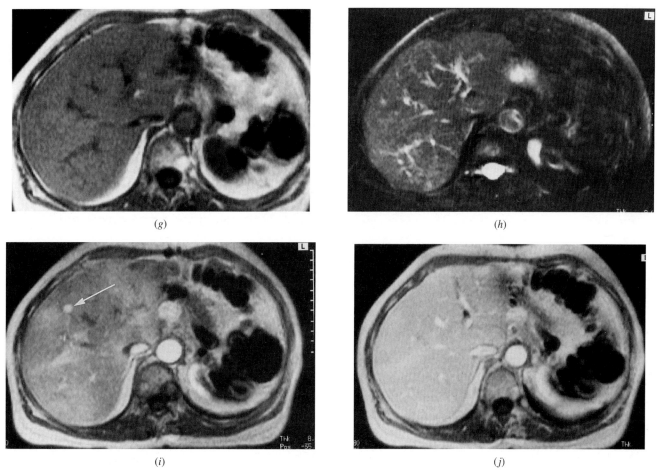

(g)   (h)

(i)   (j)

FIG. 2.91 (*Continued*) The metastasis washes out rapidly and becomes isointense with liver by 45 s (*j*). Small hypervascular malignant lesions commonly are shown only on hepatic arterial dominant phase images.

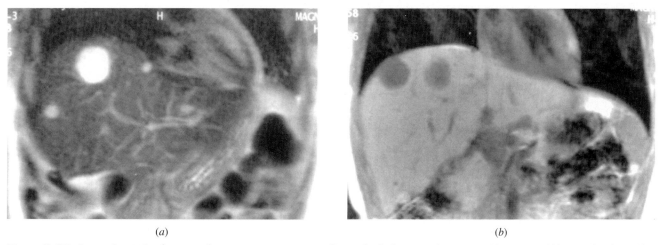

(a)   (b)

FIG. 2.92 Gastrointestinal stromal sarcoma metastases that mimic hemangiomas on T2. Coronal T2-weighted SS-ETSE (*a*), coronal, SGE (*b*), T2-weighted fat-suppressed ETSE (*c*), SGE (*d*), immediate postgadolinium SGE (*e*), and 90-s postgadolinium fat-suppressed SGE (*f*) images. There are two lesions that are well defined and demonstrate high signal on T2-weighted images (*a, c*) and low signal on T1-weighted images (*b, d*).

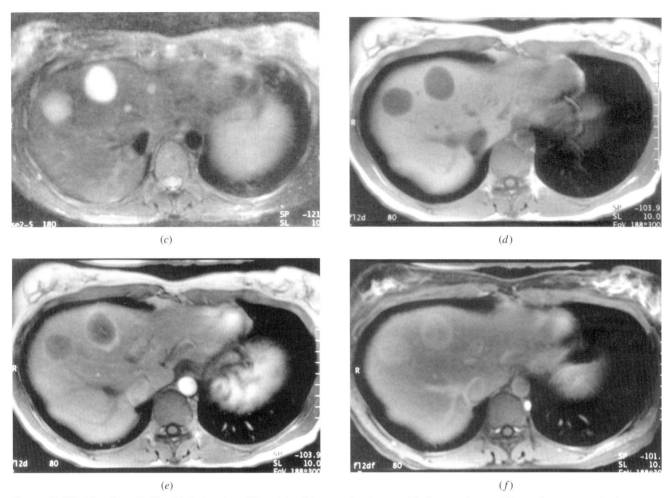

(c)   (d)

(e)   (f)

F I G . 2.92 (*Continued*) The high signal on T2-weighted images (*a, c*) resemble hemangiomas. Ring enhancement is shown on immediate postgadolinium images (*e*), diagnostic for metastases.

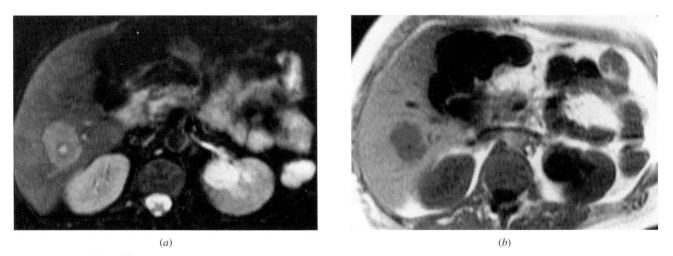

(a)   (b)

F I G . 2.93 Infected liver metastases. T2-weighted fat-suppressed SE (*a*), SGE (*b*), and immediate (*c*) and 10-min (*d*) postgadolinium SGE images. This patient with colon cancer and clinical findings of sepsis has a 4-cm infected metastasis in the right lobe of the liver. The tumor has ill-defined margins and is minimally hyperintense on T2 (*a*) with a small central focus of high signal intensity and moderately low in signal intensity on T1 (*b*) and on the immediate postgadolinium image (*c*); the infected metastasis shows ring enhancement with prominent ill-defined perilesional enhancement.

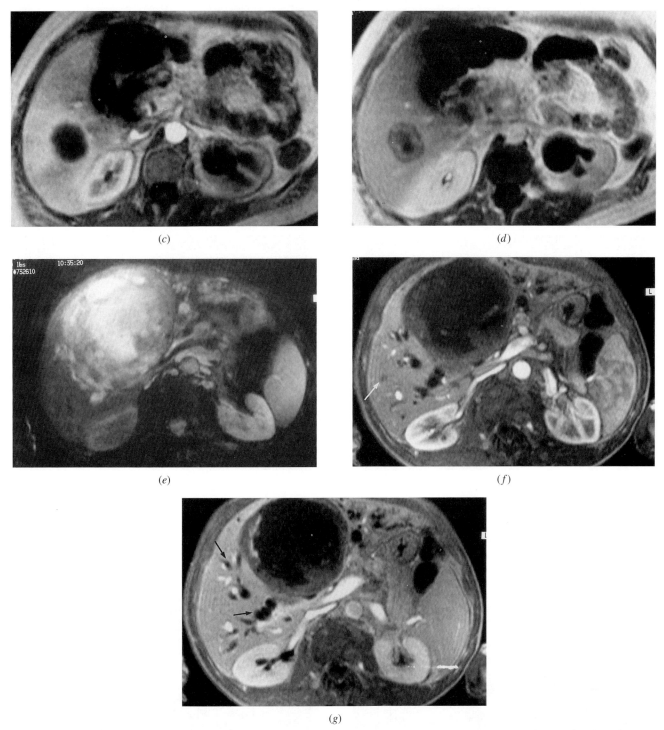

(c)

(d)

(e)

(f)

(g)

FIG. 2.93 (*Continued*) The 10-min postcontrast image (*d*) shows some centripetal enhancement with peripheral washout resulting in a low-signal intensity outer border. Chronic obstruction of the left renal collecting system is caused by entrapment of the ureter in the pelvis by the carcinoma arising in the sigmoid colon.

T2-weighted fat-suppressed ETSE (*e*) and immediate (*f*) and 2-min (*g*) postgadolinium SGE images in a second patient. A 14-cm metastasis superinfected by *Listeria* is present in the left lobe of the liver. The infected metastasis is heterogeneous and high in signal on the T2-weighted image (*e*), and demonstrates enhancement of the thick irregular wall on the immediate postgadolinium image (*f*), with progressive enhancement on the interstitial-phase image (*g*). Additional metastases smaller than 1 cm are evident only on the immediate postgadolinium images (arrow, *f*). The mass causes obstruction of the biliary tree at the level of the porta hepatis resulting in substantial intrahepatic biliary dilatation (arrows, *g*).

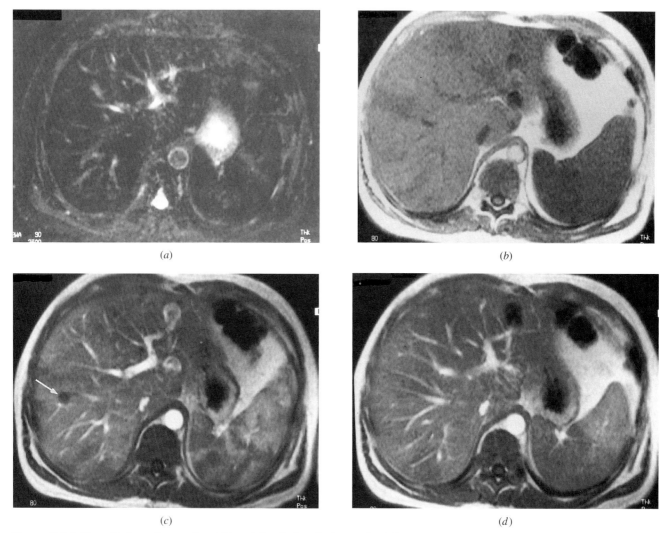

F I G . 2.94 Hepatic lymphoma, low T2-weighted signal. T2-weighted fat-suppressed SE (*a*), SGE (*b*), and immediate (*c*) and 90-s (*d*) postgadolinium SGE images. On the T2-weighted image (*a*), the liver and spleen demonstrate transfusional siderosis with low signal intensity of the liver and spleen. The SGE image (*b*) demonstrates wedge-shaped regions of low signal intensity representing increased iron deposition. On the immediate postgadolinium image (*c*), focal low-signal intensity masses (arrow, *c*) of diffuse histiocytic lymphoma are shown. These masses enhance to isointensity with hepatic parenchyma on interstitial-phase images (*d*).

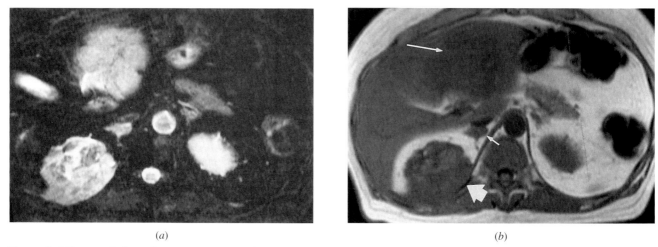

F I G . 2.95 Hepatic lymphoma, post transplant. T2-weighted fat-suppressed SE (*a*), SGE (*b*), and immediate postgadolinium SGE (*c*) images.

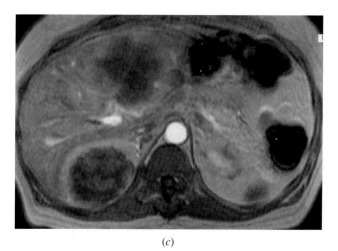

(c)

F I G . 2.95 (*Continued*) In this patient with postheart transplant lymphoma, and 8-cm hepatic mass (long arrow, *b*), a 1-cm adrenal mass (short arrow, *b*), and a 6-cm peritoneum-based mass (large arrow, *b*) are present. The hepatic mass is moderately hyperintense on the T2-weighted image (*a*), moderately hypointense on the T1-weighted image (*b*), and demonstrates predominantly peripheral enhancement on the immediate postgadolinium image (*c*). Minimal heterogeneous enhancement of the peritoneal and adrenal masses is present on the immediate postgadolinium image (*c*).

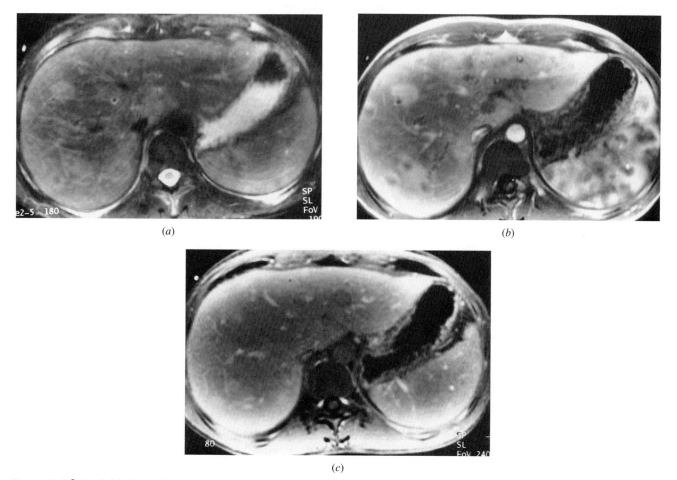

(a)

(b)

(c)

F I G . 2.96 Hodgkin lymphoma. T2-weighted fat-suppressed ETSE (*a*), immediate postgadolinium SGE (*b*), and 90-s postgadolinium fat-suppressed SGE (*c*) images. Multiple focal mass lesions smaller than 2 cm are present throughout the liver, many of which show mildly hyperintense tumor periphery on T2 (*a*) and demonstrate ring enhancement with ill-defined perilesional enhancement on immediate postgadolinium images (*b*). Arciform enhancement of the spleen is present on the immediate postgadolinium image, with no evidence of focal low-signal intensity masses (*b*). By 90 s postgadolinium (*c*) many of the hepatic masses have become isointense with liver.

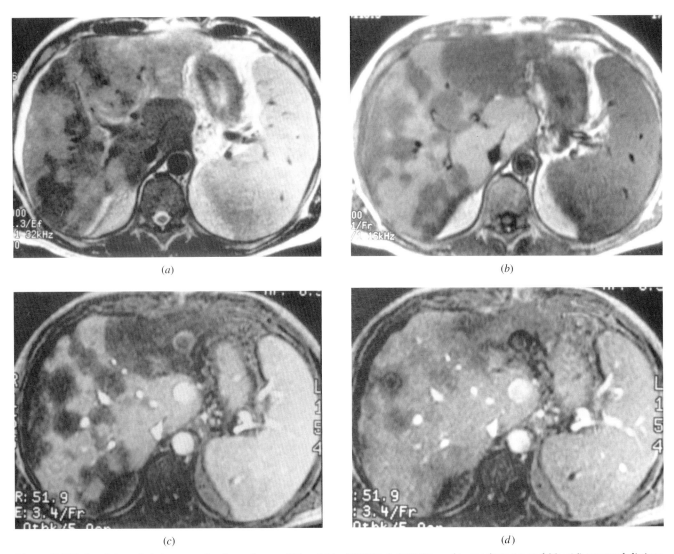

(a)   (b)

(c)   (d)

F I G . 2.97 Angiotropic intravascular lymphoma. T2-weighted ETSE (*a*), SGE (*b*), and immediate (*c*) and 90-s (*d*) postgadolinium SGE images. There is an irregular geographic pattern of liver involvement that represents angiotropic intravascular lymphoma. The vascular involvement causes moderately high signal on T2 (*a*), moderately low signal on T1 (*b*), and negligible early enhancement (*c*) with delayed enhancement (*d*). (Courtesy of Evan Siegelman, M.D., Dept. of Radiology, Hospital of the University of Pennsylvania.)

pattern may be very difficult to diagnose but is best visualized on a combination of T2-weighted fat-suppressed images and hepatic venous-phase gadolinium-enhanced fat-suppressed images. On both techniques periportal tumor is moderately high in signal intensity (fig. 2.98).

Primary hepatic lymphoma is considerably rarer than secondary involvement and histologically the majority are non-Hodgkin lymphomas. Most tumors are characterized grossly as a large solitary mass, but they may vary in appearance from multiple nodules to diffuse involvement. Tumors are moderately low in signal intensity on T1-weighted images and mild to moderately high in signal on T2-weighted images and show relatively diffuse heterogeneous enhancement on immediate postgadolinium SGE images (fig. 2.99), analogous to primary malignant hepatic tumors of other histologic types.

Multiple Myeloma. Focal deposits of multiple myeloma rarely occur in the liver and most often in the setting of disseminated disease. Pathologically, hepatic lesions are characterized by tumor cell infiltration of sinusoids and portal tracts. Focal hepatic lesions are observed most commonly in light-chain multiple myeloma. Lesions are often small, measuring approximately 1 cm in diameter. They are slightly hyperintense on T1-weighted images and minimally hyperintense on T2-weighted images (fig. 2.100) [102]. The hyperintensity on T1-weighted images may reflect the increased production of monoclonal protein.

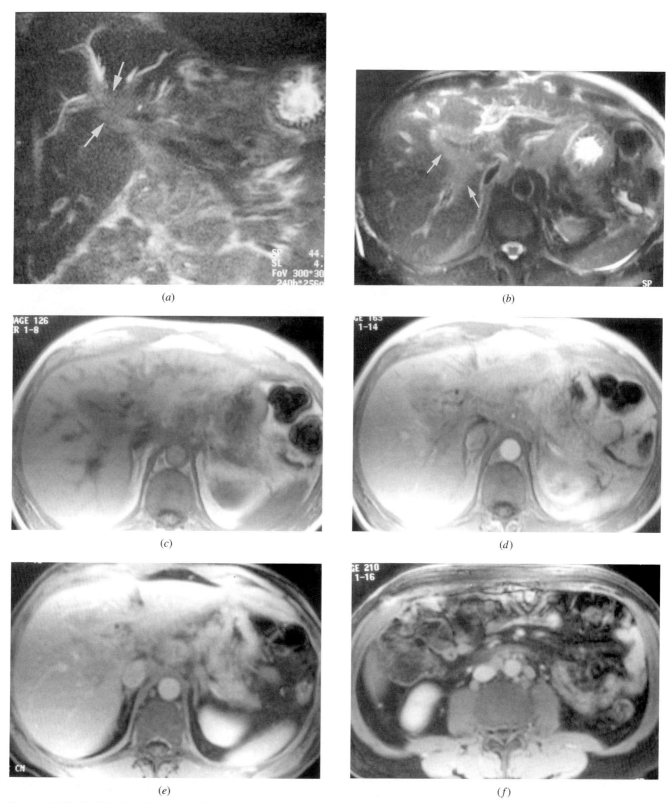

F I G . 2.98 Burkitt lymphoma with periportal infiltration. Coronal T2-weighted SS-ETSE (*a*), T2-weighted fat-suppressed SS-ETSE (*b*), SGE (*c*), immediate postgadolinium SGE (*d*), and 90-s postgadolinium fat-suppressed SGE (*e, f*) images. There is extensive soft tissue infiltration in the porta hepatis with periportal extension (arrows, *a, b*). Periportal tumor infiltration is more common with lymphoma than other form of malignant disease. Retroperitoneal nodes are also present (*f*).

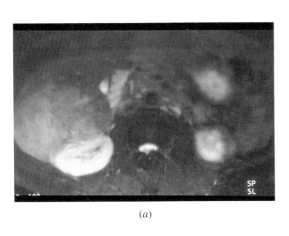

(a)

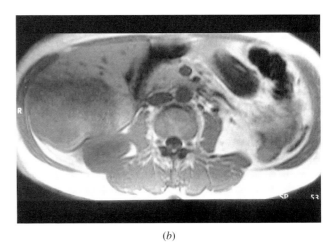

(b)

FIG. 2.99 Primary hepatic lymphoma. T2-weighted fat-suppressed ETSE (*a*), SGE (*b*), and immediate postgadolinium SGE (*c*) images. An 8-cm primary hepatic lymphoma is present in the right lobe of the liver. The tumor is mildly hyperintense on T2 (*a*), moderately hypointense on T1 (*b*), and demonstrates thick irregular multilayered peripheral enhancement on immediate postgadolinium images (*c*).

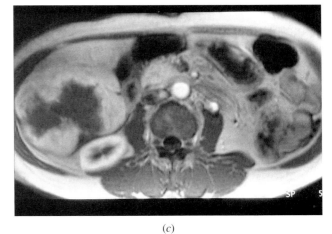

(c)

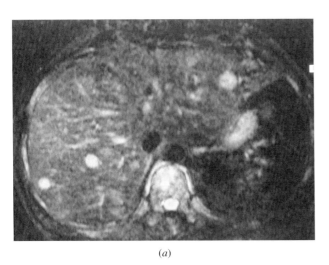

(a)

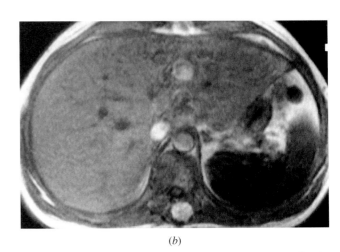

(b)

FIG. 2.100 Multiple myeloma. T2-weighted fat-suppressed ETSE (*a*), SGE (*b*), and T1-weighted fat-suppressed spin-echo (*c*) images. Multiple focal masses smaller than 1.5 cm are present in the liver that are moderately hyperintense on T2 (*a*), nearly isointense on T1-weighted image (*b*), and moderately hyperintense on the T1-weighted fat-suppressed spin-echo image (black arrows, *c*).

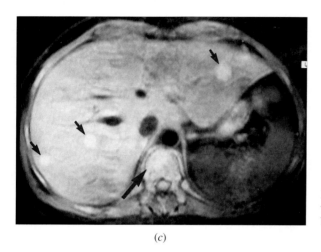

(c)

F I G . 2.100 (*Continued*) High signal intensity on T1- and T2-weighted images is also present in vertebral bodies (large arrow, *c*) because of myelomatous involvement.

Hepatocellular Carcinoma. Hepatocellular carcinoma (HCC) is the most common primary malignancy of the liver and occurs most frequently in men. In North America HCC tends to arise in a previously damaged liver and is most commonly seen in patients with cirrhosis from alcohol, viral hepatitis, chronic active hepatitis, and hemochromatosis (fig. 2.101). HCC is common in Asia because of the prevalence of viral hepatitis. Incidence in the United States is increasing because of the growing numbers of patients with chronic viral hepatitis. Hepatic architecture tends to be less distorted in patients with viral hepatitis than in patients with cirrhosis. As livers may not appear cirrhotic, a high index of suspicion for HCC is recommended in patients with focal liver masses and underlying viral hepatitis.

HCC is solitary in approximately 50% (fig. 2.102), multifocal in approximately 40% (figs. 2.103 and 2.104), and diffuse in less than 10% of cases. HCCs may arise both de novo and through progressive steps of cellular atypia [103]. Tumors are considered to arise from dysplastic nodules and to progress in a stepwise fashion from early HCC to advanced HCC. A recent multi-institutional report has proposed a new nomenclature for nodular hepatocellular lesions in which premalignant hepatocellular lesions are defined as dysplastic nodule low grade and dysplastic nodule high grade [37]. In North America, most HCCs are advanced at the time of diagnosis, although with increasing surveillance of patients with liver cirrhosis and/or viral hepatitis detection of earlier-stage neoplasm appears to be occurring more often.

Histologically, malignant cells usually form trabeculae or plates of varying thickness separated by a rich network of sinusoidal spaces filled with arterial blood. HCC are fed by hepatic arterial blood supply, but both hepatic and portal veins proliferate alongside tumors and

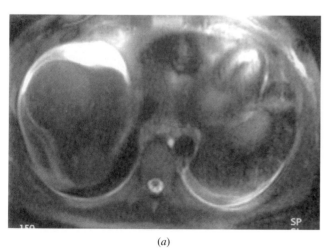

(a)

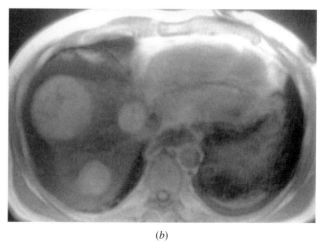

(b)

F I G . 2.101 Multifocal HCCs superimposed on idiopathic hemochromatosis. T2-weighted fat-suppressed SS-ETSE (*a*), SGE (*b*), immediate postgadolinium SGE (*c*), and 90-s postgadolinium fat-suppressed SGE (*d*) images. There are three HCC nodules that show slight increased signal on T2- (*a*) and T1-weighted (*b*) images, mildly increased enhancement immediately after gadolinium administration (*c*), and fade slight over time (*d*).

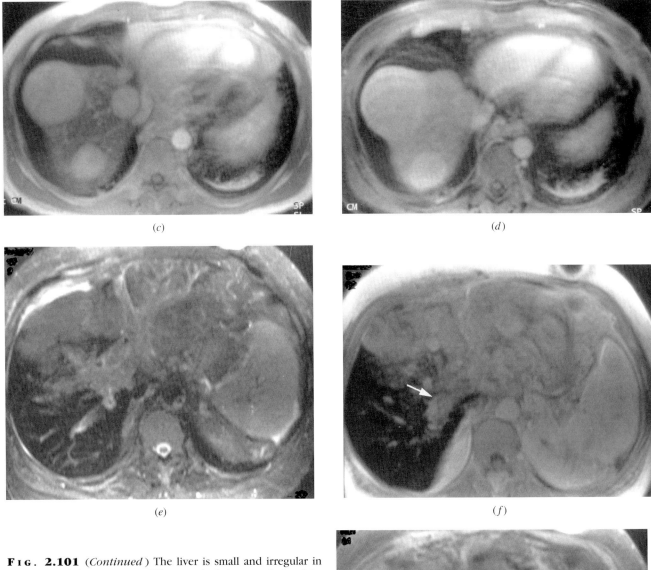

(c)

(d)

(e)

(f)

FIG. 2.101 (*Continued*) The liver is small and irregular in contour, and demonstrates diffuse marked decreased signal intensity on T2- (*a*) and T1-weighted (*b*) images, even after contrast, consistent with hepatocellular iron deposition in idiopathic hemochromatosis. Note also ascities.

Echo train-STIR (*e*), immediate postgadolinium SGE (*f*), and 90-s postgadolinium fat-suppressed SGE (*g*) images in a second patient with idiopathic hemochromatosis. There is a very large HCC involving the entire left lobe and *segments* 5 and 8 of the right lobe that demonstrates heterogeneous and moderately increased signal on T2-weighted images and heterogeneous gadolinium enhancement. The entire portal venous system is expanded and enhances after gadolinium administration (arrow, *f*) consistent with tumor thrombus. Marked decreased signal intensity of liver parenchyma reflects the iron deposition in idiopathic hemochromatosis.

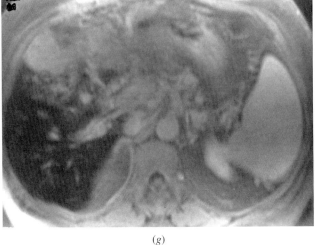

(g)

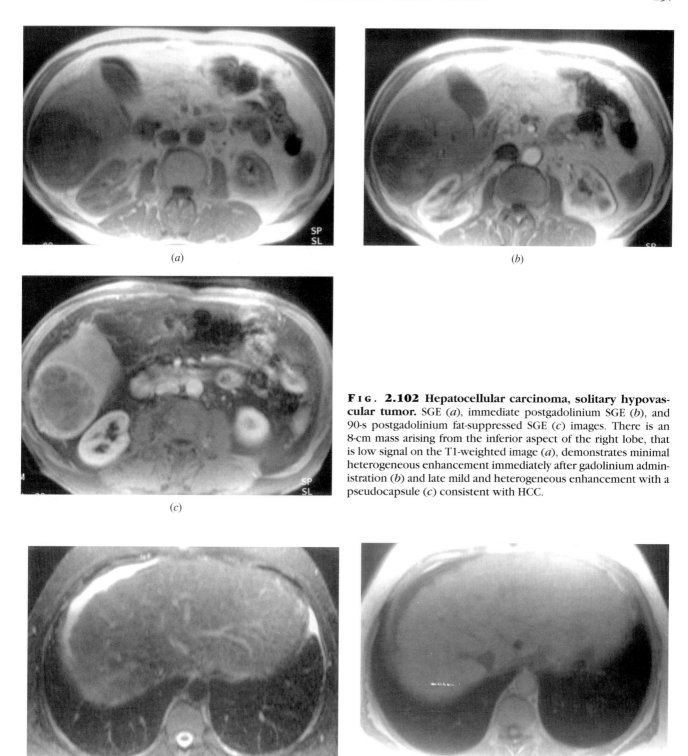

FIG. 2.102 Hepatocellular carcinoma, solitary hypovascular tumor. SGE (*a*), immediate postgadolinium SGE (*b*), and 90-s postgadolinium fat-suppressed SGE (*c*) images. There is an 8-cm mass arising from the inferior aspect of the right lobe, that is low signal on the T1-weighted image (*a*), demonstrates minimal heterogeneous enhancement immediately after gadolinium administration (*b*) and late mild and heterogeneous enhancement with a pseudocapsule (*c*) consistent with HCC.

FIG. 2.103 Multifocal small HCC. Echo-train STIR (*a*), SGE (*b*), immediate postgadolinium SGE (*c*), and 90-s postgadolinium fat-suppressed SGE (*d*) images. There are multiple small HCCs (arrows, *c*), scattered throughout the hepatic parenchyma.

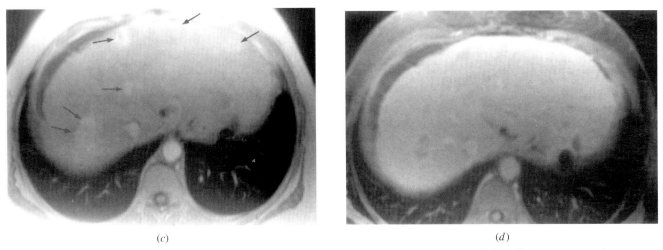

(c)   (d)

F I G . 2.103 (*Continued*) These lesions are isointense on T2 (*a*) and T1-weighted (*b*) images and show homogeneous enhancement after contrast administration (*c*), and wash-out on late images (*d*). Note the pseudocapsule enhancement on the interstitial-phase image (*d*).

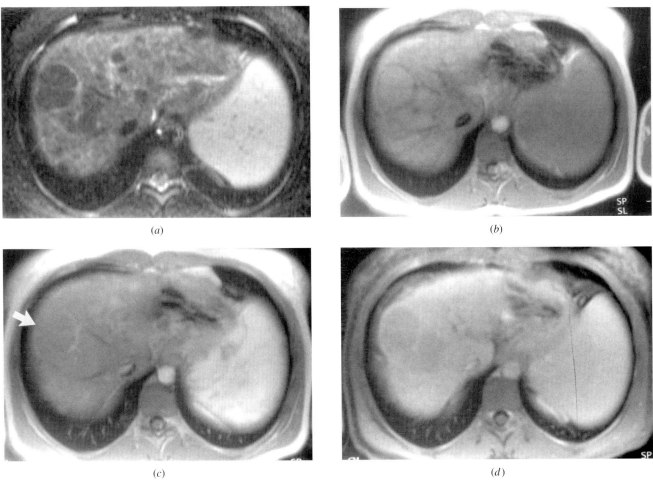

(a)   (b)

(c)   (d)

F I G . 2.104 Multifocal HCC. Echo-train STIR (*a*), SGE (*b*), immediate postgadolinium SGE (*c*), and 90-s postgadolinium fat-suppressed SGE (*d*) images. Multiple HCCs are present that are mildly hypointense on T2- (*a*) and mildly hyperintense on T1-weighted (*b*) images. The smaller lesions possess mildly intense homogeneous enhancement, and the 4-cm tumor (arrow, *c*) shows isointense enhancement immediately after gadolinium administration (*c*). Wash-out is observed on interstitial-phase images (*d*) with late pseudocapsule enhancement.

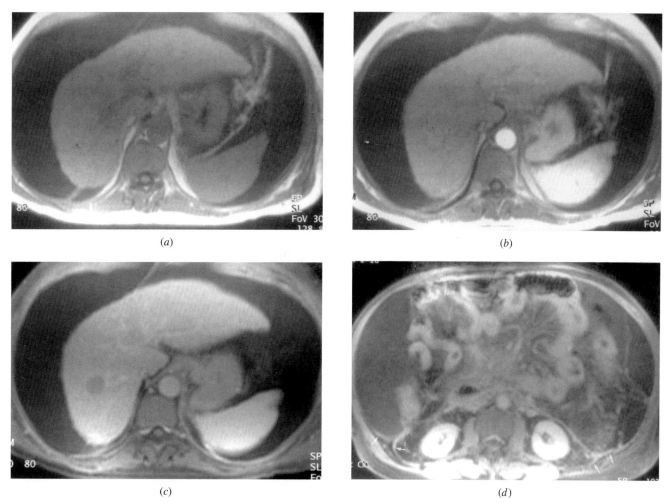

(a)

(b)

(c)

(d)

F I G . 2.105 HCC and microvarices in peritoneum. SGE (*a*), immediate postgadolinium SGE (*b*), and 90-s postgadolinium fat-suppressed (*c*, *d*) images. There is a 2-cm tumor centrally located in the right hepatic lobe that is not seen on the precontrast image (*a*) and demonstrates increased enhancement on the immediate postcontrast image (*b*) with wash-out and capsular enhancement on the late image (*c*), consistent with a small HCC. Note extensive varices throughout the peritoneal cavity (arrows, *d*). Varices typically show extension of small curvilinear structures deep to the peritoneum, as observed in this patient. Peritoneal metastases stay confined to the peritoneal surface and within the peritoneal cavity. A small well-defined central HCC, as in this patient, would also not be expected to have peritoneal metastases. Note the micronodular contour of the liver and the large-volume ascites.

cavernous structures develop in collaterals. As a consequence of these intrahepatic vascular changes, intra- and extrahepatic spread may occur by a number of routes including hepatic veins, inferior vena cava, and portal system (figs. 2.105–2.107) [104].

Imaging early after contrast injection facilitates the detection of tumor vascularity. Because of the greater sensitivity of MRI to gadolinium than CT imaging to iodine contrast, MRI frequently demonstrates HCCs, particularly tumors smaller than 1.5 cm, better than CT imaging (figs. 2.108 and 2.109). Therefore, CT imaging has a limited role for the detection of unsuspected HCC in cirrhotic patients [105].

Oi et al. [106] compared multiphase helical CT with MRI using dynamic gadolinium administration. They re-

ported that early-phase gadolinium-enhanced images detected 140 nodules compared to 106 nodules detected by early-phase helical CT. In another report, Yamashita et al. [107] reported that immediate postgadolinium SGE was superior to arterial phase helical CT for the detection of HCC using ROC analysis. In a recent report, MR imaging during arterial portography (MRPA) demonstrated 94% sensitivity for detection of HCC compared with CT during arterial portography (CTAP), which showed 83% sensitivity; however, the difference was not statistically significant [108].

HCCs have a variety of signal patterns on T1- and T2-weighted images. The most frequent appearance is minimally low signal intensity on T1-weighted images and mildly high signal intensity on T2-weighted images

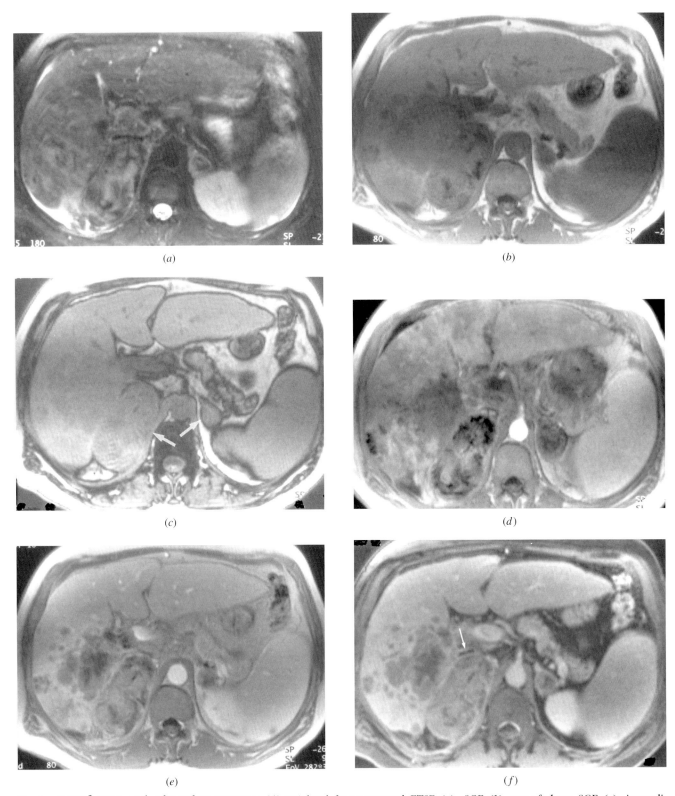

(a)

(b)

(c)

(d)

(e)

(f)

F I G . 2.106 HCC and adrenal metastases. T2-weighted fat-suppressed ETSE (*a*), SGE (*b*), out-of-phase SGE (*c*), immediate (*d*) and 45-s (*e*) postgadolinium SGE, and 90-s postgadolinium fat-suppressed SGE (*f*) images. There are multiple lesions throughout the liver, which are low signal on T1 (*b*) and high signal on T2 (*a*) and demonstrate moderately intense uniform and peripheral ring enhancement on immediate postgadolinium images (*d*), consistent with multifocal HCC, presumably with intrahepatic metastases to account for the ring enhancement in many lesions. Bilateral adrenal masses (arrows, *c*) are present that demonstrate mixed signal intensity on T1 (*b*), do not drop in signal on out-of-phase images (*c*), and enhance heterogeneously after contrast administration (*d–f*), consistent with metastases. Abnormal signal in the IVC (arrow, *f*) represents thrombus.

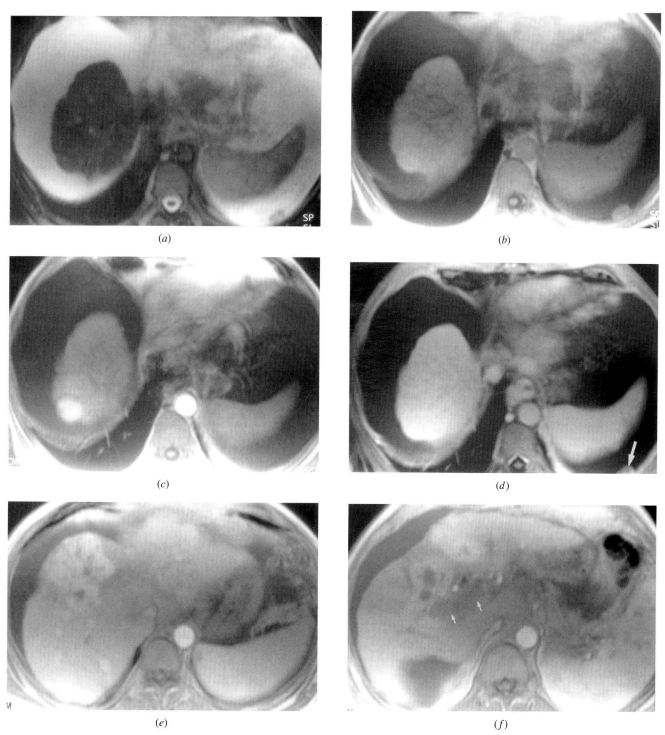

(a)

(b)

(c)

(d)

(e)

(f)

F i g . 2.107 HCC with peritoneal spread. T2-weighted fat-suppressed SS-ETSE (*a*), SGE (*b*), immediate postgadolinium SGE (*c*), and 90-s postgadolinium fat-suppressed SGE (*d*) images. The liver is small and irregular in contour compatible with cirrhosis. There is a small exophytic HCC in the right hepatic lobe that demonstrates isointensity on T2 (*a*), slight hyperintensity on T1 (*b*), intense enhancement immediately after contrast administration (*c*), and washout with capsular enhancement on the delayed image (*d*) consistent with HCC. Note the peritoneal based mass (arrow, *d*) on the left side, near the spleen consistent with peritoneal metastasis from HCC.

Immediate postgadolinium SGE (*e, f*) and 90-s postgadolinium fat-suppressed SGE (*g*) images in a second patient. The liver is nodular in contour and demonstrates a reticular pattern of enhancement compatible with cirrhosis. There is a large HCC in the dome of the liver that bulges the liver contour and shows intense heterogeneous enhancement immediately after gadolinium (*e, f*). Other smaller HCCs are also identified. Note that the main portal vein is expanded with tumor thrombus (arrows, *f*). Peritoneal thickening and enhancement is observed within the paracolic gutters (arrows, *g*), consistent with peritoneal metastases.

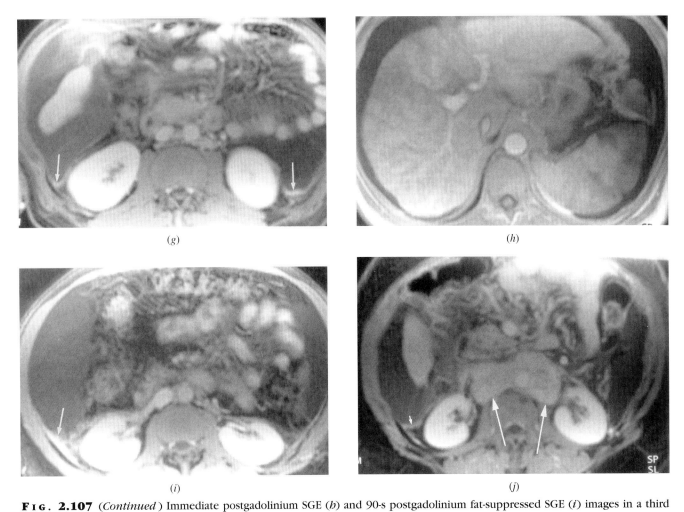

(g)

(h)

(i)

(j)

FIG. 2.107 (*Continued*) Immediate postgadolinium SGE (*h*) and 90-s postgadolinium fat-suppressed SGE (*i*) images in a third patient. There is heterogeneous mottled enhancement of the hepatic parenchyma after the administration of gadolinium consistent with diffuse HCC. Note the infiltrative peritoneal thickening and enhancement compatible with small tumoral implants (arrow, *i*).

Transverse 90-s postgadolinium fat-suppressed SGE image (*j*) in a fourth patient. This patient with HCC has thickening of the peritoneum in the right paracolic gutter (small arrow, *j*) and multiple, enlarged aortocaval and retroaortic lymph nodes (long arrows, *j*).

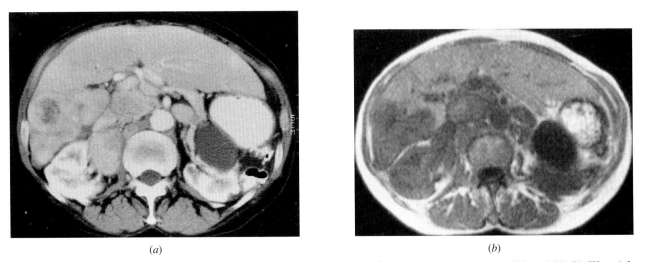

(a)

(b)

FIG. 2.108 **Multifocal HCC with adenopathy—spiral CT imaging and MRI comparison.** Spiral CT (*a*), SGE (*b*), T2-weighted fat-suppressed ETSE (*c*), immediate postgadolinium SGE (*d*), and 45-s postgadolinium SGE (*e*) images.

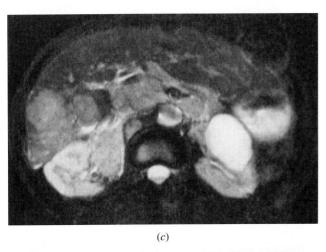

(c)

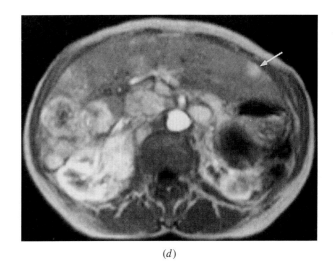

(d)

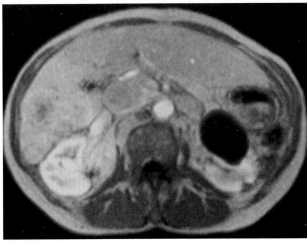

(e)

F I G . 2.108 (*Continued*) On the CT image (*a*), an HCC is identified in the right lobe with multiple nodes in the porta hepatis and retroperitoneum. Precontrast SGE image (*b*) demonstrates the HCC as a moderately low-signal intensity mass in the right lobe and the lymph nodes as moderately low in signal intensity. The T2-weighted image (*c*) demonstrates the tumor and lymph nodes as moderately high in signal intensity. On the immediate postgadolinium SGE image (*d*), the HCC in the right lobe demonstrates intense diffuse heterogeneous enhancement. Multiple additional HCCs smaller than 1 cm are also apparent (arrow, *d*) that were not visible on spiral CT images (*a*) or on noncontrast T1 (*b*) and T2-weighted (*c*) images. The small HCCs wash out to isointensity with the liver by 45 s (*e*), at a time when renal CMD is still pronounced. Intense enhancement of the associated adenopathy is also present on the immediate postgadolinium image (*d*).

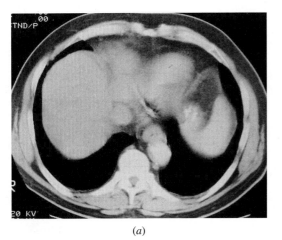

(a)

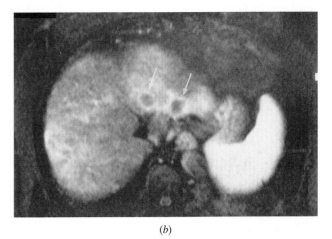

(b)

F I G . 2.109 Multifocal HCC—spiral CT and MR comparison. Spiral CT (*a*), T2-weighted fat-suppressed ETSE (*b*), and immediate postgadolinium SGE (*c*) images. The spiral CT image demonstrates a solitary HCC in a patient with 8 HCC tumors. No tumors are evident on this tomographic section (*a*).

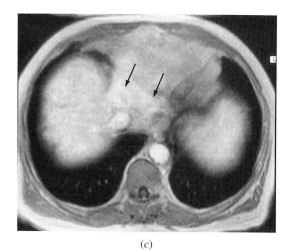

(c)

Fig. 2.109 (*Continued*) T2-weighted image (*b*) demonstrates two 1.8-cm HCCs at this level that have high-signal intensity peripheral rims and are isointense centrally (arrows, *b*). On the immediate postgadolinium image (*c*), these tumors enhance in a predominantly ring fashion (arrows, *c*).

(figs. 2.110 and 2.111) [109–117]. HCCs may, however, range from hypo- to hyperintense on T1- and T2-weighted images. Increased signal intensity on T1-weighted images correlates with a more favorable histology for well-differentiated HCC than does iso- or hypointensity [118]. A higher percentage of moderately and poorly differentiated HCCs are hyperintense on T2-weighted images [118].

Early HCC is frequently high in signal intensity on T1-weighted images and isointense on T2-weighted images [112–115]. High signal intensity on T1-weighted images may reflect the presence of fat or protein (fig. 2.112). Most of these tumors do not contain fat, and high protein content is most likely responsible for the high signal intensity of these lesions (fig. 2.113) [113, 115, 119]. In early advanced hepatocellular carcinoma,

the appearance of a low signal intensity nodule within a high-signal intensity nodule (nodule within nodule) has been described on T1-weighted images [120]. This reflects the development of a low-signal high-grade tumor within a high-signal low-grade tumor (fig. 2.114).

A multi-institutional study of appearance of HCC in North America analyzed 354 HCCs in 113 patients. They found that the combination of hypointensity on T1-weighted images, hyperintensity on T2-weighted images, and diffuse heterogeneous enhancement was the most common appearance of HCC on MR images (fig. 2.115). Small HCCs, measuring ≤1.5 cm, were frequently isointense on both T1-weighted and T2-weighted images and could be detected only on immediate gadolinium-enhanced images as diffuse, homogeneously enhancing lesions [121].

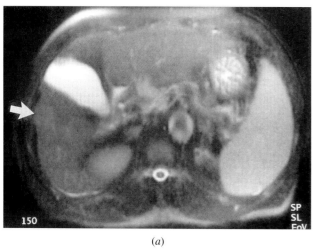

(a)

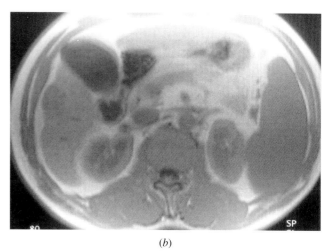

(b)

Fig. 2.110 Solitary small HCC. T2-weighted fat-suppressed SS-ETSE (*a*), SGE (*b*), immediate postgadolinium SGE (*c*), and 90-s postgadolinium fat-suppressed SGE (*d*) images. There is a 2-cm mass that bulges the liver contour slightly in the right lobe of the liver. The mass is minimally hyperintense on T2 (*a*) and mildly hypointense on T1 (*b*), demonstrates intense uniform enhancement on the immediate postgadolinium image (*c*), and fades to hypointensity by 90 s (*d*) with late enhancement of a pseudocapsule.

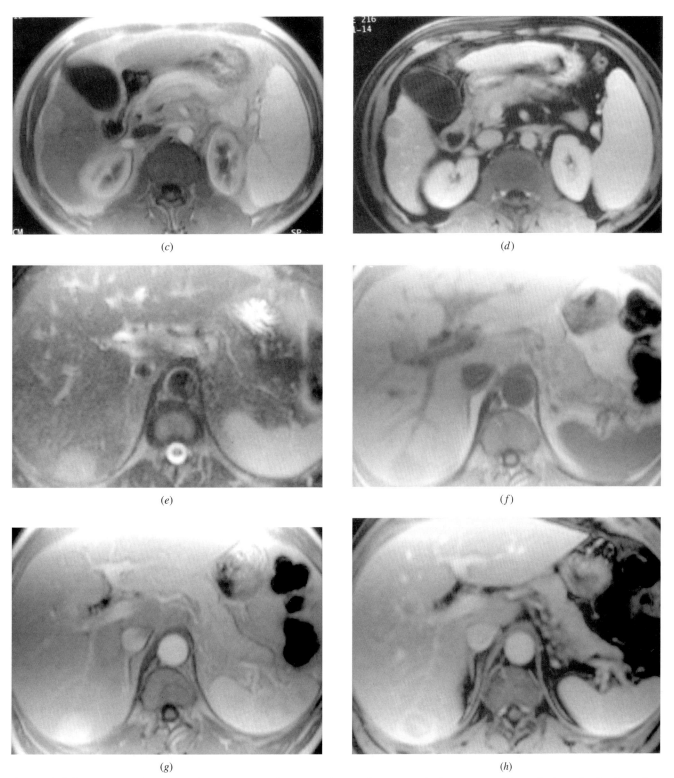

F I G . 2.110 (*Continued*) Intense hepatic arterial dominant phase enhancement is the most sensitive technique for the detection of small HCCs. Wash-out to hypointensity with late capsular enhancement is the most specific.

T2-weighted fat-suppressed SS-ETSE (*e*), SGE (*f*), immediate postgadolinium SGE (*g*), and 90-s postgadolinium fat-suppressed SGE (*h*) images in a second patient exhibit similar features for a 2.5-cm tumor.

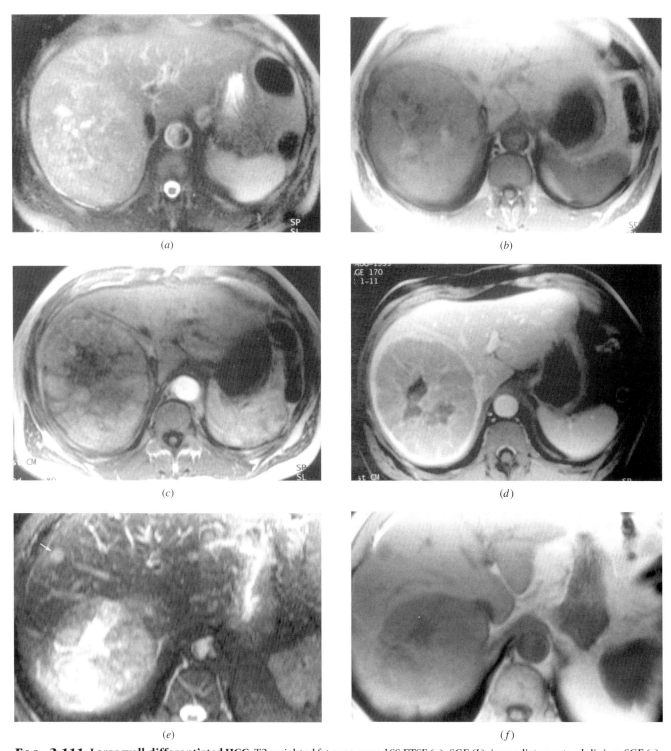

FIG. 2.111 Large well-differentiated HCC. T2-weighted fat-suppressed SS-ETSE (*a*), SGE (*b*), immediate postgadolinium SGE (*c*), and 90-s postgadolinium fat-suppressed SGE (*d*) images. There is a large well-defined mass in the right hepatic lobe that demonstrates slightly increased and heterogeneous signal intensity on T2 (*a*), moderately decreased signal intensity on T1 (*b*), heterogeneous enhancement on immediate postgadolinium images (*c*), and heterogeneous wash-out with late enhancement of a pseudocapsule (*d*).

Echo-train STIR (*e*), SGE (*f*), immediate postgadolinium SGE (*g*), and 90-s postgadolinium fat-suppressed SGE (*h*) images in a second patient. There is a large mass in the right hepatic lobe that is mildly and heterogeneously hyperintense on T2 (*e*), moderately hypointense on T1-weighted image (*f*), and demonstrates diffuse heterogeneous enhancement on immediate postgadolinium images (*g*), with heterogeneous wash-out and late enhancement of a pseudocapsule (*h*). Note a small satellite lesion (arrow, *e*) that exhibits high signal on T2 (*e*), low signal on T1 (*f*), homogeneous enhancement on hepatic arterial dominant phase (*g*), and a wash-out with pseudocapsule on delayed image (*h*). Both lesions are consistent with HCC.

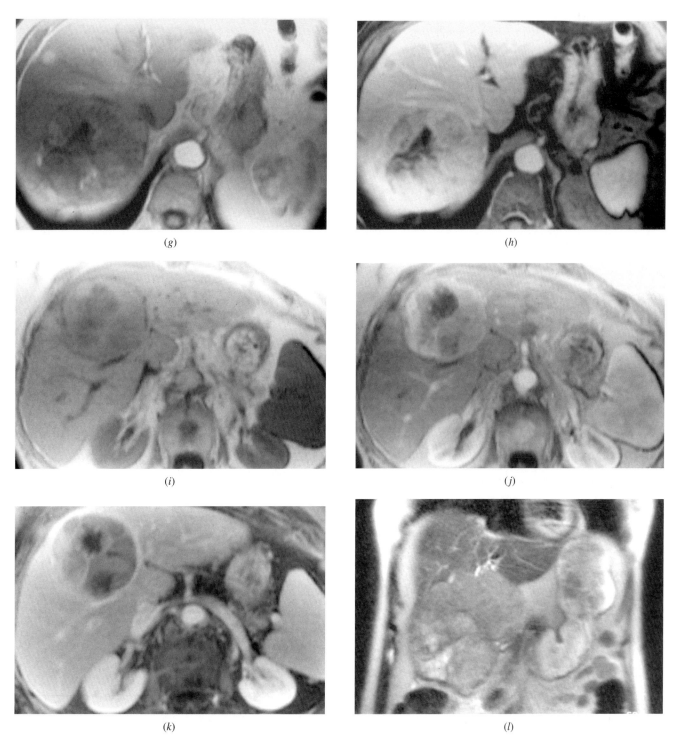

F I G. 2.111 (*Continued*) SGE (*i*), immediate postgadolinium SGE (*j*), and 90-s postgadolinium fat-suppressed SGE (*k*) images in a third patient. There is a large HCC that demonstrates heterogeneous mainly hypo to isointense signal on T1 (*i*), heterogeneous enhancement immediately after contrast administration (*j*), and wash-out with an enhanced pseudocapsule on late images (*k*), consistent with HCC.

Coronal T2-weighted SS-ETSE (*l*), coronal SGE (*m*), immediate postgadolinium SGE (*n*), and 90-s postgadolinium fat-suppressed SGE (*o*) images in a fourth patient. A large mass is present that demonstrates heterogeneous moderately high signal intensity on T2 (*l*), moderate low signal intensity on T1 (*m*), heterogeneous enhancement immediately after contrast administration (*n*), and wash-out with an enhanced pseudocapsule on interstitial-phase image (*o*).

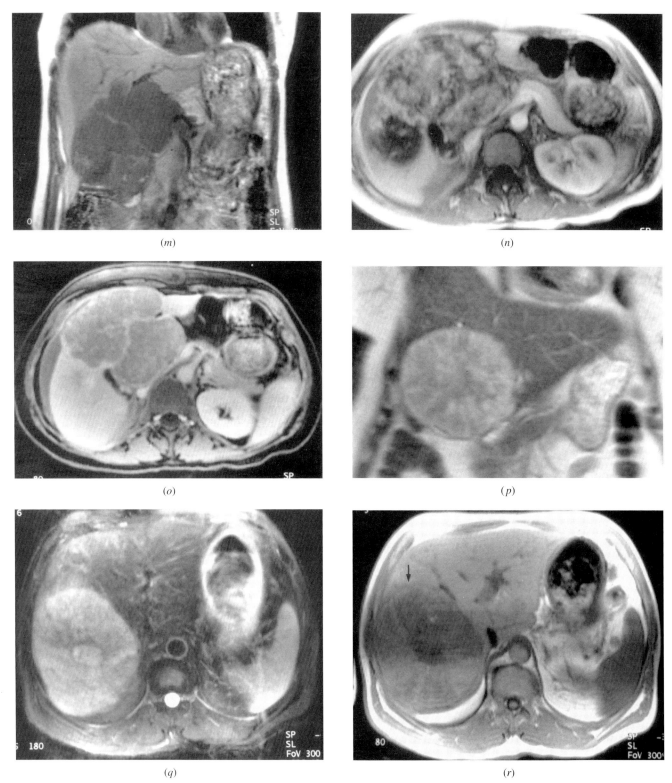

(m)

(n)

(o)

(p)

(q)

(r)

F I G . 2.111 *(Continued)* Coronal T2-weighted SS-ETSE (*p*), transverse T2-weighted fat-suppressed ETSE (*q*), SGE (*r*), immediate postgadolinium SGE (*s*), and 5-min postgadolinium SGE (*t*) images in a fifth patient. An 8-cm mass is present in the right hepatic lobe with heterogenous and moderately high signal on T2 (*p, q*), heterogeneous low signal intensity on T1-weighted images (*r*), and diffuse heterogeneous enhancement on immediate (*s*) and late (*t*) postgadolinium images.

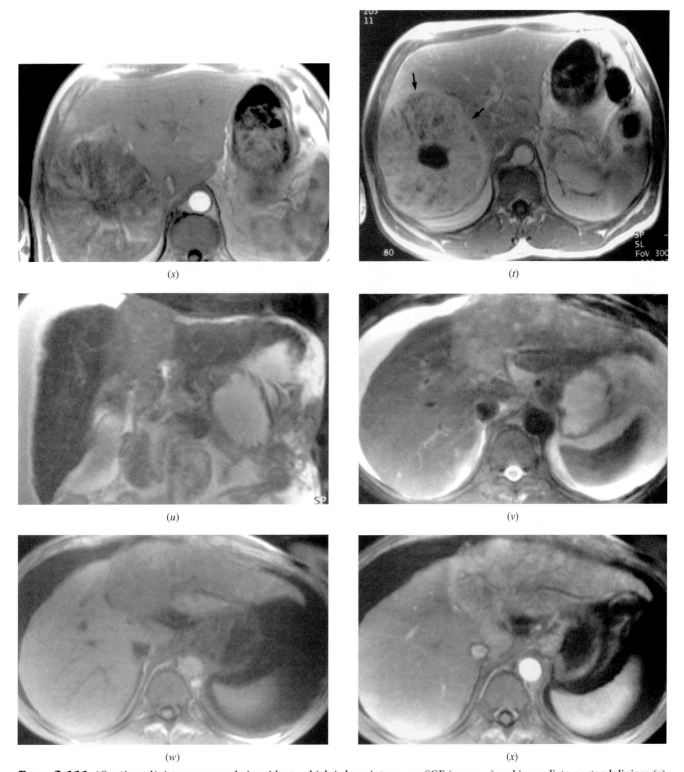

(s)

(t)

(u)

(v)

(w)

(x)

FIG. 2.111 (*Continued*) A tumor capsule is evident, which is hypointense on SGE (arrow, *r*) and immediate postgadolinium (*s*) images and enhances on late images (arrow, *t*). A large and dark central scar is best seen on the delayed image (*t*). (Reproduced with permission from Kelekis NL, Semelka RC, Worawattanakul S, Lange EE, et al.; Hepatocellular carcinoma in North America: A multiinstitutional study of appearance on T1-weighted, T2-weighted, and serial gadolinium-enhanced gradient-echo images. *Am J Roentgenol* 170: 1005–1013, 1998.)

FIG. 2.111 (*Continued*) Coronal T2-weighted SS-ETSE (*u*), transverse T2-weighted fat-suppressed ETSE (*v*), SGE (*w*), immediate postgadolinium SGE (*x*), and 90-s postgadolinium fat-suppressed SGE (*y*) images in a sixth patient. There is a large tumor mass occupying the majority of the left lobe that is mildly and heterogeneously hyperintense on T2 (*u, v*) and moderately hypointense on T1 (*w*) and shows diffuse heterogeneous enhancement on immediate postgadolinium images (*x*) and wash-out with capsular enhancement on interstitial phase images (*y*), consistent with a large HCC. Note the ascites, irregular liver contour, and varices along the lesser gastric curvature.

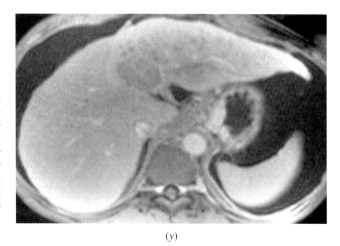

(*y*)

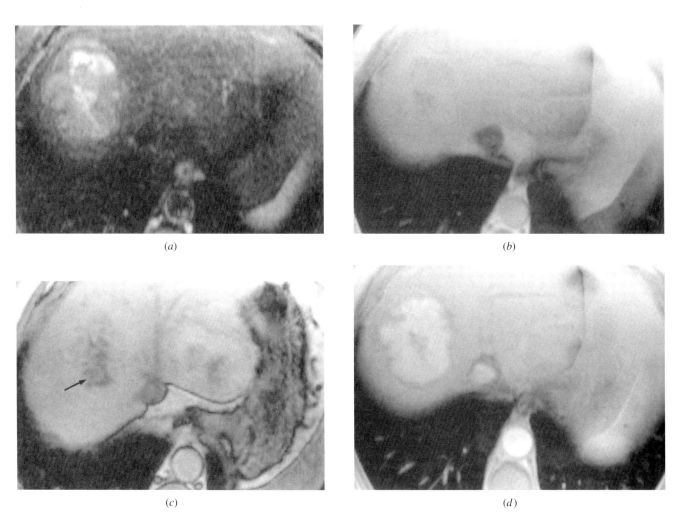

(*a*)

(*b*)

(*c*)

(*d*)

FIG. 2.112 Fat-containing well-differentiated HCC. Echo-train STIR (*a*), SGE (*b*), out-of-phase SGE (*c*), immediate postgadolinium SGE (*d*), and 90-s postgadolinium fat-suppressed SGE (*e*) images. There is a lobular mass in the right hepatic lobe that demonstrates high signal on T2 (*a*), isointensity on T1 (*b*), intense immediate enhancement after contrast (*d*) and wash-out (*e*). On late images (*e*), the pseudocapsule is high signal and well visualized. Note a small central scar that is high signal on T2 (*a*) and hypointense immediately after gadolinium (*d*) and shows late enhancement (*e*). Superficially, this well-differentiated HCC resembles an FNH. A distinguishing feature is the regions of signal heterogeneity on all MR sequences; FNH should be homogeneous on all sequences. Note also that the lesion demonstrates a peripheral region of signal loss (arrow, *c*) on the out-of-phase sequence consistent with fat.

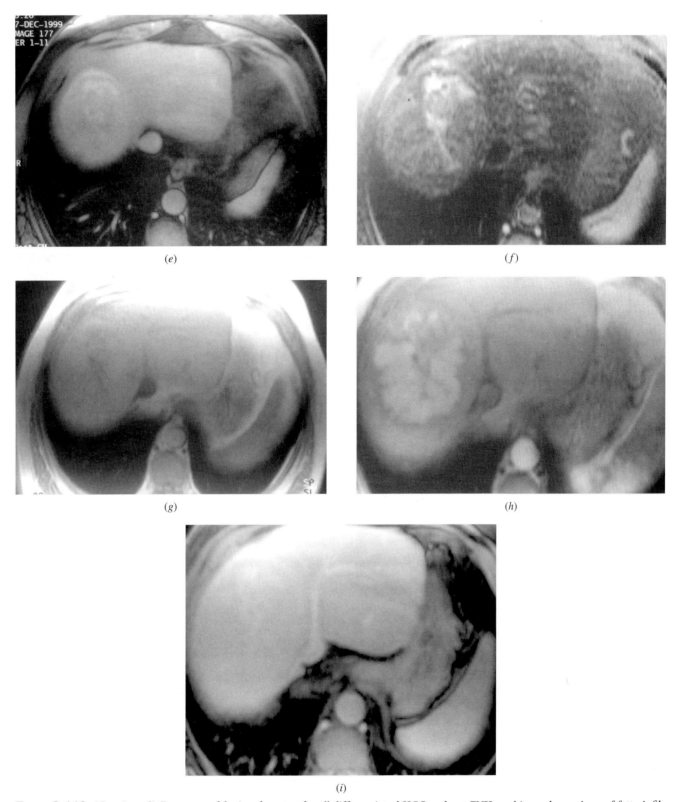

F I G . 2.112 (*Continued*) Presence of fat is a feature of well-differentiated HCC and not FNH, and irregular regions of fatty infiltration distinguish it from adenoma, which most commonly shows uniform fatty infiltration. Echo-train STIR (*f*), SGE (*g*), immediate postgadolinium SGE (*h*), and 90-s postgadolinium fat-suppressed SGE (*i*) images in the same patient, 4 months later. The lesion has increased in size, reflecting its malignant behavior.

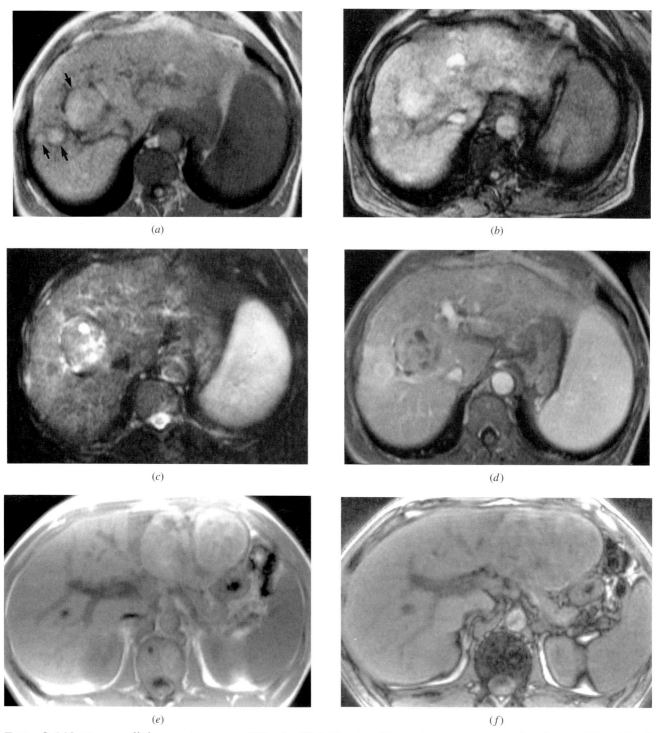

(a)   (b)

(c)   (d)

(e)   (f)

F I G . 2.113 Hepatocellular carcinoma, multifocal with high signal intensity, not representing fat, on T1-weighted images. SGE (*a*), out-of-phase SGE (*b*), T2-weighted fat-suppressed ETSE (*c*), and immediate postgadolinium SGE (*d*) images. Multiple HCCs are present that are high in signal intensity on T1 (arrows, *a*) and do not drop in signal or develop a phase-cancellation artifact on the out-of-phase image (*b*), which excludes the presence of fat. The small HCCs are isointense with liver on T2 (*c*), whereas the large tumor is heterogeneous and mildly hyperintense. On the immediate postgadolinium image (*d*) the small HCCs exhibit predominantly peripheral enhancement, whereas the larger HCC has diffuse heterogeneous enhancement. A low-signal intensity pseudocapsule is appreciated around the larger HCC on all imaging sequences.

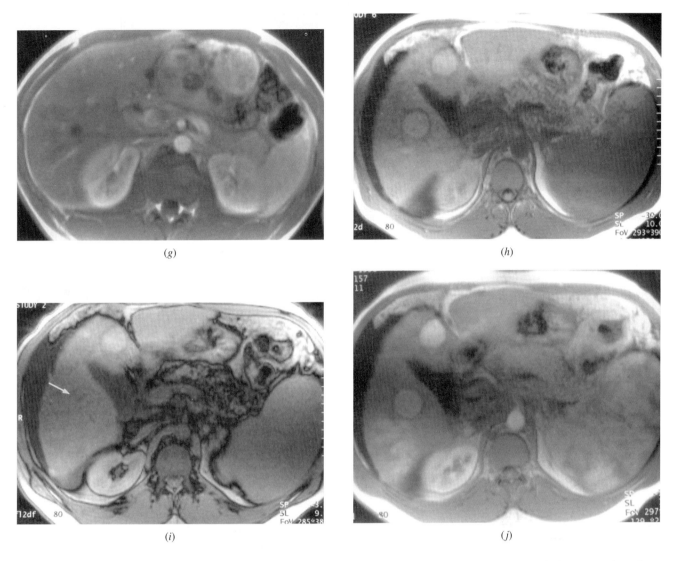

(g)

(h)

(i)

(j)

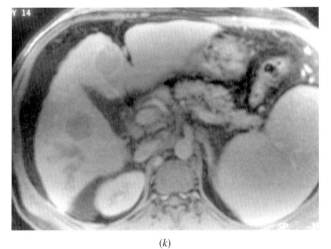

(k)

FIG. 2.113 (*Continued*) SGE (*e*), out-of-phase SGE (*f*), and immediate postgadolinium SGE (*g*) images in a second patient. There is a large HCC with high signal intensity on T1-weighted image (*e*) that does not drop in signal on out-of-phase images (*f*) and shows diffuse heterogeneous enhancement on immediate postcontrast images (*g*). This lesion is consistent with a nonfatty HCC.

SGE (*h*), out-of-phase SGE (*i*), immediate postgadolinium SGE (*j*), and 90-s postgadolinium fat-suppressed SGE (*k*) images in a third patient. There are two rounded lesions, both with high signal on in-phase images (*h*). The more posterior mass (arrow, *i*) loses signal on out-of-phase images, reflecting the presence of fat. The anterior lesion does not lose signal consistent with absence of fat. Both HCCs enhance intensely on immediate postgadolinium images (*j*) and wash out with late capsule enhancement on interstitial-phase images (*k*).

As these cases illustrate, high signal on T1-weighted images is relatively common in HCC, but in the majority of cases it does not reflect fat. The high signal is most likely on the basis of high protein content.

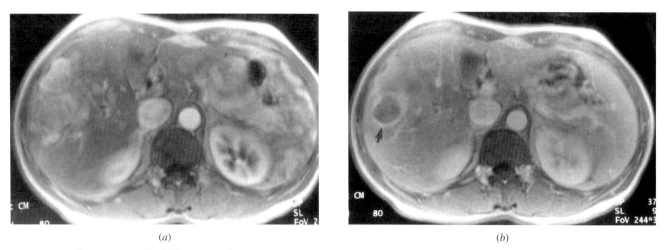

(a)   (b)

F I G . 2.114 Large poorly differentiated HCC. Immediate (*a*) and 45-s (*b*) postgadolinium SGE images demonstrate a large tumor in the right lobe of the liver. The tumor enhances in an intense heterogeneous fashion on the immediate postgadolinium images (*a*). Unlike well-differentiated HCCs, the margins are poorly defined. Capsular enhancement is present on the later postcontrast image (*b*), but of a portion (arrow, *b*) of the heterogenous tumor, unlike in well-differentiated HCCs, where the capsule circumscribes the entire lesion.

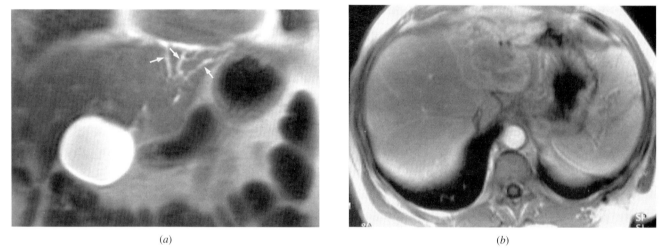

(a)   (b)

F I G . 2.115 Focal HCC with hepatic duct obstruction. Coronal T2-weighted SS-ETSE (*a*) and immediate postgadolinium SGE (*b*) images. There is a large lesion in the left hepatic lobe that demonstrates minimally hyperintense signal on T2-weighted images (*a*) and moderate heterogeneous enhancement immediately after gadolinium administration (*b*), consistent with a large HCC. Note that the mass causes ductal obstruction (arrows, *a*) of the biliary tree in *segment 2* of the left lobe.

HCCs are commonly hypervascular, and tumors >2 cm enhance in a diffuse heterogeneous fashion [54, 122, 123]. Therefore, the most sensitive sequence for detecting small HCCs is hepatic arterial dominant phase images in which small tumors will enhance intensely. However, this finding is not specific, because severely dysplastic nodules will also enhance intensely. A more specific feature is washout of tumor below the signal of liver at 2 min postcontrast with late enhancement of the pseudocapsule.

The appearance on hepatic arterial dominant phase gadolinium-enhanced images often permits distinction of HCC from metastatic disease because HCCs typically demonstrate enhancing stroma throughout the entire tumor (fig. 2.116), whereas metastases have peripheral enhancement [54]. The primary hepatic origin of HCC presumably results in a blood supply similar to and in continuity with background liver, explaining the early diffuse heterogeneous enhancement. The degree of vascularity of HCCs may vary substantially: the majority are hypervascular, but some neoplasms are very hypovascular [117]. Hypovascular tumors are variable in signal intensity on T1-weighted images but are nearly isointense on T2-weighted images, and these tumors are

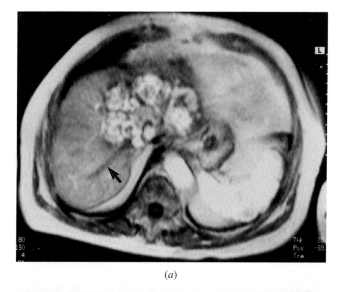

(a)

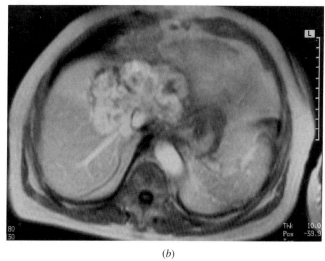

(b)

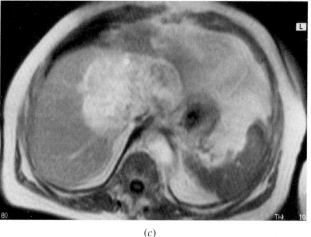

(c)

F I G . 2.116 Hepatocellular carcinoma, solitary hypervascular tumor. Immediate postgadolinium SGE (*a*), 90-s postgadolinium SGE (*b*), and 10-min postgadolinium SGE (*c*) images. An 8-cm tumor is present superiorly in the liver that demonstrates hypervascular diffuse heterogeneous enhancement on the immediate postgadolinium image (*a*). Hepatic veins are unopacified (arrow, *a*), confirming that image acquisition is in the hepatic arterial dominant phase of enhancement. On the 90-s postgadolinium image (*b*), the tumor becomes more homogeneous in enhancement. By 10 min (*c*), the tumor is homogeneously enhanced and remains high in signal intensity relative to liver. The heterogeneity of the diffuse enhancement on the immediate postcontrast image (*a*) is an important feature of malignant primary hepatocellular tumors that measure more than 3 cm in diameter and distinguishes them from benign tumors that enhance homogeneously.

frequently well differentiated [96, 117]. Lesion size and number are best evaluated on combined T1- and T2-weighted images, hepatic arterial dominant, and hepatic venous gadolinium-enhanced SGE images. All of these sequences are necessary because tumors vary in signal intensity on noncontrast images [54, 115, 117], and this combination of sequences increases observer confidence. Small tumors (<1.5 cm) are often only apparent on immediate postgadolinium SGE images (fig. 2.117). Margins in large poorly differentiated tumors are usually best seen on T2-weighted images and are less distinct on gadolinium-enhanced MR images.

Diffuse infiltration with HCC may be subtle or simulate the appearance of acute or chronic hepatitis or recent onset scarring on imaging studies. The most common appearance of diffuse infiltrative hepatocellular carcinoma is extensive hepatic parenchymal involvement with mottled, punctate high intensity on T2-weighted images and mottled, punctate intense enhancement on capillary-phase gadolinium-enhanced

images (fig. 2.118). The mottled liver texture is more readily appreciated on hepatic arterial dominant phase images. Diffuse infiltration may also appear as irregular linear strands that are hypo- to isointense on T1-weighted images and iso- to moderately hyperintense on T2-weighted images. On immediate postgadolinium images these tumor strands tend to enhance variably. Late increased enhancement of the tumor strands may reflect fibrous composition. Diffuse HCC almost always is associated with venous thrombosis. Diffuse HCC may also be invariably associated with a very high serum α-fetoprotein level.

Important ancillary features of HCC include venous thrombosis and late pseudocapsule enhancement. Tumor extension into portal veins occurs most frequently (figs. 2.119 and 2.120), but hepatic venous extension also occurs (fig. 2.121). Although, this feature is observed in fewer than 50% of cases, it is common with large and advanced tumors. Pseudocapsules are commonly observed in HCC, especially in early or well-differentiated

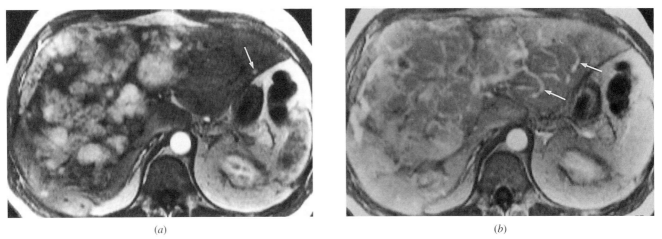

(a)   *(b)*

FIG. 2.117 Hypervascular HCC with small satellite tumors. Immediate postgadolinium SGE (*a*) and 90-s postgadolinium SGE (*b*) images. Intense diffuse heterogeneous enhancement of a 15-cm HCC is present on the immediate postgadolinium image (*a*). Multiple additional small HCCs are apparent including tumors as small as 3 mm (arrow, *a*). By 90 s after gadolinium (*b*), the large tumor has washed out in a heterogeneous fashion with prominent abnormal curvilinear hepatic veins apparent (arrows, *b*). The small HCC has become isointense with liver at this time.

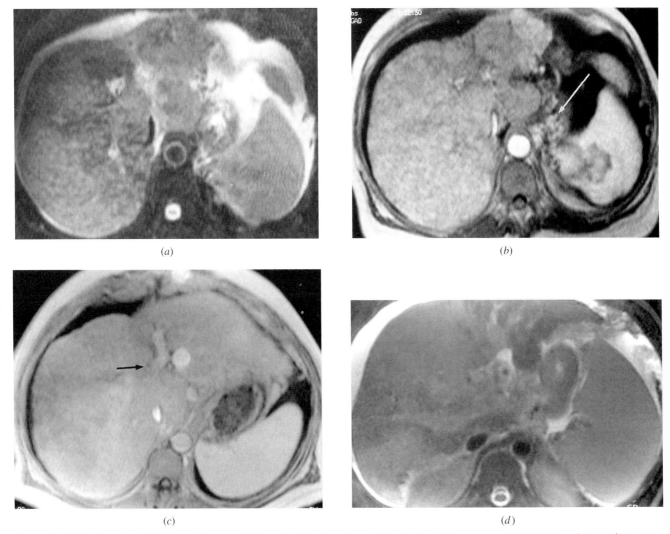

(a)   *(b)*

(c)   *(d)*

FIG. 2.118 Hepatocellular carcinoma, diffuse infiltrative type. T2-weighted fat-suppressed ETSE (*a*) and immediate post-gadolinium SGE (*b*) images. Mottled diffuse high signal intensity is present throughout the liver on the T2-weighted image (*a*).

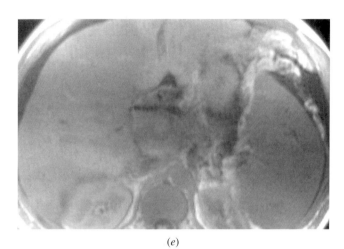
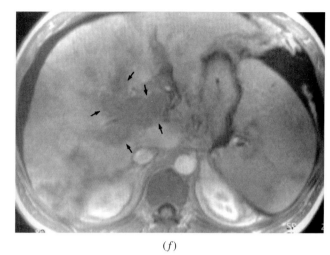

(e)   (f)

FIG. 2.118 (*Continued*) Diffuse mottled heterogeneous enhancement is appreciated on the immediate postgadolinium image (*b*). This findings represent diffuse infiltrative HCC. Mottled signal intensity is the most common MRI appearance for diffuse infiltrative HCC. Occasionally, diffuse infiltrative HCC will appear as low in signal intensity on T2-weighted images and very low in signal intensity on postgadolinium images. Prominent varices are present along the lesser curvature of the stomach (arrow, *b*).

Transverse 45-s postgadolinium SGE (*c*) in a second patient. There is a large heterogeneous region of mottled enhancement throughout the right lobe of the liver consistent with an infiltrating HCC. Note the irregularity of liver contour. Tumor thrombus of the right portal vein (arrow, *c*) is present.

Transverse T2-weighted fat-suppressed SS-ETSE (*d*), SGE (*e*), and immediate postgadolinium SGE (*f*) images in a third patient. The liver is diffusely heterogeneous in appearance with diffuse heterogeneous enhancement consistent with infiltrative HCC. The main, right, and left portal veins are distended with tumor thrombus (arrows, *f*). Note ascites and splenomegaly.

These cases illustrate the mottled heterogeneity of infiltrative HCC and that tumor thrombus in veins is almost invariably present. A third important feature is that α-fetoprotein is almost always extremely high.

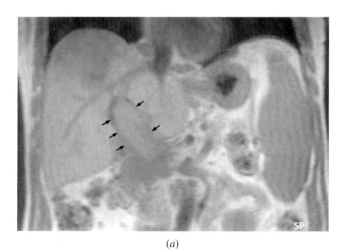
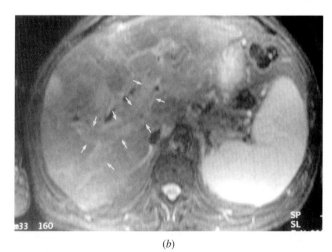

(a)   (b)

FIG. 2.119 Multifocal HCC with tumor thrombus. Coronal SGE (*a*), echo-train STIR (*b*), immediate postgadolinium SGE (*c*), and 90-s postgadolinium fat-suppressed SGE (*d*) images in a second patient. There are multiple irregular, ill-defined multifocal HCCs scattered throughout all hepatic segments that demonstrate mildly increased signal on T2 (*b*), mildly decreased signal on T1 (*a*), and heterogeneous enhancement on hepatic arterial dominant phase images (*c*), with late wash-out (*d*). The portal vein is expanded with tumor thrombus (arrows, *a, b, d*). The thrombus is not well seen on the immediate postgadolinium image (*c*), as it enhances in a comparable fashion to background liver. Late capsular enhancement of the multifocal HCCs is appreciated (*d*).

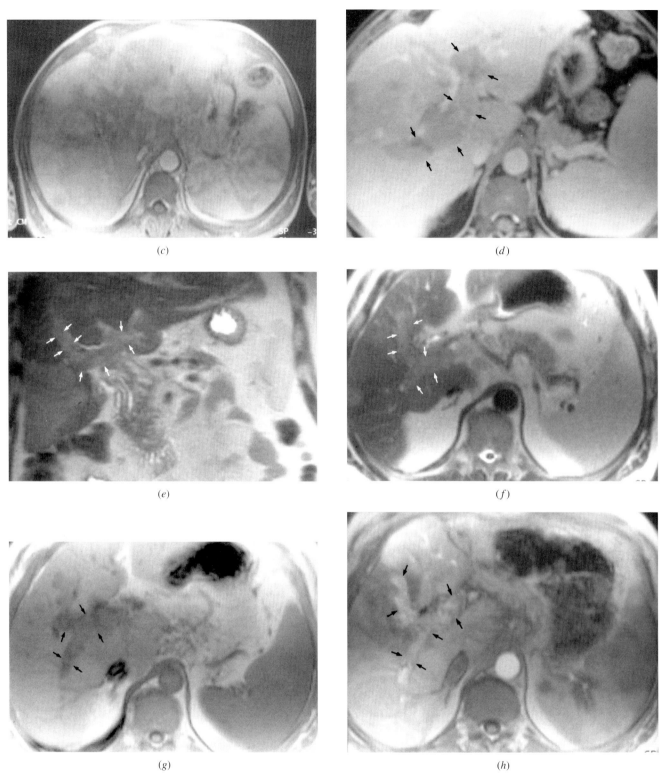

FIG. 2.119 (*Continued*) Coronal (*e*) and transverse (*f*) T2-weighted SS-ETSE, SGE (*g*), immediate postgadolinium SGE (*b*) and 90-s postgadolinium fat-suppressed SGE (*i, j, k, l*) images in a second patient. There is a large irregular mass occupying the majority of *segments* 5 and 6 of the right hepatic lobe, with tumor thrombus (small arrows, *e, f, g, b, i, j*) extending into the right, left, and main portal veins. Interstitial phase gadolinium-enhanced images clearly depict multiple lymph nodes (arrowheads, *i, j, k, l*).

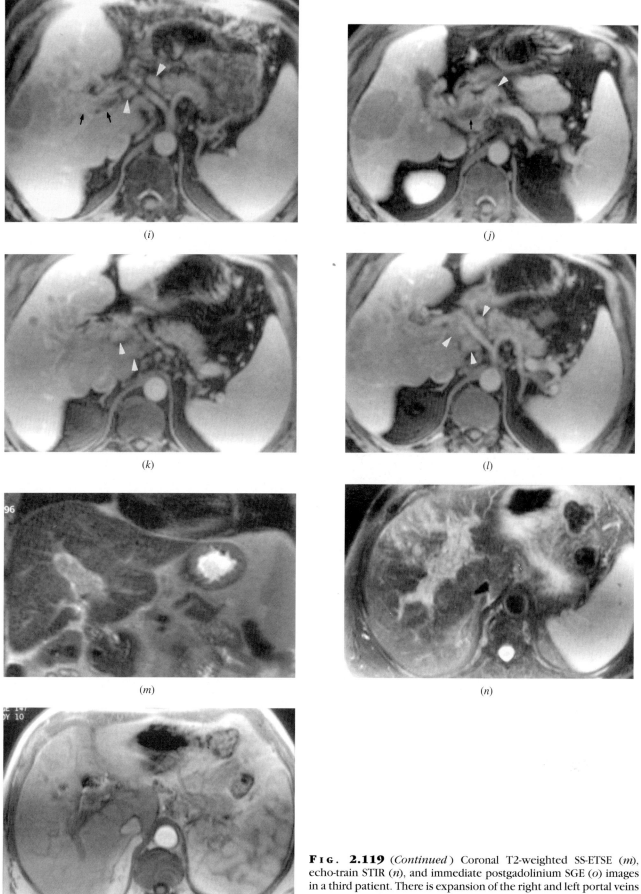

(i)

(j)

(k)

(l)

(m)

(n)

(o)

FIG. 2.119 (*Continued*) Coronal T2-weighted SS-ETSE (*m*), echo-train STIR (*n*), and immediate postgadolinium SGE (*o*) images in a third patient. There is expansion of the right and left portal veins consistent with tumor thrombus. Heterogeneous tumor is identified in *segment 4*.

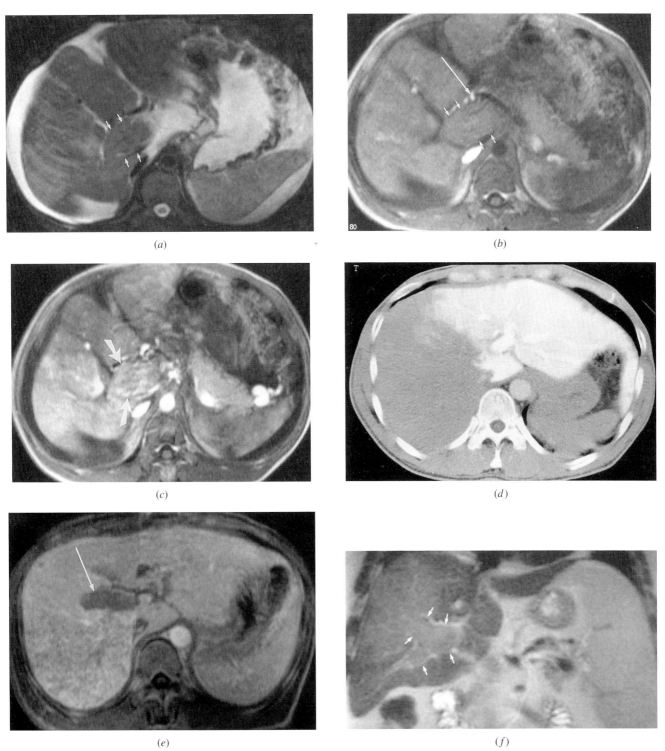

(a) *(b)*

(c) *(d)*

(e) *(f)*

F I G . 2.120 Diffuse hepatocellular carcinoma with portal vein thrombosis. T2-weighted fat-suppressed ETSE (*a*), SGE (*b*), and immediate postgadolinium SGE (*c*) images. The portal vein is expanded with tumor thrombus (small arrows, *a*, *b*), which is nearly isointense with liver on T2 (*a*) and T1 (*b*) images. Tumor thrombus enhances in a diffuse heterogeneous fashion (arrows, *c*) on the immediate postgadolinium image (*c*). The hepatic artery is identified as a small high-signal tubular structure on the precontrast and immediate postgadolinium SGE images (long arrow, *b*). Heterogeneous enhancement of the liver on the immediate postgadolinium image (*c*) reflects a combination of vascular abnormality from portal vein thrombosis and heterogeneous enhancement of diffusely infiltrative HCC. A substantial volume of ascites is present that is high in signal intensity on T2-weighted images (*a*) and low in signal intensity on pre- and postcontrast T1-weighted images (*b*, *c*).

Portal vein thrombosis in a second patient with diffuse HCC shown on spiral CTAP (*d*) and immediate postgadolinium SGE (*e*) images.

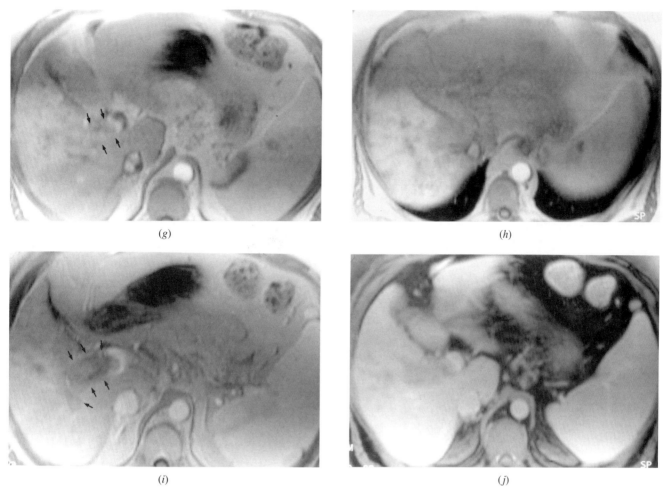

(g)

(h)

(i)

(j)

FIG. 2.120 (*Continued*) On the CTAP image (*d*), nonopacification of the right hemiliver due to thrombosis of the right portal vein is present. The immediate postgadolinium SGE image demonstrates a tumor thrombus that expands the right portal vein (arrow, *e*). Diffuse heterogeneous mottled enhancement of the right lobe of the liver is present on the MR image (*e*), which is a typical appearance for diffusely infiltrative HCC.

Coronal T2-weighted SS-ETSE (*f*), transverse immediate (*g*, *h*) and 45-s postgadolinium SGE (*i*), and 90-s postgadolinium fat-suppressed SGE (*j*) images. There is an infiltrative HCC in the right hepatic lobe that demonstrates slight high signal intensity on the T2-weighted image (*f*) and heterogeneous intense enhancement immediately after-gadolinium administration (*g*, *h*). The portal vein is expanded with tumor thrombus (arrows, *f*, *g*, *i*) that enhances in a diffuse fashion after contrast.

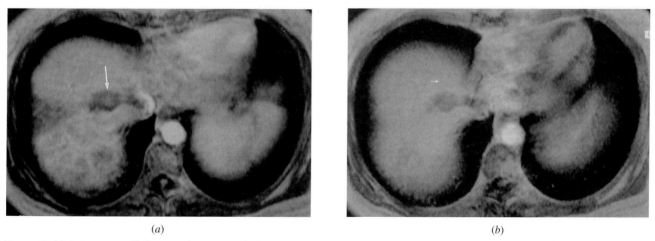

(a)

(b)

FIG. 2.121 Hepatocellular carcinoma with hepatic vein thrombosis. Transverse 45-s (*a*) and 90-s (*b*) postgadolinium SGE images. On the 45-s postgadolinium image (*a*) tumor thrombus is apparent in the middle hepatic vein as low signal intensity material that expands the vein (arrow, *a*).

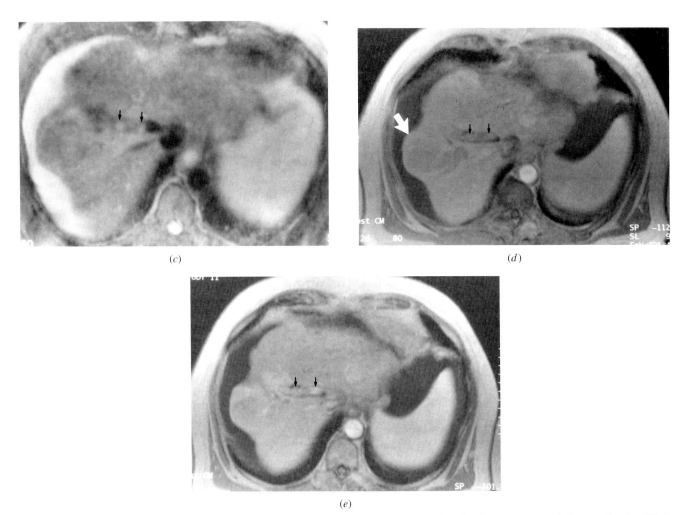

(c)

(d)

(e)

FIG. 2.121 (*Continued*) Diffuse heterogeneous enhancement is noted in the right lobe that represents diffuse infiltrative HCC. Distal to the thrombosed hepatic vein, a wedge-shaped perfusion defect is identified. On the 90-s image (*b*) the tumor thrombus maintains low signal intensity compared to liver. However, the perfusion defect resolved, and the diffuse HCC is more isointense with background liver.

T2-weighted fat-suppressed ETSE (*c*), SGE (*d*), and immediate postgadolinium SGE (*e*) images in a second patient. A 5-cm HCC (large arrow, *d*) is present in the right hepatic lobe that appears isointense on T2 (*c*) and T1 (*d*) images and exhibits minimal enhancement on hepatic arterial dominant phase images (*e*). A thin tumor capsule is identified on the precontrast T1-weighted image (*d*). In the middle hepatic vein there is an abnormal soft tissue with isointense signal intensity on T1- and T2-weighted images (arrows, *c, d, e*) and moderate enhancement after gadolinium administration (arrow, *e*). A perfusional abnormality adjacent to the middle hepatic vein is related to the presence of tumor thrombus. (Reproduced with permission from Kelekis NL, Semelka RC, Worawattanakul S, Lange EE, et al.; Hepatocellular carcinoma in North America: A multiinstitutional study of appearance on T1-weighted, T2-weighted, and serial gadolinium-enhanced gradient-echo Images. *Am J Roentgenol* 170: 1005–1013, 1998.)

tumors. The typical signal intensity of a pseudocapsule is hypointensity on T1-weighted images, minimal hyperintensity on T2-weighted images, low signal intensity on immediate postgadolinium images, and increased enhancement on delayed images [122]. Many HCCs will take up Mn-DPDP, and well-differentiated HCC may take up more Mn-DPDP than surrounding liver, reflecting persistent hepatocellular function with decreased biliary clearance [62, 75, 124].

Fibrolamellar Carcinoma. Fibrolamellar carcinoma is a distinct morphologic subtype of liver cell carcinoma. This tumor occurs in younger patients, frequently females, without underlying cirrhosis [119]. Fibrolamellar carcinoma is biologically distinct from other HCCs because it exhibits slow growth and is associated with a favorable prognosis [125]. From a pathologic viewpoint, the tumor is well defined and may show a lobular architecture with intervening fibrous septa or a central stellate scar. Microscopically, tumor cells are polygonal, large, and eosinophilic. An extensive meshwork of collagenous stroma incarcerating nests and sheets of tumor, is the sine qua non for pathologic diagnosis.

On imaging, fibrolamellar carcinomas are generally large, solitary tumors that are heterogeneous and moderately low in signal intensity on T1-weighted images and heterogeneous and moderately high in signal intensity on T2-weighted images. A huge central scar with radiating appearance is present. The central scar is vari-able in signal and has large low-signal components on T2-weighted images that enhance negligibly on delayed gadolinium-enhanced images. Enhancement of the tumor is diffuse heterogeneous and intense on immediate postgadolinium SGE images (fig. 2.122) [126]. On MR imaging, the scar is characterized by a complex arborizing pattern radiating from a central focus and extending out to tumor periphery. This profile is distinctly different from the appearance of FNH, in which the scar occupies a small central portion of the tumor and exhibits more uniform signal enhancement characteristics.

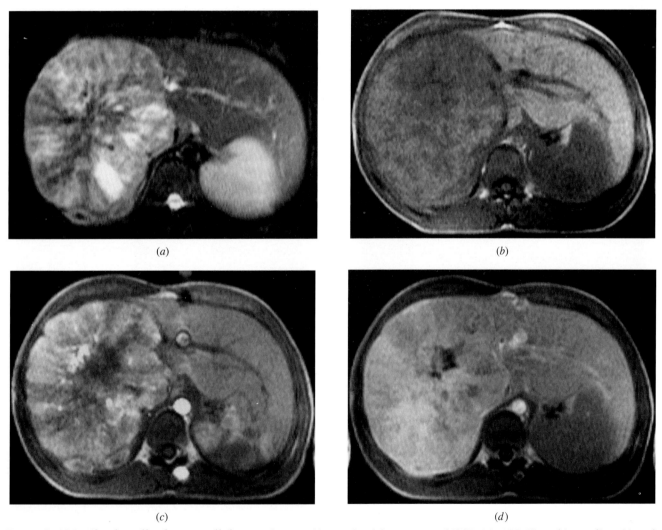

(a) (b) (c) (d)

F I G . 2.122 Fibrolamellar hepatocellular carcinoma. T2-weighted fat-suppressed ETSE (*a*), SGE (*b*) and immediate (*c*) and 10-min (*d*) postgadolinium SGE images. A 14-cm fibrolamellar hepatocellular carcinoma is present in this adolescent male with no history of liver disease and 1-yr duration of gynecomastia. The tumor is hypointense on the T1-weighted image with a low-signal intensity central scar (*b*) and heterogeneously hyperintense on the T2-weighted image (*a*) with the central radiating scar largely low in signal intensity. On the immediate postgadolinium SGE image (*c*), the tumor exhibits diffuse heterogeneous enhancement with negligible enhancement of the radiating scar. On the 10-min image (*d*), the bulk of the tumor has become isointense with background liver. Portions of the central scar are higher in signal intensity than surrounding tissue, whereas other parts remain low in signal. In contrast to FNH, the scar in fibrolamellar HCC is much larger and exhibits more heterogeneous signal on T2 and early and late postgadolinium images.

Intrahepatic or Peripheral Bile Duct Carcinoma (Cholangiocarcinoma). Intrahepatic or peripheral cholangiocarcinoma are terms applied to lesions that originate in the ducts proximal to (i.e., above) the hilum of the liver. Malignant tumors arising from the intrahepatic bile ducts are much less common than those arising from hepatocytes. Most cases of cholangiocarcinoma occur after the age of 60 years, and there is no association with cirrhosis. Pathologically, the tumor is generally better circumscribed and of firmer consistency than hepatocellular carcinoma. The microscopic picture is characterized by glandular configurations surrounded by abundant, dense fibrous stroma. The prominent sinusoidal pattern of HCC is not present. The tumor is frequently large at presentation [127]. Cholangiocarcinoma resembles HCC with low signal intensity on T1-weighted and moderate signal intensity on T2-weighted images [126]. High signal on T1-weighted images, pseudocapsule, and invasion into portal and hepatic veins are common with HCC and rarely seen with cholangiocarcinoma. Biliary and extrinsic portal vein obstruction are more common with cholangiocarcinoma. Enhancement with gadolinium varies from minimal to intense diffuse heterogeneous enhancement immediately after contrast administration (fig. 2.123). Minimal enhancement is most commonly observed. Persistent enhancement on delayed images is relatively common [128]. The intrahepatic origin of the tumor likely explains the early diffuse heterogeneous enhancement. (For a more complete description of cholangiocarcinoma, see Chapter 3, *Gallbladder and Biliary System*.)

Malignant tumors of mixed liver cell and bile duct differentiation are rare. Mixed HCC-cholangiocarcinoma may occur, and the imaging appearance is generally indistinguishable from that of HCC (fig. 2.124).

Biliary   Cystadenoma/Cystadenocarcinoma. Although rare, benign and malignant cystic tumors of biliary origin may arise in the liver. There is a peak incidence of these lesions in the fifth decade, with a great predominance of women. Pathologically, on gross inspection, tumors are typically large and multiloculated and filled with clear or mucinous fluid. Mural nodules

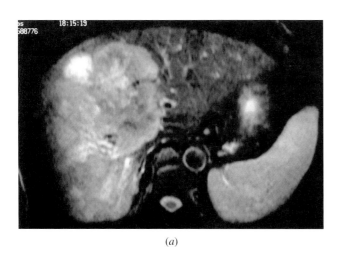

(a)

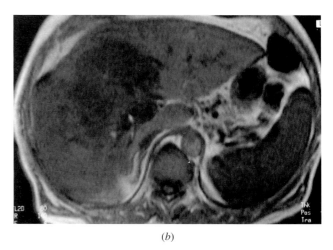

(b)

FIG. 2.123 Intrahepatic cholangiocarcinoma. T2-weighted fat-suppressed ETSE (*a*), SGE (*b*), and immediate postgadolinium SGE (*c*) images. A 14-cm tumor is present in the right lobe of the liver that is moderately high in signal intensity on the T2-weighted image (*a*) and moderately low in signal intensity on the T1-weighted image (*b*) and enhances in an intense diffuse heterogeneous fashion on the immediate postgadolinium SGE image (*c*). The appearance resembles that of an HCC.

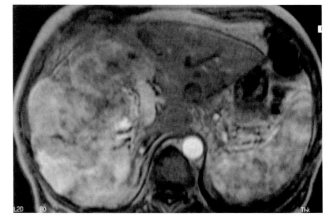

(c)

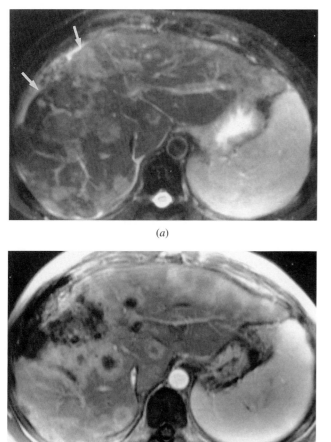

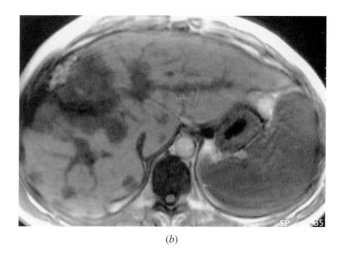

(a)

(b)

(c)

F I G . 2.124 Mixed HCC-cholangiocarcinoma. T2-weighted fat-suppressed ETSE (*a*), SGE (*b*), and immediate postgadolinium SGE (*c*) images. A large 14-cm tumor is centered in the medial segment, and multiple small satellite lesions are scattered throughout the remainder of the liver. The tumors are moderately high in signal on the T2-weighted image (*a*) and moderately low in signal intensity on the T1-weighted image (*b*) and enhance intensely immediately after gadolinium administration (*c*). Capsular retraction is also noted (arrows, *a*).

may be a component of some cysts. Histologically, cystic and stromal components are present to variable degrees. Malignant lesions will exhibit pronounced cytologic atypia with evidence of stromal invasion [61, 129–131].

On imaging, these tumors frequently have solid nodules associated with cystic components (fig. 2.125) [132]. Occasionally, mucin content renders these tumors high in signal intensity on T1-weighted images [61, 131]. Solid components of the tumor demonstrate early heterogeneous enhancement in a pattern consistent with tumors of hepatic origin. Enhancement is often minimal in intensity, distinguishing these tumors from the extensive enhancement of HCC.

Angiosarcoma. Angiosarcoma is the most common sarcoma arising in the liver and accounts for 1.8% of all liver cancers. An increased risk for the development of this tumor in adults has been documented in the following settings: 1) cirrhosis, 2) vinyl chloride exposure, 3) thorium dioxide exposure (thorotrast) for ra-

diographic purposes, and 4) arsenic exposure [133]. This tumor is usually encountered in middle-aged patients and occurs more commonly in men. Pathologically, angiosarcomas appear most commonly as multicentric nodules diffusely involving the liver. Occasionally, tumor may present as a solitary, large mass. Microscopically, angiosarcoma is characterized by ill-defined clusters of malignant endothelial cells lining and expanding the sinusoids. Internal hemorrhage is relatively common. Angiosarcoma may be high signal intensity on T2-weighted images [134] and demonstrate peripheral nodular enhancement with centripetal progression, mimicking the appearance of hemangioma (fig. 2.126). The frequent presence of hemorrhage, which results in heterogeneous low signal intensity on T2-weighted images, and lack of central enhancement due to hemorrhage are distinguishing features [135].

Hemangioendothelioma. **Infantile hemangioendothelioma** are congenital lesions and the most common mesenchymal tumor of the liver in childhood

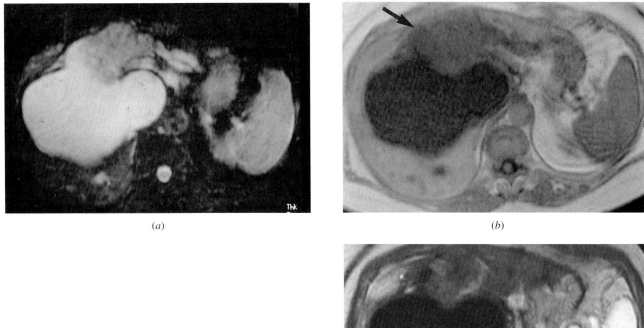

(a)

(b)

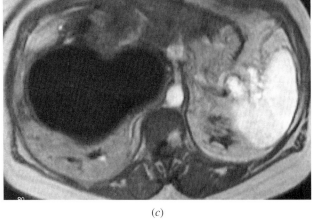

(c)

F I G . 2.125 Biliary cystadenoma. T2-weighted fat-suppressed ETSE (*a*), SGE (*b*), and immediate postgadolinium SGE (*c*) images. A large cystic mass with a 5-cm solid nodular component (arrow, *b*) is present in the liver. The nodular component is moderately hyperintense on the T2-weighted image (*a*) and slightly hypointense on the T1-weighted image (*b*) and enhances in a diffuse heterogeneous fashion on the immediate postgadolinium image (*c*). Diffuse heterogeneous enhancement on immediate postgadolinium images is a feature of tumors of hepatic origin.

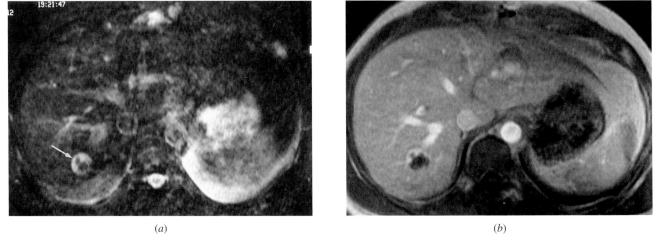

(a)

(b)

F I G . 2.126 Angiosarcoma. T2-weighted fat-suppressed ETSE (*a*) and 90-s (*b*) and 10-min (*c*) postgadolinium SGE images. A 2-cm angiosarcoma is present in the right lobe of the liver. The mass is well defined and largely hyperintense on the T2-weighted image (arrow, *a*) with a central region of low signal intensity due to hemorrhage. On the 90-s postgadolinium image (*b*), peripheral nodular enhancement is present. By 10 min after contrast (*c*), nodular enhancement has progressed centripetally, with a central nonenhanced area that corresponds to the region of hemorrhage on the T2-weighted image. Angiosarcomas mimic the appearance of hemangiomas.

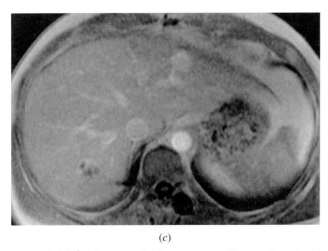

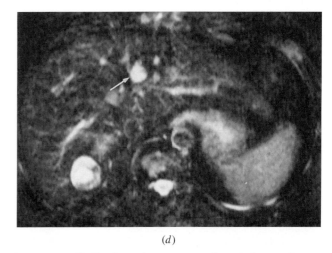

(c)   (d)

F i g . 2.126 (*Continued*) The presence of hemorrhage in this case is a common finding in angiosarcomas and rare in hemangiomas. Interval increase in size of this tumor is identified on a follow-up study obtained 1 month later, shown on T2-weighted fat-suppressed SS-ETSE (*d*). Increase in size of a second tumor is also present. Rapid growth is compatible with angiosarcomas and not with hemangiomas. A change in the signal intensity of the larger mass on the T2-weighted image (*d*) is also noted between studies because of aging of the central hemorrhage.

[1–36]. Although infantile hemangioendothelioma are histologically benign, they frequently lead to death within 6 months secondary to heart or liver failure. Spontaneous regression of the lesions tend to occur after 8 months of age [59, 137]. Pathologic examination shows a multicentric tumor involving both lobes. Microscopically, numerous dilated vascular channels are lined by

multiple layers of plump endothelial cells. Cavernous, vascular channels are frequent.

On imaging, these lesions tend to be numerous similar-size tumors that are uniformly hyperintense on T2-weighted images and enhance homogeneously on interstitial-phase gadolinium-enhanced images (fig. 2.127).

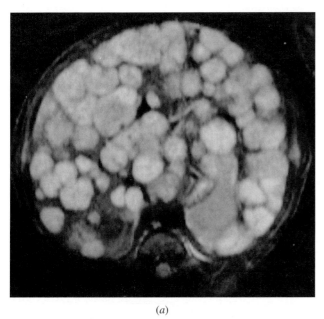

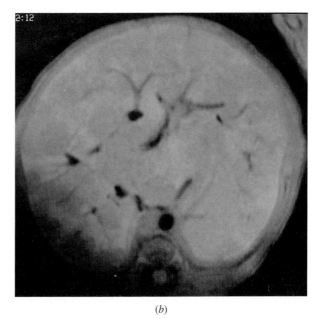

(a)   (b)

F i g . 2.127 Infantile hemangioendothelioma. T2-weighted fat-suppressed ETSE (*a*), T1-weighted fat-suppressed SE (*b*), and T1-weighted interstitial-phase gadolinium-enhanced fat-suppressed SE (*c*) images. The liver in this 9-month-old boy is extensively replaced with focal mass lesions, smaller than 1 cm, that are high in signal intensity on the T2-weighted image (*a*) and mildly low in signal intensity on the T1-weighted image (*b*) and that enhance homogeneously on the interstitial-phase gadolinium-enhanced image (*c*). This appearance is characteristic for hemangioendothelioma in neonatal patients.

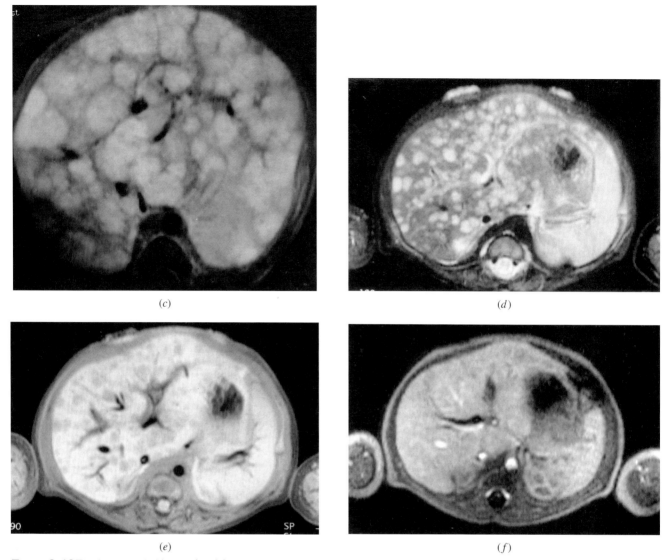

(c)

(d)

(e)

(f)

FIG. 2.127 (*Continued*) T2-weighted fat-suppressed ETSE (*d*), T1-weighted fat-suppressed SE (*e*), and T1-weighted immediate postgadolinium magnetization-prepared gradient-echo (*f*) images in a second patient who is 2 years old. The liver has multiple small foci of increased signal on T2-weighted images (*d*), decreased signal on T1-weighted images (*e*), and intense uniform or nodular enhancement after administration of gadolinium, consistent with infantile hemangioendothelioma.

Epithelioid hemangioendotheliomas are malignant, slow-growing tumors, usually occurring in middle-aged patients. Pathologically, lesions tend to be multiple, distributed throughout the liver [134]. Microscopically, malignant tumor cells infiltrate the sinusoids, central vein, and portal vein branches. Tumors tend to be low-grade malignancies. These tumors are heterogeneous in signal intensity on T2-weighted images and demonstrate irregular rim or diffuse heterogeneous enhancement on immediate postgadolinium images. The appearance is similar to that of hepatocellular carcinoma, particularly in tumors with aggressive growth patterns (fig. 2.128).

Hepatoblastoma. Hepatoblastoma is the most common primary malignant tumor of the liver in children and may occur in the newborn to adolescent patient and older. The tumor is most often detected or 3 years of age, with a median age of 1 year. In the mid-teens, the most common primary malignant tumor changes from hepatoblastoma to hepatocellular carcinoma. Hepatoblastoma occurs more often in boys than in girls with a ratio of 3:2. On gross inspection, hepatoblastoma is a solid, well-defined, occasionally lobulated mass surrounded by a pseudocapsule. Although it is usually solitary, multiple lesions can be seen in less than 20%

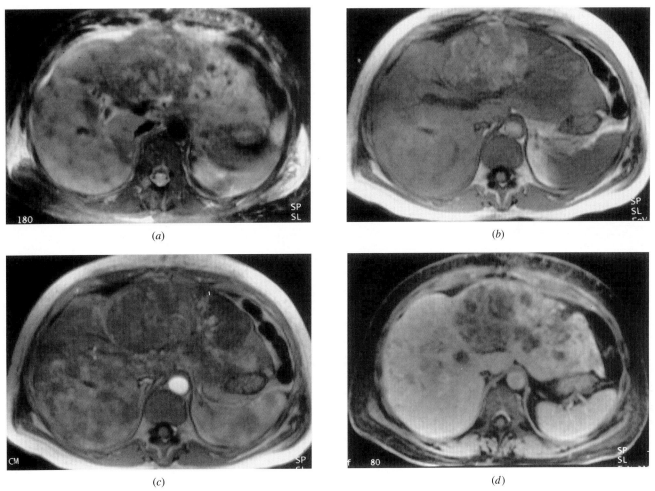

(a)

(b)

(c)

(d)

F I G. 2.128 Epithelioid hemangioendotheliosarcoma. T2-weighted fat-suppressed ETSE (*a*), SGE (*b*), immediate postgadolinium SGE (*c*), and 90-s postgadolinium fat-suppressed SGE (*d*) images in an adult patient with epithelioid hemangioendotheliosarcoma. Extensive liver involvement with a multifocal malignant epithelioid hemangioendotheliosarcoma is present. The tumor is heterogeneous and isointense to minimally hyperintense on the T2-weighted image (*a*). Regions of high signal intensity are present in the largest mass on the T1-weighted image (*b*). Enhancement is diffuse heterogeneous on the immediate postgadolinium image (*c*), with heterogeneous wash-out on the 90-s postcontrast image (*d*). The MRI appearance of this epitheloid hemangioendotheliosarcoma resembles HCC.

of cases. Areas of necrosis and calcifications are frequently present [137].

On MR imaging, hepatoblastoma resembles hepatocellular carcinoma in that tumors show diffuse heterogeneous enhancement on immediate postgadolinium images (fig. 2.129)

Posttreatment Malignant Liver Lesions

Malignant liver lesions may be treated by a number of interventions, including surgical resection, intravenous chemotherapy, intra-arterial chemotherapy, alcohol injection, cryotherapy, radiofrequency ablation,

and chemoembolization [138–156]. The appearance of hepatic parenchyma and malignant liver lesions after therapeutic interventions has been described. However, studies involving large series and serial posttreatment imaging are few in number [140–147, 149, 151–155] and have not included dynamic gadolinium-enhanced SGE imaging. In the evaluation of the posttreatment liver, the time course of benign posttreatment tissue changes, primarily tissue injury and granulation tissue, and the appearance of persistent or recurrent disease must be ascertained. As with postradiation or postsurgical changes in other tissues and organ systems, the distinction between benign and malignant disease usually can be

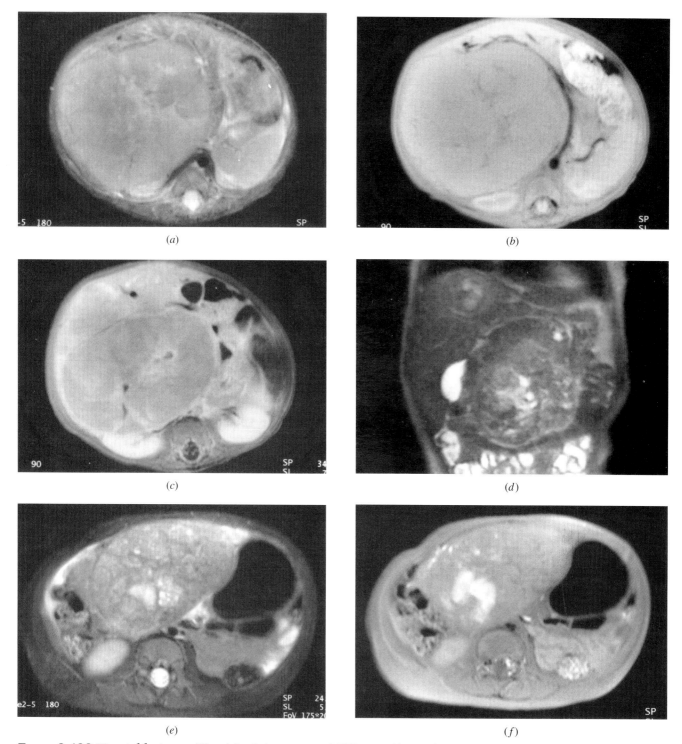

(a)

(b)

(c)

(d)

(e)

(f)

FIG. 2.129 Hepatoblastoma. T2-weighted fat-suppressed ETSE (*a*), T1-weighted fat-suppressed SE (*b*), and T1-weighted interstitial-phase gadolinium-enhanced fat-suppressed SE (*c*) images in a 2-month-old boy. There is a large, slightly lobulated mass arising from the liver, which demonstrates slightly increased signal intensity on T2 (*a*), mildly decreased signal intensity on T1 (*b*), and mildly heterogeneous enhancement on interstitial-phase gadolinium-enhanced images (*c*). Note that the mass displaces the celiac axis, the right kidney, aorta, inferior vena cava, and pancreas.

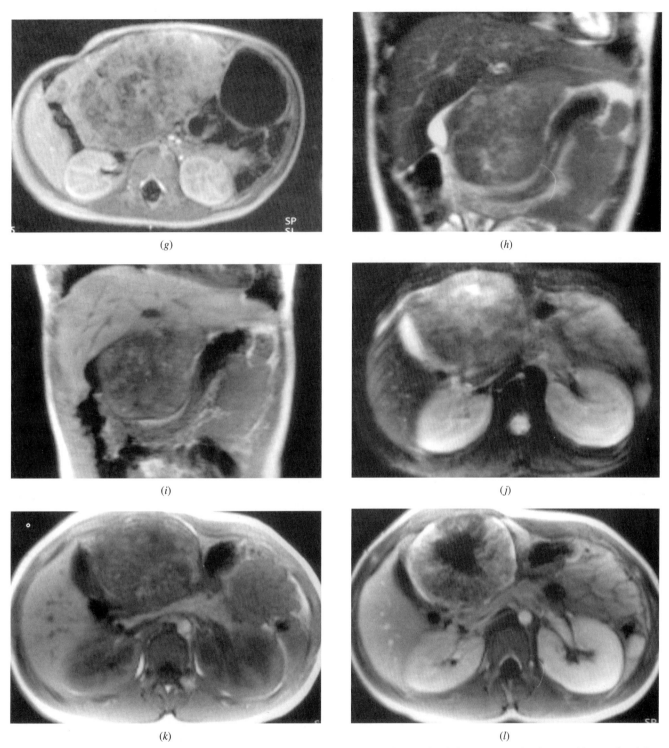

F I G . 2.129 (*Continued*) Coronal T2-weighted SS-ETSE (*d*), transverse T2-weighted fat-suppressed ETSE (*e*), T1-weighted fat-suppressed SE (*f*) and immediate postgadolinium SE (*g*) images in a second patient with hepatoblastoma, who is 1 year old. There is a large mass arising from the left hepatic lobe inferiorly, which demonstrates heterogeneous signal on T2 (*d, e*) and T1 (*f*) images. On the T1-weighted image (*f*) there are also several focal areas of high signal consistent with hemorrhage. The tumor enhances in a diffuse heterogeneous fashion (*g*).

Coronal T2-weighted SS-ETSE (*h*), coronal SGE (*i*), T2-weighted fat-suppressed SS-ETSE (*j*), SGE (*k*), immediate postgadolinium SGE (*l*), and 90-s postgadolinium fat-suppressed SGE (*m*) in a 14-year-old girl. There is a large tumor that is heterogeneous and moderately hyperintense on T2 (*h, j*). The tumor shows diffuse heterogeneous enhancement on immediate postgadolinium images (*l*), which fades by 90 s (*m*). The central region does not enhance, consistent with fibrous tissue.

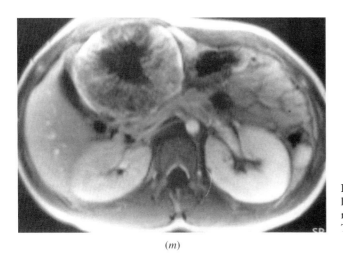

(m)

FIG. 2.129 (*Continued*) The most common primary liver malignancy changes from hepatoblastoma to hepatocellular carcinoma in the adolescent period between 14 and 16 years of age. This last patient is at the upper age range of hepatoblastoma.

made with certainty beyond 1 year after treatment. At this time point, benign disease usually exhibits regular or linear margins, low signal intensity on T2-weighted images, and minimal enhancement. In comparison, malignant disease tends to appear more irregular, nodular, or masslike, with moderately high signal intensity on T2-weighted images and moderate enhancement. Immediate postgadolinium images effectively define pathophysiological changes that reflect successful response or recurrence. Certain features of treatment-related changes depend on the form of therapy. The following discussion describes some of those features.

Resection

After resection, malignancy may recur along the margin of resection or separate focal lesions may develop in the remainder of the liver [146, 147, 149, 151–155].

Tumor development along the resection margin is a common mode of recurrence of hepatocellular carcinoma or metastases after resection (figs. 2.130 and 2.131). After approximately 3 months, the immediate postsurgical changes of moderately high signal intensity on T2-weighted images and mild ill-defined enhancement on early postgadolinium SGE images, present in a linear distribution along the resection margin, begin to resolve. Tumor recurrence, in distinction, has a nodular margin that is moderately high in signal intensity on T2-weighted images and exhibits moderately intense early enhancement on postgadolinium images. These features progress over time.

Development of separate focal lesions occurs more commonly in the setting of surgical resection for metastatic disease. These lesions appear identical to untreated malignant lesions.

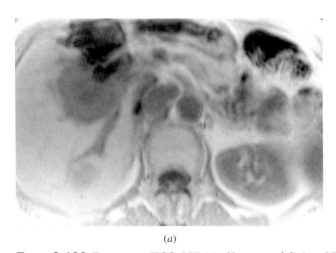

(a)

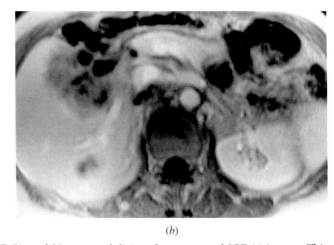

(b)

FIG. 2.130 Recurrent HCC. SGE (*a*), 45-s postgadolinium SGE (*b*), and 90-s postgadolinium fat-suppressed SGE (*c*) images. This patient had previously undergone a left hepatic lobe resection for HCC. There are multiple lesions throughout the right lobe, all of which appear low signal on T1-weighted images (*a*) and exhibit peripheral enhancement after-gadolinium (*b*, *c*) consistent with recurrent disease. Note the large volume of tumor along the resection margin consistent with incomplete excision.

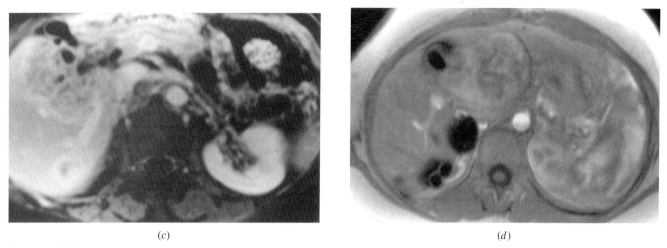

(c) (d)

F I G . 2.130 (*Continued*) Immediate postgadolinium SGE (*d*) image in a second patient with a history of HCC and left hepatectomy. There is a large mass that enhances heterogeneously on immediate postgadolinium images consistent with recurrent HCC. The recurrence is along the resection margin compatible with incomplete excision. Note the surgical clips along the free liver edge from prior resection.

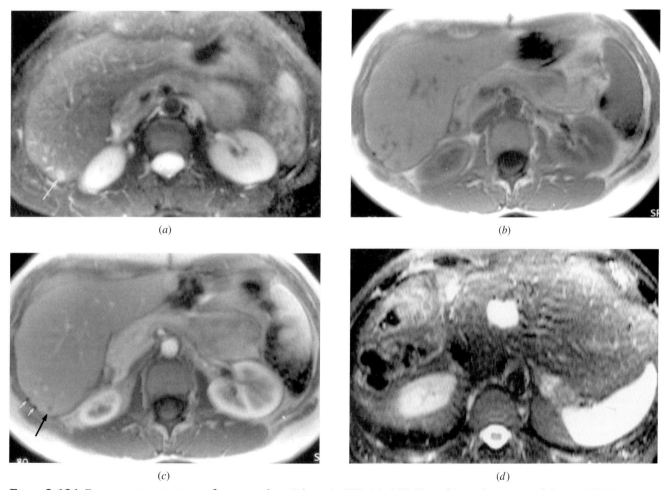

(a) (b)

(c) (d)

F I G . 2.131 Recurrent metastases after resection. Echo-train STIR (*a*), SGE (*b*), and immediate postgadolinium SGE (*c*) images in a patient who has a history of colon cancer and previous resection of liver metastases. There is a small lesion that demonstrates moderately high signal on T2 (arrow, *a*), mildly low signal on T1 (*b*), and ring enhancement (arrow, *c*) after gadolinium administration, consistent with a recurrent metastasis. Note the surgical clips (small arrows, *c*) adjacent to the lesion.

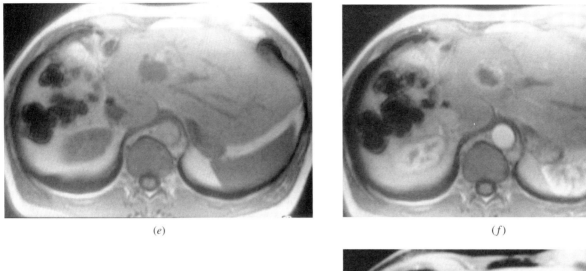

(e)   (f)

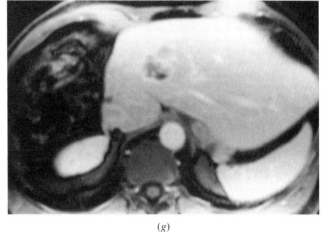

Fig. 2.131 (*Continued*) Echo-train STIR (*d*), SGE (*e*), immediate postgadolinium SGE (*f*), and 90-s postgadolinium fat-suppressed SGE (*g*) images in a second patient, who has a history of gastrointestinal stromal sarcoma and right hepatectomy 15 months prior for liver metastasis. There is a lesion in the left lobe that demonstrates high signal on T2 (*d*), low signal on T1 (*e*), peripheral ring enhancement immediately after gadolinium administration (*f*), and slight progression of enhancement on the late image (*g*).

(g)

Intravenous Chemotherapy

A number of chemotherapeutic agents are currently utilized in the treatment of focal liver lesions. The number of agents and their cytotoxic effectiveness for the treatment of malignant disease continue to progress dramatically. At present, commonly used chemotherapeutic regimens for the treatment of liver metastases are 5-fluorouracil based. The mechanisms of tumor cell control are complex and probably involve a number of pathways. Recent research has focused on the antiangiogenesis of some of these agents.

The time course and variation in appearance of metastases that have responded to chemotherapy have not been fully elucidated. One report described the appearance of liver metastases treated by intravenous chemotherapy in 34 patients on serial MRI studies [141]. In that report, a good prognosis was associated with increased signal intensity of the lesions on T1-weighted images and decreased signal intensity on T2-weighted images, essentially approaching the signal intensity of liver. A poor prognosis was reflected by decreased signal intensity on T1-weighted images and increased signal intensity on T2-weighted images. Metastases that do not respond grow in size. Features of mild response may be stability of lesion size and signal intensity on T2-weighted, precontrast, and postcontrast T1-weighted images.

We have previously described the appearance of liver metastases 2–7 months after initiation of chemotherapy [108]. In that report, liver metastases became more well-defined and higher in signal intensity on T2-weighted images, showing peripheral nodular enhancement with progressive enhancement and hyperintensity relative to liver on 10-min delayed images (figs. 2.132–2.134). The appearance was considered to mimic that of hemangiomas. Explanations for this change in appearance are related to altered physiology and blood supply of metastatic tumors treated with chemotherapy. The less aggressive enhancement patterns of metastasis postchemotherapy might be ascribed to

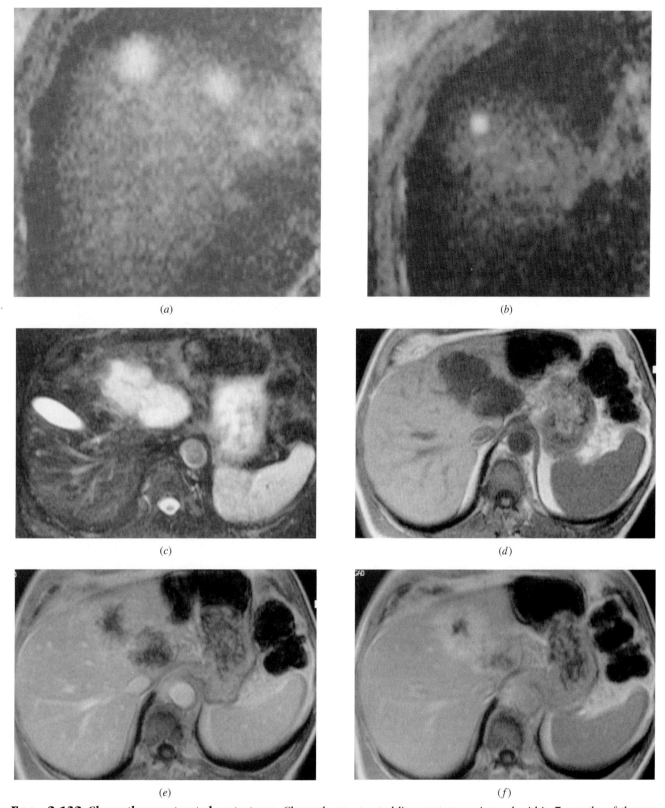

F I G . 2.132 Chemotherapy-treated metastases. Chemotherapy-treated liver metastases imaged within 7 months of therapy initiation. T2-weighted fat-suppressed ETSE image before chemotherapy (*a*) and T2-weighted fat-suppressed ETSE image 3 months after initiation of chemotherapy (*b*).

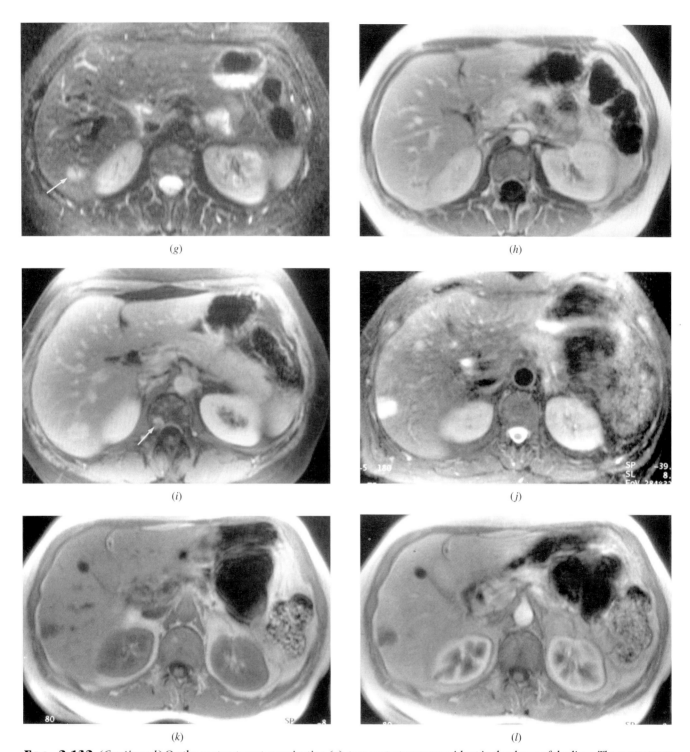

(g)

(h)

(i)

(j)

(k)

(l)

F I G . 2.132 (*Continued*) On the pretreatment examination (*a*), two metastases are evident in the dome of the liver. The metastases have slightly ill-defined margins and are moderate in signal intensity. The large metastasis measures 1.5 cm and the smaller 1 cm. Three months after initiation of chemotherapy, the larger metastasis has decreased in size to 4 mm, has well-defined margins, and is hyperintense on the T2-weighted image (*b*).

T2-weighted fat-suppressed SS-ETSE (*c*), SGE (*d*), 90-s (*e*), and 10-minute postgadolinium SGE (*f*) images in a second patient demonstrate two 4 cm metastases. The metastases are well defined, high in signal intensity on the T2-weighted image (*c*), and low in signal intensity on the T1-weighted image (*d*), and demonstrate peripheral irregular enhancement (*e*) that progresses centripetally. The lesions appear hyperintense relative to the liver with a low-signal intensity central scar at 10 min (*f*).

In both patients, the appearance of these subacute treated metastases (2–7 months after initiation of chemotherapy) mimics the appearance of hemangiomas. History of chemotherapy treatment for liver metastasis is critical to obtain in patients with lesions that resemble hemangiomas.

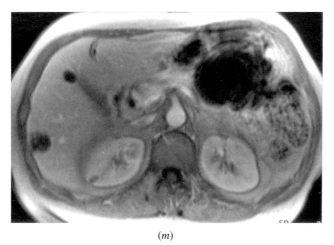

(m)

FIG. 2.132 (*Continued*) Echo-train STIR (*g*), 45-s postgadolinium SGE (*h*), and 90-s postgadolinium fat-suppressed SGE (*i*) images in a patient who has a history of liver metastases from breast cancer, treated with chemotherapy 2 years before MR imaging. There is a lesion in the right hepatic lobe that demonstrates high signal on T2 (arrow, *g*), peripheral ring enhancement on the 45-s image (*h*), and complete fill-in on the delayed image (*i*), consistent with a subacute chemotherapy treated metastasis with features suggestive of hemangioma. Note also multiple bone metastases (arrow, *i*).

Echo-train STIR (*j*), SGE (*k*), and immediate (*l*) and 45-s postgadolinium SGE (*m*) images in a patient who has liver metastases from ovarian cancer. A lobular high-signal lesion is present in the right hepatic lobe that demonstrates high signal on T2 (*j*), low signal intensity on T1-weighted image (*k*), negligible enhancement immediately after gadolinium administration (*l*), and small central nodules on the 45-s image (*m*).

chemo-induced tumor antiangiogenesis. Continued resolution of metastatic lesions results in a progressive decrease in a signal intensity on T2-weighted images and progressive decrease in contrast enhancement (fig. 2.135).

The appearance of chronic healed metastases is comparable to the appearance of treated focal lesions of other causes, such as infection. The chronic healed phase of lesion response usually develops at least 1.5 years after initiation of treatment. Chronic healed

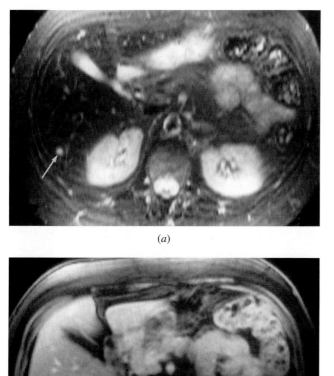

(a)

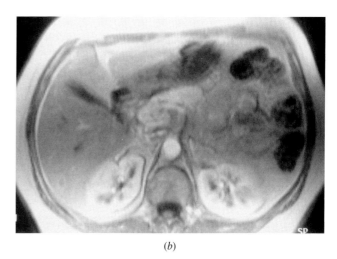

(b)

(c)

FIG. 2.133 Metastases from breast cancer—postchemotherapy. Echo-train STIR (*a*), immediate postgadolinium SGE (*b*), and 90-s postgadolinium fat-suppressed SGE (*c*) images. There is a small lesion in the right lobe that exhibits high signal on T2 (arrow, *a*) and ring enhancement on the immediate postgadolinium image (*b*), and persists on the late image (*c*). High signal on T2-weighted images is an early response (<1 year) to chemotherapy.

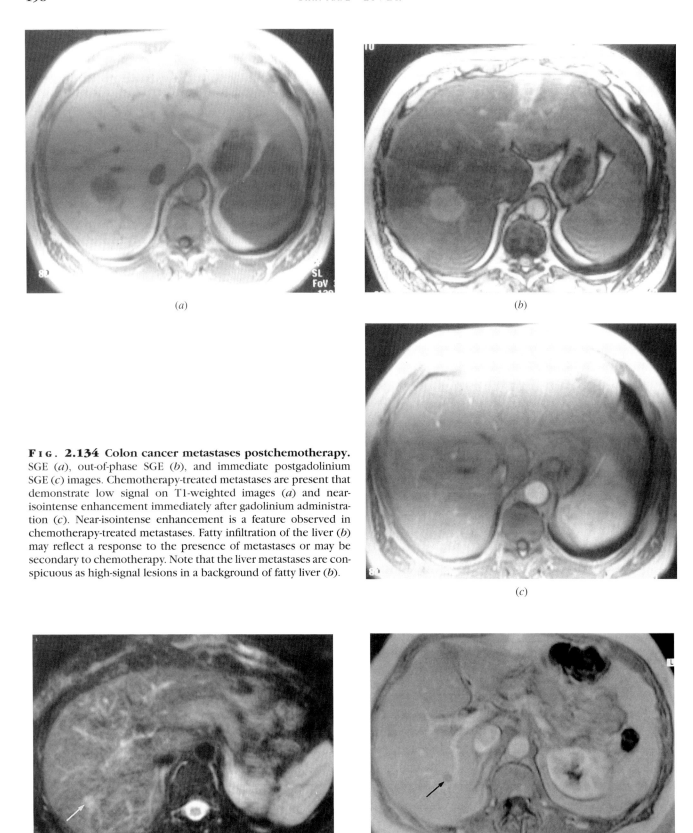

FIG. 2.134 Colon cancer metastases postchemotherapy. SGE (*a*), out-of-phase SGE (*b*), and immediate postgadolinium SGE (*c*) images. Chemotherapy-treated metastases are present that demonstrate low signal on T1-weighted images (*a*) and near-isointense enhancement immediately after gadolinium administration (*c*). Near-isointense enhancement is a feature observed in chemotherapy-treated metastases. Fatty infiltration of the liver (*b*) may reflect a response to the presence of metastases or may be secondary to chemotherapy. Note that the liver metastases are conspicuous as high-signal lesions in a background of fatty liver (*b*).

FIG. 2.135 Liver metastases, chronic, (11 years) postchemotherapy treatment. T2-weighted fat-suppressed ETSE (*a*) and immediate postgadolinium SGE (*b*) images. A 7-mm lesion is present in the right lobe of the liver that is minimally hyperintense on the T2-weighted image (arrow, *a*) and that demonstrates negligible enhancement on the immediate postgadolinium SGE image (arrow, *b*).

lesions possess an irregular, angular, polygonal margin frequently associated with retraction of surrounding liver parenchyma. In superficial lesions, capsule retraction may develop, creating a puckered appearance on imaging studies. Chronic healed lesions contain mature fibrous tissue that has a low fluid content and is hypovascular. These lesions appear as low signal intensity on T1-weighted images (moderately hypointense with liver) and low signal intensity on T2-weighted images (negligibly hypointense to isointense with liver). They exhibit negligible early enhancement (substantially hypointense to liver) with progressive enhancement on later postcontrast images (isointense to moderately hyperintense). The fibrotic process of chronic healed metastases may be very extensive in the presence of numerous liver metastases, such that a hepatic cirrhosis-type liver appearance may develop [145, 147]. The fact that this is most commonly observed in breast cancer reflects that metastases can be extremely numerous with a diffuse miliary pattern as well as fact that breast cancer metastases are among the metastases that respond best to chemotherapy (fig. 2.136).

During the course of chemotherapy, lesions develop acute granulation tissue that may mask the appearance of coexistent viable tumor. Successful resolution of metastases should not be considered until lesions are in the chronic healed phase.

Alcohol Injection/Cryotherapy/Radiofrequency Ablation

Alcohol injection, cryotherapy, and radiofrequency ablation (figs. 2.137–2.139) have been employed to ablate focal lesions by localized nonspecific cytotoxicity [142]. Immediately after treatment, a necrotic cavity is created, which develops an enhancing rim of granulation tissue. With successful treatment, shrinkage of the cavity develops in the subacute phase by tissue retraction and gradual growth of granulation tissue into the space. Response to alcohol injection has been described using MRI [140, 142, 144]. On MR images, tumors that are successfully ablated exhibit a regular, smoothly contoured thin rim of inflammatory tissue that enhances substantially on immediate postgadolinium images (fig. 2.140). This appearance persists for approximately 3 months, after which progressive decrease in rim enhancement and lesion size occurs. In contrast, residual tumor is manifested as a thickened, irregularly

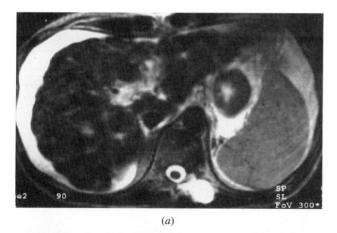

(a)

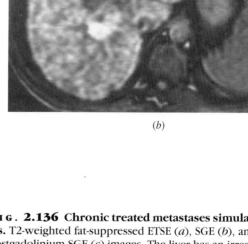

(b)

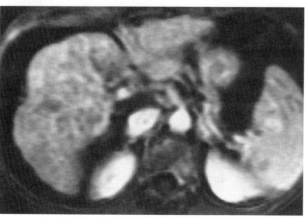

(c)

F I G . 2.136 Chronic treated metastases simulating cirrhosis. T2-weighted fat-suppressed ETSE (*a*), SGE (*b*), and immediate postgadolinium SGE (*c*) images. The liver has an irregular contour and contains multiple irregular linear structures that are high in signal on T2 (*a*) and T1 (*b*) images and enhance after contrast administration (*c*). Ascites is also present. The extensive hepatic fibrosis resembles cirrhosis. This appearance is most commonly observed in patients with breast cancer who have a miliary pattern of liver metastases that have responded to chemotherapy, resulting in extensive fibrous tissue (Courtesy of Susan M. Ascher, M.D., Dept. of Radiology, Georgetown University Medical Center.)

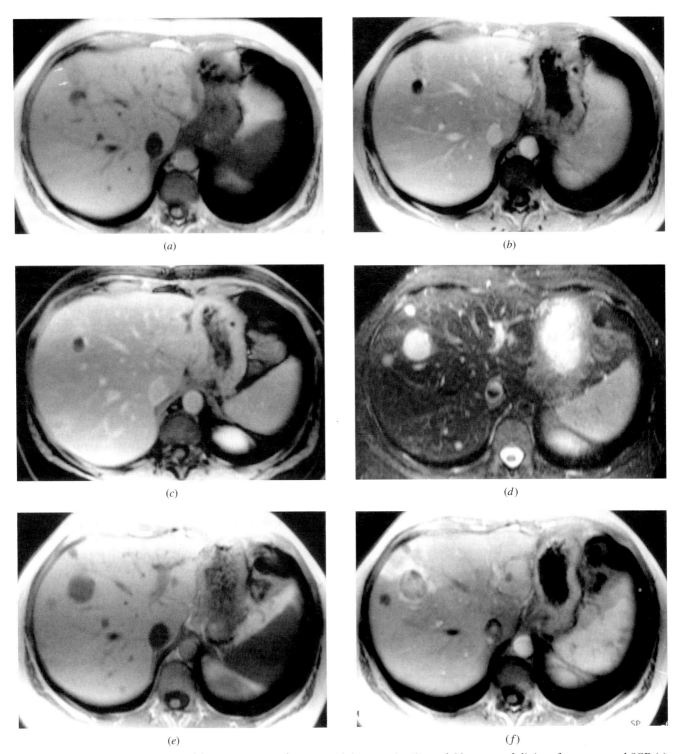

(a)

(b)

(c)

(d)

(e)

(f)

F I G . 2.137 Radiofrequency ablation. SGE (*a*), 45-s postgadolinium SGE (*b*), and 90-s postgadolinium fat-suppressed SGE (*c*) images in a patient, who has a history of liver metastasis from retroperitoneal leiomyosarcoma and has been treated with radiofrequency ablation. There is a rounded lesion in the right hepatic lobe that demonstrates low signal on T1 (*a*), negligible enhancement immediately after gadolinium administration (*b*), and a thin rim of enhancement on the late image (*c*). Note that the track of the radiofrequency probe is visible as a linear defect extending from liver surface to lesion (arrows, *a*).

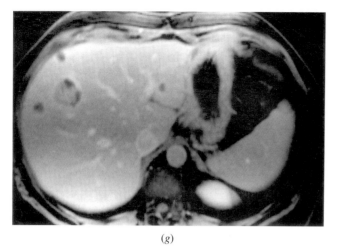

(g)

F I G . 2.137 (*Continued*) Echo-train STIR (*d*), SGE (*e*), immediate postgadolinium SGE (*f*), and 90-s postgadolinium fat-suppressed SGE (*g*) images in the same patient 2 months later. More lesions are appreciated in the hepatic parenchyma. The largest lesion, which was present on the first exam, demonstrates diffuse heterogeneous enhancement on the immediate postgadolinium image (*f*) that persists on the later image (*g*), in comparison to the findings from the earlier study in which no central lesion enhancement was observed. Note the presence of perilesional enhancement on the immediate postgadolinium image (*f*).

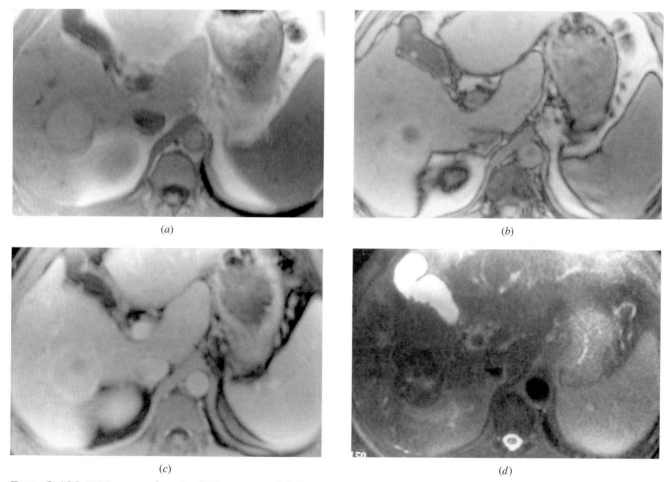

(a)

(b)

(c)

(d)

F I G . 2.138 **HCC pre- and postradiofrequency ablation.** SGE (*a*), out-of-phase SGE (*b*), and 90-s postgadolinium fat-suppressed SGE (*c*) images. There is an HCC in the right hepatic lobe that is isointense on T1 (*a*), contains a central focus that drops in signal on out-of-phase (*b*), and demonstrates heterogeneous enhancement on interstitial-phase images. The central focus that loses signal on the out-of-phase image represents fat.

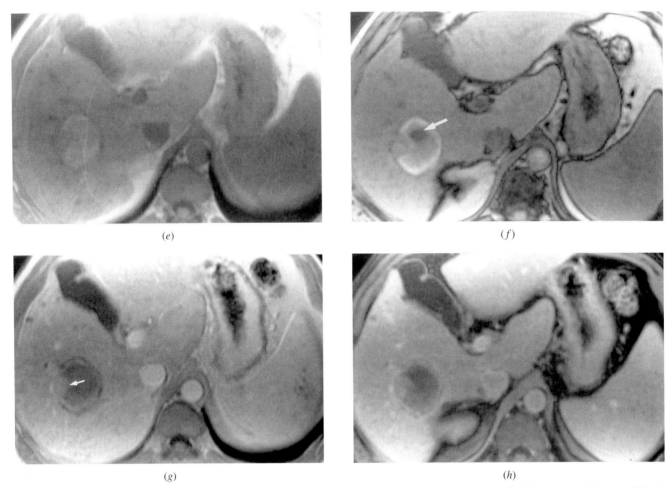

(e)

(f)

(g)

(h)

FIG. 2.138 (*Continued*) T2-weighted fat suppressed SS-ETSE (*d*), SGE (*e*), out-of-phase SGE (*f*), 45-s postgadolinium SGE (*g*) and 90-s postgadolinium fat-suppressed SGE (*h*) images in the same patient 5 months later, after radiofrequency ablation. The HCC has increased in size, is isointense on T2 (*d*) and slightly hypertense on T1 (*e*), and contains a small focus that drops in signal on the out-of-phase image (arrow, *f*). After gadolinium administration there is a thin rim of enhancement surrounding the entire lesion with lack of enhancement of the majority of the lesion on early (*g*) and late (*h*) images. A mural nodule (arrow, *g*) is present along the lateral wall of the lesion that demonstrates contrast enhancement consistent with residual tumor.

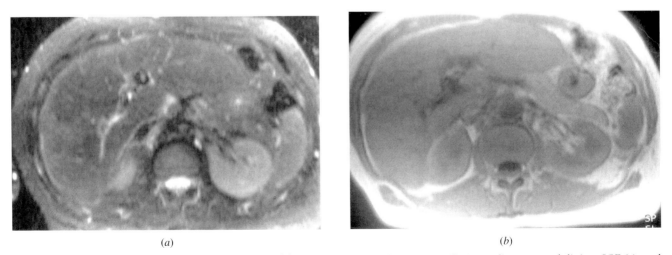

(a)

(b)

FIG. 2.139 HCC pre- and postradiofrequency ablation. Echo-train STIR (*a*), SGE (*b*), immediate postgadolinium SGE (*c*), and 90-s postgadolinium fat-suppressed SGE (*d*) images.

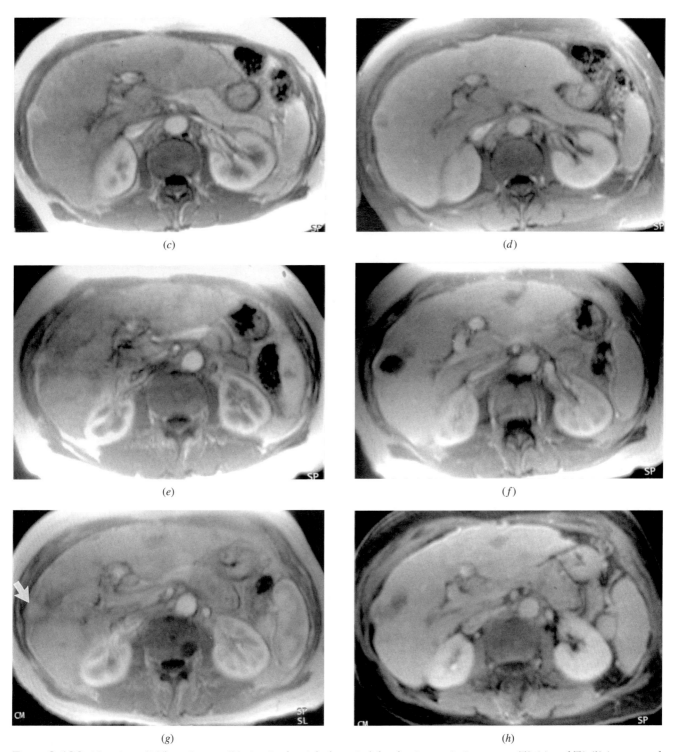

F I G . 2.139 (*Continued*) There is a small lesion in the right hepatic lobe that is near isointense on T2 (*a*) and T1 (*b*) images and demonstrates early heterogeneous enhancement (*c*) and wash-out with pseudocapsule enhancement on the late image (*d*), consistent with a small HCC. Immediate (*e*) and 45-s (*f*) postgadolinium SGE images in the same patient 1 week postradiofrequency ablation shows a necrotic lesion with ring enhancement on the 45-s postcontrast administration (*f*). Immediate postgadolinium SGE (*g*) and 90-s postgadolinium fat-suppressed SGE (*h*) images 2 months postradiofrequency ablation. In the interval a soft tissue mass (arrow, *g*) has developed on the lateral aspect of the tumor consistent with recurrence. The recurrent nodule shows internal enhancement on the immediate postgadolinium images (*g*) that wash out in a heterogeneous fashion by 90 s (*h*).

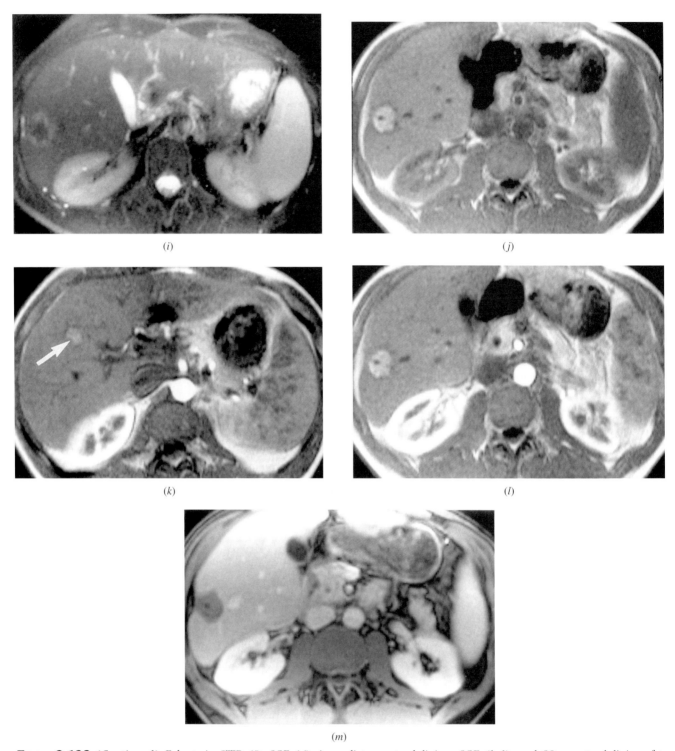

(i)

(j)

(k)

(l)

(m)

FIG. 2.139 (*Continued*) Echo-train STIR (*i*), SGE (*j*), immediate postgadolinium SGE (*k, l*), and 90-s postgadolinium fat-suppressed SGE (*m*) images in a second patient. There is a metastasis in *segment 6* of the right hepatic lobe that demonstrates isointensity on T2 (*i*), hyperintensity on T1 (*j*), and negligible enhancement immediately after administration of gadolinium, consistent with a hemorrhagic nonviable lesion post-RF ablation. Note the puckering of the liver capsule.

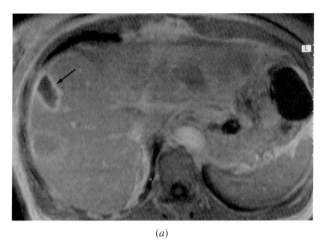

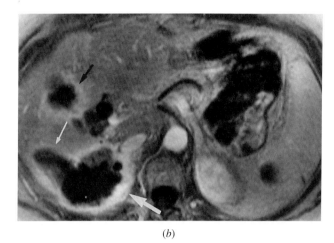

(a)   (b)

F I G . 2.140 Liver metastases, postcryotherapy, acute changes. Transverse 90-s postgadolinium SGE images (*a*, *b*) in two patients. In the first patient (*a*), a cryotherapy defect is present in the right lobe (arrow, *a*) that has a uniform-thickness enhancing wall in continuity with enhancing liver capsule of similar thickness. In the acute stage this appearance is compatible with tumor ablation and formation of acute granulation tissue along the cavity wall. The oblong shape of the defect corresponds to the direction of placement of the cryotherapy device. In the second patient (*b*), a cryotherapy tract (thin white arrow, *b*) is noted in continuity with a necrotic cavity. Portions of the cavity wall are thick and irregular (large white arrow, *b*). A second cryotherapy defect is noted in a more anterior location (black arrow, *b*). The cavity wall is thick and irregular. The presence of thick irregular walls after treatment is consistent with persistent disease.

contoured cavity wall (see fig. 2.140) [140, 142–144]. Residual tumor appears moderate in signal intensity and on T2-weighted images and demonstrates moderately intense enhancement on immediate post-gadolinium images (fig. 2.141).

Chemoembolization

Chemoembolic therapy is based on the pathophysiologic premise that hypervascular malignant tumors receive a disproportionately greater blood supply from hepatic arteries than surrounding intact liver and thus cytotoxic agents are preferentially delivered to malignant cells (figs. 2.142–2.146) [149]. Within one month postchemoembolization complete response is evidenced by the lack of enhancing tumor stroma. Changes on T2-weighted images depend on the fluid content of the lesions, which is diminished after successful treatment, because therapy is directed at inflowing blood and results in ischemic necrosis. Successfully treated lesions enhance negligibly on immediate postgadolinium SGE

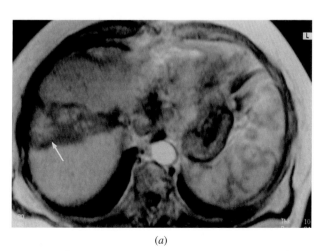

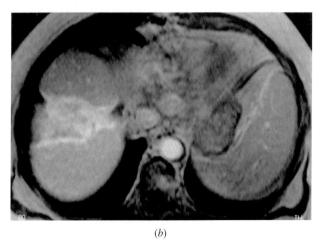

(a)   (b)

F I G . 2.141 Liver metastases, postcryotherapy, chronic changes with recurrent disease. Immediate (*a*) and 10-min (*b*) postgadolinium SGE images. A large wedge-shaped defect is present in the superior aspect of the liver that enhances minimally on the immediate postgadolinium image (*a*) and shows delayed enhancement at 10 min (*b*). This enhancement pattern is consistent with fibrosis. Focal irregular regions of soft tissue are identified within the wedge-shaped tissue (arrow, *a*) that represent adenocarcinoma.

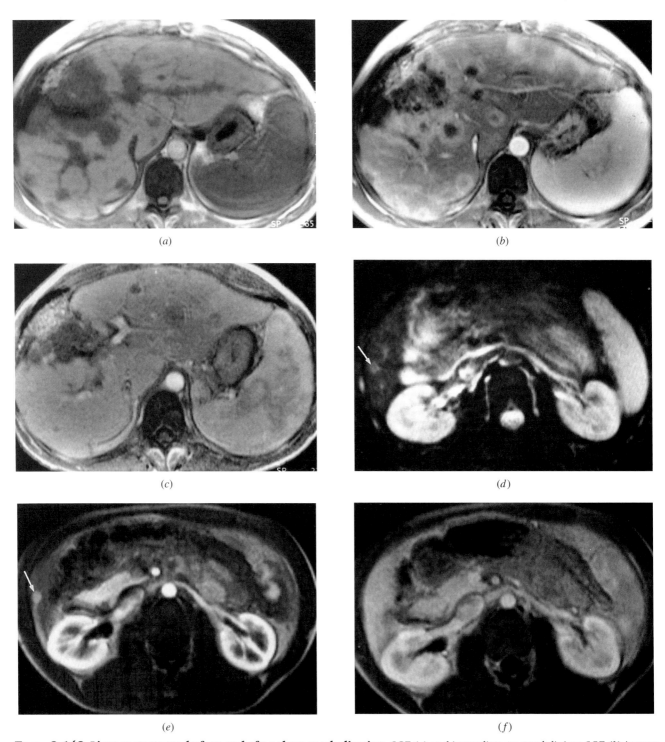

(a)

(b)

(c)

(d)

(e)

(f)

F IG. 2.142 Liver metastases, before and after chemoembolization. SGE (*a*) and immediate postgadolinium SGE (*b*) images before chemoembolization and immediate postgadolinium SGE image (*c*) 1 month after chemoembolization. On the pretreatment images (*a*, *b*), an 8-cm tumor and multiple tumors smaller than 2.5 cm are present throughout the liver. Prominent ring enhancement is present in these tumors (*b*). One month after chemoembolization (*c*), lesions have decreased in size and number and mural enhancement has markedly diminished (*c*).

T2-weighted fat-suppressed ETSE (*d*), immediate (*e*), and 45-s postgadolinium SGE (*f*) images in a second patient before chemoembolization.

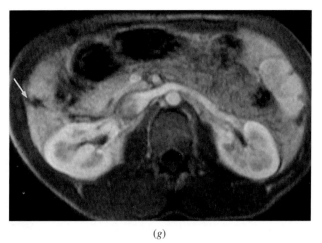

(g)

F I G . 2.142 (*Continued*) This patient with recurrent fibrolamellar HCC possesses multiple liver lesions that are modestly high in signal intensity on T2-weighted images (arrow, *d*), show intense uniform enhancement immediately after gadolinium administration (arrow, *e*), and fade rapidly to isointensity with liver by 45 s (*f*). Immediate postgadolinium SGE image acquired 1 month after chemoembolization (*g*) shows complete lack of enhancement of the lesion that now has polygonal angular margins (arrow, *g*), consistent with scarring.

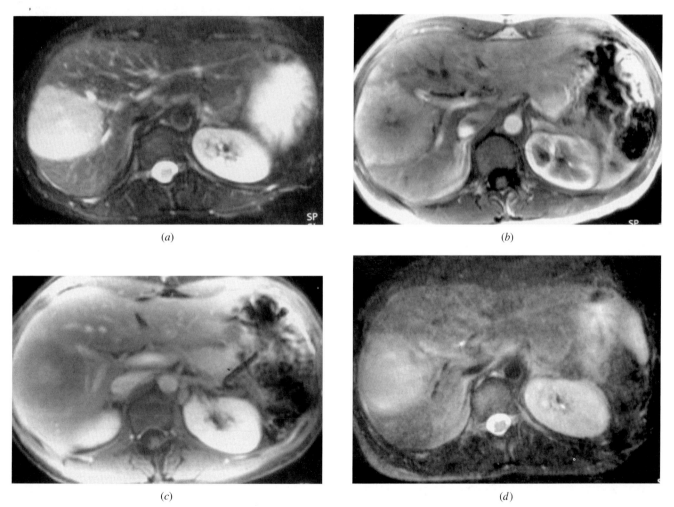

(a)

(b)

(c)

(d)

F I G . 2.143 Metastases from gastrinoma—pre- and postchemoembolization. Echo-train STIR (*a*), immediate postgadolinium SGE (*b*), and 90-s postgadolinium fat-suppressed SGE (*c*) images. There is a large mass in the right hepatic lobe that demonstrates high signal on the T2-weighted image (*a*) and intense enhancement after contrast administration (*b*) with wash-out on interstitial-phase image (*c*), consistent with a hypervascular metastasis.

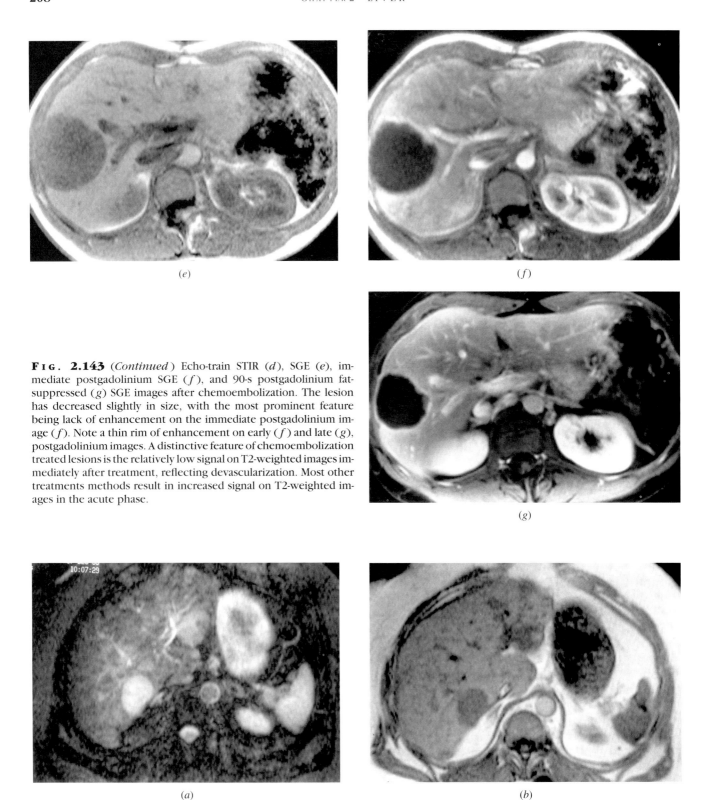

(e)

(f)

(g)

FIG. 2.143 (*Continued*) Echo-train STIR (*d*), SGE (*e*), immediate postgadolinium SGE (*f*), and 90-s postgadolinium fat-suppressed (*g*) SGE images after chemoembolization. The lesion has decreased slightly in size, with the most prominent feature being lack of enhancement on the immediate postgadolinium image (*f*). Note a thin rim of enhancement on early (*f*) and late (*g*), postgadolinium images. A distinctive feature of chemoembolization treated lesions is the relatively low signal on T2-weighted images immediately after treatment, reflecting devascularization. Most other treatments methods result in increased signal on T2-weighted images in the acute phase.

(a)

(b)

FIG. 2.144 Metastases from carcinoid—pre- and postchemoembolization. T2-weighted fat-suppressed ETSE (*a*), SGE (*b*), and immediate postgadolinium SGE (*c*) images. A 4-cm metastasis is present in the right lobe, and a second 4-cm lesion in the lateral segment. They appear moderately high signal intensity on T2 (*a*) and low signal intensity on T1 (*b*) and show intense enhancement immediately after contrast administration (*c*).

SGE (*d*), immediate postgadolinium (*e*), and 45-s postgadolinium SGE (*f*) images in the same patient after chemoembolization. Note that the lesion has decreased in size and shows minimal enhancement on the immediate postgadolinium image (*e*), with progressive enhancement on later images.

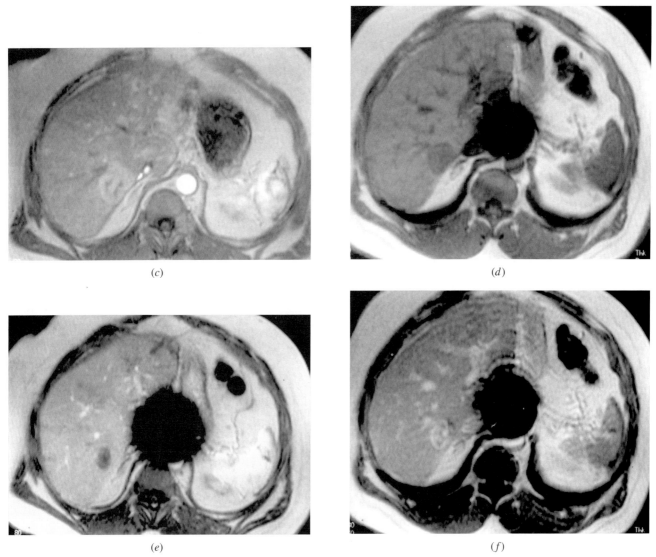

(c)

(d)

(e)

(f)

FIG. 2.144 (*Continued*) This enhancement pattern is consistent with fibrosis. Note the large metal artifact in the porta hepatis that represents a metal coil placed at the time of chemoembolization.

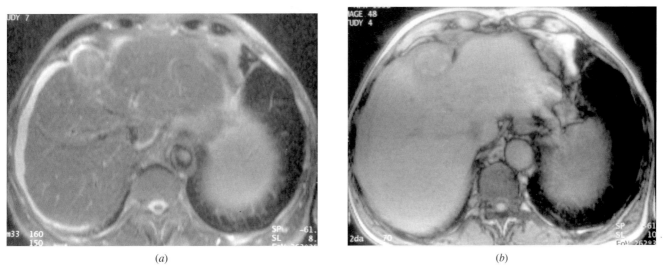

(a)

(b)

FIG. 2.145 HCC and chemoembolization. Echo-train STIR (*a*), out-of-phase SGE (*b*), 45-s postgadolinium SGE (*c*), and 90-s postgadolinium fat-suppressed SGE (*d*), images.

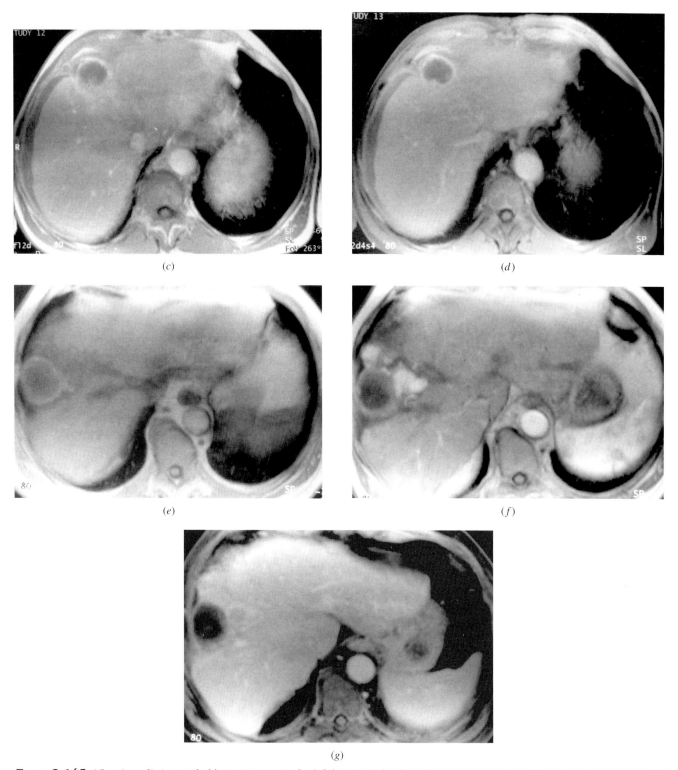

(c)

(d)

(e)

(f)

(g)

F IG . 2.145 *(Continued)* A rounded lesion is seen in the left hepatic lobe that demonstrates minimal high signal intensity on T2 (*a*), minimal low signal intensity with a high signal rim on T1 (*b*), and capsular enhancement postgadolinium (*c, d*) with lack of tumor enhancement. The combination of isointensity on T2 with lack of central enhancement on postgadolinium T1-weighted images is consistent with devascularization of tumor, which occurs with chemoembolization.

SGE (*e*), immediate postgadolinium SGE (*f*), and 90-s postgadolinium fat-suppressed SGE (*g*) images in a second patient. There is an oval lesion located in the right hepatic lobe that shows decreased signal intensity centrally and increased signal intensity peripherally on the noncontrast T1-weighted image (*e*). On the immediate postgadolinium image (*f*) there is intense enhancement surrounding the well-defined lesion consistent with persistent tumor in the lesion periphery. This persistent tumor fades on interstitial-phase images (*g*). The central devascularized portion does not enhance on early or late postcontrast images. The peripheral high-signal rim on the precontrast image represents extracellular methemoglobin.

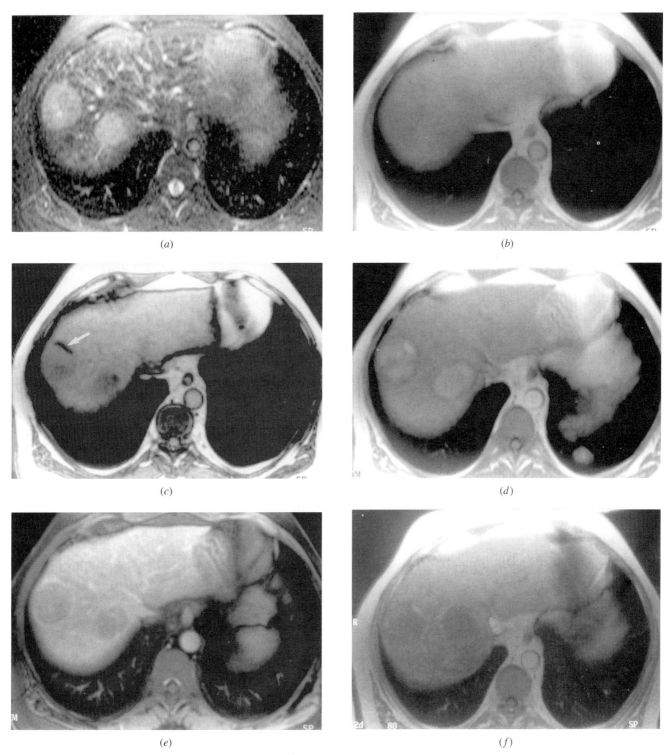

F I G . 2.146 HCC postchemoembolization. Echo-train STIR (*a*), SGE (*b*), out-of-phase SGE (*c*), immediate postgadolinium SGE (*d*), and 90-s postgadolinium fat-suppressed SGE (*e*), images. There are two rounded lesions that are mildly high signal on T2 (*a*) and minimally low signal on T1 (*b*) and demonstrate intense heterogeneous enhancement immediately postgadolinium (*d*), with wash-out and capsular enhancement on the late image (*e*), consistent with HCC. Note that one of the lesions, demonstrates a small focus (arrow, *c*) that exhibits signal drop on the out-of-phase sequence consistent with fat.

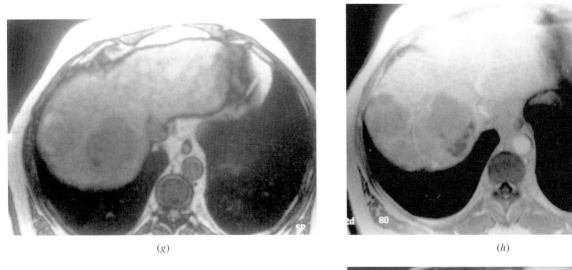

(g)

(h)

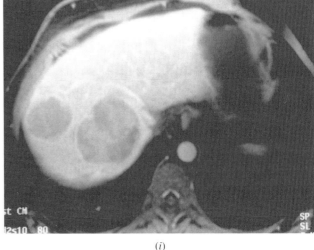

FIG. 2.146 (*Continued*) SGE (*f*), out-of-phase SGE (*g*), immediate postgadolinium SGE (*h*), and 90-s postgadolinium fat-suppressed SGE (*i*) images in the same patient 7 months later. Note the increased size of the lesions. The lesions demonstrate diminished enhancement on early (*h*) and late (*i*) images reflecting central desvascularization from chemoembolization.

(i)

images (see fig. 2.142). In one report, 27 tumors treated with chemoembolization were low in signal on T2-weighted and postgadolinium T1-weighted images [139]. All of these tumors were necrotic at biopsy. Partial response appears as a decrease in tumor size, with residual tumor showing increased signal intensity on T2-weighted images and enhancement on immediate postgadolinium images (fig. 2.147). Substantial variation does occur, reflecting variation in the degree of response and the time course of healing. One series correlated serial changes of liver lesions on T1, T2, and dynamic postgadolinium images pre- and postchemoembolization (figs. 2.142–2.144) [157]. Homogeneous intense enhancement on hepatic arterial dominant phase images combined with small malignant lesion size on pretreatment MR studies were the best predictors of successful response. Lesions that showed good response became low signal on T2-weighted images immediately after treatment, reflecting the devascularization of tumor. This differs from local therapy techniques that result in

high T2 signal early after therapy. The best indication of good response is negligible enhancement on hepatic arterial dominant phase images after chemoembolization.

The evaluation of treatment response of malignant liver lesions using MRI is an important clinical tool and holds great promise for future applications. Immediate postgadolinium SGE is particularly effective at demonstrating response, presumably because it reflects changes in tumor angiogenesis and demonstrates patterns of granulation tissue enhancement that vary with age. Further investigation is required to evaluate interval changes throughout the course of therapy and to correlate these changes with clinical response to therapy.

Blood pool contrast agents are currently under development. One report demonstrated the relationship between contrast enhancement and capillary permeability after liver irradiation, with the implication that the physiologic effects of increased capillary permeability may have an impact on the timing of therapeutic regimens [150].

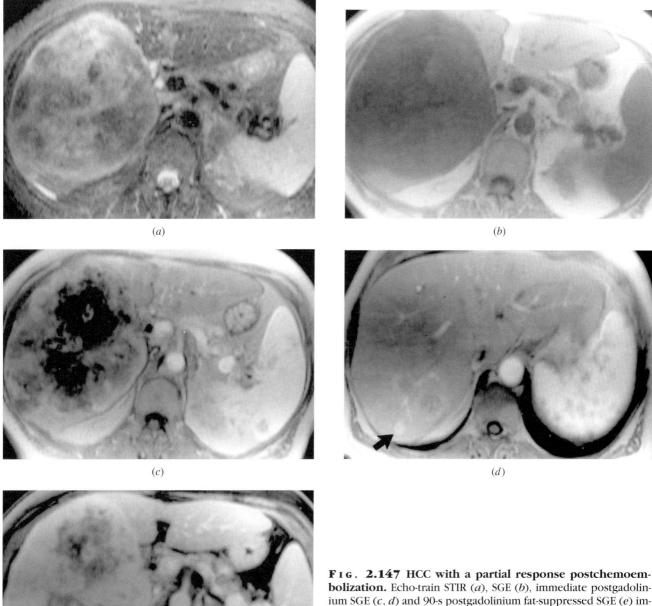

(a)

(b)

(c)

(d)

(e)

FIG. 2.147 HCC with a partial response postchemoembolization. Echo-train STIR (*a*), SGE (*b*), immediate postgadolinium SGE (*c*, *d*) and 90-s postgadolinium fat-suppressed SGE (*e*) images. There is a large mass that shows hyperintense signal on T2 (*a*) and hypointense signal on T1 (*b*). Immediately after gadolinium it shows intense heterogeneous enhancement (*c*) with large regions of low signal centrally within the tumor consistent with necrosis, reflecting a partial response to chemoembolization. On a higher tomographic section a small satellite HCC (arrow, *d*), is present, which demonstrates intense uniform enhancement.

Diffuse Liver Parenchymal Disease

Chronic Liver Disease

A variety of hereditary congenital or familial disorders will result in chronic liver disease, including Wilson disease (fig. 2.148), primary biliary cirrhosis (fig. 2.149), α-1 antitrypsin deficiency, and primary sclerosing cholangitis (PSC). All of these entities will progress to chronic liver disease and cirrhosis. At the present time, with the exception of PSC, these disorders do not appear to show recognizable or specific patterns of liver injury by MR imaging.

The morphologic changes of PSC on pathologic evaluation consist of fibrosing cholangitis of bile ducts with progressive obliteration of their lumens. In between areas of scarring, bile ducts become ectatic. The disease

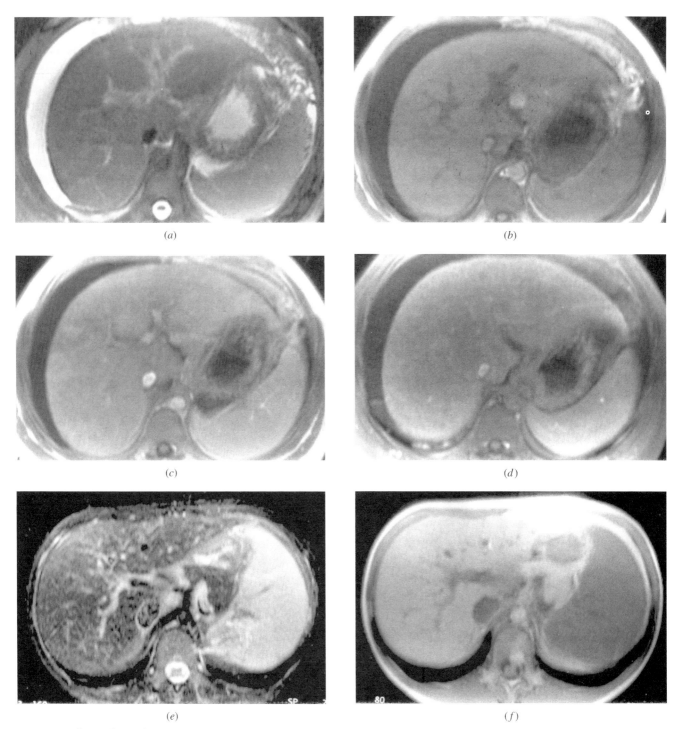

(a)   *(b)*

(c)   *(d)*

(e)   *(f)*

F I G . 2.148 Wilson disease. Echo-train STIR (*a*), SGE (*b*), immediate postgadolinium SGE (*c*), and 90-s postgadolinium fat-suppressed SGE (*d*), images in a patient with Wilson disease and acute presentation in fulminant liver failure. Early patchy enhancement (*c*) compatible with acute severe hepatitis and late linear stromal enhancement (*d*) are both present, consistent with acute on chronic hepatitis.

Echo-train STIR (*e*), SGE (*f*), out-of-phase SGE (*g*), immediate postgadolinium SGE (*h*), and 90-s postgadolinium fat-suppressed SGE (*i*) images in a second patient. There are multiple regenerative nodules present, best shown on out-of-phase image (*g*) because decrease in signal of background fatty liver. Splenomegaly is present.

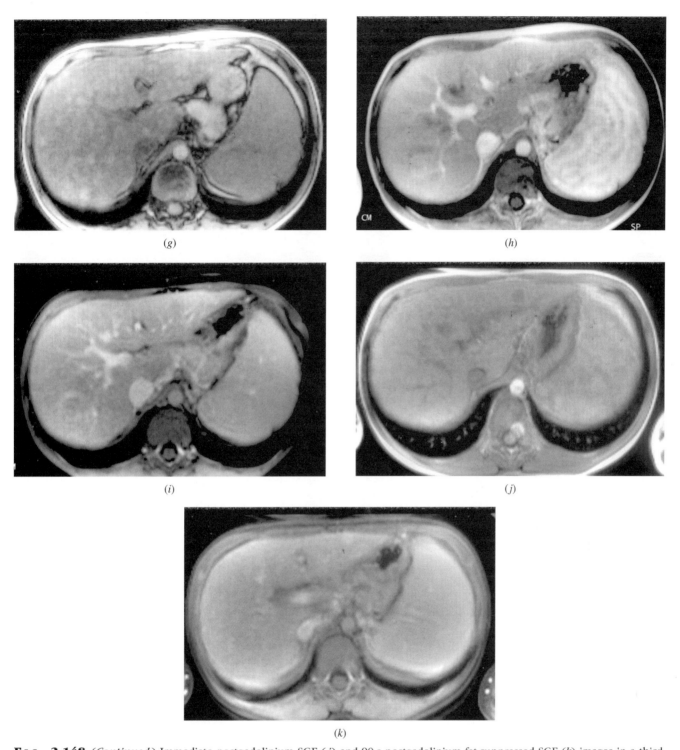

F ɪ ɢ . 2.148 (*Continued*) Immediate postgadolinium SGE (*j*) and 90-s postgadolinium fat-suppressed SGE (*k*) images in a third patient with Wilson disease and changes of cirrhosis, including thin reticular fibrous stroma, perigastric varices, and splenomegaly.

The MR features of Wilson disease do not at present appear to show characteristic features that distinguish it from other forms of chronic hepatic disease.

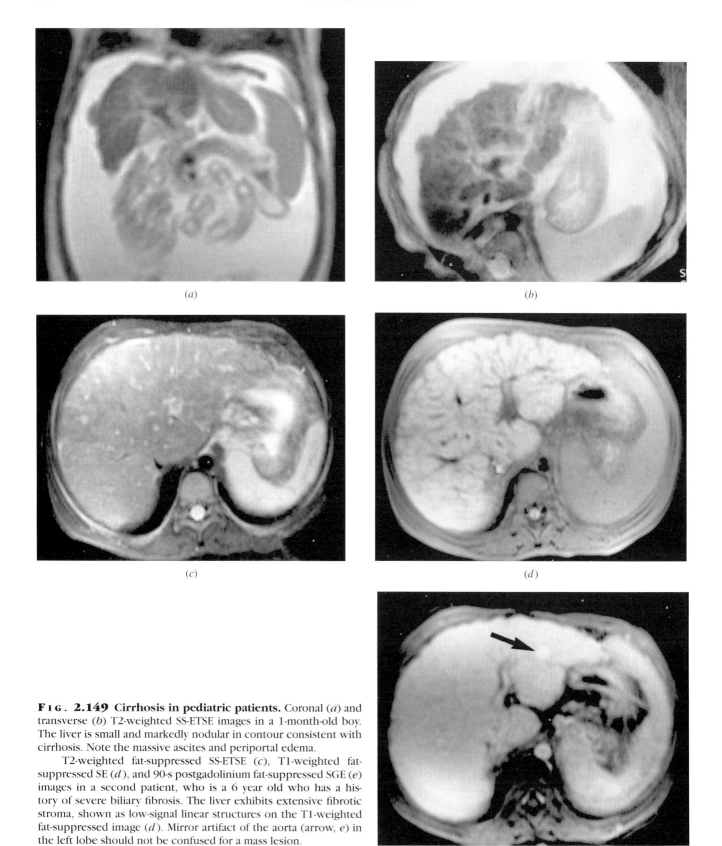

(a)

(b)

(c)

(d)

(e)

FIG. 2.149 Cirrhosis in pediatric patients. Coronal (*a*) and transverse (*b*) T2-weighted SS-ETSE images in a 1-month-old boy. The liver is small and markedly nodular in contour consistent with cirrhosis. Note the massive ascites and periportal edema.

T2-weighted fat-suppressed SS-ETSE (*c*), T1-weighted fat-suppressed SE (*d*), and 90-s postgadolinium fat-suppressed SGE (*e*) images in a second patient, who is a 6 year old who has a history of severe biliary fibrosis. The liver exhibits extensive fibrotic stroma, shown as low-signal linear structures on the T1-weighted fat-suppressed image (*d*). Mirror artifact of the aorta (arrow, *e*) in the left lobe should not be confused for a mass lesion.

culminates in biliary cirrhosis. On imaging, changes of cirrhosis in PSC are associated with central macroregenerative nodules that cause peripheral biliary ductal dilatation and peripheral liver atrophy. This pattern appears to be both relatively common and distinctive for PSC (fig. 2.150).

Cirrhosis

Although there have been many definitions of cirrhosis, perhaps the most concise and descriptive definition states that cirrhosis is "a diffuse process characterized by fibrosis and a conversion of normal architecture into structurally abnormal nodules" [158]. Cirrhosis is a stage in the evolution of many chronic diseases including viral infections, alcohol abuse, hemochromatosis, autoimmune disease, Wilson disease, and primary sclerosing cholangitis. The most common underlying causes in North America include alcoholism and viral hepatitis [159]. From a clinicopathologic perspective, cirrhosis is not a static phenomenon but a dynamic process that runs the gamut of inflammation, cell injury and death, fibrosis, and regeneration. Pathologic gross inspection of cirrhotic livers generally shows two types of patterns: 1) micronodular cirrhosis, in which parenchymal nodules are small (<3 mm diameter) and separated by thin fibrous septa, and 2) macronodular cirrhosis, in which parenchymal nodules are large and variably sized, and separated by fibrous septa sometimes reaching proportions of large scars. Because of the underlying pathophysiology of the disease, the conversion from micro-to macronodular cirrhosis is claimed to be a general phe-

nomenon. The Copenhagen Study Group for Liver Disease studied 156 cirrhotic patients and observed a conversion ratio of micronodular to macronodular cirrhosis of 90% in 10 years [160].

By MR imaging, a variety of morphologic changes are observed in cirrhotic livers. Atrophy of the right lobe and the medial segment of the left lobe is common in cirrhotic livers. Relative sparing of the caudate lobe and lateral segment of the left lobe is often present. In fact, these segments may undergo hypertrophy. The combination of scarring, atrophy, and parenchymal regenerative activity may involve any segment of the liver and occasionally may result in a bizarre hepatic contour that can simulate tumor mass (fig. 2.151). Often the hypertrophic region in the liver possesses imaging and enhancement features comparable to those in the remainder of the liver, thus facilitating a correct diagnosis. Central large regenerative nodules may be most characteristic of cirrhosis due to PSC. In these cases, regions of atrophic, cirrhotic liver and obstructed bile ducts may be compressed at the periphery of massively expanded, centrally located regenerative nodules.

Morphologic changes of the liver are seen less frequently in early compensated cirrhosis, impairing diagnosis by imaging. Enlargement of the hilar periportal space was visible in 98% of patients with early cirrhosis, whereas this finding was seen in only 11% of patients with normal livers. Expansion of the major interlobar fissure is seen frequently, causing extrahepatic fat to fill the space between the left medial and lateral segments, presenting the expanded gallbladder fossa sign [161]. The expanded gallbladder fossa sign had high specificity and

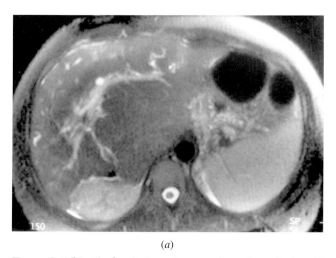

(a)

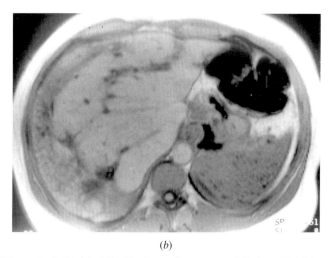

(b)

F I G . 2.150 Cirrhosis in primary sclerosing cholangitis. Echo-train STIR (*a*), SGE (*b*), immediate postgadolinium SGE (*c*), and 90-s postgadolinium fat-suppressed SGE (*d*) images. The liver shows distorted anatomy with heterogeneous signal. The caudate lobe is massively enlarged by large macroregenerative nodules that cause atrophy of the peripheral liver, resulting in signal changes of increased signal on T2 (*a*), decreased signal on T1 (*b*), and early negligible (*c*), and late progressive enhancement (*d*). There is ductal dilatation in the peripheral liver due to obstruction from the central hypertrophy. These findings are consistent with cirrhosis due to primary sclerosing cholangitis.

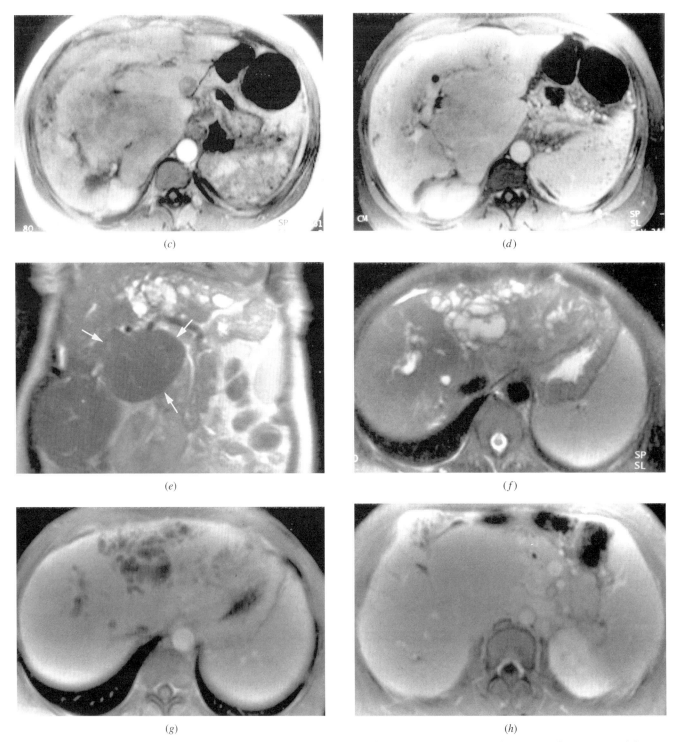

FIG. 2.150 (*Continued*) Coronal T2-weighted SS-ETSE (*e*), T2-weighted fat-suppressed SS-ETSE (*f*), and 90-s postgadolinium fat-suppressed SGE (*g*, *h*) images in a second patient. Note the massive enlargement of the caudate lobe (arrows, *e*), which causes distal obstruction of the biliary tree.

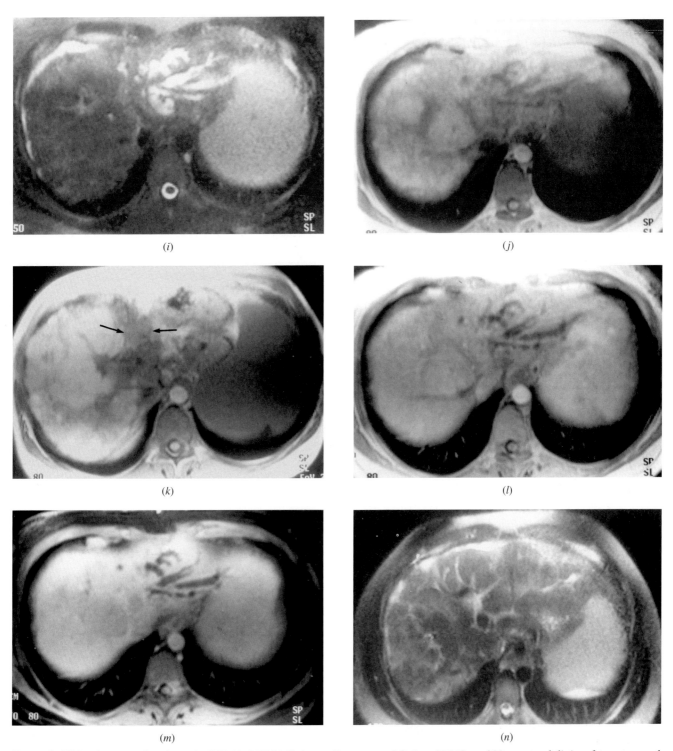

FIG. 2.150 (*Continued*) Echo-train STIR (*i*), SGE (*j*, *k*), immediate postgadolinium SGE (*l*), and 90-s postgadolinium fat-suppressed SGE (*m*) images in a third patient with PSC. The liver demonstrates a shrunken fibrotic appearance with multiple macroregenerative nodules, which are more widely distributed than the first two patients. Severe lateral segment intrahepatic biliary ductal dilatation is present from obstruction by dense fibrous tissue (arrows, *k*).

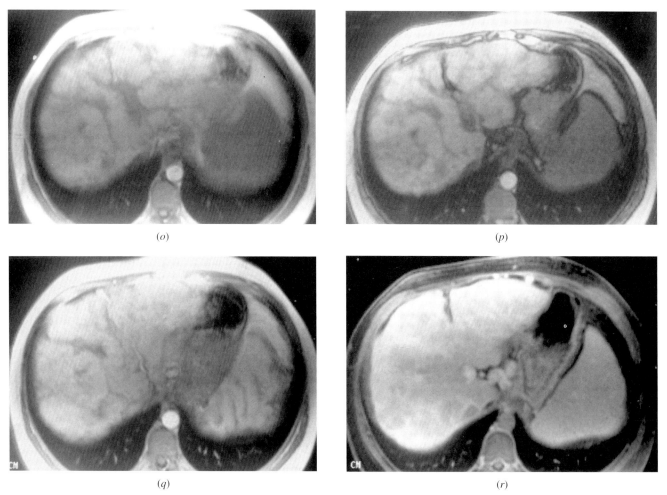

(o)   (p)

(q)   (r)

FIG. 2.150 (*Continued*) Echo-train STIR (*n*), SGE (*o*), out-of-phase SGE (*p*), immediate postgadolinium SGE (*q*), and 90-s post-gadolinium fat-suppressed SGE (*r*) images in a fourth patient with PSC. The liver is heterogeneous in signal on T2- (*n*) and T1-weighted (*o, p*) images with multiple macronodules and fibrotic bands present. This patient does not have the characteristic central macron-odular pattern found in PSC.

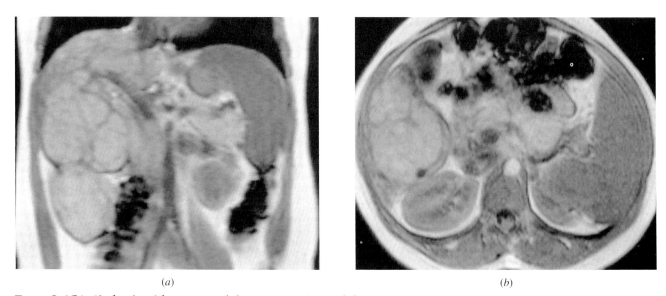

(a)   (b)

FIG. 2.151 Cirrhosis with macronodular regenerative nodule. Coronal SGE (*a*), SGE (*b*), T2-weighted fat-suppressed ETSE (*c*), and immediate (*d*) and 90-s (*e*) postgadolinium SGE images.

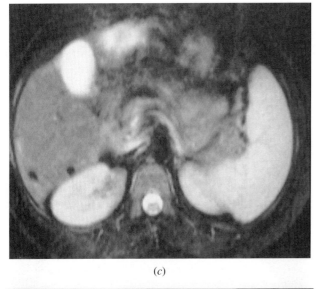

(c)

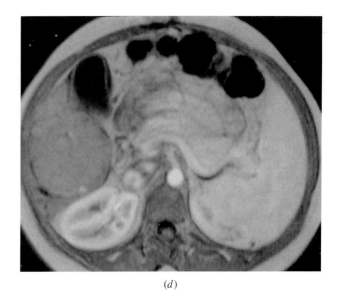

(d)

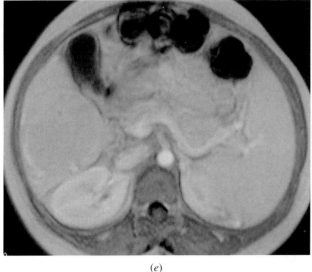

(e)

FIG. 2.151 (*Continued*) Prominent linear bands that are low in signal intensity on T1-weighted images (*a, b*) are present throughout the liver, a finding consistent with scarring. The inferior portion of the right lobe has a bulbous contour that simulated a mass lesion on CT examination. The focal enlargement possesses the same signal intensity features as the remainder of the liver (*a*), which include fibrotic markings apparent on T1-weighted images (*a, b*), homogeneous intermediate signal intensity on T2-weighted images (*c*), early diminished enhancement of scar tissue (*d*), and more uniform enhancement on interstitial-phase images (*e*).

positive predictive value (98% for each) for diagnosing cirrhosis [161]. Enlargement of the hilar periportal space containing increased fatty tissue is considered a consequence of atrophy of the medial segment of the left hepatic lobe [159].

The most consistent morphological feature of cirrhosis is the demonstration of fibrous tissue that appears on imaging as a reticular network of linear stroma of varying thickness (fig. 2.152). On T1-weighted images fibrous tissue is low signal: on T2-weighted images fibrous tissue varies from high signal to low signal, depending on chronicity, with acute fibrous tissue having a higher fluid content and therefore higher signal. On hepatic arterial dominant phase images, fibrous tissue enhances negligibly and demonstrates late enhancement on hepatic venous phase images. Fibrous tissue is most consistently shown on short TE T1-weighted SGE images, that out-of-phase imaging may further facilitate

(TE = 2 ms) and as late-enhancing stroma on 2-min postgadolinium fat-suppressed SGE images (fig. 2.153 and 2.154) [162].

Many cirrhotic livers contain regions of low signal intensity on T1-weighted images and high signal intensity on T2-weighted images secondary to hepatocellular damage, inflammation, or both [163, 164]. Acute-on-chronic liver inflammation is shown as regions of transient increased enhancement on immediate postgadolinium images (fig. 2.155) [162]. Usually regions of enhancement are small with irregular margins. In these cases, distinction from tumor is not problematic. Occasionally, patchy areas of enhancement are large and persist on later postcontrast images. Under these circumstances distinction from diffuse HCC can be problematic. In the setting of HCC, an important distinguishing feature is the association with tumor thrombus. This finding is rare with acute-on-chronic hepatitis. Serum α-fetoprotein

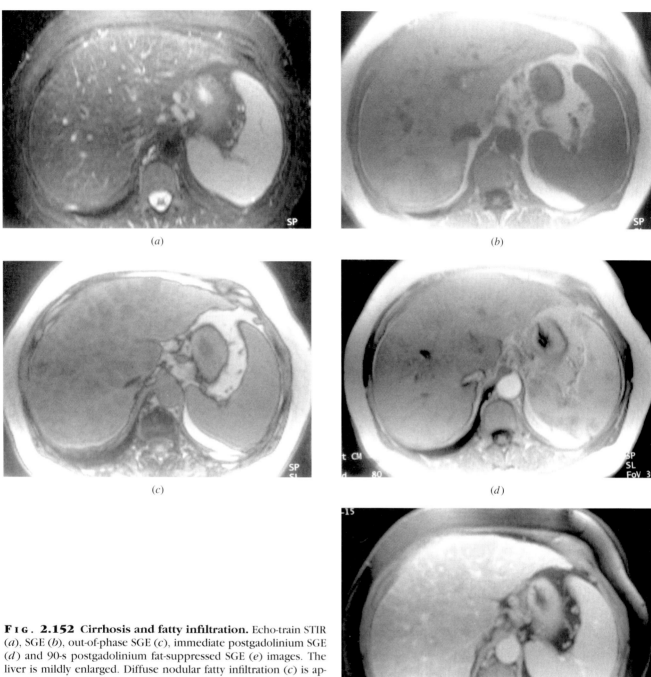

F I G . 2.152 Cirrhosis and fatty infiltration. Echo-train STIR (*a*), SGE (*b*), out-of-phase SGE (*c*), immediate postgadolinium SGE (*d*) and 90-s postgadolinium fat-suppressed SGE (*e*) images. The liver is mildly enlarged. Diffuse nodular fatty infiltration (*c*) is appreciated with foci of liver losing signal on out-of-phase and intervening bands of fibrosis tissue retaining signal. Note that the fibrous tissue enhances on delayed images (*e*), creating a reticular appearance.

level may support the diagnosis because it is typically very elevated with diffuse HCC and not substantially elevated with acute-on-chronic hepatitis.

Tiny peribiliary cysts also occur in cirrhotic livers [165–167]. These cysts typically measure 5 mm or less in size.

In cirrhotic livers, parenchymal nodules are created by the regenerative activity of hepatocytes and the net-

work of scars. The formation of regenerative nodules (RNs) results in gross distortion of hepatic architecture. Micronodular cirrhosis, common in alcoholic liver disease and hemochromatosis, displays regenerative nodules of 3 mm or less, ensheathed by thin fibrous septa. In patients with virus-induced cirrhosis (mainly hepatitis B), the regenerative nodules are 3–15 mm with thick fibrous septa; this pattern is classified as macronodular

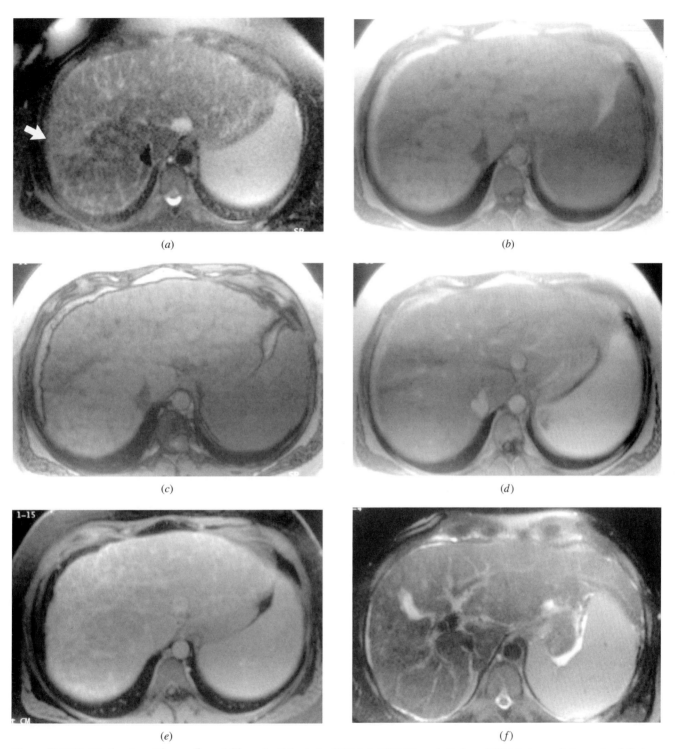

F I G . 2.153 Cirrhosis with confluent fibrosis. Echo-train STIR (*a*), SGE (*b*), out-of-phase SGE (*c*), immediate postgadolinium SGE (*d*) and 90-s postgadolinium fat-suppressed SGE (*e*) images. There is a linear pattern of fibrosis throughout the liver with a focal region of confluent fibrosis (arrow, *a*) that is mildly high in signal on T2 (*a*) and mildly low in signal on T1-weighted image (*b*) and demonstrates negligible enhancement on early postcontrast (*d*) and late mild enhancement (*e*). Note that the fine pattern of fibrosis present throughout the liver is particularly well shown on the short TE out-of-phase image (*c*) as low signal linear structures and on late postgadolinium as linear enhancing structures (*e*).

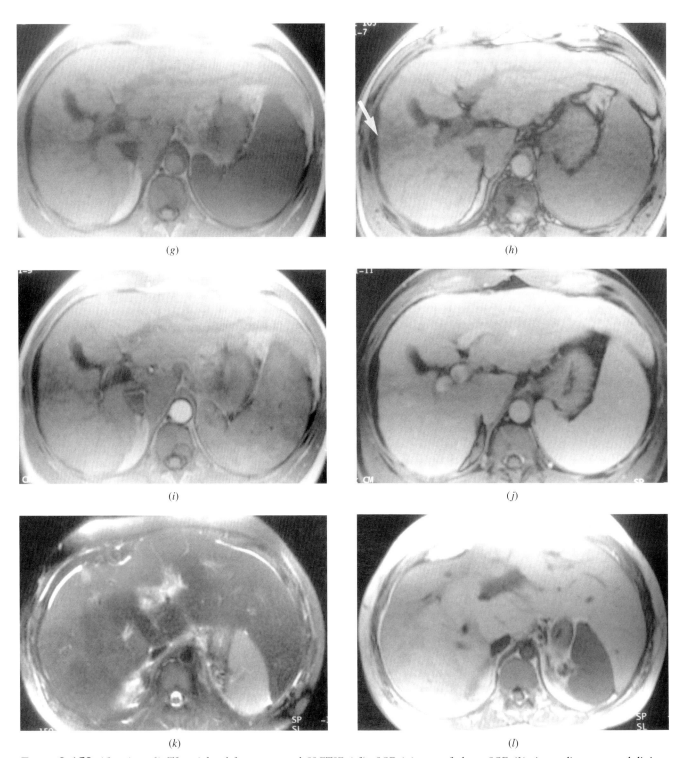

(g)

(h)

(i)

(j)

(k)

(l)

FIG. 2.153 (*Continued*) T2-weighted fat-suppressed SS-ETSE (*f*), SGE (*g*), out-of-phase SGE (*h*), immediate postgadolinium SGE (*i*), and 90-s postgadolinium fat-suppressed SGE (*j*) images in a second patient. The liver is small and nodular in contour and demonstrates a reticular heterogeneous enhancement pattern consistent with cirrhosis. A confluent region of fibrosis is evident in segment 8 peripherally (arrow, *h*). No focal lesion is identified within the liver. Note the presence of splenomegaly.

T2-weighted fat-suppressed SS-ETSE (*k*), SGE (*l*), out-of-phase (*m*), immediate postgadolinium SGE (*n*), and 90-s postgadolinium fat-suppressed SGE (*o*) images in a third patient.

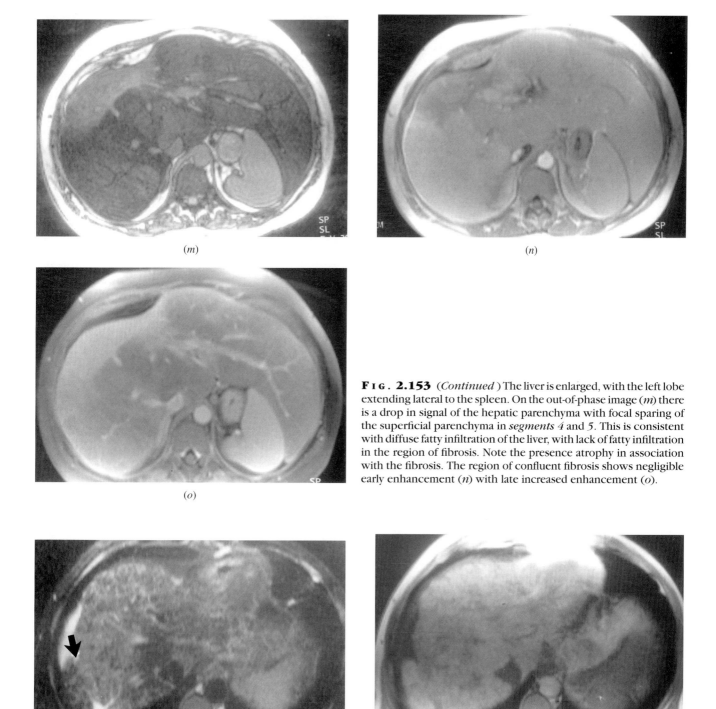

(m)

(n)

(o)

FIG. 2.153 (*Continued*) The liver is enlarged, with the left lobe extending lateral to the spleen. On the out-of-phase image (*m*) there is a drop in signal of the hepatic parenchyma with focal sparing of the superficial parenchyma in *segments 4* and *5*. This is consistent with diffuse fatty infiltration of the liver, with lack of fatty infiltration in the region of fibrosis. Note the presence atrophy in association with the fibrosis. The region of confluent fibrosis shows negligible early enhancement (*n*) with late increased enhancement (*o*).

(a)

(b)

FIG. 2.154 Cirrhosis with extensive and confluent fibrosis. Echo-train STIR (*a*), SGE (*b*), immediate postgadolinium SGE (*c*), and 90-s postgadolinium fat-suppressed SGE (*d*); echo-train STIR (*e*), SGE (*f*), out-of-phase SGE (*g*), immediate postgadolinium SGE (*h*), and 90-s postgadolinium fat-suppressed SGE (*i*) images in two different patients with cirrhosis. In both cases, the liver is diminutive in size and demonstrates nodular and irregular contour with distorted anatomy.

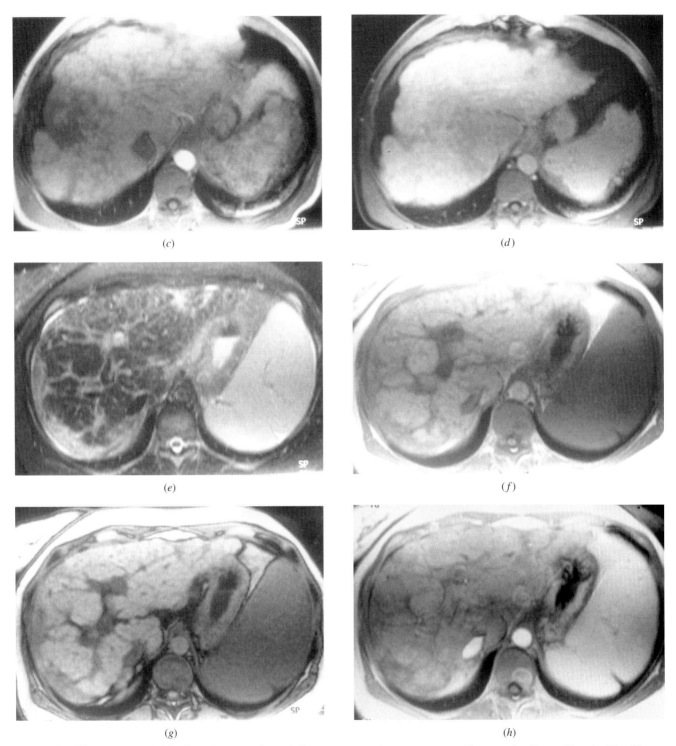

(c)

(d)

(e)

(f)

(g)

(h)

FIG. 2.154 (*Continued*) The hepatic parenchyma is heterogeneous in appearance with extensive linear fibrosis. The fibrous stroma is best shown on the short TE out-of-phase sequence (*g*) as low-signal reticular strands and on the late postgadolinium fat-suppressed SGE as enhancing tissue.

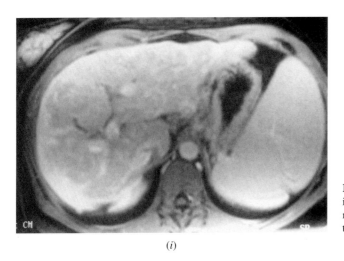

(i)

F I G . 2.154 (*Continued*) Confluent areas of fibrosis are present in both patients. Parenchymal atrophy associated with the scarring results in an unusual-appearing exophytic region of hypertrophy in the first patient (arrow, *a*).

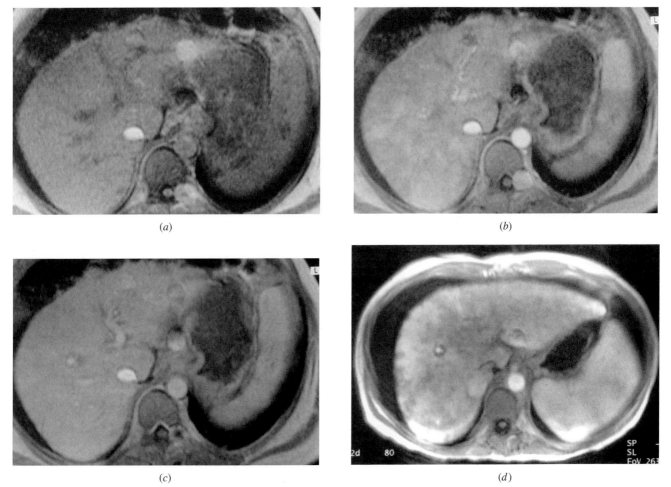

(a)

(b)

(c)

(d)

F I G . 2.155 Cirrhosis, acute hepatitis resulting in transient early enhancement. SGE (*a*), immediate postgadolinium SGE (*b*), and 45-s postgadolinium SGE (*c*) images. Normal signal intensity of the liver is present on the T1-weighted image (*a*). Ill-defined, <2-cm regions of blotchy enhancement are present on the immediate postgadolinium image (*b*), which resolve by 45 s (*c*). The presence of enhancing tissue immediately after contrast raises the concern of HCC in a cirrhotic patient. Diffuse HCC usually results in a mottled enhancement pattern with smaller foci of enhancing tissue. Diffuse HCC also is associated with venous tumor thrombus. The underlying cause for this enhancement abnormality in this patient is superimposed acute hepatitis on chronic hepatitis.

Immediate postgadolinium SGE image (*d*) in a second patient demonstrates patchy transient increased enhancement throughout the liver.

cirrhosis [159]. Although some diseases are classically associated with one pattern or another, most cirrhotic livers are mixed [118]. MRI demonstrates RNs with greater conspicuity than other imaging modalities. Because RNs have a portal venous blood supply with minimal contribution from hepatic arteries, RNs do not enhance substancially on hepatic arterial dominant phase images [118]. On T2-weighted images, RNs are low in signal intensity relative to high-signal intensity inflammatory fibrous septa or damaged liver (figs. 2.156–2.158) [168]. Approximately 25% of RNs accumulate more iron than the surrounding hepatic parenchyma, facilitating their identification as low signal on T2-weighted and T2*-weighted gradient-echo images, and low signal on postgadolinium SGE images because hepatic parenchyma

enhances greater than iron-containing nodules [169, 170] (fig. 2.159).

Dysplastic nodules (DNs) are defined as neoplastic, clonal lesions that represent an intermediate step in the pathway of carcinogenesis of hepatocytes in cirrhotic livers [171]. Dysplastic nodules are diagnosed as low or high grade according to the current classification system for nodular hepatocellular lesions by the International Working Party [37]. They are considered as premalignant nodules and are found in 15–25% of cirrhotic livers [118]. Studies have documented the development of HCC within a DN in a short as a 4-month period [118]. On gross pathologic examination, DNs can usually be distinguished from ordinary RNs based on larger size (usually >8 mm), although some may be smaller. The blood

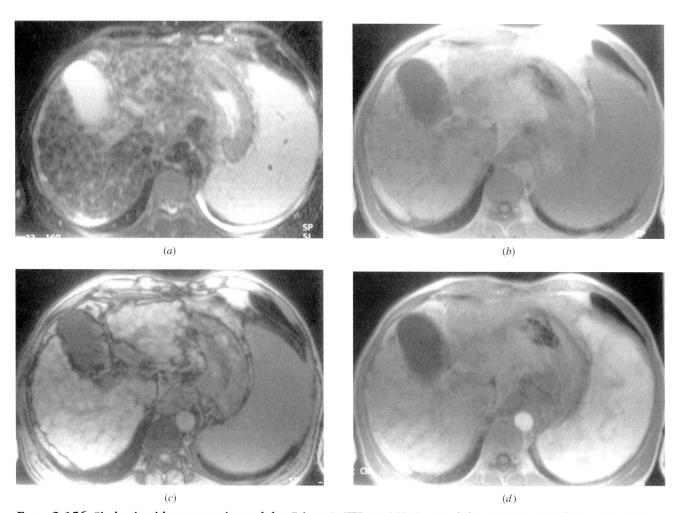

(a)   (b)

(c)   (d)

F I G . 2.156 Cirrhosis with regenerative nodules. Echo-train STIR (*a*), SGE (*b*), out-of-phase SGE (*c*), immediate postgadolinium SGE (*d*), and 90-s postgadolinium fat-suppressed SGE (*e*) images. The liver is small with an extensive nodular pattern. A reticular pattern of fibrosis in present which is well shown on out-of-phase images (*c*) as low-signal intensity linear tissue and demonstrates negligible enhancement on immediate postgadolinium images (*d*) with progressive enhancement on late images (*e*). Multiple regenerative nodules appear as rounded <1-cm masses best seen as high-signal lesions on out-of-phase images (*c*). Ascites, splenomegaly, and paraesophageal varices are present.

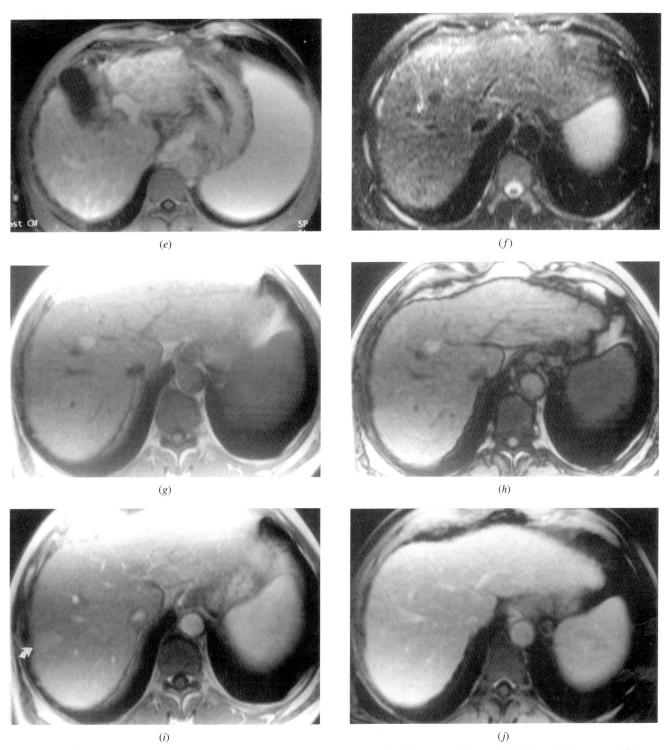

FIG. 2.156 (*Continued*) Echo-train STIR (*f*), SGE (*g*), out-of-phase SGE (*h*), 45-s postgadolinium SGE (*i*), and 90-s postgadolinium fat-suppressed SGE (*j*) images in a second patient. There are multiple scattered rounded foci throughout the liver that show decreased signal on T2 (*f*) and increased signal on noncontrast T1-weighted (*g*) and out-of-phase (*h*) images. Lesions are not apparent on early (*i*) or late (*j*) postgadolinium images, consistent with regenerative or mildly dysplastic nodules. Note also the fine reticular pattern on postgadolinium images (*i, j*) with progressive enhancement, consistent with fibrotic change associated with cirrhosis. A small transiently enhancing focus (curved arrow, *i*) is present in *segment 8* that reflects a vascular phenomenon.

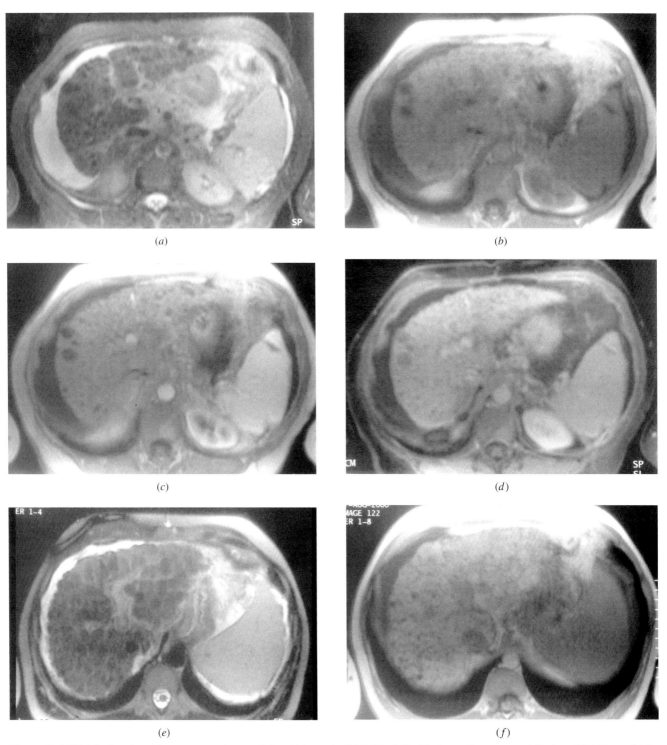

FIG. 2.157 Cirrhosis with regenerative nodules. Echo-train STIR (*a*), SGE (*b*), immediate postgadolinium SGE (*c*), and 90-s postgadolinium fat-suppressed SGE (*d*); echo-train STIR (*e*), SGE (*f*), out-of-phase SGE (*g*), immediate postgadolinium SGE (*h, i*), and 90-s postgadolinium fat-suppressed SGE (*j*) images in two different patients. The livers are diminutive in size and show irregular nodular contours consistent with cirrhosis. Multiple varying sized siderotic nodules are appreciated throughout the hepatic parenchyma that demonstrate low signal on both T2- (*a, e*) and T1-weighted (*b, f*) images and negligible enhancement after gadolinium administration, compatible with regenerative nodules.

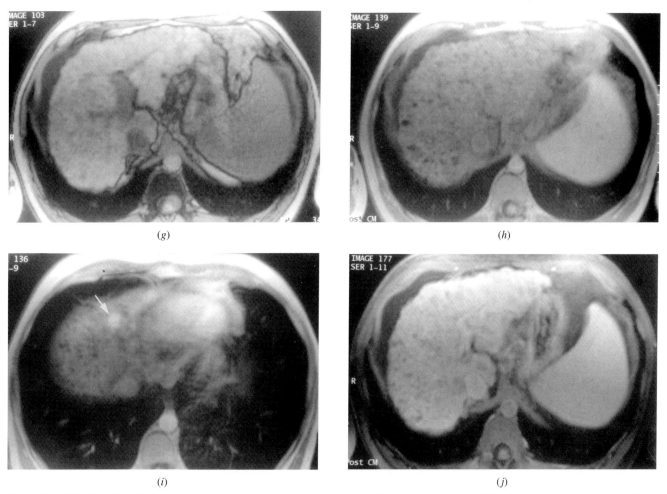

(g)

(h)

(i)

(j)

FIG. 2.157 (*Continued*) In the second patient, an intensely enhancing 1-cm nodule (arrow, *i*) is present in the dome of the liver, consistent with a severely dysplastic nodule.

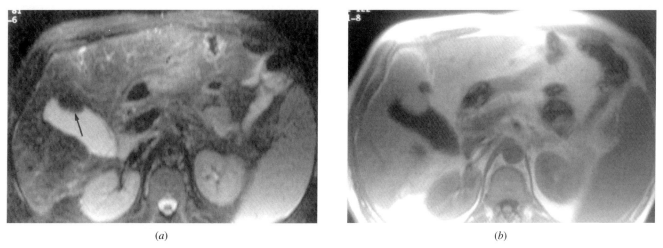

(a)

(b)

FIG. 2.158 Cirrhosis and regenerative nodules. Echo-train STIR (*a*), SGE (*b*), immediate postgadolinium SGE (*c*), and 90-s postgadolinium fat-suppressed SGE (*d*) images. The liver demonstrates mild diffuse heterogeneous signal on all sequences.

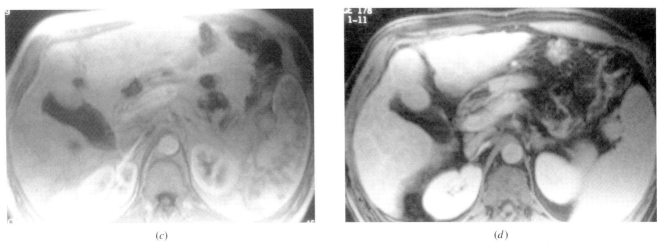

F I G . 2.158 (*Continued*) There is a hepatic nodule (arrow, *a*) that indents the anterior wall of the gallbladder that arises from the tip of *segment 4* that demonstrates near isointensity with liver on all sequences compatible with a regenerative nodule.

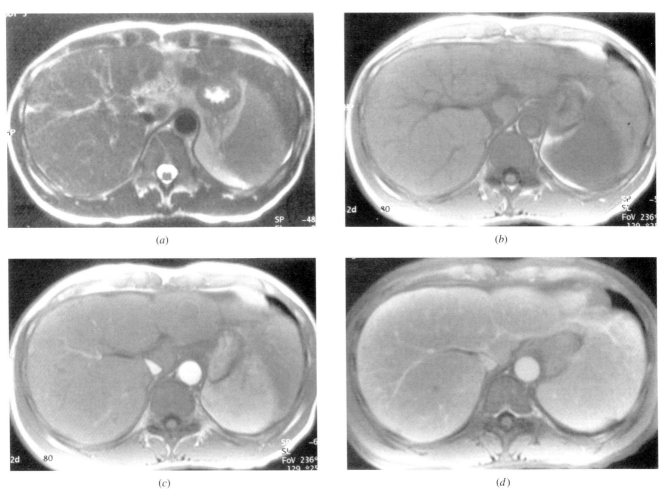

F I G . 2.159 Iron-containing regenerative nodule. T2-weighted ETSE (*a*), SGE (*b*), immediate postgadolinium SGE (*c*), and 90-s postgadolinium fat-suppressed SGE (*d*) images. There are multiple tiny lesions scattered throughout the liver that demonstrate mild hypointensity to background liver on T2- (*a*) and T1-weighted (*b*) images and negligible enhancement after contrast administration (*c*), consistent with regenerative nodules. Lesions are best seen on the postgadolinium images. Note the fine reticular linear pattern of enhancement on the delayed image (*d*).

supply to DNs is usually from the portal venous system, but a minority may also be fed by hepatic arteries. The signal intensity characteristics of DNs overlap with those of small HCCs. A common pattern is homogeneous hyperintensity on T1-weighted images and hypointensity on T2-weighted images. They are almost never hyperintense on T2-weighted images, unlike HCC. Other characteristics that distinguish HCC from DNs are lesion size larger than 3 cm, intense enhancement on hepatic arterial dominant phase images, presence of a capsule, tumor washout, and rapid interval growth [118].

DNs that develop foci of HCC appear as a high-signal intensity focus within a low-signal intensity nodule on T2-weighted images—a nodule within a nodule. The central nodule represents the focus of HCC (fig. 2.160) [118].

Portal hypertension results from obstruction at presinusoidal (e.g., portal vein), sinusoidal (e.g., cirrhosis),

postsinusoidal (e.g., hepatic vein), or multiple levels [172]. The most common cause of portal hypertension is cirrhosis. Portal hypertension causes or exacerbates complications of cirrhosis such as variceal bleeding, ascites, and splenomegaly. Portosystemic shunts may be identified using 2D time-of-flight techniques or gadolinium-enhanced SGE sequences. Gadolinium-enhanced 3D GE imaging, alone or with fat suppression, is a particularly effective technique. Direction of flow may be determined by using 2D phase-contrast techniques, or directional information may be derived by observing time-of-flight effects in the main portal vein and correlating it with time-of-flight effects in the aorta and inferior vena cava (IVC). The latter technique is best performed by acquiring superior and inferior multislice slabs, the bottom and top respectively, of the two slabs obtained at the level of the porta hepatis.

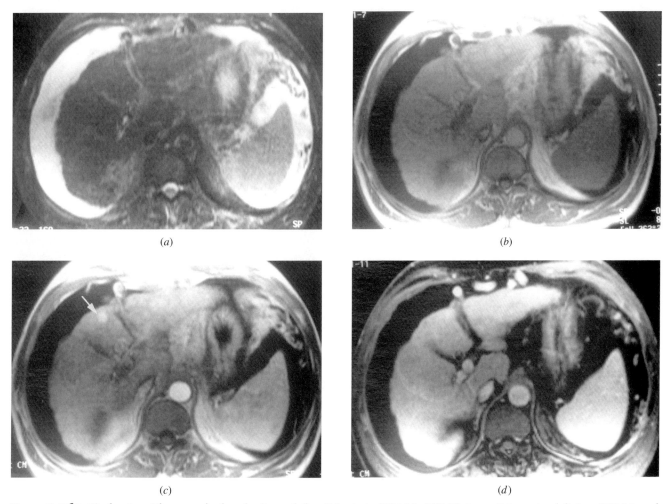

(a)   (b)

(c)   (d)

F I G . 2.160 Cirrhosis with severely dysplastic nodules. Echo-train STIR (*a*), SGE (*b*), immediate postgadolinium SGE (*c*), and 90-s postgadolinium fat-suppressed SGE (*d*) images. The liver is small and nodular, compatible with cirrhosis. There is a 1-cm lesion (arrow, *c*) in *segment 4* that is not evident on T2- (*a*) or T1-weighted (*b*) images but displays intense enhancement on the immediate postgadolinium image (*c*) and fades to isointensity on the late image (*d*), consistent with a severely dysplastic nodule. Note also the presence of ascites and collateral vessels.

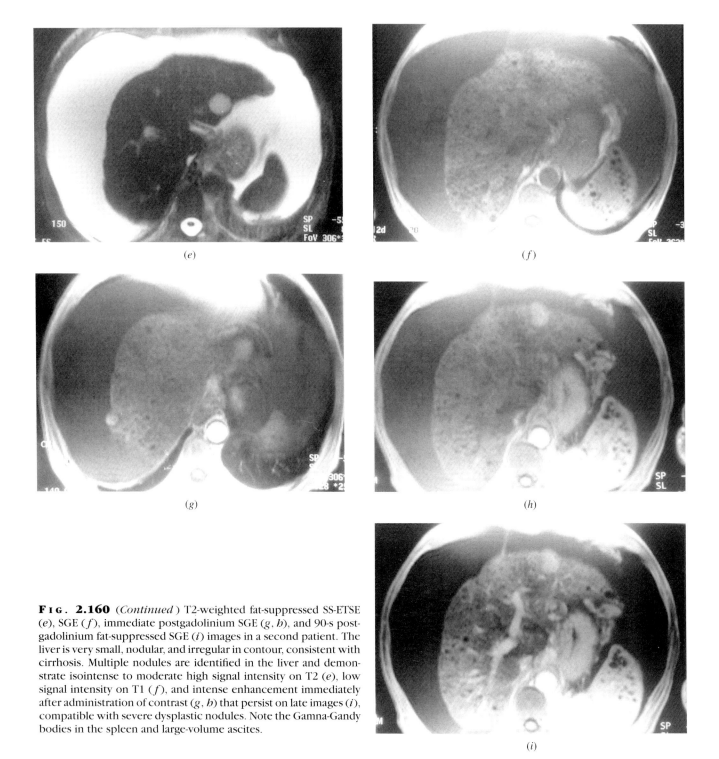

(e)

(f)

(g)

(h)

(i)

FIG. 2.160 *(Continued)* T2-weighted fat-suppressed SS-ETSE (*e*), SGE (*f*), immediate postgadolinium SGE (*g*, *h*), and 90-s post-gadolinium fat-suppressed SGE (*i*) images in a second patient. The liver is very small, nodular, and irregular in contour, consistent with cirrhosis. Multiple nodules are identified in the liver and demonstrate isointense to moderate high signal intensity on T2 (*e*), low signal intensity on T1 (*f*), and intense enhancement immediately after administration of contrast (*g*, *h*) that persist on late images (*i*), compatible with severe dysplastic nodules. Note the Gamna-Gandy bodies in the spleen and large-volume ascites.

In the early stages of portal hypertension, the portal venous system dilates, but flow is maintained. Later, substantial portosystemic shunting develops, reducing the volume of flow to the liver and decreasing the size of the portal vein. With advanced portal hypertension, portal flow may reverse and become hepatofugal. Thrombosis of the portal veins may develop with development of collaterals referred to as cavernous transformation (figs. 2.161 and 2.162).

Mesenteric, omental and retroperitoneal edema occur commonly in patients with cirrhosis because of portal hypertension (figs. 2.163 and 2.164). The appearance of mesenteric edema varies from a mild infiltrative haze to a severe masslike sheath that engulfs the mesenteric

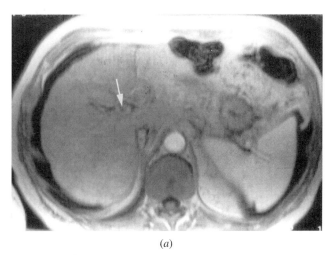

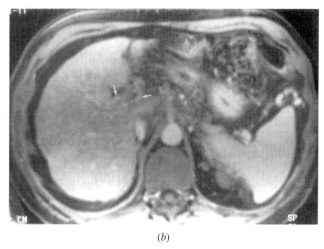

(a)   (b)

FIG. 2.161 Cavernous transformation of portal vein. Immediate postgadolinium SGE (*a*) and 90-s postgadolinium fat-suppressed SGE (*b*) images in a patient with cirrhosis. Thrombus (arrow, *a*) is present in a diminutive portal vein, and multiple small serpiginous collateral vessels (arrows, *b*) are identified in the porta hepatis consistent with cavernous transformation. Note also ascites and splenomegaly.

vessels [159, 173]. Gastrointestinal wall thickening is seen in as many as 25% of patients with end-stage cirrhosis also secondary to portal hypertension. Many of these patients do not have specific or focal bowel symptoms [159].

Portal varices arise from increased portal pressure, and portal blood is shunted into systemic veins, bypassing hepatic parenchyma. Nutrients absorbed from the gastrointestinal (GI) tract are metabolized less effectively, and hepatic function decreases. Toxic metabolites such as ammonia accumulate in the blood and result

in clinical manifestations such as hepatic encephalopathy. Diminished portal flow to the liver parenchyma is a major factor in the production of liver atrophy and prevention of regeneration [174], and portosystemic shunting may play a role in the development of hepatic atrophy in advanced cirrhosis. Major sites of portosystemic collateralization include gastroesophageal junction, paraumbilical veins (figs. 2.165 and 2.166), retroperitoneal regions, perigastric, splenorenal, omentum, peritoneum and hemorrhoidal veins [159]. Esophageal varices are a serious complication because they may rupture and

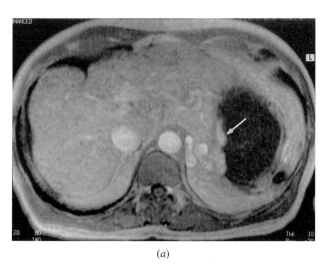

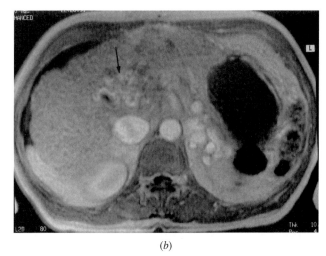

(a)   (b)

FIG. 2.162 Cirrhosis, varices. Transverse 45-s postgadolinium SGE images (*a, b*) demonstrate a cirrhotic liver with irregular contour and multiple low-signal intensity regenerative nodules smaller than 5 mm. Prominent varices are present along the lesser curvature, which are well shown on portal-phase postgadolinium images. Multiple small serpiginous enhancing structures are present in the porta hepatis (arrow, *b*) that reflect cavernous transformation of the portal vein. A prominent varix is also present within the gastric wall along the lesser curvature (arrow, *a*). Signal-void small-volume ascites is also present (*a, b*).

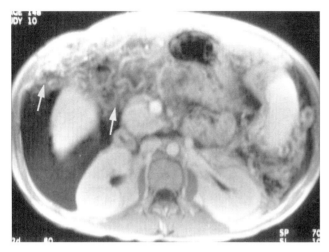

FIG. 2.163 Intraperitoneal and omental varices. Transverse 1-min postgadolinium SGE image demonstrates a tangle of small caliber varices in the right intraperitoneal space with involvement of the omentum (arrows) and in a perisplenic location.

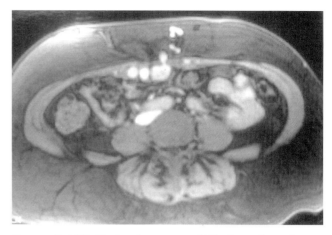

FIG. 2.165 Cirrhosis, paraumbilical varices (caput medusa). Transverse 90-s postgadolinium SGE image demonstrates large varices along the right paramedian peritoneum. Multiple subcutaneous paraumbilical varices are present, which are rendered very conspicuous because of removal of the competing high signal of fat.

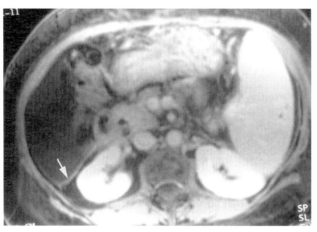

FIG. 2.164 Cirrhosis and peritoneal enhancement. Interstitial-phase gadolinium-enhanced fat-suppressed SGE image demonstrates mild linear peritoneal enhancement (arrow) consistent with microvarices in the peritoneal lining.

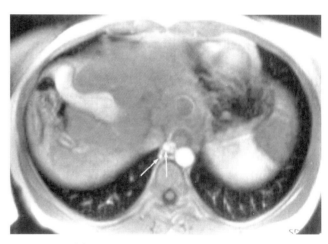

FIG. 2.166 Cirrhosis, varices, recanalized umbilical vein. Transverse 45-s postgadolinium SGE image demonstrates recanalization of a very large umbilical vein. Note that small paraesophageal varices (arrows) are also present.

produce life-threatening hemorrhage (fig. 2.167). Flow-sensitive gradient echo or gadolinium-enhanced SGE images effectively demonstrate varices as high-signal tubular structures (fig. 2.168). Varices are particularly conspicuous using fat suppression with gadolinium enhancement on SGE images as the competing high signal intensity of fat is removed. Gadolinium-enhanced water excitation SGE is another approach to demonstrate varices, as the excitation pulse possesses time-of-flight effects that accentuates the high signal in vessels produced by gadolinium enhancement. These sequences are more sensitive than contrast angiography, endoscopy, or contrast-enhanced CT imaging for detecting varices [175].

Porta Hepatis Lymphadenopathy

Porta hepatis lymphadenopathy is a common finding in benign and malignant liver disease. Porta hepatis lymphadenopathy is almost invariably present in chronic liver disease. The detection of malignant porta hepatis lymph nodes is also crucial in decision making for management of patients with malignant disease. The most effective approach for the detection of lymph nodes is the combined use of a fat-suppressed T2-weighted sequence and interstitial-phase gadolinium-enhanced T1-weighted fat-suppressed imaging. On the T2 sequence lymph nodes are moderately high signal and both liver and background fat are relatively low signal, rendering excellent conspicuity. Definition of the rounded

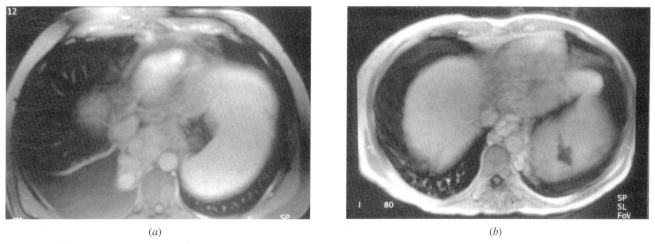

(a)   *(b)*

F I G . 2.167 Cirrhosis, paraesophageal varices. Transverse 45-s postgadolinium SGE (*a, b*) in two patients demonstrate large paraesophageal varices.

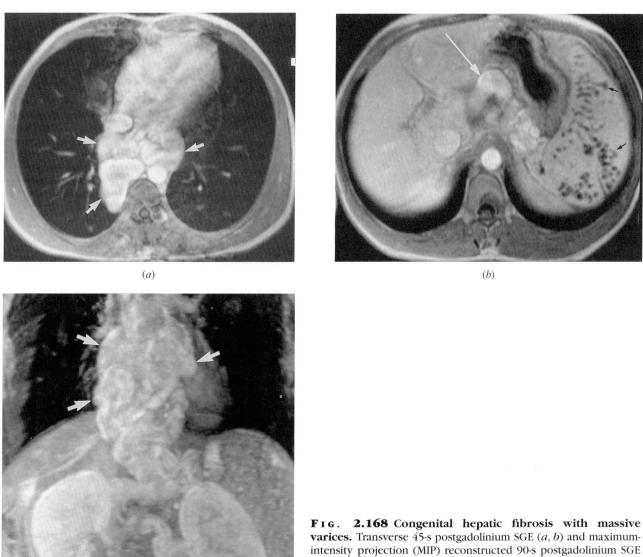

(a)   *(b)*

(c)

F I G . 2.168 Congenital hepatic fibrosis with massive varices. Transverse 45-s postgadolinium SGE (*a, b*) and maximum-intensity projection (MIP) reconstructed 90-s postgadolinium SGE (*c*) images. Massive esophageal varices (arrows, *a*) and large varices along the lesser curvature of the stomach (large arrow, *b*) are present. The 3D reconstructed SGE images demonstrate the craniocaudal extent of esophageal varices (arrows, *c*). Gamna-Gandy bodies are present in the spleen (small arrows, *b*).

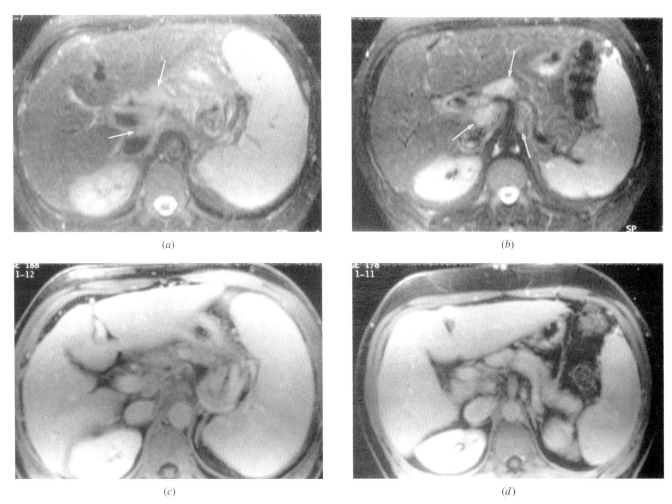

(a)

(b)

(c)

(d)

F I G . 2.169 Porta hepatis lymph nodes. Echo-train STIR (*a, b*), 90-s postgadolinium fat-suppressed SGE (*c, d*); echo-train STIR (*e*) and 90-s postgadolinium fat-suppressed SGE (*f*); and 90-s postgadolinium fat-suppressed SGE (*g, h*) images in three patients with porta hepatis lymph nodes (arrows, *a, b, g, h*). The lymph nodes in the porta hepatis are best detected by the combination of identification of high-signal tissue on T2-weighted fat-suppressed images (*a, b, e*) and demonstration that the high-signal tissue has definable convex margins on interstitial-phase gadolinium-enhanced fat-suppressed SGE images (*c, d, f, g, h*). All of these patients have chronic hepatitis or cirrhosis. Enlarged porta hepatis lymph nodes are common in patients with chronic liver disease.

contour of lymph nodes is optimal with the gadolinium-enhanced T1-weighted fat-suppressed technique and thereby distinguishes rounded lymph nodes from ill-defined inflammatory tissue, which is also high signal on T2 (fig. 2.169).

Iron Overload
Primary (Idiopathic Hemochromatosis)

■ GENETIC HEMOCHROMATOSIS

Genetic hemochromatosis (GH) is the most common genetic disorder among the caucasian population in the United States; 1 in every 250–300 persons is homozygous for the hemochromatosis mutation, and at least 1 in

every 10 persons is a carrier for the mutation [176]. GH results from excessive gastrointestinal absorption and deposition of iron in tissues such as liver, heart, pancreas, anterior pituitary, joints, and skin. Serologic abnormalities and mild symptoms may occur earlier in life, but the clinical signs and symptoms do not appear until the fifth or sixth decade of life [176]. Untreated, it results in end-organ damage, which may include cirrhosis and HCC; HCC arises in up to 36% of cases and often is the cause of death [176, 177]. Pathologic features of hemochromatosis in the liver include iron deposition as hemosiderin pigment granules in hepatocytes. Iron is a direct hepatotoxin. Fibrous septa develop slowly, leading to micronodular cirrhosis. Bile duct epithelium, Kupffer cell (RES) uptake of hemosiderin pigment is not marked. Early in the disease process, iron accumulation

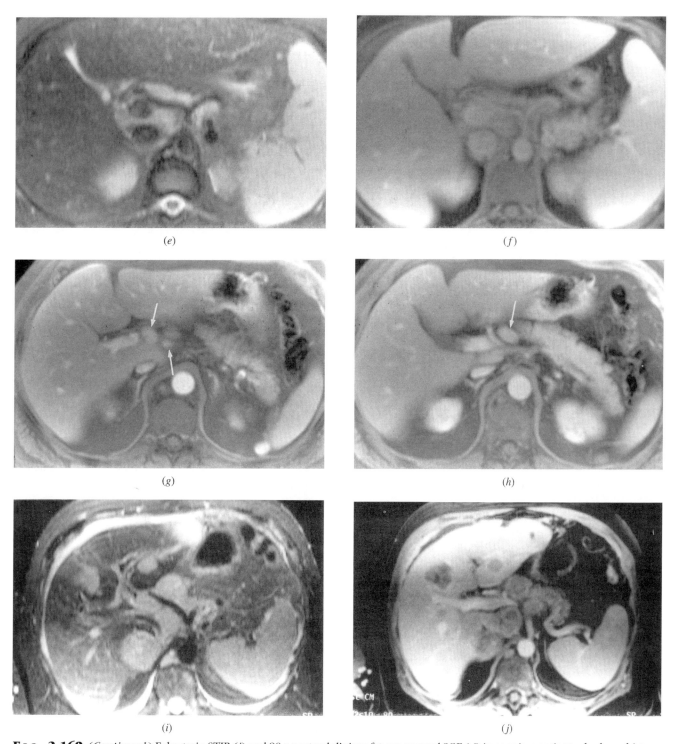

(e)

(f)

(g)

(h)

(i)

(j)

F i g . 2.169 (*Continued*) Echo-train STIR (*i*) and 90-s postgadolinium fat-suppressed SGE (*j*) images in a patient who has a history of squamous cell skin cancer. Multiple enlarged lymph nodes are present in the porta hepatis and celiac axis regions consistent with malignant lymphadenopathy. Note also the presence of liver metastases. The combined use of fat-suppressed T2-weighted sequence and gadolinium-enhanced T1-weighted fat-suppressed images is the most consistent method to demonstrate porta hepatis lymphadenopathy.

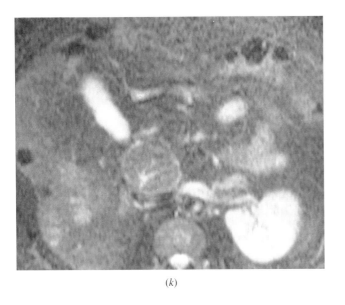

(k)

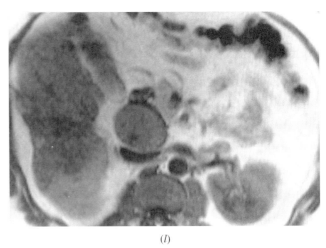

(l)

FIG. 2.169 (*Continued*) Echo-train STIR (*k*), SGE (*l*), and 90-s postgadolinium fat-suppressed SGE (*m*) images in a patient who has a history of HCC. There is a portal caval lymph node that demonstrates intermediate signal on T2 (*k*) and low signal on T1-weighted images (*l*) and moderate enhancement after administration of contrast (*m*). Malignant lymph nodes tend to have a rounded configuration, as in this case. These three MR techniques all maximize contrast between lymph nodes and background tissue.

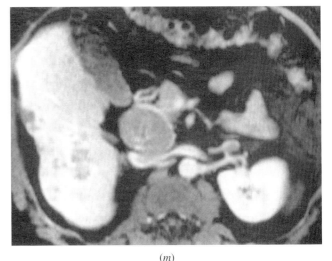

(m)

is restricted to the liver (fig. 2.170) [178]. Disease detection at this stage, with institution of phlebotomy therapy, may result in a normal life expectancy. Over time, iron deposition progresses to involve other organs, primarily the pancreas and heart. In advanced disease, decreased signal intensity of the liver and pancreas occurs. A diagnostic feature of idiopathic hemochromatosis is that signal intensity of the spleen is not substantially decreased on T2-weighted or T2*-weighted images (fig. 2.171). This finding is due to accumulation of iron within the parenchyma of the liver and pancreas and lack of selective uptake by the RES in the spleen. The presence of iron deposition in the pancreas correlates with irreversible changes of cirrhosis in the liver.

Some patients who present with HCC have previously unsuspected GH [179]. Because tumor cells do not contain excess iron [180, 181] they are well shown as high-signal intensity masses relative to iron-overloaded liver on MR images. In a patient with hemochromatosis, nonsiderotic nodules that are not hemangiomas or cysts are highly suspicious for HCC, because regenerative nodules in these patients contain iron. Dysplastic nodules in patients with increased hepatic iron may contain a different concentration of iron than surrounding hepatic parenchyma.

Secondary Hemochromatosis

■ TRANSFUSIONAL IRON OVERLOAD

Transfusional iron overload is the most common form of excess iron deposition in North America. Fibrosis is usually mild despite even heavy iron stores, and cirrhosis

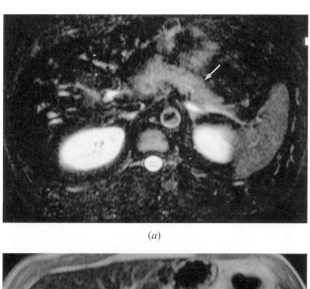

(a)

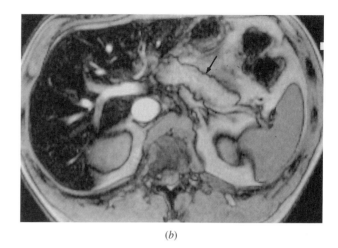

(b)

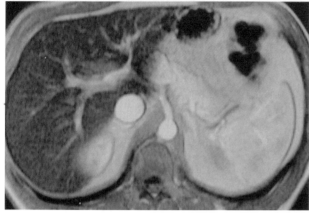

(c)

F I G . 2.170 Idiopathic hemochromatosis, early disease. T2-weighted fat-suppressed ETSE (*a*), out-of-phase SGE (*b*), and immediate postgadolinium SGE (*c*) images. The liver is low in signal intensity on noncontrast T2-weighted (*a*) and T1-weighted (*b*) images consistent with substantial iron deposition. The spleen is relatively normal in signal intensity on these sequences, reflecting that iron is not in the RES but in hepatocytes. The pancreas (arrow, *a*, *b*) is normal in signal intensity on noncontrast images and enhances normally with gadolinium. Iron deposition limited to the liver is consistent with early precirrhotic disease.

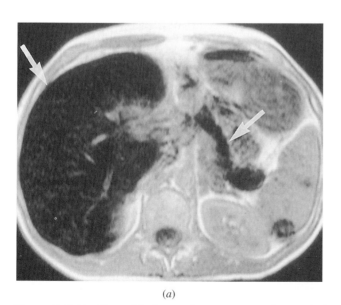

(a)

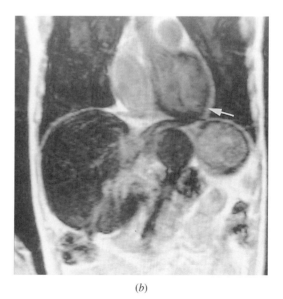

(b)

F I G . 2.171 Idiopathic hemochromatosis, advanced disease. Transverse (*a*) and coronal SGE (*b*), and coronal 45-s postgadolinium SGE (*c*) images. The precontrast T1-weighted image (*a*) demonstrates signal void liver and pancreas (arrows, *a*). The coronal SGE image (*b*) also demonstrates low-signal intensity left ventricular myocardium (arrow, *b*).

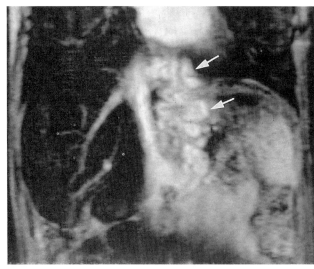

(c)

FIG. 2.171 (*Continued*) On the 45-s postgadolinium image (*c*), multiple enhanced varices are shown (arrows, *c*), which reflect portal hypertension secondary to cirrhosis.

is rare. Iron deposition in the RES results in low signal intensity of the spleen, liver, and bone marrow on MR images, best shown on T2- or T2*-weighted images.

Iron overload from multiple transfusions may be distinguished from genetic hemochromatosis in that large amounts of iron accumulate primarily within the RES of the liver (Kupffer cells) and spleen (monocytes/macrophages) in transfusional overload, with relative sparing of the functional cells within the parenchyma.

Evaluation of pancreatic and splenic signal intensity allows this distinction. Signal intensity of the spleen is usually normal with genetic hemochromatosis, whereas signal intensity of the pancreas is normal with most cases of transfusional overload.

In mild forms of transfusional siderosis, signal loss is appreciated only on T2- and T2*-weighted images, and signal intensity on T1-weighted images appears relatively normal (fig. 2.172). In moderate to severe forms of iron deposition the T2-shortening effect of iron results in low signal on T1-weighted images as well (fig. 2.173). If liver and spleen are gray on TE = 4 SGE we consider iron deposition moderate, and if liver and spleen are near signal void iron deposition is severe. In massive iron overload (e.g., >100 units) direct tissue deposition may occur in other cells and tissues, notably the pancreas (figs. 2.174 and 2.175) [178, 179].

Regional variation in iron deposition in the liver parenchyma may occur. Focal iron sparing or focal iron

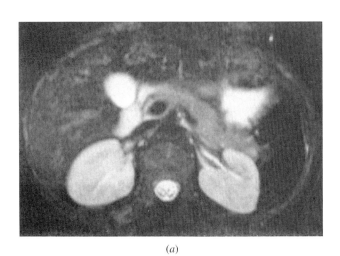

(a)

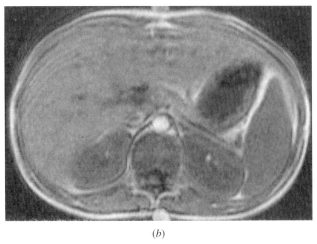

(b)

FIG. 2.172 Transfusional siderosis, mild. T2-weighted fat-suppressed ETSE (*a*) and SGE (*b*) images. On the T2-weighted image (*a*), the liver and spleen are low in signal intensity and the pancreas is normal in signal intensity. Signal intensity of the liver, spleen, and pancreas appear normal on the T1-weighted image (*b*). Iron deposition in the liver and spleen that results in signal loss appreciable only on T2-weighted images, and not on T1-weighted images, is compatible with mild transfusional siderosis.

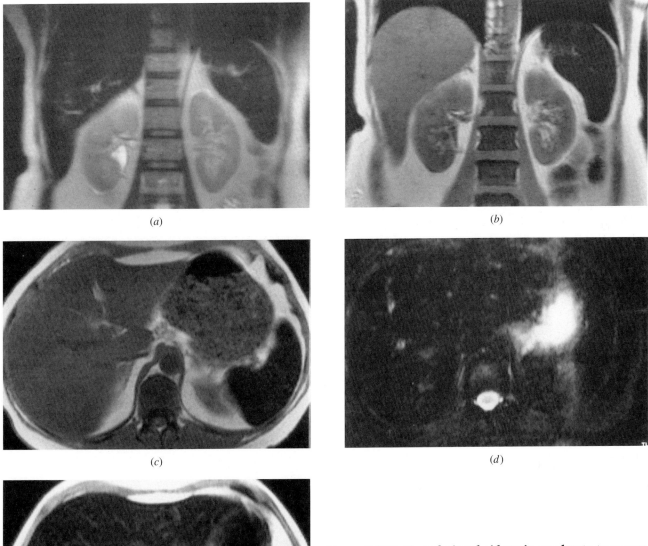

(a)

(b)

(c)

(d)

(e)

F I G. 2.173 Transfusional siderosis, moderate to severe. Coronal T2-weighted SS-ETSE (*a*), coronal SGE (*b*), and transverse SGE (*c*) images. Low signal intensity of the liver and spleen is present on T2-weighted images (*a*). Mildly low signal intensity of the liver and moderately low signal intensity of the spleen are observed on T1-weighted images (*b, c*) consistent with moderate iron deposition.

T2-weighted fat-suppressed ETSE (*d*) and SGE (*e*) images in a second patient demonstrate very low signal intensity of the liver and spleen on T1 (*e*) and T2-weighted (*d*) images consistent with severe iron deposition.

deposition may occur (fig. 2.176). Observation of magnetic susceptibility effects in areas of greater iron deposition establish the diagnosis.

■ HEMOLYTIC ANEMIA

Hepatic signal intensity in patients with hemolytic anemia varies, based on the rate of reincorporation of iron into the bone marrow, the rate of absorption of oral iron, and the transfusional history. Patients with thalassemia vera have increased absorption of oral iron and, in the absence of blood transfusions, will develop erythrogenic hemochromatosis primarily affecting the liver [182]. The appearance is generally indistinguishable from idiopathic hemochromatosis. Patients with heterozygous forms of hemolytic anemias may not have low enough red blood cell counts or hemoglobin levels to necessitate transfusion and may therefore develop this pattern

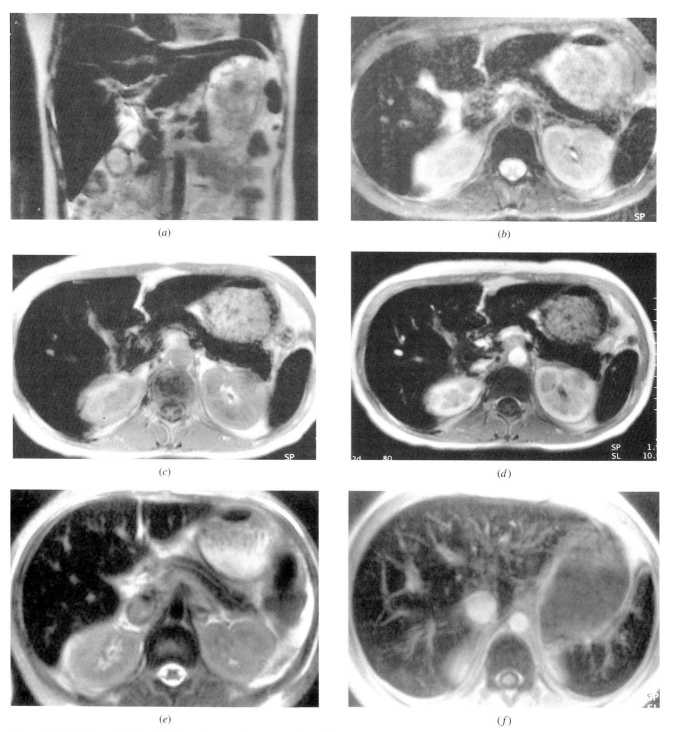

(a)   (b)

(c)   (d)

(e)   (f)

FIG. 2.174 Transfusional siderosis, massive. Coronal SS-ETSE (*a*), T2-weighted fat-suppressed ETSE (*b*), SGE (*c*), and immediate postgadolinium SGE (*d*) images. Massive iron deposition is present in the liver, spleen and pancreas (*a–c*), demonstrated by signal-void liver, spleen, and pancreas. Blooming artifact is apparent surrounding the pancreas (*c*). These organs remain signal void after gadolinium administration (*d*).

T2-weighted SS-ETSE (*e*) and 1-min postgadolinium SGE (*f*) images in a second patient with massive iron deposition demonstrate dark liver, spleen and pancreas on T2-weighted (*e*) and postgadolinium T1-weighted (*f*) images.

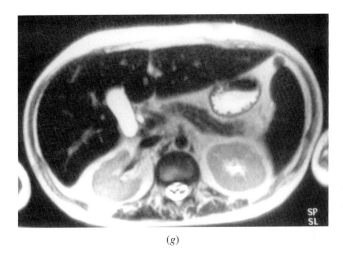

(g)

FIG. 2.174 (*Continued*) T2-weighted SS-ETSE (*g*) in a third patient, who is 8 years old and has a history of lymphoma. There is decreased signal intensity of the liver, spleen, and pancreas on T2-weighted images. The decreased signal intensity in the pancreas reflects multiple blood transfusions.

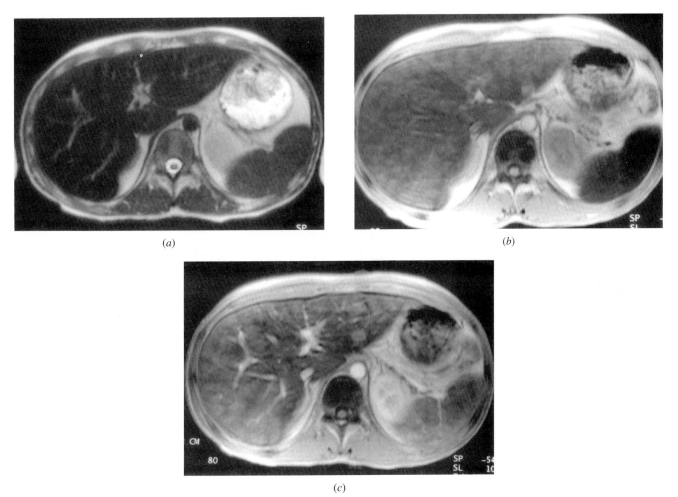

(a)

(b)

(c)

FIG. 2.175 Transfusional siderosis, heterogeneous iron deposition. T2-weighted SS-ETSE (*a*), SGE (*b*), and immediate postgadolinium SGE (*c*) images in a patient who has a history of acute leukemia. The liver and the spleen are low signal intensity on T2 (*a*) and T1-weighted (*b*) images consistent with iron deposition. On pre- and postcontrast T1-weighted images, there is a heterogeneous appearance consistent with heterogeneous distribution of iron deposition, in the setting of transfusional siderosis.

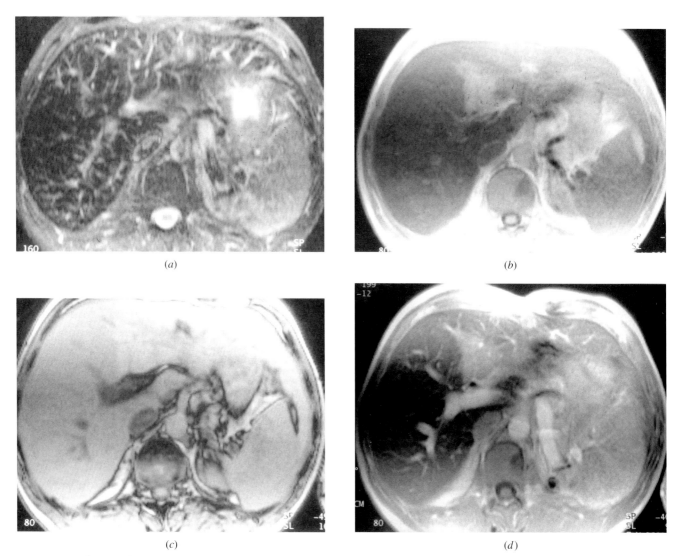

(a)

(b)

(c)

(d)

FIG. 2.176 Transfusional siderosis with focal sparing. Echo-train STIR (*a*), SGE (*b*), out-of-phase SGE (*c*), and immediate postgadolinium SGE (*d*) images. The liver is enlarged and demonstrates decreased signal reflecting iron deposition. There is a region in *segment 4* with increased signal intensity on the T1-weighted image. On the short-TE out-of-phase image (*c*) the susceptibility artifact from iron diminishes, resulting in a decrease in the signal intensity difference between iron-deposited and normal liver. This is virtually the opposite effect that is seen in focal normal liver in the setting of fat infiltration. Normal vessels are appreciated extending through the focal normal liver on the postgadolinium image.

of iron overload (fig. 2.177). The majority of patients with hemolytic anemias have received blood transfusions and therefore also develop coexisting transfusional iron overload (fig. 2.178).

Patients with sickle cell anemia have rapid turnover of hepatic iron and will have normal hepatic signal intensity unless they have undergone recent blood transfusions [182]. Renal cortical signal intensity may be decreased because of filtration and tubular absorption of free hemoglobin, the severity of which is not dependent on transfusional history (see Chapter 9, *Kidneys*) [178]. Iron overload in the liver and renal cortex is typically seen in patients with paroxysmal nocturnal hemoglobinuria [179].

CIRRHOSIS

Hepatocellular iron is commonly increased mildly in patients with cirrhosis, particularly those with cirrhosis secondary to ethanol abuse. The cause of the excess iron deposition is not well understood but may be related to anemia, pancreatic insufficiency, or decreased transferrin synthesis [176]. The degree of signal loss of the liver is not as great as that seen with idiopathic hemochromatosis or transfusional siderosis.

Coexisting Fat and Iron Deposition
Fat and iron deposition may occur concurrently within the liver. Coexisting fat and iron deposition may be

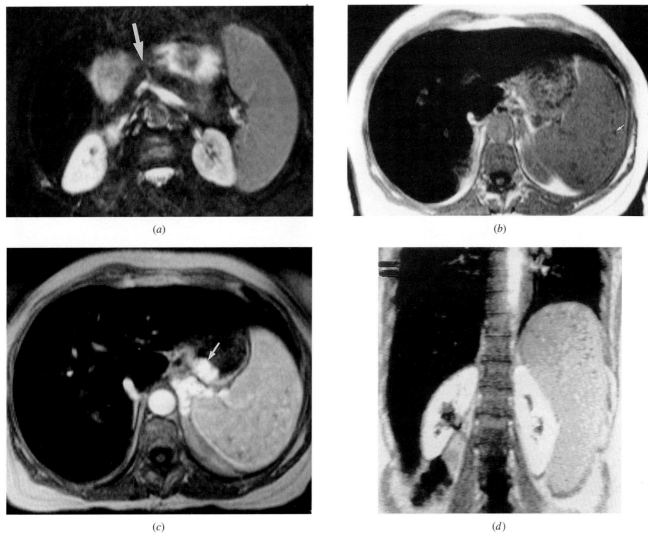

(a)

(b)

(c)

(d)

F I G . 2.177 Heterozygous thalassemia. T2-weighted fat-suppressed ETSE (*a*), SGE (*b*), and 45-s (*c*) and coronal 90-s (*d*) post-gadolinium SGE images. The liver demonstrates severe iron deposition and is signal void on T2-(*a*) and T1-weighted (*b*) images. The spleen is greatly enlarged and shows negligible iron deposition but does contain Gamna-Gandy bodies (arrow, *b*). The pancreas is modestly low in signal intensity (arrow, *a*). Varices along the lesser curvature and within the gastric wall (arrow, *c*) are clearly shown on the 45-s postgadolinium images. Splenomegaly (*d*), Gamma-Gandy bodies, and varices are secondary to portal hypertension. The pattern of iron deposition reflects increased intestinal absorption without transfusional siderosis, which is a common appearance for heterozygous hemolytic anemias, as these patients often do not require blood transfusions.

demonstrated by using several gradient-echo MR sequences with differing in-phase and out-of-phase echo times. In the presence of iron, signal intensity of the liver will decrease steadily as echo time increases because of $T2^*$ effects. At out-of-phase echo times both higher than and lower than the echo time for in-phase images, a disproportionate drop of liver signal intensity will occur relative to spleen because of fat-water phase cancellation. The combined observations that liver and spleen are nearly signal void on T2-weighted images, reflecting iron deposition, and that liver drops in signal intensity relative to spleen comparing out-of-phase to in-phase SGE images, reflecting fat deposition, are also diagnostic for coexistent iron and fat deposition (fig. 2.179).

Fatty Liver

Fatty liver, or steatosis, is defined as accumulation of lipid within hepatocytes. It constitutes one of the commonest abnormalities in liver surgical or autopsy specimens. Fat (primarily triglyceride) accumulates within hepatocytes in patients with a variety of conditions, including diabetes mellitus, obesity, and malnutrition, or after exposure to ethanol or other chemical toxins. Fatty change may be uniform, patchy, focal, or spare foci of normal liver. At times focal fatty infiltration or geographic regions of normal liver within fatty liver may mimic the appearance of mass lesions.

Fatty liver may interfere with the detection of focal liver masses on CT images or sonography [183].

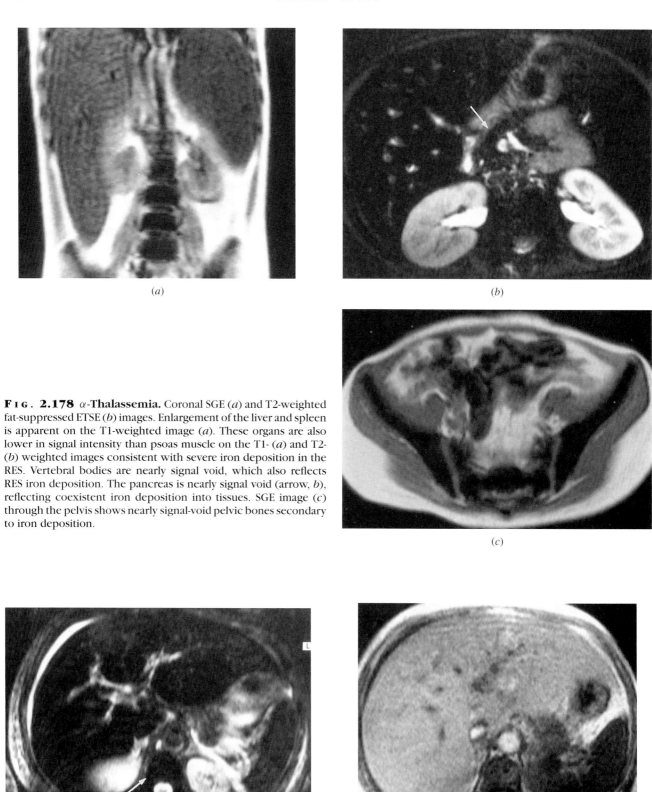

F I G . 2.178 *α*-**Thalassemia.** Coronal SGE (*a*) and T2-weighted fat-suppressed ETSE (*b*) images. Enlargement of the liver and spleen is apparent on the T1-weighted image (*a*). These organs are also lower in signal intensity than psoas muscle on the T1- (*a*) and T2- (*b*) weighted images consistent with severe iron deposition in the RES. Vertebral bodies are nearly signal void, which also reflects RES iron deposition. The pancreas is nearly signal void (arrow, *b*), reflecting coexistent iron deposition into tissues. SGE image (*c*) through the pelvis shows nearly signal-void pelvic bones secondary to iron deposition.

F I G . 2.179 Coexistent iron and fatty deposition. T2-weighted fat-suppressed SS-ETSE (*a*), SGE (*b*), and out-of-phase SGE (*c*) images. On T2 (*a*), the liver, spleen, and bone marrow (arrow, *a*) are nearly signal void, which is consistent with coexistent iron deposition.

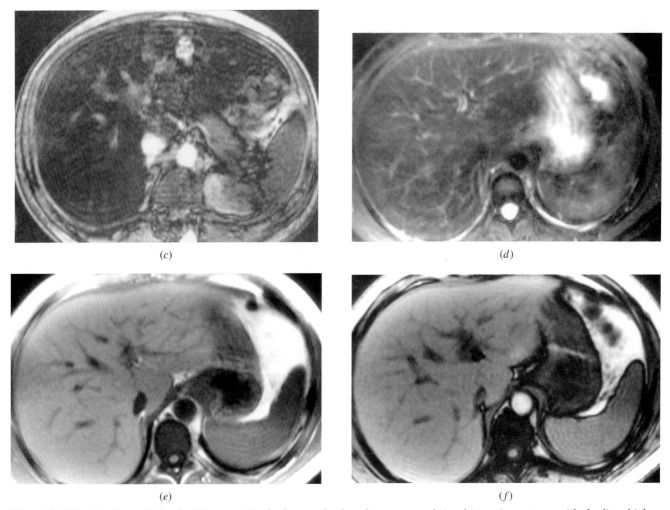

(c)   (d)

(e)   (f)

F I G. 2.179 (*Continued*) On the T1 image (*b*), the liver and spleen have a normal signal intensity pattern, with the liver higher in signal intensity than the spleen. On the longer-echo-time out-of-phase image (*c*), the liver drops in signal intensity below that of spleen, which is consistent with fatty infiltration. Ascites is well shown as high-signal intensity fluid along the liver margin on the T2-weighted image (*a*).

Echo-train STIR (*d*), in-phase SGE (*e*), and out-of-phase SGE (*f*) images in a second patient demonstrate iron deposition and mild fatty infiltration in the liver. Iron deposition is shown by the low signal on T2 (*d*), and fat is shown by the loss of liver-spleen contrast on the shorter-TE out-of-phase sequence (*f*).

These cases illustrate the effect of iron on T2. It is essential to be aware that T1-weighted gradient-echo sequences demonstrate out-of-phase effects, which cycle with in-phase and out-of-phase times, and susceptibility effects, which increase with increase in TE.

MRI is particularly effective in evaluating the liver of patients with fatty liver for the presence of focal lesions such as metastases. In this setting, non-fat-suppressed T1-weighted images and fat-suppressed T2-weighted images maximize the contrast between the liver and lesions. On non-fat-suppressed T1-weighted images, the liver may be higher in signal intensity than normal liver, maximizing the contrast with low-signal intensity masses, whereas on fat-suppressed T2-weighted images fatty liver is lower in signal intensity than normal liver, maximizing the contrast with moderately high-signal intensity masses.

Out-of-phase SGE imaging is a highly accurate technique to examine for fatty liver and to distinguish focal fat from neoplastic masses [184, 185]. Comparing out-of-phase to in-phase SGE images, the presence of fatty metamorphosis results in signal loss. The spleen is generally used as the organ of reference for signal loss. As fat content approaches 50% of the voxel element in the liver, the liver appears blacker relative to the spleen. For lesser amounts of fat (<15%) signal of liver on a TE = 2 out-of-phase sequence appears near equivalent to the signal of spleen, whereas the TE = 4 in-phase sequence demonstrates some higher signal of the liver relative to the spleen. In cases of focal fat, reference is usually to surrounding hepatic parenchyma. Demonstration that a lesion, which is isointense or hyperintense to liver on in-phase SGE images, loses signal homogeneously on

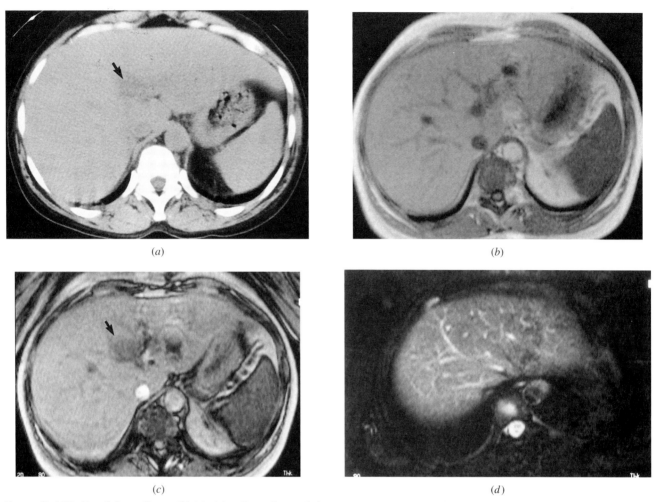

(a)   (b)

(c)   (d)

F I G . 2.180 Focal fatty liver. CT (*a*), SGE (*b*), and out-of-phase SGE (*c*) images. A CT image acquired in a patient with breast cancer demonstrates a low-density lesion in the medial segment (arrow, *a*). The in-phase T1-weighted image (*b*) shows no lesion in this location, whereas on the out-of-phase image (*c*), signal drop occurs in the central region of the medial segment (arrow, *c*), which is diagnostic for focal fatty infiltration when combined with the information that enhancement was isointense on the hepatic arterial dominant phase images.

out-of-phase images is highly diagnostic for focal fat (figs. 2.180–2.182). Focal normal liver in the setting of diffuse fatty infiltration of the liver is shown by a focus of high signal intensity in a background of diminished signal intensity liver on out-of-phase images (figs. 2.183 and 2.184). An important ancillary observation is that uncomplicated fatty deposition within the liver enhances with gadolinium usually indistinguishably from normal liver. This feature pertains to the hepatic arterial dominant phase images as well. Focal masses that contain fat generally have different enhancement, as described below.

The morphology of focal fatty infiltration most often permits distinction from fat within tumors, such as HCC, adenoma, regenerative nodule, angiomyolipoma, or lipoma. Focal fat usually has angular, wedge-shaped margins that are usually relatively well defined. Common locations for focal fat are adjacent to the ligamentum

teres, the central tip of segment IV and, less commonly, along the gallbladder. The central tip of segment IV is also a common location for focal fatty sparing. Variations in blood supply from the remainder of the liver may account for this. Masses that contain fat usually have a rounded configuration.

Although some well-differentiated HCCs contain lipid, most HCCs with high signal intensity on T1-weighted images do not [186]. Hemorrhage, melanin, and protein may be associated with nonfatty masses with high signal intensity on T1-weighted images. Out-of-phase images distinguish between these tumors and lipid-containing masses or focal fatty infiltration. HCC that contains lipid tends to be more well defined than focal fatty infiltration. HCC is often encapsulated and is most commonly not homogeneously fatty. It usually contains some elements with high signal intensity on

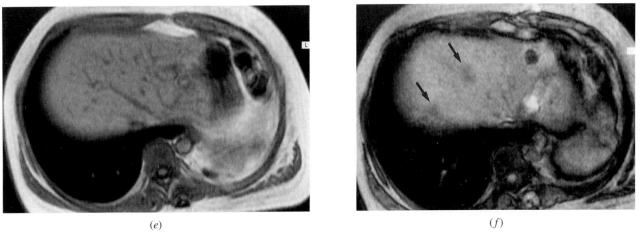

(e)   (f)

F I G . 2.180 (*Continued*) T2-weighted fat-suppressed ETSE (*d*), SGE (*e*), and out-of-phase SGE (*f*) images in a second patient. Previous ultrasound study in this young boy with acute myelogeneous leukemia demonstrated two liver lesions. No liver lesions are apparent on the in-phase T1-weighted image (*e*). On the out-of-phase image (*f*), two focal low-signal rounded masses are apparent (arrows, *f*). The T2-weighted image (*d*) does not reveal any lesions. No tumor blush was apparent on immediate postgadolinium images (not shown). The identification of lesions on only out-of-phase SGE images is diagnostic for fatty infiltration.

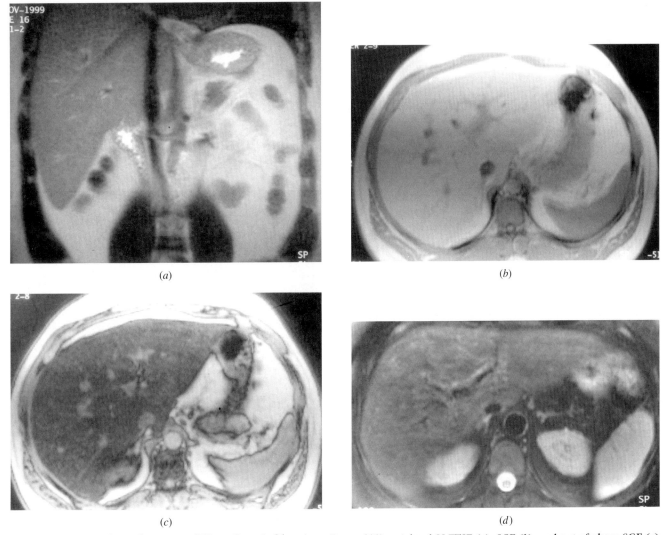

(a)   (b)

(c)   (d)

F I G . 2.181 Moderately severe diffuse fatty infiltration. Coronal T2-weighted SS-ETSE (*a*), SGE (*b*), and out-of-phase SGE (*c*) images. The liver is high in signal on the echo-train T2-weighted image (*a*) which reflects the fact that fat, including fatty liver, is high signal on long-echo-train sequences.

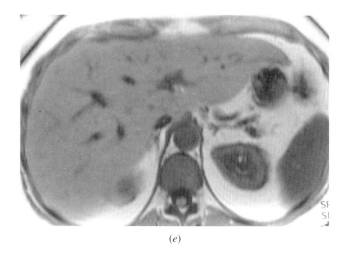

(e)

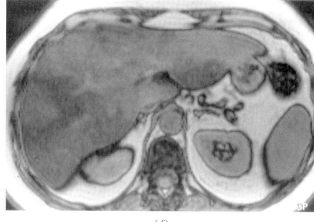

(f)

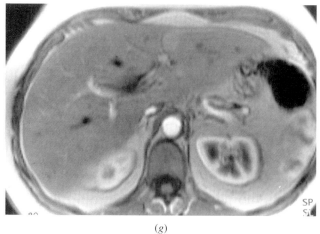

(g)

FIG. 2.181 (*Continued*) A useful internal comparison is the psoas muscle: liver should be of comparable signal. Note in this patient that the liver is considerably higher in signal than psoas. In-phase (b) and out-of-phase (c) images confirm moderately severe fatty infiltration.

T2-weighted fat-suppressed ETSE (d), SGE (e), out-of-phase SGE (f), and immediate postgadolinium SGE (g) images in a second patient. The liver demonstrates moderately severe heterogeneous drop in signal on the out-of-phase image (f) with respect to in-phase (e) image, consistent with severe diffuse patchy fatty infiltration. Note that enhancement of fatty liver is generally indistinguishable from normal when an in-phase echo time is used for gadolinium-enhanced imaging.

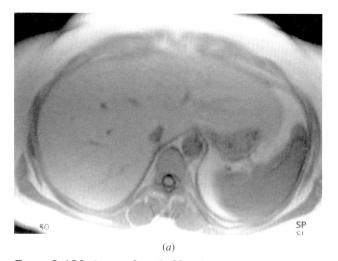

(a)

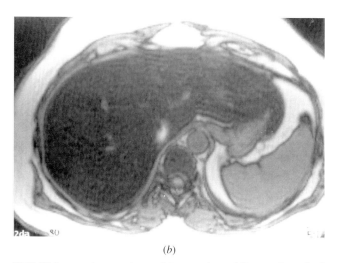

(b)

FIG. 2.182 Severe fatty infiltration. SGE (a) and out-of-phase SGE (b) images in a patient with an enlarged liver and marked fatty infiltration.

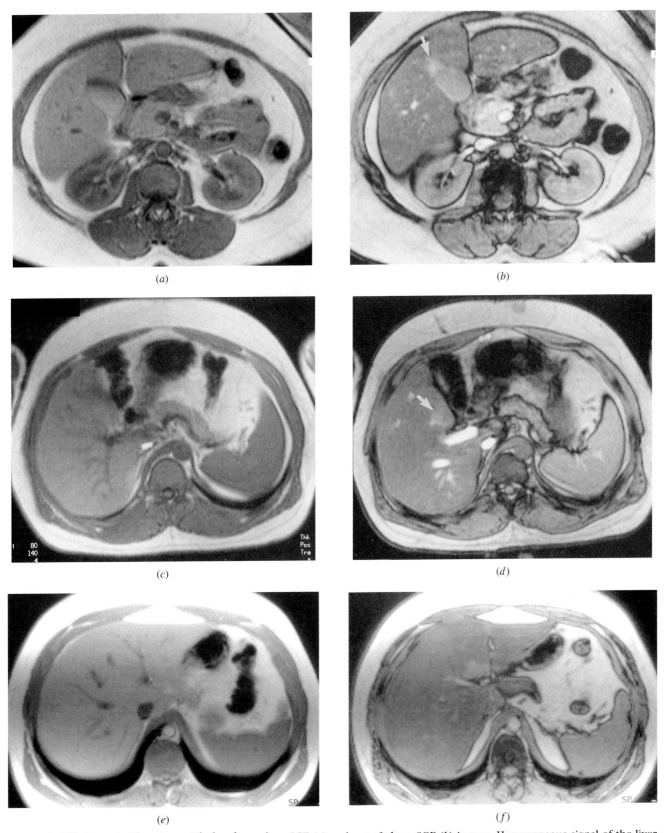

(a)

(b)

(c)

(d)

(e)

(f)

F I G . 2.183 Fatty infiltration with focal sparing. SGE (*a*) and out-of-phase SGE (*b*) images. Homogeneous signal of the liver is present on the T1-weighted image (*a*). On the out-of-phase image (*b*), the liver drops in signal with a focus of higher signal liver adjacent to the gallbladder (arrow, *b*) representing focal normal liver.

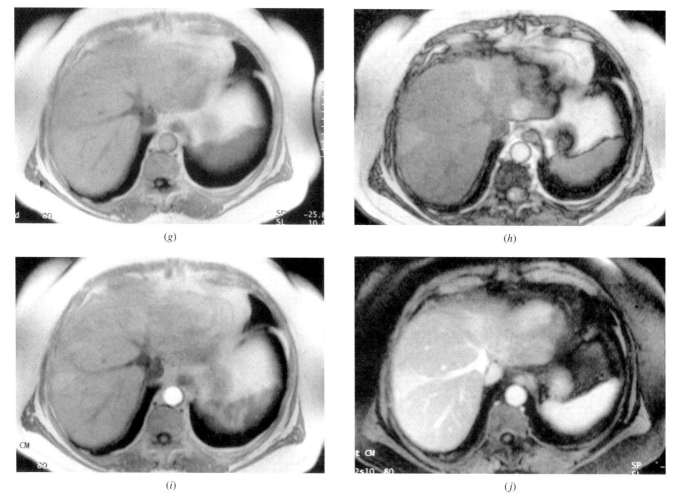

(g)

(h)

(i)

(j)

FIG. 2.183 (*Continued*) SGE (*c*) and out-of-phase SGE (*d*) images in a second patient. The liver is normal in signal intensity on the in-phase image (*c*). On the out-of-phase image (*d*), the liver drops in signal intensity relative to the spleen, with focal sparing present in the tip of *segment 4* (arrow, *d*).

SGE (*e*) and out-of-phase SGE (*f*) images in a third patient. There is a mild fatty infiltration of the liver with focal sparing of the tip of *segment 4* (*f*)

SGE (*g*), out-of-phase SGE (*h*), immediate postgadolinium SGE (*i*), and 90-s postgadolinium fat-suppressed SGE (*j*) images in a fourth patient. Wedge-shaped regions of focal normal liver in a fatty deposited liver are present. Note that on 90-s postgadolinium image (*j*) these same regions are identified as higher signal. This reflects a fat suppression effect of the remainder of the liver rather than a gadolinium-enhanced effect of the regions of normal liver.

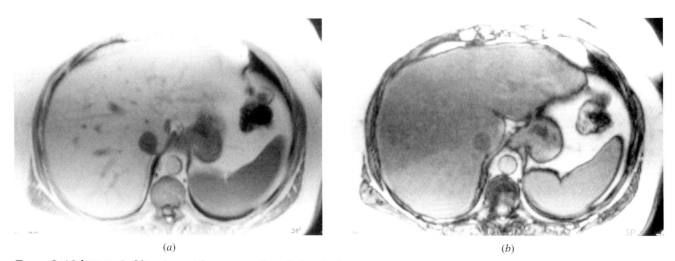

(a)

(b)

FIG. 2.184 Fatty infiltration with segmental variation in fat content. SGE (*a*), out-of-phase SGE (*b*), immediate postgadolinium SGE (*c*), and 90-s postgadolinium fat-suppressed SGE (*d*) images.

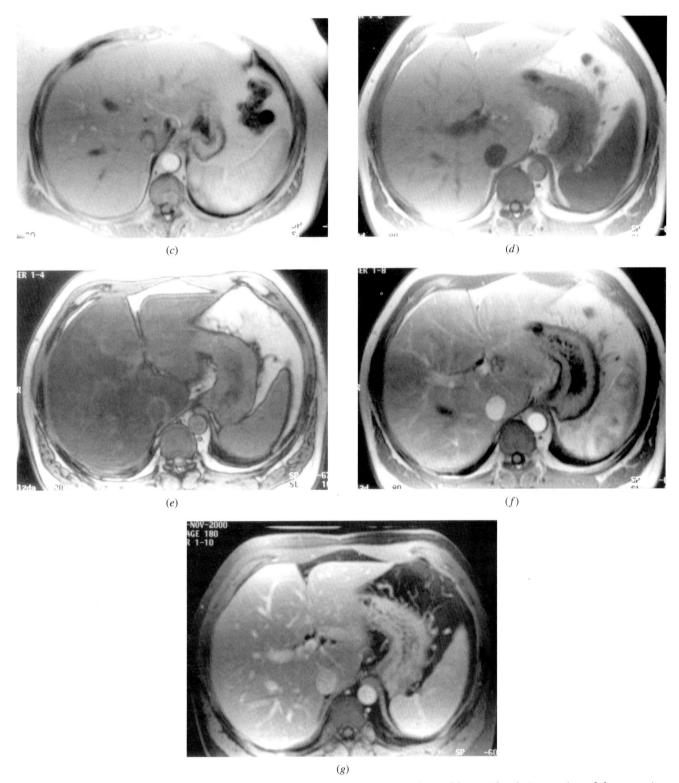

(c)

(d)

(e)

(f)

(g)

F I G . 2.184 (*Continued*) On the out-of-phase (*b*) image there is trisegmental signal loss with relative sparing of the posterior segment of the right lobe. Signal intensity on postgadolinium images is unremarkable for the entire liver.

SGE (*d*), out-of-phase SGE (*e*), immediate postgadolinium SGE (*f*), and 90-s postgadolinium fat-suppressed SGE (*g*) images in a second patient. There is slightly less fatty infiltration of the left lobe compared to the right, reflected by relatively lesser drop in signal on the out-of-phase image (*e*).

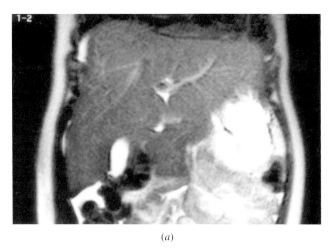

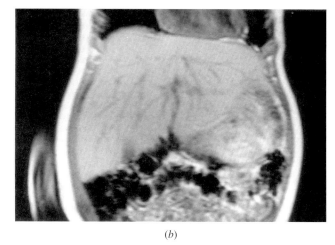

(a)   (b)

F I G . 2.185 Storage disease. Coronal T2-weighted SS-ETSE (*a*) and SGE (*b*) images in a patient who has a history of mucopolysaccharidosis. The liver is enlarged.

fat-suppressed T2-weighted images. Of all focal hepatic lesions, hepatic adenoma may most closely resemble focal fatty infiltration as these tumors may have relatively uniform fat content. Demonstration of a capillary blush on immediate postgadolinium SGE images establishes the diagnosis of adenoma. Angiomyolipoma and lipoma may be composed of fat and therefore will not drop in signal intensity on out-of-phase images; however, these lesions will demonstrate a phase-cancellation artifact along their margin with liver. Angiomyolipoma and lipoma will lose signal when fat-suppressed techniques are used.

Mucopolysaccharidoses

The mucopolysaccharidoses are a group of inherited disorders caused by incomplete degradation and storage of acid mucopolysaccharides (glycosaminoglycans). The clinical manifestations result from the accumulation of mucopolysaccharides in somatic and visceral tissues. Mucopolysaccharides are major components of the extracellular substance of connective tissue. Because of widespread accumulation of incompletely degraded mucopolysaccharides, many organ system are affected. Hepatosplenomegaly, skeletal deformities, valvular lesions, subendothelial arterial deposits, particularly in the coronary arteries, and CNS abnormalities are common. Pathologic postmortem examination of six cases of mucopolysaccharidoses revealed a unique finding of diffuse fibrosis throughout the liver in each case [187]. Extensive hepatocyte and Kupffer cell vacuolization is a microscopic finding. The degree of disability and overall prognosis in each of the mucopolysaccharidoses are determined by extent of the physical and mental involvement [188]

On MR images, hepatotomegaly is commonly observed (fig. 2.185). More specific MR imaging features are yet to be elucidated.

Hepatic Vascular Disorders

Arteriovenous Fistulas

Abnormal arterial-venous communications or fistulas may occur in the liver secondary to injury, tumor, or congenital disease. Clinically, important or symptomatic hepatic vascular fistulas are uncommon but are usually caused by trauma, including iatrogenic trauma (fig. 2.186) [189]. Fistulas are well shown employing gadolinium-enhanced technique, either as 2D technique or as 3D MRA technique (fig. 2.187).

Congenital vascular fistulas are rare. One of the more common conditions is hereditary hemorrhagic telangiectasia (Rendu-Osler-Weber syndrome). Telangiectasias, aneurysms and arteriovenous shunts occur frequently in several internal organs in this condition. Visceral involvement has been documented in the liver, GI tract, lungs, spleen, brain, kidneys, and genital tracts [190].

On imaging, the liver may be filled with numerous variably sized abnormal arterial-venous communications. Lesions may appear as multiple well-defined enhancing masses (fig. 2.188).

Portal Venous Obstruction/Thrombosis

Obstruction of the portal vein may be insidious and well tolerated or may be an acute, potentially life-threatening event. Most cases fall in between these two extremes. Blockage of the portal vein may be extrahepatic or intrahepatic. Common causes of extrahepatic portal vein

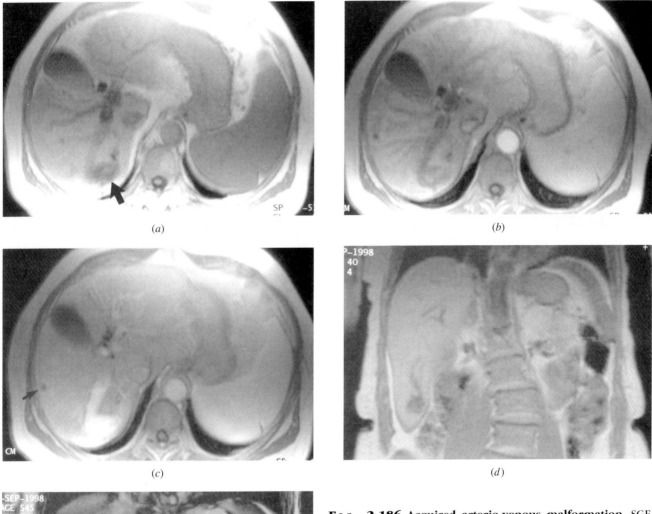

(a)

(b)

(c)

(d)

(e)

F I G . 2.186 Acquired arterio-venous malformation. SGE (*a*), immediate postgadolinium SGE (*b*), and 45-s postgadolinium SGE (*c*) images. There is a 2-cm rounded structure (arrow, *a*) in the posterior segment of the right lobe, with a prominent posterior branch of the right portal vein entering the lesion. After contrast administration there is early minimal enhancement (*b*) and 45-s intense enhancement (*c*) of this lesion in continuity with the portal vein (*c*). Note also the tiny hepatic cyst or biliary hamartoma (arrow, *c*), nodular contour of the liver, and splenomegaly.

Coronal SGE (*d*) and gadolinium-enhanced refocused gradient-echo (*e*) images in a second patient. There is a lesion in the inferior aspect of the right lobe that demonstrates large paired vessels leading into and away from it. This lesion shows decreased signal on the precontrast image (*d*) and intense enhancement after gadolinium administration (*e*) consistent with arterio-venous malformation.

obstruction include 1) massive hilar lymphadenopathy due to metastatic abdominal cancer, 2) phlebitis resulting from peritoneal sepsis (e.g., appendicitis), 3) propagation of splenic vein thrombosis secondary to pancreatitis and 4) postsurgical thrombosis following abdominal procedures. Cirrhosis of the liver is the most common intrahepatic cause of portal venous obstruction. Intravas-

cular invasion by primary or secondary cancer in the liver may occur [191].

On imaging, portal vein thrombosis may be demonstrated by using black-blood techniques (e.g., spin-echo techniques with superior and inferior saturation pulses) and bright-blood techniques (e.g., time-of-flight gradient-echo or gadolinium-enhanced SGE). A

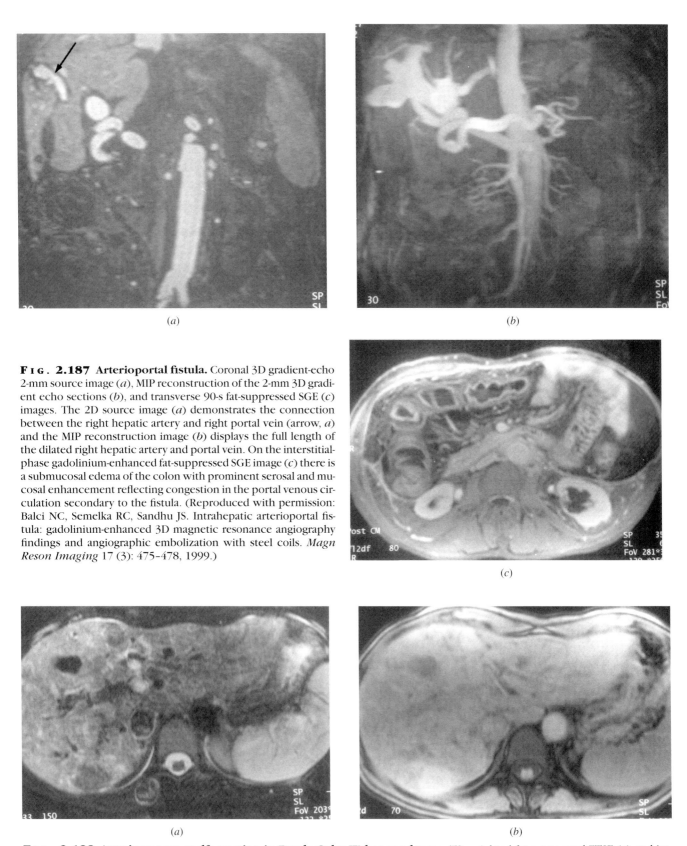

(a)

(b)

FIG. 2.187 Arterioportal fistula. Coronal 3D gradient-echo 2-mm source image (*a*), MIP reconstruction of the 2-mm 3D gradient echo sections (*b*), and transverse 90-s fat-suppressed SGE (*c*) images. The 2D source image (*a*) demonstrates the connection between the right hepatic artery and right portal vein (arrow, *a*) and the MIP reconstruction image (*b*) displays the full length of the dilated right hepatic artery and portal vein. On the interstitial-phase gadolinium-enhanced fat-suppressed SGE image (*c*) there is a submucosal edema of the colon with prominent serosal and mucosal enhancement reflecting congestion in the portal venous circulation secondary to the fistula. (Reproduced with permission: Balci NC, Semelka RC, Sandhu JS. Intrahepatic arterioportal fistula: gadolinium-enhanced 3D magnetic resonance angiography findings and angiographic embolization with steel coils. *Magn Reson Imaging* 17 (3): 475–478, 1999.)

(c)

(a)

(b)

FIG. 2.188 Arterio-venous malformation in Rendu-Osler-Weber syndrome. T2-weighted fat-suppressed ETSE (*a*) and immediate postgadolinium SGE (*b*) images in a patient with Osler-Weber-Rendu syndrome. There are multiple varying size liver lesions, many of which demonstrate intense enhancement on immediate postgadolinium images (*b*) representing arterio-venous malformation. Some lesions are low signal on T2 (*a*) and postgadolinium images consistent with hemorrhage and thrombosis.

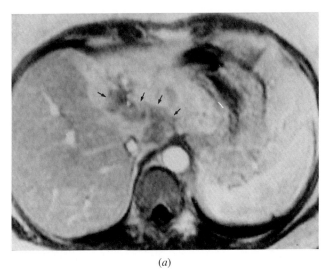 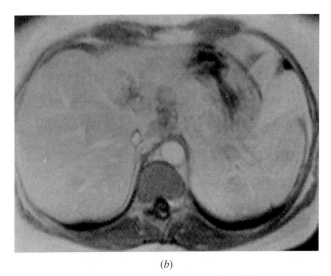

(a)　　　　　　　　　　　　　　　　　　(b)

FIG. 2.189 Portal vein thrombosis, secondary to tumor. Immediate postgadolinium SGE (*a*) and 90-s postgadolinium SGE (*b*) images. A liver metastasis is present in the caudate lobe and the lateral segment associated with heterogeneously enhancing thrombus extending into the left portal vein (arrows, *a*). On the immediate postgadolinium image (*a*), there is increased enhancement of the left lobe, which equilibrates by 90-s (*b*).

combination of both approaches is often useful to increase diagnostic confidence. Portal veins may be occluded by tumor thrombus, bland thrombus, or extrinsic compression. MRI usually is able to distinguish between these entities. Tumor and bland thrombus may be distinguished from each other by the observation that tumor thrombus is higher in signal intensity on T2-weighted images, is soft-tissue signal intensity on time-of-flight gradient-echo images, and enhances with gadolinium (fig. 2.189). Bland thrombus is low in signal

intensity on T2-weighted and time-of-flight gradient-echo images and does not enhance with gadolinium (figs. 2.190 and 2.191). Tumor thrombus is most often observed with hepatocellular carcinoma, although it may also occur with metastases. Bland thrombus may be observed in the setting of cirrhosis and various inflammatory/infectious processes involving organs in the portal circulation, with pancreatitis being the most common. Increased enhancement of the vein wall is appreciated in the setting of infected bland thrombus.

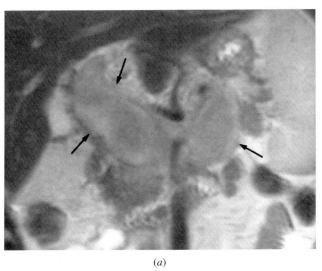 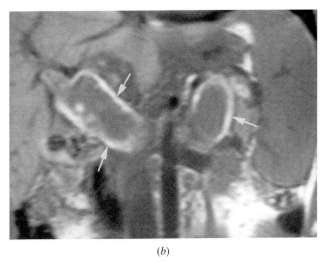

(a)　　　　　　　　　　　　　　　　　　(b)

FIG. 2.190 Portal and splenic vein thrombosis—subacute blood thrombus. Coronal T2-weighted SS-ETSE (*a*), coronal SGE (*b*), T2-weighted fat-suppressed SS-ETSE (*c*), SGE (*d*), fat-suppressed SGE (*e*), and 90-s postgadolinium fat-suppressed SGE (*f, g, h*) images in a 21-yr-old man who has a history of spontaneous retroperitoneal hematoma associated with portal and splenic vein thrombosis.

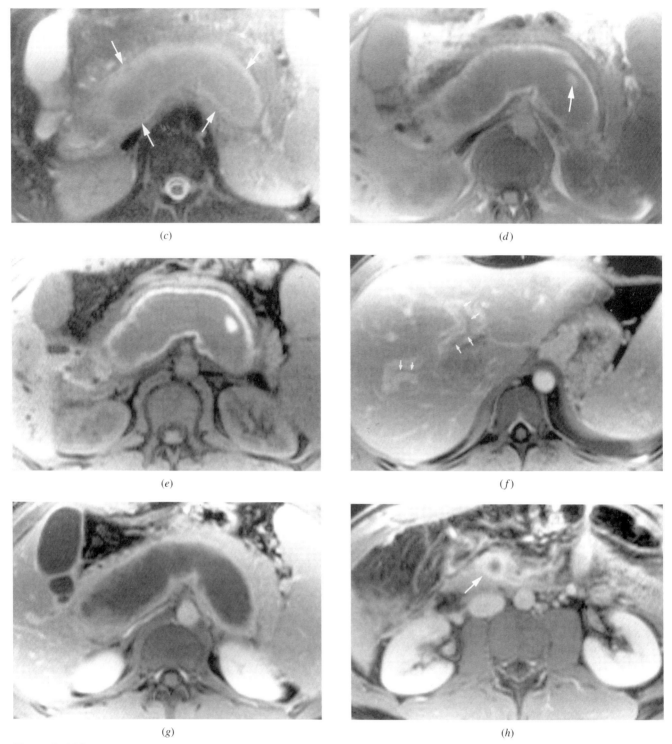

(c)

(d)

(e)

(f)

(g)

(h)

F I G . 2.190 (*Continued*) There is marked dilatation of the splenic vein, portal vein, and proximal superior mesenteric vein, which contains an expansive thrombus (arrows, *a–c*) extending throughout this venous system. The thrombus demonstrates an increased signal intensity rim on T1-weighted images (*b, d, e*) and a small focus of increased signal intensity (arrow, *d*) within the thrombus, consistent with blood products at different stages of breakdown. Fat-suppressed postgadolinium images (*f, g*) demonstrate no evidence of enhancement within the thrombus. Thrombus is present in normal caliber intrahepatic portal vein branches (*f*). Substantially increased enhancement of tissues surrounding the thrombosed SMV (arrow, *b*) suggests an underlying inflammatory process.

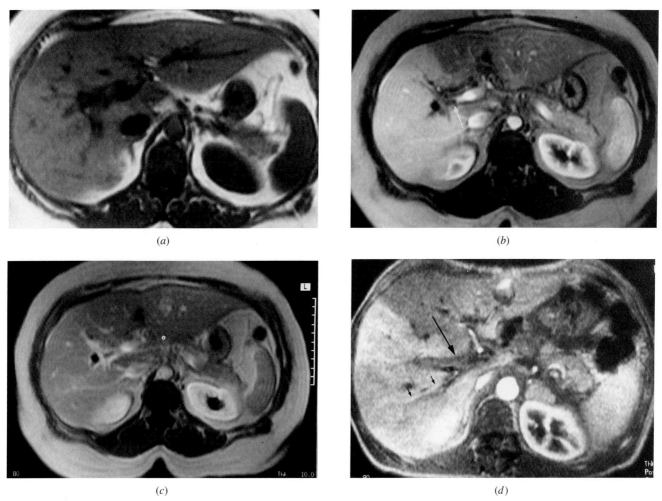

(a)

(b)

(c)

(d)

F I G . 2.191 Portal vein thrombosis—blood thrombus. SGE (*a*) and immediate (*b*) and 2-min (*c*) postgadolinium SGE images in a patient who has ascending cholangitis. The SGE image (*a*) demonstrates a normal-signal intensity liver. On the immediate postgadolinium image (*b*), increased enhancement of the right lobe of the liver is apparent, with signal void thrombus (arrow, *b*) identified in continuity with the gadolinium-containing high-signal right portal vein. Liver parenchymal enhancement equilibrates by 2 min (*c*).

Immediate postgadolinium SGE image (*d*) in a second patient, who has pancreatitis, demonstrates transient increased enhancement of the right lobe of the liver. A patent high-signal right hepatic artery is seen (small arrows, *d*); a low-signal intensity thrombus is present in the right portal vein (long arrow, *d*).

Extrinsic compression of portal veins is most commonly caused by malignant tumors but may also occur with benign tumors such as hemangiomas. Cholangiocarcinoma, in particular, has a propensity to cause extrinsic compression and obstruction of portal veins. Lobar or segmental portal vein obstruction caused by tumor may result in discrete wedge-shaped regions of increased signal intensity on T2-weighted images and on immediate postgadolinium SGE images [184, 192–196]. Increased signal intensity on T2-weighted images may reflect some degree of hepatocellular injury. Decreased blood supply results in decreased size of hepatocytes, which increases the proportion of liver volume occupied by the vascular and interstitial spaces. Obstruction of the portal vein may also cause atrophy, with compensatory hypertrophy of

other segments [184, 192]. Collateral periportal veins may maintain portal perfusion when the main portal vein is thrombosed. In time, this network of collateral venous channels dilates and the thrombosed portal vein retracts, producing cavernous transformation [197, 198].

After administration of intravenous gadolinium, transient increased enhancement of hepatic parenchyma may be apparent in areas with decreased portal perfusion during the hepatic arterial dominant phase of enhancement (see figs. 2.189, and 2.190) [88, 199]. We reported exact correlation between perfusion defects on CTAP with regions of transient high signal intensity on immediate postgadolinium SGE images in eight patients (fig. 2.192) [199]. These findings showed that regions with absent or diminished portal venous supply received

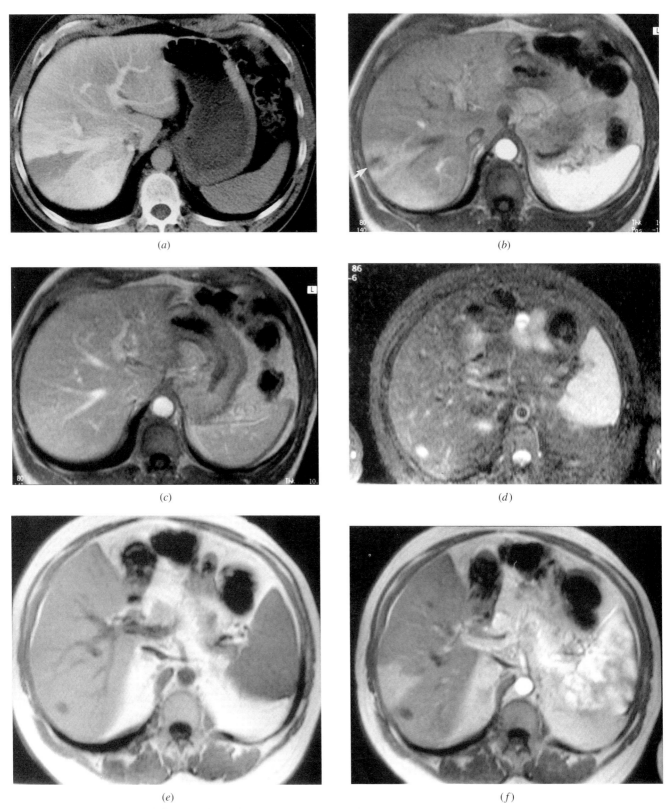

(a)

(b)

(c)

(d)

(e)

(f)

FIG. 2.192 Perfusional abnormality related to colon cancer liver metastasis. Spiral CTAP (*a*), immediate postgadolinium SGE (*b*), and 90-s postgadolinium SGE (*c*) images. The CTAP image (*a*) demonstrates a wedge-shaped perfusion defect in the right lobe of the liver. On the immediate postgadolinium SGE image (*b*), wedge-shaped increased enhancement is present surrounding a peripheral 2-cm liver metastasis (arrow, *b*). By 90-s after gadolinium (*c*), both the perfusion defect and the metastases have equilibrated with liver. (Reproduced with permission from [89]). Semelka RC, Schlund JF, Molina PL, Willms AG, Kahlenberg M, Mauro MA, Weeks SM, Cance WG: Malignant liver lesions: Comparison of spiral CT arterial portography and MR imaging for diagnostic accuracy, cost, and effect on patient management. *J Magn Reson Imaging* 6: 39–43, 1996.

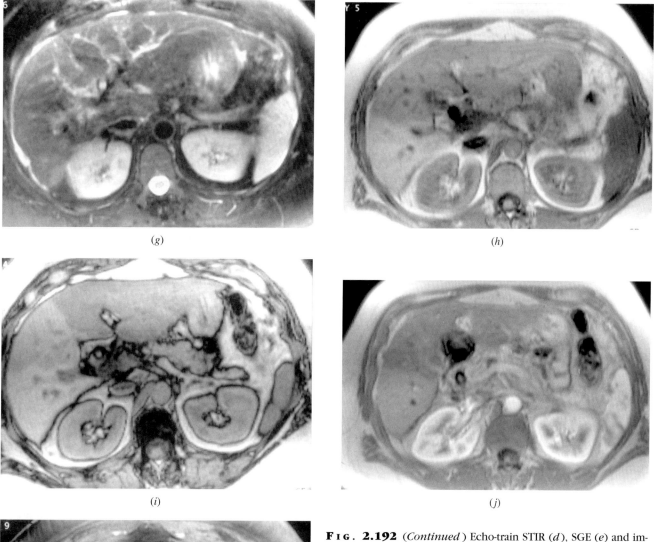

(g)

(h)

(i)

(j)

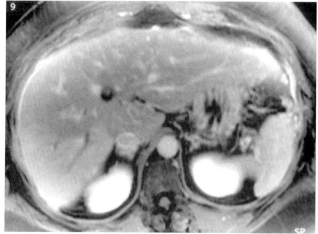

(k)

F I G . 2.192 (*Continued*) Echo-train STIR (*d*), SGE (*e*) and immediate postgadolinium SGE (*f*) images in a second patient, show a perfusional abnormality of transient increased enhancement seen on the immediate postgadolinium image (*f*), in a patient who has a history of colon cancer. Note the small cyst adjacent to the abnormal area. Perfusional abnormalities of transient increased enhancement are not uncommon in patients with colon cancer liver metastases. Many are related to metastases, but in some their cause is not clear, as in this case.

T2-weighted fat-suppressed ETSE (*g*), SGE (*h*), out-of-phase SGE (*i*), immediate postgadolinium SGE (*j*), and 90-s postgadolinium fat-suppressed SGE (*k*) images in a third patient with a history of colon cancer. There is a segmental signal intensity difference in liver, seen on T1-weighted images before and after gadolinium. Note also the thickening and enhancement of the peritoneum from peritoneal metastases, best seen on interstitial-phase fat-suppressed T1-weighted images (*k*).

increased hepatic arterial supply. This paradoxical increased enhancement of hepatic parenchyma distal to an obstructed portal vein branch largely reflects increased hepatic arterial supply due to an autoregulatory mechanism. Segments with obstructed portal venous supply and increased hepatic arterial supply will display early intense enhancement after contrast administration. Gadolinium delivered in the first pass is more concentrated in hepatic arteries than in portal veins and is delivered earlier by hepatic arteries than by portal veins. On later images, concentration of gadolinium in hepatic arteries and portal veins equilibrates, which explains the transient nature of the increased enhancement.

Hepatic Venous Thrombosis

Budd-Chiari Syndrome. Although originally described for acute, usually fatal, thrombotic occlusion of the hepatic veins, the definition of Budd-Chiari syndrome has been broadened to include subacute and chronic occlusive syndromes.

Obstruction of venous outflow from the liver results in portal hypertension, ascites, and progressive hepatic failure. Budd-Chiari syndrome is more common in women, and an underlying thrombotic tendency is present in up to one-half of patients. Causes include polycythemia vera, pregnancy, postpartum state, and intra-abdominal cancer, especially HCC [200]. Pathologically, acute changes after hepatic vein thrombosis show dilatation of veins and congestion of sinusoids. As disease advances, sinusoids become collagenized and hepatocytes become atrophic with loss of parenchyma.

Usually, hepatic venous outflow is not completely eliminated because a variety of accessory hepatic veins may drain above or below the site of obstruction. In some cases, obstruction may be segmental or subsegmental. Although the disease most commonly involves major hepatic veins, demonstration of patent central hepatic veins may be observed as small or intermediate-sized veins may be occluded in isolation [201]. In the chronic setting, regions with completely obstructed hepatic venous outflow will develop shunting of blood from hepatic arteries to portal veins, producing reversed portal venous flow [195, 202–204]. The involved liver parenchyma is thereby deprived of portal vein supply. Hepatic regeneration, hypertrophy, and atrophy depend in part on the degree of portal perfusion [174]. Budd-Chiari syndrome most often results in atrophy of peripheral liver, which experiences severe venous obstruction, and hypertrophy of the caudate lobe and central liver, which are relatively spared.

Absence of hepatic veins may be demonstrated by techniques in which flowing blood is signal void or by techniques in which flowing blood is high in signal intensity such as time-of-flight techniques or portal-phase gadolinium-enhanced SGE sequences. Generally, a combination of both approaches results in the highest diagnostic accuracy, although bright-blood techniques are the most accurate and usually suffice.

On dynamic gadolinium-enhanced MR images, the peripheral atrophic liver in Budd-Chiari syndrome may enhance to a greater or lesser extent than normal or hypertrophied liver. A recent study found that dynamic enhancement patterns differed for acute, subacute, and chronic Budd-Chiari syndrome, with combinations of enhancement patterns present when acute is superimposed on subacute disease [205]. In acute-onset Budd-Chiari syndrome the peripheral liver enhances less than central liver, presumably because of acute increased tissue pressure with resultant diminished blood supply from both hepatic arterial and portal venous systems. The liver demonstrates a dramatic appearance of increased central enhancement compared to decreased enhancement of liver that persists on later postcontrast images. This is associated with low signal on T1 and moderately high signal on T2-weighted images reflecting associated edema (figs. 2.193 and 2.194) [206].

In subacute Budd-Chiari syndrome, reversal of flow in portal veins and development of small intra- and extrahepatic venovenous collaterals occur. Many of the collaterals are capsule based. On dynamic gadolinium-enhanced MR images the enhancement of subacute disease differs substantially from the acute syndrome. Mildly increased and heterogeneous enhancement is apparent in the peripheral liver relative to central liver on hepatic arterial dominant phase images that, over time, becomes more homogeneous with the remainder of the liver. Signal of the peripheral liver is mildly low on T1 and mildly increased on T2, similar to acute Budd-Chiari syndrome. Caudate lobe hypertrophy is mild to moderate, and collateral vessels are not prominent in the subacute setting (fig. 2.195).

In chronic Budd-Chiari syndrome, hepatic edema is not a prominent feature and fibrosis develops. Fibrosis results in decreased signal of peripheral liver on T1- and T2-weighted images. Enhancement differences between peripheral and central liver on serial postgadolinium images become more subtle. Venous thrombosis, appreciated in acute and subacute disease, is usually not observed in chronic disease. Massive caudate lobe hypertrophy, massive enlarged bridging intrahepatic collaterals, extrahepatic collaterals, and mildly dysplastic and regenerative nodules are all features observed in chronic Budd-Chiari syndrome.

In the chronic setting, hepatic venous obstruction produces hepatic ischemia, which may result in the development of nodular regenerative hyperplasia [207, 208]. The nodules are usually round and of variable size, having high signal intensity on T1-weighted images and intermediate or low signal intensity on T2-weighted im-

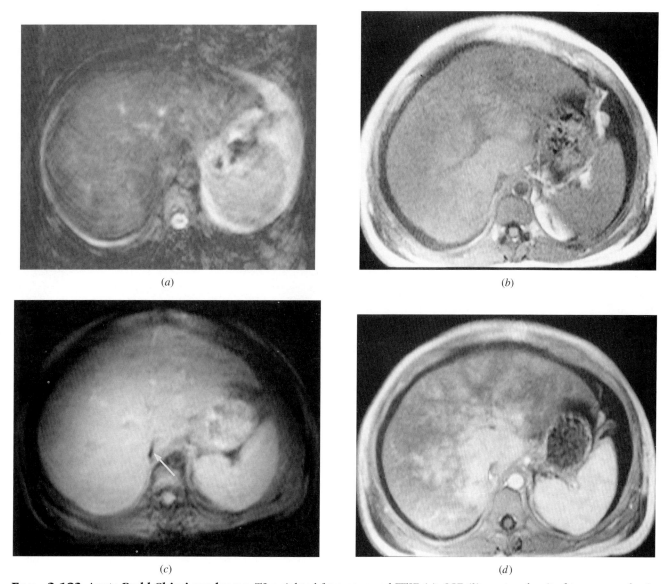

(a)

(b)

(c)

(d)

FIG. 2.193 Acute Budd-Chiari syndrome. T2-weighted fat-suppressed ETSE (*a*), SGE (*b*), proton-density fat-suppressed spin-echo (*c*), and immediate postgadolinium SGE (*d*) images. The T2-weighted image (*a*) shows normal signal intensity of the caudate lobe and central liver and heterogeneous higher signal intensity of the peripheral liver. On the precontrast T1-weighted image (*b*), the caudate lobe and central portion of the liver are normal in signal intensity, whereas the peripheral liver is low in signal intensity. The proton-density image (*c*), acquired at the expected level of the hepatic veins, demonstrates absence of hepatic veins and a compressed IVC (arrow, *c*). On the immediate postgadolinium SGE image (*d*), the caudate lobe and central liver enhance intensely, whereas peripheral liver is low in signal intensity. (Reproduced with permission from Noone T, Semelka RC, Woosley JT, Pisano ED: Ultrasound and MR findings in acute Budd-Chiari syndrome with histopathologic correlation. *J Comput Assist Tomogr* 20: 819–822, 1996).

ages, similar to macroregenerative nodules (fig. 2.196) [209]. However, nodules tend to possess intense enhancement on immediate postgadolinium SGE images.

Varices are usually prominent in chronic Budd-Chiari syndrome and are well shown on gadolinium-enhanced SGE images. These vessels tend to be most intensely enhanced on portal-phase images. Extensive portosystemic varices, as observed in other chronic liver diseases, are also present. Curvilinear intrahepatic collat-

erals and capsule-based collaterals are characteristic of chronic Budd-Chiari syndrome (see fig. 2.196).

Hepatic vein thrombosis may occur in the setting of malignant disease. HCC is the cancer most commonly associated with hepatic vein thrombosis. HCC involvement of the major hepatic veins has been reported in 6–23% of cases [210]. Tumor thrombosis demonstrates gadolinium enhancement, whereas bland thrombus does not enhance. As with Budd-Chiari syndrome, the degree of

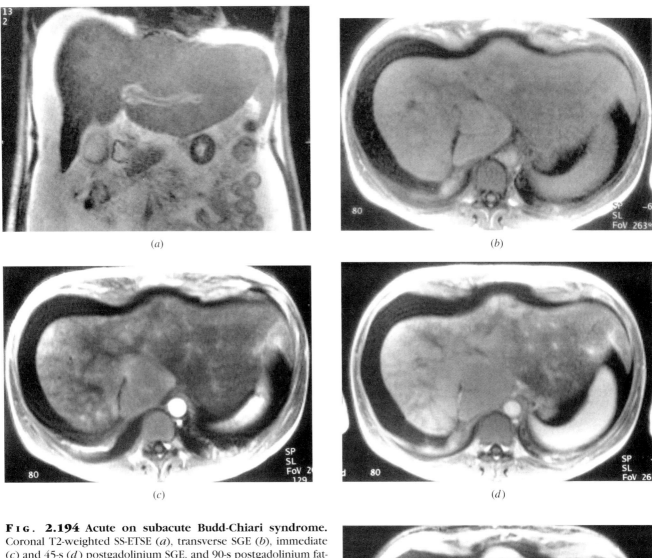

(a)

(b)

(c)

(d)

FIG. 2.194 Acute on subacute Budd-Chiari syndrome.
Coronal T2-weighted SS-ETSE (*a*), transverse SGE (*b*), immediate
(*c*) and 45-s (*d*) postgadolinium SGE, and 90-s postgadolinium fat-
suppressed SGE (*e*) images. The coronal T2-weighted image (*a*)
shows high signal of the lateral segment relative to the right lobe.
On the T1-weighted image (*b*), moderately diminished signal is
identified in the enlarged lateral segment of the left lobe, with mild
diminished signal of the right lobe. The enlarged caudate lobe possesses a more normal signal intensity. The immediate postgadolinium image (*c*) reveals markedly diminished enhancement of the
lateral segment, consistent with acute changes of Budd-Chiari, and
mildly heterogeneous and increase signal of the right lobe, consistent with subacute changes of Budd-Chiari. The caudate lobe has a
mild heterogeneity with signal intensity intermediate between the
acutely affected lateral segment and subacutely affected right lobe.
Enchancement abnormalities diminish but persist on late postcontrast images (*d*, *e*).

(e)

enhancement of liver parenchyma that has thrombosed
hepatic veins depends on the acuity of the thrombosis.
In acute thrombosis, involved parenchyma enhances less
than surrounding liver. In chronic thrombosis, enhancement is more variable and may be increased.

Hepatic Arterial Obstruction

Hepatic arterial obstruction is much less common than
either portal vein or hepatic vein obstruction. Hepatic
arterial obstruction is most commonly seen in the setting
of liver transplantation. In patients without transplants,

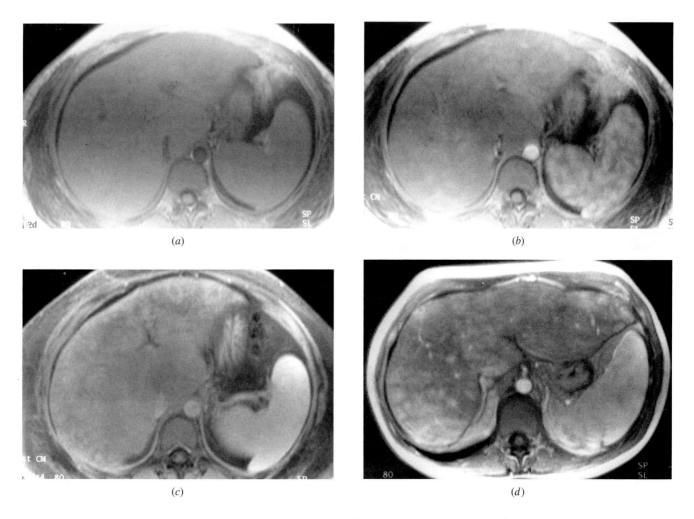

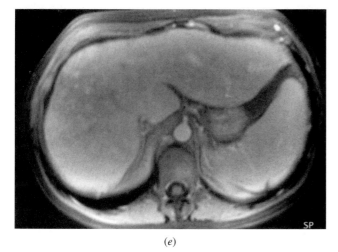

FIG. 2.195 Subacute Budd-Chiari syndrome. SGE (*a*), immediate postgadolinium SGE (*b*), and 90-s postgadolinium fat-suppressed SGE (*c*) images. Peripheral liver is diminished in signal on T1-weighted image (*a*) and demonstrates a diffuse, heterogeneous mildly increased enhancement on immediate postgadolinium image (*b*) that persists on later image (*c*), consistent with hepatic vascular compensation to venous thrombosis as observed in subacute Budd-Chiari syndrome. (Reproduced with permission from Noone TC, Semelka RC, Siegelman ES, Balci NC, Hussain SM, Kim PN, Mitchell DG. Budd-Chiari Syndrome: Spectrum of appearances of acute, subacute, and chronic disease with magnetic resonance imaging. *J Magn Reson Imaging* 11: 44–50, 2000.)

Immediate postgadolinium SGE (*d*) and 90-s postgadolinium fat-suppressed SGE (*e*) images in a second patient. The liver is enlarged with an irregular contour. There is mild hypertrophy of the caudate lobe. After administration of contrast (*d*), the liver enhances in a diffusely heterogeneous pattern and becomes more homogeneous on the later image (*e*).

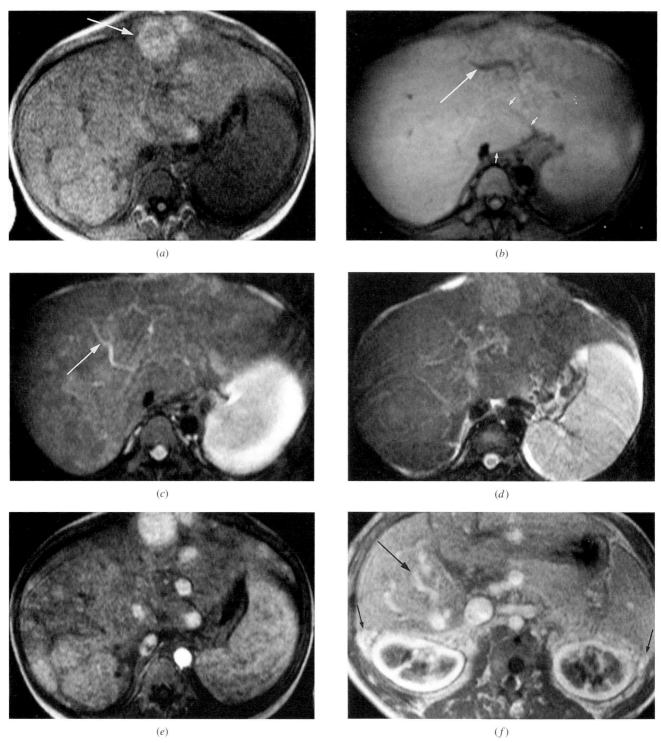

(a)   (b)

(c)   (d)

(e)   (f)

F I G . 2.196 Chronic Budd-Chiari syndrome. SGE (*a*), proton-density fat-suppressed spin-echo (*b*), T2-weighted fat-suppressed ETSE (*c, d*), and immediate postgadolinium SGE (*e*) images. On T1-weighted images (*a*), multiple well-defined high-signal intensity mass lesions representing adenomatous hyperplasia are identified, the largest measuring 3.5 cm in diameter (arrow, *a*). The proton-density image at the expected level of the hepatic veins (*b*), demonstrates absence of hepatic veins, with intrahepatic curvilinear venous collaterals in their stead (arrow, *b*). Enlargement of the caudate lobe is shown (small arrows, *b*). The T2-weighted image (*c*) taken from a slightly higher tomographic section demonstrates curvilinear intrahepatic collaterals (arrow, *c*) with absence of hepatic veins. The immediate postgadolinium image (*e*) acquired at the same tomographic level as the precontrast images (*a, d*) shows intense enhancement of the adenomatous hyperplastic nodules, with multiple enhancing nodules apparent that were not visualized on precontrast images. Slight heterogeneity of hepatic enhancement is present. However, the enhancement pattern is distinctly different from that of acute Budd-Chiari syndrome.

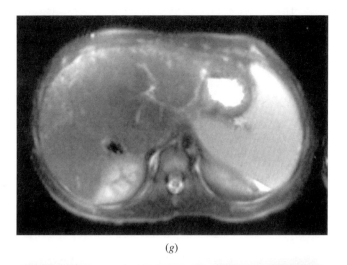

(g)

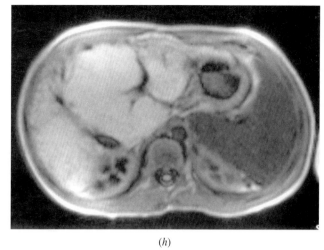

(h)

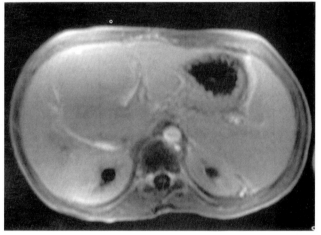

(i)

FIG. 2.196 (*Continued*) Immediate postgadolinium SGE image (*f*) in a second patient with chronic Budd-Chiari syndrome. Extensive abdominal collaterals are present (arrows, *f*) including curvilinear intrahepatic collaterals (long arrow, *f*).

T2-weighted fat-suppressed SS-ETSE (*g*), magnetization-prepared gradient-echo (*h*) and immediate postgadolinium magnetization-prepared gradient-echo (*i*) images in an 8-yr-old boy. Massive enlargement of the caudate lobe is present with relative atrophy and peripheral nodularity of the peripheral liver consistent with chronic Budd-Chiari syndrome.

embolic occlusion is the most common cause of hepatic arterial compromise. Diminished enhancement of involved hepatic parenchyma is apparent on early postcontrast images (fig. 2.197).

Preeclampsia-Eclampsia

Hepatic disease is common in preeclampsia and may result in the hemolytic anemia, elevated Liver function tests, and low platelets (HELLP) syndrome, which may cause peripheral vascular occlusions of the liver or hepatic hematoma [211]. Microscopically, sinusoids contain fibrin deposits with hemorrhage into the subendothelial space. Blood may dissect through portal connective tissue to form lakes of blood. MR images show peripheral wedgelike defects on regions of increased enhancement on postgadolinium images and heterogeneous high signal intensity on T2-weighted images from edema and, in more severe disease, infarction (figs. 2.198 and 2.199). Hematoma appears as a peripheral fluid collection with signal intensity depending on the age of the blood products, usually deoxyhemoglobin or intracellular methemoglobin reflecting the acute nature of the disease process.

Congestive Heart Failure

Patients with congestive heart failure may present with hepatomegaly and hepatic enzyme elevations. On early dynamic contrast-enhanced CT or MR images, the liver may enhance in a mosaic fashion with a reticulated pattern of low-signal intensity linear markings. By 1 min postcontrast the liver becomes more homogeneous. The suprahepatic IVC is frequently enlarged with enlargement of the hepatic veins. Contrast injected in a brachial vein may appear earlier in the hepatic veins and suprahepatic IVC than in the portal veins and infrahepatic IVC, reflecting reflux of contrast from the heart (fig. 2.200).

Portal Venous Air

Portal venous air, a serious condition associated with bowel ischemia, appears as signal-void foci within distal branches of the portal vein in the nondependent portion of the liver (typically the left lobe) on all imaging

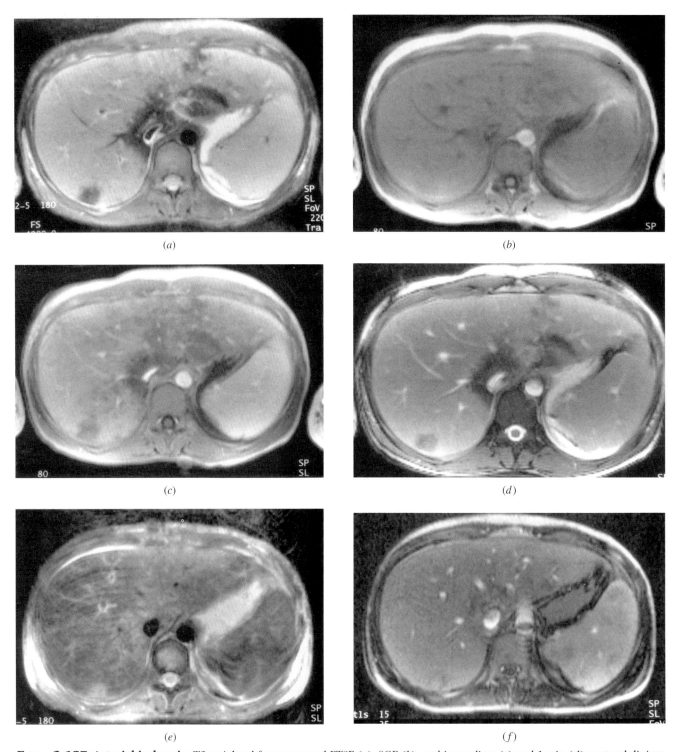

(a)

(b)

(c)

(d)

(e)

(f)

F I G . 2.197 Arterial ischemia. T2-weighted fat-suppressed ETSE (*a*), SGE (*b*), and immediate (*c*) and 1-min (*d*) postgadolinium SGE images. The liver is enlarged with diffuse increased signal intensity on T2-weighted images (*a*) consistent with edema. There is a 2-cm focus in the right hepatic lobe and irregular central region that demonstrate decreased signal intensity on both T2- (*a*) and T1- (*b*) weighted images, most pronounced on T2, and negligible enhancement on early (*c*) and late (*d*) postgadolinium images. These features are consistent with arterial ischemia.

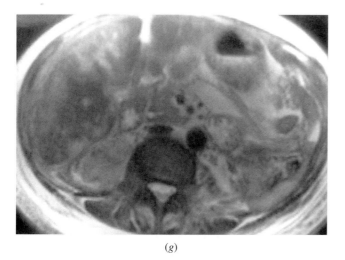

(g)

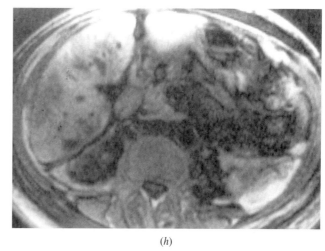

(h)

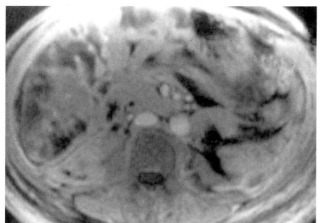

(i)

FIG. 2.197 (*Continued*) T2-weighted fat-suppressed ETSE (*e*) and immediate postgadolinium magnetization-prepared gradient-echo (*f*) images in the same patient 15 days later show a slight increased signal intensity involving the focus in the right lobe and central liver on the T2-weighted image associated with diffuse low signal of the liver secondary to intervening blood transfusion. Note that the previously ischemic areas in the right lobe and central liver demonstrate enhancement on early postgadolinium images (*f*). These findings are consistent with reperfusion of ischemic regions, which matched the clinical picture.

T2-weighted fat-suppressed SS-ETSE (*g*), SGE (*h*), and 90-s postgadolinium fat-suppressed SGE (*i*) images in a second patient demonstrate irregular peripheral regions in the right lobe inferiorly that are high signal on T2 (*g*) and low signal on T1 (*h*) and show negligible enhancement on late images (*i*) consistent with ischemic or infarcted regions caused by small-branch arterial occlusion.

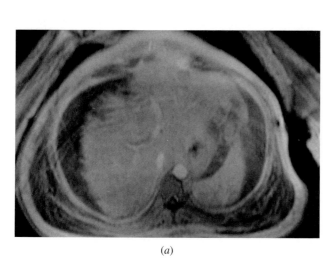

(a)

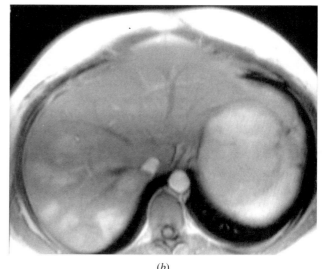

(b)

FIG. 2.198 HELLP syndrome. Transverse 45-s postgadolinium SGE image (*a*) demonstrates an abnormal serrated margin of the liver and massive ascites. Liver changes reflect ischemic injury.

Immediate postgadolinium image (*b*) in a second patient with HELLP syndrome shows an early patchy enhancement of the liver.

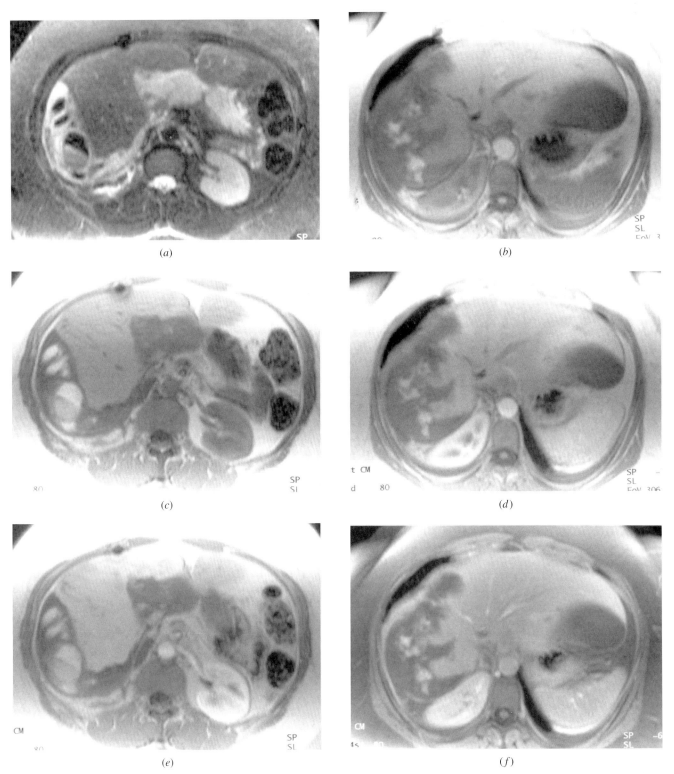

(a)

(b)

(c)

(d)

(e)

(f)

FIG. 2.199 Spontaneous intra-hepatic hemorrhage. Echo-train STIR (*a*), SGE (*b*, *c*), immediate postgadolinium SGE (*d*, *e*), and 90-s postgadolinium fat-suppressed SGE (*f*, *g*) images in a 34-yr-old female patient who has a history of spontaneous intrahepatic hematoma. There is a large complex subcapsular collection that demonstrates mixed signal intensity consistent with blood of different ages.

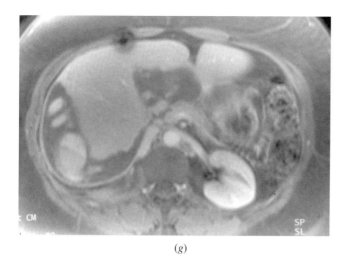

(g)

Fig. 2.199 (*Continued*) Spontaneous intrahepatic hematoma occurs most commonly in patients who are on anticoagulant therapy. Hepatic adenomas are the most common cause in women of child-bearing age who are not on anticoagulation therapy and are taking birth control pills. Note the jagged peripheral margin of the liver (*b, d, f*), which is an appearance also observed in spontaneous hepatic hemorrhage in the HELLP syndrome.

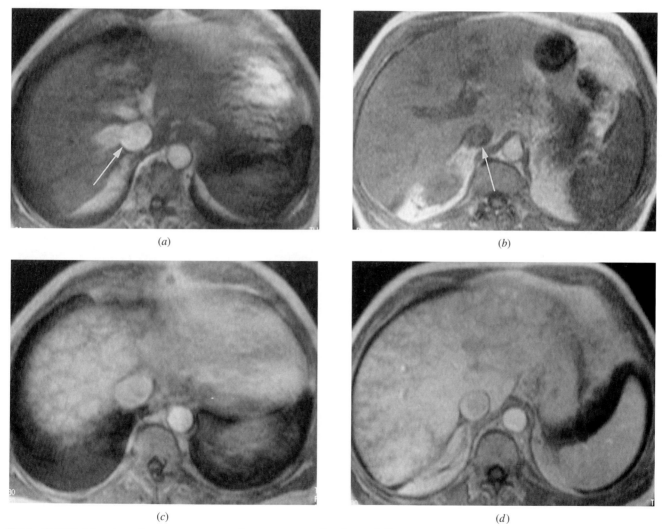

(a)   (b)

(c)   (d)

Fig. 2.200 Mosaic enhancement secondary to congestive heart failure. Immediate (*a, b*), 45-s postgadolinium (*c, d*), and 90-s postgadolinium SGE (*e*) images. The immediate postgadolinium images (*a, b*) demonstrate the presence of gadolinium in the superior IVC early in the arterial phase of enhancement with no enhancement of the abdominal organs, because of the low cardiac output state of the patient. Reflux of gadolinium into the dilated suprahepatic IVC and hepatic veins is present (arrow, *a*) with no contrast present in the infrahepatic IVC (arrow, *b*). On the 45-s postgadolinium images (*c, d*) a mosaic enhancement pattern is present throughout the liver reflecting hepatic congestion. This mosaic enhancement resolves on the 90-s postgadolinium image (*e*).

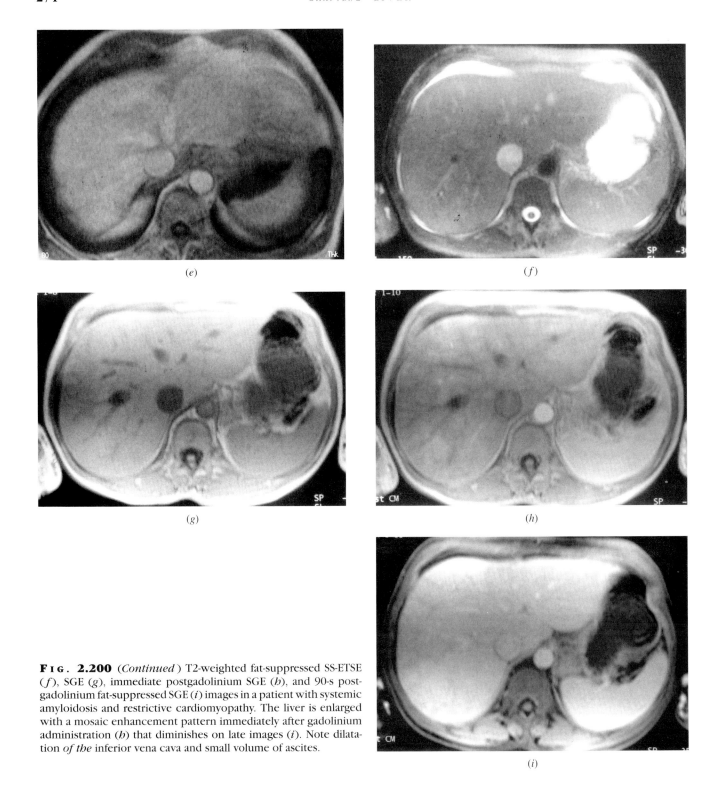

(e)

(f)

(g)

(h)

(i)

FIG. 2.200 (*Continued*) T2-weighted fat-suppressed SS-ETSE (*f*), SGE (*g*), immediate postgadolinium SGE (*h*), and 90-s postgadolinium fat-suppressed SGE (*i*) images in a patient with systemic amyloidosis and restrictive cardiomyopathy. The liver is enlarged with a mosaic enhancement pattern immediately after gadolinium administration (*h*) that diminishes on late images (*i*). Note dilatation *of the* inferior vena cava and small volume of ascites.

sequences. Magnetic susceptibility artifact may also be identified. Air is best appreciated using a combination of high-resolution T2-weighted echo-train spin-echo and postgadolinium T1-weighted images in which air will be signal void on both sets of images. The air is most clearly shown on the postcontrast T1-weighted images (fig. 2.201). The T2-weighted images confirm the fact

that the tubular structures that are dark on T1-weighted images are also dark on T2, reflecting signal-void air rather than high-signal fluid.

Air in the Biliary Tree
Air in the biliary tree is usually a relatively benign condition. Air in the biliary tree is less peripheral than air in

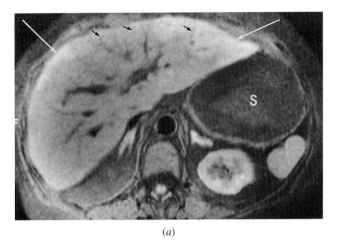
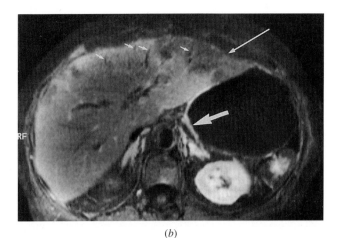

(a)   *(b)*

F I G . 2.201 Portal venous air. T1-weighted fat-suppressed SE (*a*) and 90-s postgadolinium fat-suppressed SE (*b*) images. On the precontrast T1-weighted fat-suppressed image (*a*), subtle, linear, signal-void, short, vertically oriented markings are present (small arrows, *a*). Regions of peripheral hepatic high signal intensity are present reflecting hemorrhage (long arrows, *a*). The stomach (s) is dilated. On the gadolinium-enhanced T1-weighted fat-suppressed spin-echo image (*b*), the vertically oriented peripheral collections of portal venous air are more clearly defined (small arrows, *b*). Regions that were hyperintense on the precontrast image are shown to have diminished enhancement (long arrow, *b*). The dilated stomach shows increased mural enhancement (large arrow, *b*) consistent with ischemic changes. Portal venous air is signal void and poorly seen on T2-weighted images (not shown); fluid would be high in signal intensity and well shown on T2-weighted images.

the portal veins and is more clearly observed as branching tubular structures conforming to the biliary tree. Air is most commonly observed in the left biliary ducts, reflecting the patient's supine position in the bore of the magnet. Air in the biliary tree is signal void on all MR sequences (fig. 2.202).

Heterogeneous Hepatic Parenchymal Enhancement

Heterogeneous hepatic parenchymal enhancement is usually observed as a transient phenomenon on hep-

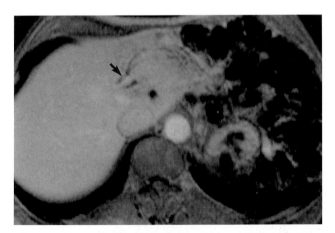

F I G . 2.202 Biliary tree air. Transverse 90-s postgadolinium SGE image in a patient with a choledochojejunostomy shows signal-void, tubular structures with an arborized pattern (arrow). This biliary tree air is more central in location than the portal venous air. The T2-weighted image (not shown) demonstrates signal-void, poorly shown bile ducts consistent with air-containing rather than fluid-containing ducts.

atic arterial dominant phase images. This entity must be distinguished from diseases that have a definable cause. Common disease processes that result in increased hepatic parenchymal enhancement include portal vein thrombosis or compression and acute hepatitis. These disease processes should be excluded based on imaging findings and clinical history. In the absence of pathophysiologic causes, regional imbalance in hepatic arterial and portal venous supply may also result from anomalous hepatic arterial origins.

Heterogeneous hepatic parenchymal enhancement often occurs in a generalized patchy fashion, with the presence of wedge-shaped regions of increased enhancement that usually conform to subsegmental distributions (fig. 2.203). The etiology of this abnormality is presently unknown but is presumed to reflect an imbalance between hepatic arterial and portal venous blood supply with increased hepatic arterial supply to subsegments of increased enhancement. This is frequently not related to focal fatty infiltration but may be associated with homogeneous enhancement of the spleen on immediate postgadolinium images. Minor liver enzyme elevations may be observed [212]. The concomitant splenic enhancement abnormality may imply an underlying immunologic basis for this phenomenon.

Inflammatory Parenchymal Disease

Viral Hepatitis

Viral hepatitis may cause severe disease, resulting in acute hepatitis, chronic hepatitis, and progression to cirrhosis. Hepatitis B, C, and D are parenterally transmitted,

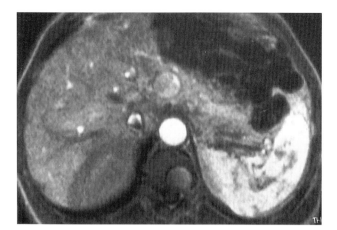

F I G .   2.203 Transient heterogeneous enhancement. Immediate postgadolinium SGE image demonstrates transient heterogeneous hepatic enhancement. Transient heterogeneous enhancement is commonly associated with homogeneous enhancement of the spleen, which is not, however, present in this case. (Reproduced with permission from Semelka RC, Shoenut JP, Greenburg, HM, Micflikier AB. The liver In: Semelka RC, Shoenut JP, eds. *MRI of the Abdomen with CT Correlation.* New York: Raven p. 13–41, 1993.)

and all may result in these conditions. Acute hepatitis is diagnosed by clinical and serologic studies. Pathologically, in acute viral hepatitis, major histologic findings are focal hepatocyte necrosis, inflammatory infiltrates, and evidence of hepatocyte regeneration during the recovery phase. Imaging studies are generally not performed unless the clinical picture is complicated. Acute hepatitis may result in heterogeneous hepatic signal intensity, which is most apparent on T2-weighted images and immediate postgadolinium images (fig. 2.204). Periportal edema may be identified. Periportal lymph nodes are usually present in chronic disease.

The microscopic changes of chronic viral hepatitis show chronic inflammation that extends out from the portal tracts into the adjacent parenchyma with associated necrosis of hepatocytes. Fibrous septum formation, hepatocyte regeneration, and cirrhosis may eventuate. In patients with chronic hepatitis, imaging studies are more commonly obtained, usually to detect the presence of cirrhosis or HCC. On T2-weighted images, chronic active hepatitis often has periportal high signal intensity, corresponding to inflammation (fig. 2.205), enlarged lymph nodes, or both. This is a nonspecific finding observed in a number of hepatobiliary and pancreatic diseases [213]. Focal inflammatory changes or fibrosis may develop in chronic active hepatitis, resulting in diffuse or regional high signal intensity on T2-weighted images [214, 215] and heterogeneous increased enhancement on SGE images most often appreciated as late increased enhancement of linear stroma (fig. 2.206).

Radiation-Induced Hepatitis

The liver may be included in radiation portals for a variety of malignancies, metastases in adjacent vertebra, or pancreatic ductal adenocarcinoma. Edema may develop within 6 months of radiation injury. Edema appears as decreased signal intensity on T1-weighted images and increased signal intensity on T2-weighted images [216, 217]. Fat is usually decreased within the radiation portal in patients with fatty liver (fig. 2.207) [218, 219]. This reflects decreased delivery of triglycerides due to diminished portal flow. Increased enhancement is apparent on delayed postgadolinium SGE images in radiation-damaged liver. Increased enhancement is more conspicuous when fat suppression techniques are used (see fig. 2.207). This increased enhancement is related to

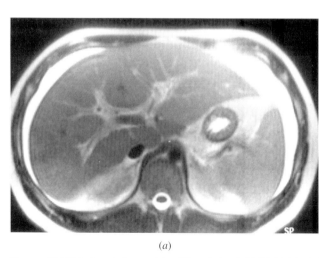

(a)

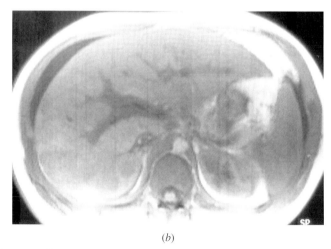

(b)

F I G .   2.204 Acute hepatitis. T2-weighted SS-ETSE (*a*), SGE (*b*), immediate postgadolinium SGE (*c*), and 90-s postgadolinium fat-suppressed SGE (*d*) images in a patient who has a history of leukemia. The liver is enlarged and demonstrates a mild heterogeneous signal on both T2- (*a*) and T1-weighted (*b*) images.

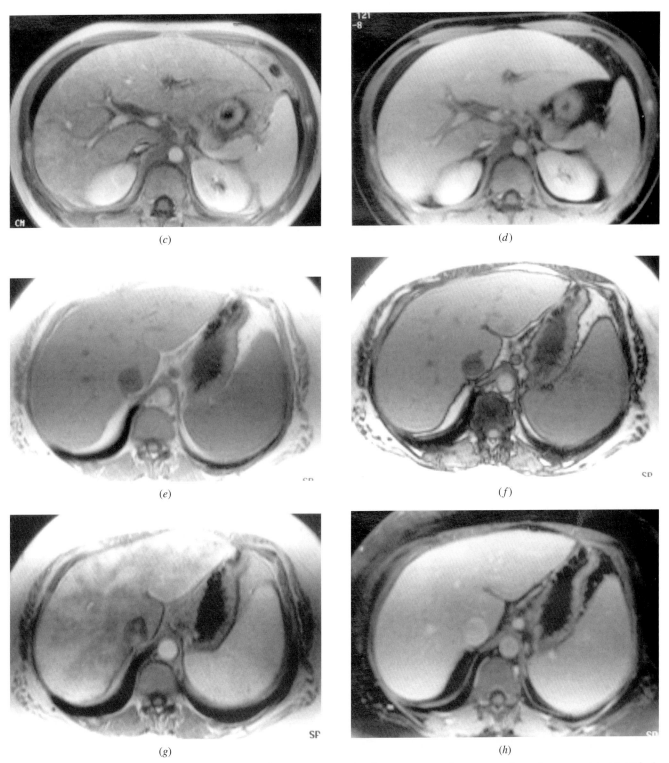

F I G . 2.204 (*Continued*) On immediate postgadolinium images (*c*), heterogeneous intense patchy enhancement is identified, which is transient. The liver becomes more uniform in signal intensity on the late images (*d*). Periportal edema, which appears high signal on T2 (*a*) and does not enhance on postgadolinium images (*c, d*), is present. Moderately large-volume ascites is shown.

SGE (*e*), out-of-phase SGE (*f*), immediate postgadolinium SGE (*g*), and 90-s postgadolinium fat-suppressed SGE (*h*) images in a second patient. The liver is mildly greater in signal intensity on the in-phase image (*e*), with signal intensity of liver and spleen becoming more comparable on the shorter-TE out-of-phase sequence. This appearance of subtle loss of signal of the liver is consistent with mild fat infiltration. There are multiple patchy regions of enhancement after administration of contrast (*g*) throughout the liver consistent with acute on chronic hepatitis.

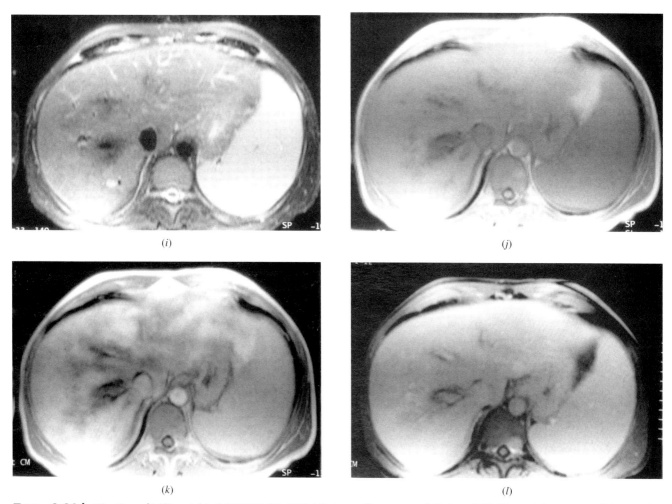

(i)

(j)

(k)

(l)

FIG. 2.204 (*Continued*) T2-weighted SS-ETSE (*i*), SGE (*j*), immediate postgadolinium SGE (*k*), and 90-s postgadolinium fat-suppressed SGE (*l*) images in a third patient. The liver demonstrates a markedly heterogeneous early enhancement pattern with low signal in a perihepatic vein distribution (*k*). Low signal intensity in a perihepatic vein distribution is appreciated on the T2-weighted image (*i*).

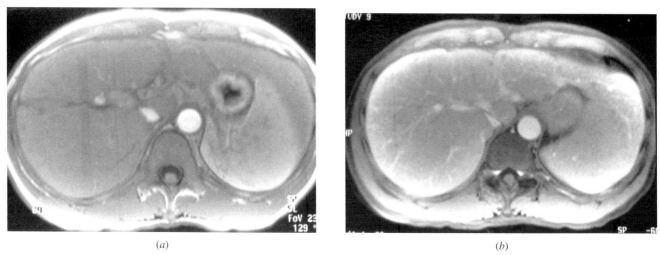

(a)

(b)

FIG. 2.205 Chronic hepatitis. Immediate postgadolinium SGE (*a*) and 90-s postgadolinium fat-suppressed SGE (*b*) images show delayed enhancement of liver fibrous tissue on late postgadolinium images (*b*) consistent with fibrosis.

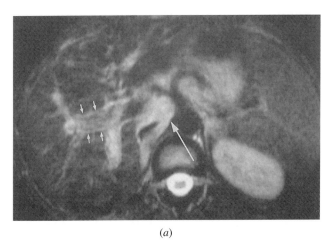

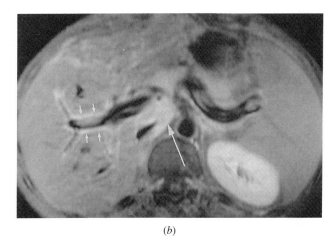

(a)   (b)

F I G . 2.206 Viral hepatitis. T2-weighted fat-suppressed SE (*a*) and 90-s postgadolinium fat suppressed SE (*b*) images in a patient with HIV infection and positive serology for hepatitis B and C. On the fat-suppressed T2-weighted sequence (*a*) porta hepatis and para-aortic lymph nodes (arrow, *a*) are clearly shown as high-signal intensity masses in lower-signal intensity background. High signal within the liver in a periportal distribution is also present (small arrows, *a*). This periportal abnormality identified on the T2-weighted image is shown to be enhancing tissue (small arrows, *b*) on the gadolinium-enhanced T1-weighted fat-suppressed image (*b*). Gadolinium enhancement distinguishes periportal inflammatory or neoplastic tissue from edema that would appear signal void after contrast. Enhancement of adenopathy (arrow, *b*) is also appreciated.

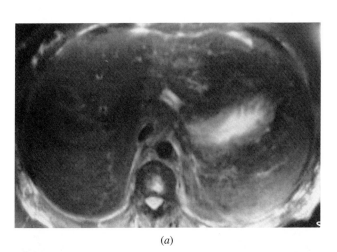

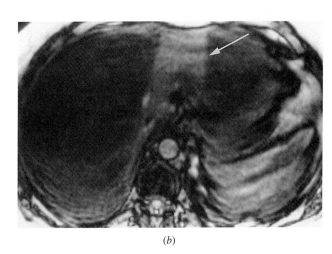

(a)   (b)

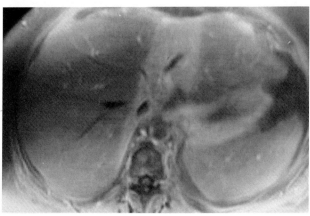

F I G . 2.207 Radiation damage. T2-weighted fat-suppressed SE (*a*), out-of-phase SGE (*b*), and interstitial-phase gadolinium-enhanced T1-weighted fat-suppressed SE (*c*) images in a patient who had undergone radiation therapy for a vertebral body metastasis. The out-of-phase image (*b*) shows low-signal intensity fatty replaced liver with a central, vertically oriented band of higher signal intensity nonfatty liver (arrow, *b*). Similar findings are apparent on the fat-suppressed T2-weighted image (*a*), with subtle higher signal intensity of the central band of nonfatty liver. The gadolinium-enhanced T1-weighted fat-suppressed image (*c*) demonstrates increased enhancement of the radiation damaged liver that may reflect radiation-induced vasculitis.

(c)

leaky capillaries in early radiation injury and represents granulation tissue in late injury.

Sarcoidosis

Sarcoidosis, a systemic granulomatous disease of unknown etiology, is one of the most common causes of hepatic noncaseating granulomas [220]. The liver follows lymph nodes and lung in the frequency of involvement, and the liver is involved histologically in 60–90% of patients [221]. The majority of patients show minimal evidence of clinical or biochemical hepatic dysfunction. Granulomas are characterized pathologically by compact aggregates of plump epithelioid cells, sometimes with multinucleated giant cells, surrounded by a cuff of lymphocytes and macrophages. Focal involvement of the liver and spleen in sarcoidosis with noncaseating

granulomas is well demonstrated on MR images. Sarcoid granulomas are small (approximately 1 cm in diameter), rounded lesions low in signal intensity on T1- and T2-weighted images, that enhance in a diminished, delayed fashion on gadolinium-enhanced SGE images (fig. 2.208) [222, 223]. The diminished enhancement reflects the hypovascular nature of the granuloma. Occasionally, the spleen may be lower in signal intensity than liver on T2-weighted images [222]. Concomitant retroperitoneal lymph nodes are often present, exhibiting a distinctive, feathery, moderately high signal on T2-weighted images.

Inflammatory Pseudotumor

Inflammatory pseudotumor of the liver is a rare hepatic lesion that presents macroscopically as a tumor-like mass but reveals a mixed inflammatory infiltrate on

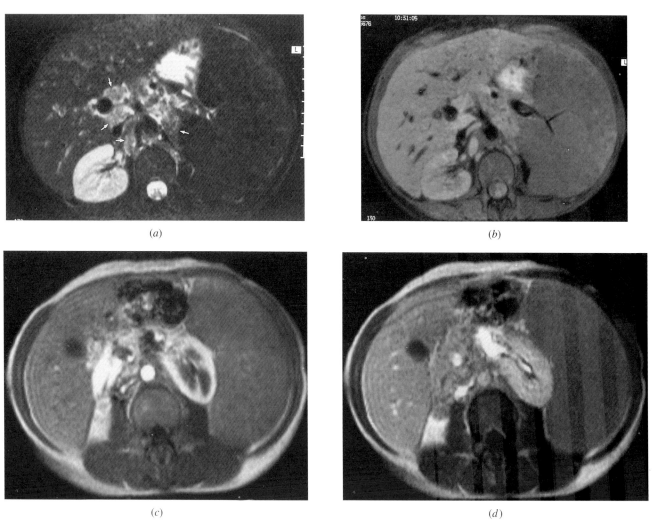

(a)

(b)

(c)

(d)

F I G . 2.208 **Hepatosplenic sarcoidosis.** T2-weighted fat-suppressed SE (*a*), T1-weighted fat-suppressed SE (*b*), and immediate (*c*) and 5-min (*d*) postgadolinium SGE images. The spleen is massively enlarged, and contains multiple <1-cm nodules which are moderately low signal intensity on precontrast T2 (*a*) and T1 (*b*) weighted images, and demonstrate negligible enhancement on early postgadolinium images (*c*) with gradual enhancement over time (*d*). Extensive retroperitoneal, celiac, and periportal lymphadenopathy is also present (*a*, *b*), which has a speckled appearance on the T2-weighted image (arrows, *a*). A speckled signal on T2 has been described for lymph nodes affected by sarcoidosis.

microscopic inspection. The mixed inflammatory infiltrate consists of chronic inflammation, plasma cells, and histiocytes; special immunologic studies show polyclonal, and therefore, nonmalignant populations of cells. Focal fibrosis, areas of necrosis, and obliteration of blood vessels may occasionally be noted. Inflammatory pseudotumor of the liver may result in systemic symptoms, including fever, weight loss, malaise, and right upper quadrant pain [224]. The lesion is often mistaken for hepatic malignancy. Although the disease responds to steroid administration and the prognosis is usually good, fatal outcome has been reported [225]. Inflammatory pseudotumors are usually solitary, although in 20% of the cases they are multiple [224]. Masses are generally less than 2 cm in diameter and are slightly ill defined. Tumors are mildly hyperintense on T2-weighted images and are best shown as patchy, rounded regions of transient increased enhancement on immediate postgadolinium images (fig. 2.209) [226]. Occasionally tumors may be large and the diffuse heterogeneous enhancement may mimic the appearance of HCC (fig. 2.209).

Infectious Parenchymal Disease

Abscesses

Pyogenic Abscess. Pyogenic abscesses are the most frequent form of focal hepatic infections resulting from an infectious process of bacterial origin. Pathologically, pyogenic liver abscesses may occur as solitary or multiple lesions ranging from millimeters to massive lesions. Microscopically, in early stages, lesions are ill defined with intense acute inflammation, purulent debris, and devastation of hepatic parenchyma and stroma. In later stages, the abscesses becomes circumscribed, surrounded by a shell of granulation tissue consisting of abundant, newly formed blood vessels, fibroblasts, and chronic inflammation. End stages show complete fibrous encapsulation. The pathways of infectious agents are

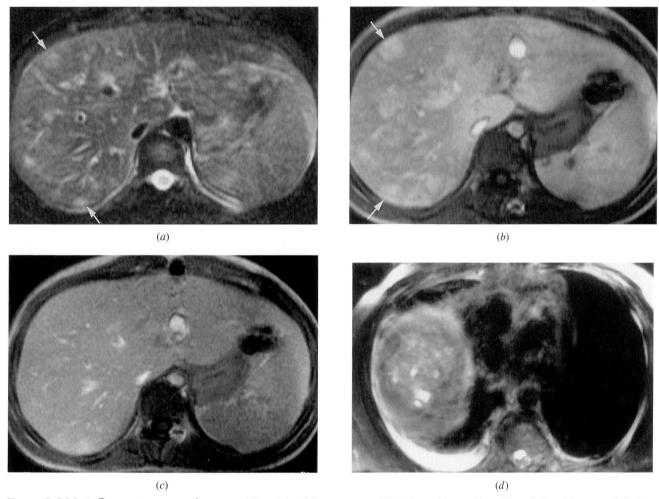

(a)

(b)

(c)

(d)

F I G . 2.209 Inflammatory pseudotumor. T2-weighted fat-suppressed SE (*a*), and immediate (*b*) and 90-s (*c*) postgadolinium SGE images. No definite lesions are apparent on the precontrast T1-weighted image (not shown). Occasional, mildly hyperintense ill-defined lesions are present on the T2 image (arrows, *a*). Multiple small, irregular enhancing foci are demonstrated throughout the liver on the immediate postgadolinium image (arrows, *b*), which fade to isointensity by 90 s (*c*).

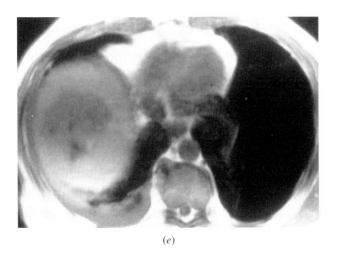

(e)

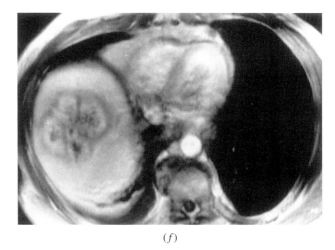

(f)

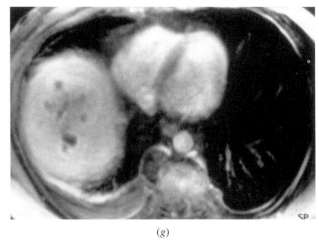

(g)

FIG. 2.209 (*Continued*) T2-weighted fat-suppressed SS-ETSE (*d*), SGE (*e*), immediate postgadolinium SGE (*f*), and 90-s postgadolinium fat-suppressed SGE (*g*) images in a second patient. A 6-cm mass lesion is present in the liver, which is minimally high in signal intensity on T2 (*d*) and moderately low in signal intensity on T1 (*e*), enhances in an intense diffuse heterogeneous fashion immediately after gadolinium (*f*), and becomes more homogeneous and lower signal intensity on later images (*g*). The appearance resembles HCC; however, the liver is not cirrhotic. The patient also presented with fever and malaise, which are symptoms often observed with inflammatory pseudotumor.

via the biliary tract (figs. 2.210 and 2.211), portal vein, hepatic artery, and direct extension from contiguous organs. Blunt or penetrating injuries can also cause infection in the liver with abscess formation [227]. Abscesses may occur in the context of recent surgery, Crohn's disease, appendicitis, and diverticulitis [228]. Characteristic gadolinium-enhanced MRI findings are low-signal lesions with enhancing capsules [229]. The abscess wall reveals intense enhancement on immediate postgadolinium images, which persists on intermediate- and late-phase images. Some pyogenic abscess contain internal septations, which enhance early and demonstrate persistent enhancement on serial postgadolinium images (fig. 2.212) [227]. Abscesses typically have perilesional enhancement with indistinct outer margins on immediate postgadolinium SGE images caused by a surrounding rim of granulation tissues and a hyperemic inflammatory response in adjacent liver (figs. 2.213 and 2.214) [230]. The higher sensitivity of MRI to gadolinium chelates than of CT imaging to iodinated agents renders dynamic gadolinium-enhanced MRI a useful technique for patients in whom a distinction between simple cysts and multiple abscesses cannot be made on the basis of CT imaging. Metastases may mimic the appearance of hepatic abscesses because both may have prominent rim enhancement. Metastases may also mimic abscesses clinically if they become secondarily infected. The diagnosis of infected metastases should be considered when the lesion wall is thicker than 5 mm and has nodular components. Bacterial abscesses commonly are associated with portal vein thrombosis (see fig. 2.215). A recent report described characteristic features of hepatic abscesses on MRI [230]. Pyogenic abscesses revealed moderate enhancement of stromal and fibrous elements on immediate postgadolinium images with persistent enhancement on hepatic venous images and no enhancement of additional stroma or progressive fill-in of the lesion over time. This feature of abscesses is distinctly diffent from the appearance of the vast majority of metastases, which show progressive internal enhancement on late-phase postgadolinium images [230].

Nonpyogenic Abscess

Amebic Abscess. Amebic liver abscesses are caused by a protozoan parasite, *Entamoeba histolytica*, and are not uncommon in developing tropical countries

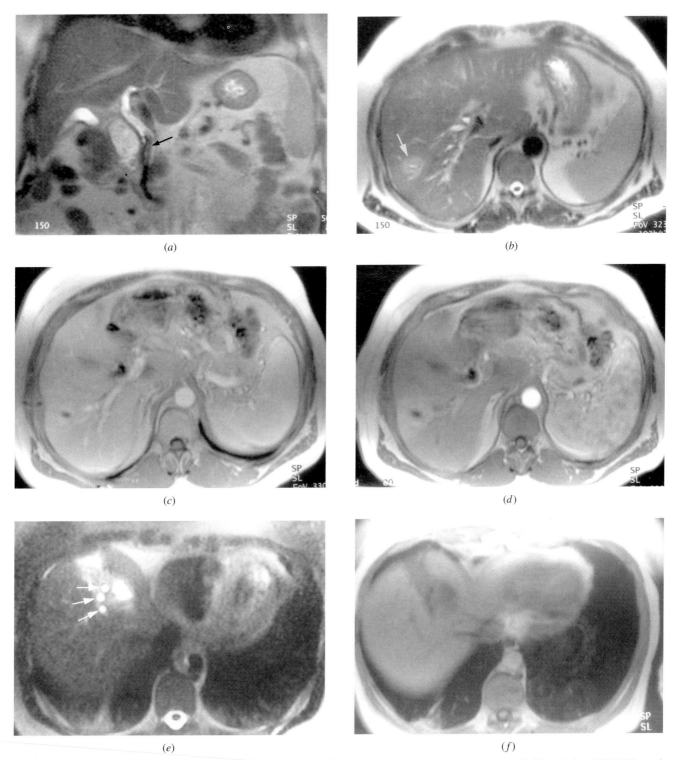

F I G . 2.210 Liver abscesses secondary to infective cholangitis. Coronal (*a*) and transverse (*b*) T2-weighted SS-ETSE, and immediate (*c*) and 45-s (*d*) postgadolinium SGE images. There is a lesion in the right hepatic lobe (arrow, *b*) that demonstrates increased signal intensity on T2 (*b*), decreased signal on T1 (not shown), and circumferential ill-defined perilesional and capsular enhancement on immediate postgadolinium images (*c*), with fading of the perilesional enhancement and persistent capsular enhancement on 45-s images (*d*). There is no enhancement of internal stroma or fill-in of the lesion with time. Note the biliary stent (arrow, *a*) situated in the common bile duct (*a*).

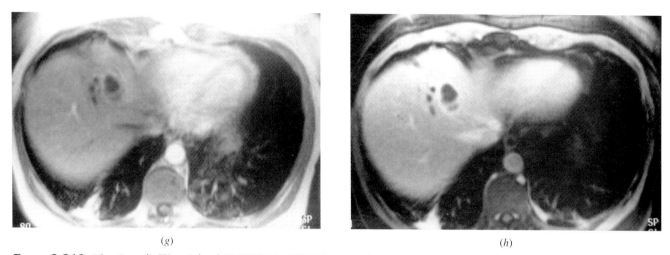

(g)   (h)

F I G . 2.210 (*Continued*) T2-weighted SS-ETSE (*e*), SGE (*f*), immediate postgadolinium SGE (*g*) and 90-s postgadolinium fat-suppressed SGE (*h*) images in a second patient. There is an irregular region of increased signal on T2 (*e*) and decreased signal on T1 (*f*) in the dome of the liver. Adjacent to this area, there are multiple rounded structures (arrows, *e*) that demonstrate increased signal on T2 (*e*) and decreased signal on T1 (*f*), which represent dilated ducts. After gadolinium administration (*g*, *h*), a cystic mass with a thickened, enhancing wall and internal septations is identified, consistent with an abscess secondary to segmental infective cholangitis.

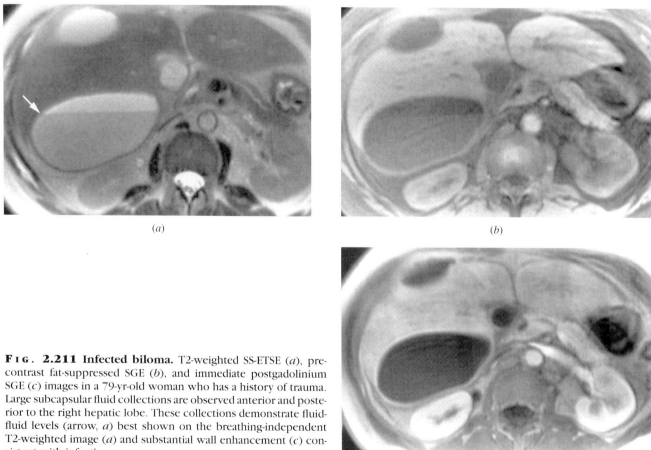

(a)

(b)

F I G . 2.211 Infected biloma. T2-weighted SS-ETSE (*a*), pre-contrast fat-suppressed SGE (*b*), and immediate postgadolinium SGE (*c*) images in a 79-yr-old woman who has a history of trauma. Large subcapsular fluid collections are observed anterior and posterior to the right hepatic lobe. These collections demonstrate fluid-fluid levels (arrow, *a*) best shown on the breathing-independent T2-weighted image (*a*) and substantial wall enhancement (*c*) consistent with infection.

(c)

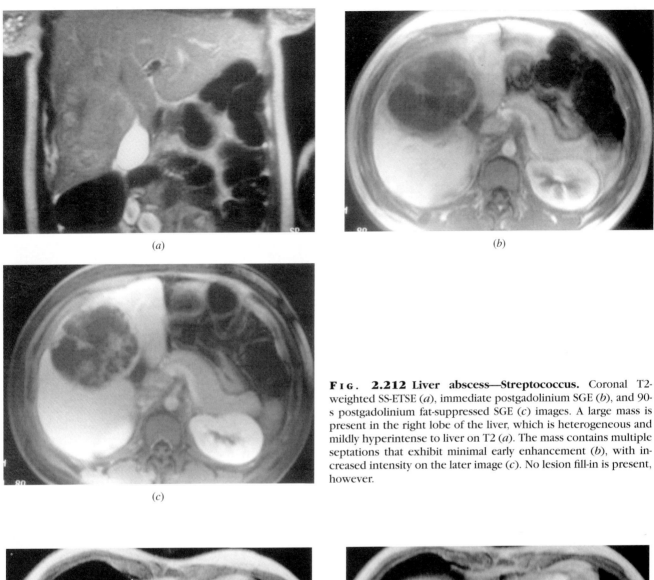

(a)

(b)

(c)

FIG. 2.212 Liver abscess—Streptococcus. Coronal T2-weighted SS-ETSE (*a*), immediate postgadolinium SGE (*b*), and 90-s postgadolinium fat-suppressed SGE (*c*) images. A large mass is present in the right lobe of the liver, which is heterogeneous and mildly hyperintense to liver on T2 (*a*). The mass contains multiple septations that exhibit minimal early enhancement (*b*), with increased intensity on the later image (*c*). No lesion fill-in is present, however.

(a)

(b)

FIG. 2.213 Pyogenic abscesses. SGE (*a*) and immediate postgadolinium SGE (*b*) images in a patient with *Fusibacterium* liver abscesses. Two slightly ill-defined low-signal intensity masses are present in the liver (arrows, *a*) on the precontrast T1-weighted image (*a*). Immediately after gadolinium administration (*b*), the lesions demonstrate substantial perilesional enhancement. The larger lesion demonstrates a thin outer low-signal rim surrounding an enhancing ring.

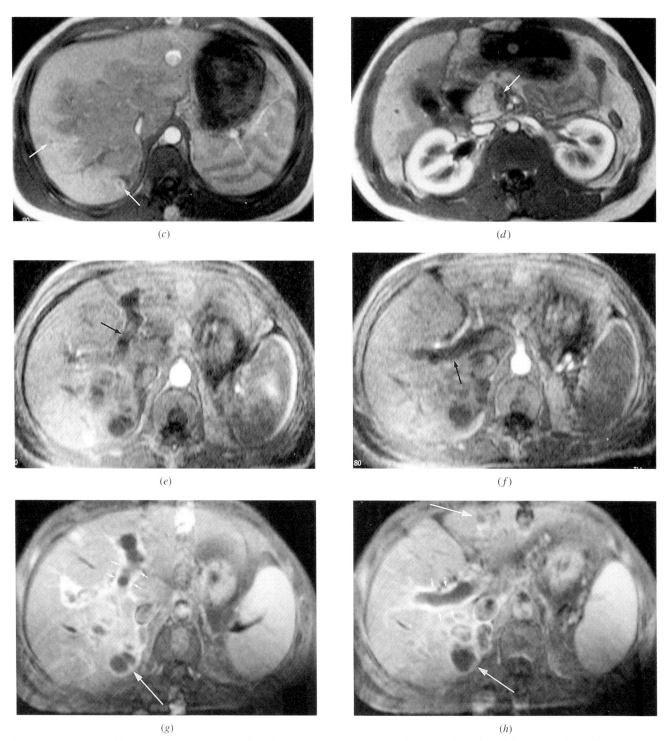

(c)

(d)

(e)

(f)

(g)

(h)

F I G . 2.213 (*Continued*) Immediate postgadolinium SGE images from cranial (*c*) and caudal (*d*) locations through the liver in a second patient. Abnormal diminished central enhancement is present in the liver (*c*) because of portal vein thrombosis. Small abscesses with enhancing rings (arrows, *c*) are present. On the more inferior tomographic image (*d*), thrombus is identified in the SMV with enhancement of the vein wall (arrow, *d*) reflecting infection of the thrombus.

Immediate postgadolinium SGE images (*e*, *f*) and interstitial phase gadolinium-enhanced T1-weighted fat-suppressed SE images (*g*, *h*) in a third patient obtained at the level of the left portal vein (*e*, *g*) and right portal vein (*f*, *h*). The left (arrow, *e*) and right (arrow, *f*) portal veins are expanded with low-signal thrombus on the immediate postgadolinium images. On the gadolinium-enhanced fat-suppressed images enhancement of the walls of the portal veins is present (small arrows, *g*, *h*) reflecting the infected nature of the thrombus. The abscesses in the right and left lobes of the liver are well seen on the interstitial phase images as low-signal intensity irregular-shaped cystic masses with enhancing rims (long arrows, *g*, *h*).

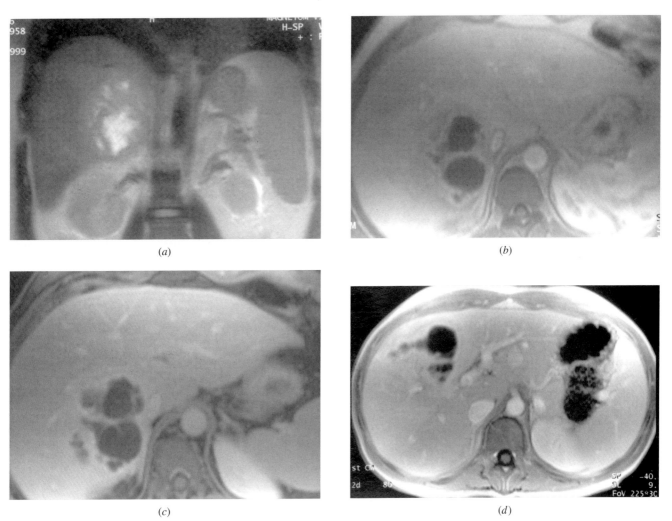

F I G . 2.214 Pyogenic liver abscesses. Coronal T2-weighted SS-ETSE (*a*), immediate postgadolinium SGE (*b*), and 90-s post-gadolinium fat-suppressed SGE (*c*) images. A large septated lesion is present, which is heterogenous and high signal intensity on T2 (*a*), low signal intensity on postgadolinium T1-weighted images (*b, c*), with intense capsular and internal septa enhancement on immediate postgadolinium image (*b*) that persists on the late images (*c*). A characteristic feature of abscesses is that the capsule and septa enhance on immediate postgadolinium images and persist in enhancement on 90-s images (*c*), with no progressive internal stromal enhancement. Metastases, in distinction, tend to exhibit progressive stromal enhancement.

Transverse 45-s postgadolinium SGE image (*d*) in a second patient demonstrates a lesion with intense mural enhancement consistent with abscess.

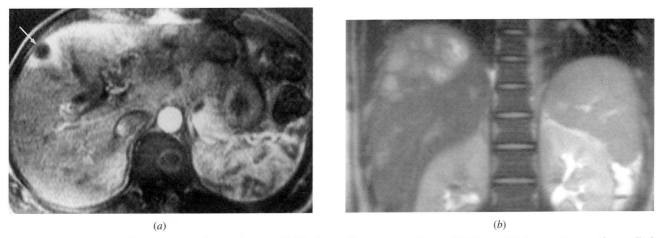

F I G . 2.215 Hepatic abscess secondary to appendicitis. Immediate postgadolinium SGE image (*a*) demonstrates a thin-walled cystic lesion in the liver (arrow, *a*) with prominent perilesional enhancement, consistent with an abscess.

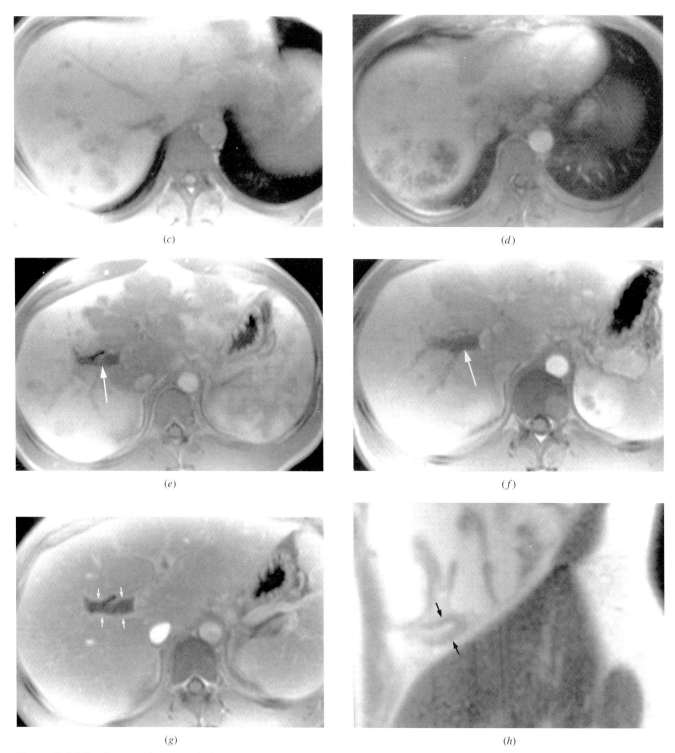

(c)

(d)

(e)

(f)

(g)

(h)

Fig. 2.215 (*Continued*) Coronal T2-weighted SS-ETSE (*b*), transverse SGE (*c*), immediate (*d, e*) and 45-s (*f*) postgadolinium SGE, and 90-s fat-suppressed postgadolinium SGE (*g*) of the abdomen, and sagittal T2-weighted SS-ETSE (*h*) and 90-s postgadolinium fat-suppressed SGE (*i*) images of the pelvis in a second patient. There are multiple lesions with a cluster appearance in the right hepatic lobe that demonstrate high signal intensity on T2-weighted images (*b*), low signal intensity on T1-weighted images (*c*), and enhancement of the abscess wall and septations with perilesional enhancement immediately after administration of contrast (*d*). Abnormal enhancement of the liver on the immediate postgadolinium image reflects the presence of portal vein thrombosis, with increased enhancement of the right lobe due to increased hepatic arterial supply.

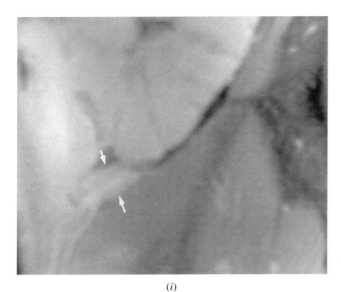

(i)

FIG. 2.215 (*Continued*) The portal vein is expanded with thrombus (arrow *e*, *f*) that is low signal on T1-weighted image and does not enhance after administration of contrast, consistent with a bland thrombus. The portal vein wall enhances (small arrows, *g*) on the interstitial-phase fat-suppressed images, reflecting that the thrombus is infected. Note on the sagittal images (*h*, *i*) that the appendix (arrows, *h*, *i*) is thick-walled with increased enhancement consistent with acute appendicitis.

[227]. Amebic abscess may arise in patients who live in or have traveled to tropical climates. Amebic abscesses may develop secondary to small ischemic necrotic areas caused by obstruction of small venules by the trophosites and their byproducts [227]. Presenting features includes pain, fever, weight loss, nausea and vomiting, diarrhea, and anorexia [231]. Lesions are usually solitary, affect the right lobe more often than the left lobe [227], and are prone to invade the diaphragm with development of pulmonary consolidation and empyema [232]. Lesions are encapsulated and thick walled (5–10 mm) and demonstrate substantial enhancement of the capsule on gadolinium-enhanced images, which permits differentiation from liver cysts (fig. 2.216).

Echinococcal Disease

Echinococcal disease is a worldwide zoonosis produced by two main types of larval forms of equinococus tapeworms: *E. granulosus* and *E. alveolaris* [227].

Echinococcus granulosus is the causative organism for hydatid cysts and is the type of echinococcus indigenous in North America. Pathologically, the typical hydatid cyst is spherical with a fibrous rim. Surrounding liver reaction to the abscess is minimal with small volume granulation tissue. Rupture of a cyst may provoke an intense inflammatory and granulomatous reaction in surrounding tissue. The typical imaging appearance is reappearance in an intrahepatic encapsulated multicystic lesion with daughter cysts arranged peripherally within the larger cyst. Satellite cysts located exterior to the fibrinous membrane of the main hepatic cyst are not uncommon and have been reported in 16% of hydatid cysts in a series of 185 patients [231]. The fibrous capsule and internal septations are well shown on T2-weighted images and gadolinium-enhanced T1-weighted images.

Single-shot echo-train spin-echo is particularly effective at showing the architectural detail of cystic lesions. Lesions are frequently complex, with mixed low signal intensity on T1-weighted images and mixed high signal intensity on T2-weighted images due to the presence of proteinaceous and cellular debris (fig. 2.217). Calcification of the cyst wall and internal calcifications are frequently identified on CT images but may not be distinguishable from the fibrous tissue of the capsule on MR images.

Echinococcus alveolaris is the causative organism for hepatic alveolar echinococcosis (HAE), a rare parasitic disease in which the fox is the main host of the adult parasite, with dogs and cats being less frequently cited hosts. Pathologically, HAE is characterized grossly by multilocular or confluent cystic, necrotic cavities. A fibrous rim is not present. Balci et al. described the MR appearance of HAE in 13 patients [233]. All lesions were large (mean 9.7 cm), solitary, and with irregular margins. Tumors were heterogeneous in signal with mixed cystic/solid components on postgadolinium images (fig. 2.218). Because HAE does not form membranes, or capsules, it tends to involve extensive regions in the liver, with a propensity to involve the porta hepatis. The infiltration causes stenoses of intrahepatic bile ducts, hepatic veins, and portal veins, which commonly result in portal hypertension. Cystic and necrotic areas are common findings in HAE. Calcification is also common, and appears as clusters of microcalcifications or large calcified foci. The differential diagnosis of HAE includes various infiltrative lesions of the liver, such as HCC and metastases: the presence of enhancement in primary and metastatic neoplasms may help in differentiation. HAE can be differentiated from hydatid disease, because the latter process shows well-defined cyst walls and regular contours.

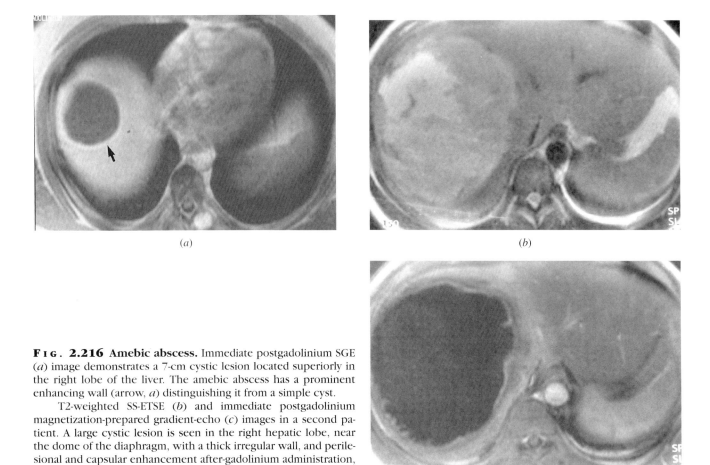

(a)

(b)

(c)

F I G . 2.216 Amebic abscess. Immediate postgadolinium SGE (*a*) image demonstrates a 7-cm cystic lesion located superiorly in the right lobe of the liver. The amebic abscess has a prominent enhancing wall (arrow, *a*) distinguishing it from a simple cyst.

T2-weighted SS-ETSE (*b*) and immediate postgadolinium magnetization-prepared gradient-echo (*c*) images in a second patient. A large cystic lesion is seen in the right hepatic lobe, near the dome of the diaphragm, with a thick irregular wall, and perilesional and capsular enhancement after-gadolinium administration, consistent with abscess.

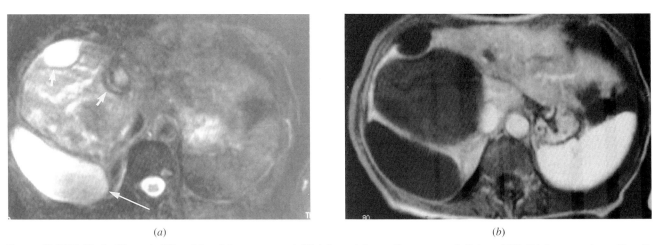

(a)

(b)

F I G . 2.217 Hydatid cyst. T2-weighted fat-suppressed SE (*a*), and immediate postgadolinium SGE (*b*) images. A multicystic lesion is present, with the large cyst appearing heterogenous and moderate in signal intensity on T2 (*a*), and contains peripherally arranged daughter cysts (arrows, *a*). A satellite cyst is also present (long arrow, *a*). The hydatid cyst walls enhance after gadolinium administration (*b*). This appearance is typical for a hydatid cyst.

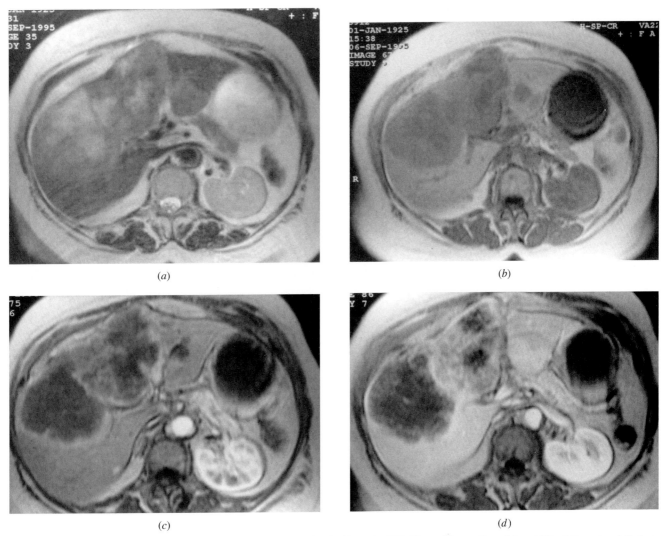

F I G . 2.218 Hepatic Alveolar echinococcosis. T2-weighted ETSE (*a*), SGE (*b*), and immediate (*c*) and 90-s (*d*) postgadolinium SGE images. A large lesion with irregular margins is present in the liver that demonstrates mildly high signal on T2 (*a*), low signal on T1 (*b*), and a peripheral rim of enhancement immediately after gadolinium administration (*c*) that persists on late images (*d*). There is a substantial solid component within the large infective lesion. (Courtesy of N. Cem Balci, MD, Dept. of Radiology, Florence Nightingale Hospital, Istanbul, Turkey)

Mycobacterial Infection

Mycobacterium tuberculosis. *Mycobacterium tuberculosis* is the most common cause of infectious hepatic granulomas [227]. The incidence of hepatic infection caused by tuberculosis is increasing, reflecting in part an increase in numbers of patients who are immunocompromised, such as patients with HIV infection. Abdominal tuberculosis mainly involves abdominal lymph nodes and the ileocecal junction. Hepatic tuberculosis occurs secondary to dissemination of the bacilli [227]. Focal hepatic lesions are typically small and multiple with an appearance similar to that of fungal lesions (see next section). Infection has a propensity to involve the portal triads and spreads in a superficial infiltrating fashion. This can be visualized as periportal high signal intensity on T2-weighted fat-suppressed images and gadolinium-enhanced T1-weighted fat-suppressed images. Associated porta hepatis nodes are common.

Mycobacterium Avium Intracellulare (MAI).

Nontuberculous mycobacterial hepatic infections are common and represent the most common hepatic infection in AIDS [234]. MAI infection is found in 50% of livers of patients dying with AIDS [235]. Microscopically, hepatic MAI lesions may show a spectrum of appearances ranging from loose aggregates of histiocytes to tight, well-formed granulomas. CT findings reported to be suggestive of disseminated MAI infection include enlarged mesenteric and/or retroperitoneal lymph nodes, hepatosplenomegaly, and diffuse jejunal wall thickening

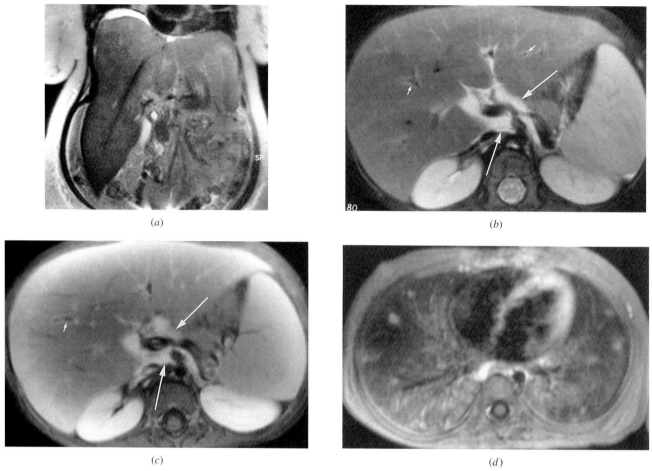

FIG. 2.219 Mycobacterium avium intracellulare (MAI) hepatic infection. Coronal T2-weighted SS-ETSE (*a*), transverse T2-weighted fat-suppressed ETSE (*b*), and interstitial-phase gadolinium-enhanced T1-weighted fat-suppressed SE (*c*) images. The coronal image (*a*) demonstrates hepatomegaly. On the fat-suppressed T2-weighted image (*b*), high-signal intensity soft tissue is present in the porta hepatis (long arrows, *b*) that extends along periportal tracks (short arrows, *b*). After gadolinium administration (*c*), enhancing porta hepatis tissue is clearly shown on the fat-suppressed image (long arrows, *c*), and enhancement is also noted of the periportal tissue (short arrow, *c*). Periportal distribution is a common pattern of involvement with MAI. Gadolinium-enhanced, gated T2-weighted fat-suppressed SE image (*d*) of the lungs demonstrates a ground-glass appearance with irregularly marginated 1-cm enhancing nodules consistent with MAI lung infection.

(fig. 2.219) [236]. Low-density centers of involved lymph nodes are considered a characteristic feature on CT images. Similar findings may be appreciated on MR images.

Fungal Infection

Hepatosplenic or visceral candidiasis is a form of invasive fungal infection that has emerged as a serious complication of the immunocompromised state, especially in AIDS patients, patients on medical therapy for acute myelogeneous leukemia (AML), and patients with bone marrow transplantation [237–239]. Prolonged duration of neutropenia is thought to be the most important risk factor for hepatosplenic candidiasis [239]. The most common infecting organism is *Candida albicans*, but other fungi may be found. Acute hepatosplenic candidiasis involves the liver and spleen, with renal involve-

ment occurring in less than 50% of patients. Disseminated *Candida albicans* infects the liver in a high proportion of cases, leading to development of multifocal microabscesses or granulomas. Although definitive diagnosis requires microbiologic or histologic evidence of infection, the absence of organisms on liver biopsy tissue or negative culture findings in the presence of clinical suspicion does not rule out the diagnosis. Therefore, cross-sectional imaging is necessary for diagnosis [240]. Patient survival depends on early diagnosis. Liver lesions are frequently smaller than 1 cm and subcapsular in location. The small size and peripheral nature of these lesions make them difficult to detect with CT imaging or standard spin-echo MR sequences. Patients with AML undergo multiple blood transfusions, so the liver and spleen are low in signal intensity on T1-weighted and

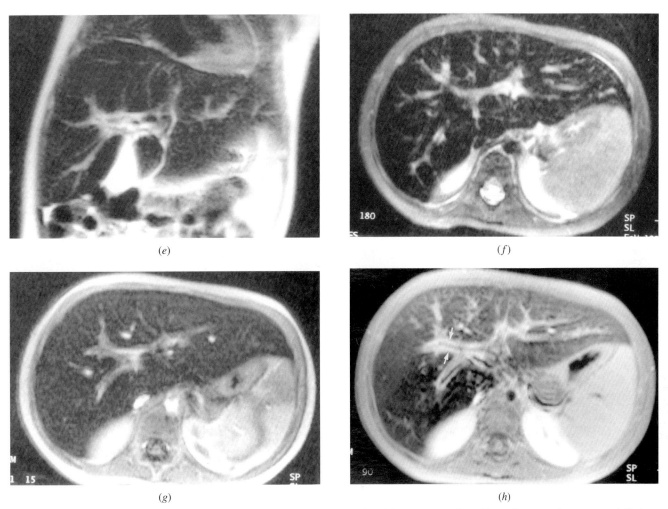

F I G . 2.219 (*Continued*) Coronal T2-weighted SS-ETSE (*e*), T2-weighted fat-suppressed SS-ETSE (*f*), immediate postgadolinium SGE (*g*), and 90-s postgadolinium fat-suppressed SGE (*h*) images in a second patient, who has a history of hereditary blood dyscrasia and has currently MAI infection, demonstrates tissue in the porta hepatis and periportal tracks that is high signal on T2 (*e*, *f*), and enhances on late gadolinium-enhanced fat-suppressed T1-weighted images (arrows, *h*). Note also the iron deposition in the liver from transfusional siderosis.

T2-weighted images [241, 242]. T2-weighted fat-suppressed spin-echo sequences are effective at demonstrating these lesions, because of the high conspicuity of this sequence for small lesions and the absence of chemical shift artifact that may mask small peripheral lesions. STIR images also show these lesions well because of the fat-nulling effect of this sequence [241]. MRI employing T2-weighted fat suppression and dynamic gadolinium-enhanced SGE images has been shown to be more sensitive for the detection of hepatosplenic candidiasis than contrast-enhanced CT imaging [240, 243].

Because acute lesions of fungal disease are abscesses, they are high in signal intensity on T2-weighted images. They also may be seen on gadolinium-enhanced T1-weighted images as signal-void foci with no appreciable abscess wall enhancement (figs. 2.220 and 2.221). It has been observed that patients with hepatosplenic candidiasis who are immunocompetent possess abscesses that demonstrate mural enhancement. The absence of abscess wall enhancement may reflect the patient's neutropenic state. Overall sensitivity of MRI is 100%, and specificity is 96% [240].

After institution of antifungal antibiotics, successful response may be demonstrated. Central high signal develops within lesions on T1-weighted and T2-weighted images that enhances with gadolinium, representing granuloma formation. In addition, a distinctive dark perilesional ring is observed on all sequences, representing collections of iron-laden macrophages throughout granulation tissue at the periphery of lesions (fig. 2.222) [244]. This represents the subacute treated phase, which may represent a good prognostic finding, reflecting the patient's ability to mount an immune response.

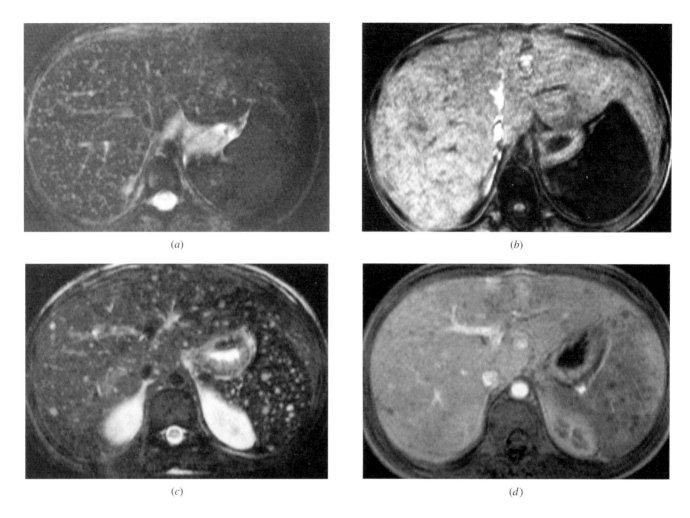

(a) (b)

(c) (d)

F I G . 2.220 Acute hepatosplenic candidiasis. T2-weighted fat-suppressed ETSE (*a*) and immediate postgadolinium SGE (*b*) images. On the T2-weighted images (*a*), multiple well-defined <1-cm high-signal intensity foci are scattered throughout the hepatic parenchyma with a smaller number of similar lesions apparent in the spleen. On the immediate postgadolinium image (*b*) the liver lesions are near signal void and do not show ring or perilesional enhancement.

T2-weighted fat-suppressed SS-ETSE (*c*) and immediate postgadolinium SGE (*d*) images in a second patient. Multiple well-defined <1-cm high-signal intensity lesions are scattered throughout the liver and spleen on the T2-weighted image (*c*). Lesions are near signal void and do not show ring or perilesional enhancement on the immediate postgadolinium image (*d*).

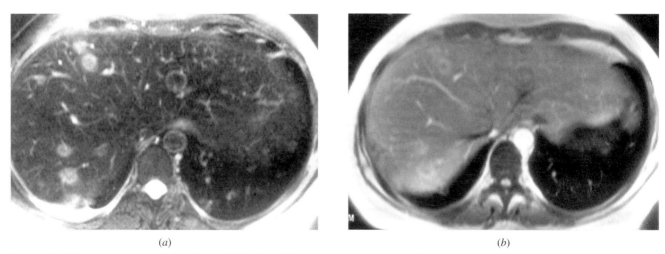

(a) (b)

F I G . 2.221 Acute hepatosplenic candidiasis with ring enhancement. T2-weighted fat-suppressed SS-ETSE (*a*) and 45-s postgadolinium SGE (*b, c*) images.

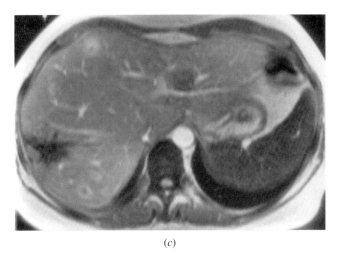

(c)

FIG. 2.221 (*Continued*) There are multiple small, rounded lesions scattered throughout the liver that show high signal intensity on T2 (*a*) and decreased signal intensity on T1-weighted images (not shown), with postgadolinium ring enhancement (*b, c*). Acute candidiasis was present at histopathology and microbiology. The presence of ring enhancement reflects that the patient is able to mount an immune response and therefore is not severely immunocompromised.

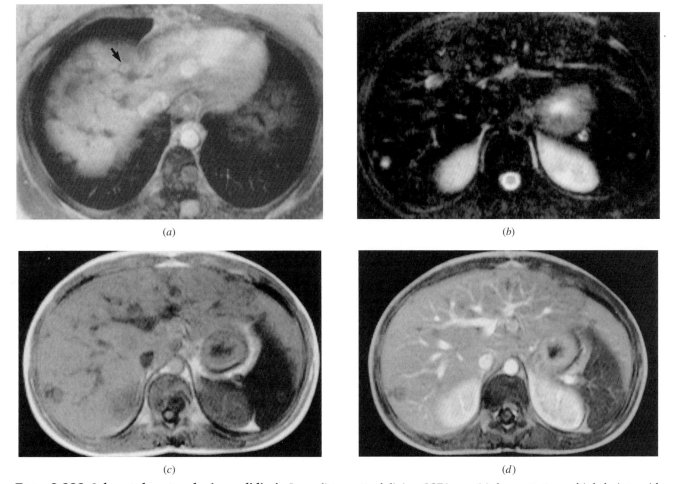

(a)

(b)

(c)

(d)

FIG. 2.222 Subacute hepatosplenic candidiasis. Immediate postgadolinium SGE image (*a*) demonstrates multiple lesions with a concentric ring pattern with an outer irregular signal void rim, inner high signal ring, and central low signal dot (arrow, *a*).

T2-weighted fat-suppressed SE (*b*) SGE (*c*) and immediate postgadolinium SGE (*d*) images in a second patient. Multiple concentric ring lesions are evident that are best shown on precontrast and immediate postgadolinium SGE images (*c, d*). The outer low-signal intensity ring is not appreciated on T2-weighted images (*b*) because the perilesional iron deposition blends in with the background RES iron deposition.

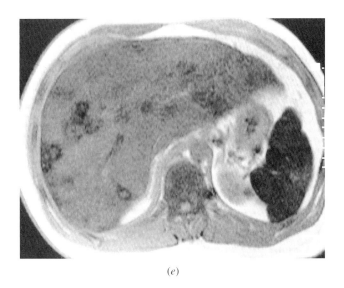

(e)

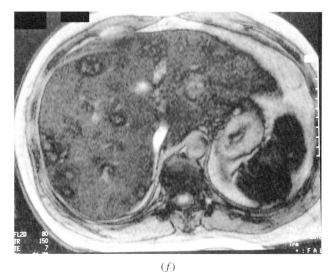

(f)

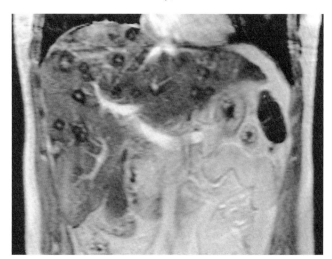

(g)

FIG. 2.222 (*Continued*) SGE (*e*), out-of-phase SGE (*f*), and coronal 45-s postgadolinium SGE (*g*) images in a third patient. Multiple concentric ring lesions are scattered throughout the liver on the SGE image (*e*). The outer signal-void ring becomes more prominent on the longer TE out-of-phase image (*f*) because of a magnetic susceptibility artifact from iron. Lesion appearance is largely unchanged on the postgadolinium image (*g*).

MRI also demonstrates chronic healed lesions that have responded to antifungal therapy [243]. These lesions are irregularly shaped and low in signal. Chronic healed lesions are hypointense on T1-weighted images and are generally isointense and poorly shown on T2-weighted images (fig. 2.223). The lesions are most conspicuous as low-signal intensity defects with angular margins on immediate postgadolinium SGE images. Capsular retraction may also be observed adjacent to the lesions. This constellation of imaging features is consistent with chronic scar formation.

TRAUMA

Hepatic trauma may be well shown on MR images. Hemoperitoneum may be shown as peritoneal fluid with blood products of varying age and signal intensity on T1-weighted and T2-weighted images. Deoxyhemoglobin and intracellular hemoglobin in acute/early subacute hemorrhage appear near signal void on T2-weighted images, which is a very distinctive finding [245]. The specific appearance of subacute hemorrhage is high-signal intensity on T1-weighted and T2-weighted images due to the presence of extracellular methemoglobin. Active bleeding can be shown as progressive accumulation of high-signal gadolinium on serial post-gadolinium images in a fluid-containing space [246].

Liver lacerations are demonstrated as linear hepatic defects. Intraparenchymal hemorrhage will appear as intraparenchymal fluid with varying signal intensity on T1-weighted and T2-weighted images, reflecting the above-described hemoglobin breakdown products (figs. 2.224–2.226).

HEPATIC TRANSPLANTATION

Liver disease is the tenth leading cause of death in the United States, and transplantation has become the

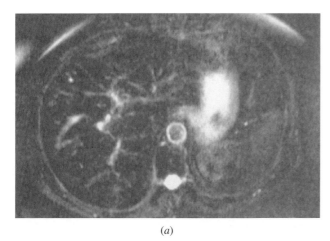
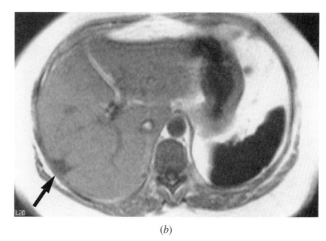

(a)   (b)

F I G . 2.223 Chronic healed candidiasis. T2-weighted fat-suppressed SE (*a*) and SGE (*b*) images. On T2-weighted image (*a*) the area of fibrosis has similar signal intensity to background liver and is not definable. On T1-weighted image (arrow, *b*), an irregular, polygonal low-signal lesion is present in the right lobe of the liver.

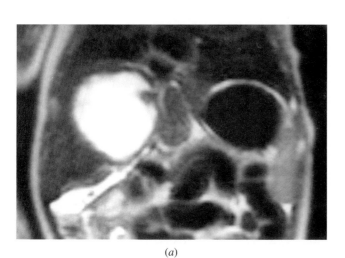
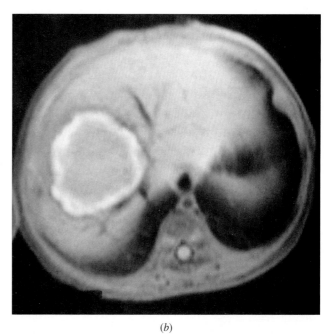

(a)   (b)

F I G . 2.224 Liver Hematoma. Coronal T2-weighted SS-ETSE (*a*) and T1-weighted fat-suppressed SE (*b*) images in an 8-wk-old girl who has a history of malpositioned umbilical venous catheter and subsequent liver hematoma. There is a fluid collection in the right lobe of the liver that is hyperintense on T2-weighted images (*a*) and isointense centrally with a hyperintense peripheral ring on the fat-suppressed T1-weighted image (*b*), consistent with hematoma. The appearance on the T1-weighted image, with the high-signal peripheral ring, is diagnostic for a hematoma.

Coronal T2-weighted SS-ETSE (*c*), transverse T2-weighted fat-suppressed SS-ETSE (*d*), T1-weighted fat-suppressed SE (*e*), and T1-weighted interstitial phase postgadolinium fat-suppressed SE (*f*) images in a newborn patient with disseminated intravascular coagulation.

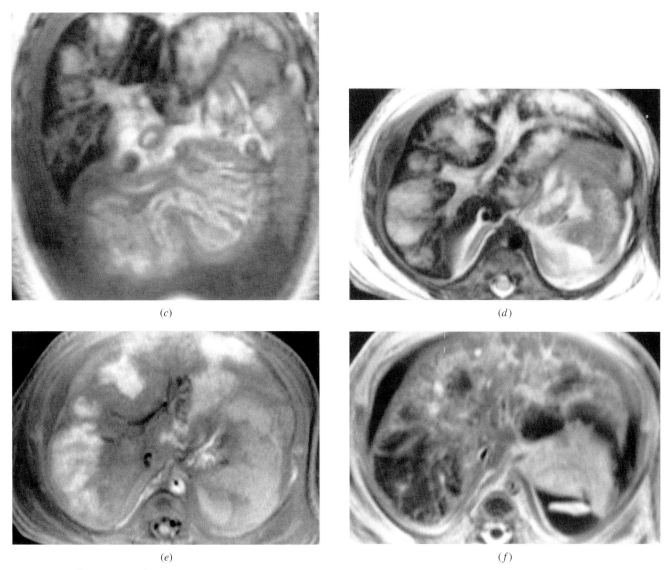

(c)

(d)

(e)

(f)

Fig. 2.224 (*Continued*) There are abnormal patchy areas throughout the hepatic parenchyma that exhibit high signal intensity on T2 (*c, d*) and T1-weighted images (*e*) consistent with subacute blood (extracellular methemoglobin). After contrast, these areas demonstrate negligible enhancement (*f*) compatible with ischemia.

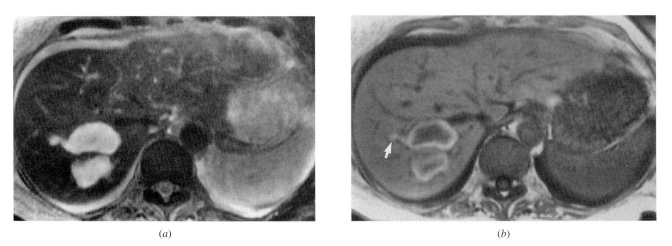

(a)

(b)

Fig. 2.225 Hepatic trauma. T2-weighted fat-suppressed ETSE (*a*), SGE (*b*), and 45-s postgadolinium SGE (*c*) images. Two hematomas are present in the liver that demonstrate minimally heterogeneous hyperintense signal on T2-weighted image (*a*), and a peripheral ring of high signal intensity on precontrast T1-weighted image (*b*), which is diagnostic for subacute hematomas.

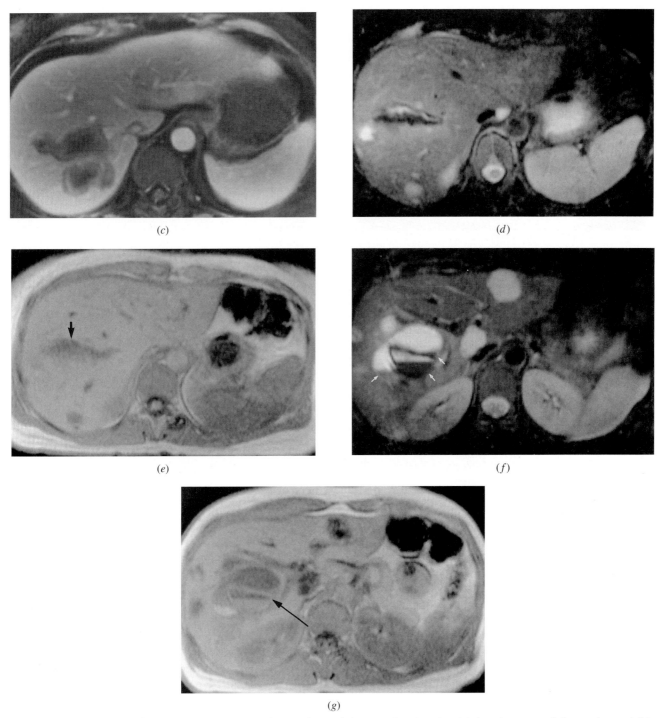

F I G . 2.225 (*Continued*) These lesions do not enhance after gadolinium administration (*c*), but the extracellular methemoglobin ring remains hyperintense. A high-signal intensity laceration tract is also noted (arrow, *a*).

T2-weighted fat-suppressed ETSE images (*d*, *f*) and T1-weighted noncontrast SGE (*e*, *g*) images acquired in a second patient, from two tomographic levels (*d*, *e* and *f*, *g*). An acute liver laceration is present (arrow, *f*) through the right lobe of the liver, which contains fluid that is dark and bright (oxyhemoglobin) and dark and dark (deoxyhemoglobin) on T1-and T2-weighted images, respectively. Hemorrhage has extended into two liver cysts that contain a combination of acute blood products including oxyhemoglobin (dark on T1-weighted and bright on T2-weighted images; thin arrow, *g*) and intracellular methemoglobin (bright on T1-weighted and dark on T2-weighted images; short arrows, *f*).

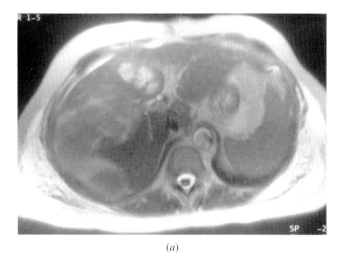

(*a*)

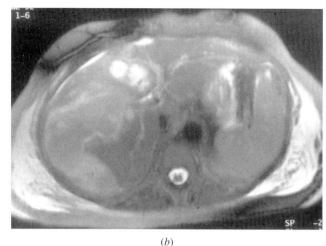

(*b*)

FIG. 2.226 Intrahepatic hemorrage post surgery. T2-weighted SS-ETSE (*a*), T2-weighted fat-suppressed SS-ETSE (*b*), and single-shot magnetization-prepared gradient-echo (*c*) images in a patient after laparoscopic cholecystectomy, who has a history of end-stage renal disease. There is a large area in the right hepatic lobe extending into the subcapsular space, which demonstrates increased signal intensity on both T2 (*a*, *b*) and T1 (*c*) weighted images consistent with intrahepatic hematoma. Note the peripheral rim of high signal on the T1-weighted image (*c*). Subcutaneous edema is more readily appreciated on the fat-suppressed T2-weighted image (*b*) than on the nonsuppressed image (*a*) because of removal of the competing high signal of fat on these long-echo-train sequences.

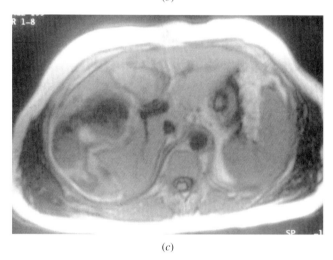

(*c*)

treatment of choice for end-stage disease [247, 248]. Major recent advances and technical progress in liver surgery and transplantation have been based, in large part, on improved understanding of the internal architecture of the liver. Toward this end, MRI provides valuable information for preoperative and postoperative liver evaluation of both donors and recipients. The increased utilization of adult-to-adult living related hemiliver donation has resulted in an increased role for MRI in the preoperative evaluation, reflecting the comprehensive nature of the information provided by MRI. Donors routinely undergo a liver MR protocol with MRCP and MRA (figs. 2.227–2.229). The usual surgical procedure involves resecting the right lobe for donation and retaining the left lobe in the donor. The precise amount of liver required to sustain an adult has not been quantified; it is postulated that 1% of the recipient's body mass should be sufficient [248]. The resection plane is approximately 1 cm into the right lobe from the middle hepatic vein and extends inferiorly to the bifurcation between the right and left portal veins [248], so that the donor retains the middle hepatic vein. Evaluation is made of relative size of right and left lobes and anomalies of the biliary or vascular system. Contraindications for transplantation include focal mass lesions, depending on size and type (e.g., malignant), or preexistent diffuse liver disease that may be the same type as the recipient (e.g., chronic hepatitis, primary sclerosing cholangitis). After surgery, donors are assessed for surgical complications of transplantation (e.g., abscess, biloma, transection or stenosis of vessels on bile duct) and for hypertrophy of the left lobe (fig. 2.230).

In recipients, preoperatively, patency of the inferior vena cava, portal vein, hepatic artery, and common bile duct are evaluated, and the presence of malignant disease is determined [175, 249]. Patients with malignant tumors evaluated for possible transplantation are evaluated for extent of hepatic involvement and for the presence of porta hepatis nodes or distant disease. Recipients may receive living related partial livers (lateral segment for small pediatric patients, right lobe for adult-to-adult recipients) (fig. 2.231) or cadaveric whole or partial livers (fig. 2.232).

The most common cause of early liver graft failure is rejection. The incidence of rejection is as high as 64% in some published series [250]. Early diagnosis is

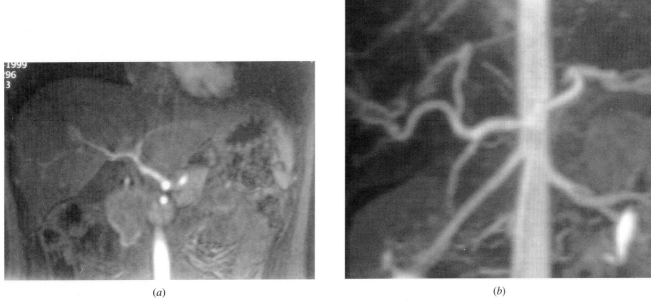

FIG. 2.227 Liver donor MRA. Coronal 3D gradient-echo 2-mm source image (*a*) and MIP reconstruction of the 2-mm 3D gradient-echo sections (*b*) in two different patients shows the hepatic artery arising from the celiac axis.

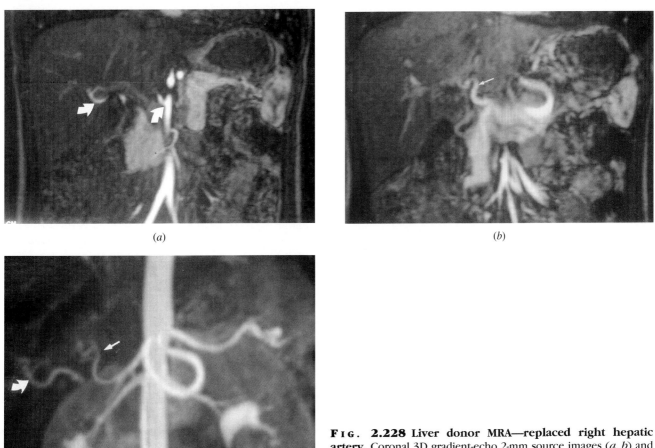

FIG. 2.228 Liver donor MRA—replaced right hepatic artery. Coronal 3D gradient-echo 2-mm source images (*a, b*) and MIP reconstruction of the 2-mm 3D gradient-echo sections (*c*) images that demonstrate the left hepatic artery arising from the celiac trunk (short arrow, *b, c*) and the right hepatic artery (curved arrows, *a, c*) arising from the SMA.

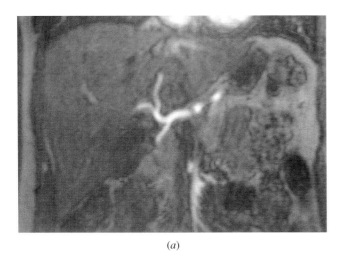

(a)

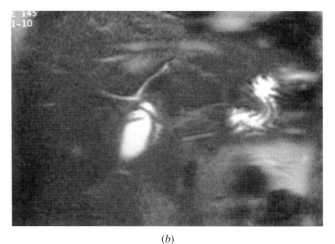

(b)

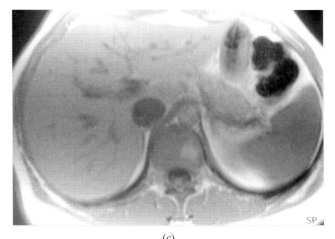

(c)

FIG. 2.229 **Liver donor evaluation (pretransplant).** Coronal 3D gradient-echo 2-mm source image (a), source image from a MRCP study (b), and transverse SGE (c) images demonstrate three MR techniques used to evaluate liver donors: MRA, MRCP and tissue imaging sequences.

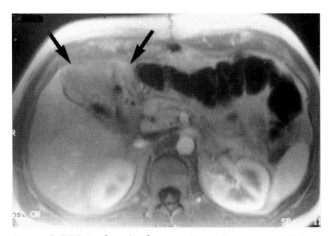

FIG. 2.230 **Ischemic changes.** Immediate postgadolinium image in a lateral segment liver donor patient demonstrates heterogeneous areas with diminished enhancement in *segment 4* (arrows) reflecting postsurgical injury.

essential to allow modification of immunosuppressive therapy [251]. The differential diagnosis of rejection in-

cludes biliary obstruction, cholangitis, ischemic injury, viral infection, and drug toxicity.

Vascular complications are important causes of graft failure [252]. Hepatic artery thrombosis is the most frequent and severe complication, occurring in 4–12% of adult patients and up to 42% of pediatric patients [253]. Hepatic artery stenosis has an estimated incidence of 11% and, presumably, eventually leads to hepatic artery thrombosis if left untreated [253]. Hepatic artery patency can be documented by MRI in most cases. Technical modification of the gadolinium-enhanced 3D FISP technique to demonstrate small-vessel stenosis is undergoing continued refinement. A recent report compared 3D gadolinium-enhanced MR angiograms with conventional angiography and ultrasound. The results indicate that gadolinium-enhanced 3D MR angiography achieved accurate results in 34 (89%) of the 38 examinations. The incidence of venous complications—portal vein and inferior vena cava thrombosis/stenosis—is lower than that of arterial complication [253] and does not necessarily lead to graft failure. Portal vein and IVC patency can be diagnosed reproducibly on MR images (fig. 2.233) [254].

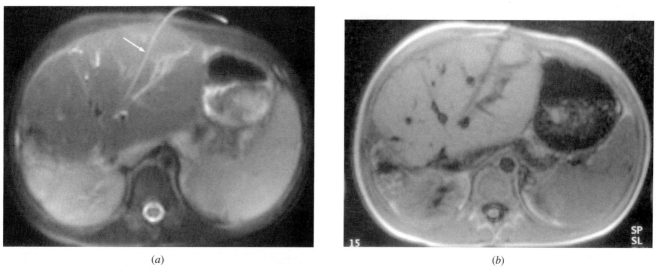

(a)   (b)

F I G . 2.231 Transplanted liver recipient—lateral segment. T2-weighted fat-suppressed SS-ESTE (*a*) and SGE (*b*) images in a pediatric patient who had undergone liver transplantation of a lateral segment 6 years earlier. The liver has developed a rounded configuration through hyperplasia. Note a percutaneous biliary drain (arrow, *a*).

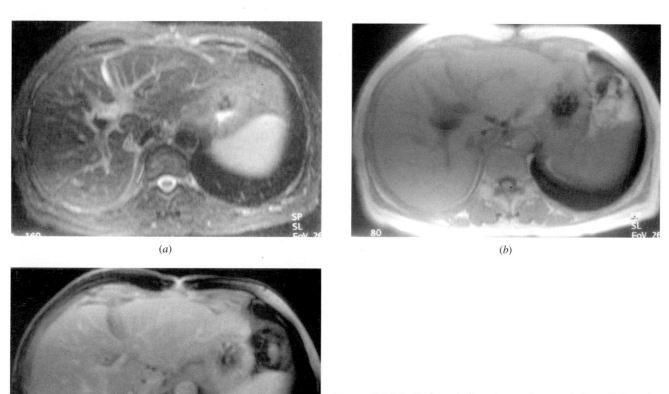

(a)   (b)

(c)

F I G . 2.232 Cadaveric liver transplant recipient. Echo-train STIR (*a*), SGE (*b*), and 90-s postgadolinium fat-suppressed SGE (*c*) images in a patient after transplant of a cadaveric liver. The liver showed normal signal without evidence for mass lesions or abnormal enhancement. No perihepatic fluid is identified. Note the clip artifacts in the porta hepatis and adjacent to the IVC, which are observed in patients with cadaveric liver transplant.

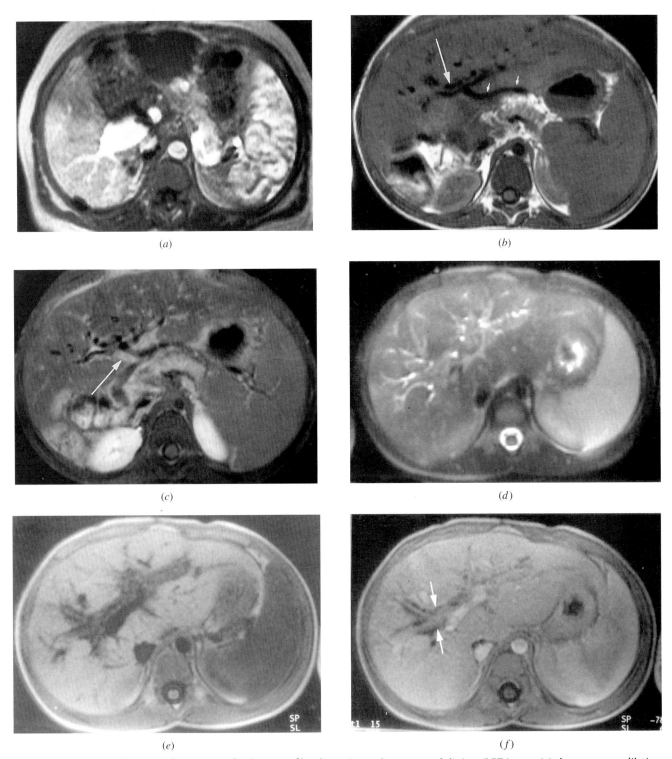

(a)   *(b)*   *(c)*   *(d)*   *(e)*   *(f)*

FIG. 2.233 Hepatic transplant—portal vein complications. Immediate postgadolinium SGE image (*a*) demonstrates dilation of the right portal vein secondary to anastomotic stenosis.

T1-weighted SE (*b*) and interstitial-phase gadolinium-enhanced T1-weighted fat-suppressed SE (*c*) images in a pediatric patient with a trisegmental transplant. Patent hepatic arterial graft (small arrows, *b*) and biliary ducts (long arrow, *b*) are evident. There is no evidence of a patent portal vein. Enhancing inflammatory tissue is present in the porta hepatis and in the expected location of the portal vein (long arrow, *c*).

Echo-train STIR (*d*), SGE (*e*), and 90-s postgadolinium fat-suppressed SGE (*f*) images in a 6-yr-old girl, 14 months after transplant. There is an abnormal decreased signal intensity seen in the distal right portal vein (arrows, *f*) on the interstitial-phase image with slight expansion of the portal vein and patchy enhancement to this segment of the liver. These features are consistent with thrombosis of the right portal vein. Note also that mild intrahepatic ductal dilatation is present (*d*).

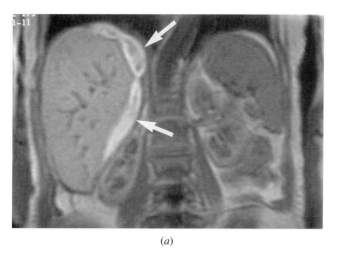 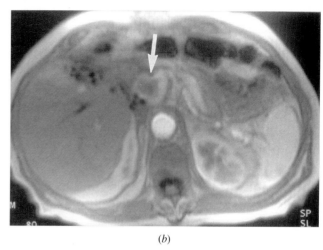

(a)   (b)

FIG. 2.234 Hematoma in recipient hemiliver. Coronal SGE (*a*) and transverse immediate postgadolinium SGE (*b*) images in a patient who is the recipient of a right hepatic lobe transplant. There is a perihepatic fluid collection (arrows, *a*, *b*) that demonstrates a high-signal peripheral rim on noncontrast T1-weighted images (*a*), consistent with hematoma.

Fluid collections are commonly observed after hepatic transplantation and include hematomas (fig. 2.234), seromas, bilomas (fig. 2.235), abscesses, and simple ascites. Bile leaks may develop at the anastomosis for technical reasons or may be secondary to bile duct necrosis in those patients with hepatic artery thrombosis [255].

Strictures of the biliary tree are often a late complication of liver transplant and usually occur at the anastomosis secondary to scar formation. Stenosis or obstruction of the biliary tree (fig. 2.236) may be shown using techniques that render bile low in signal, high in signal (MR cholangiography), or using a combination of both. Mucocele of the cystic duct remnant

is a rare cause of biliary obstruction and may appear as a focal fluid collection adjacent to the hepatic duct [256]. MRI is able to distinguish between hematomas and other fluid collections in hepatic transplants. In the acute postoperative phase, deoxyhemoglobin and extracellular methemoglobin have distinctive very low signal on T2-weighted images. In the period spanning several days to several months postsurgery, intra- or extracellular methemoglobin in subacute hematomas is higher in signal on T1-weighted images than other fluid.

Periportal signal abnormalities are frequently present in transplanted livers. The typical appearance is tissue that is low in signal intensity on T1-weighted images and high in signal intensity on T2-weighted images.

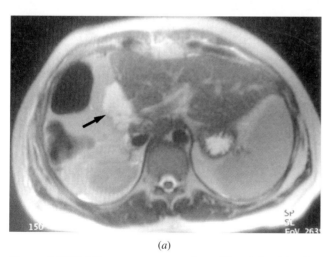 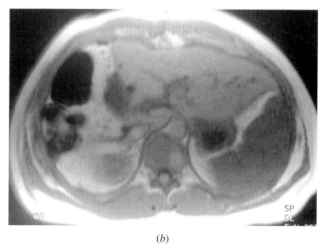

(a)   (b)

FIG. 2.235 Biloma, posttransplant. T2-weighted SS-ETSE (*a*) and SGE (*b*) images in a living-related right hemiliver donor after transplant. There is a fluid collection (arrow, *a*) along the resection margin of the liver that demonstrates high signal on T2- (*a*) and low signal on T1-weighted (*b*) images, consistent with biloma.

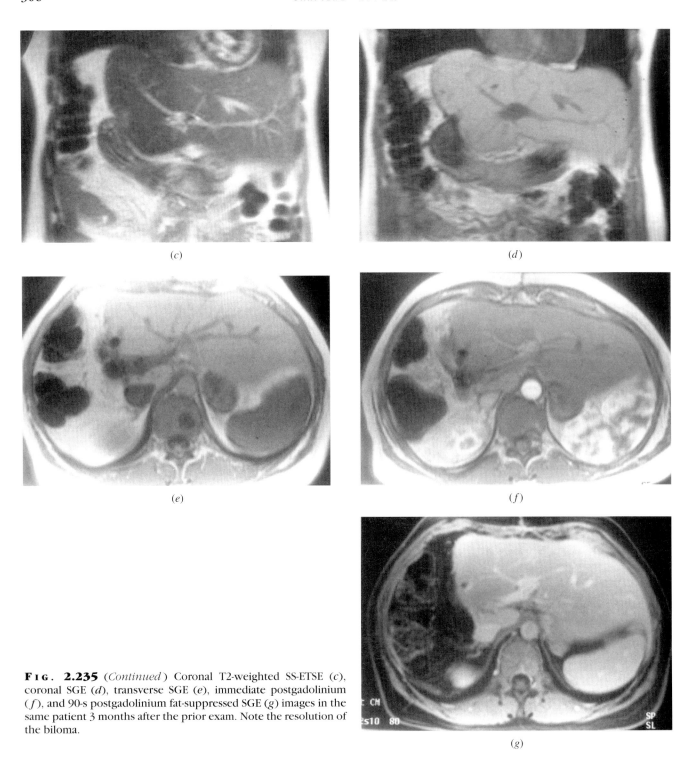

FIG. 2.235 (*Continued*) Coronal T2-weighted SS-ETSE (*c*), coronal SGE (*d*), transverse SGE (*e*), immediate postgadolinium (*f*), and 90-s postgadolinium fat-suppressed SGE (*g*) images in the same patient 3 months after the prior exam. Note the resolution of the biloma.

Abnormal tissue is most substantial in the porta hepatis and extends along the branching portal tracts into the liver parenchyma (fig. 2.237) [257]. In many cases, periportal signal abnormalities may represent lymphocytic infiltration due to rejection; however, other causes such as dilated lymphatics due to impaired drainage after surgery must be considered [258]. Beyond the immediate transplant period, expansion of the periportal tissue in a masslike fashion may be a harbinger of posttransplant lymphoproliferative disorder (PTLD) (fig. 2.238). PTLD occurs in transplant recipients whose immune systems are compromised. Most cases can be linked to infection with Epstein-Barr virus and may involve any organ in the body. Lymph nodes, lungs, and GI tract are most

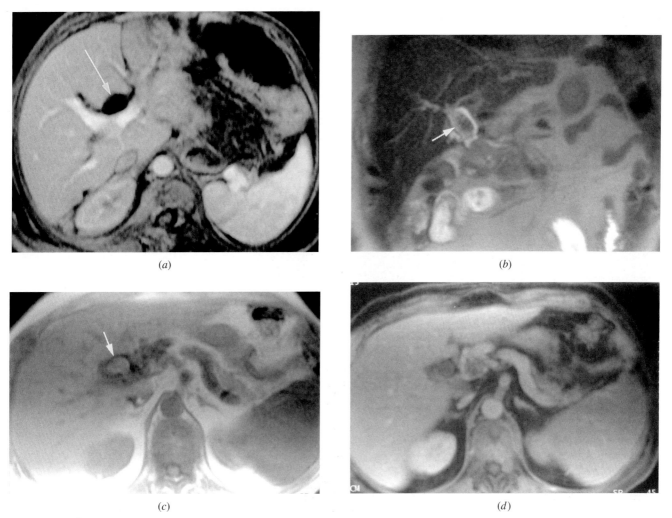

F I G . 2.236 Liver transplant, biliary duct stenosis. Transverse 90-s postgadolinium fat-suppressed SGE image (*a*). Dilation of the common hepatic duct (arrow, *a*) is present, secondary to anastomotic stenosis.

Coronal T2-weighted SS-ETSE (*b*), SGE (*c*), and 90-s postgadolinium fat-suppressed SGE (*d*) images in a second patient. There is an anastomotic stricture associated with a filling defect within the common bile duct consistent with a sludge ball or stone (arrow, *b*, *c*). Note the mild intrahepatic biliary ductal dilatation (*b*). The findings were confirmed by ERCP.

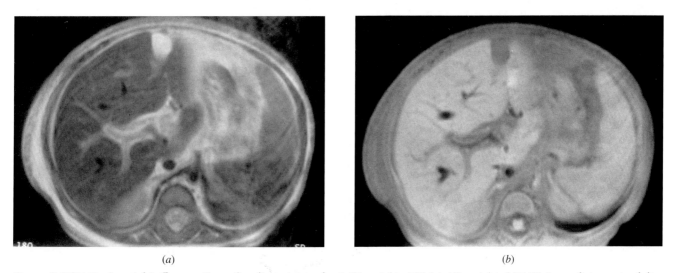

F I G . 2.237 Periportal inflammation after liver transplant. T2-weighted SE (*a*), T1-weighted SE (*b*), immediate postgadolinium magnetization-prepared gradient-echo (*c*), and T1-weighted interstitial-phase postgadolinium fat-suppressed SE (*d*) images in a 17-month-old patient after liver transplant.

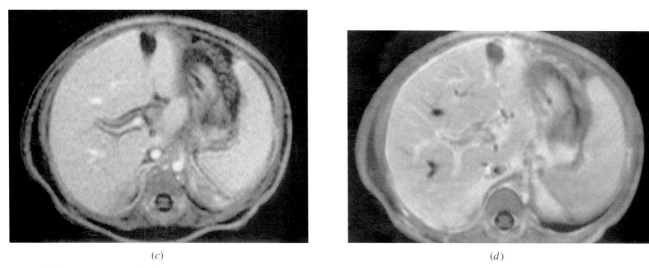

(c)   (d)

F I G . 2.237 (*Continued*) There is a moderate amount of periportal inflammatory change, which appears high signal on T2 (*a*) and enhances on interstitial-phase postgadolinium fat-suppressed images (*c*), likely postsurgical changes.

commonly involved with PTLD [240, 255]. PTLD is varied in presentation, ranging from polyclonal (nonmalignant) B cell proliferations to conventional malignant lymphoma, usually B cell [259]. Inflammatory periportal tissue also may be observed in acute hepatitis after biliary surgery, in various benign or malignant diseases, and in portal adenopathy [213].

Hepatocellular carcinoma may develop in the transplanted liver. This is an important complication in patients who were diagnosed with hepatocellular carcinoma pretransplantation, or in whom focal hepatocellular carcinoma was found incidentally in the pathologic evaluation of the recipient's resected liver (fig. 2.239) [260].

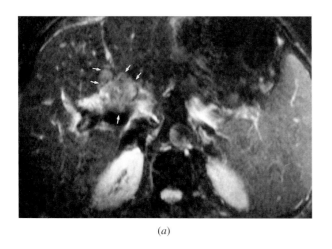

(a)

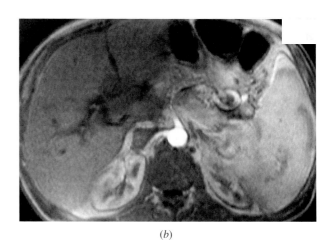

(b)

F I G . 2.238 Lymphoproliferative disorder. T2-weighted fat-suppressed ETSE (*a*) and immediate postgadolinium SGE (*b*) images. A 3-cm mass is present in the porta hepatis that is moderate in signal on the T2-weighted image (arrows, *a*) and enhances minimally with gadolinium (*b*).

Interstitial-phase gadolinium-enhanced fat-suppressed SGE (*c*) image in a second patient with posttransplant lymphoproliferative disorder. A mass (arrows, *c*) in the porta hepatis is appreciated with negligible enhancement on the late postcontrast image (*c*).

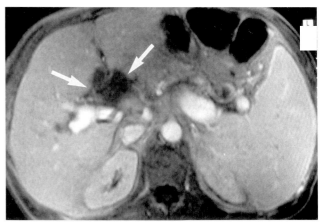

(c)

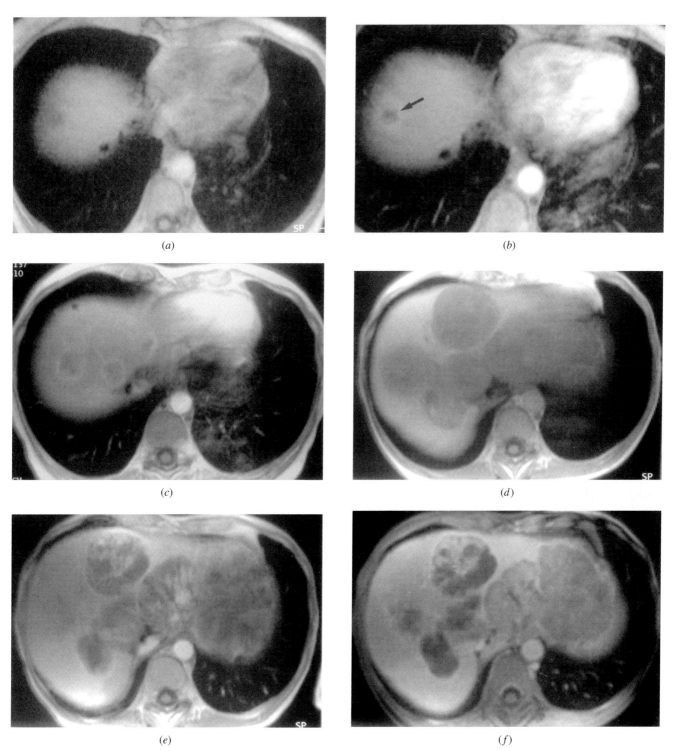

(a)

(b)

(c)

(d)

(e)

(f)

F i g . 2.239 Recurrent HCC in liver transplant. SGE (*a*) and immediate postgadolinium SGE (*b*) images in a patient who has developed HCC within a transplanted liver. Multiple small masses involve the dome of the right lobe of the liver that demonstrate mildly low-signal intensity on T1-weighted images (*a*) and rim enhancement on the immediate postgadolinium image (arrow, *b*). Three months later the lesions have increased in size and number, as shown on the immediate postgadolinium SGE image (*c*). One year later, SGE (*d*), immediate postgadolinium SGE (*e*), and 90-s postgadolinium fat-suppressed SGE (*f*) images demonstrate massive increase in size and number of HCCs. This represents metastases to a liver transplant in a patient who had HCC in her native liver.

MRI demonstrates a variety of morphologic abnormalities in transplanted livers and is able to identify various causes of graft failure. At present, however, no specific MRI findings have been identified to establish or quantify transplant rejection or hepatocellular function. In the future, hepatocyte specific contrast agents or MR spectroscopy may play a role in this determination.

CONCLUSIONS

MRI is an excellent imaging modality in the detection and characterization of both focal and diffuse liver disease. MRI exceeds spiral CT imaging for many of these evaluations: however, comparisons with multidetector CT are lacking. Among all focal liver lesions, MRI has greater impact on patient management than CT imaging in the evaluation of hypervascular malignant lesions such as hepatocellular carcinoma or metastases from hypervascular primary tumors. MRI may be the most accurate nonoperative imaging modality for evaluating patients with suspected limited involvement of the liver with malignant disease who are considered candidates for partial hepatic resection. MRI is also the imaging modality of choice for the detection of hepatosplenic candidiasis. No other imaging modality can exceed the accuracy of MRI for the evaluation of diffuse liver disease, so MRI should be used to investigate patients with suspected iron deposition, fatty infiltration, or cirrhosis. In many settings, however, MRI may be adequately employed as a problem-solving modality to characterize and determine the extent of focal liver lesions. It is also clear that patients who are not candidates for contrast-enhanced CT examination (e.g., patients with poor renal function or contrast allergy) should be studied with MRI.

REFERENCES

1. Couinaud C: *Le Foie. Etudes Anatomiques et Chirurgicales.* Paris: Masson 1957.
2. Heiken JP: Chapter 12. Liver in: Lee JKT, Sagel SS, Stanley RJ, Heiken JP. *Computed Body Tomography with MR correlation*, p. 701–777. 3rd edition. Lippincott-Raven Philadelphia. 1998.
3. MacSween RNM, Scathorne RJ. Chapter 1. Developmental anatomy and normal structure. In: MacSween RNM, Anthony PP, Scheuer PJ, Burt AD, Portamann BC, eds.: *Pathology of the Liver.* P. 1–49. 3rd edition. Churchill Livingstone, London, 1994.
4. Chiu CYV, Semelka RC: Contrast enhanced MR imaging of the abdomen. *J Hong Kong Coll Radiologists* 3(4): 433–442, 2000.
5. Semelka RC, Heimberger TKG: Contrast agents for MR imaging of the liver. *Radiology* 218: 227–238, 2001.
6. Caudana R, Morana G, Pirovano GP, Nicoli N, Portuese A, Spinazzi A, Di Rito R, Pistolesi GF: Focal malignant hepatic lesions: MR imaging enhanced with gadolinium benzoxypropionictetraacetate (BOPTA)—preliminary results of phase II clinical application. *Radiology* 199: 513–520, 1996.
7. Kettritz U, Schlund JF, Wilbur K, Eisenberg LB, Semelka RA: Comparison of gadolinium chelates with Manganese-DPDP for liver lesion detection and characterization: preliminary results. *Magn Reson Imag* 14(10): 1185–1190, 1996.
8. Hamm B, Staks T, Muhler A, Bollow M, Taupitz M, Frenzel T, Wolf KJ, Weinmann HJ, Lange L: Phase I clinical evaluation of Gd-EOB-DTPA as a hepatobiliary MR contrast agent: Safety, pharmacokinetics, and MR imaging. *Radiology* 195: 785–792, 1995.
9. Hagspiel KD, Neidl KF, Eichenberger AC, Weder W, Marincek B: Detection of liver metastases: Comparison of superparamagnetic iron oxide-enhanced and unenhanced MR imaging at 1.5 T with dynamic CT, intraoperative US, and percutaneous US. *Radiology* 196: 471–478, 1995.
10. Ros PR, Freeny PC, Marms SE, et al.: Hepatic MR imaging with ferumoxides: A multicenter clinical trial of the safety and efficacy in the detection of focal hepatic lesions. *Radiology* 196: 481–488, 1995.
11. Yamamoto H, Yamashita Y, Yoshimatsu S, Baba Y, Hatanaka Y, Murakami R, Nishiharu T, Takahashi M, Higashida Y, Moribe N: Hepatocellular carcinoma in cirrhotic livers: Detection with unenhanced and iron oxide-enhanced MR imaging. *Radiology* 195: 106–112, 1995.
12. Saini S, Edelman RR, Sharma P, Li W, Mayo-Smith W, Slater GJ, Eisenberg PJ, Hahn PF: Blood-pool MR contrast material for detection and characterization of focal hepatic lesions: Initial clinical experience with ultrasmall superparamagnetic iron oxide (AMI-227). *Am J Roentgenol* 164: 1147–1152, 1995.
13. Mitchell DG. Liver I: Currently available gadolinium chelates. *Magn Reson Imaging Clin N Am. Contrast Agents for Body MR Imaging.* WB Saunders. 4: 37–51, 1996
14. Yamashita Y, Hantanaka Y, Yamammoto H., et al.: Differential diagnosis of focal liver lesions. Role of spin-echo and contrast-enhanced dynamic MR imaging. *Radiology* 193: 59–65, 1994.
15. Whitney WS, Herfkens RJ, Jeffrey RB, McDonnell CH, Li KC, VanDalsem WJ, Low RN, Francis IR, Dabatin JF, Glazer GM: Dynamic breath-hold multiplanar spoiled gradient recalled MR imaging with gadolinium enhancement for differentiating hepatic hemangiomas from malignancies at 1.5 T. *Radiology* 189: 863–870, 1993.
16. Martin DR, Semelka RC, Chung JJ, Balci NC, Wilber K: Sequential use of gadolinium chelate and mangafodipir trisodium for the assessment of focal liver lesions: Initial observations. *Magn Reson Imaging* 18: 955–963,2000.
17. Semelka RC, Lee JKT, Worawattanakul S, Noone TC, Patt RH, Asher SM: Sequential use of ferumoxide particles and gadolinium chelate for the evaluation of focal liver lesions on MRI. *J Magn Reson Imaging* 8: 670–674, 1998.
18. Vogl TJ, Kummel S, Hammerstingl R, Schellenbeck M, Schumacher G, Balzer T, Schwarz W, Muller PK, Bechstein WO, Mack MG, Sollner O, Felix R: Liver tumors: Comparison of MR imaging with Gd-EOB-DTPA and Gd-DTPA. *Radiology* 200: 59–67, 1996.
19. Weissleder R, Lee AS, Fischman AJ, Reimer P, Shen T, Wilkinson R, Callahan RJ, Brady TJ: Polyclonal human immunoglobulin G labeled with polymeric iron oxide: Antibody MR imaging. *Radiology* 181: 245–249, 1991.
20. Vogl TJ, Hammerstingl R, Schwarz W, et al.: Superparamagnetic iron oxide-enhanced versus godolinium-enhanced MR imaging for differential diagnosis of focal liver lesions. *Radiology* 198: 881–887, 1996.
21. Sherlock S, Dooley J: *Diseases of the Liver and Biliary System.* Blackwell Science. 10th edition, p.4. 1997.
22. Rossai J: *Ackerman's Surgical Pathology.* Vol.1 8th edition. Mosby, St Louis, p. 898 1995.
23. Barnes PA, Thomas JL, Bernardino ME: Pitfalls in the diagnosis of hepatic cysts by computed tomography. *Radiology* 141: 129–133, 1981.

24. Semelka RC, Shoenut JP, Greenberg HM, Mickflickier AB: The liver. In: Semelka RC, Shoenut JP (eds.). *MRI of the Abdomen with CT Correlation*. New York: Raven, p. 13–41, 1993.

25. Kadoya M, Matsui O, Nakanuma Y, Yoshikawa J, Arai K, Takashima T, Amano M, Kimura M: Ciliated hepatic foregut cyst: Radiologic features. *Radiology* 175: 475–477, 1990.

26. Shoenut JP, Semelka RC, Levi C, Greenberg H: Ciliated hepatic foregut cysts: US, CT, and contrast-enhanced MR imaging. *Abdom Imaging* 19: 150–152, 1994.

27. Itai Y, Ebihara R, Eguchi N, Saida Y, Kurosaki Y, Minami M, Araki T: Hepatobiliary cysts in patients with autosomal dominant polycystic kidney disease: Prevalence and CT findings. *Am J Roentgenol* 164: 339–342, 1995.

28. Semelka RC, Hussain SM, Marcos HB, Woosley JT: Biliary hamartomas: solitary and multiple lesions shown on current MR techniques including gadolinium enhancement. *J Magn Reson Imaging* 10: 196–201, 1999.

29. Semelka RC: Letter of response. *Radiology* 219: 299–300, 2001.

30. Aytaç S, Fitoz S, Akyar S, Atasoyç, Erekul S: Focal intrahepatic extramedullary hematopoiesis: color Doppler US and CT findings. *Abdom Imaging* 24: 366–368, 1999.

31. Navarro M, Crespo C, Perez L, Martinez C, Galant J, Gonzalez I. Massive intrahepatic extramedullary hematopoiesis in myelofibrosis. *Abdom Imaging* 25: 184–186, 2000.

32. Nonomura A, Mizukami Y, Cadoya M. Angiomyolipoma of the Liver: a collective review. *J Gastroenterol* 29(1): 95–105, 1994.

33. Worawattanakul S, Kelekis NL, Semelka RC, Woosley JT: Hepatic angiomyolipoma with minimal fat content: MR demonstration. *Magn Reson Imaging* 14: 687–689, 1996.

34. Morton KM, Bluemke DA, Hruban RH, Soyer P, Fishman EK. CT and MR imaging of benign hepatic and biliary tumors. *Radiographics* 19: 431–451, 1999.

35. Craig J, Peters R, Edmondson H: Tumors of the liver and intrahepatic bile ducts. In: Hartman H, Sobin L (eds.). *Atlas of Tumor Pathology*. Second series, fascicle 26. Washington, DC: Armed Forces Institute of Pathology, 1989.

36. Karhunen PJ. Benign hepatic tumours and tumour like conditions in men. *J Clin Pathol* 39: 183–188, 1986.

37. International Working Party: Terminology of nodular hepatocellular lesions. International Working Party. *Hepatology* 22: 983–993, 1995.

38. Mitsuodo K, Watanabe Y, Saga T, et al.: Nonenhanced hepatic cavernous hemangioma with multiple calcifications: CT and pathologic correlation. *Abdom Imaging* 20: 459–461, 1995.

39. Li KC, Glazer GM, Quint LE, Francis IR, Aisen AM, Ensminger WD, Bookstein FL: Distinction of hepatic cavernous hemangioma from hepatic metastases with MR imaging. *Radiology* 169: 409–415, 1988.

40. Lombardo DM, Baker ME, Spritzer CE, Blinder R, Meyers W, Herfkens RJ: Hepatic hemangiomas vs. metastases: MR differentiation at 1.5 T. *Am J Roentgenol* 155: 55–59, 1990.

41. Semelka RC, Shoenut JP, Kroeker MA, Greenberg HM, Simm FC, Minuk GY, Kroeker RM, Micflikier AB: Focal liver disease: Comparison of dynamic contrast-enhanced CT and T2-weighted fat-suppressed, FLASH, and dynamic gadolinium-enhanced MR imaging at 1.5 T. *Radiology* 184: 687–694, 1992.

42. Schmiedl U, Kolbel G, Hess CF, Klose U, Kurtz B: Dynamic sequential MR imaging of focal liver lesions: Initial experience in 22 patients at 1.5 T. *J Comput Assist Tomogr* 14: 600–607, 1990.

43. Quinn SF, Benjamin GG: Hepatic cavernous hemangiomas: Simple diagnostic sign with dynamic bolus CT. *Radiology* 182: 545–548, 1992.

44. Low RN. MRI of the Liver using gadolinium chelates. *Magn Reson Imaging Clin N Am* (in press)

45. Hamm B, Thoeni RF, Gould RG, Bernardino ME, Luning M, Saini S, Mahfouz AE, Taupitz M, Wolf KJ: Focal liver lesions: Characterization with nonenhanced and dynamic contrast material-enhanced MR imaging. *Radiology* 190: 417–423, 1994.

46. Semelka RC, Brown ED, Ascher SM, Patt RH, Bagley AS, Li W, Edelman RR, Shoenut JP, Brown JJ: Hepatic hemangiomas: A multi-institutional study of appearance on T2-weighted and serial gadolinium-enhanced gradient-echo MR images. *Radiology* 192: 401–406, 1994.

47. Kim TK, Choi BI, Han JK, Jang H, Han MC: Optimal MR imaging protocol for hepatic hemangiomas: Comparison of T2-weighted fast and conventional SE and serial Gd-DTPA-enhanced GRE techniques. *Radiology* 197(P): 175, 1995.

48. Semelka RC, Sofka CM. Hepatic hemangiomas. *Magn Reson Imaging Clin N Am* 5(2): 241–253, 1997.

49. Jeong MG, Yu JS, Kim KW: Hepatic cavernous hemangioma: Temporal peritumoral enhancement during multiphase dynamic MR imaging. *Radiology* 216: 692–697, 2000.

50. Choi BI, Han MC, Park JH, Kim SH, Han MH, Kim CW: Giant cavernous hemangioma of the liver: CT and MR imaging in 10 cases. *Am J Roentgenol* 152: 1221–1226, 1989.

51. Mitchell DG, Saini S, Weinreb J, De Lange EE, Runge VM, Kuhlman JE, Parisky Y, Johnson CD, Brown JJ, Schnall M, et al.: Hepatic metastases and cavernous hemangiomas: Distinction with standard- and triple-dose gadoteridol-enhanced MR imaging. *Radiology* 193: 49–57, 1994.

52. Burdeny DA, Semelka RC, Kelekis NL, Kettritz U, Woosley JT, Cance WG, Lee JKT: Chemotherapy treated liver metastases mimicking hemangiomas on MR images. *Abdom Imag* 24: 378–382, 1999.

53. Semelka RC, Cance WG, Marcos HB, Mauro MA: Liver metastases: comparison of current MR techniques and spiral CT during arterial portography for detection in 20 surgically staged cases. *Radiology* 213: 86–91, 1999.

54. Larson RE, Semelka RC, Bagley AS, Molina PL, Brown ED, Lee JK: Hypervascular malignant liver lesions: Comparison of various MR imaging pulse sequences and dynamic CT. *Radiology* 192: 393–399, 1994.

55. McFarland EG, Mayo-Smith WW, Saini S, Hahn PF, Goldberg MA, Lee MJ: Hepatic hemangiomas and malignant tumors: improved differentiation with heavily T2-weighted conventional spin-echo MR imaging. *Radiology* 193: 43–47, 1994.

56. Kerlin P, Davis GL, McGill DB, Weiland LH, Adson MA, Sheedy PFD: Hepatic adenoma and focal nodular hyperplasia: Clinical, pathologic, and radiologic features. *Gastroenterology* 84: 994–1002, 1983.

57. Shortell CK, Schwartz SI: Hepatic adenoma and focal nodular hyperplasia. *Surg Gynecol Obstet* 173: 426–431, 1991.

58. Meissner K: Hemorrhage caused by ruptured liver cell adenoma following long-term oral contraceptives: a case report. *Hepatogastroenterology* 45(19): 224–225, 1998.

59. Klatskin G, Conn HO. *Histopathology of the Liver*. Oxford University Press. New York, p. 368. 1993.

60. Paulson EK, McClellan JS, Washington K, Spritzer CE, Meyers WC, Baker ME: Hepatic adenoma: MR characteristics and correlation with pathologic findings. *Am J Roentgenol* 163: 113–116, 1994.

61. Powers C, Ros PR, Stoupis C, Johnson WK, Segel KH: Primary liver neoplasms: MR imaging with pathologic correlation. *Radiographics* 14: 459–482, 1994.

62. Hamm B, Vogl TJ, Branding G, Schnell B, Taupitz M, Wolf KJ, Lissner J: Focal liver lesions: MR imaging with Mn-DPDP-initial clinical results in 40 patients. *Radiology* 182: 167–174, 1992.

63. Flejou JF, Barge J, Menu Y, et al.: Liver adenomatosis: an entity distinct from liver adenoma? *Gastroenterology* 83: 1132–1138, 1985.

64. Grazioli L, Federle MP, Ichikawa T, Balzano E, Nalesnik M, Madariaga J: Liver adenomatosis: clinical, histopathologic, and imaging findings in 15 patients. *Radiology* 216: 395–402, 2000.

65. Mortelé KJ, Praet M, Vlierberghe HV, Kunnen M, Ros PR: CT and MR imaging findings in focal nodular hyperplasia of the liver: Radiologic-pathologic correlation. *Am J Roentgenol* 175: 687–692, 2000.

66. Wanless IR, Albrecht S, Bilbao J, Frei JV, Heathcote EJ, Roberts EA, Chiasson D: Multiple focal nodular hyperplasia of the liver associated with vascular malformations of various organs and neoplasia of the brain: A new syndrome. *Mod Pathol* 2: 456–462, 1989.

67. Eisenberg LB, Warshauer DM, Woosley JT, Cance WG, Bunzendahl H, Semelka RC: CT and MRI of hepatic focal nodular hyperplasia with peripheral steatosis. *J Comput Assist Tomogr* 19: 498–500, 1995.

68. Lee MJ, Saini S, Hamm B, Taupitz M, Hahn PF, Seneterre E, Ferrucci JT: Focal nodular hyperplasia of the liver: MR findings in 35 proved cases. *Am J Roentgenol* 156: 317–320, 1991.

69. Vilgrain V, Flejou JF, Arrive L, Belghiti J, Najmark D, Menu Y, Zins M, Vullierme MP, Nahum H: Focal nodular hyperplasia of the liver: MR imaging and pathologic correlation in 37 patients. *Radiology* 184: 699–703, 1992.

70. Schiebler ML, Kressel HY, Saul SH, Yeager BA, Axel L, Gefter WB: MR imaging of focal nodular hyperplasia of the liver. *J Comput Assist Tomogr* 11: 651–654, 1987.

71. Haggar AM, Bree RL: Hepatic focal nodular hyperplasia: MR imaging at 1.0 and 1.5 T. *J Magn Reson Imaging* 2: 85–88, 1992.

72. Wanless IR, Mawdsley C, Adams R: On the pathogenesis of focal nodular hyperplasia of the liver. *Hepatology* 5(6): 1194–1200, 1985.

73. Mahfouz AE, Hamm B, Taupitz M, Wolf KJ: Hypervascular liver lesions: Differentiation of focal nodular hyperplasia from malignant tumors with dynamic gadolinium-enhanced MR imaging. *Radiology* 186: 133–138, 1993.

74. Mathieu D, Vilgrain V, Mahfouz AE, Anglade MC, Vullierme MP, Denys A: Benign liver tumor. *Magn Reson Imaging Clin N Am* 5(2): 255–288, 1997.

75. Vogl TJ, Hamm B, Schnell B, McMahon C, Branding G, Lissner J, Wolf KJ: Mn-DPDP enhancement patterns of hepatocellular lesions on MR images. *J Magn Reson Imaging* 3: 51–58, 1993.

76. Rummeny EJ, Wernecke K, Saini S, Vassallo P, Wiesmann W, Oestmann JW, Kivelitz D, Reers B, Reiser MF, Peters PE: Comparison between high-field-strength MR imaging and CT for screening of hepatic metastases: A receiver operating characteristic analysis. *Radiology* 182: 879–886, 1992.

77. Nelson RC, Chezmar JL, Sugarbaker PH, Murray DR, Bernardino ME: Preoperative localization of focal liver lesions to specific liver segments: Utility of CT during arterial portography. *Radiology* 176: 89–94, 1990.

78. Sugarbaker PH, Kemeny N: Management of metastatic cancer to the liver. *Adv Surg* 22: 1–56, 1989.

79. Hughes KS, Rosenstein RB, Songhorabodi S, Adson MA, Ilstrup DM, Fortner JG, Maclean BJ, Foster JH, Daly JM, Fitzherbert D, et al.: Resection of the liver for colorectal carcinoma metastases: A multi-institutional study of long-term survivors. *Dis Colon Rectum* 31: 1–4, 1988.

80. Semelka RC, Shoenut JP, Ascher SM, Kroeker MA, Greenberg HM, Yaffe CS, Micflikier AB: Solitary hepatic metastasis: Comparison of dynamic contrast-enhanced CT and MR imaging with fat-suppressed T2-weighted, breath-hold T1-weighted FLASH, and dynamic gadolinium-enhanced FLASH sequences. *J Magn Reson Imaging* 4: 319–323, 1994.

81. Stark DD, Wittenberg J, Butch RJ, Ferrucci JT Jr: Hepatic metastases: Randomized, controlled comparison of detection with MR imaging and CT. *Radiology* 165: 399–406, 1987.

82. Zeman RK, Dritschilo A, Silverman PM, Clark LR, Garra BS, Thomas DS, Ahlgren JD, Smith FP, Korec SM, Nauta RJ, et al.: Dynamic CT vs. 0.5 T MR imaging in the detection of surgically proven hepatic metastases. *J Comput Assist Tomogr* 13: 637–644, 1989.

83. Vassiliades VG, Foley WD, Alarcon J, Lawson T, Erickson S, Kneeland JB, Steinberg HV, Bernardino ME: Hepatic metastases: CT versus MR imaging at 1.5 T. *Gastrointest Radiol* 16: 159–163, 1991.

84. Semelka RC, Hricak H, Bis KG, Werthmuller WC, Higgins CB: Liver lesion detection: Comparison between excitation-spoiling fat suppression and regular spin-echo at 1.5 T. *Abdom Imaging* 18: 56–60, 1993.

85. De Lange EE, Mugler JP III, Bosworth JE, DeAngelis GA, Gay SB, Hurt NS, Berr SS, Rosenblatt JM, Merickel LW, Harris EK: MR imaging of the liver: Breath-hold T1-weighted MP-GRE compared with conventional T2-weighted SE imaging-lesion detection, localization, and characterization. *Radiology* 190: 727–736, 1994.

86. Jones EC, Chezmar JL, Nelson RC, Bernardino ME: The frequency and significance of small (less than or equal to 15 mm) hepatic lesions detected by CT. *Am J Roentgenol* 158: 535–539, 1992.

87. Bruneton JN, Raffaelli C, Maestro C, Padovani B: Benign liver lesions: Implications of detection in cancer patients. *Eur Radiol* 5: 387–390, 1995.

88. Noone TC, Semelka RC, Balci NC, Graham ML: Common occurrence of benign liver lesions in patients with newly diagnosed breast cancer investigated by MRI for suspected liver metastases. *J Magn Reson Imaging* 10: 165–169, 1999.

89. Semelka RC, Schlund JF, Molina PL, Willms AG, Kahlenberg M, Mauro MA, Weeks SM, Cance WG: Malignant liver lesions: Comparison of spiral CT arterial portography and MR imaging for diagnostic accuracy, cost, and effect on patient management. *J Magn Reson Imaging* 6: 39–43, 1996.

90. Semelka RC, Martin DR, Balci C, Lance T: Focal liver lesions: comparison of dual phase CT and multisequence multiplanar MR imaging including dynamic gadolinium enhancement. *J Magn Reson Imaging* 13: 397–401, 2001.

91. Semelka RC, Cumming MJ, Shoenut JP, Magro CM, Yaffe CS, Kroeker MA, Greenberg HM: Islet cell tumors: Comparison of dynamic contrast-enhanced CT and MR imaging with dynamic gadolinium enhancement and fat suppression. *Radiology* 186: 799–802, 1993.

92. Soyer P, Riopel M, Bluemke DA, Scherrer A: Hepatic metastases from leiomyosarcoma: MR features with histopathologic correlation. *Abdom Imaging* 22(1): 67–71, 1997.

93. Mahfouz AE, Hamm B, Wolf KJ: Peripheral washout: A sign of malignancy on dynamic gadolinium-enhanced MR images of focal liver lesions. *Radiology* 190: 49–52, 1994.

94. Semelka RC, Hussain SM, Marcos HB, Woosley JT. Perilesional enhancement of hepatic metastases: correlation between MR imaging and histopathologic findings—initial observations. *Radiology* 215: 89–94, 2000.

95. Outwater E, Tomaszewski JE, Daly JM, Kressel HY: Hepatic colorectal metastases: Correlation of MR imaging and pathologic appearance. *Radiology* 180: 327–332, 1991.

96. Semelka RC, Bagley AS, Brown ED, Kroeker MA: Malignant lesions of the liver identified on T1- but not T2-weighted MR images at 1.5 T. *J Magn Reson Imaging* 4: 315–318, 1994.

97. Semelka RC, Worawattanakul S, Kelekis NL, John G, Woosky JT, Graham M, Cance WG, et al.: Liver lesion detection, characterization, and effect on patient management: comparison of single-phase spiral CT and current MR techniques. *J Magn Reson Imaging* 7: 1040–1047, 1997.

98. Trump DL, Fahnstock R, Cloutier CT, Dickman MD: Anaerobic liver abscess and intrahepatic metastases—a case report and review of the literature. *Cancer* 41(2): 682–686, 1978.

99. Ackel F, Lersch C, Huber W, et al.: Multimicrobial sepsis including clostridium perfringens after chemoembolization of a single liver

metastases from common bile duct cancer. *Digestion* 62: 208–212, 2000.

100. Scheimberg IB, Pollock DJ, Collins PW, et al.: Pathology of the liver in leukemia and lymphoma. A study of 110 autopsies. *Histopathology* 26: 311–322, 1995.

101. Kelekis NL, Semelka RC, Siegelman ES, Ascher SM, Outwater EK, Woosley TJ, Reinhold C, Mitchell DG: Focal hepatic lymphoma: MR demonstration using current techniques including gadolinium enhancement. *J Magn Reson Imaging* 15(6): 625–636, 1997.

102. Kelekis NL, Warshauer DM, Semelka RC, Sallah AS: Nodular liver involvement in light chain multiple myeloma: Appearance on US and MRI. *Clin Imaging* 21: 207–209, 1997.

103. Choi BI, Takayasu K, Han MC: Small hepatocellular carcinomas and associated nodular lesions of the liver: Pathology, pathogenesis, and imaging findings. *Am J Roentgenol* 160: 1177–1187, 1993.

104. Terada T, Hoso M, Nakanuma Y. Development of cavernous vasculatures in liver with hepatocellular carcinoma. An autopsy study. *Liver* 9: 172–178, 1999.

105. Miller WJ, Baron RL, Dodd GD III, Federle MP: Malignancies in patients with cirrhosis: CT sensitivity and specificity in 200 consecutive transplant patients. *Radiology* 193: 645–650, 1994.

106. Oi H, Murakami T, Kim T, Matsushita M, Kishimoto H, Nakamura H: Dynamic MR imaging and early-phase helical CT for detecting small intrahepatic metastases of hepatocellular carcinoma. *Am J Roentgen* 166: 369–374, 1996.

107. Yamashita Y, Mitsuzaki K, Yi T, et al.: Small heptacellular carcinoma in patients with chronic liver damage: Prospective comparison of detection with dynamic MR imaging and helical CT of the whole liver. *Radiology* 200: 79–84, 1996.

108. Kelekis NL, Semelka RC, Worawattanakul S, et al.: Hepatocellular carcinoma in North America: A multiinstitutional study of appearance on T1-weighted, T2-weighted, and serial gadolinium-enhanced gradient-echo images. *Am J Roentgenol* 170: 1005–1013, 1998.

109. Rummeny E, Weissleder R, Stark DD, Saini S, Compton CC, Bennett W, Hahn PF, Wittenberg J, Malt RA, Ferrucci JT: Primary liver tumors: Diagnosis by MR imaging. *Am J Roentgenol* 152: 63–72, 1989.

110. Matsui O, Kadoya M, Kameyama T, Yoshikawa J, Arai K, Gabata T, Takashima T, Nakanuma Y, Terada T, Ida M: Adenomatous hyperplastic nodules in the cirrhotic liver: Differentiation from hepatocellular carcinoma with MR imaging. *Radiology* 173: 123–126, 1989.

111. Rosenthal RE, Davis PL: MR imaging of hepatocellular carcinoma at 1.5 tesla. *Gastrointest Radiol* 17: 49–52, 1992.

112. Hirai K, Aoki Y, Majima Y, Abe H, Nakashima O, Kojiro M, Tanikawa K: Magnetic resonance imaging of small hepatocellular carcinoma. *Am J Gastroenterol* 86: 205–209, 1991.

113. Kadoya M, Matsui O, Takashima T, Nonomura A: Hepatocellular carcinoma: Correlation of MR imaging and histopathologic findings. *Radiology* 183: 819–825, 1992.

114. Muramatsu Y, Nawano S, Takayasu K, Moriyama N, Yamada T, Yamasaki S, Hirohashi S: Early hepatocellular carcinoma: MR imaging. *Radiology* 181: 209–213, 1991.

115. Ebara M, Watanabe S, Kita K, Yoshikawa M, Sugiura N, Ohto M, Kondo F, Kondo Y: MR imaging of small hepatocellular carcinoma: Effect of intratumoral copper content on signal intensity. *Radiology* 180: 617–621, 1991.

116. Itoh K, Nishimura K, Togashi K, Fujisawa I, Noma S, Minami S, Sagoh T, Nakano Y, Itoh H, Mori K, et al.: Hepatocellular carcinoma: MR imaging. *Radiology* 164: 21–25, 1987.

117. Yamashita Y, Fan ZM, Yamamoto H, Matsukawa T, Yoshimatsu S, Miyazaki T, Sumi M, Harada M, Takahashi M: Spin-echo and dynamic gadolinium-enhanced FLASH MR imaging of hepatocel-

lular carcinoma: Correlation with histopathologic findings. *J Magn Reson Imaging* 4: 83–90, 1994.

118. Krinsky GA, Lee VS: MR imaging of cirrhotic nodules. *Abdom Imaging* 25: 471–482, 2000.

119. Kelekis NL, Semelka RC, Woosley JT: Malignant lesions of the liver with high signal intensity on T1-weighted MR images. *J Magn Reson Imaging* 6: 291–294, 1996.

120. Winter TC III, Takayasu K, Muramatsu Y, Furukawa H, Wakao F, Koga H, Sakamoto M, Hirohashi S, Freeny PC: Early advanced hepatocellular carcinoma: Evaluation of CT and MR appearance with pathologic correlation. *Radiology* 192: 379–387, 1994.

121. Yu JS, Kim KW, Lee JT, Yoo HS. MR imaging during arterial portography for assessment of hepatocellular carcinoma: Comparison with CT during arterial portography. *Am J Roentgenol* 170: 1501–1506, 1998.

122. Mahfouz AE, Hamm B, Wolf KJ: Dynamic gadopentetate dimeglumine-enhanced MR imaging of hepatocellular carcinoma. *Eur Radiol* 3: 453–458, 1993.

123. Yoshida H, Itai Y, Ohtomo K, Kokubo T, Minami M, Yashiro N: Small hepatocellular carcinoma and cavernous hemangioma: Differentiation with dynamic FLASH MR imaging with Gd-DTPA. *Radiology* 171: 339–342, 1989.

124. Liou J, Lee JK, Borrello JA, Brown JJ: Differentiation of hepatomas from nonhepatomatous masses: Use of MnDPDP-enhanced MR images. *Magn Reson Imaging* 12: 71–79, 1994.

125. Craig JR, Peters RL, Edmondson HA, Omata M: Fibrolamellar carcinoma of the liver: A tumor of adolescents and young adults with distinctive clinico-pathologic features. *Cancer* 46: 372–379, 1980.

126. Corrigan K, Semelka RC: Dynamic contrast-enhanced MR imaging of fibrolamellar hepatocellular carcinoma. *Abdom Imaging* 20: 122–125, 1995.

127. Hamrick-Turner J, Abbitt PL, Ros PR: Intrahepatic cholangiocarcinoma: MR appearance. *Am J Roentgenol* 158: 77–79, 1992.

128. Low RN, Sigeti JS, Francis IR, Weinman D, Bower B, Shimakawa A, Foo TK: Evaluation of malignant biliary obstruction: Efficacy of fast multiplanar spoiled gradient-recalled MR imaging vs. spin-echo MR imaging, CT, and cholangiography. *Am J Roentgenol* 162: 315–323, 1994.

129. Choi BI, Lim JH, Han MC, Lee DH, Kim SH, Kim YI, Kim CW: Biliary cystadenoma and cystadenocarcinoma: CT and sonographic findings. *Radiology* 171: 57–61, 1989.

130. Kokubo T, Itai Y, Ohtomo K, Itoh K, Kawauchi N, Minami M: Mucin-hypersecreting intrahepatic biliary neoplasms. *Radiology* 168: 609–614, 1988.

131. Palacios E, Shannon M, Solomon C, Guzman M: Biliary cystadenoma: Ultrasound, CT, and MRI. *Gastrointest Radiol* 15: 313–316, 1990.

132. Buetow PC, Buck JL, Pantongrag-Brown L, Ros PR, Devaney K, Goodman ZD, Cruess DF: Biliary cystadenoma and cystadenocarcinoma: Clinical-imaging-pathologic correlations with emphasis on the importance of ovarian stroma. *Radiology* 196: 805–810, 1995.

133. Rossai J. *Ackerman's Surgical pathology*. Vol.1 8th edition. Mosby, St. Louis, p. 918, 1995.

134. Buetow PC, Buck JL, Ros PR, Goodman ZDLC: Malignant vascular tumors of the liver: Radiologic-pathologic correlation. *Radiographics* 14: 153–166, quiz 167–158, 1994.

135. Woraqattanakul S, Semelka RC, Kelekis NL, Woosley JT: Angiosarcoma of the liver: MR imaging pre- and post-chemotherapy. *Magn Reson Imaging* 15(5): 613–617, 1997.

136. Siegel MJ. MR imaging of pediatric abdominal neoplasms. *Magn Reson Imaging Clin N Am* 8: 837–851, 2000.

137. Buetow PC, Rao P, Marshall H. Imaging of pediatric liver tumors. *MR Clin N Am* 5(2): 397–413, 1997.

138. Arrive L, Hricak H, Goldberg HI, Thoeni RF, Margulis ARLC: MR appearance of the liver after partial hepatectomy. *Am J Roentgenol* 152: 1215–1220, 1989.

139. Bartolozzi C, Lencioni R, Caramella D, Falaschi F, Cioni R, DiCoscio G: Hepatocellular carcinoma: CT and MR features after transcatheter arterial embolization and percutaneous ethanol injection. *Radiology* 191: 123–128, 1994.

140. Bartolozzi C, Lencioni R, Caramella D, Mazzeo S, Ciancia EM: Treatment of hepatocellular carcinoma with percutaneous ethanol injection: Evaluation with contrast–enhanced MR imaging. *Am J Roentgenol* 162: 827–831, 1994.

141. Giovagnoni A, Paci E, Terilli F, Cellerino R, Piga A: Quantitative MR imaging data in the evaluation of hepatic metastases during systemic chemotherapy. *J Magn Reson Imaging* 5: 27–32, 1995.

142. Lee MJ, Mueller PR, Dawson SL, Gazelle SG, Hahn PF, Goldberg MA, Boland GWLC: Percutaneous ethanol injection for the treatment of hepatic tumors: Indications, mechanism of action, technique, and efficacy. *Am J Roentgenol* 164: 215–220, 1995.

143. Nagel HS, Bernardino MELC: Contrast-enhanced MR imaging of hepatic lesions treated with percutaneous ethanol ablation therapy. *Radiology* 189: 265–270, 1993.

144. Sironi S, De Cobelli F, Livraghi T, Villa G, Zanello A, Taccagni G, DelMaschio ALC: Small hepatocellular carcinoma treated with percutaneous ethanol injection: Unenhanced and gadolinium-enhanced MR imaging follow-up. *Radiology* 192: 407–412, 1994.

145. Shirkhoda A, Baird S: Morphologic changes of the liver following chemotherapy for metastatic breast carcinoma: CT findings. *Abdom Imaging* 19: 39–42, 1994.

146. Soyer P, Bluemke DA, Zeitoun G, Marmuse JP, Levesque MLC: Detection of recurrent hepatic metastases after partial hepatectomy: Value of CT combined with arterial portography. *Am J Roentgenol* 162: 1327–1330, 1994.

147. Young ST, Paulson EK, Washington K, Gulliver DJ, Vredenburgh JJ, Baker ME: CT of the liver in patients with metastatic breast carcinoma treated by chemotherapy: Findings simulating cirrhosis. *Am J Roentgenol* 163: 1385–1388, 1994.

148. Harned RK, II, Chezmar JL, Nelson RC: Recurrent tumor after resection of hepatic metastases from colorectal carcinoma: Location and time of discovery as determined by CT. *Am J Roentgenol* 163: 93–97, 1994.

149. Lang EK, Brown CL Jr: Colorectal metastases to the liver: Selective chemoembolization. *Radiology* 189: 417–422, 1993.

150. Scwickert HC, Stiskal M, Roberts TPL, van Dijke CF, Mann J, Muehler A, Shames DM, Demsar F, Disston A, Brasch RC: Contrast–enhanced MR imaging assessment of tumor capillary permeability: Effect of irradiation on delivery of chemotherapy. *Radiology* 198: 893–898, 1996.

151. Matsumoto R, Selig AM, Colucci VM, Jolesz FALC: MR monitoring during cryotherapy in the liver: Predictability of histologic outcome. *J Magn Reson Imaging* 3: 770–776, 1993.

152. Matsumoto R, Oshio K, Jolesz FALC: Monitoring of laser and freezing-induced ablation in the liver with T1-weighted MR imaging. *J Magn Reson Imaging* 2: 555–562, 1992.

153. Vogl TJ, Muller PK, Hammerstingl R, et al.: Malignant liver tumors treated with MR imaging-guided laser-induced thermotherapy: Technique and prospective results. *Radiology* 196: 257–265, 1995.

154. Kuszyk BS, Choti MA, Urban BA, Chambers TP, Bluemke DA, Sitzmann JV, Fishman EKLC: Hepatic tumors treated by cryosurgery: Normal CT appearance. *Am J Roentgenol* 166: 363–368, 1996.

155. McLoughlin RF, Saliken JF, McKinnon G, Wiseman D, Temple W: CT of the liver after cryotherapy of hepatic metastases: Imaging findings. *Am J Roentgenol* 165: 329–332, 1995.

156. Marn CS, Andrews JC, Francis IR, Hollett MD, Walker SC, Ensminger WD: Hepatic parenchymal changes after intraarterial Y–90 therapy: CT findings. *Radiology* 187: 125–128, 1993.

157. Semelka RC, Worawattanakul S, Mauro M, Bernard SA, Cance WG. Malignant hepatic tumors: changes on MRI after hepatic arterial chemoembolization–preliminary findings. *J Magn Reson Imaging* 8(1): 48–56, 1998.

158. Anthony PP, Ishak KG, Nayak NC, at al.: The morphology of cirrhosis. *J Clin Pathol* 31: 395–414, 1978.

159. Gore RM: Diffuse liver disease. In: Gore RM, Levine NS, Laufer I, Eds. *Textbook of Gastrointestinal Radiology*. Philadelphia, PA: Saunders, p. 1968–2017, 1994.

160. Fauerholdt L, Schlichting P, Christensen E, et al.: Conversion of micronodular cirrhosis into macronodular cirrhosis. *Hepatology* 3: 928–931, 1983.

161. Ito K, Mitchell DG, Gabata T, Hussain SM: Expanded gallbladder fossa: simple MR imaging sign of cirrhosis. *Radiology* 211: 723–726, 1999.

162. Semelka RC, Chung JJ, Hussain SM, Marcos HB, Woosley JT: Chronic hepatitis: correlation of early patchy and late linear enhancement patters on gadolinium-enhanced MR images with histopathology—initial experience. *J Magn Reson Imaging* 13: 385–391, 2001.

163. Lehmann B, Fanucci E, Gigli F, Uhlenbrock D, Bartolozzi C: Signal suppression of normal liver tissue by phase corrected inversion recovery: A screening technique. *J Comput Assist Tomogr* 13: 650–655, 1989.

164. Marti-Bonmati L, Talens A, del Olmo J, de Val A, Serra MA, Rodrigo JM, Ferrandez A, Torres V, Rayon M, Vilar JS: Chronic hepatitis and cirrhosis: Evaluation by means of MR imaging with histologic correlation. *Radiology* 188: 37–43, 1993.

165. Baron RL, Campbell WL, Dodd GD: Peribiliary cysts associated with severe liver disease: Imaging-pathologic correlation. *Am J Roentgenol* 162: 631–636, 1994.

166. Itai Y, Ebihara R, Tohno E, Tsunoda HS, Kurosaki Y, Saida Y, Doy M: Hepatic peribiliary cysts: Multiple tiny cysts within the larger portal tract, hepatic hilum, or both. *Radiology* 191: 107–110, 1994.

167. Terayama N, Matsui O, Hoshiba K, Kadoya M, Yoshikawa J, Gabata T, Takashima T, Terada T, Nakanuma Y, Shinozaki K, et al.: Peribiliary cysts in liver cirrhosis: US, CT, and MR findings. *J Comput Assist Tomogr* 19: 419–423, 1995.

168. Ohtomo K, Itai Y, Ohtomo Y, Shiga J, Iio M: Regenerating nodules of liver cirrhosis: MR imaging with pathologic correlation. *Am J Roentgenol* 154: 505–507, 1990.

169. Terada T, Nakanuma Y: Survey of iron-accumulative macroregenerative nodules in cirrhotic livers. *Hepatology* 10: 851–854, 1989.

170. Mitchell DG, Lovett KE, Hann HW, Ehrlich S, Palazzo J, Rubin R: Cirrhosis: Multiobserver analysis of hepatic MR imaging findings in a heterogeneous population. *J Magn Reson Imaging* 3: 313–321, 1993.

171. Hytiroglou P, Theise NH. Differential diagnosis of hepatocellular nodular lesions. *Semin Diag Pathol* 15: 285–299, 1998.

172. Groszmann RJ, Atterbury CE: The pathophysiology of portal hypertension: A basis for classification. *Semin Liver Dis* 2: 177–186, 1982.

173. Chopra S, Dodd GD, Chintapalli KN, Esola CC, Ghiatas AA: Mesenteric, omental, and retroperitoneal edema in cirrhosis: frequency and spectrum of CT findings. *Radiology* 211: 737–742, 1999.

174. Starzl TE, Francavilla A, Halgrimson CG, Francavilla FR, Porter KA, Brown TH, Putnam CW: The origin, hormonal nature, and action of hepatotrophic substances in portal venous blood. *Surg Gynecol Obstet* 137: 179–199, 1973.

175. Finn JP, Edelman RR, Jenkins RL, Lewis WD, Longmaid HE, Kane RA, Stokes KR, Mattle HP, Clouse ME: Liver transplantation: MR angiography with surgical validation. *Radiology* 179: 265–269, 1991.

176. Brandhagen DJ, Fairbanks VF, Batts KP, Thebodeau SN. Update on hereditary hemochromatosis and the HFE gene. *Mayo Clin Proc* 74: 917–9121, 1999.

177. McLaren G, Muir W, Kellermeyer R: Iron overload disorders: Natural history, pathogenesis, diagnosis and therapy. *Crit Rev Clin Lab Sci* 19: 205–226, 1984.

178. Siegelman ES, Mitchell DG, Semelka RC: Abdominal iron deposition: Metabolism, MR findings, and clinical importance. *Radiology* 199: 13–22, 1996.

179. Siegelman ES, Mitchell DG, Rubin R, Hann HW, Kaplan KR, Steiner RM, Rao VM, Schuster SJ, Burk DL Jr, Rifkin MD: Parenchymal versus reticuloendothelial iron overload in the liver: Distinction with MR imaging. *Radiology* 179: 361–366, 1991.

180. Terada T, Kadoya M, Nakanuma Y, Matsui O: Iron-accumulating adenomatous hyperplastic nodule with malignant foci in the cirrhotic liver. Histopathologic, quantitative iron, and magnetic resonance imaging in vitro studies. *Cancer* 65: 1994–2000, 1990.

181. Terada T, Nakanuma Y: Iron-negative foci in siderotic macroregenerative nodules in human cirrhotic liver. A marker of incipient neoplastic lesions. *Arch Pathol Lab Med* 113: 916–920, 1989.

182. Siegelman ES, Outwater E, Hanau CA, Ballas SK, Steiner RM, Rao VM, Mitchell DG: Abdominal iron distribution in sickle cell disease: MR findings in transfusion and nontransfusion dependent patients. *J Comput Assist Tomogr* 18: 63–67, 1994.

183. Yates CK, Streight RA: Focal fatty infiltration of the liver simulating metastatic disease. *Radiology* 159: 83–84, 1986.

184. Mitchell DG: Focal manifestations of diffuse liver disease at MR imaging. *Radiology* 185: 1–11, 1992.

185. Mitchell DG, Kim I, Chang TS, Vinitski S, Consigny PM, Saponaro SA, Ehrlich SM, Rifkin MD, Rubin R: Fatty liver. Chemical shift phase-difference and suppression magnetic resonance imaging techniques in animals, phantoms, and humans. *Invest Radiol* 26: 1041–1052, 1991.

186. Mitchell DG, Palazzo J, Hann HW, Rifkin MD, Burk DL Jr, Rubin R: Hepatocellular tumors with high signal on T1-weighted MR images: Chemical shift MR imaging and histologic correlation. *J Comput Assist Tomogr* 15: 762–769, 1991.

187. Parfrey NA, Hutchins GN. Hepatic fibrosis in the mucopolysaccharises. The *Am J Med* 81: 825–829, 1986.

188. *Nelson Textbook of Pediatrics*, 14th edition. Philadelphia: Saunders, p. 372–377, 1992.

189. Sharlock S, Dooley J: *Diseases of the Liver and Biliary System* 10th edition. Blackwell Science, p. 1086, 1997.

190. Guttmacher AE, Marchuk DA, White RI: Hereditary hemorrhagic telangiectasia. *N Engl J Med* 333: 918–924, 1995.

191. Cotran RS, Cumar V, Robbins SL: *Pathologic Basis of Disease*. 5th edition. Philadelphia: Saunders, p. 872, 1994.

192. Itai Y, Ohtomo K, Kokubo T, Okada Y, Yamauchi T, Yoshida H: Segmental intensity differences in the liver on MR images: A sign of intrahepatic portal flow stoppage. *Radiology* 167: 17–19, 1988.

193. Lorigan JG, Charnsangavej C, Carrasco CH, Richli WR, Wallace S: Atrophy with compensatory hypertrophy of the liver in hepatic neoplasms: Radiographic findings. *Am J Roentgenol* 150: 1291–1295, 1988.

194. Carr DH, Hadjis NS, Banks LM, Hemingway AP, Blumgart LH: Computed tomography of hilar cholangiocarcinoma: A new sign. *Am J Roentgenol* 145: 53–56, 1985.

195. Itai Y, Murata S, Kurosaki Y: Straight border sign of the liver: Spectrum of CT appearances and causes. *Radiographics* 15: 1089–1102, 1995.

196. Schlund JF, Semelka RC, Kettritz U, Eisenberg LB, Lee JKT: Transient increased segmental hepatic enhancement distal to portal vein obstruction on dynamic gadolinium-enhanced gradient echo MR images. *J Magn Reson Imaging* 5: 375–377, 1995.

197. De Gaetano AM, Lafortune M, Patriquin H, De Franco A, Aubin B, Raradis K: Cavernous transformation of the portal vein: Patterns of intrahepatic and splachnic collateral circulation detected with Doppler sonography. *Am J Roentgenol* 165: 1151–1156, 1995.

198. Nakao N, Miura K, Takahashi H, Miura T, Ashida H, Ishikawa Y, Utsunomiya J: Hepatic perfusion in cavernous transformation of the portal vein: Evaluation by using CT angiography. *Am J Roentgenol* 152: 985–986, 1989.

199. Schlund JF, Semelka RC, Kettritz U, Weeks SM, Kahlenberg M, Cance WG: Correlation of perfusion abnormalities on CTAP and immediate postintravenous gadolinium-enhanced gradient echo MRI. *Abdom Imaging* 21: 49–52, 1996.

200. Shearman DJC, Finlayson NDC, Camilleri M: *Diseases of the Gastrointestinal Tract and Liver*. 3nd edition. New York: Churchill Livingstone, p. 1079, 1997.

201. Miller WJ, Federle MP, Straub WH, Davis PL: Budd-Chiari syndrome: Imaging with pathologic correlation. *Abdom Imaging* 18: 329–335, 1993.

202. Mathieu D, Vasile N, Menu Y, Van Beers B, Lorphelin JM, Pringot J: Budd-Chiari syndrome: Dynamic CT. *Radiology* 165: 409–413, 1987.

203. Murata S, Itai Y, Hisashi K, Nakajima K, et al.: Effect of temporary occlusion of the hepatic vein on dual blood supply in the liver: Evaluation with spiral CT. *Radiology* 195: 351–356, 1995.

204. Pollard JJ, Nebesar RA: Altered hemodynamics in the Budd-Chiari syndrome demonstrated by selective hepatic and selective splenic angiography. *Radiology* 89: 236–243, 1967.

205. Noone TC, Semelka RC, Siegelman ES, Balci NC, Hussain SM, et al.: Budd-Chiari syndrome: Spectrum of appearances of acute, subacute, and chronic disease with magnetic resonance imaging. *J Magn Reson Imaging* 11: 44–50, 2000.

206. Noone T, Semelka RC, Woosley JT, Pisano ED: Ultrasound and MR findings in acute Budd-Chiari syndrome with histopathologic correlation. *J Comput Assist Tomogr* 20: 819–822, 1996.

207. Castellano G, Canga F, Solis-Herruzo JA, Colina F, Martinez-Montiel MP, Morillas JD: Budd-Chiari syndrome associated with nodular regenerative hyperplasia of the liver. *J Clin Gastroenterol* 11: 698–702, 1989.

208. De Sousa JM, Portmann B, Williams R: Nodular regenerative hyperplasia of the liver and the Budd-Chiari syndrome. Case report, review of the literature and reappraisal of pathogenesis. *J Hepatol* 12: 28–35, 1991.

209. Soyer P, Lacheheb D, Caudron C, Levesque M: MRI of adenomatous hyperplastic nodules of the liver in Budd-Chiari syndrome. *J Comput Assist Tomogr* 17: 86–89, 1993.

210. Nakashima T, Okuda K, Kojiro M, et al.: Pathology of hepatocellular carcinoma in Japan. 232 consecutive cases autopsied in 10 years. *Cancer* 51: 863–877, 1983.

211. Rooholamini SA, Au AH, Hansen GC, Kioumehr F, Dadsetan MR, Chow PP, Kurzel RB, Mikhail G: Imaging of pregnancy-related complications. *Radiographics* 13: 753–770, 1993.

212. Brown JJ, Borrello JA, Raza HS, Balfe DM, Baer AB, Pilgram TK, Atilla S: Dynamic contrast-enhanced MR imaging of the liver: Parenchymal enhancement patterns. *Magn Reson Imaging* 13: 1–8, 1995.

213. Matsui O, Kadoya M, Takashima T, Kameyama T, Yoshikawa J, Tamura S: Intrahepatic periportal abnormal intensity on MR images: An indication of various hepatobiliary diseases. *Radiology* 171: 335–338, 1989.

214. Itai Y, Ohtomo K, Kokubo T, Minami M, Yoshida H: CT and MR imaging of postnecrotic liver scars. *J Comput Assist Tomogr* 12: 971–975, 1988.

215. Stark DD, Goldberg HI, Moss AA, Bass NM: Chronic liver disease: Evaluation by magnetic resonance. *Radiology* 150: 149–151, 1984.

216. Unger EC, Lee JK, Weyman PJ: CT and MR imaging of radiation hepatitis. *J Comput Assist Tomogr* 11: 264–268, 1987.

217. Yankelevitz DF, Knapp PH, Henschke CI, Nisce L, Yi Y, Cahill P: MR appearance of radiation hepatitis. *Clin Imaging* 16: 89–92, 1992.

218. Cutillo DP, Swayne LC, Cucco J, Dougan H: CT and MR imaging in cystic abdominal lymphangiomatosis. *J Comput Assist Tomogr* 13: 534–536, 1989.

219. Garra BS, Shawker TH, Chang R, Kaplan K, White RD: The ultrasound appearance of radiation-induced hepatic injury. Correlation with computed tomography and magnetic resonance imaging. *J Ultrasound Med* 7: 605–609, 1988.

220. MacSween RNM, Burt AD. Chapter 17. Liver pathology associated with diseases of other organs. In: MacSween RNM, Anthony PP, Scheuer PJ, Burt AD, Portmann BC, eds.: *Pathology of the Liver.* 3nd edition. New York: Churchill Livingstone, p. 713–764, 1994.

221. Gitlin N: *The Liver and Systemic disease.* New York: Churchill Livingstone, p. 30. 1997.

222. Kessler A, Mitchell DG, Israel HL, Goldberg BB: Hepatic and splenic sarcoidosis: Ultrasound and MR imaging. *Abdom Imaging* 18: 159–163, 1993.

223. Warshauer DM, Semelka RC, Ascher SM: Nodular sarcoidosis of the liver and spleen: Appearance on MR images. *J Magn Reson Imaging* 4: 553–557, 1994.

224. Shek TW, Ng IO, Chan KW: Inflammatory pseudotumor of the liver. Report of four cases and review of the literature. *Am J Surg Pathol* 17: 231–238, 1993.

225. Horiuchi R, Uchida T, Kojima T, Shikata T: Inflammatory pseudotumor of the liver. Clinicopathologic study and review of the literature. *Cancer* 65: 1583–1590, 1990.

226. Kelekis NL, Warshauer DM, Semelka RC, Eisenberg LB, Woosley JT: Inflammatory pseudotumor of the liver: Appearance on contrast enhanced helical CT and dynamic MR images. *J Magn Reson Imaging* 5: 551–553, 1995.

227. Oto A, Akhan O, Ozmen M. Focal inflammatory diseases of the liver. *Eur J Radiol* 32: 61–75, 1999.

228. Bertel CK, van Heerden JA, Sheedy PF: Treatment of pyogenic hepatic abscesses. Surgical vs. percutaneous drainage. *Arch Surg* 121: 554–558, 1986.

229. Mendez RJ, Schiebler ML, Outwater EK, Kressel HY: Hepatic abscesses: MR imaging findings. *Radiology* 190: 431–436, 1994.

230. Balci NC, Semelka RC, Noone TC, Siegelman ES, Beeck BO, Brown JJ, Lee MG: Pyogenic hepatic abscesses: MRI findings on T1– and T2-weighted and serial gadolinium-enhanced gradient-echo images. *J Magn Reson Imaging* 9: 285–290, 1999.

231. Ralls PW, Henley DS, Colletti PM, Benson R, Raval JK, Radin DR, Boswell WD, Jr., Halls JM: Amebic liver abscess: MR imaging. *Radiology* 165: 801–804, 1987.

232. Landay MJ, Setiawan H, Hirsch G, Christensen EE, Conrad MR: Hepatic and thoracic amaebiasis. *Am J Roentgenol* 135: 449–454, 1980.

233. Balci NC, Tunaci A, Semelka RC, Tunaci M, Özden I, Rezanu, I. B., Hepatic alveolar echinococcosis: MRI findings. *Magn Reson Imaging* 18: 537–541, 2000.

234. Lebovics E, Thung SN, Schaffner F: The liver in the acquired immunodeficiency syndrome: a clinical and histologic study. *Hepatology* 5: 293–298, 1995

235. Schneiderman DJ, Arenson DM, Cello JP: Hepatic disease in patients with acquired immune deficiency syndrome (AIDS). *Hepatology* 7: 925–930, 1987.

236. Pantongrag-Brown L, Krebs TL, Daly BD, et al.: Frequency of abdominal CT findings in AIDS patients with *M. Avium* complex bacteraemia. *Clin Radiol* 53: 816–819, 1998.

237. Shirkhoda A, Lopez-Berestein G, Holbert JM, Luna MA: Hepatosplenic fungal infection: CT and pathologic evaluation after treatment with liposomal amphotericin B. *Radiology* 159: 349–353, 1986.

238. Lewis JH, Patel HR, Zimmerman HJ: The spectrum of hepatic candidiasis. *Hepatology* 2: 479–487, 1982.

239. Sallah S, Semelka RC, Kelekis N, Worawattanakul S, Sallah W. Diagnosis and monitoring response of treatment of hepatosplenic candidiasis in patients with acute leukemia using magnetic resonance imaging. *Acta Haematol* 100: 77–81, 1998.

240. Semelka RC, Kelekis NL, Sallah S, Worawattanakul S, Ascher SM. Hepatosplenic fungal disease: diagnostic accuracy and spectrum of appearance on MR imaging. *Am J Roentgenol* 169(5): 1311–6, 1997.

241. Cho JS, Kim EE, Varma DG, Wallace S: MR imaging of hepatosplenic candidiasis superimposed on hemochromatosis. *J Comput Assist Tomogr* 14: 774–776, 1990.

242. Lamminen AE, Anttila VJ, Bondestam S, Ruutu T, Ruutu PJ: Infectious liver foci in leukemia: Comparison of short-inversion-time inversion-recovery, T1-weighted spin-echo, and dynamic gadolinium-enhanced MR imaging. *Radiology* 191: 539–543, 1994.

243. Semelka RC, Shoenut JP, Greenberg HM, Bow EJ: Detection of acute and treated lesions of hepatosplenic candidiasis: Comparison of dynamic contrast-enhanced CT and MR imaging. *J Magn Reson Imaging* 2: 341–345, 1992.

244. Kelekis NL, Semelka RC, Jeon HJ, Sallah AS, Shea TC, Woosley JT: Dark ring sign: Finding in patients with fungal liver lesions and transfusional hemosiderosis undergoing treatment with antifungal antibiotics. *Magn Reson Imaging* 14: 615–618, 1996.

245. Balci NC, Semelka RC, Noone TC, Ascher SM: Acute and subacute liver-related hemorrhage: MRI findings. *Magn Reson Imaging* 17(2): 207–211, 1999.

246. Hasegawa S, Eisenberg LB, Semelka RC: Active intrahepatic gadolinium extravasation following TIPS. *Magn Reson Imaging.* 16: 851–855, 1998.

247. Center for disease control, National Center of Health Statistics (NCHS): *Vital Statistics System*, 1998.

248. Bassignani M, Fulcher AS, Szucs RA, Chong WK, Prasad UR, Marcos A: Use of imaging for living donor liver transplantation. *Radiographics* 21: 39–52, 2001.

249. Nghiem HV, Winter TC III, Mountford MC, Mack LA, Yuan C, Coldwell DM, Althaus SJ, Carithers RL Jr, McVicar JP, Freeny PC: Evaluation of the portal venous system before liver transplantation: Value of phase-contrast MR angiography. *Am J Roentgenol* 164: 871–878, 1995.

250. Weisner R, Demetris A, Belle S, et al.: Acute hepatic allograft rejection: incidence risk factor and impact on outcome. *Hepatology* 28: 638–645, 1998.

251. Demetris AJ, Lasky S, Van Thiel DH, Starzl TE, Dekker A: Pathology of hepatic transplantation: A review of 62 adult allograft recipients immunosuppressed with a cyclosporine/steroid regimen. *Am J Pathol* 118: 151–161, 1985.

252. Wozney P, Zajko AB, Bron KM, Point S, Starzl TE: Vascular complications after liver transplantation: A 5-year experience. *Am J Roentgenol* 147: 657–663, 1986.

253. Glockner JF, Forauer AR, Solomon H, Varma CR, Perman WH: Three-dimensional gadolinium-enhanced MR angiography of vascular complications after liver transplantation. *Am J Roentgenol* 174: 1447–1452, 2000.

254. Dalen K, Day DL, Ascher NL, Hunter DW, Thompson WM, Castaneda-Zuniga WR, Letourneau JG: Imaging of vascular complications after hepatic transplantation. *Am J Roentgenol* 150: 1285–1290, 1988.

255. Ito K, Siegelman ES, Stolpen AH, Mitchell DG: MR imaging of complications after liver transplantation. *Am J Roentgenol* 175: 1145–1149, 2000.

256. Zajko AB, Bennett MJ, Campbell WL, Koneru B: Mucocele of the cystic duct remnant in eight liver transplant recipients: Findings at cholangiography, CT, and US. *Radiology* 177: 691–693, 1990.

257. Lang P, Schnarkowski P, Grampp S, van Dijke C, Gindele A, Steffen R, Neuhaus P, Felix R: Liver transplantation: Significance of the periportal collar on MRI. *J Comput Assist Tomogr* 19: 580–585, 1995.

258. Marincek B, Barbier PA, Becker CD, Mettler D, Ruchti C: CT appearance of impaired lymphatic drainage in liver transplants. *Am J Roentgenol* 147: 519–523, 1986.

259. Pickhardt PJ, Siegel MJ: Posttransplantation lymphoproliferative disorders of the abdomen: CT evaluation in 51 patients. *Radiology* 213: 73–78, 1999.

260. Dupuy D, Costello P: Cross-sectional imaging of liver transplantation. *Semin Ultrasound CT MR* 13: 399–409, 1992.

GALLBLADDER AND BILIARY SYSTEM

TILL R. BADER, M.D., RICHARD C. SEMELKA, M.D.,
AND CAROLINE REINHOLD, M.D.

INTRODUCTION

Significant technical improvements of MRI hardware and software during recent years have led to the development of new and faster imaging sequences that are capable of demonstrating soft tissue well and visualizing the biliary and pancreatic ductal systems with excellent image quality, sharpness, and resolution previously only known from endoscopic retrograde cholangiopancreatography (ERCP). In several studies, these MR techniques, termed magnetic resonance cholangiopancreatography (MRCP), have been shown to be comparable with ERCP in the diagnosis of choledocholithiasis, malignant obstruction of the biliary and pancreatic ducts, congenital anomalies, and chronic pancreatitis [1–7]. The advantages of MRCP over other imaging techniques include a) the examination is noninvasive and requires no anesthesia; b) the examination is not operator dependent, and high-quality images can be obtained consistently; c) no administration of intraductal or intravenous contrast agent is necessary; d) no ionizing radiation is employed; e) visualization of ducts proximal to an obstruction is superior to that achieved by ERCP; f) MRCP can be successfully performed in the presence of biliary-enteric anastomoses (e.g., hepaticojejunostomy, choledochojejunostomy, Billroth II anastomosis); g) combina-tion with conventional MR sequences is possible and helpful for the evaluation of duct wall and extraductal disease. A significant advantage of ERCP is that it allows therapeutic interventions at the time of initial diagnosis. Although generally considered a safe procedure, ERCP is associated with morbidity and mortality rates of 8% and 1%, respectively [8]. In addition, unsuccessful cannulation of the common bile duct (CBD) or pancreatic duct occurs in 3–10% of cases [9, 10]. Therefore, in some institutions MRCP is gradually becoming the primary imaging modality for a number of diagnostic purposes for the biliary system, with ERCP reserved for therapeutic interventions (e.g., sphincterotomy, stone removal, dilatation of strictures, stent placement) [1]. Ultrasound, because of its lesser costs, remains the modality of choice for the evaluation of cholecystolithiasis, which accounts for 90% of gallbladder diseases.

NORMAL ANATOMY

The intrahepatic bile ducts are a component of the intrahepatic portal triad. They follow the course of portal venous branches along their ventral aspect. Subsegmental branches join to form segmental branches that join to form the right and left hepatic biliary ducts, which join to form the common hepatic duct (CHD). The confluence of both hepatic ducts is usually at the level of the porta hepatis, but it can be substantially lower. The gallbladder is situated in the gallbladder fossa, located between the right and left lobe of the liver, between Couinauld segments four and five. Anatomically, the gallbladder is composed of the fundus, body, and neck. The gallbladder is usually oval in shape, measuring approximately 7–10 cm in length and 2–3.5 cm in width, which can vary substantially depending on the dietary status. The wall thickness of a normal, well-filled gallbladder does not exceed 3 mm. The gallbladder is connected to the CHD via the cystic duct, which has a mucosal endoluminal fold (called the spiral fold or valve). The confluence of the cystic duct and the CHD is typically located superior to the head of the pancreas to form the CBD. The CBD enters the head of the pancreas and usually joins with the main pancreatic duct (Wirsung) just before it enters the duodenum through the sphincter of Oddi in the major papilla (papilla of Vater).

MRI TECHNIQUE

T2-weighted Sequences/MRCP

Magnetic resonance cholangiopancreatography (MRCP) is based on the acquisition of heavily T2-weighted images to provide visualization of stationary or slow-moving fluids (e.g., bile) with high signal intensity. Because of the heavy T2 weighting of these sequences, the signal from the pancreatico-biliary system appears hyperintense, whereas the signal from background tissue (e.g., hepatic and pancreatic tissue, peritoneal fat, fast-flowing blood) is either very low or signal void, resulting in excellent contrast and depiction of the pancreatico-biliary system. The use of phased-array surface coil imaging, small field of view, and fat suppression techniques has resulted in higher signal-to-noise and contrast-to-noise ratios, allowed the acquisition of thinner sections, measurement of T2- rather than T2* decay, decreased susceptibility artifacts, and diminished sensitivity to motion artifacts and slow flow [11–14].

Current MRCP techniques are based on echo-train spin-echo techniques that allow two-dimensional (2D) and three-dimensional (3D) approaches. Multiple 180° pulses with successive echoes (echo train) are acquired with a separate phase-encoding gradient applied before each echo. Each of these detected echoes represents a different line within k-space. Ultrafast single-shot echo-train spin-echo techniques are capable of acquiring images in less than 1 s [15, 16]. After a single 90° excitation pulse, an extremely long echo train of 100–150 refocusing 180° pulses is applied as a single-shot technique. After acquiring slightly more than half of k-space after the

single 90° pulse, the remainder of k-space is filled by extrapolation, because of the intrinsic symmetry of k-space (half-Fourier technique). The extremely long echo train leads to diminution of echo signal intensity as the echo train progresses and, consequently, to decreased signal-to-noise and contrast-to-noise ratios. However, this effect is counteracted by the ultrashort acquisition time (<1 s) that "freezes" any physiological motion and avoids misregistration and by the very low signal intensity from background tissue, which is an effect of the very long TE (600–1000). Overall, this leads to a reduction of noise and increase of contrast. The half-Fourier single-shot echo-train spin-echo sequences that are currently most widely used are half-Fourier RARE (rapid acquisition with relaxation enhancement) and HASTE (half-Fourier acquisition single-shot turbo spin echo) [17–19]. Acquiring images with a very long TE renders very little signal from tissue with short TE such as fat and parenchymal organs, which makes the application of fat suppression techniques unnecessary. Fluids with relatively short TE, such as concentrated bile or mucinous fluid, however, will also give very little signal, which may hinder the depiction of small biliary ducts or mucinous lesions. An intermediate TE (80–100 ms) results in images where all fluid, including concentrated bile and mucinous fluid, is bright and even small ducts are well depicted. The use of fat suppression to diminish the signal from surrounding tissue is advisable and makes maximum intensity projection (MIP) postprocessing possible (fig. 3.1).

Single-shot echo-train spin-echo sequences, such as HASTE and RARE techniques, can be applied as breath-hold or breathing-independent sequences. The breathing-independent approach is the fastest technique and is especially useful in patients who are uncooperative or cannot hold their breath (e.g., infant, very sick, and old patients). A thick-collimation single section of up to 3-cm thickness is acquired in a right anterior oblique coronal plane, obtained in less than 2 s (fig. 3.2). Several slabs can be acquired in various rotations to view the ducts from different angles. The images resemble conventional ERCP images and are particularly useful to provide an overview of the pancreatico-biliary system and to visualize nondilated ducts. However, this technique is not appropriate to investigate intraductal pathologies because visualization of small intraductal signal void structures (e.g., calculi) is masked by partial volume averaging with intraductal high signal from fluid (e.g., bile). Therefore, the additional acquisition of thin-collimation multisection images performed as breath-hold technique in a right anterior oblique plane provides a cholangiographic display capturing the bifurcation of the CHD into right and left hepatic ducts (fig. 3.3). An additional acquisition in the axial plane provides a useful evaluation of the distal CBD and the pancreatic duct. Alternatively, thick slab images in the coronal and axial planes can

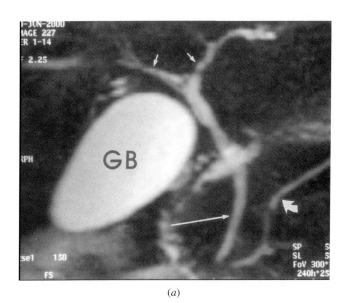

(a)

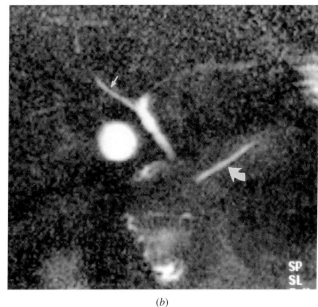

(b)

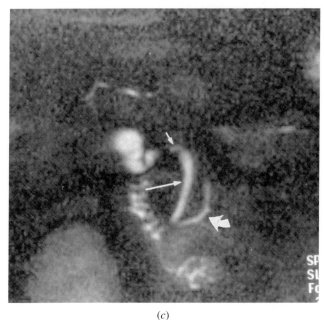

(c)

F I G . 3.1 Normal biliary system, MRCP. 3D maximum intensity projection (MIP) reconstruction image (*a*) of a series of T2-weighted fat-suppressed thin-section single-shot echo-train spin-echo images (*b*, *c*). The 3D MIP reconstruction image (*a*) gives an overview of the intra- and extrahepatic biliary tree and the pancreatic duct. Fluid in the duodenum partly overlays the midportion of the CBD (*a*). Thin-section source images (*b*, *c*) allow exact evaluation of the lumen and walls of the bile ducts without overlay. The right and left main hepatic ducts (short arrows, *a*, *b*), the CHD, the CBD (long arrow, *a*, *c*), the entry of the cystic duct (short arrow, *c*), the pancreatic duct (curved arrows, *a–c*), and the gallbladder (GB) are clearly depicted as high-signal structures.

be used as localizers to focus the acquisition of thin-collimation images on the middle and distal CBD in the coronal plane. Thin-collimation images can be obtained as multiple single-section acquisitions with no gap in an interleaved fashion to avoid cross talk. Slice thickness of 3–4 mm provides sufficient signal to obtain good-quality images and is sufficiently thin to detect small calculi (figs. 3.1 and 3.3). Three-dimensional reconstruction can be performed using a maximum-intensity projection (MIP) algorithm on the thin-collimation source images that generates images that closely resemble conventional cholangiograms (figs. 3.1–3.3). However, volume-averaging effects degrade spatial and contrast resolution, which makes it necessary to use the source images for

the evaluation of pathology, in particular for the detection of small stones and subtle mural irregularity.

T1-weighted Sequences

T1-weighted sequences are useful for the evaluation of duct walls and parenchymal lesions. These can be acquired as SGE sequences, obtained before and after gadolinium administration. Fat suppression techniques are essential as they improve the delineation of enhancing duct walls, inflammatory tissue, small lymph nodes, and tumor infiltration from surrounding fatty tissue [20]. The use of breath-hold SGE sequences after gadolinium administration also provides information on the blood

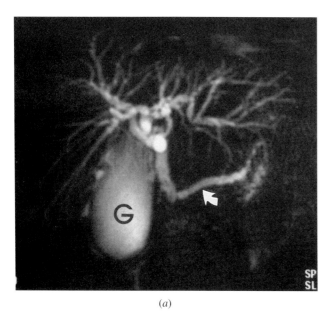

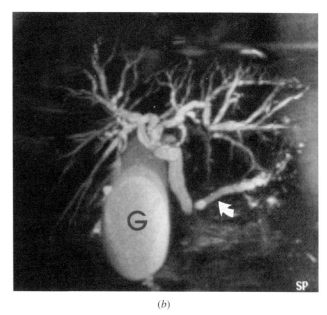

(a)

(b)

F I G . 3.2 Thick-section MRCP versus 3D MIP reconstruction image. T2-weighted fat-suppressed thick-section MRCP single-shot echo-train spin-echo (a) and 3D MIP reconstruction image (b) from a series of thin-section single-shot echo-train spin-echo images. A pancreatic head carcinoma obstructs the preampullary CBD and pancreatic duct. The entire biliary tree and the pancreatic duct (curved arrow, a, b) are dilated. Note the finer resolution and detail of the 3D MIP image (b). G = gallbladder.

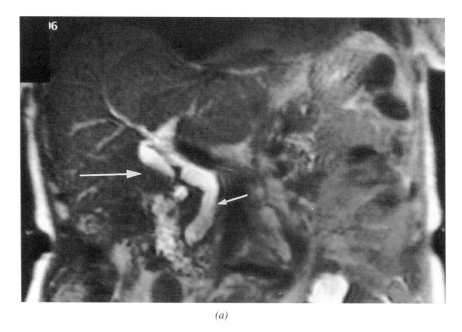

(a)

F I G . 3.3 Thin-section MRCP versus 3D MIP reconstruction image. MRCP 3D MIP reconstruction (a) and coronal T2-weighted fat-suppressed thin-section single-shot echo-train spin-echo (b) images. On the MIP image (a), severe dilation of the CBD (short arrow, a) is shown, but no CBD calculus is visualized. Multiple signal-void calculi are demonstrated in the gallbladder (long arrow, a). The coronal thin-section image (b) reveals a 5-mm preampullary CBD stone (arrow, b).

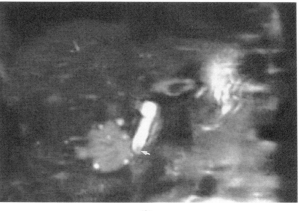

(b)

322

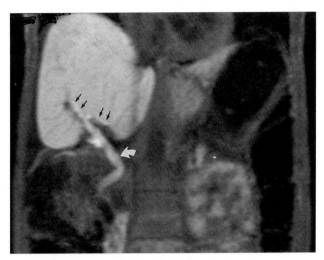

FIG. 3.4 Manganese(Mn)-DPDP-enhanced normal biliary tree. T1-weighted coronal Mn-DPDP-enhanced SGE image with fat suppression. The normal intrahepatic (small arrows) and extrahepatic (curved arrow) bile ducts demonstrate high signal intensity due to the T1 shortening of Mn-DPDP, which is excreted in the bile. Note also the enhancement of normal liver parenchyma.

supply and interstitial space of diseased tissue that facilitates characterization.

In addition to standard nonspecific extracellular gadolinium chelates, T1-shortening intravenous contrast agents that are partly eliminated in bile have been used for the evaluation of the biliary system; these include manganese(Mn)-DPDP and gadolinium(Gd)-EOB-DTPA [21, 22]. Owing to their lipophilic character, these contrast agents are taken up by hepatocytes and secreted into the biliary ductal system. On T1-weighted images, this leads to bright signal of contrasted bile in biliary ducts and gallbladder (fig. 3.4). Bright bile images can be generated using 2D or 3D T1-weighted gradient-echo techniques. However, in the presence of high-grade biliary obstruction, the bile ducts distal to the obstruction may remain noncontrasted, and in patients with diminished hepatocyte function, the biliary system may be poorly opacified. Clinical rules for evaluating the biliary system with biliary excretion contrast agents have yet to be established.

NORMAL APPEARANCE AND VARIANTS

Gallbladder

On T2-weighted sequences, the walls of the gallbladder and bile ducts are of low signal intensity, and normal bile shows high signal intensity (fig. 3.5). On T1-weighted images, the wall of the gallbladder is of in-

termediate signal intensity, comparable to adjacent soft tissue such as liver. Bile within the gallbladder may vary from very low to high signal intensity on T1-weighted images because of variations in the concentration of water, cholesterol, and bile salts (fig. 3.5) [23]. Nonconcentrated bile accumulates in the gallbladder and demonstrates low signal intensity on T1-weighted sequences, similar to water. With reabsorption of water and increased cholesterol and bile salt concentration, the T1 relaxation time decreases and the signal from concentrated bile becomes increasingly high with increased concentration (fig. 3.6) [23]. In the presence of concentrated bile (e.g., in prolonged fasting state), a layering effect is often appreciated with the concentrated hyperintense bile in the dependent portion of the gallbladder fundus (fig. 3.7). After i.v. gadolinium administration, the normal gallbladder wall enhances homogeneously comparable to the enhancement of adjacent liver parenchyma (fig. 3.5). Variations of the gallbladder include phrygian cap configuration, ectopic location (i.e., intrahepatic, retrohepatic, or beneath the left lobe), and septations. Septations are best visualized on single-shot T2-weighted sequences, in which they appear low signal in a background of high-signal fluid.

Bile Ducts

With MRCP sequences, the intrahepatic ducts can be visualized as an arborizing system of high signal intensity that can be followed into the outer third of the liver in over 90% of patients (fig. 3.1) [24]. The clinically most important variants are aberrant intrahepatic ducts that may join the common hepatic duct (CHD), common bile duct (CBD), cystic duct, or the gallbladder, or an anomalous right hepatic duct that joins the CBD, all of which place the patient at increased risk for bile duct injury at endoscopic cholecystectomy [25]. The role of MRCP in the preoperative evaluation of the biliary tree is still in evolution [5, 26].

The extrahepatic ducts (CHD, cystic duct, CBD) are consistently well evaluated (fig. 3.8). Occasionally, surgical clips, metallic stents, or pneumobilia may render segments of the ducts signal void. The cystic duct can be visualized in its full extent including its insertion into the CBD (fig. 3.1). A number of variations of its insertion are of clinical significance for laparoscopic cholecystectomy because they also have been shown to increase the risk of bile duct injury. Such variants include a low or medial duct insertion, insertion into the right hepatic duct, a long parallel course of the cystic and common hepatic ducts, and a short cystic duct [5, 27].

The CBD empties into the duodenum through the major papilla. This is a small mucosal protrusion into the duodenum resulting from the muscles that surround the distal CBD and ventral pancreatic duct. Its signal

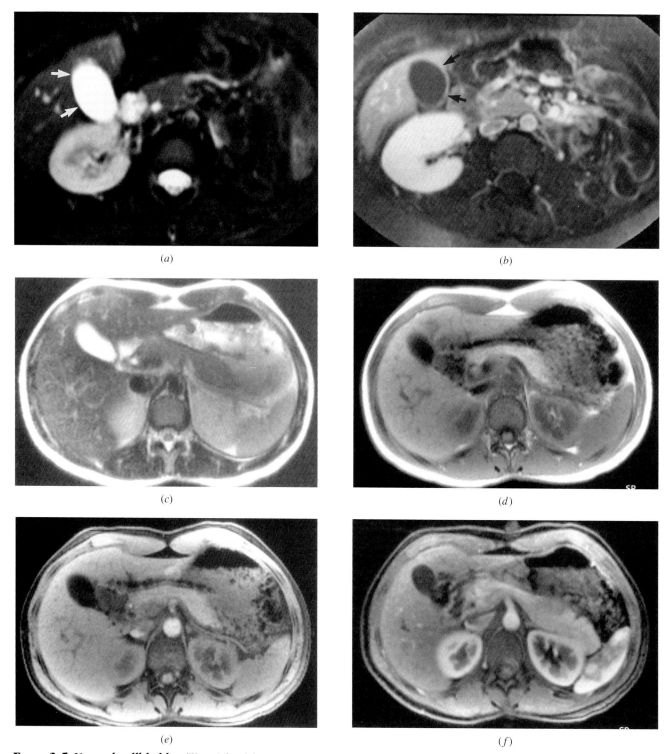

(a)

(b)

(c)

(d)

(e)

(f)

F I G . 3.5 Normal gallbladder. T2-weighted fat-suppressed spin-echo (*a*) and gadolinium-enhanced T1-weighted fat-suppressed spin-echo (*b*) images. On the T2-weighted image (*a*), the gallbladder content is high signal intensity and the gallbladder wall (arrows) is not well visualized. On the gadolinium-enhanced T1-weighted fat-suppressed spin-echo image (*b*), the gallbladder wall (arrows) is well shown as a thin enhancing structure. The gallbladder wall adjacent to the liver is not clearly defined because the enhancement of gallbladder wall and liver are similar.

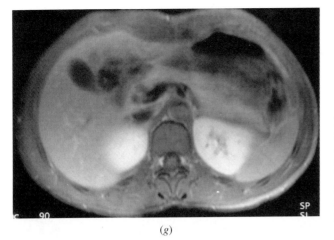

(g)

FIG. 3.5 (*Continued*) T2-weighted spin-echo (*c*), T1-weighted SGE (*d*), fat-suppressed SGE (*e*), immediate postgadolinium fat-suppressed SGE (*f*), and 2-min postgadolinium fat-suppressed spin-echo (*g*) images in a second patient with normal gallbladder. The bile is high in signal on the T2-weighted image (*c*) and low in signal on the T1-weighted images (*d–g*). The normal gallbladder wall is barely perceptible as a thin line, best shown on the immediate postgadolinium image (*f*).

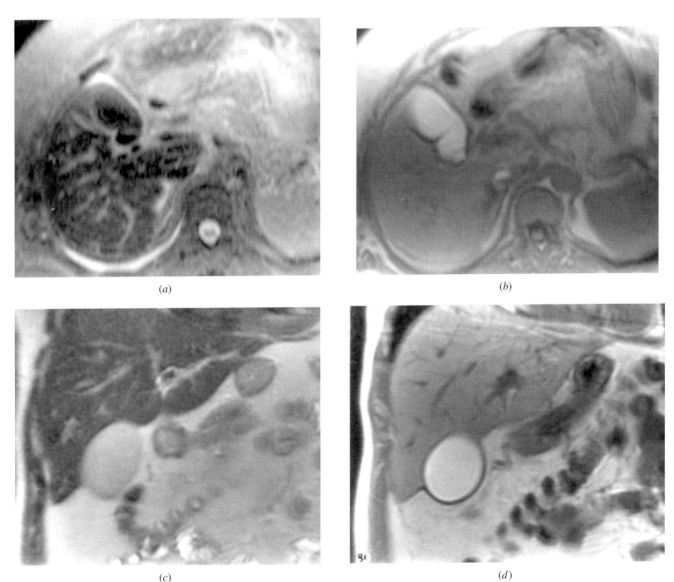

(a)

(b)

(c)

(d)

FIG. 3.6 Abnormal signal of bile. T2-weighted fat-suppressed spin-echo (*a*) and T1-weighted SGE (*b*) images in a patient with primary biliary cirrhosis. The bile in the gallbladder is highly concentrated, resulting in low signal on the T2-weighted image (*a*) and high signal on the T1-weighted image (*b*). A small pleural effusion is present in the right posterior pleural recess showing high signal on the T2-weighted image (*a*).

Coronal T2-weighted single-shot echo-train spin-echo (*c*) and coronal T1-weighted SGE (*d*) images in a second patient with concentrated bile in the gallbladder showing moderately high signal on the T2-weighted image (*c*) and high signal on the T1-weighted image (*d*). Note that on the T2-weighted image (*c*), both fluid and fat are higher signal than bile.

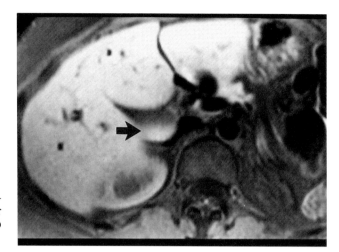

FIG. 3.7 Layering of gallbladder bile. T1-weighted fat-suppressed spin-echo image. Layering of the bile in the gallbladder is observed with the more concentrated, hyperintense bile (arrow) in the dependent portion of the gallbladder.

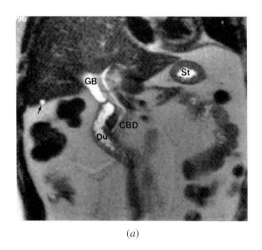

(*a*)

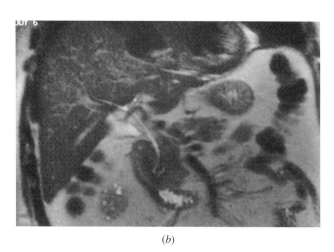

(*b*)

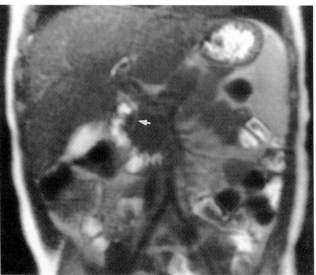

(*c*)

FIG. 3.8 Normal biliary tree. Coronal T2-weighted single-shot echo-train spin-echo images (*a, b, c*) in three patients. In the first patient (*a*), the biliary tree is visualized with high signal allowing clear depiction of normal anatomy. The second part of the duodenum (Du) is outlined by a small amount of physiologic fluid in this fasting patient (*a*) (CBD, common bile duct; GB, gallbladder; St, stomach). A small liver cyst (arrow, *a*) is present in the right lobe. In a second adult patient (*b*), the right and left hepatic, common hepatic, and common bile duct are demonstrated. A short portion of the pancreatic duct is also seen. In a 1-year-old child (*c*), the CBD (arrow) is well visualized despite the lack of patient cooperation.

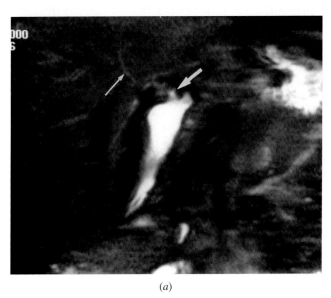 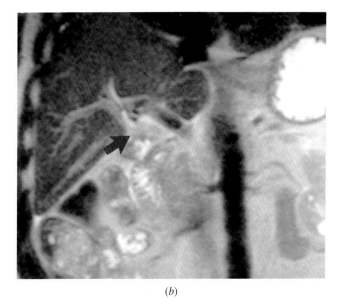

(a)   (b)

F I G . 3.9 Biliary anastomosis. Coronal T2-weighted fat-suppressed thin-section MRCP single-shot echo-train spin-echo image (*a*) in a patient with hepatico-porto-enterostomy (after Kasai operation) showing the normal anastomosis between a bowel loop and the porta hepatis (arrow). Intrahepatic non-dilated bile ducts are also well depicted (thin arrow).

Coronal T2-weighted single-shot echo-train spin-echo image (*b*) in a patient with normal Roux-en-Y anastomosis (arrow, *b*). The intrahepatic bile ducts, the anastomosis, and the connecting bowel loop are well visualized. The presence of a biliary-enteric anastomosis is suspected when small bowel is noted tucked into the porta hepatis, as observed in this patient.

intensity is isointense to duodenal wall on T1- and T2-weighted images. Along the superior aspect of the major papilla is the superior papillary fold, which often forms a hood over the papilla that may be quite prominent. Inferior to the papilla is the longitudinal fold. The shape and size of the major papilla can vary with reported average diameters of 15 × 7 mm (longitudinal × transverse) [28]. The minor papilla is the orifice of the dorsal pancreatic duct and is located proximal to the major papilla. With MRCP, Taourel et al. [29] visualized the major papilla in 40% of cases. The minor papilla was seen less frequently.

On T1-weighted sequences, the signal of bile in intrahepatic ducts is usually low because of its high water content. In the CBD, however, the signal can be variable, reflecting the concentration of bile, although concentrated bile is observed much less frequently in the CBD compared with the gallbladder. On postgadolinium fat-suppressed images acquired approximately 2 min after gadolinium administration, the bile duct walls are best depicted and show moderate enhancement that may be slightly higher than that of normal liver parenchyma.

Biliary Anastomoses

In the presence of end-to-end anastomosis (e.g., after orthotopic liver transplantation), Roux-en-Y, or other choledochoenteric anastomoses, ERCP is technically very difficult to perform or contraindicated. In such in-

stances, MRCP is the imaging modality of choice and may be particularly useful to exclude strictures (e.g., at the anastomosis) and to demonstrate the morphology and diameter of the bile ducts distal and proximal to the anastomosis (fig. 3.9).

DISEASES OF THE GALLBLADDER

Nonneoplastic Disease

Gallstone Disease

Predisposing factors for cholelithiasis can be summarized as "female, forty, fat, fair, fertile," preexisting cholestasis, inflammatory bowel disease, and metabolic disorders (e.g., diabetes mellitus, pancreatic disease, hypercholesterolemia, cystic fibrosis). The primary imaging modality for cholecystolithiasis is sonography. However, because of the high prevalence of this disease, gallstones frequently are encountered incidentally and familiarity with their MRI appearance is essential.

MRCP sequences are highly sensitive and accurate in depicting cholecystolithiasis and can outperform ultrasound and computed tomography [1]. Gallstones generally present as intraluminal, signal-void, round, or faceted structures on both T1- and T2-weighted images (fig. 3.10). Occasionally, areas of high signal intensity will be present in gallstones on T1- and T2-weighted sequences, or, less commonly, the stones will appear largely hyperintense on T1-weighted sequences

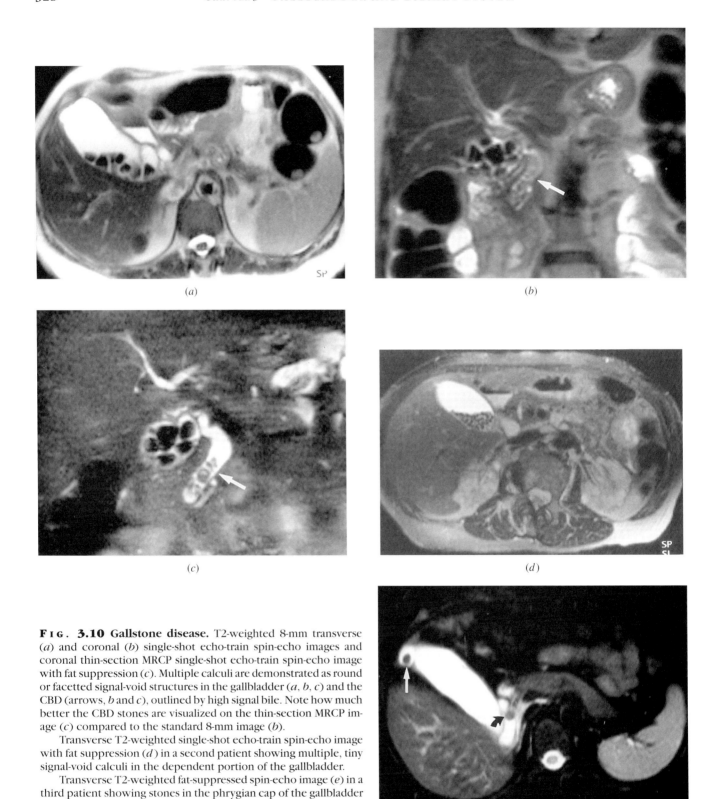

F I G . 3.10 Gallstone disease. T2-weighted 8-mm transverse (*a*) and coronal (*b*) single-shot echo-train spin-echo images and coronal thin-section MRCP single-shot echo-train spin-echo image with fat suppression (*c*). Multiple calculi are demonstrated as round or facetted signal-void structures in the gallbladder (*a*, *b*, *c*) and the CBD (arrows, *b* and *c*), outlined by high signal bile. Note how much better the CBD stones are visualized on the thin-section MRCP image (*c*) compared to the standard 8-mm image (*b*).

Transverse T2-weighted single-shot echo-train spin-echo image with fat suppression (*d*) in a second patient showing multiple, tiny signal-void calculi in the dependent portion of the gallbladder.

Transverse T2-weighted fat-suppressed spin-echo image (*e*) in a third patient showing stones in the phrygian cap of the gallbladder (straight arrow, *e*) and in the cystic duct (curved arrow, *e*).

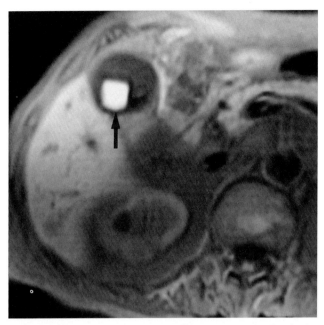

F I G . 3.11 Hyperintense gallstone. T1-weighted fat-suppressed spin-echo image showing a gallstone (arrow) of uniform high signal intensity of its central portion with a signal-void peripheral rim. (Courtesy of Caroline Reinhold, MD, Dep. of Radiology, McGill University.)

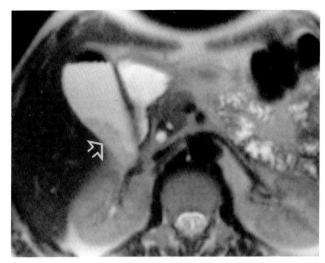

F I G . 3.12 Floating gallstones. Transverse T2-weighted single-shot echo-train spin-echo image demonstrating multiple small, signal-void calculi floating in the nondependent portion of the gallbladder. Concentrated bile (sludge) is shown, and appears as moderately hypointense material in the dependent portion of the gallbladder (open arrow).

(fig. 3.11) [30, 31]. The exact cause for the increased signal intensity has not yet been established. It has been shown, using spectroscopy and chemical analysis of gallstones, that it is not caused by high lipid content [31]. Therefore, the presence of protein macromolecules or dispersed calcium microparticles, which shorten T1-relaxation times, may be a reasonable explanation [32, 33]. Occasionally, the specific weight of a gallstone is lower than that of bile and the gallstone will float in the nondepending portion of the gallbladder (fig. 3.12). In this case, a gallstone can be differentiated from a gallbladder polyp by the lack of enhancement on T1-weighted postgadolinium images.

Acute Cholecystitis
Acute inflammation of the gallbladder is caused by obstruction of the cystic duct (e.g., by cystic duct stones) in 80–95% of patients. Morphologic criteria to establish the diagnosis have been described in the ultrasound literature. A combination of gallbladder wall thickening (>3 mm), three-layered appearance of the wall, hazy delineation of the gallbladder, localized pain (Murphy's sign), presence of gallstones, gallbladder hydrops, and fluid surrounding the gallbladder indicate a high probability of acute cholecystitis. In the presence of acalculous cholecystitis, or if many of these signs are absent, establishing the correct diagnosis with ultrasound is challenging and findings can be equivocal.

Acute cholecystitis results in increased blood flow and capillary leakage due to inflammatory changes, which is reflected on MRI by increased enhancement on postgadolinium images. The high sensitivity of MRI for gadolinium enhancement, especially with the use of fat suppression techniques, makes it an effective technique for the diagnosis of acute cholecystitis, demonstrating higher sensitivity and accuracy than ultrasound [34]. On T1-weighted immediate postgadolinium images, the enhancement is most pronounced along the mucosal layer of the gallbladder wall and progresses to involve the entire thickness of the wall on more delayed images (fig. 3.13). The percentage of contrast enhancement of the gallbladder wall has been shown to correlate well with the presence of acute cholecystitis and was more accurate than wall thickness in distinguishing acute from chronic cholecystitis and gallbladder malignancy [35]. An important finding in acute cholecystitis is the transient increased enhancement of adjacent liver tissue on immediate postgadolinium images, which can be observed in approximately 70% of patients (figs. 3.13–3.15) [35]. This reflects a hyperemic inflammatory response to the adjacent acute inflammation in the gallbladder wall. Thus findings that are indicative of acute cholecystitis on postgadolinium T1-weighted images are a) increased wall enhancement, b) transient increased enhancement of adjacent liver parenchyma on immediate postgadolinium images, and c) increased thickness of the gallbladder wall [36]. Findings on T2-weighted images that are helpful to establish the diagnosis are a) presence of gallstones, b) presence of pericholecystic fluid, c) presence of intramural abscesses appearing as hyperintense foci

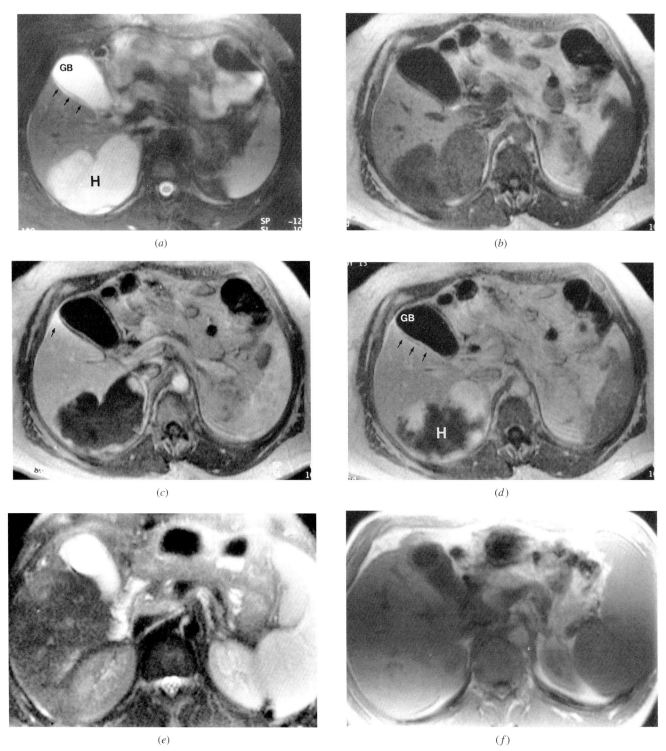

(a)   (b)

(c)   (d)

(e)   (f)

F I G . 3.13 Acute cholecystitis. Transverse T2-weighted fat-suppressed echo-train spin-echo (*a*), T1-weighted SGE (*b*), immediate postgadolinium SGE (*c*), and 90-s postgadolinium SGE (*d*) images. The wall of the gallbladder (GB) is mildly thickened (4 mm) and shows increased signal intensity on the T2-weighted image (arrows, *a*). A giant hemangioma (H) is seen in *segment 6* of the liver. On the immediate postgadolinium image (*c*), increased enhancement of the gallbladder mucosa and transient increased enhancement of liver parenchyma adjacent to the gallbladder is apparent (arrow, *c*). On the 90-s postgadolinium image (*d*), increased enhancement of the entire gallbladder wall (arrows, *d*) is shown. Also note the peripheral nodular enhancement of the hemangioma (H).

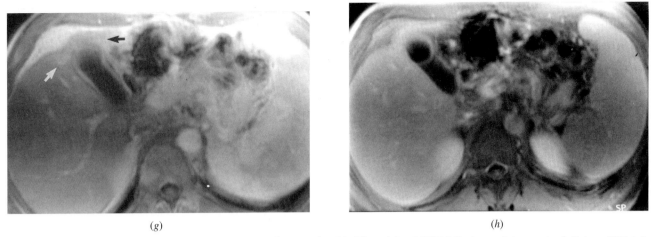

(g)   (h)

F I G . 3.13 (*Continued*) T2-weighted fat-suppressed spin-echo (*e*), T1-weighted SGE (*f*), immediate postgadolinium SGE (*g*), and 2-min postgadolinium fat-suppressed SGE (*b*) images in another patient. The gallbladder wall shows increased signal and wall thickening on the T2-weighted image (*e*). Increased enhancement of the gallbladder mucosa and transient increased enhancement of adjacent liver parenchyma (arrows, *g*) are seen on the immediate postgadolinium image (*g*).

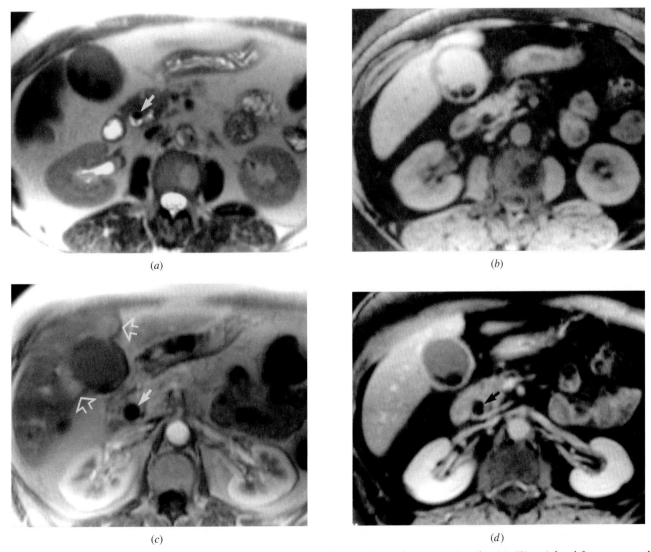

(a)   (b)

(c)   (d)

F I G . 3.14 Acute cholecystitis with gallstones. T2-weighted single-shot echo-train spin-echo (*a*), T1-weighted fat-suppressed SGE (*b*), immediate postgadolinium SGE (*c*), and 2-min postgadolinium fat-suppressed SGE (*d*) images. The bile in the gallbladder is highly concentrated, showing low signal on the T2-weighted image (*a*) and high signal on the T1-weighted image (*b*). Several low-signal gallstones are visualized in the gallbladder and the CBD (arrows, *a, c, d*). The gallbladder wall is thickened. On the immediate postagadolinium image (*c*), the adjacent liver parenchyma demonstrates transient increased enhancement (open arrows, *c*).

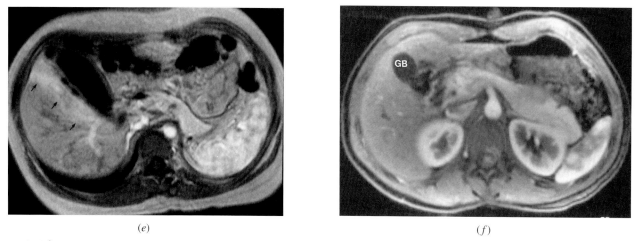

(e)   (f)

F I G . 3.14 (*Continued*) Immediate postgadolinium SGE image (*e*) in another patient demonstrating transient hyperemic enhancement of the liver (arrows, *e*) adjacent to the gallbladder.

Immediate postgadolinium fat-suppressed SGE image (*f*) in a normal subject for comparison, demonstrating homogeneous enhancement of the liver. GB, gallbladder.

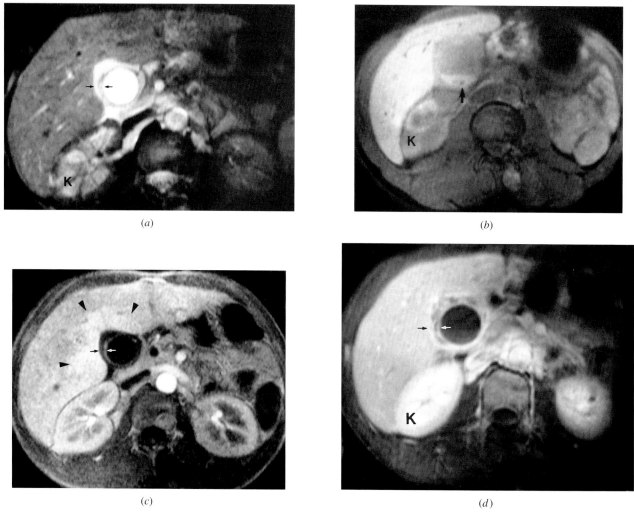

(a)   (b)

(c)   (d)

F I G . 3.15 Acute on chronic cholecystitis. T2-weighted fat-suppressed echo-train spin-echo (*a*), T1-weighted fat-suppressed spin-echo (*b*), immediate postgadolinium SGE (*c*), and 2-min postgadolinium fat-suppressed spin-echo (*d*) images. The gallbladder wall is thickened (arrows, *a*, *c*, *d*) with increased mural signal intensity on the T2-weighted image (*a*). On the T1-weighted image (*b*), layering of high-signal concentrated bile in the dependent portion and a small, hypointense, gallbladder stone (arrow, *b*) are shown. On the immediate postgadolinium image (*c*), moderate enhancement of the gallbladder mucosa and transient increased enhancement of adjacent liver parenchyma (arrowheads, *c*) are suggestive of acute cholecystitis. Delayed heterogeneous enhancement of the markedly thickened gallbladder wall, demonstrated on the 2-min postgadolinium image (*d*), is suggestive of chronic inflammatory changes. The low signal intensity of the renal cortex is due to iron deposition in this patient with sickle cell anemia. K, kidney.

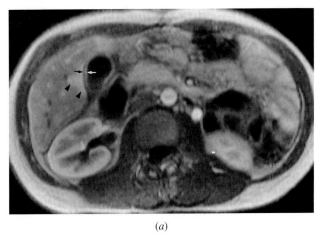

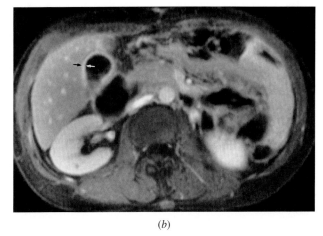

(a)   *(b)*

FIG. 3.16 Chemoembolization-induced acute cholecystitis. Immediate (*a*) and 90-s (*b*) postgadolinium SGE images. Transient pericholecystic enhancement of the liver parenchyma (arrowheads, *a*) is noted on the immediate postgadolinium image (*a*). Homogeneous enhancement is observed after 90 s (*b*). The thickened gallbladder wall (arrows, *a*, *b*) shows progressive enhancement from *a* to *b*.

in the gallbladder wall, and d) increased wall thickness (figs. 3.13–3.15) [35]. Periportal high signal intensity may be observed but is a nonspecific finding.

Acute acalculous cholecystitis comprises about 5–15% of all acute cholecystitis cases. It can be caused by depressed motility (e.g., in patients with severe trauma/surgery, burns, shock, anesthesia, diabetes mellitus), by decreased blood flow in the cystic artery due to extrinsic obstruction or embolization (fig. 3.16), or by bacterial infection.

Hemorrhagic Cholecystitis

Hemorrhagic cholecystis is more prevalent in patients with acalculous cholecystitis than in patients with calculous cholecystitis. Blood breakdown products in the gallbladder wall and lumen can be clearly identified with precontrast MRI sequences. Because of the specific signal intensity characteristics of these blood breakdown products on T1- and T2-weighted sequences, the age of the hemorrhage may be determined (fig. 3.17).

Chronic Cholecystitis

Chronic cholecystitis is more common than acute cholecystitis. Because of the longstanding inflammatory process, a variable degree of fibrosis occurs causing wall thickening and shrinkage of the gallbladder. In contrast to acute cholecystitis, mural gadolinium enhancement is mild and most prominent on delayed postgadolinium images. Pericholecystic enhancement is minimal or absent, because of the lesser severity of the inflammatory process (fig. 3.18). The adjacent liver parenchyma usually does not show increased enhancement [37]. The wall of the gallbladder may calcify, resulting in porcelain gallbladder (fig. 3.19). On MR images, calcifications may appear as signal-void foci. Patients with porcelain

gallbladder may be at increased risk for gallbladder carcinoma. Therefore, enhancing nodular tissue arising from the gallbladder wall, best shown on fat-suppressed late postgadolinium images, should raise suspicion of malignant disease in these patients. A uniform wall of less than 4 mm, however, excludes the presence of malignancy (fig. 3.19).

Xanthogranulomatous Cholecystitis

Xanthogranulomatous cholecystitis (fibroxanthogranulomatous inflammation) is a rare, focal or diffuse, destructive inflammatory disease of the gallbladder that is assumed to be a variant of chronic cholecystitis. The pathogenesis is thought to be occlusion of mucosal outpouchings (Rokitansky-Aschoff sinuses) with subsequent rupture and intramural extravasation of inspissated bile and mucin, which causes an inflammatory reaction with multiple intramural xanthogranulomatous nodules. The importance of this disease is that it mimics gallbladder carcinoma both clinically and radiologically [38]. The MRI findings are focal or diffuse gallbladder wall thickening with contrast enhancement. Small intramural abscesses may be demonstrated as foci of high signal on T2-weighted images and low signal on T1-weighted images [39].

Diffuse Gallbladder Wall Thickening

Diffuse gallbladder wall thickening may be present in a number of hepatic, biliary, and pancreatic diseases. Among nontumorous causes are hepatitis, liver cirrhosis, hypoalbuminemia, renal failure, systemic or hepatic venous hypertension, AIDS cholangiopathy, and graft-versus-host disease. Important features to discriminate these conditions from cholecystitis are minimal enhancement of the gallbladder wall and lack of increased

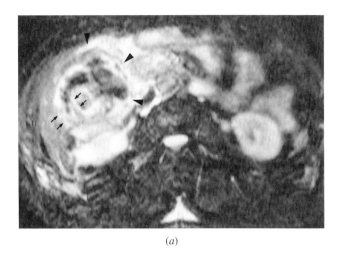

(a)

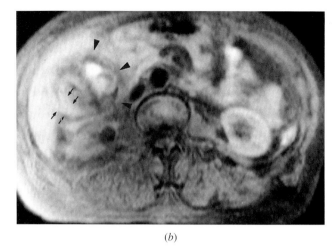

(b)

FIG. 3.17 Hemorrhagic cholecystitis. T2-weighted fat-suppressed echo-train spin-echo (a), T1-weighted fat-suppressed spin-echo (b), and immediate postgadolinium SGE (c) images. On the T2-weighted image (a), the thickened gallbladder wall (small arrows, a) shows areas of high and low signal. A pericholecystic area of predominantly low signal (arrowheads, a) is located antero-medially. On the T1-weighted image (b) areas of high signal intensity consistent with hemorrhage are noted within the substantially thickened gallbladder wall (small arrows, b). The large complex anteromedial area (arrowheads, b) is predominantly of high signal, which in combination with the low signal on the T2-weighted image is consistent with intracellular methemoglobin in an area of hemorrhage. The delayed postgadolinium SGE image (c) shows to better advantage the thick gallbladder wall (small arrows, c) and the hemorrhagic pericholecystic fluid collection (arrowheads, c). A calculus (long arrow, c) is incidentally shown in the right renal collecting system.

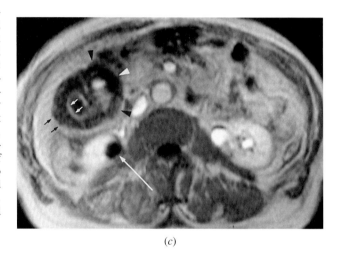

(c)

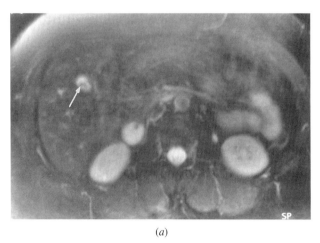

(a)

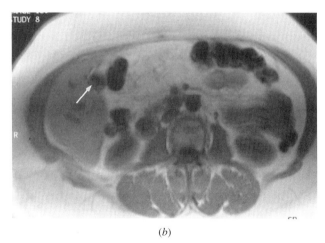

(b)

FIG. 3.18 Chronic cholecystitis. T2-weighted fat-suppressed spin-echo (a), T1-weighted SGE (b), immediate postgadolinium SGE (c), and 90-s postgadolinium fat-suppressed SGE (d) images. On the T2-weighted image (a), the gallbladder is shrunken and irregular in shape with poorly defined walls and a low-signal gallstone (arrow, a). On the precontrast T1-weighted image (b), the gallbladder wall is partly hyperintense (arrow, b). It enhances mildly on the immediate postgadolinium image (c), but no increased enhancement is noted in the adjacent liver parenchyma. On the 90-s postgadolinium fat-suppressed image (d), the gallbladder wall shows progressive enhancement.

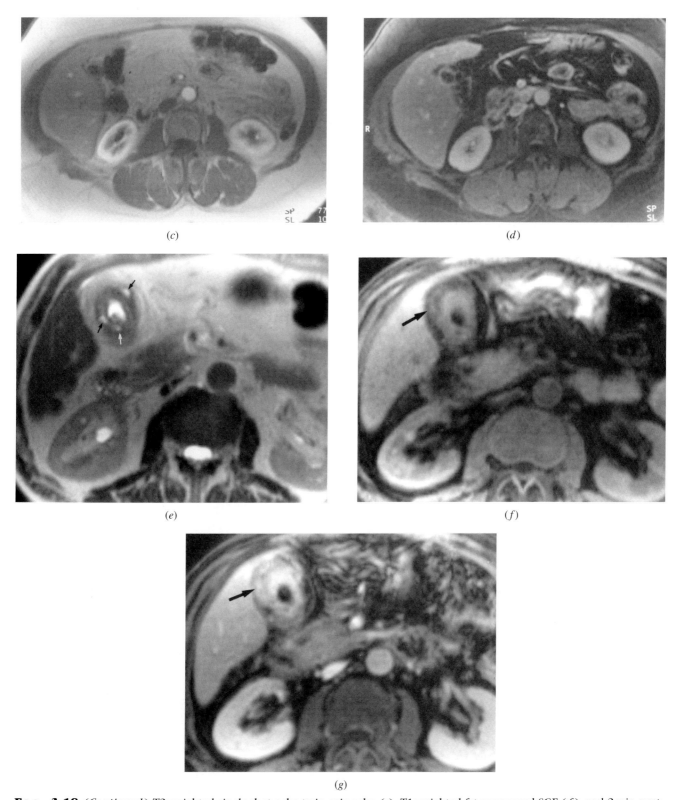

(c)   *(d)*

(e)   *(f)*

(g)

F I G . 3.18 (*Continued*) T2-weighted single-shot echo-train spin-echo (*e*), T1-weighted fat-suppressed SGE (*f*), and 2-min post-gadolinium fat-suppressed SGE (*g*) images in a second patient with chronic cholecystitis. The gallbladder is shrunken and irregular in shape and shows pronounced wall thickening. On the T2-weighted image (*e*), small hyperintense foci (short arrows, *e*) represent intramural fluid collections. The gallbladder shows enhancement on the 2-min postgadolinium image (*g*). In the pericholecystic space, complex septations (arrows, *f*, *g*) demonstrating enhancement on the postgadolinium image (*g*) are suggestive of fibrous inflammatory tissue. Small low-signal calculi are seen in the gallbladder lumen (*e–g*).

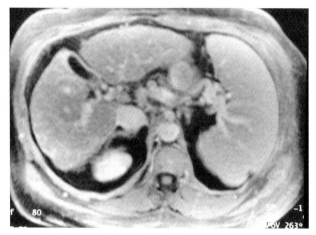

F I G . 3.19 Porcelain gallbladder. Diffuse calcification of the gallbladder wall was seen on a CT examination (not shown). The T1-weighted 2-min postgadolinium fat-suppressed SGE image demonstrates uniform enhancement of a smooth 3-mm-thick gallbladder wall, which excludes superimposed malignancy.

enhancement of adjacent structures on postgadolinium images, in particular the lack of transient increased enhancement of adjacent liver parenchyma (fig. 3.20).

NEOPLASTIC DISEASE

Gallbladder Polyps

Gallbladder polyps are often incidentally identified arising from the gallbladder wall and are either sessile or pedunculated. They comprise a wide spectrum of histologic types; however, the vast majority are benign. Nevertheless, gallbladder polyps pose a dilemma with respect to diagnosis of potential malignancy and the determination of proper long-term management. The majority are cholesterol polyps that do not have malignant potential. Approximately 10% of gallbladder polyps, however, are adenomas that are thought to have malignant potential [40]. However, this determination may be

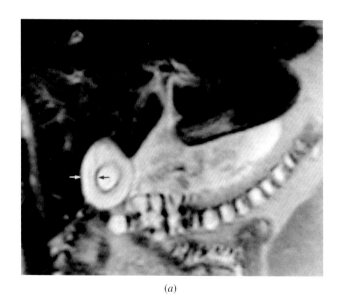

(a)

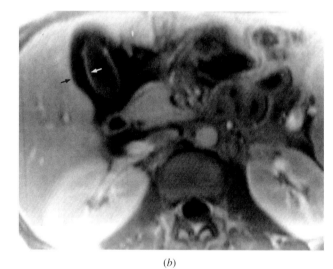

(b)

F I G . 3.20 Gallbladder wall edema. Coronal T2-weighted fat-suppressed single-shot echo-train spin-echo (a), T1-weighted immediate postgadolinium SGE (b), and 2-min postgadolinium fat-suppressed SGE (c) images. In this patient after bone marrow transplantation, the gallbladder wall is markedly edematous and thickened (arrows, a–c). Because of the high fluid content of the wall, the signal intensity is high on the T2-weighted image (a) and low on the T1-weighted images (b, c). The gallbladder mucosa shows moderate early and late enhancement (b, c). The adjacent liver parenchyma is normal.

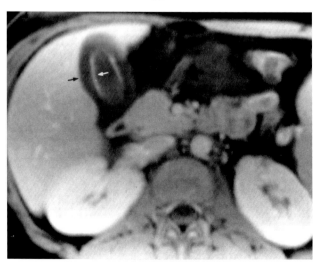

(c)

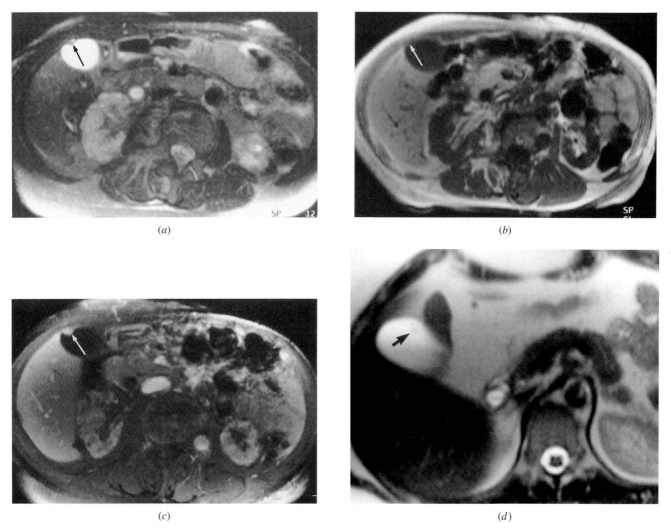

F I G . 3.21 Gallbladder polyps. T2-weighted fat-suppressed single-shot echo-train spin-echo (*a*), T1-weighted SGE (*b*), and 2-min postgadolinium fat-suppressed SGE (*c*) images. A 1-cm polyp (arrows, *a–c*) is shown on the nondependent surface of the gallbladder. The polyp is intermediate signal on the T2-weighted image (*b*), showing high contrast against bile. The polyp is low signal on the T1-weighted image (*a*) and can barely be seen. Intense uniform enhancement of the polyp is appreciated on the 2-min postgadolinium image (*c*). Enhancement and nondependent location distinguish the polyp from a gallbladder calculus. T2-weighted single-shot echo-train spin-echo (*d*) and T1-weighted 60-s postgadolinium SGE (*e*) images in a second patient.

reliably established only by histology. Polyps are typically homogeneously low to intermediate in signal intensity on T1- and T2-weighted MR images. On T1-weighted postgadolinium images, they show moderate homogeneous enhancement that is most pronounced on delayed images (fig. 3.21). Polyps can be readily distinguished from calculi on the basis of gadolinium enhancement or by location, if the polyp is located on the nondependent surface of the gallbladder wall, because calculi generally layer on the dependent surface or float horizontally within the gallbladder. Polyp size may be used as an indicator for malignant potential: polyps 1 cm or smaller have minimal risk for malignancy and can be managed by imaging follow-up [41]. Symptomatic lesions, polyps larger than 1 cm, or interval increase in size

are worrisome for malignancy, and cholecystectomy is indicated [42].

Gallbladder Adenomyomatosis

Adenomyomatosis is a relatively common disease with a reported incidence of up to 5% [43]. This disease entity is characterized by hyperplasia of epithelial and muscular elements with mucosal outpouching of epithelium-lined cystic spaces into a thickened muscularis layer. These changes can involve the entire gallbladder or may be focal. The mucosal outpouchings are termed Rokitansky-Aschoff sinuses, and they form small intramural diverticula that are pathognomonic. On MR images, these fluid-filled sinuses appear as small intramural foci of low

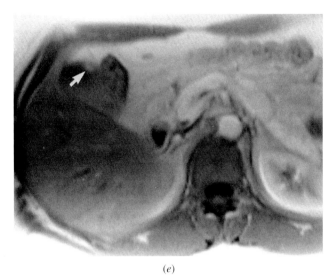

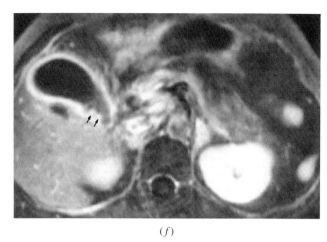

(e)   (f)

F I G . 3.21 (*Continued*) A polyp (arrows, *d*, *e*) is demonstrated in the nondependent portion of the gallbladder, showing intermediate signal on the T2-weighted image (*d*) and enhancement on the postgadolinium image (*e*). Layering of concentrated bile in the dependent portion of the gallbladder is seen on both sequences (*d*, *e*).

Transverse interstitial-phase gadolinium-enhanced fat-suppressed SE image (*f*) in a third patient, with coexistent acute acalculous cholecystitis, demonstrates two small enhancing polyps (arrows, *f*). Note the intense enhancement of the acutely inflamed and thickened gallbladder wall.

signal intensity on T1-weighted images and of high signal intensity on T2-weighted images [43, 44]. After gadolinium administration, early mucosal enhancement and late homogeneous enhancement can be observed (fig. 3.22) [43]. Demonstration of Rokitansky-Aschoff sinuses using a breath-hold or breathing-independent T2-weighted sequence has been shown to be a useful imaging finding to differentiate adenomyomatosis from gallbladder carcinoma [43]. However, this differentiation may be difficult on the basis of imaging.

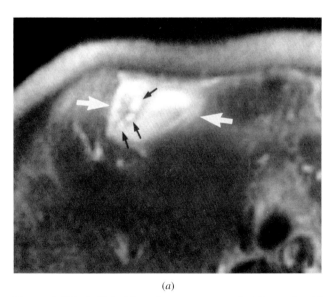

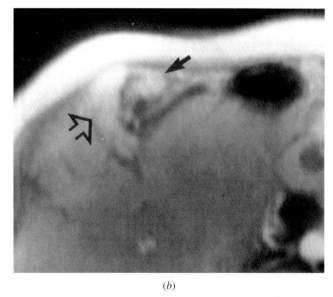

(a)   (b)

F I G . 3.22 Gallbladder adenomyomatosis. T2-weighted fat-suppressed single-shot echo-train spin-echo (*a*) and immediate postgadolinium T1-weighted SGE (*b*) images. The gallbladder (large arrows, *a*) has a phrygian cap configuration, is shrunken, and shows partial severe wall thickening. Layering of low-signal concentrated bile in the dependent portion is demonstrated on the T2-weighted image (*a*). Rokitansky-Aschoff sinuses (small arrows, *a*) are visualized as high-signal foci in the gallbladder wall on the T2-weighted image (*a*). On the postgadolinium image (*b*), the gallbladder (arrow, *b*) and the adjacent liver parenchyma (open arrow, *b*) show increased enhancement, reflecting inflammation. In this patient who also has primary sclerosing cholangitis, the liver is cirrhotic with nodular enlargement of the caudate lobe.

Gallbladder Carcinoma

Gallbladder carcinoma is the most common biliary malignancy and occurs predominantly in the sixth and seventh decades with a slight female predominance [45]. Porcelain gallbladder has been considered a predisposing factor for gallbladder carcinoma. A recent large series has cast doubt on this supposition [46]. In a review of 10,741 cholecystectomies, 15 specimens were porcelain gallbladder, and none of these 15 had gallbladder carcinoma [46]. Other diseases that are associated with gallbladder carcinoma are cholecystolithiasis, inflammatory bowel disease (predominantly ulcerative colitis), and chronic cholecystitis. However, less than 1% of patients with gallstones develop gallbladder carcinoma, and the risk for carcinoma is minimal if the stones are small and asymptomatic. The risk of developing car-

cinoma is increased if the stones are large and symptomatic, warranting prophylactic cholecystectomy. The most common histologic type of gallbladder carcinoma is adenocarcinoma, with squamous cell tumor being far less common [47]. The 5-year survival rate is very poor (approximately 6%), reflecting that up to 75% of tumors are unresectable at initial presentation because local invasion of adjacent organs.

Findings at MRI that are suggestive of gallbladder carcinoma are 1) a mass either protruding into the gallbladder lumen or replacing the lumen completely, 2) focal or diffuse thickening of the gallbladder wall greater than 1 cm, and 3) soft tissue (tumor) invasion of adjacent organs such as the liver, duodenum, and pancreas, which occurs frequently (fig. 3.23) [45, 48]. On T1-weighted MR images, the tumor is hypo- or

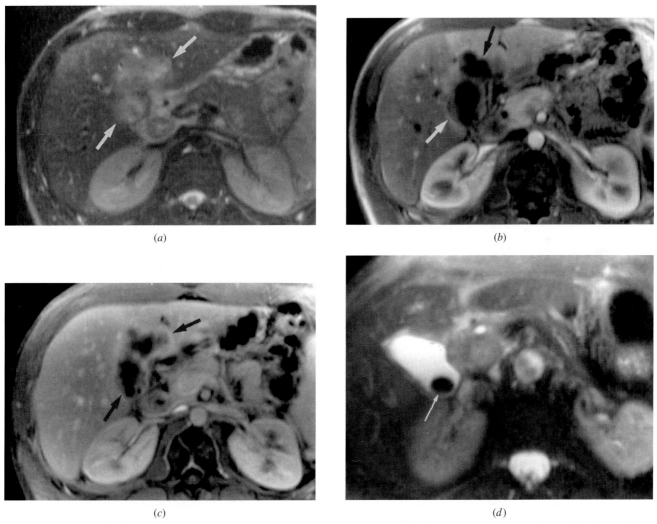

(a)

(b)

(c)

(d)

F I G . 3.23 Gallbladder carcinoma. T2-weighted fat-suppressed single-shot echo-train spin-echo (*a*), T1-weighted immediate postgadolinium SGE (*b*), and 2-min postgadolinium fat-suppressed SGE (*c*) images. The gallbladder (arrows, *a–c*) has a masslike appearance and shows an irregular and markedly thickened wall (arrows) that is moderately hyperintense on the T2-weighted image (*a*). Intense, slightly heterogeneous enhancement is demonstrated on the immediate and 2-min postgadolinium images (*b*, *c*), showing poor delineation from liver parenchyma.

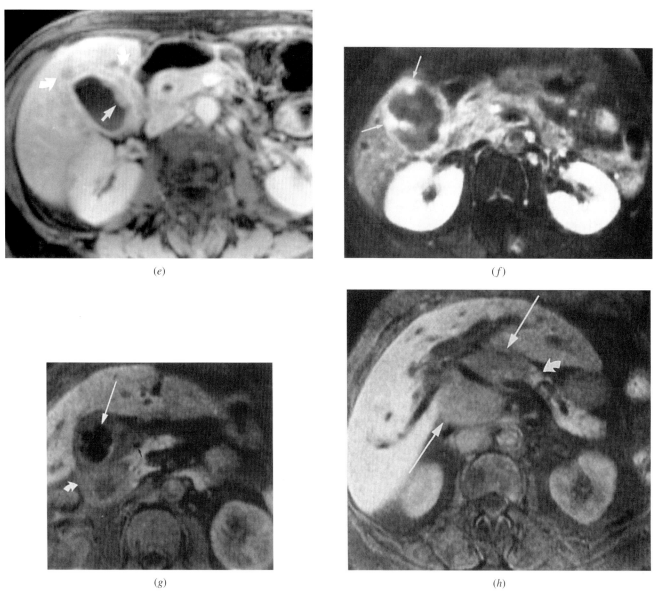

(e)

(f)

(g)

(h)

F I G . 3.23 (*Continued*) T2-weighted fat-suppressed single-shot echo-train spin-echo (*d*) and T1-weighted 2-min postgadolinium fat-suppressed SGE (*e*) images in a second patient with adenocarcinoma of the gallbladder. A signal-void stone is shown on the T2-weighted image (*d*). The gallbladder wall demonstrates partial irregular thickening (arrow, *e*), best visualized on the postgadolinium image (*e*). Small hypoenhancing areas in the adjacent liver parenchyma (curved arrows, *e*) are suggestive of metastases to the liver.

Transverse T1-weighted 2-min postgadolinium fat-suppressed SGE image (*f*) in a third patient with gallbladder cancer demonstrates irregular nodular thickening of the gallbladder wall (arrows, *f*).

T1-weighted fat-suppressed spin-echo images (*g, h*) in a fourth patient demonstrating gallbladder cancer, which is intermediate in signal intensity and infiltrates along the duodenal wall (curved arrow, *g*) and head of the pancreas encasing the gastroduodenal artery (short arrow, *g*). Signal-void calculi are present within the gallbladder (long arrow, *g*). On a more superior image at the level of the porta hepatis (*h*), a large tumor (straight arrows, *h*) is demonstrated. Good contrast is observed between intermediate-signal tumor and high-signal pancreas (curved arrow, *h*).

isointense compared to adjacent liver. On T2-weighted sequences, it is usually hyperintense relative to the liver and poorly delineated (fig. 3.23) [48, 49]. The tumor usually enhances on T1-weighted immediate post-gadolinium images in a heterogeneous fashion, which facilitates differentiation from chronic cholecystitis [50]. However, superimposed infection or perforation of gall-

bladder carcinoma may be indistinguishable from severe acute cholecystitis. Invasion of the tumor into adjacent organs and the presence of lymph node metastases are features of advanced disease and can be best visualized using a combination of a T2-weighted fat-suppressed sequence, T1-weighted immediate postgadolinium SGE, and 2-min postgadolinium fat-suppressed SGE sequence

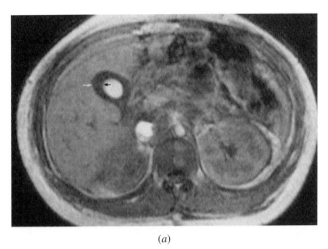
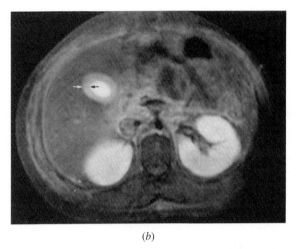

(a)   (b)

F I G . 3.24 Burkitt lymphoma of the gallbladder. T1-weighted SGE (*a*) and 2-min postgadolinium fat-suppressed spin-echo (*b*) images. The gallbladder wall (arrows, *a*, *b*) is diffusely thickened because of infiltration by lymphoma. Note the uniform moderate enhancement of the wall after contrast administration (*b*), which is less than that observed for acute cholecystitis.

(fig. 3.23) [48]. Preservation of a fat plane between tumor and surrounding structures excludes invasion. Delayed fat-suppressed gadolinium-enhanced images are particularly useful to delineate tumor spread along bile ducts and into the mesenteric fatty tissue.

Metastases to the Gallbladder

A number of malignant diseases can metastasize to the gallbladder. Among the most common primary malignancies are breast carcinoma, melanoma, and lymphoma. Breast cancer and melanoma more commonly show focal gallbladder involvement, whereas lymphoma more commonly presents with diffuse mural involvement and thickening (fig. 3.24).

DISEASES OF THE BILE DUCTS

One of the main indications for MRCP and/or conventional MRI of the biliary system is to reveal the cause for biliary obstruction and to characterize the lesion process as benign or malignant. In patients in whom ERCP is difficult to perform or contraindicated (e.g., in patients who have undergone liver transplantation or biliary-enteric anastomosis), MRCP is the modality of choice to evaluate biliary obstruction. Common causes for benign obstruction are gallstone disease or strictures as a sequel to inflammation or surgery. Malignant causes are pancreatic head tumors, primary biliary tumors, ampullary tumors, and compression from adjacent malignancies. In all cases it is necessary to define the level, grade, and cause of the biliary obstruction. Therefore, demonstration of the lumen and the walls of the bile ducts, as well as the surrounding tissue, is required. This can be

achieved with a combination of MRCP and conventional MRI sequences acquired before and after intravenous administration of gadolinium.

The normal maximal diameter of the CBD as visualized with MRCP (measured on coronal source images) is considered 7 mm in patients with the gallbladder in place and 10 mm in patients after cholecystectomy. Duct diameter, however, increases slightly with increasing patient age. Normal intrahepatic bile ducts show smooth walls that taper slowly toward the periphery.

BENIGN DISEASE

Choledocholithiasis

Calculi in the biliary ducts, although less frequent than in the gallbladder, are the most common cause of extrahepatic obstructive jaundice. With the increase of laparoscopic cholecystectomy over recent years, the interest in preoperative diagnosis of choledocholithiasis has surged, because the presence of bile duct stones renders laparoscopic procedures extremely difficult. Ultrasound and CT imaging are not well suited for the diagnosis of choledocholithiasis because of their relatively low sensitivity and accuracy [51–54]. ERCP is still considered the gold standard technique for the evaluation of the biliary ductal system and allows therapeutic interventions such as sphincterotomy for the release of CBD stones. However, significant complications (e.g., pancreatitis) after sphincterotomy occur in 6–13% of patients with an overall mortality rate up to 1.5% [55–57]. Even with diagnostic ERCP alone, the rate of major complications or death is 5–8% and the rate of failed ERCP is 5–20% [8, 58, 59].

MRCP is a noninvasive technique that is ideally suited for detecting bile duct stones owing to the high

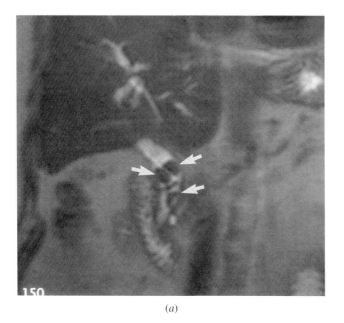

(a)

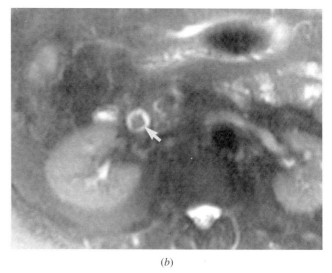

(b)

FIG. 3.25 Choledocholithiasis, MRCP. T2-weighted single-shot echo-train spin-echo images in the coronal (*a*) and transverse plane with fat suppression (*b*) and coronal thin-section MRCP single-shot echo-train spin-echo image with fat suppression (*c*). Multiple faceted low-signal calculi (arrows, *a*, *b*) are shown in the dilated CBD with good contrast against surrounding high signal bile. On the thin-section MRCP image (*c*), the dilated intrahepatic ducts (short arrows, *c*) and a stone in the CHD (long arrow, *c*) are visualized more clearly. The normal pancreatic duct (curved arrow, *c*) is also well depicted.

(c)

contrast of calculi as intraluminal low-signal intensity or signal-void structures against high-signal intensity bile (fig. 3.25). A number of studies have shown that MRCP is superior to CT or ultrasound and comparable or superior to ERCP in detecting choledocholithiasis [1, 4, 17, 60]. At MRI, ductal biliary stones typically have a rounded or oval-shaped configuration with a meniscus of fluid above their proximal edge (fig. 3.26). On thin-section source images, stones consistently appear as signal-void foci and can be detected as small as 2 mm in dilated and nondilated ducts [1]. On thick-section images, however, the detection rate of stones depends on their size. Large or medium-sized stones in normal-caliber ducts are readily detectable as signal-void structures, but small stones that are completely surrounded by fluid may escape detection because of volume-averaging effects. Another potential missed diagnosis is an impacted stone in

the ampulla, not surrounded by fluid, that may be misinterpreted as a stricture (fig. 3.27). A recent study by Soto et al. [61] compared the performance of thick-slab, thin-slab, and 3D fast-SE MRCP sequences with ERCP for detecting choledocholithiasis in 49 patients. They found sensitivity and specificity rates exceeding 92% and 92%, respectively, for all sequences. There was 100% agreement between MRCP and ERCP in the detection of ductal dilatation.

Pitfalls of MRCP. A common pitfall in the diagnosis of choledocholithiasis are intraductal air bubbles (pneumobilia), which can be differentiated from stones by observing that air filling defects lie on the nondependent portion of the bile duct against the wall or by recognition of an air-fluid level (fig. 3.28). Blood clots,

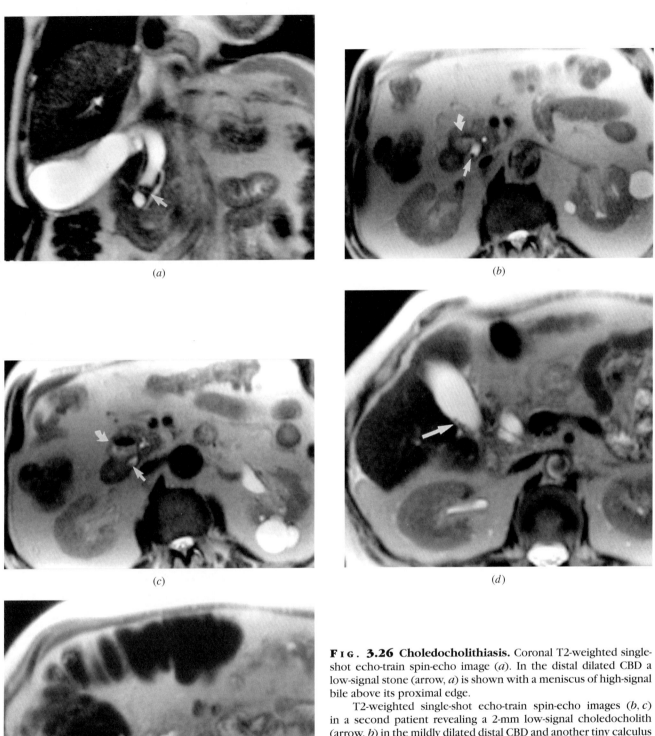

(a)

(b)

(c)

(d)

(e)

FIG. 3.26 Choledocholithiasis. Coronal T2-weighted single-shot echo-train spin-echo image (*a*). In the distal dilated CBD a low-signal stone (arrow, *a*) is shown with a meniscus of high-signal bile above its proximal edge.

T2-weighted single-shot echo-train spin-echo images (*b, c*) in a second patient revealing a 2-mm low-signal choledocholith (arrow, *b*) in the mildly dilated distal CBD and another tiny calculus more caudally (*c*) in the preampullary CBD (arrow, *c*). A duodenal diverticulum (curved arrows, *b, c*) is shown with high-signal fluid content in the dependent and a signal-void air bubble in the non-dependent portions. High-signal cortical renal cysts are present in the left kidney.

Transverse T2-weighted single-shot echo-train spin-echo images (*d, e*) in a third patient demonstrating several low-signal 2-mm calculi in the gallbladder (arrow, *d*) and in the preampullary CBD (arrow, *e*).

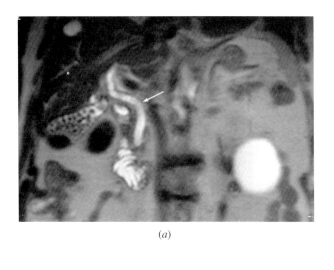

(a)

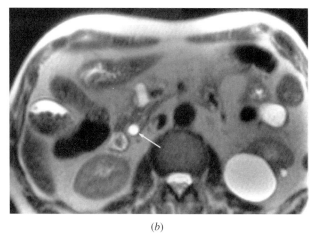

(b)

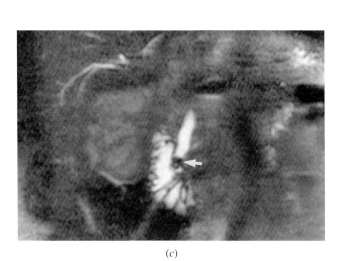

(c)

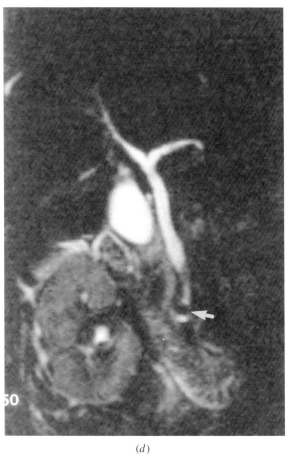

(d)

FIG. 3.27 Ampullary choledocholithiasis. Coronal (*a*) and transverse (*b*) T2-weighted single-shot echo-train spin-echo images and coronal thin-section MRCP single-shot echo-train spin-echo image with fat suppression (*c*). Multiple small low-signal calculi are demonstrated in the gallbladder (*a*, *b*). The CHD and CBD (arrows, *a*, *b*) are dilated, but no intraductal stone is visualized on the 8-mm coronal and transverse images (*a*, *b*). The thin-section MRCP image (*c*) reveals a small choledocholith (arrow, *c*) that is lodged in the ampulla and obstructs the CBD. The duodenum is filled with fluid outlining its folds (*a*, *c*). High-signal cysts are incidentally revealed in the dome of the liver (*a*) and the left kidney (*a*, *b*).

Coronal thin-section MRCP single-shot echo-train spin-echo images with fat suppression (*d*, *e*) in a second patient revealing a small stone (arrow, *d*) in the ampullary portion of the CBD, barely outlined by high-signal bile. A second stone (arrow, *e*) in the distal CBD is fully surrounded by fluid.

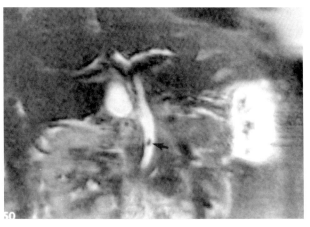

(e)

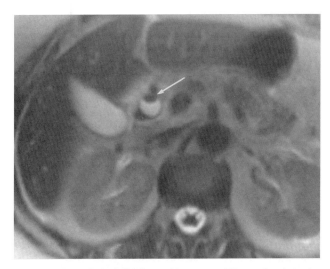

F I G . 3.28 Air in bile ducts. Transverse T2-weighted single-shot echo-train spin-echo image in a patient after ERCP showing a signal-void air bubble (arrow) floating in the nondependent portion of the CBD.

however, may be indistinguishable from biliary stones. Other pitfalls that may mimic calculi include a) tortuosity of the bile duct that results in the duct traveling in and out of the imaging plane; b) insertion of the cystic duct into the CBD that, when observed en face on coronal

images, may appear as a round hypointense focus mimicking a stone; c) metallic clips; and d) external compression artifact from the right hepatic or the gastroduodenal artery, which may result in a signal-void focus (fig. 3.29) [2, 62]. Careful attention to exact location of these defects (e.g., air in a nondependent location, continuation of the cystic duct or right hepatic or gastroduodenal arteries on adjacent images, clips in the gallbladder fossa) and interpretation of MRCP MIP reconstruction images in conjunction with thin-section source images most often permits correct exclusion of these entities as representing stones.

Ampullary Stenosis

The clinical symptoms of ampullary stenosis include recurrent, intermittent upper abdominal pain, abnormal liver tests, and dilatation of the common bile duct.

Ampullary Fibrosis. The most common cause of benign ampullary stenosis is fibrosis, which occurs most frequently as a sequel to stone passage in the context of choledocholithiasis. The degree of biliary ductal dilatation is usually mild to moderate but can be severe. In the acute phase, swelling and edema of the ampulla may be present, shown as enlarged prominence of the ampulla

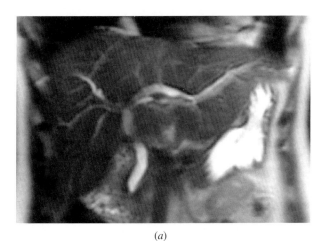

(a)

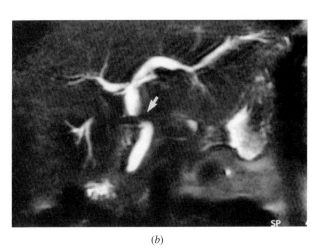

(b)

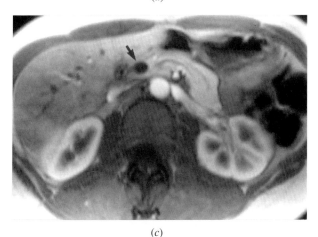

(c)

F I G . 3.29 Ampullary fibrosis, imaging artifacts. Coronal T2-weighted single-shot echo-train spin-echo image (*a*), thin-section MRCP single-shot echo-train spin-echo image with fat suppression (*b*), and transverse T1-weighted immediate postgadolinium SGE image (*c*). The intrahepatic and extrahepatic bile ducts are dilated. The signal-void area in the proximal CBD (arrow, *b*) is caused by the crossing hepatic artery and does not represent an intraductal stone. The tubular nature of the vessel is better depicted on the MRCP image (*b*) than on the standard T2-weighted image (*a*). On the postgadolinium image (*c*), the pancreas is well delineated against the dilated CBD (arrow, *c*) and shows normal enhancement. The diagnosis of ampullary fibrosis was confirmed by ERCP.

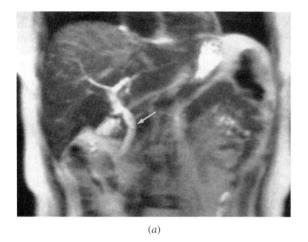

(a)

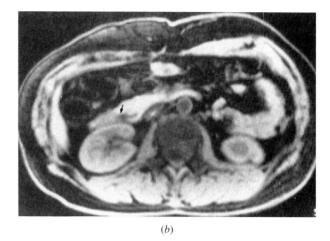

(b)

FIG. 3.30 Ampullary fibrosis. Coronal T2-weighted thin-section MRCP single-shot echo-train spin-echo image (*a*) shows the entire dilated CBD (arrow, *a*), excluding ductal calculi.

Transverse T1-weighted fat-suppressed SGE (*b*) and immediate postgadolinium SGE (*c*) images in a second patient with ampullary fibrosis. The pancreas and ampulla appear normal on the fat-suppressed SGE image (*b*) at the level of the ampulla (arrow, *b*), with no evidence of a mass. This is confirmed on the immediate postgadolinium image (*c*), which shows homogeneous enhancement of the pancreas at the level of the ampulla (arrow, *c*), excluding tumor.

(c)

and increased signal intensity on T2-weighted images. In the chronic stage, fibrosis of the ampulla appears as low signal intensity on T2-weighted images without enlargement of the ampulla. Rarely, these fibrotic changes are proliferative and lead to pronounced enlargement of the ampulla that may give the impression of an obstructing tumor. T1-weighted immediate postgadolinium images are a useful tool to show normal enhancement of the periampulary pancreatic parenchyma to exclude pancreatic tumor (figs. 3.29 and 3.30). Nevertheless, endoscopic biopsy may sometimes be necessary to establish the correct diagnosis.

Papillary Dysfunction. Functional stenosis of the sphincter of Oddi includes spasm of the sphincter of Oddi and abnormalities of the sequencing or frequency rate of sphincteric contraction waves [63]. This results in delayed drainage of the CBD with clinical symptoms and radiologic signs of biliary obstruction at the level of the papilla. MRI can aid in establishing the diagnosis by ruling out morphologic causes for biliary ductal dilatation (fig. 3.31). To visualize the function of the sphincter of Oddi, the use of serial thin-section MRCP single-shot echo-train spin-echo images ("functional MRCP") with-

out or with prior administration of secretin ("pharmacodynamic MRCP") is under investigation [63].

Sclerosing Cholangitis

Inflammation and obliterative fibrosis of intrahepatic and extrahepatic bile ducts characterize this disease entity. Progressive periductal fibrosis eventually leads to disappearance of small ducts and strictures of larger ducts. The anatomic changes in the biliary tract and the hepatic histologic changes are nonspecific and can either be secondary to infection or hepatic arterial damage or "primary" when immune factors are thought to underlie the disease [64].

Primary Sclerosing Cholangitis. Approximately 71% of patients with primary sclerosing cholangitis (PSC) also have inflammatory bowel disease [65]. Approximately 87% of these patients have ulcerative colitis, and 13% have Crohn disease [65]. PSC results in cholestasis with progression to secondary biliary cirrhosis and hepatic failure. Current hypotheses hold immune factors or toxic bacterial products that cross the inflamed colonic mucosa and enter the portal venous bloodstream accountable for PSC by inducing pericholangitic

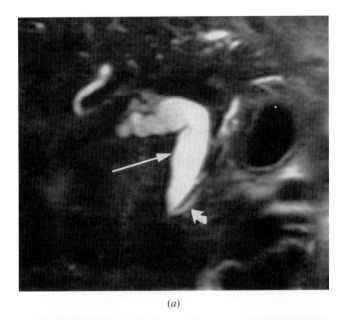

(a)

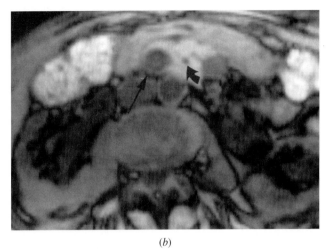

(b)

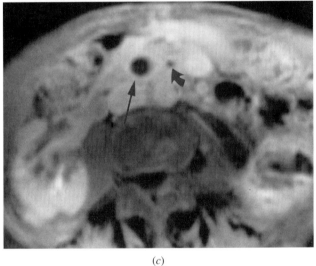

(c)

FIG. 3.31 Papillary dysfunction. Coronal T2-weighted thin-section MRCP single-shot echo-train spin-echo image with fat suppression (*a*) and transverse T1-weighted fat-suppressed SGE (*b*) and 2-min postgadolinium fat-suppressed SGE (*c*) images. The CBD (straight arrows, *a–c*) is severely dilated without evidence of an intraductal stone on the thin-section MRCP image (*a*). The pancreatic duct (curved arrow, *a–c*) is also mildly dilated. The pancreas and region of the ampulla show no evidence of a tumor on the precontrast (*b*) and postgadolinium (*c*) images. Papillary dysfunction was diagnosed on ERCP.

inflammation and fibrosis [64]. The diagnosis of PSC is made using cholangiographic findings supported by histologic results. Clinical features, such as ulcerative colitis or cholestasis, may be supportive but are not diagnostic.

The imaging appearance of PSC is characterized by multifocal, irregular strictures and dilatations of segments of the intra- and extrahepatic biliary tree. The strictures are usually short and annular, alternating with normal or slightly dilated segments, producing a beaded appearance (fig. 3.32). Because of fibrosis of higher-order intrahepatic bile ducts the biliary tree has the appearance of cut-off peripheral ducts, described as pruning. The disease may involve intrahepatic ducts or extrahepatic ducts alone or both, with the cystic duct usually spared. All of these findings are not pathognomonic for primary sclerosing cholangitis and can be found in secondary forms as well. If the intrahepatic ducts are involved in isolation, differentiation must be made from primary bil-

iary cirrhosis, which can be distinguished clinically from PSC. The conventional imaging modality to establish the diagnosis of PSC is endoscopic retrograde cholangiopancreatography (ERCP). However, this method is associated with risks of pancreatitis and perforation and has been shown to result in progression of cholestasis in patients with PSC [58, 66]. MRCP has shown to be an adequate method for the diagnosis and follow-up of PSC [67, 68]. The imaging features that can be depicted in PSC are identical to the findings described for ERCP. In a prospective, comparative study with ERCP involving 102 patients, MRCP showed a sensitivity and specificity to depict PSC of 85–88% and 92–97%, respectively [68]. Factors that led to difficulties in interpreting the MR images and to false-positive and false-negative diagnoses were a) the presence of liver cirrhosis and b) PSC limited to the peripheral intrahepatic ducts. Cirrhosis may lead to distortion of the biliary tree that may mimic PSC

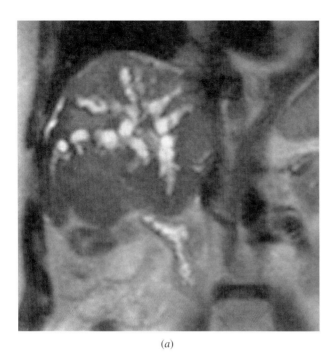
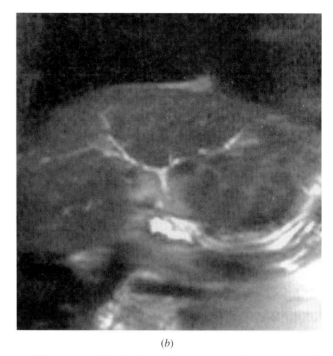

(a)   (b)

F I G . 3.32 Primary sclerosing cholangitis (PSC), beading. Coronal T2-weighted single-shot echo-train spin-echo images without (*a*) and with fat suppression (*b*) in two different patients (*a*, *b*, respectively). The high-signal intrahepatic bile ducts demonstrate beading caused by short strictures alternating with dilated (*a*) or normal-caliber (*b*) segments.

even on ERCP images. If PSC is limited to the peripheral ductal system, the higher image resolution of ERCP makes this a more sensitive test compared with current MRCP sequences. However, a limitation of ERCP is that the presence of severe strictures may lead to inadequate opacification of proximal bile ducts and to false-negative diagnoses [68]. MRCP provides visualization of bile ducts proximal to even severe stenoses and demonstrates bile duct stones in these locations, where they often escape detection with ERCP. In fact, visualization of bile ducts is considered easier with MRCP in the presence of severe ductal obstruction because of the expanded fluid-filled state of the obstructed ducts. In our experience, however, subtle changes of mild PSC can be difficult to detect using current MR techniques.

The use of conventional MR sequences and intravenous gadolinium provides information on the liver parenchyma and bile duct walls, which is valuable for a thorough evaluation [69]. In a study of patients with PSC by Revelon et al. [70], peripheral, wedge-shaped zones of hyperintense signal on T2-weighted images were found in the liver in 72% of patients. These triangular areas ranged from 1 to 5 cm in diameter (fig. 3.33). Periportal edema or inflammation, seen as high signal intensity along the porta hepatis on T2-weighted images, was present in 40% of patients. A study by Ito et al. [71] evaluated the imaging features of PSC on dynamic gadolinium-enhanced MRI. Thickening of bile duct walls and wall enhancement were seen in 50% and 67% of patients, respectively (fig. 3.33). On pregadolinium T1-weighted images, 23% of patients showed areas of in-creased signal intensity in the liver that did not represent focal fatty infiltration. On immediate postgadolinium images, 56% of all patients showed areas of increased parenchymal enhancement that were patchy, peripheral, segmental, or a combination of these patterns. These regions remained mildly or markedly hyperintense on delayed-phase images in 90% of patients. Other findings occasionally associated with PSC are atrophy of liver segments, periportal lymphadenopathy, and findings attributable to liver cirrhosis and portal hypertension, such as hypertrophy of the caudate lobe, regenerative nodules, and abdominal varices. In our experience, cirrhosis secondary to PSC often results in large central regenerative nodules that may cause periportal obstruction of bile ducts and, eventually, segmental atrophy of peripheral liver (fig. 3.33).

PSC is associated with an increased malignant potential, and the most important and common malignant entity that may occur in these patients is cholangiocarcinoma. Cholangiocarcinoma is the second most common cause of death, after liver failure, in patients with PSC, occurring in up to 20% of patients [72]. The diagnosis of superimposed cholangiocarcinoma in patients with PSC is difficult because of the underlying morphological bile duct changes. The MR appearance of cholangiocarcinoma is described below.

Infectious Cholangitis
Infectious, bacterial, or ascending cholangitis is a clinically defined syndrome caused by complete or partial biliary obstruction with associated ascending infection

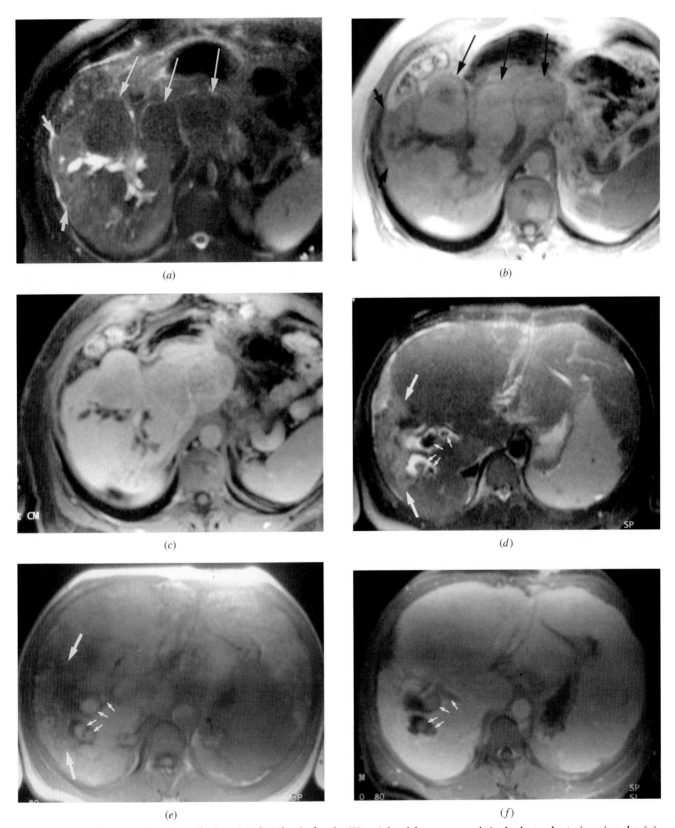

FIG. 3.33 Primary sclerosing cholangitis (PSC), cirrhosis. T2-weighted fat-suppressed single-shot echo-train spin-echo (*a*), T1-weighted SGE (*b*), and 2-min postgadolinium fat-suppressed SGE (*c*) images. The intrahepatic bile ducts are dilated and demonstrate beading. The liver is nodular and cirrhotic in this patient with late-stage PSC. Three large macroregenerative nodules (long arrows, *a*, *b*) located in the central portion of the liver appear to obstruct the bile ducts centrally. The nodules are slightly hypoenhancing on the 2-min postgadolinium image (*c*). A subsegmental distal area of atrophic liver parenchyma (short arrows, *a*, *b*) appears slightly hyperintense on the T2-weighted image (*a*) and hypointense on the T1-weighted image (*b*).

FIG. 3.33 (*Continued*) T2-weighted fat-suppressed single-shot echo-train spin-echo (*d*), T1-weighted SGE (*e*), and 2-min postgadolinium fat-suppressed SGE (*f*) images in a second patient. The liver shows multiple large macroregenerative nodules. The bile ducts in the right lobe of the liver are severely dilated and contain several calculi (small arrows, *d-f*) that are high signal on the T1-weighted image (*e*). A wedge-shaped peripheral area of liver parenchyma (arrows, *d*, *e*) is atrophic, showing high signal on the T2-weighted image (*d*) and low signal on the T1-weighted image (*e*) with late enhancement on the 2-min postgadolinium image (*f*).

T1-weighted 2-min postgadolinium SGE image with fat suppression (*g*) in a third patient demonstrating a beaded appearance of the intrahepatic bile ducts (arrows, *g*). The branches of the portal vein (V, *g*) are enhanced, facilitating differentiation from low-signal dilated intrahepatic bile ducts. The liver demonstrates a mildly irregular surface and enlargement of the left lobe.

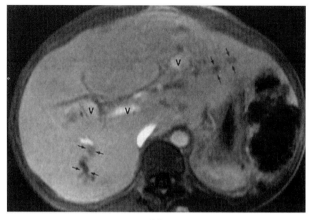

(*g*)

from the intestine. It encompasses a wide spectrum of clinical manifestations ranging from a mild to a fulminating form that constitutes a life-threatening surgical emergency. Prerequisite conditions are the presence of microorganisms in the bile and presence of partial or complete biliary obstruction. The typical clinical symptoms that lead to the diagnosis of ascending cholangitis are jaundice, abdominal pain, and sepsis (chills and fever), referred to as Charcot's triad. This triad is present in approximately 70% of patients.

The distribution of inflammatory changes may be diffuse or segmental. The most consistent imaging finding in infectious cholangitis is generalized or segmental biliary dilatation that can be mild or severe but does not correlate well with the severity or stage of the disease [73]. Bile duct walls are commonly mild to moderately thickened and show increased enhancement, which can be best appreciated on T1-weighted fat-suppressed 2-min postgadolinium images (fig. 3.34). Imaging findings on T2-weighted images are streaky increased signal in the periportal area and wedge-shaped hyperintense regions in the liver parenchyma (fig. 3.34). On pregadolinium T1-weighted images, these wedge-shaped regions in the liver are usually hypointense but may also show increased signal intensity. On immediate postgadolinium images, increased focal parenchymal enhancement can frequently be observed, consistent with inflammation (fig. 3.34). The greater inflammatory nature of infectious cholangitis compared to PSC is reflected by the more common occurrence of regions of increased enhancement on immediate postgadolinium images in the former condition. Liver abscesses may complicate infectious cholangitis and are best visualized on T2-weighted and T1-weighted dynamic postgadolinium images. Thrombosis of the portal vein is not uncommonly associated with infectious cholangitis (fig. 3.35) and aids in the distinction from sclerosing cholangitis, in which this occurrence is uncommon.

A particular form of infectious cholangitis is recurrent pyogenic cholangitis (oriental cholangitis), which is caused by infestation of the biliary tract by *Clonorchis sinensi* or other parasites. This leads to inflammatory infiltration of bile ducts, proliferative fibrosis, periductal abscesses, and calculi (pigment stones). MR imaging findings are disproportionally severe dilatation of the extrahepatic bile ducts proximal and distal to calculi, stricture of bile ducts, thickening of duct walls, and hepatic abscesses [74]. Liver segments that contain biliary duct stones frequently undergo atrophy. Absence of a tumor mass helps to differentiate this condition from cholangiocarcinoma. However, cautious interpretation of findings is essential because cholangiocarcinoma has an increased incidence in these patients [74].

AIDS Cholangiopathy

In HIV-positive patients, involvement of the pancreaticobiliary tract may be an early feature of AIDS (acquired immunodeficiency syndrome) [75]. Inflammation and edema of the biliary mucosa resulting in mucosal thickening and irregularity are the hallmark of AIDS cholangiopathy. This may lead to strictures, dilatations, and pruning resembling sclerosing cholangitis [1, 75]. When the papilla of Vater is involved, ampullary stenosis with common bile duct dilatation may result. The gallbladder may also be involved and show acalculous cholecystitis with imaging features similar to acute cholecystitis. Furthermore, patients have a predisposition for superimposed infectious cholangitis, often by unusual pathogens (e.g., cytomegalovirus, cryptosporidium, mycobacteriae, *Candida albicans*) [75].

Cystic Diseases of Bile Ducts

Congenital biliary cysts comprise choledochal cysts, diverticula originating from extrahepatic ducts, choledochocele, Caroli disease, and segmental cysts, depending on the location of the dilatation of the biliary tract. MRCP with 3D MIP reconstructions can display the anatomical extent and degree of these lesions, diagnose associated findings such as stone disease, and, in combination with gadolinium-enhanced T1-weighted images, evaluate for

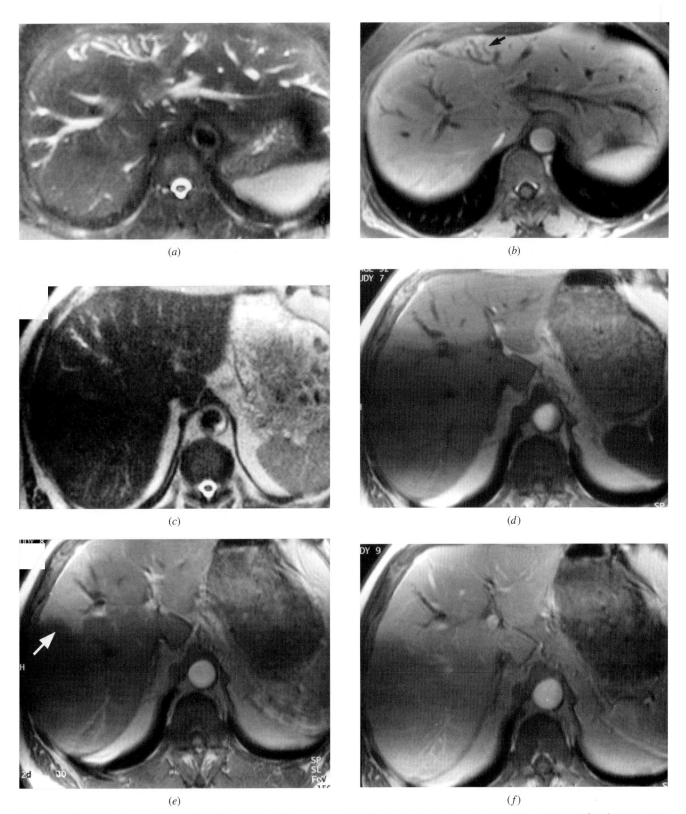

(a)   *(b)*

(c)   *(d)*

(e)   *(f)*

F I G . 3.34 Infectious cholangitis. T2-weighted fat-suppressed single-shot echo-train spin-echo (*a*) and T1-weighted 2-min post-gadolinium fat-suppressed SGE (*b*) images. The entire intrahepatic biliary tree is severely dilated, visualized as high signal on the T2-weighted image (*a*). On the T1-weighted image (*b*), the low-signal ducts are well differentiated from gadolinium-enhanced vessels. The walls of the bile ducts show increased enhancement that is most pronounced in *segment 4* of the liver (arrow, *b*).

T2-weighted single-shot echo-train spin-echo (*c*), T1-weighted SGE (*d*), immediate postgadolinium SGE (*e*), and 2-min postgadolinium fat-suppressed SGE (*f*) images in a second patient. A peripheral wedge-shaped area of liver parenchyma between *segments 4* and *8* shows moderate biliary ductal dilatation. The liver parenchyma in this area demonstrates increased signal on both the T2- (*c*) and T1-weighted (*d*) images, consistent with inspissated bile. Increased enhancement of this area (arrow, *e*) is demonstrated on the postgadolinium images (*e, f*), reflecting local inflammation and hyperemia in the liver parenchyma. The bile duct walls show increased enhancement, best visualized on the 2-min postgadolinium image (*f*).

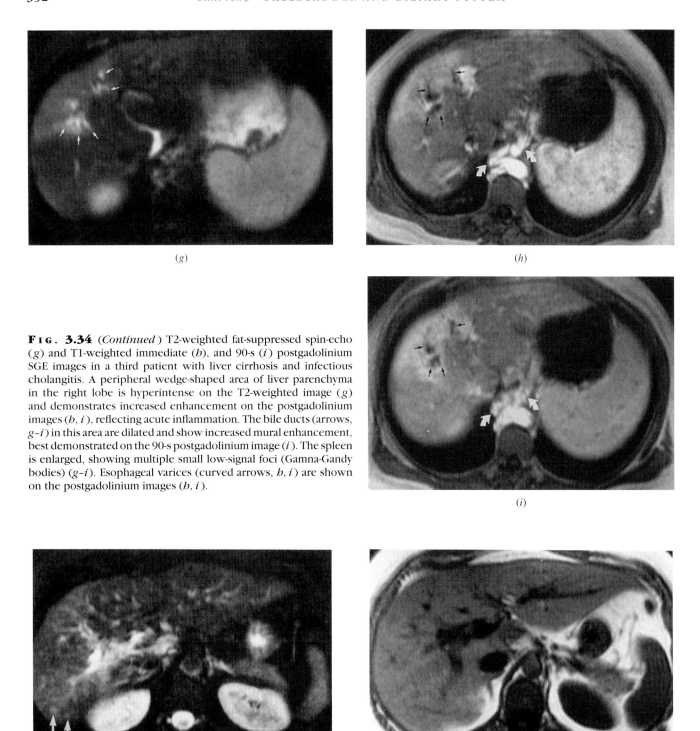

(g)

(h)

FIG. 3.34 (*Continued*) T2-weighted fat-suppressed spin-echo
(*g*) and T1-weighted immediate (*h*), and 90-s (*i*) postgadolinium
SGE images in a third patient with liver cirrhosis and infectious
cholangitis. A peripheral wedge-shaped area of liver parenchyma
in the right lobe is hyperintense on the T2-weighted image (*g*)
and demonstrates increased enhancement on the postgadolinium
images (*h, i*), reflecting acute inflammation. The bile ducts (arrows,
g–i) in this area are dilated and show increased mural enhancement,
best demonstrated on the 90-s postgadolinium image (*i*). The spleen
is enlarged, showing multiple small low-signal foci (Gamna-Gandy
bodies) (*g–i*). Esophageal varices (curved arrows, *h, i*) are shown
on the postgadolinium images (*h, i*).

(i)

(a)

(b)

FIG. 3.35 Infectious cholangitis with portal vein thrombosis. T2-weighted fat-suppressed spin-echo (*a*), T1-weighted SGE
(*b*), immediate postgadolinium SGE (*c*), and 1-min postgadolinium SGE (*d, e*) images. The right lobe of the liver is hyperintense
on both the T2- (*a*) and T1-weighted (*b*) images, consistent with edema and inspissated bile. On the T2-weighted image (*a*), small
hyperintense areas (arrows, *a*) likely represent foci of infection. The liver parenchyma shows increased enhancement of the right lobe
on the postgadolinium SGE images (*c, d*) due to thrombosis of the right portal vein (arrow, *d*) and consequent arterial hyperperfusion.
The thrombus (arrow, *d*) is best visualized as a near signal-void filling defect of the right portal vein on the 1-min postgadolinium
image (*d*). Increased enhancement of bile duct walls is demonstrated on the 1-min postgadolinium SGE images (arrow, *e*).

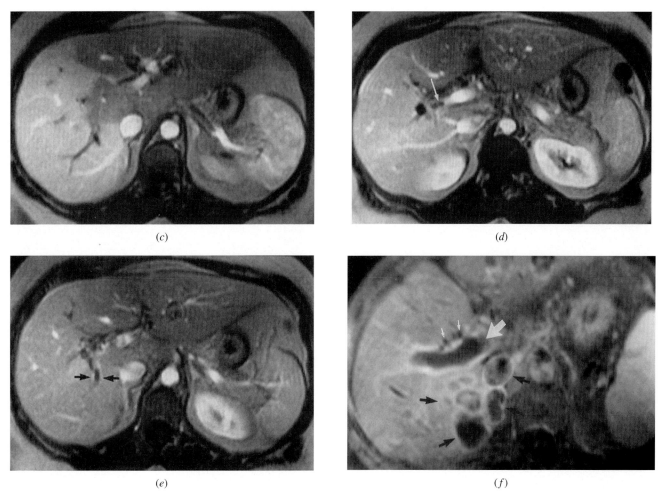

(c)

(d)

(e)

(f)

FIG. 3.35 (*Continued*) T1-weighted 2-min postgadolinium fat-suppressed SGE image (*f*) in a second patient. The portal vein (large white arrow, *f*) is dilated and shows lack of central enhancement with increased enhancement of the vessel walls, consistent with thrombosis. Several liver abscesses (black arrows, *f*) are visualized as round hypointense lesions with enhancing rims. Several bile ducts (small white arrows, *f*) are moderately dilated.

malignancy. A classification system that groups all types of biliary cystic diseases together has been introduced by Todani et al. [76]: Type I, choledochal cyst; Type II, diverticulum of extrahepatic ducts; Type III choledochocele; Type IV, multiple segmental cysts; Type V, Caroli disease. It is, however, unclear whether they represent variations of the same disease or they are separate entities with distinct etiologies. For clinical purposes, however, description of morphology and location is usually adequate.

Choledochal Cyst. The most common cystic dilatations are choledochal cysts (77–87%) that present before the age of 10 in approximately 50% of cases. Choledochal cysts are segmental aneurysmal dilatations of the CBD alone or the CBD and CHD (fig. 3.36). The etiology is an anomalous junction of the CBD and the pancreatic duct proximal to the major papilla, where there is no ductal sphincter. This allows a free reflux of pan-

creatic enzymes into the biliary system, weakening the walls of the bile ducts. Choledochal cysts are associated with an increased incidence of other biliary anomalies, gallstone disease, pancreatitis, and cholangiocarcinoma. Choledochal cysts may also be coexistent with intrahepatic bile duct cysts (multiple segmental cysts) (fig. 3.37).

Choledochocele. Choledochoceles are cystic dilatations of the distal CBD that herniate into the lumen of the duodenum and create a "cobra head" appearance on cholangiographic images (fig. 3.38).

Caroli Disease. Caroli disease is an uncommon form of congenital dilatations of intrahepatic bile ducts with normal extrahepatic ducts. Demonstration that these multiple cystic spaces communicate with the biliary tree is mandatory for the differentiation from cystic

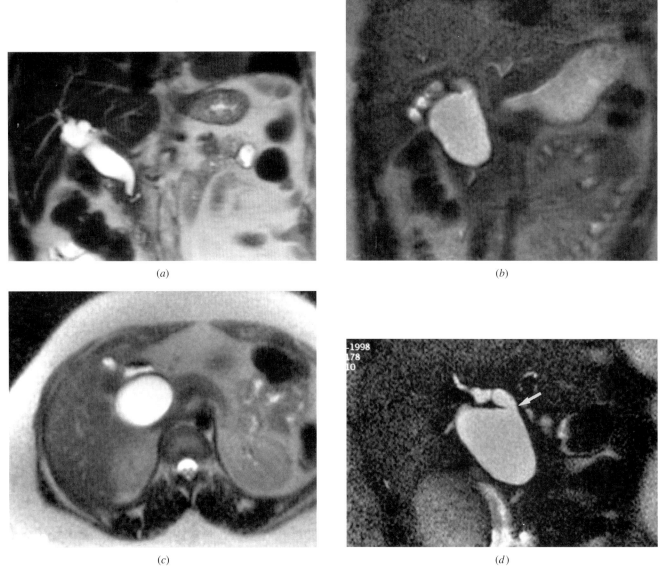

(a)

(b)

(c)

(d)

F I G. 3.36 Choledochal cyst. Coronal T2-weighted single-shot echo-train spin-echo image (*a*) showing a high-grade cylindrical dilatation of the CHD and CBD. The intrahepatic bile ducts are normal.

T2-weighted coronal (*b*) and transverse (*c*) single-shot echo-train spin-echo images and coronal thin-section MRCP single-shot echo-train spin-echo image with fat suppression (*d*) in a child demonstrating a saccular choledochal cyst arising from the CHD. The MRCP image (*d*) shows the origin of the choledochal cyst (arrow, *d*).

disease of the liver and abscesses. This can be best demonstrated with thin-section T2- or T1-weighted images, where Caroli disease presents with rounded cystic dilatations of equivalent signal intensity compared to bile (bright on T2- and low on T1-weighted images) communicating with bile ducts (fig. 3.39) [77].

Mass Lesions

Benign tumors that involve the biliary tract are relatively uncommon. Tumors can be solitary or multiple. Benign mass lesions can result in ductal obstruction and hepatic atrophy, possessing an imaging appearance comparable to malignant disease, as illustrated by a rare benign tumor, giant cell tumor of the bile duct (fig. 3.40).

Papillary adenomas of the biliary tract are rare benign epithelial tumors that have an increased risk for malignant transformation. Multiple small papillomas scattered throughout the biliary tree are characteristic of biliary papillomatosis. This condition is associated with an irregular pattern of intrahepatic bile duct dilatation caused by obstruction by the papillomas. These small tumors are best visualized on 2-min postgadolinium fat-suppressed SGE images as tiny enhancing mass lesions (fig. 3.41).

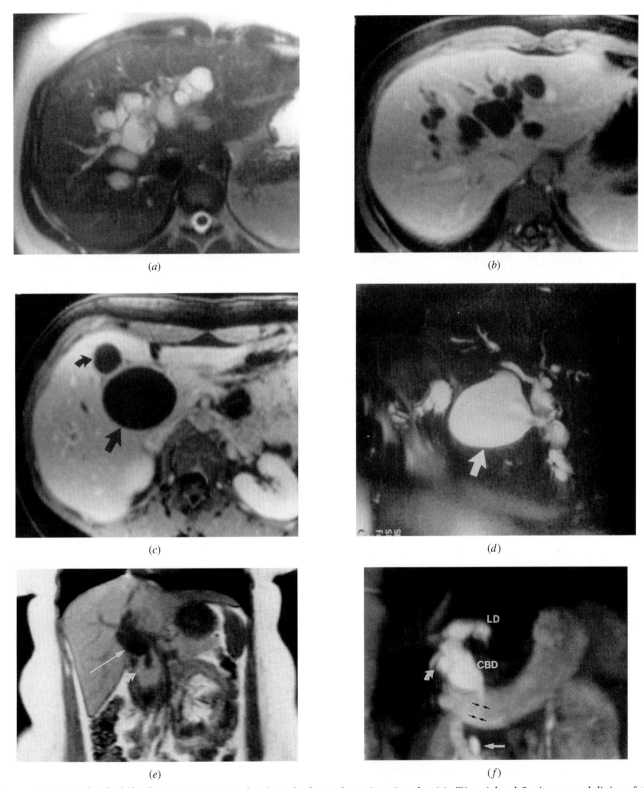

(a)

(b)

(c)

(d)

(e)

(f)

FIG. 3.37 Multiple bile duct cysts. T2-weighted single-shot echo-train spin-echo (*a*), T1-weighted 2-min postgadolinium fat-suppressed SGE (*b*, *c*) images, and coronal T2-weighted thin-section MRCP single-shot echo-train spin-echo image with fat suppression (*d*). Multiple intrahepatic bile duct cysts are demonstrated showing high signal on the T2-(*a*) and low signal on the T1-weighted (*b*) images. A large choledochal cyst (straight arrow, *c*, *d*) is revealed abutting the gallbladder (curved arrow, *c*). The MRCP image (*d*) nicely demonstrates the intra- and extrahepatic extent of biliary cystic disease.

Coronal T1-weighted SGE (*e*) and MRCP MIP reconstruction (*f*) images in a second patient. A cystic dilatation of the proximal CBD (long arrow, *e*) above the head of the pancreas (curved arrow, *e*) is appreciated on the SGE image (*e*). The left hepatic duct (LD, *f*) shown with high signal on the MRCP MIP image (*f*) also demonstrates fusiform dilatations. Cystic dilatations are also visualized in the cystic duct at its insertion into the CHD (curved arrow, *f*) and of the preampullary CBD (straight arrow, *f*). The mid-CBD (small arrows, *f*) is of normal caliber.

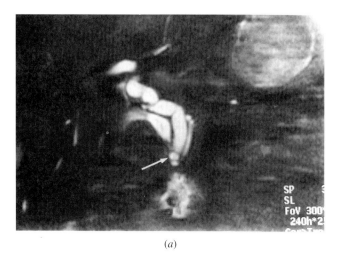

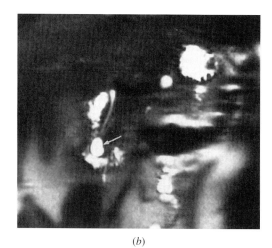

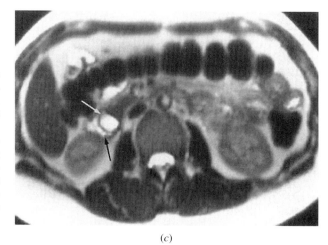

F I G . 3.38 Choledochocele. Coronal thin-section MRCP single-shot echo-train spin-echo image with fat suppression (*a*). The ampullary section of the CBD shows a small cystic dilatation (arrow, *a*) that protrudes into the lumen of the duodenum. The rest of the CBD is also dilated.

T2-weighted single-shot echo-train spin-echo images in the coronal plane with fat suppression (*b*) and the transverse plane without fat suppression (*c*) in a second patient. The CBD shows a cystic expansion (white arrows, *b*, *c*) of its ampullary section. The transverse image (*c*) demonstrates that the choledochocele (white arrows, *c*) bulges into the duodenum (black arrow, *c*), which contains high-signal intensity intraluminal fluid.

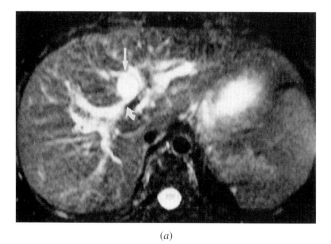

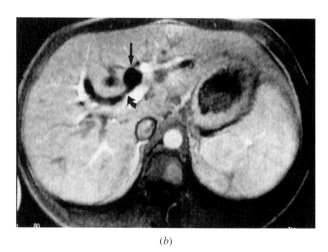

F I G . 3.39 Caroli disease. T2-weighted fat-suppressed spin-echo (*a*) and immediate postgadolinium SGE (*b*, *c*) images. Cystic intrahepatic biliary dilatation (straight arrows, *a*–*c*) is present in the left (*a*, *b*) and right (*c*) lobes of the liver.

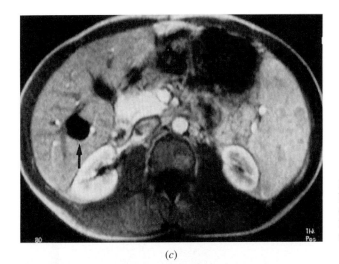

(c)

FIG. 3.39 (*Continued*) Differentiation from liver cysts is made by demonstration of continuity with a mildly dilated bile duct (curved arrow, *a*, *b*). Differentiation of bile ducts from portal vein branches is facilitated on the postgadolinium images (*b*, *c*), where the latter demonstrate enhancement.

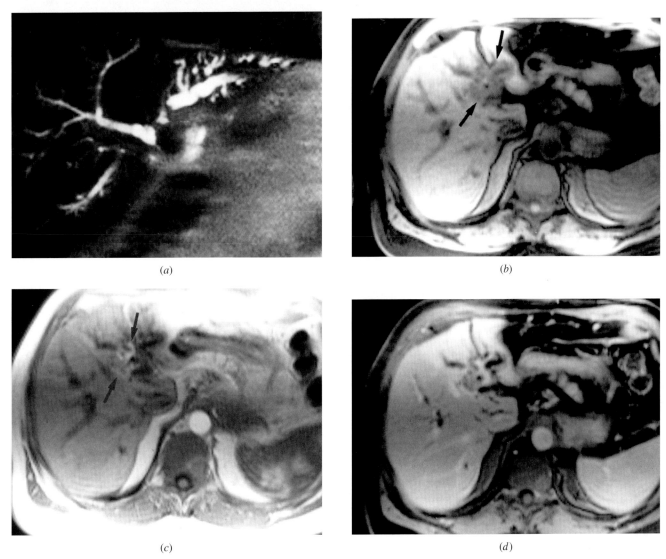

(a)

(b)

(c)

(d)

FIG. 3.40 Giant cell tumor of the bile duct. Coronal thin-section MRCP single-shot echo-train spin-echo image with fat suppression (*a*), transverse T1-weighted fat-suppressed SGE (*b*), immediate postgadolinium SGE (*c*), and 2-min postgadolinium fat-suppressed SGE (*d*) images. An obstruction at the confluence of the right and left main hepatic ducts is visualized on the MRCP image (*a*) with dilatation of the right and left intrahepatic biliary system. The tumor (arrow, *b*) appears moderately low signal intensity on the T1-weighted image (*b*). On the immediate postgadolinium image (*c*), the tumor demonstrates increased enhancement (arrow, *c*), with persistent enhancement on the 2-min postgadolinium image (*d*). The liver parenchyma distal to the tumor shows delayed increased enhancement (*d*). The tumor mimics the MRI appearance of Klatskin tumor but was diagnosed giant cell tumor of the left hepatic duct at histopathology.

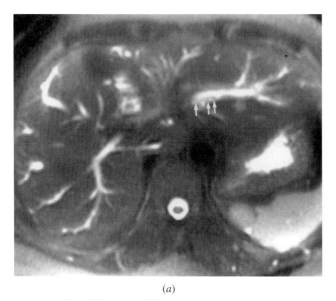
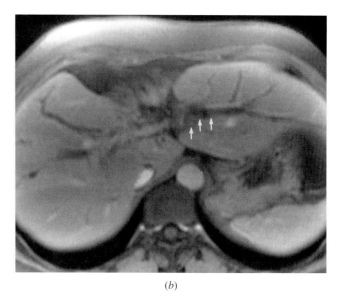

(a)   (b)

F I G . 3.41 Biliary papillomatosis. T2-weighted single-shot echo-train spin-echo (*a*) and T1-weighted 2-min postgadolinium fat-suppressed SGE (*b*) images. Several small, biliary intraductal, papillary tumors (arrows, *a, b*) are revealed showing enhancement on the postgadolinium image (*b*). The entire biliary tree is moderately dilated because of obstruction by papillomas in the CHD and CBD.

Postsurgical Biliary Complications

Benign biliary strictures are a sequel of surgical injury (e.g., laparoscopic cholecystectomy, gastric and hepatic resection, biliary-enteric anastomosis, biliary reconstruction after liver transplantation) in 90–95% of cases [78, 79]. The remainder are secondary to penetrating or blunt trauma, inflammation associated with gallstone disease, chronic pancreatitis, ampullary fibrosis, toxic or ischemic lesions of the hepatic artery, or primary infection. The advent of minimally invasive therapeutic procedures, performed by interventional radiology or endoscopy, have greatly increased the need for preoperative diagnosis and imaging to plan the optimal therapeutic approach. The major advantage of MRCP is the ability to visualize the biliary tree above and below a high-grade stricture or complete obstruction. The bile ducts distal to a stenosis, however, may be collapsed and nonvisualized on MIP reconstruction images leading to overestimation of the stricture. Thin-section source images must be used to evaluate the extent of high-grade stenoses, as even minimal amounts of fluid in collapsed ducts can be depicted on these images.

Other biliary complications of cholecystectomy are retained bile duct stones, biliary leak, and biliary fistula. In a study of such complications by Coakley et al. [80], two readers correctly categorized postsurgical complications in 88% and 76%, respectively. However, high-grade biliary stricture and transsection of bile ducts both presented as abrupt termination of a dilated duct, and, consequently, MRCP failed to distinguish between those entities but grouped them together as occlusion.

In patients with biliary-enteric anastomoses, ERCP often cannot be performed. MRCP, however, is very effective in visualizing the anatomy of the anastomosis, strictures of the anastomosis or of intrahepatic ducts, and biliary tract stones proximal to the anastomosis, in up to 100% of patients (figs. 3.9 and 3.41) [1, 81]. Close scrutiny of the thin-section source images is mandatory because the biliary-enteric anastomosis and stones can be obscured on thick-section and MIP reconstruction images by the high signal intensity of surrounding bile and bowel fluid (fig. 3.42). Metallic surgical clips and pneumobilia can also produce artifacts that should not be mistaken as stones or strictures.

MALIGNANT DISEASE

Cholangiocarcinoma

Cholangiocarcinomas are well-differentiated sclerosing adenocarcinomas in two-thirds of cases; the remainder are anaplastic, squamous cell, or cystadenocarcinomas. The most common predisposing diseases in Western countries are ulcerative colitis and sclerosing cholangitis. In Far Eastern countries, recurrent pyogenic cholangitis (caused by clonorchis sinensis infestation) is the most common cause. Other predisposing

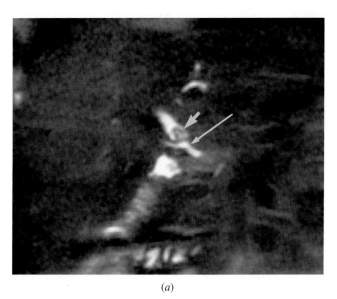 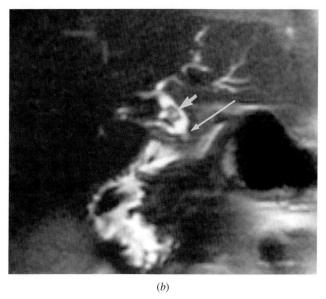

(a)   (b)

F I G . 3.42 MRCP after liver transplantation. Coronal thin-section MRCP single-shot echo-train spin-echo images with fat suppression (a, b). Slight narrowing of the anastomosis (long arrows, a, b) between the graft CBD and the host CBD is observed. A low-signal stone (short arrows, a, b) is visualized in the dilated graft CBD immediately proximal to the anastomosis.

factors are Caroli disease, choledochal cysts, α-1-antitrypsin deficiency, and autosomal dominant polycystic kidney disease. Cholangiocarcinoma is typically a malignancy of older patients (>50 years). Patients usually present with jaundice and weight loss. Three types of cholangiocarcinomas can be differentiated on the basis of anatomical distribution: the peripheral (or intrahepatic) type arising from peripheral bile ducts in the liver, the hilar type (Klatskin tumor) with its origin at the confluence of the right and left hepatic ducts, and the extrahepatic type arising from the CHD or CBD [82, 83].

The peripheral type constitutes approximately 10% of all cholangiocarcinomas and is the second most common primary liver tumor after hepatocellular carcinoma (HCC). Peripheral cholangiocarcinomas usually present as masslike lesions that do not obstruct the central bile ducts [84]. Therefore, they can obtain a large size and show intrahepatic metastases before they cause clinical symptoms. Their typical MR imaging appearance is a mass lesion that is mildly heterogeneous with moderately low signal intensity on T1-weighted images and mildly to moderately hyperintense signal on T2-weighted images (fig. 3.43) [69]. On immediate post-gadolinium images, they usually show mild to moderate enhancement that is usually diffuse heterogeneous in pattern. Progressive enhancement may be observed on late fat-suppressed images, reflecting a high content of fibrous tissue (fig. 3.43). This feature, if present, may suggest the type of tumor and differentiate it from

hepatocellular carcinoma, which typically shows intense diffuse heterogenous enhancement on immediate post-gadolinium images and wash-out on delayed images [85]. Additional features that help differentiate cholangiocarcinomas from HCC are lack of vascular invasion and rare occurrence of cholangiocarcinoma in cirrhotic livers [85]. Peripheral cholangiocarcinoma is also described in Chapter 2, *Liver*.

Klatskin tumors are usually small-volume superficial spreading tumors that result in early biliary obstruction and dilatation of proximal ducts (fig. 3.44). These tumors may uncommonly present as masslike lesions similar to peripheral tumors. Most often, they show circumferential growth and spread along bile ducts with poor conspicuity on noncontrast MR images (fig. 3.45). Biliary dilatation can involve one or both lobes of the liver, depending on the location of the tumor. Lobar atrophy of the liver combined with marked biliary dilatation should raise suspicion of cholangiocarcinoma (fig. 3.46), but this feature is not pathognomonic [86].

Extrahepatic cholangiocarcinomas usually grow in a circumferential pattern similar to Klatskin tumors. They arise in the CBD and result in biliary obstruction in the vast majority of patients. The imaging features of Klatskin tumors and extrahepatic cholangiocarcinomas at MRCP are dilatation of the proximal biliary tree with stricture or abrupt termination at the tumor, typically showing a shoulder sign (fig. 3.47) [87]. Irregularity of the ductal wall is indicative of infiltration

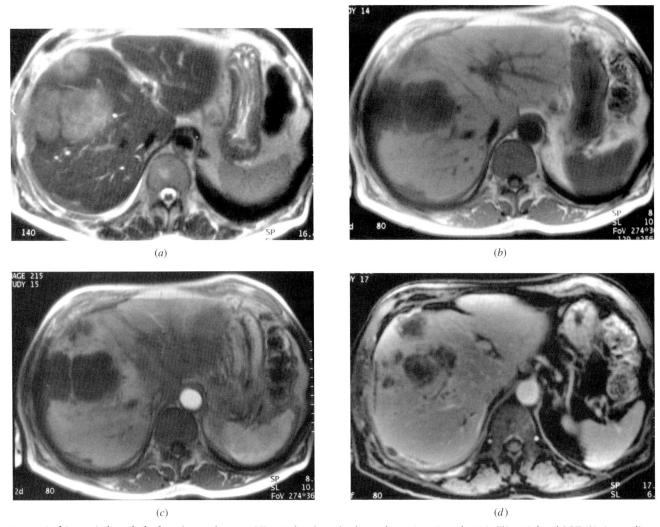

(a)　　　　　　　　　　　　(b)

(c)　　　　　　　　　　　　(d)

F I G . 3.43 Peripheral cholangiocarcinoma. T2-weighted single-shot echo-train spin-echo (*a*), T1-weighted SGE (*b*), immediate postgadolinium SGE (*c*), and 2-min postgadolinium fat-suppressed SGE (*d*) images. A large tumor with intrahepatic metastases is observed in the right lobe of the liver. The signal is moderately hyperintense on the T2-weighted image (*a*) and hypointense on the T1-weighted image (*b*). On the immediate postgadolinium image (*c*) the tumors are hypoenhancing and demonstrate mild perilesional enhancement. Progressive heterogeneous enhancement of the tumors is observed on the 2-min postgadolinium image (*d*).

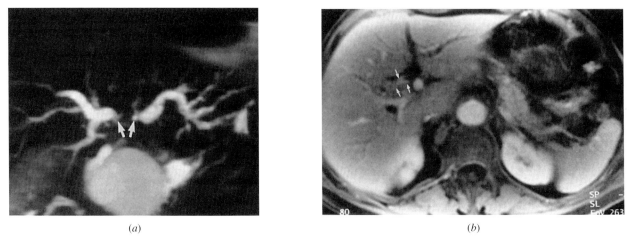

(a)　　　　　　　　　　　　(b)

F I G . 3.44 Klatskin tumor. Coronal MRCP MIP reconstruction (*a*), transverse T1-weighted 2-min postgadolinium fat-suppressed SGE (*b*), and ERCP (*c*) images. Obstruction of the right and left main hepatic ducts (arrows, *a*) at the level of the porta hepatis with dilatation of peripheral ducts is visualized on the MRCP image (*a*).

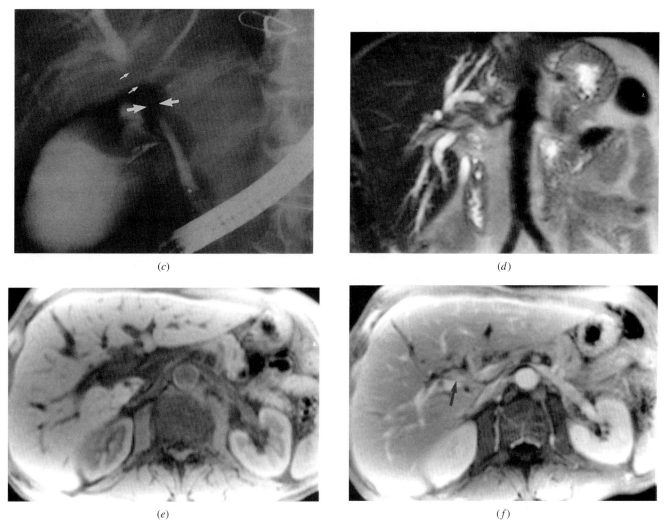

(c)

(d)

(e)

(f)

F IG. 3.44 (*Continued*) A small enhancing tumor (small arrows, *b*), measuring 4 mm in diameter, extends from the CHD into the right main hepatic duct, as shown on the postgadolinium image (*b*). ERCP (*c*) also shows the obstruction (arrows, *c*) at the level of the porta hepatis and the extension of the tumor into the right main hepatic duct (small arrows, *c*). Note the poor visualization of the left biliary ductal sytem on the ERCP image (*c*) because of underfilling.

Coronal T2-weighted single-shot echo-train spin-echo (*d*), transverse T1-weighted fat-suppressed SGE (*e*), and 2-min postgadolinium fat-suppressed SGE (*f*) images in a second patient. Dilatation of the right and left intrahepatic biliary tree is observed on the T2-weighted image (*d*). The tumor shows poor conspicuity on the precontrast SGE image (*e*). On the 2-min postgadolinium image (*f*), the small Klatskin tumor (arrow, *f*) in the porta hepatis demonstrates enhancement and can be well differentiated from surrounding structures.

and raises a high suspicion of malignancy. Occasionally, tumors can show intraluminal papillary growth presenting as a filling defect on MRCP images. ERCP may on occasion poorly evaluate tumors because of incomplete biliary opacification. An advantage of MRCP in combination with conventional MRI is that it can also visualize the biliary tree proximal to an occlusion, which often is not possible or advisable with ERCP, as well as detect distant disease such as liver metastases or lymph node involvement.

On T1-weighted MR images with or without fat suppression, cholangiocarcinomas appear mildly to moderately hypointense but may also be isointense relative to liver parenchyma. On T2-weighted images, they are isointense or mildly hyperintense (figs. 3.43–3.45) [85]. Thickening of bile duct walls greater than 5 mm is highly suggestive of cholangiocarcinoma [69]. However, this measurement is not sensitive, as at least 50% of tumors show thinner wall diameters [85]. The finding of relatively minor increase of wall thickness

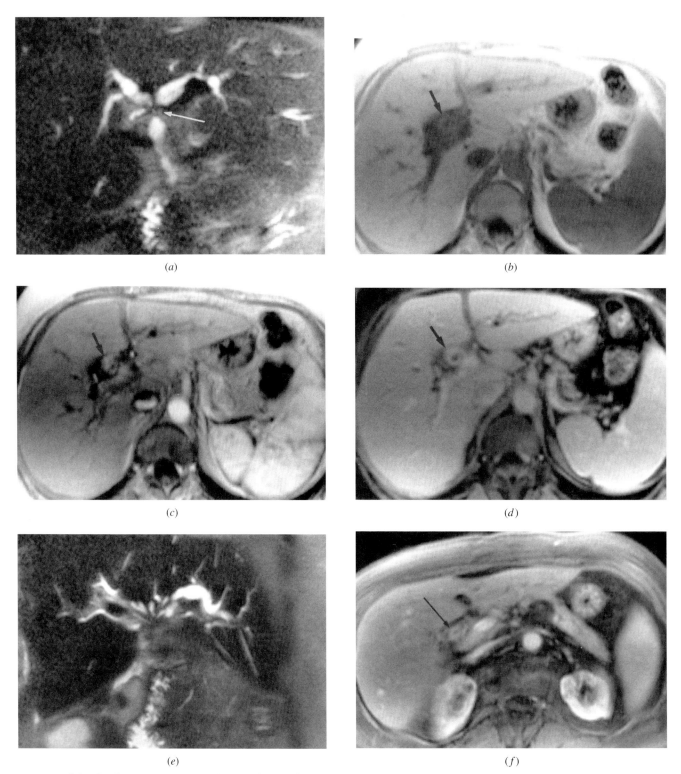

(a)

(b)

(c)

(d)

(e)

(f)

FIG. 3.45 Klatskin tumor, circumferential growth. Coronal T2-weighted thin-section MRCP single-shot echo-train spin-echo image with fat suppression (*a*), transverse T1-weighted SGE (*b*), immediate postgadolinium SGE (*c*), and 2-min postgadolinium fat-suppressed SGE (*d*) images. A short obstruction at the confluence of the right and left main hepatic ducts (arrow, *a*) is revealed on the MRCP image (*a*). It is difficult to delineate the tumor (arrow, *b*) from surrounding structures on the T1-weighted precontrast image (*b*). After gadolinium administration, the tumor shows intense enhancement (arrows, *c*, *d*) on the immediate (*c*) and late (*d*) postgadolinium images. Note the circumferential growth and small volume of the Klatskin tumor, best visualized on the postgadolinium images (*c*, *d*).

Coronal T2-weighted thin-section MRCP single-shot echo-train spin-echo image with fat suppression (*e*) and transverse T1-weighted 2-min postgadolinium fat-suppressed SGE image (*f*) in a second patient. The Klatskin tumor obstructs the intrahepatic biliary system at the porta hepatis, demonstrated on the MRCP image (*e*). The tumor shows circmferential growth in the CHD (arrow, *f*) and increased enhancement on the late postgadolinium image (*f*).

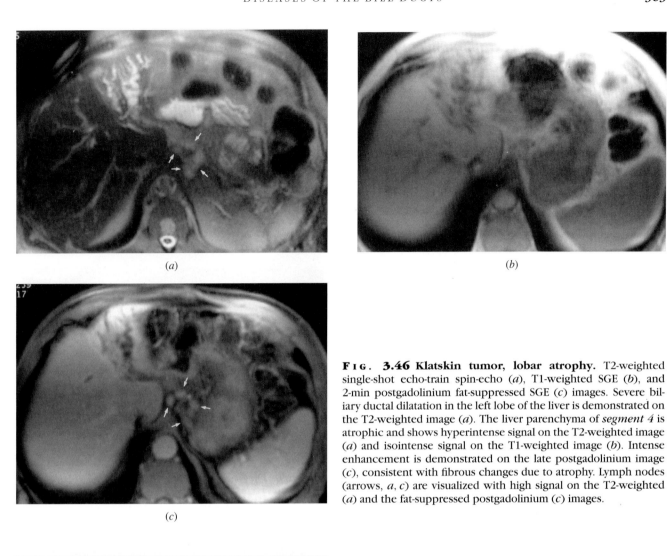

(a)

(b)

(c)

FIG. 3.46 Klatskin tumor, lobar atrophy. T2-weighted single-shot echo-train spin-echo (*a*), T1-weighted SGE (*b*), and 2-min postgadolinium fat-suppressed SGE (*c*) images. Severe biliary ductal dilatation in the left lobe of the liver is demonstrated on the T2-weighted image (*a*). The liver parenchyma of *segment 4* is atrophic and shows hyperintense signal on the T2-weighted image (*a*) and isointense signal on the T1-weighted image (*b*). Intense enhancement is demonstrated on the late postgadolinium image (*c*), consistent with fibrous changes due to atrophy. Lymph nodes (arrows, *a, c*) are visualized with high signal on the T2-weighted (*a*) and the fat-suppressed postgadolinium (*c*) images.

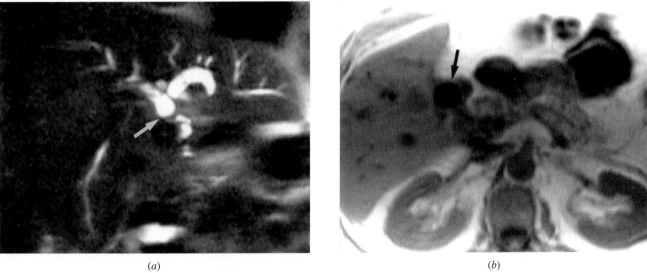

(a)

(b)

FIG. 3.47 Extrahepatic cholangiocarcinoma. Coronal T2-weighted thin-section MRCP single-shot echo-train spin-echo image with fat suppression (*a*), transverse T1-weighted SGE (*b*) and 2-minute postgadolinium fat-suppressed SGE (*c*) images.

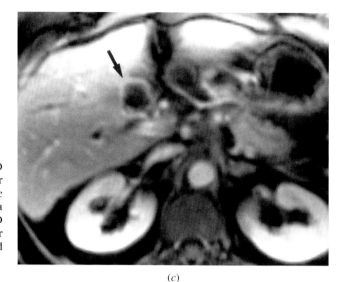

(c)

F I G . 3.47 (*Continued*) Obstruction of the proximal CBD (arrow, *a*) is present, showing an abrupt cut-off ("shoulder sign") on the MRCP image (*a*). The intrahepatic biliary tree is markedly dilated (*a*). The extrahepatic cholangiocarcinoma shows circumferential growth along the dilated proximal CBD (arrows, *b, c*). On the late postgadolinium image (*c*), the tumor shows intense enhancement (arrows, *c*) and can be differentiated from adjacent liver parenchyma.

(3–4 mm) in association with high-grade biliary obstruction is highly suggestive of cholangiocarcinoma in patients without a history of recent gallbladder surgery. On immediate postgadolinium images, cholangiocarcinomas are usually hypovascular, showing minimal or moderate enhancement that intensifies on delayed images (figs. 3.43–3.45) [85]. A combination of early and late fat-suppressed gadolinium-enhanced images is very helpful to identify these tumors. Fat suppression also reduces the signal of fatty tissue in the porta hepatis, which improves the conspicuity of cholangiocarcinomas and facilitates the evaluation of the extent of tumor and infiltration into adjacent tissues and organs.

Findings that indicate that a tumor is unresectable are vascular encasement and direct invasion of liver parenchyma. Most cholangiocarcinomas are unresectable at the time of initial diagnosis and can be treated only with palliative biliary drainage. Biliary stent placement results in mild inflammation of bile duct walls, which appears as increased gadolinium enhancement with an appearance indistinguishable from superficial spread of cholangiocarcinoma (fig. 3.48). If feasible, it is preferable to image patients suspected of biliary tumor before stent placement to avoid the problem of misstaging the tumor because of inflammatory changes secondary to the presence of the stent. Lymphadenopathy

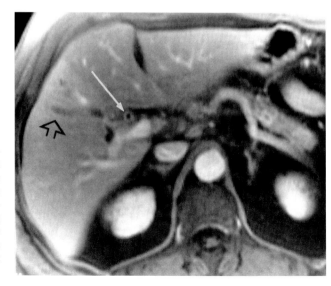

F I G . 3.48 Klatskin tumor and biliary stent. Transverse 2-min postgadolinium fat-suppressed SGE image. A biliary stent (arrow) is present in this patient with Klatskin tumor of the right hepatic duct. The bile duct walls around the stent show intense enhancement that makes differentiation between reactive inflammation caused by the stent placement and tumor spread along the bile duct impossible. *Segment 8* of the liver (open arrow) shows biliary dilatation with increased enhancement of bile duct walls and increased parenchymal enhancement, which may reflect inflammatory changes.

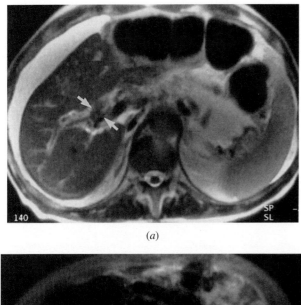

(a)

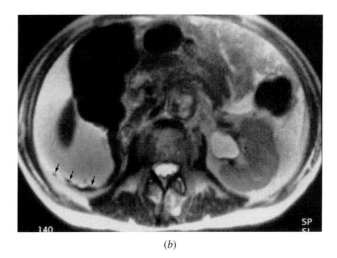

(b)

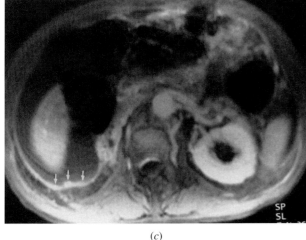

(c)

FIG. 3.49 Cholangiocarcinoma with peritoneal metastases. T2-weighted single-shot echo-train spin-echo (a, b) and 2-min postgadolinium fat-suppressed SGE (c) images. In the porta hepatis (a), a tumor (arrows, a) is shown that is isointense compared to liver. Ascites surrounding the liver is demonstrated with high signal on the T2-weighted (a, b) and low signal on the T1-weighted (c) images. More caudally (b, c), nodular peritoneal implants (arrows, b, c) are visualized, demonstrating intense enhancement on the 2-min postgadolinium fat-suppressed image (c).

with portocaval and porta hepatis nodes is an associated finding in up to 73% of patients with cholangiocarcinoma (fig. 3.46). This is best demonstrated using a combination of T2-weighted fat-suppressed and T1-weighted 2-min postgadolinium fat-suppressed images [85]. On these late postgadolinium images, fine tumor strands are frequently observed, and 5-mm or smaller lymph nodes are consistent with tumor extension, if three or more of them are clustered in the region of the tumor. In advanced cholangiocarcinoma, intraperitoneal tumor spread may occasionally be found and is also best seen on late postgadolinium fat-suppressed images (fig. 3.49).

Periampullary and Ampullary Carcinoma

Carcinomas arising from the ampulla of Vater, periampullary duodenum, or distal CBD are grouped together and termed periampullary carcinomas. Their presentation is similar to that of pancreatic head ductal adenocarcinoma including obstruction of both the CBD and pancreatic duct. The prognosis of periampullary carcinoma is significantly better than that of pancreatic carcinoma, with a 5-year survival rate up to 85% [88]. Periampullary carcinomas can cause ampullary obstruction and become clinically symptomatic even when they are only a few millimeters in size. Therefore, signs and symptoms of dilatation of the biliary tree and the pancreatic duct are observed relatively early in the course of these tumors, which likely accounts in part for their better prognosis. MRCP is very effective for the visualization of biliary and pancreatic ductal dilatation and the determination of the level of obstruction. On T1-weighted fat-suppressed images, periampullary carcinomas typically appear as low-signal intensity masses (fig. 3.50). Obstruction of the pancreatic duct eventually results in chronic pancreatitis. Chronic pancreatitis results in a reduced signal intensity of the pancreas on precontrast T1-weighted images, which diminishes the conspicuity

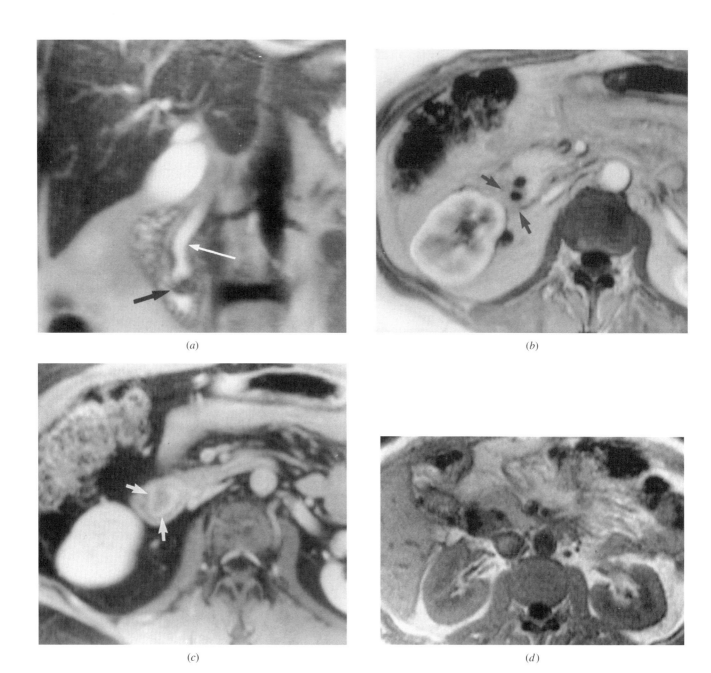

(a)

(b)

(c)

(d)

FIG. 3.50 Ampullary carcinoma. Coronal T2-weighted single-shot echo-train spin-echo (*a*), transverse T1-weighted immediate postgadolinium SGE (*b*), and 2-min postgadolinium fat-suppressed SGE (*c*) images. The ampullary carcinoma (black arrow, *a*) obstructs the CBD (white arrow, *a*), as visualized on the T2-weighted image (*a*). On the immediate postgadolinium image (*b*), the tumor (arrows, *b*) is hypoenhancing compared to normal pancreas and is well delineated. It surrounds the CBD completely and the pancreatic duct partially, which are both dilated and visualized as signal-void structures. Note the peripheral rim enhancement of the tumor (arrows, *c*) on the 2-min postgadolinium image (*c*) on a more inferior section where the tumor protrudes into the duodenum.

T1-weighted SGE (*d*) and immediate postgadolinium SGE (*e*) images in a second patient demonstrating a 2.5-cm ampullary carcinoma of low signal intensity, that shows good contrast against high-signal pancreas on the precontrast image (*d*). The tumor is hypoenhancing compared to pancreatic parenchyma (*e*), surrounds the distal CBD (straight arrow, *e*), and protrudes into the duodenum (curved arrow, *e*).

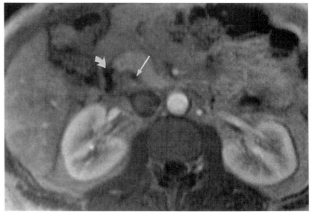

(e)

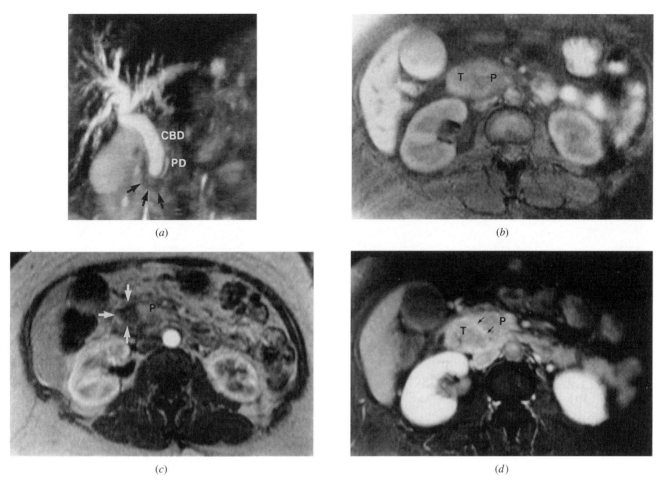

F I G . 3.51 Ampullary carcinoma. Coronal MRCP MIP reconstruction (*a*), T1-weighted fat-suppressed spin-echo (*b*), immediate postgadolinium SGE (*c*), and 2-min postgadolinium fat-suppressed spin-echo (*d*) images. On the MRCP image (*a*), an obstructing mass (arrows, *a*) is visualized at the level of the ampulla resulting in severe dilatation of the intra- and extrahepatic biliary system and moderate dilatation of the pancreatic duct. On the precontrast T1-weighted image (*b*), the tumor (T, *b*) cannot be differentiated from the pancreas (P, *b*), which shows abnormal low signal intensity due to pancreatitis. On the immediate postgadolinium image (*c*), the tumor (arrows, *c*) is well visualized, demonstrating decreased enhancement compared to pancreas. Note a peripheral rim of enhancement (arrows, *d*) of the tumor on the 2-min postgadolinium image (*d*). CBD, common bile duct; GB, gallbladder; PD, pancreatic duct.

of periampullary carcinomas on this sequence. On immediate postgadolinium T1-weighted images, pancreatic parenchyma enhances greater than tumor, even in presence of chronic pancreatitis. Periampullary carcinomas enhance minimally on early postgadolinium images because of their hypovascular character (figs. 3.50 and 3.51) [89]. On 2-min postgadolinium fat-suppressed images, a thin rim of enhancement is commonly observed along the periphery of these tumors, which may be a relatively specific finding (figs. 3.50 and 3.51) [5]. Combining MRCP techniques with T1-weighted precontrast fat-suppressed and immediate and 2-min postgadolinium sequences is a very effective approach for the noninvasive evaluation of biliary obstructions [90].

Periampullary carcinomas may arise in the setting of choledochocele, fostered by longstanding chronic inflammation. A sudden change in clinical status or sudden development of jaundice may indicate the presence of cancer even if the tumor volume is small (fig. 3.52).

Metastases to the Bile Ducts and Ampulla
Metastases to the bile ducts or ampulla may occur in rare instances. Breast cancer, melanoma, and lymphoma are the most common malignancies to do so. They result in biliary obstruction and resemble the appearance of primary tumors of the bile ducts and ampulla.

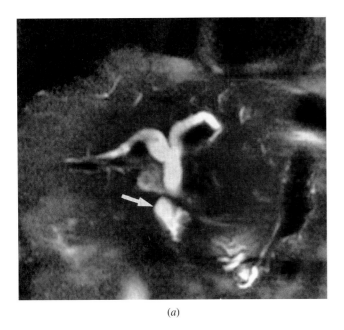

(a)

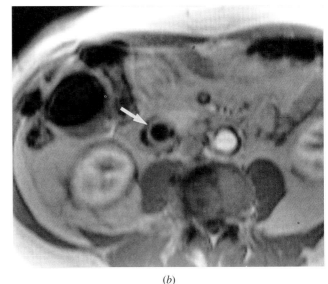

(b)

FIG. 3.52 Ampullary carcinoma superimposed on chole-dochocele. Coronal T2-weighted thin-section MRCP single-shot echo-train spin-echo image with fat suppression (*a*), transverse T1-weighted SGE (*b*), and 2-min postgadolinium fat-suppressed SGE (*c*) images in a patient with a choledochocele. The choledochocele (arrows, *a–c*) is visualized protruding into the duodenal lumen biliary obstruction with dilated intra- and extrahepatic ducts is observed on the MRCP image (*a*). The walls of the choledochocele are minimally thickened and show intense enhancement on the 2-min postgadolinium image (*c*). On surgical resection, this was found to represent cholangiocarcinoma in the wall of the choledochocele. This patient had sudden development of jaundice and abdominal pain. Sudden development of these symptoms in the absence of stone disease should raise clinical suspicion of malignancy.

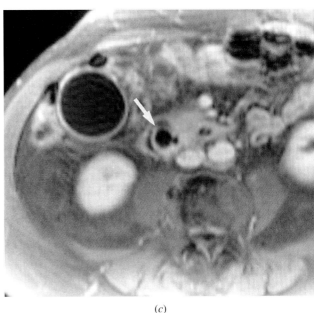

(c)

REFERENCES

1. Fulcher AS, Turner MA, Capps GW, Zfass AM, Baker KM: Half-Fourier RARE MR cholangiopancreatography: experience in 300 subjects. *Radiology* 207(1): 21–32, 1998.

2. Holzknecht N, Gauger J, Sackmann M, Thoeni RF, Schurig J, Holl J, Weinzierl M, Helmberger T, Paumgartner G, Reiser M: Breath-hold MR cholangiography with snapshot techniques: prospective comparison with endoscopic retrograde cholangiography. *Radiology* 206(3): 657–664, 1998.

3. Reinhold C, Taourel P, Bret PM, Cortas GA, Mehta SN, Barkun AN, Wang L, Tafazoli F. Choledocholithiasis: evaluation of MR cholangiography for diagnosis. *Radiology* 209(2): 435–442, 1998.

4. Guibaud L, Bret PM, Reinhold C, Atri M, Barkun AN: Bile duct obstruction and choledocholithiasis: Diagnosis with MR cholangiography. *Radiology* 197: 109–115, 1995.

5. Taourel P, Bret PM, Reinhold C, Barkun AN, Atri M: MR cholangiography of anatomical variants of the biliary tree. *Radiology* 199: 521–527, 1996.

6. Soto JA, Barish MA, Yucel EK, et al.: Pancreatic duct: MR cholangiopancreatography with a three-dimensional fast spin-echo technique. *Radiology* 196: 459–464, 1995.

7. Hirohashi S, Hirohashi R, Uchida H, et al.: Pancreatitis: evaluation with MR cholangiopancreatography in children. *Radiology* 203: 411–415, 1997.

8. Cohen SA, Siegel JH, Kasmin FE: Complications of diagnostic and therapeutic ERCP. *Abdom Imaging* 21: 385–394, 1996.

9. Rieger R, Wayand W: Yield of prospective, noninvasive evaluation of the common bile duct combined with selective ERCP/sphincterotomy in 1,930 consecutive laparoscopic cholecystectomy patients. *Gastrointest Endosc* 42: 6–12, 1995.

10. Soto JA, Yucel EK, Barish MA, Chuttani R, Ferrucci JT: MR cholangiopancreatography after unsuccessful or incomplete ERCP. *Radiology* 199: 91–98, 1996.

11. Ichikawa T, Nitatori T, Hachiya J, Mizutani Y: Breath-held MR cholangiopancreatography with half-averaged single shot hybrid rapid acquisition with relaxation enhancement sequence: Comparison of fast GRE and SE sequences. *J Comput Assist Tomogr* 20(5): 798–802, 1996.

12. Outwater EK: MR cholangiography with a fast-spin echo sequence (Abstract). *J Magn Reson Imaging* 3(P): 131, 1993.

13. Takehara Y, Ichijo K, Tooyama N, Kodaira N, Yamamoto H, Tatami M, Saito M, Watahiki H, Takahashi M: Breath-hold MR cholangiopancreatography with a long-echo-train fast spin-echo sequence and a surface coil in chronic pancreatitits. *Radiology* 192: 73–78, 1994.

14. Reinhold C, Guibaud L, Genin G, Bret PM: MR cholangiopancreatography: Comparison between two-dimensional fast spin-echo and three-dimensional gradient-echo pulse sequences. *J Magn Reson Imaging* 4: 379–384, 1995.

15. Hennig J, Nauerth A, Friedburg H: RARE imaging: a fast imaging method for clinical MR. *Magn Reson Med* 3: 823–833; 1986.

16. Kiefer B, Grassner J, Hausmann R: Image acquisition in a second with half-Fourier acquisition single shot turbo spin echo. *J Magn Reson Imag* 4(P): 86–87, 1994.

17. Regan F, Fradin J, Khazan R, Bohlmann M, Magnuson T: Choledocholithiasis: evaluation with MR cholangiography. *Am J Roentgenol* 167: 1441–1445, 1996.

18. Miyazaki T, Yamashita Y, Tsuchigame T, Yamamoto H, Urata J, Takahasi M: MR cholangiopancreatography using HASTE (half-fourier acquisition single-shot turbo spin-echo) sequences. *Am J Roentgenol* 166: 1297–1303, 1996.

19. Soto JA, Alvarez O, Munera F, Velez SM, Valencia J, Ramirez N: Diagnosing bile duct stones: Comparison of unenhanced helical CT, oral contrast-enhanced CT cholangiography, and MR cholangiography. *Am J Roentgenol* 175(4): 1127–1134, 2000.

20. Semelka RC, Shoenut JP, Greenberg HM, Mickflickier AB: The liver. In: Semelka RC, Shoenut JP (eds.). *MRI of the Abdomen with CT Correlation.* New York: Raven Press, p. 13–41, 1993.

21. Hamm B, Staks T, Muhler A, Bollow M, Taupitz M, Frenzel T, Wolf KJ, Weinmann HJ, Lange L: Phase I clinical evaluation of Gd-EOB-DTPA as a hepatobiliary MR contrast agent: Safety, pharmacokinetics, and MR imaging. *Radiology* 195: 785–792, 1995.

22. Vogl TJ, Hamm B, Schnell B, McMahon C, Branding G, Lissner J, Wolf KJ: Mn-DPDP enhancement patterns of hepatocellular lesions on MR images. *Magn Reson Imaging* 3: 51–58, 1993.

23. Demas BE, Hricak H, Moseley M, Wall SD, Moon K, Goldberg HI, Margulis AR: Gallbladder bile: An experimental study in dogs using MR imaging and proton MR spectroscopy. *Radiology* 157: 453–455, 1985.

24. Macaulay SE, Schulte SJ, Sekijima JH, Obregon RG, Simon HE, Rohrmann CA Jr, Freeny PC, Schmiedl UP: Evaluation of a nonbreath-hold MR cholangiography technique. *Radiology* 196: 227–232, 1995.

25. Strasberg SM, Hertl M, Soper NJ: An analysis of the problem of biliary surgery during laparoscopic cholecystectomy. *J Am Coll Surg* 180: 101–125, 1995.

26. Hirao K, Miyazaki A, Fujimoto T, Isomoto I, Hayashi K: Evaluation of aberrant bile ducts before laparoscopic cholecystectomy: helical CT cholangiography versus MR cholangiography. *Am J Roentgenol* 175(3): 713–720, 2000.

27. Soper NJ, Brunt LM: The case for routine operative cholangiography during laparoscopic cholecystectomy. *Surg Clin N Am* 74: 953–959, 1994.

28. Sterling JA: The common channel for bile and pancreatic ducts. *Surg Gynecol Obstet* 98: 420–424, 1954.

29. Taourel P, Reinhold C, Bret PM, Barkun AN, Atri M: Biliary and pancreatic ductal anatomy: Normal findings and variants demonstrated with MR cholangiopancreatography (Abstract). *RSNA* 197(P): 502, 1995.

30. Moeser PM, Julians, Karstaedt N, Sterchi M: Unusual presentation of cholelithiasis on T1-weighted MR imaging. *J Comput Assist Tomogr* 12: 150–152, 1988.

31. Baron RL, Shuman WP, Lee SP, Rohrmann CA Jr, Golden RN, Richards TL, Richardson ML, Nelson JA: MR appearance of gallstones in vitro at 1.5 T: Correlation with chemical composition. *Am J Roentgenol* 153: 497–502, 1989.

32. Dell LA, Brown MS, Orrison WW, Eckel CG, Matwiyoff NA: Physiologic intracranial calcification with hyperintensity on MR imaging: case report and experimental model. *Am J Neuroradiol* 9(6): 1145–1148, 1988.

33. Bangert BA, Modic MT, Ross JS, Obuchowski NA, Perl J, Ruggieri PM, Masaryk TJ: Hyperintense disks on T1-weighted MR images: correlation with calcification. *Radiology* 195(2): 437–443, 1995.

34. Hakansson K, Leander P, Ekberg O, Hakansson HO: MR imaging in clinically suspected acute cholecystitis. A comparison with ultrasonography. *Acta Radiol* 41(4): 322–328, 2000.

35. Loud PA, Semelka RC, Kettritz U, Brown JJ, Reinhold C: MRI of acute cholecystitis: Comparison with the normal gallbladder and other entities. *Magn Reson Imaging* 14(4): 349–355, 1996.

36. Semelka RC, Shoenut JP, Mickflickier AB: The gallbladder and biliary tree. In: Semelka RC, Shoenut JP (eds.). *MRI of the Abdomen with CT Correlation.* New York: Raven Press, p. 43–52, 1993.

37. Kelekis NL, Semelka RC. MR imaging of the gallbladder. *Top Magn Res Imaging* 8(5): 312–320, 1996.

38. Chun KA, Ha HK, Yu ES, Shinn KS, Kim KW, Lee DH, Kang SW, Auh YH: Xanthogranulomatous cholecystitis: CT features with emphasis on differentiation from gallbladder carcinoma. *Radiology* 203: 93–97, 1997.

39. Furuta A, Ishibashi T, Takahashi S, Sakamoto K: MR imaging of xanthogranulomatous cholecystitis. *Radiat Med* 14(6): 315–319, 1996.

40. Roa I, Araya JC, Villaseca M, De Aretxabala X, Riedemann P, Endoh K, Roa J: Preneoplastic lesions and gallbladder cancer: An estimate of the period required for progression. *Gastroenterology* 111: 232–236, 1996.

41. Chijiiwa K, Tanaka M: Polypoid lesion of the gallbladder: Indications of carcinoma and outcome after surgery for malignant polypoid lesion. *Int Surg* 79: 106–109, 1994.

42. Kubota K, Bandai Y, Noie T, Ishizaki Y, Teruya M, Makuuchi M: How should polypoid lesions of the gallbladder be treated in the era of laparoscopic cholecystectomy? *Surgery* 117: 481–487, 1995.

43. Yoshimitsu K, Honda H, Jimi M, Kuroiwa T, Hanada K, Irie H, Tajima T, Takashima M, Chijiiwa K, Shimada M, Masuda K: MR diagnosis of adenomyomatosis of the gallbladder and differentiation from gallbladder carcinoma: Importance of showing Rokitansky-Aschoff sinuses. *Am J Roentgenol* 172(6): 1535–1540, 1999.

44. Kim MJ, Oh YT, Park YN, Chung JB, Kim DJ, Chung JJ, Mitchell DG: Gallbladder adenomyomatosis: Findings on MRI. *Abdom Imaging* 24(4): 410–413, 1999.

45. Rooholamini SA, Tehrani NS, Razavi MK, Au AH, Hansen GC, Ostrzega N, Verma RC: Imaging of gallbladder carcinoma. *Radiographics* 14: 291–306, 1994.

46. Towfigh S, MCfadden DW, Cortina GR, Thompson JE, Tompkins RK, Chandler C, Hines OJ. Porcelain gallbladder is not associated with gallbladder carcinoma. *Am Surg* 67(1): 7–10, 2001.

47. Roa I, Araya JC, Villaseca M, Roa J, de Aretxabala X, Ibacache G: Gallbladder cancer in a high risk area: Morphological features and spread patterns. *Hepatogastroenterology* 46(27): 1540–1546, 1999.

48. Sagoh T, Itoh K, Togashi K, Shibata T, Minami S, Noma S, Yamashita K, Nishimura K, Asato R, Mori K, Nishikawa T, Kakano Y, Konishi J: Gallbladder carcinoma: Evaluation with MR imaging. *Radiology* 174: 131–136, 1990.

49. Rossman MD, Friedman AC, Radecki PD, Caroline DF: MR imaging of gallbladder carcinoma. *Am J Roentgenol* 148: 143–144, 1987.

50. Demachi H, Matsui O, Hoshiba K, Kimura M, Miyata S, Kuroda Y, Konishi K, Tsuji M, Miwa A: Dynamic MRI using a surface coil in chronic cholecystitis and gallbladder carcinoma: Radiologic and histopathologic correlation. *J Comput Assist Tomogr* 21(4): 643–651, 1997.

51. Panasen P, Partanen K, Pikkarainen P, Alhava E, Pirinen A, Janatuinen E: Ultrasonography, CT, and ERCP in the diagnosis of choledochal stones. *Acta Radiol* 33: 53–56, 1992.

52. O'Connor HJ, Hamilton I, Ellis WR, Watters J, Lintott DJ, Axon AT: Ultrasound detection of choledocholithiasis: Prospective comparison with ERCP in the postcholecystectomy patient. *Gastrointest Radiol* 11: 161–164, 1986.

53. Cronan JJ: US diagnosis of choledocholithiasis: A reappraisal. *Radiology* 161: 133–134, 1986.

54. Stott MA, Farrand PA, Guyer PB, Dewbury KC, Browning JJ, Sutton R: Ultrasound of the common bile duct in patients undergoing cholecystectomy. *J Clin Ultrasound* 19: 73–76, 1991.

55. Cotton PB, Lehman G, Vennes J, Geenen JE, Russell RCG, Meyers WC, Liguory C, Nicki N: Endoscopic sphincterotomy complications and their management: An attempt at consensus. *Gastrointest Endosc* 37(3): 383–393, 1991.

56. Cohen SA, Kasim FE, Rutkovsky FD, et al.: Endoscopic sphincterotomy techniques and complications. *Am J Gastroenterol* 87: 1282, 1992.

57. Mehta SN, Pavone E, Barkun AN. Outpatient therapeutic ERCP: a series of 262 consecutive cases. *Gastrointest Endosc* 44(4): 443–449, 1996.

58. Duncan HD, Hodgkinson L, Deakin M, Green JR: The safety of diagnostic and therapeutic ERCP as a daycase procedure with a selective admission policy. *Eur J Gastroenterol Hepatol* 9(9): 905–908, 1997.

59. Loperfido S, Angelini G, Benedetti G, Chilovi F, Costan F, De Berardinis F, De Bernardin M, Ederle A, Fina P, Fratton A: Major early complications from diagnostic and therapeutic ERCP: A prospective multicenter study. *Gastrointest Endosc* 48(1): 1–10, 1998.

60. Holzknecht N, Gauger J, Sackmann M, Thoeni RF, Schurig J, Holl J, Weinzierl M, Helmberger T, Paumgartner G, Reiser M: Breath-hold MR cholangiography with snapshot techniques: prospective comparison with endoscopic retrograde cholangiography. *Radiology* 206(3): 657–664, 1998.

61. Soto JA, Barish MA, Alvarez O, Medina S. Detection of choledocholithiasis with MR cholangiography: Comparison of three-dimensional fast spin-echo and single- and multisection half-Fourier rapid acquisition with relaxation enhancement sequences. *Radiology* 215(3): 737–745, 2000.

62. Irie H, Honda H, Kuroiwa T, Yoshimitsu K, Aibe H, Shinozaki K, Masuda K: Pitfalls in MR cholangiopancreatographic interpretation. *RadioGraphics* 21: 23–37, 2001.

63. Takehara Y: Fast MR imaging for evaluating the pancreaticobiliary system. *Eur J Radiol* 29: 211–232, 1999.

64. Sherlock S: Pathogenesis of sclerosing cholangitis: The role of non-immune factors. *Semin Liver Dis* 11(1): 5–10, 1991.

65. Lee YM, Kaplan MM: Primary sclerosing cholangitis. *N Engl J Med* 332: 924–932, 1995.

66. Beuers U, Spengler U, Sackmann M, Paumgartner G, Sauerbruch T: Deterioration of cholestasis after endoscopic retrograde cholangiography in advanced primary sclerosing cholangitis. *J Hepatol* 15: 140–143, 1992.

67. Ernst O, Asselah T, Sergent G, et al.: MR cholangiography in primary sclerosing cholangitis. *Am J Roentgenol* 171: 1027–1030, 1998.

68. Fulcher AS, Turner MA, Franklin KJ, Shiffman ML, Sterling RK, Luketic VA, Sanyal AJ: Primary sclerosing cholangitis: evaluation with MR cholangiography—a case-control study. *Radiology* 215(1): 71–80, 2000.

69. Semelka RC, Shoenut JP, Kroeker MA, Hricak H, Minuk GY, Yaffe CS, Micflikier AB: Bile duct disease: Prospective comparison of ERCP, CT, and fat suppression MRI. *Gastrointest Radiol* 17: 347–352, 1992.

70. Revelon G, Rashid A, Kawamoto S, Bluemke DA. Primary sclerosing cholangitis: MR imaging findings with pathologic correlation. *Am J Roentgenol* 173(4): 1037–1042, 1999.

71. Ito K, Mitchell DG, Outwater EK, Blasbalg R: Primary sclerosing cholangitis: MR imaging features. *Am J Roentgenol* 172(6): 1527–1533, 1999.

72. LaRusso NF, Wiesner RH, Ludwig J, MacCarty RL: Current concepts. Primary sclerosing cholangitis. *N Engl J Med* 310: 899–903, 1984.

73. Balthazar EJ, Birnbaum BA, Naidich M: Acute cholangitis: CT evaluation. J Comput Assist Tomogr 17(2): 283–289, 1993.

74. Kim MJ, Cha SW, Mitchell DG, Chung JJ, Park S, Chung JB: MR imaging findings in recurrent pyogenic cholangitis. *Am J Roentgenol* 173(6): 1545–1549, 1999.

75. Miller FH, Gore RM, Nemcek AA Jr, Fitzgerald SW: Pancreaticobiliary manifestations of AIDS. *Am J Roentgenol* 166(6): 1269–1274, 1996.

76. Todani T, Watanabe Y, Narusue M, Tabuchi K, Okajima K: Congenital bile duct cysts: Classification, operative procedures, and review of thirty-seven cases including cancer arising from choledochal cyst. *Am J Surg* 134(2): 263–269, 1977.

77. Pavone P, Laghi A, Catalano C, Materia A, Basso N, Passariello R: Caroli's disease: evaluation with MR cholangiopancreatography (MRCP). *Abdom Imaging* 21: 117–119, 1996.

78. Lillemoe KD, Pitt HA, Cameron JL: Current management of benign bile duct strictures. *Adv Surg* 25: 119–173, 1992.

79. Laghi A, Pavone P, Catalano C, Rossi M, Panebianco V, Alfani D, Passariello R: MR cholangiography of late biliary complications after liver transplantation. *Am J Roentgenol* 172(6): 1541–1546, 1999.

80. Coakley FV, Schwartz LH, Blumgart LH, Fong Y, Jarnagin WR, Panicek DM. Complex post-cholecystectomy biliary disorders: Preliminary experience with evaluation by breath-hold MR cholangiography. *Radiology* 209: 141–146, 1998.

81. Pavone P, Laghi A, Catalano C, Broglia L, Panebianco V, Messina A, Salvatori FM, Passariello R: MR cholangiography in the examination of patients with biliary-enteric anastomoses. *Am J Roentgenol* 169(3): 807–811, 1997.

82. Soyer P, Bluemke DA, Reichle R, Calhoun PS, Bliss DF, Scherrer A, Fishman EK: Imaging of intrahepatic cholangiocarcinoma. 1. Peripheral cholangiocarcinoma. *Am J Roentgenol* 165: 1427–1431, 1995.

83. Soyer P, Bluemke DA, Reichle R, Calhoun PS, Bliss DF, Scherrer A, Fishman EK: Imaging of intrahepatic cholangiocarcinoma. 2. Hilar cholangiocarcinoma. *Am J Roentgenol* 165: 1433–1436, 1995.

84. Hamrick-Turner J, Abbitt PL, Ros PR: Intrahepatic cholangiocarcinoma: MR appearance. *Am J Roentgenol* 158: 77–79, 1992.

85. Worawattanakul S, Semelka RC, Noone TC, Calvo BF, Kelekis NL, Woosley JT: Cholangiocarcinoma: Spectrum of appearances on MR images using current techniques. *Magn Reson Imaging* 16(9): 993–1003, 1998.

86. Soyer P: Capsular retraction of the liver in malignant tumor of the biliary tract: MRI findings. *Clin Imaging* 18: 255–257, 1994.

87. Fulcher AS, Turner MA: HASTE MR cholagiography in the evaluation of hilar cholangiocarcinoma. *Am J Roentgenol* 169: 1501–1505, 1997.

88. Yamaguchi K, Enjoji M: Carcinoma of the ampulla of Vater: A clinicopathologic study and pathologic staging of 109 cases of carcinoma and 5 cases of adenoma. *Cancer* 59: 506–515, 1987.

89. Semelka RC, Kelekis NL, John G, Ascher SM, Burdeny DA, Siegelman ES: Ampullary carcinoma: demonstration by current MR techniques. *J Magn–Reson Imaging* 7: 153–156, 1997.

90. Pavone P, Laghi A, Passariello R: MR cholangiopancreatography in malignant biliary obstruction. *Semin Ultrasound CT MR* 20(5): 317–323, 1999.

PANCREAS

RICHARD C. SEMELKA, M.D., LARISSA L. NAGASE, M.D.,
DIANE ARMAO, M.D., AND N. CEM BALCI, M.D.

That sweetbread gazing up at me
Is not what it purports to be.
Says Webster in one paragraph,
It is the pancreas of a calf.
Since it is neither sweet nor bread,
I think I'll take a bun instead.
Ode to sweet bread
Ogden Nash

The pancreas, meaning "all flesh", was probably named by early Greek anatomists circa 300 BC. To the ancient Greeks, the term "flesh" referred to animal meat used as food and suggests the possibility that the pancreas, still today one of the organs prized as "sweet bread", may have been a delicacy.

NORMAL ANATOMY

The pancreas is a soft, fleshy, lobulated gland located retroperitoneally against the posterior body wall. The anatomic divisions of the pancreas include the head, uncinate process, neck, body, and tail. The broad head is embraced by the curve of the duodenum. An extension of the head, the uncinate process hooks behind the superior mesenteric artery and vein. The border between the head and body is a slightly narrowed region, the neck. On the posterior aspect of the neck is a shallow groove marking the passage of the superior mesenteric vein and the beginning of the portal vein. The body is oriented in an oblique fashion extending to the left of midline, and the tail is located in the region of the splenic hilum. The anatomic relationship of the head of the pancreas includes the second portion of the duodenumv laterally, the gastroduodenal artery anteriorly, the inferior vena cava posterolaterally, the third portion of the duodenum posteroinferiorly, and the superior mesenteric vessels medially.

The splenic vein lies along the posterior surface of the body and tail of the pancreas. This constant relationship is an important landmark for the identification of the pancreatic body. The left adrenal gland is seated posterior to the splenic vein. The tail of the pancreas often drapes over the left kidney and terminates in the splenic hilum. The tail may be folded anteriorly over the body of the pancreas. The stomach lies anterior to the pancreas and is separated from it by parietal peritoneum and the lesser sac. The transverse mesocolon forms the inferior boundary of the lesser sac and is formed by the fusion of leaves of the parietal peritoneum, which covers the anterior surface of the pancreas. The lesser sac and transverse mesocolon are common pathways for the tracking and accumulation of fluid in acute pancreatitis.

In elderly patients, fatty replacement of the pancreas occurs frequently as a normal degenerative process and results in a feathery, lobulated appearance on imaging. The posterior aspect of the pancreas does not have a serosal covering, which accounts for the extensive dissemination of fluid in pancreatitis and the early spread of pancreatic ductal cancer into retroperitoneal fat.

The pancreatic duct measures 1–2 mm in diameter in normal subjects. Although considerable variation in the size of the head occurs, the normal pancreatic head is 2–2.5 cm in diameter, with the remainder of the gland approximately 1–2 cm thick. The main pancreatic duct extends from the tail of the pancreas through the head and empties via the sphincter of Oddi into the second part of the duodenum at the major papilla. The main duct is termed the duct of Wirsung. A smaller accessory duct, the duct of Santorini, is frequently present and extends from the body of the pancreas through the neck and enters separately into the duodenum in a more proximal location at the minor papilla.

The pancreas is a mixed exocrine and endocrine gland. The main mass of pancreatic microstructure is exocrine in nature, composed of acinar cells, which store and release digestive enzymes. Embedded in acinar tissue are small, scattered islets of Langerhans composed of endocrine cells that synthesize hormones.

The major hormones released by the pancreas are insulin and glucagon.

MRI TECHNIQUE

New MRI techniques that limit artifacts in the abdomen have increased the role of MRI in detection and characterization of pancreatic disease. Breath-hold spoiled gradient-echo (SGE) techniques, fat suppression techniques, and dynamic administration of gadolinium chelate have resulted in image quality of the pancreas sufficient to detect and characterize focal pancreatic mass lesions smaller than 1 cm in diameter, and to evaluate diffuse pancreatic disease [1–4].

MR cholangiopancreatography (MRCP) permits good demonstration of the biliary and pancreatic ducts to assess ductal obstruction, dilatation, and abnormal duct pathways [5–7]. The combination of tissue-imaging sequences and MRCP provides comprehensive information to evaluate the full range of pancreatic disease.

MRI of the pancreas is optimal at high field (≥1.0 T) because of a good signal-to-noise (S/N) ratio, which facilitates breath-hold imaging, and increased fat-water frequency shift, which facilitates chemically selective excitation-spoiling fat suppression. T1-weighted chemically selective fat suppression and T1-weighted breath-hold SGE are effective techniques for imaging pancreatic parenchyma. The normal pancreas is high in signal intensity (SI) on T1-weighted fat-suppressed images because of the presence of aqueous protein in the acini of the pancreas [1]. Normal pancreas is well shown using this technique (fig. 4.1) [8, 9]. In elderly patients, the signal intensity of the pancreas may diminish and be lower than that of liver [2]. This may reflect changes of fibrosis secondary to the aging process.

Our standard MR protocol includes T1-weighted fat-suppressed imaging (either SGE or spin-echo), SGE, and postgadolinium imaging in the capillary phase (immediate postcontrast) and the interstitial phase (1–10 min postcontrast) [4]. T2-weighted single-shot echo-train spin-echo sequences such as T2-weighted half-Fourier acquisition snapshot turbo spin-echo (HASTE) provide a sharp anatomic display of the common bile duct (CBD) on coronal plane images and of the pancreatic duct on transverse plane images. MRCP images can be acquired oriented in the plane of the pancreatic duct, in an oblique coronal projection, to delineate longer segments of the pancreatic duct in continuity [10]. T2-weighted fat-suppressed images are useful for demonstrating liver metastases and islet cell tumors. T2-weighted images also provide information on the complexity of the fluid in pancreatic pseudocysts, which may reflect the presence of complications such as necrotic debris or infection. Regarding gadolinium enhancement, the pancreas demonstrates a uniform capillary blush on immediate postcontrast images, which renders it higher in signal intensity than liver, neighboring bowel, and adjacent fat (fig. 4.2) [4]. By 1 min after contrast, the pancreas becomes approximately isointense with fat, and beyond 2 min the pancreas is lower in signal intensity than background fat. Pancreatic head is readily distinguished from duodenum on immediate postgadolinium images because the pancreas enhances substantially greater than bowel (fig. 4.2). MRI combining T1, T2, early and late postgadolinium images, MRCP, and MRA generate comprehensive information on the pancreas [11].

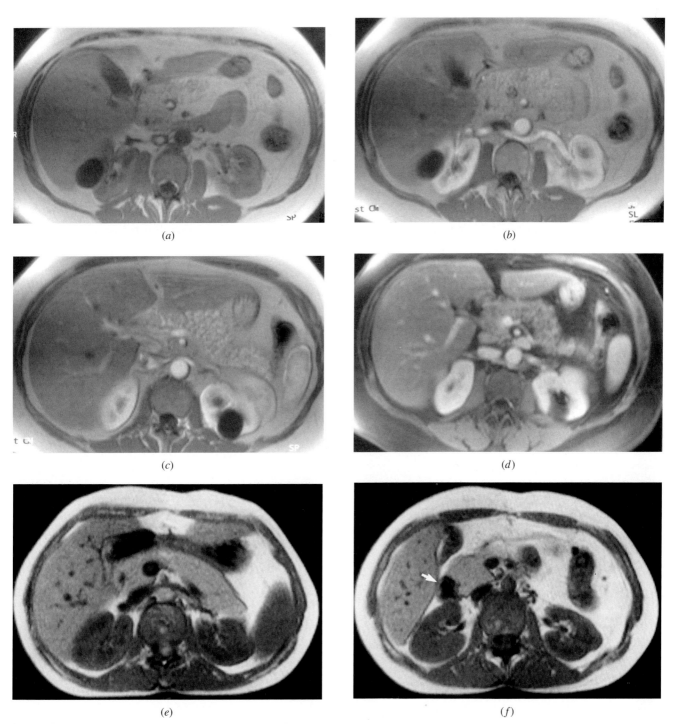

F I G . 4.1 Normal pancreas. T1-weighted SGE (*a*), immediate postgadolinium T1-weighted SGE (*b*, *c*), and 90-s postgadolinium fat-suppressed SGE (*d*) images. The pancreas has a marbled appearance, which is a normal finding associated with aging.

T1-weighted SGE (*e*, *f*), T1-weighted fat-suppressed spin-echo (*g*, *h*), and immediate postgadolinium T1-weighted SGE images (*i*, *j*) in a second patient. Images of the pancreatic body (*e*, *g*, *i*) and head (*f*, *h*, *j*) illustrate the appearance of normal pancreas. Lack of breathing artifact renders the pancreas well shown on T1-weighted SGE images (*e*, *f*). The normal pancreas is high in signal intensity on T1-weighted fat-suppressed images (*g*, *h*) because of the presence of aqueous protein in the acini of the pancreas. A uniform capillary blush is apparent on the immediate postgadolinium images (*i*, *j*). The head of the pancreas is clearly distinguishable from duodenum (arrow, *f*, *h*, *j*). Small bowel has a feathery appearance and is moderate in signal intensity on T1-weighted fat-suppressed images (long arrow, *h*), which is clearly different from the homogeneous or marbled high signal intensity of the pancreas.

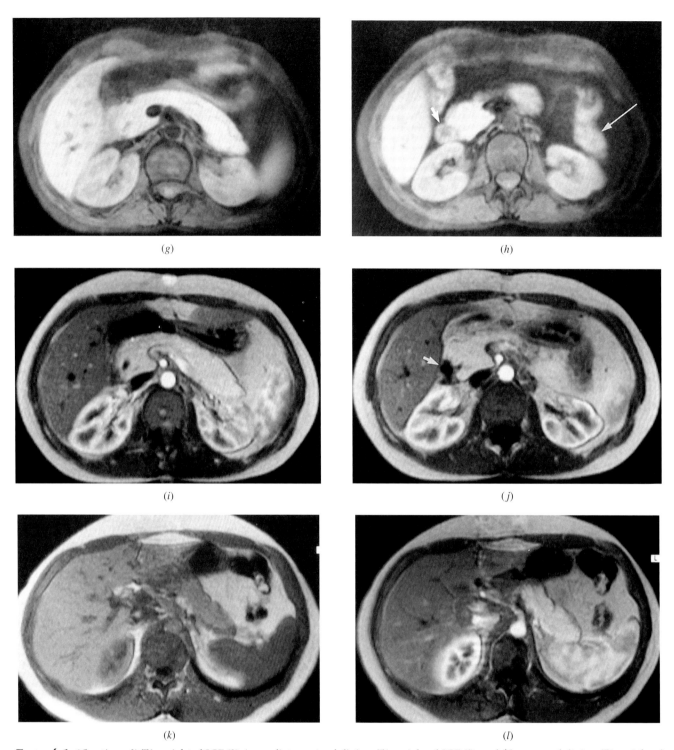

(g)   *(h)*

(i)   *(j)*

(k)   *(l)*

F i g . 4.1 (*Continued*) T1-weighted SGE (*k*), immediate postgadolinium T1-weighted SGE (*l*), and 45-s postgadolinium T1-weighted SGE (*m*) images in a third patient. Normal pancreas has lower signal intensity than background fat on T1-weighted images (*k*), enhances with a uniform capillary blush resulting in a signal intensity greater than background fat on immediate postgadolinium images (*l*), and fades in signal intensity to isointense with background fat by 45 s (*m*).

Immediate postgadolinium images through the mid- (*n*) and inferior (*o*) pancreatic head in a fourth patient. Enhancement of the pancreas is more intense than that of normal bowel on immediate postgadolinium images. The inferior aspect of the pancreatic head (small arrow, *o*) can be distinguished from lesser-enhancing adjacent duodenum (long arrows, *o*).

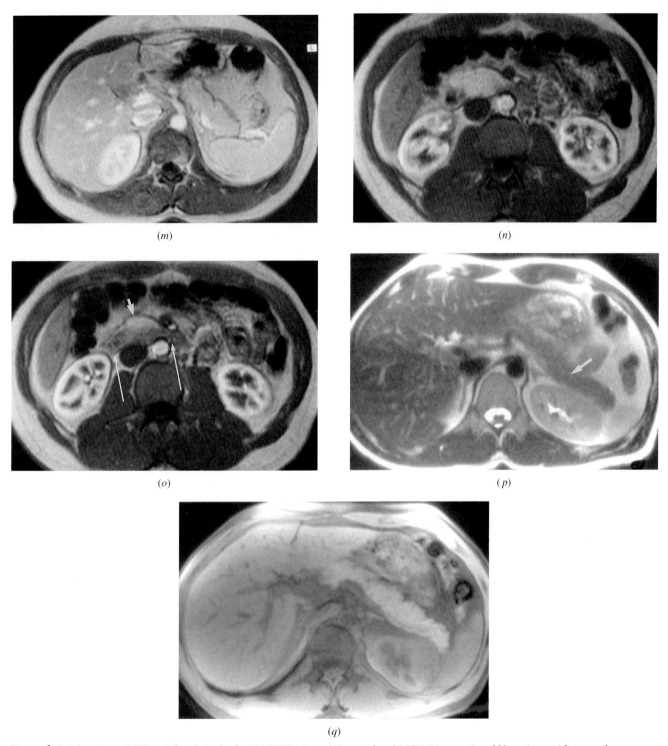

(m)

(n)

(o)

(p)

(q)

F I G . 4.1 *(Continued)* T2-weighted single-shot SS-ETSE (*p*) and T1-weighted SGE (*q*) images in a fifth patient with normal pancreas. The pancreatic body and tail show lobulated and well-delineated contour, and the parenchyma has homogeneous signal intensity. Note that the normal caliber pancreatic duct is well shown (arrow, *p*) on the breathing-independent T2-weighted sequence.

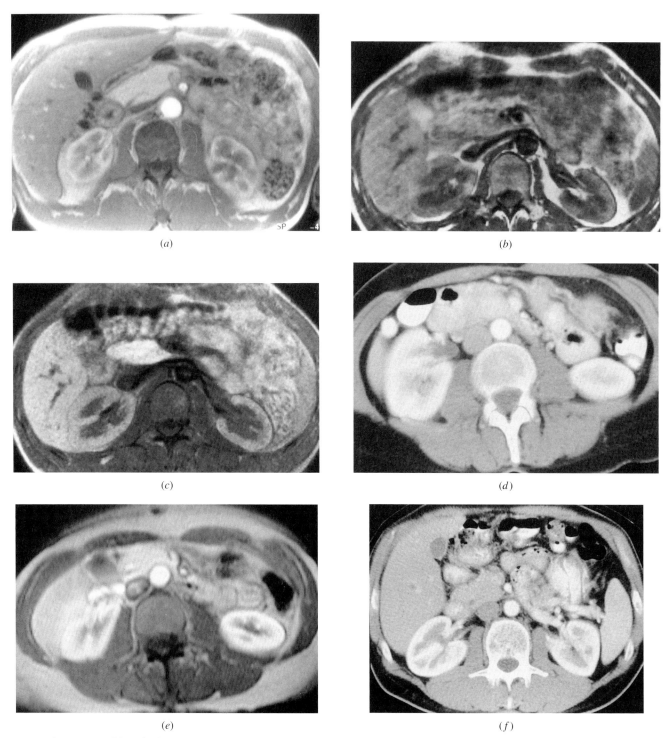

(a)

(b)

(c)

(d)

(e)

(f)

FIG. 4.2 Normal head of pancreas. Immediate postgadolinium T1-weighted SGE image of a normal prominent pancreatic head (*a*). Note the characteristic homogeneous and intense enhancement of the normal pancreatic parenchyma.

T1 spin-echo (T1-SE) (*b*) and T1-weighted fat-suppressed spin-echo (*c*) images in a second patient. The normal pancreatic head is poorly visualized on the T1-SE image (*b*) because of ghosting artifact and minimal signal difference between pancreas and background tissue. On the T1-weighted fat suppressed image (*c*), the head is clearly visualized because of minimal phase artifact and good conspicuity of high-signal intensity pancreatic tissue.

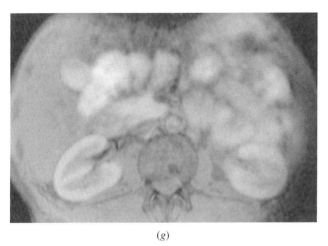

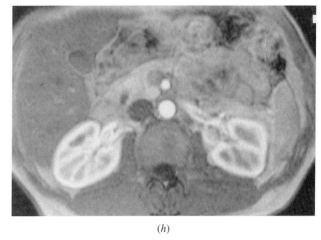

(g)   (h)

F I G . 4.2 (*Continued*) Spiral CT (*d*) and immediate postgadolinium T1-weighted SGE (*e*) images in a third patient. The head of the pancreas appears large and heterogeneous on the spiral CT image (*d*), which was considered indeterminate for pancreatic cancer. On the immediate postgadolinium T1-weighted SGE image (*e*), the head of the pancreas enhances in a normal uniform pattern, which excludes the presence of cancer.

Spiral CT (*f*), T1-weighted fat-suppressed spin-echo (*g*) and immediate postgadolinium T1-weighted SGE image (*h*) in a fourth patient. The head of the pancreas appears large with a bulbous contour of the uncinate process, findings that were considered inconclusive for pancreatic cancer. Normal high signal intensity on the precontrast T1-weighted fat-suppressed spin-echo image (*g*) and uniform moderately intense enhancement on the immediate postgadolinium T1-weighted SGE image (*h*) excludes the presence of cancer.

Recognition of the characteristic high signal intensity of normal pancreas on precontrast T1-weighted fat-suppressed and immediate postgadolinium images is useful in circumstances of abnormalities of position. After left nephrectomy, the tail of the pancreas falls into the renal fossa, which can simulate recurrent disease on CT examination. Normal pancreas can be readily distinguished by its high signal intensity (fig. 4.3).

DEVELOPMENTAL ANOMALIES

Pancreas Divisum

Pancreas divisum is the most clinically important and common major anatomic variant. Although a misleading term, pancreas divisum is, by definition, a superficially normal-appearing pancreas in which no communication has developed between the duct of the dorsally derived pancreas and the duct of the embryonic ventral pancreas, which normally forms most of the main pancreatic duct [12]. The result of this congenital abnormality is that portions of the pancreas have separate ductal systems: a very short ventral duct of Wirsung drains only the lower portion of the head while the dorsal duct of Santorini drains the tail, body, neck, and upper aspect of the head. The incidence of this anomaly varies between 1.3 and 6.7% of the population [13]. One study described 108 patients who underwent both endoscopic retrograde cholangiopancreatography (ERCP) and MRCP and reported exact correlation between these modalities for the detection and exclusion of pancreas divisum [6]. On MRCP images, separate entries of the ducts of Santorini and Wirsung into the duodenum are consistently demonstrated because of the good conspicuity of the linear high-signal intensity tubular structures (fig. 4.4). Variations in pancreas divisum are also shown, which include the dominant dorsal duct syndrome.

Although a controversial topic, pancreas divisum may be a predisposing factor in recurrent pancreatitis [14, 15]. It is postulated that in some subjects the disproportion between the small caliber of the minor papilla and the large amount of secretions from the dorsal part of the gland leads to a relative outflow obstruction from the dorsal pancreas, resulting in pain or pancreatitis [16]. Compared with patients with pancreatitis and normal duct anatomy, the pancreas in pancreas divisum may appear normal in signal intensity on T1-weighted fat-suppressed images and immediate postgadolinium SGE images because the attacks of recurrent pancreatitis tend to be less severe and changes of chronic pancreatitis may not develop.

Annular Pancreas

Annular pancreas is an uncommon congenital anomaly in which glandular pancreatic tissue, in continuity with the head of the pancreas, encircles the duodenum. In

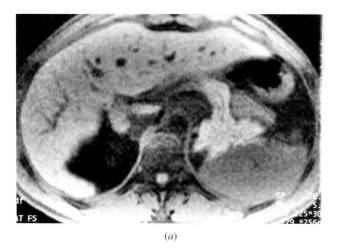

(a)

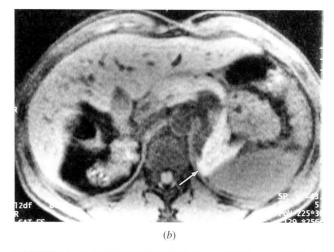

(b)

FIG. 4.3 Pancreatic tail seated in the left renal fossa after left nephrectomy. T1-weighted fat-suppressed SGE images (a, b) demonstrate normal high-signal intensity pancreas situated in the left renal fossa (arrow, b).

T1-weighted fat-suppressed SGE image (c) in a second patient who underwent a bilateral nephrectomy shows the pancreatic tail seated posteriorly, filling the space in the renal fossa.

(c)

most cases, the annular portion surrounds the second part of the duodenum. Patients may present with duodenal obstruction. On MR images, pancreatic tissue is identified encasing the duodenum. Noncontrast T1-weighted fat-suppressed and/or immediate post-gadolinium SGE images are particularly effective at demonstrating this entity because of the high signal intensity of pancreatic tissue, which is readily distinguished from the lower signal intensity of adjacent tissue and duodenum (fig. 4.5) [17].

Congenital Absence of the Dorsal Pancreatic Anlage

Congenital absence of the dorsal pancreatic anlage is a very rare congenital anomaly. This congenital abnormality predisposes to recurrent attacks of pancreatitis with eventual exocrine and endocrine pancreatic failure [12]. The head of the pancreas terminates with a rounded contour, unlike surgical or posttraumatic absence of the distal pancreas, which has more squared-off or irregular terminations (fig. 4.6).

Short Pancreas in the Polysplenia Syndrome

Polysplenia syndrome is a congenital syndrome characterized by multiple, misplaced small spleens characteristic in the right upper quadrant and isomerism (bilateral left sidedness) [18]. In a study involving adults with polysplenia syndrome, discovered incidentally, four of eight patients evaluated with CT showed a short pancreas. The short pancreas may also have an abnormal orientation (fig. 4.7). Possible explanation for the anomaly is disturbance in the blood supply to the pancreas-spleen region during embryonal life [19].

GENETIC DISEASE

Cystic Fibrosis

Cystic fibrosis is the most common lethal genetic disease affecting Caucasians, with an incidence of 1 in 2000 live births. It is an autosomal recessive multisystem disease

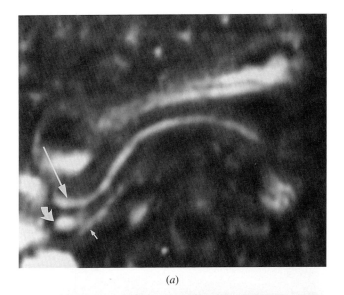

(a)

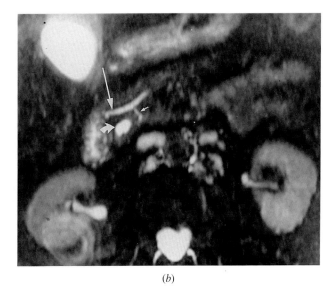

(b)

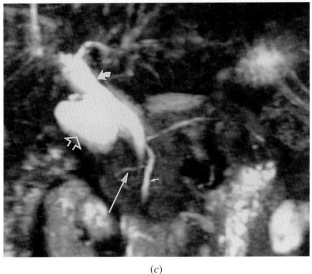

(c)

FIG. 4.4 Pancreas divisum. MRCP image (*a*) formatted in an oblique tranverse plane demonstrates separate entry of the ducts of Santorini (long arrow, *a*) and Wirsung (short arrow, *a*) into the duodenum with no communication between the ductal systems. MRCP image (*b*) in a second patient with dominant dorsal duct syndrome shows a large duct of Santorini (long arrow, *b*) and a small communication with a diminutive duct of Wirsung (short arrow, *b*). The common bile duct (curved arrow, *a, b*) is identified between the ducts of Santorini and Wirsung. Oblique coronal MRCP (*c*) in a patient with normal ductal anatomy shows a small duct of Santorini (long arrow, *c*) and a larger duct of Wirsung (short arrow, *c*). The common bile duct (curved arrow, *c*) and gallbladder (hollow arrow, *c*) are also shown. MR pancreatography has the advantage of being a noninvasive diagnostic method for pancreas divisum. (Courtesy of Caroline Reinhold, MD, Dept. of Radiology, Mc Gill University.)

with an abnormality of the long arm of chromosome 7, and homozygotes express the disease fully. The disease is characterized by dysfunction of the secretory process of all exocrine glands and reduced mucociliary transport, which results in mucous plugging of the exocrine glands. The diagnosis is made during childhood when the patient has clinical manifestations of recurrent bronchopulmonary infections lending to chronic lung disease, malabsorption secondary to pancreatic insufficiency, and an increased sweat sodium concentration. MRI has proven to be an effective modality in demonstrating pancreas changes in patients with cystic fibrosis [20–22]. In the demonstration of fatty infiltration, MRI is superior to ultrasound and avoids ionizing radiation used in computed tomography. A slight drawback of MRI in this setting is the failure to demonstrate calcifications, which are encountered in a small percentage of patients with cystic fibrosis.

Pathologic examination of the pancreas in patients who have survived until early adulthood shows a spectrum of changes involving atrophy and fibrosis of the exocrine pancreas. There are varying degrees of fatty replacement with residual islet cells surrounded by fibrofatty stroma. Three basic imaging patterns of pancreatic abnormalities have been described: pancreatic enlargement with complete fatty replacement with or without loss of the lobulated contour, atrophic pancreas with partial fatty replacement (fig. 4.8), and diffuse atrophy of the pancreas without fatty replacement [20–22]. Pancreatic enlargement with complete fatty replacement is the most common pattern observed in cystic fibrosis [22]. Fatty replacement is high in signal intensity on T1-weighted images and demonstrates loss of signal intensity on T1-weighted fat-suppressed images. These findings correlate with the pathologic description of mature adipose tissue and isolated foci of

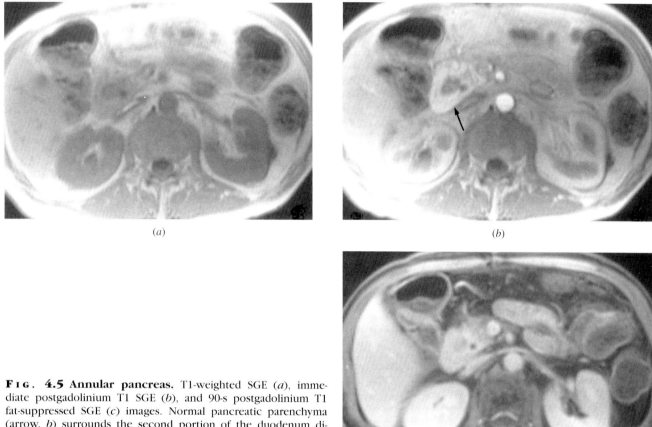

(a)

(b)

FIG. 4.5 Annular pancreas. T1-weighted SGE (*a*), immediate postgadolinium T1 SGE (*b*), and 90-s postgadolinium T1 fat-suppressed SGE (*c*) images. Normal pancreatic parenchyma (arrow, *b*) surrounds the second portion of the duodenum diagnostic for annular pancreas. This is best shown on noncontrast T1-weighted fat-suppressed and immediate postgadolinium (*b*) images.

(c)

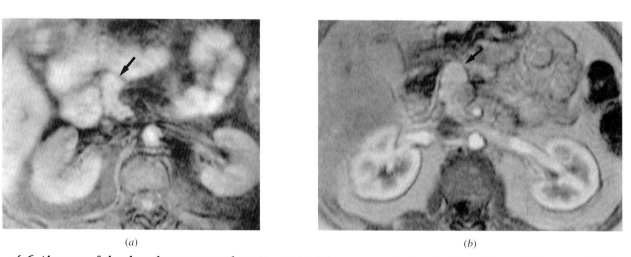

(a)

(b)

FIG. 4.6 Absence of the dorsal pancreas anlage. T1-weighted fat-suppressed spin-echo (*a*) and immediate postgadolinium T1-weighted SGE (*b*) images. A normal appearing head of the pancreas is apparent. The pancreas terminates with a rounded contour (arrow, *a, b*) at the level of the pancreatic neck.

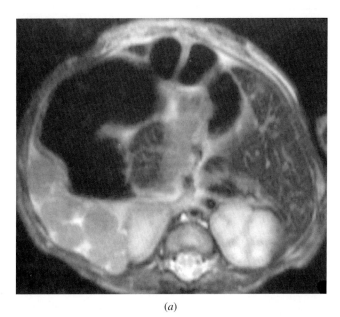

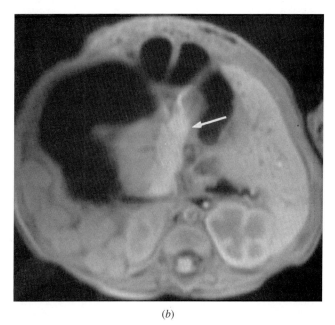

(a)

(b)

F I G . 4.7 Short pancreas in the polysplenia syndrome. T2-weighted fat-suppressed SS-ETSE (*a*) and T1-weighted fat-suppressed spin-echo (*b*) images in a 9-week-old boy with polysplenia syndrome. The pancreas has an abnormal anterior posterior orientation and appears short (arrow, *b*), but the parenchyma signal intensity is normal. The most common pancreatic finding in polysplenia syndrome is short pancreas. Note situs inversus and multiple small spleens.

Langerhans cell islets in the pancreas of cystic fibrosis patients.

Other manifestations of cystic fibrosis include the formation of pancreatic cysts secondary to duct obstruction by inspissated mucus secretions. MRCP is valuable in demonstrating pancreatic duct abnormalities, namely, narrowing, dilatation, stricture, and beading.

Primary Hemochromatosis

Primary hemochromatosis is a homozygous recessive heritable disease in which there is excessive accumulation of body iron, most of which is deposited in the parenchyma of various organs. The liver, pancreas, and heart are primarily affected. Iron deposition results in a loss of signal intensity that is more pronounced on T2- or T2*-weighted sequences (fig. 4.9), but in severe deposition a loss of signal intensity is also apparent on T1-weighted images. Iron deposition in primary hemochromatosis is most substantial in the liver. Deposition of iron in the pancreas tends to occur late in the course of disease after liver damage is irreversible [23, 24].

von Hippel-Lindau Syndrome

von Hippel-Lindau Syndrome is an autosomal dominant condition with variable penetration. This condi-

tion is characterized by tumors in the cerebellum and retina. Patients may have cysts of the liver and kidney, with a strong propensity to develop renal cell carcinoma. Patients with von Hippel-Lindau Syndrome may develop pancreatic cysts, islet cell tumors, or microcystic cystadenoma. In one series, cysts were the most common pancreatic lesions and were present in 19 of 52 patients in whom no other pancreatic lesions were present (fig. 4.10) [25].

MASS LESIONS

Pancreatic mass lesions can be detected and successfully characterized using a pattern recognition approach employing T1, T2, and immediate and late postgadolinium images. Table 4.1 summarizes a pattern recognition approach for the most common pancreatic tumors.

Lipoma

Lipoma is the most common benign solid tumor that affects the pancreas. Rounded morphology and larger size distinguish this tumor from prominent fat within the interstices of the pancreas. The diagnosis is readily made employing nonsuppressed and fat-attenuating techniques (fig. 4.11)

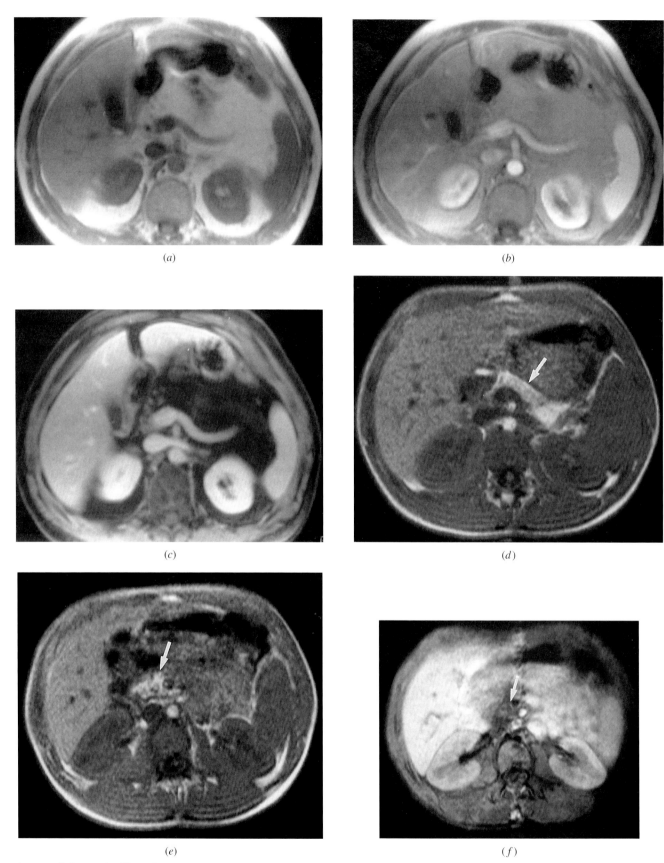

(a)

(b)

(c)

(d)

(e)

(f)

F I G . 4.8 Cystic fibrosis. T1-weighted SGE (*a*), immediate postgadolinium T1-weighted SGE (*b*), and 90-s postgadolinium T1-weighted fat-suppressed SGE (*c*) images in a patient with cystic fibrosis. The pancreas is markedly enlarged and hyperintense on T1-weighted image (arrows, *a*) and hypointense on fat-suppressed (*c*) images, consistent with fatty replacement of the pancreatic parenchyma by adipose tissue. The complete fatty replacement of the pancreas is the most common manifestation of cystic fibrosis.

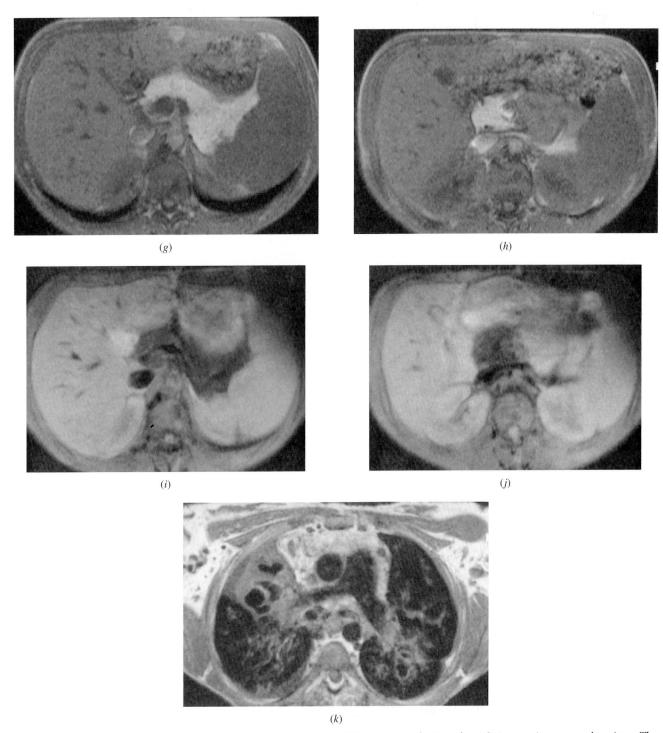

(g)

(h)

(i)

(j)

(k)

FIG. 4.8 (*Continued*) T1-weighted SGE (*d, e*) and T1-weighted fat-suppressed spin-echo (*f*) images in a second patient. The pancreas is atrophic and demonstrates fatty replacement.

T1-weighted SGE (*g, h*), T1-weighted fat-suppressed spin-echo (*i, j*), and gated T1-SE (*k*) images in a third patient, who has an enlarged fatty replaced pancreas. Extensive pulmonary fibrosis is present (*k*).

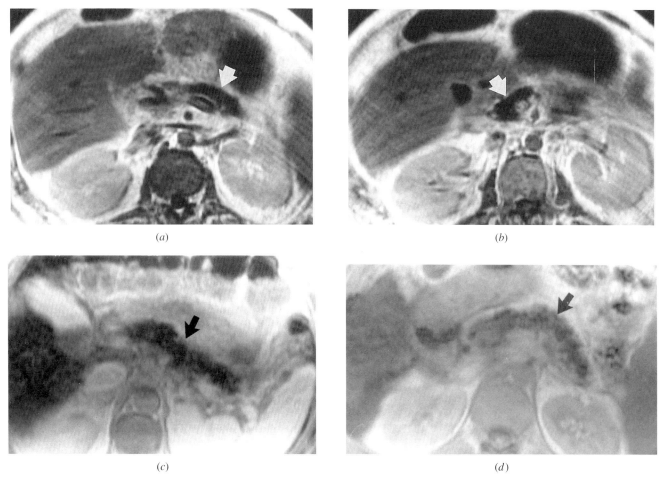

(a)   (b)

(c)   (d)

F I G . 4.9 Iron deposition in the pancreas from primary hemochromatosis. T1-weighted SGE (*a, b*) images. The pancreas (arrow, *a, b*) is signal void on T1-weighted images because of the susceptibility effect of iron. The liver is a transplanted liver and therefore has not sustained iron deposition. Transverse 1-min postgadolinium SGE image (*c*) in a second patient with primary hemochromatosis. Both the pancreas (arrow, *c*) and liver show decreased signal intensity. Gallstones are also present. T1-weighted SGE (*d*) image in a third patient with primary hemochromatosis shows a low-signal pancreas (arrow, *d*).

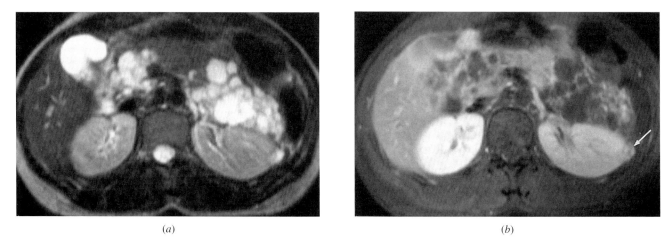

(a)   (b)

F I G . 4.10 Pancreatic cysts in von Hippel-Lindau disease. T2-weighted SS-ETSE (*a*) and gadolinium-enhanced T1-weighted fat-suppressed spin-echo (*b*) images. Multiple pancreatic cysts are scattered throughout the pancreas, which are high in signal intensity on T2-weighted images (*a*) and low in signal intensity on gadolinium-enhanced images (*b*). Thick septations are present between many of the clustered cysts. A small renal cancer is identified in the left kidney (arrow, *b*).

Table 4.1 Pattern Recognition: Focal Pancreatic Lesions

	T1	T2	Early Gd	Late Gd	Other Features
Ductal adeno Ca (small)	↓	Ø	↓	↓–↑	Usually no background chronic pancreatitis, so tumor is well seen on precontrast T1.
Ductal adeno Ca (large)					Usually causes background chronic pancreatitis; tumor is not well seen on precontrast T1.
	↓–Ø	Ø–↑	↓	↓	Focal mass with definable margins shown on early post-Gd images is the most common imaging characteristic.
Islet cell tumors Insulinoma	↓	↑	↑, homogeneous and benign	Ø–↑	Tumors are usually <1 cm.
Gastrinoma					Tumors are usually located in the region of the pancreatic head.
					Approximately 50% have metastases at initial diagnosis.
	↓	↑	↑, ring	Ø–↑	Liver metastases tend to be a uniform population of numerous smooth ring-enhancing tumors shown on immediate post-Gd images that exhibit peripheral washout on delayed images.
Somastostatinoma, Glucagonoma, Untyped	↓	↑	↑, diffuse heterogeneous	Ø, heterogeneous	Tumors are usually large at initial diagnosis, with the majority having liver metastases. Liver metastases are numerous and vary in size with irregular ring enhancement.
VIPoma	↓	↑	↑	Ø	Primary tumor is usually small at initial diagnosis with few varying size liver metastases with irregular ring enhancement.
Microcystic cystadenoma	↓	↑↑	Ø–↑	Ø	Small cysts best seen on single-shot T2 sequences. Thin and regular septations, but may measure up to 4 mm in thickness with regular thickness. Septations may enhance moderately on immediate post-Gd images of larger tumors with thicker septations, and these tumors may possess a central scar that shows delayed enhancement.
Microcystic cystadenoma	↓	↑↑	Ø–↑	Ø	Septations are uniform in thickness, and there is no evidence of irregular tumor tissue or nodule.
Macrocystic cystadenocarcinoma					Septations are irregular in thickness with irregular-shaped tumor tissue and tumor nodule.
	↓	↑	Ø–↑	Ø–↑	Tumor may be very locally aggressive and may have liver metastases.
					Liver metastases may be high signal on T1 weighted images because of presence of mucin.

↓↓ moderately to markedly decreased signal intensity
↓ mildly decreased signal intensity
Ø isointense
↑ mildly increased signal intensity
↑↑ moderately to markedly increased signal intensity

Adenocarcinoma

Adenocarcinoma of the pancreas refers to carcinoma arising in the exocrine portion of the gland. Pancreatic ductal adenocarcinoma accounts for 95% of the malignant tumors of the pancreas. Pancreatic adenocarcinoma is the fourth most common cause of cancer death in the United States [26]. The lesion is more common in men and Blacks [27]. The age range for tumor occurrence is the fourth through the eighth decade, with tumor incidence peaking in the eighth decade [28]. The tumor has a poor prognosis, with a 5-year survival of 5% [27].

Approximately 60–70% of pancreatic adenocarcinomas occur in the head (figs. 4.12–4.19), 15% in the body (figs. 4.20 and 4.21), 5% in the tail (fig. 4.22), and 10–20% with a diffuse involvement (fig. 4.23) [29]. Tumors in the head of the pancreas are in a strategic position to encroach upon the common bile duct, major papilla, and duodenum. They tend to present smaller in size than tumors in the body or tail because of the development of jaundice secondary to obstruction of the common bile duct. Painless jaundice is the classical presenting feature of carcinomas within the pancreatic head.

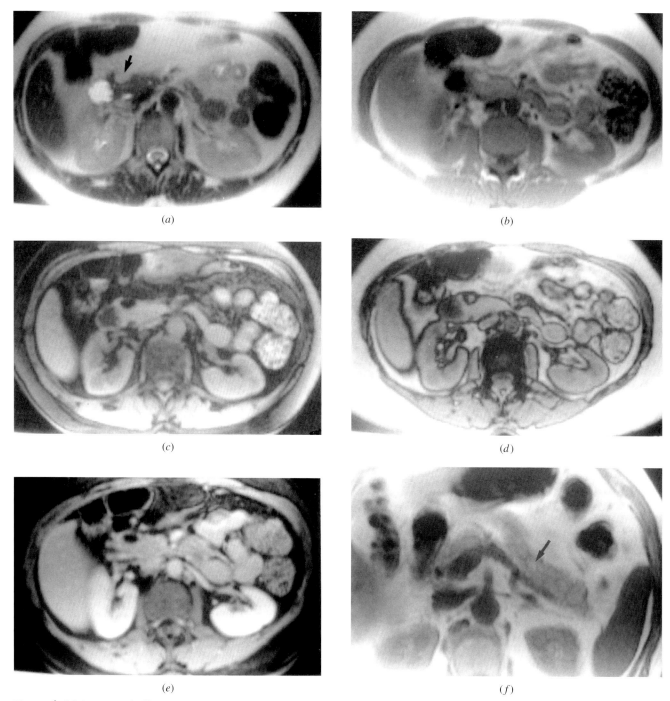

(a)

(b)

(c)

(d)

(e)

(f)

F I G . 4.11 Pancreatic lipoma. T2-weighted SS-ETSE (*a*), T1-weighted SGE (*b*), T1-weighted fat-suppressed SGE (*c*), T1-weighted out-of-phase SGE (*d*) and 90-s postgadolinium T1-weighted fat-suppressed SGE (*e*) images. There is a small lesion in the anterior aspect of the head of the pancreas (arrow, *a*), which appears isointense with adjacent intraperitoneal fat on T1- (*b*) and T2-weighted (*a*) images with drop in signal intensity on fat-suppressed images (*c*, *e*). A phase-cancellation artifact surrounds the lesion on the T1 out-of-phase image (*d*). These findings are diagnostic for a pancreatic lipoma.

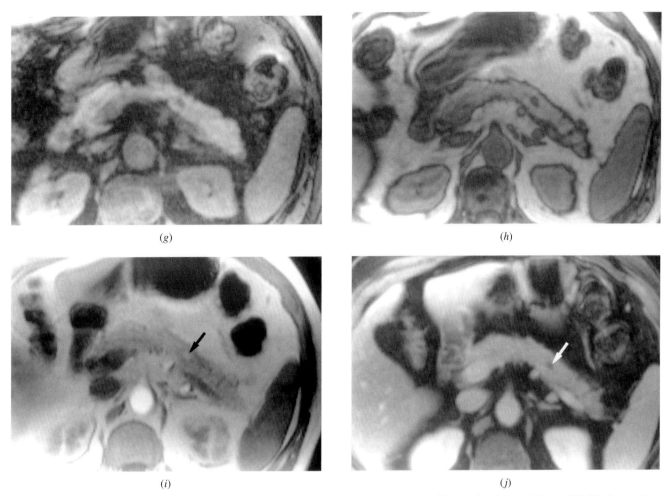

(g)

(h)

(i)

(j)

F I G. 4.11 (*Continued*) T1-weighted SGE (*f*), T1-weighted fat-suppressed SGE (*g*), T1-weighted out-of-phase SGE (*h*), immediate postgadolinium T1-weighted SGE (*i*), and 90-s postgadolinium fat-suppressed SGE (*j*) images in a second patient with a small lipoma (arrow, *f*) in the pancreatic body/tail. An important reason to correctly identify a lesion as a lipoma is not to misinterpret high signal on immediate postgadolinium nonsuppressed images as consistent with enhancement (arrow, *i*), nor to misinterpret low signal on interstitial-phase gadolinium-enhanced fat-suppressed images as consistent with wash-out (arrow, *j*).

In general, the diagnosis of pancreatic adenocarcinoma is made when the tumor is relatively large (about 5 cm) and has extended beyond the pancreas (85% of cases). Carcinoma involving the body and tail of the pancreas grows insidiously and usually has already metastasized widely at the time of diagnosis [30]. The most common sites of metastases, in order of decreasing frequency, are liver, regional lymph nodes, peritoneum, and lungs [29]. The rich lymphatic supply and lack of a capsule account for the early spread of cancer to regional lymph nodes. The nodal groups involved include parapancreatic, para-aortic, paracaval, paraportal, and celiac. Calcification is a rare constituent of the mass itself, although adenocarcinoma may occur in a pancreas containing background calcification.

Pancreatic cancer arising in the head of the pancreas may cause obstruction of the CBD and pancreatic duct [31]. This appearance on MRCP studies results in the "double duct sign," which was originally described on ERCP (fig. 4.15). A characteristic imaging appearance of pancreatic carcinoma consists of enlargement of the head of the pancreas with dilatation of the pancreatic and common bile duct and atrophy of the body and tail of the pancreas. However, enlargement of the head of the pancreas with obstruction of both ducts is not a feature unique to pancreatic cancer, as this same appearance may be appreciated, although less commonly, in patients with focal pancreatitis. Other features that assist in the diagnosis of pancreatic cancer include the presence of lymphadenopathy, encasement of the celiac axis or superior mesenteric artery, and liver metastases (figs. 4.24 and 4.25) [29, 32]. On tomographic images, vascular encasement is observed as a loss of the fat plane around vessels [33]. Liver metastases are the only absolute indication of malignancy, as lymphadenopathy and vascular encasement may rarely occur in inflammatory disease.

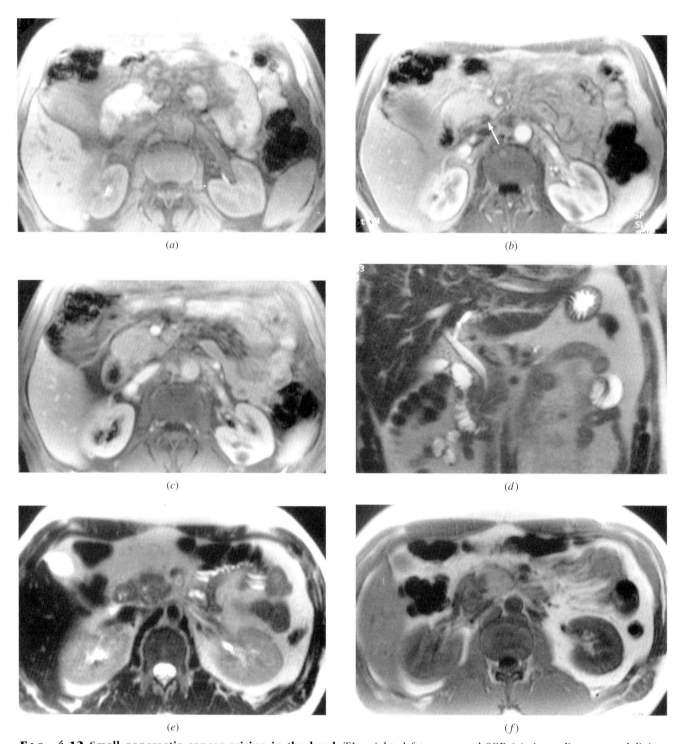

(a)

(b)

(c)

(d)

(e)

(f)

FIG. 4.12 Small pancreatic cancer arising in the head. T1-weighted fat-suppressed SGE (*a*), immediate postgadolinium T1-weighted SGE (*b*), and 90-s postgadolinium fat-suppressed SGE (*c*) images. A 6-mm tumor (arrow, *b*) is present in the uncinate process of the pancreas, which does not result in ductal obstruction because of its small size and location. Note that the mass is most clearly shown on the immediate postgadolinium image (*b*) as a small hypoenhancing lesion. Coronal (*d*) and transverse (*e*) T2-weighted SS-ETSE, T1-weighted SGE (*f*), T1-weighted fat-suppressed SGE (*g*), and immediate (*h*) and 45-s (*i*) postgadolinium T1-weighted SGE and 90-s postgadolinium fat-suppressed SGE (*j*) images in a second patient with moderately differentiated adenocarcinoma. There is a 1.5-cm mass arising in the lateral aspect of the pancreatic head, which invades the duodenal wall and causes biliary ductal dilatation.

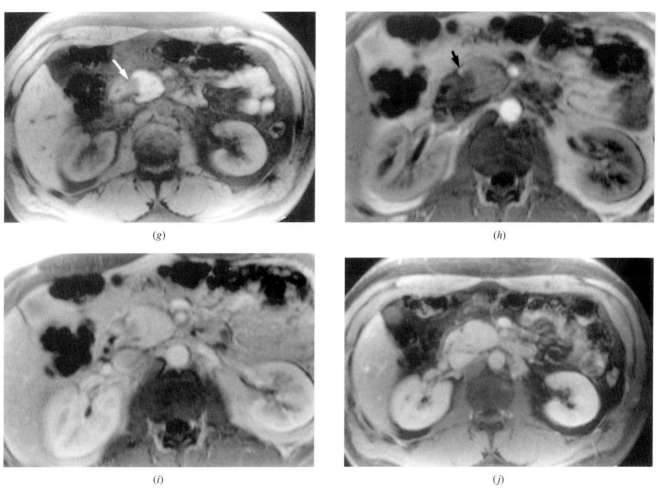

(g)

(h)

(i)

(j)

F I G. 4.12 (*Continued*) On the T2-weighted images (*d, e*) CBD obstruction is well shown, but the tumor itself is almost imperceptible. The tumor (arrow, *g*) is most clearly appreciated on the noncontrast T1-weighted fat suppressed SGE image (*g*) and the immediate postgadolinium SGE image (*h*). Progressive tumor enhancement and pancreatic parenchyma wash-out over time (*i, j*) diminishes the tumor-pancreas contrast, which is most problematic with small tumors. The gastroduodenal artery (arrow, *h*) is well shown on the immediate postgadolinium image as an enhancing structure. The tumor is shown to abut this vessel. Approximately one-quarter of all pancreas head cancers exhibit some degree of duodenal wall invasion.

Because liver metastases are not always present on initial evaluation, the most useful imaging feature for the diagnosis of pancreatic cancer is the demonstration of a focal hypovascular mass within pancreatic parenchyma.

Detection of carcinoma is best performed by immediate postgadolinium SGE images [1, 4, 34, 35]. Pancreatic tissue is well delineated from tumors, and tumor margins are clearly shown using this sequence in all regions of the pancreas. Small tumors or tumors of the pancreatic tail are also well demonstrated on noncontrast T1-weighted fat-suppressed images. Larger tumors in the pancreatic head are revealed less consistently with noncontrast T1-weighted fat-suppressed images, as explained below. Conventional spin-echo images are generally limited in the detection of pancreatic cancer [36]. Tumors are usually minimally hypointense relative to pancreas on T2-weighted images and are therefore difficult to visualize. Semelka et al. published a study comparing single-phase spiral CT imaging with MRI including noncontrast T1-weighted fat-suppressed spin-echo and immediate postgadolinium SGE for the detection or exclusion of pancreatic cancer in 16 patients with findings indeterminate for cancer on spiral CT imaging (fig. 4.13) [35]. Immediate postgadolinium SGE was found to be the most sensitive approach to detect pancreatic cancer, particularly in the head of the pancreas. Both immediate postgadolinium SGE and noncontrast T1-weighted fat-suppressed imaging performed well at excluding cancer and both were significantly superior to spiral CT imaging. These findings are similar to those reported by Gabata et al. [34], who compared these MR techniques to dynamic contrast-enhanced CT imaging.

Because of their abundant fibrous stroma and relatively sparse vascularity, pancreatic cancers enhance

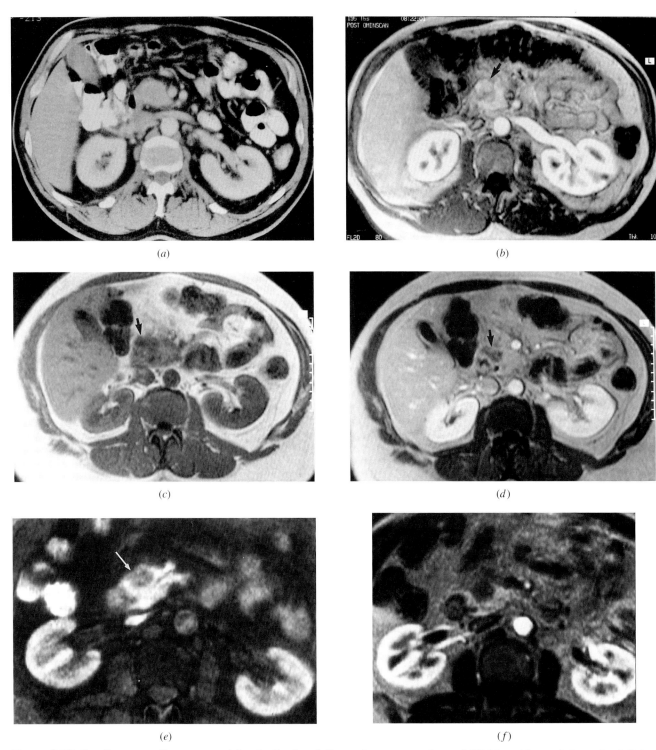

FIG. 4.13 Small pancreatic cancer arising in the head. Dynamic contrast-enhanced CT (*a*) and immediate postgadolinium T1-weighted SGE (*b*) images. The non-organ-deforming cancer is not apparent on the CT image (*a*). On the immediate postgadolinium image (*b*), a heterogeneous low-signal intensity tumor (arrow, *b*) is identified in the head of the pancreas, clearly demarcated from uniform enhancing pancreatic tissue.

to a lesser extent than surrounding normal pancreatic tissue on early postcontrast images [34]. It is therefore critical to exploit this difference in vascularity in contrast-enhanced studies by imaging in the dynamic capillary phase of enhancement (fig. 4.13) [34, 35]. Thin section thickness is also helpful, but 8-mm-thick sections may be sufficiently thin to detect even small (<1 cm) cancers because of the high contrast resolution on SGE images.

An adequate signal-to-noise ratio may be achieved with section thickness of 5 mm by using a phased-array

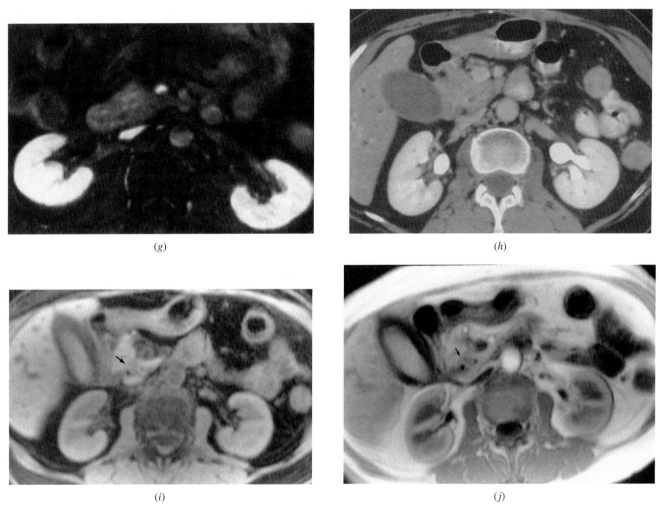

(g)

(h)

(i)

(j)

F I G . 4.13 (*Continued*) T1-weighted SGE (*c*) and 45-s postgadolinium T1-weighted SGE (*d*) images in a second patient. A 2-cm pancreatic cancer is present that is minimally lower in signal intensity than pancreas on the precontrast image (*c*) and enhances substantially less than pancreas on the early postgadolinium image (arrow, *d*). T1-weighted fat-suppressed spin-echo (*e*), immediate postgadolinium T1-weighted SGE (*f*), and interstitial-phase gadolinium-enhanced T1-weighted fat-suppressed spin-echo (*g*) images in a third patient. A small non-organ-deforming cancer is present in the head of the pancreas (arrow, *e*). The tumor does not obstruct the main pancreatic duct, so background pancreas remains high in signal intensity on T1-weighted fat-suppressed images (*e*). The immediate postgadolinium T1-weighted SGE image (*f*) demonstrates normal capillary enhancement of the pancreas with minimal enhancement of the cancer. The interstitial-phase gadolinium-enhanced T1-weighted fat-suppressed image (*g*) demonstrates minimally higher signal intensity of the tumor compared to the background pancreas, reflecting a greater accumulation of gadolinium by the tumor and obscuring the cancer.

Spiral CT (*h*), T1-weighted fat-suppressed SGE (*i*), and immediate postgadolinium T1-weighted SGE (*j*) images in a fourth patient. The pancreatic cancer is not visualized on the spiral CT image (*h*). On the T1-weighted fat-suppressed image, the tumor is low in signal intensity (arrow, *i*) relative to background pancreas. On the immediate postgadolinium image (*j*), the tumor (arrow, *j*) enhances less than background pancreas.

surface coil. SGE acquired as a three-dimensional (3D) technique may maintain a sufficient signal-to-noise ratio with even thinner section thickness (3–4 mm). Although pancreatic cancers are lower in signal intensity than pancreas on immediate postgadolinium (capillary phase) images, the appearance of cancers on ≥1-min postgadolinium (interstitial phase) images is variable [34]. The enhancement of cancer relative to pancreas reflects the volume of extracellular space and venous drainage of cancers compared with pancreatic tissue. In general, large pancreatic tumors tend to remain low in signal

intensity on later images (fig. 4.17), whereas smaller tumors may range from hypointense to hyperintense.

Pancreatic cancers appear as low-signal intensity masses on noncontrast T1-weighted fat-suppressed images and are clearly separated from normal pancreatic tissue, which is high in signal intensity [4, 34, 35]. Pancreatic tissue distal to pancreatic cancer is often lower in signal intensity than normal pancreatic tissue [34, 35]. This phenomenon may be explained by tumor-associated chronic pancreatitis occurring distal to the tumor because of obstruction of the main pancreatic

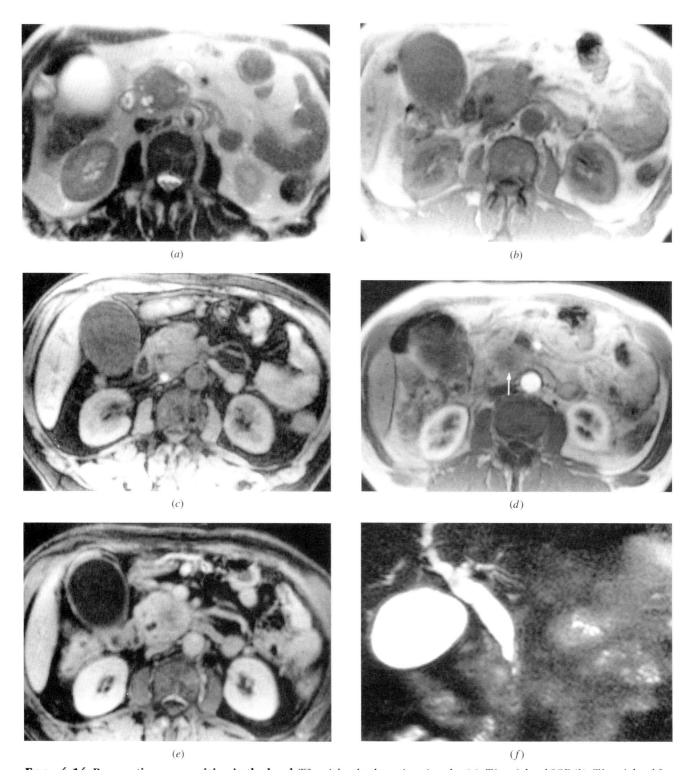

(a)

(b)

(c)

(d)

(e)

(f)

F I G . 4.14 Pancreatic cancer arising in the head. T2-weighted echo-train spin-echo (*a*), T1-weighted SGE (*b*), T1-weighted fat-suppressed SGE (*c*), immediate postgadolinium T1-weighted SGE (*d*), and 90-s postgadolinium fat-suppressed SGE (*e*) images. There is a 4-cm tumor arising in the pancreatic head, which appears hypointense on T1- (*b, c*) and T2-weighted (*a*) images. On immediate postgadolinium images (*c*), the tumor exhibits diminished enhancement compared to normal adjacent pancreatic parenchyma, with demarcation of the tumor edges (arrow, *d*) with background pancreas.

MRCP (*f*), immediate postgadolinium T1-weighted SGE (*g*), and 90-s postgadolinium fat-suppressed SGE (*h*) images in a second patient with poorly differentiated pancreatic adenocarcinoma. The pancreatic cancer appears as a hypoenhancing mass (arrow, *g*) on the immediate postgadolinium image (*g*) with demarcated margins. Relationship to the superior mesenteric vessels, which are spared, is well shown on the interstitial phase gadolinium-enhanced fat-suppressed image (*h*).

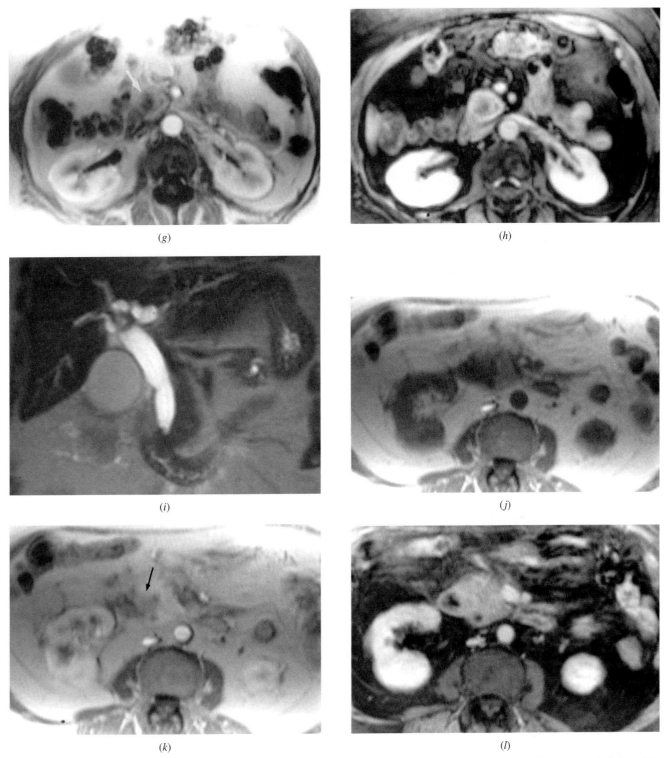

(g)

(h)

(i)

(j)

(k)

(l)

FIG. 4.14 (*Continued*) Coronal T2-weighted echo-train spin-echo (*i*), T1-weighted SGE (*j*), immediate postgadolinium T1-weighted SGE (*k*), and 90-s postgadolinium fat-suppressed SGE (*l*) images. A 2-cm moderately differentiated adenocarcinoma of the pancreatic head is present (arrow, *k*), which is most clearly depicted on the immediate postgadolinium image (*k*). On the interstitial-phase gadolinium-enhanced fat-suppressed image, the tumor has decreased in conspicuity because of progressive tumor enhancement and pancreatic parenchymal wash-out. Invasion of the medial duodenal wall is shown by contiguous extension of tumor to the wall.

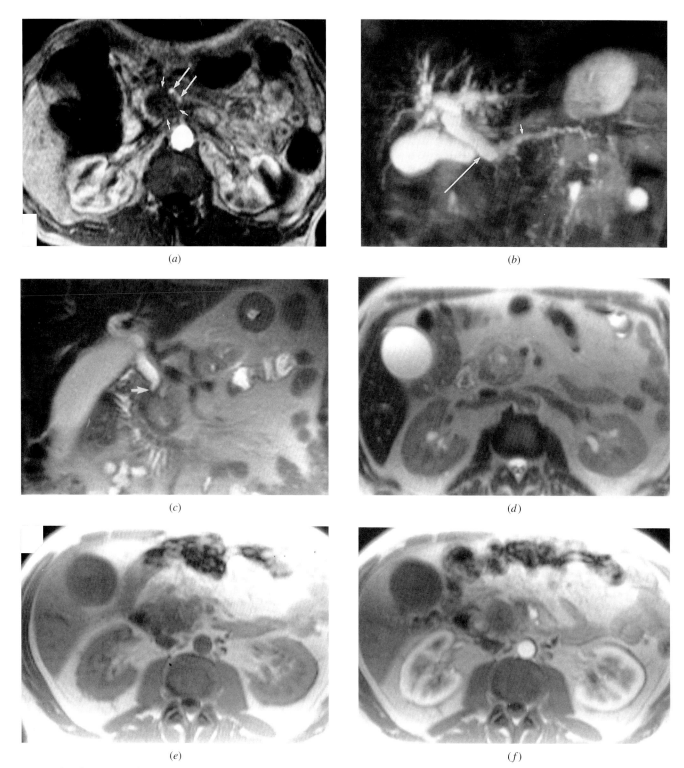

F I G . 4.15 Pancreatic cancer arising in the head with biliary tree dilatation. Immediate postgadolinium T1-weighted SGE (*a*) and non-breath-hold 3D MIP MRCP (*b*) images. A 3.5-cm cancer arises from the head of the pancreas. On the immediate postcontrast image (*a*), the tumor is well shown as a low-signal intensity mass (small arrows, *a*) that is closely applied to the superior mesenteric vein and superior mesenteric artery (arrows, *a*). The MRCP image (*b*) demonstrates obstruction of the CBD (long arrow, *b*) and pancreatic duct (small arrow, *b*) creating the "double duct" sign.

Coronal (*c*) and transverse (*d*) T2-weighted SS-ETSE, T1-weighted SGE (*e*), immediate (*f*) and 45-s (*g*) postgadolinium T1-weighted SGE, and transverse (*h*) and coronal (*i*) interstitial-phase gadolinium-enhanced fat-suppressed SGE images in a second patient with a poorly differentiated pancreatic adenocarcinoma arising in the head. Obstruction of the CBD (arrow, *e*) by the pancreatic head cancer is clearly shown on the coronal image (*c*). The pancreatic mass is mildly heterogeneous and hyperintense on T2-weighted (*c*, *d*) images with minimal enhancement on early postcontrast images (*f*) and progressive enhancement on later images (*h*).

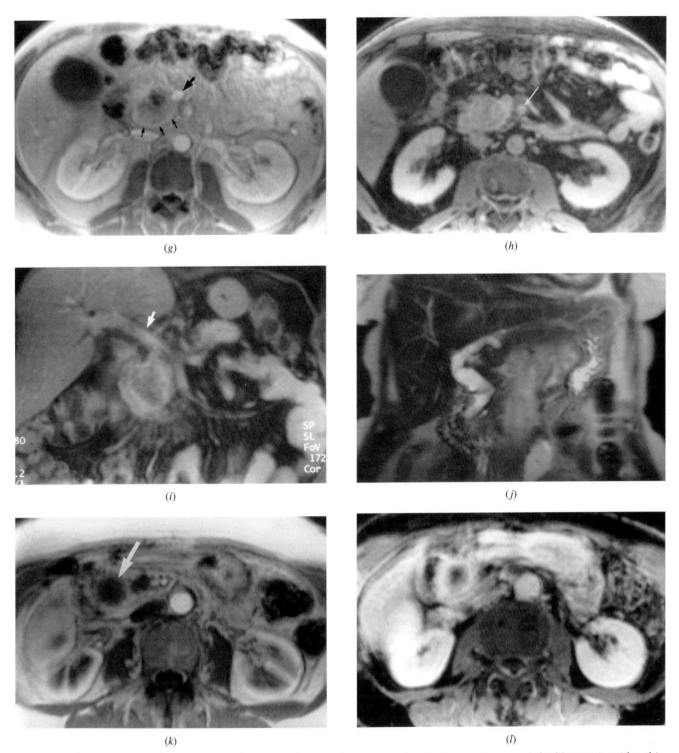

F I G. 4.15 (*Continued*) The tumor partially encases the superior mesenteric vein (arrow, *h*), and a definable margin with a thin rim of adjacent pancreas (small arrows, *g*) is appreciated. Duskiness of the fat around the superior mesenteric artery (arrow, *h*) is shown on the interstitial-phase gadolinium-enhanced fat-suppressed image (*h*). The coronal gadolinium-enhanced fat-suppressed image shows a patent portal vein (arrow, *i*) and its relationship with the cancer.

Coronal T2-weighted SS-ETSE (*j*), immediate postgadolinium T1-weighted SGE (*k*), and 90-s postgadolinium fat-suppressed SGE (*l*) images in a third patient with pancreatic cancer. Obstruction of the CBD is present. A hypoenhancing tumor (arrow, *k*) with definable margins with adjacent pancreas is clearly shown on the immediate postgadolinium image (*k*), which has central necrotic areas and causes biliary tree dilatation.

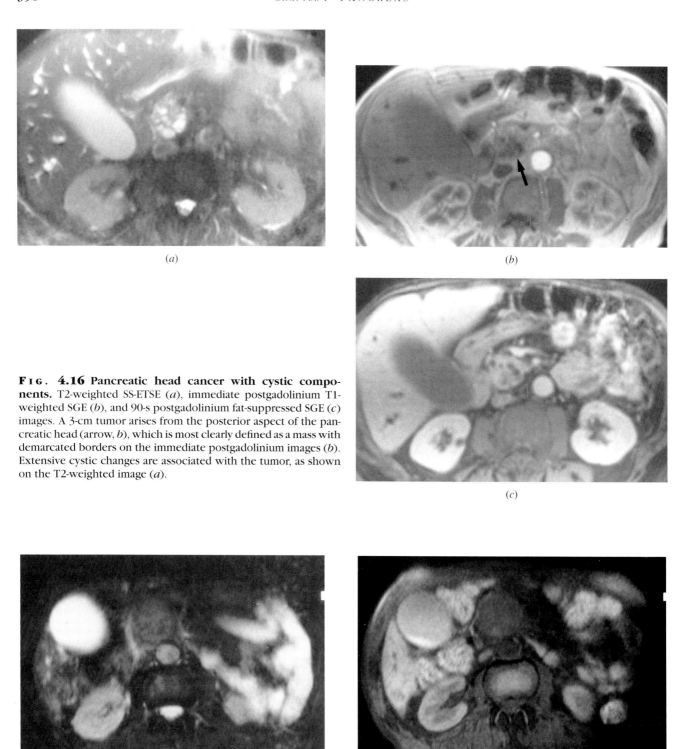

F I G . 4.16 Pancreatic head cancer with cystic compo-nents. T2-weighted SS-ETSE (*a*), immediate postgadolinium T1-weighted SGE (*b*), and 90-s postgadolinium fat-suppressed SGE (*c*) images. A 3-cm tumor arises from the posterior aspect of the pan-creatic head (arrow, *b*), which is most clearly defined as a mass with demarcated borders on the immediate postgadolinium images (*b*). Extensive cystic changes are associated with the tumor, as shown on the T2-weighted image (*a*).

F I G . 4.17 Large pancreatic cancer arising in the head. T2-weighted fat-suppressed SS-ETSE (*a*), T1-weighted fat-suppressed spin-echo (*b*), immediate postgadolinium T1-weighted SGE (*c*), and interstitial-phase gadolinium-enhanced T1-weighted fat-suppressed spin-echo (*d*) images. A large 5-cm cancer is present in the head of the pancreas that is low in signal intensity on T1-weighted images (*b*) and low in signal intensity on T2-weighted images (*a*) and enhances minimally on early (*c*) and late (*d*) postgadolinium images. This represents the typical appearance of a large pancreatic ductal cancer. Liver metastases are present and are most clearly defined on immediate postgadolinium images as focal low-signal intensity masses with irregular rim enhancement (arrows, *c*). The liver is the most common site for metastatic lesions from primary pancreatic cancer.

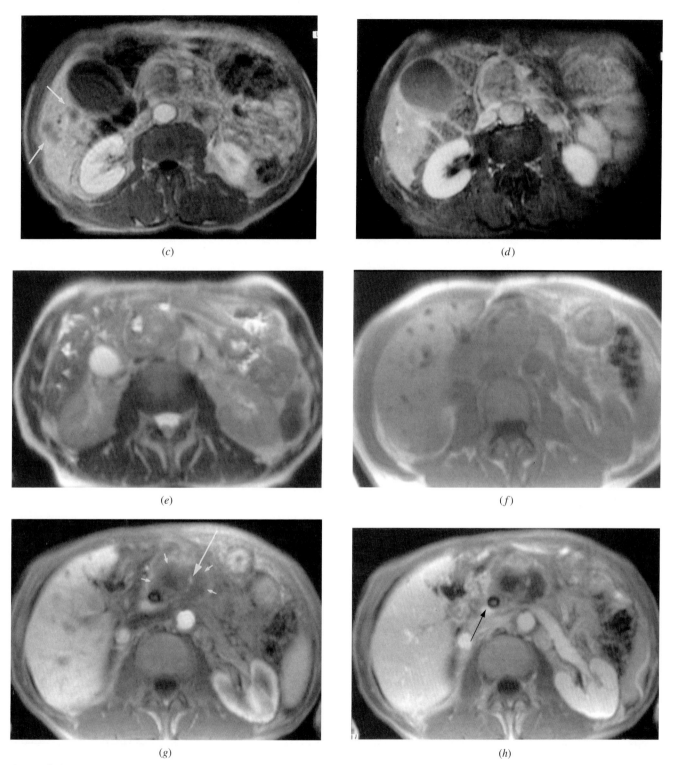

(c)

(d)

(e)

(f)

(g)

(h)

FIG. 4.17 (*Continued*) T2-weighted SS-ETSE (*e*), T1-weighted SGE (*f*), immediate postgadolinium T1-weighted SGE (*f*), and 90-s postgadolinium fat-suppressed T1-weighted SGE (*g*) images in a second patient. There is a 5.5-cm adenocarcinoma (small arrows, *g*) arising in the pancreatic head, which encases the superior mesenteric artery (long arrow, *g*). The superior mesenteric vein is thrombosed and not visualized. There is a stent in the CBD that causes susceptibility artifact (arrow, *h*).

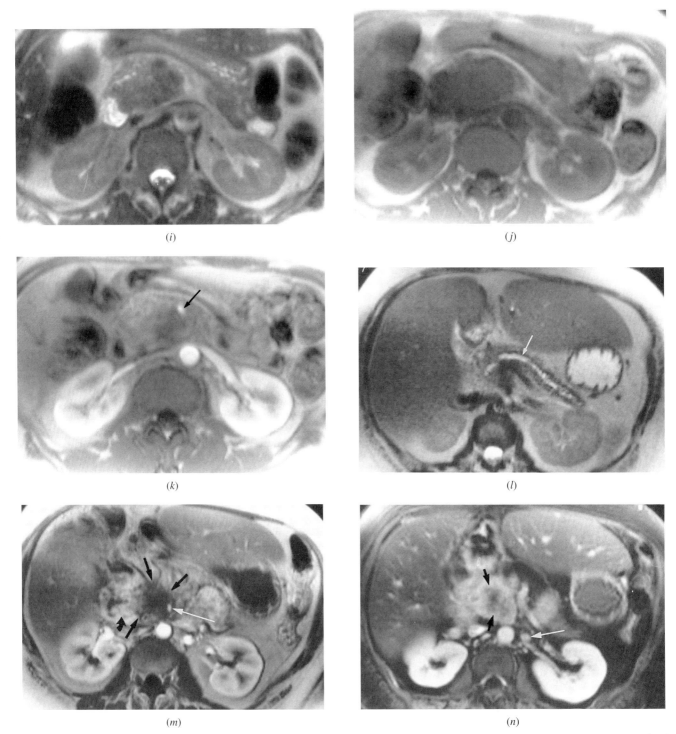

(i)

(j)

(k)

(l)

(m)

(n)

F I G . 4.17 (*Continued*) T2-weighted SS-ETSE (*i*), T1-weighted SGE (*j*), and immediate postgadolinium SGE (*k*) images in a third patient. A 6 × 5-cm cancer arises in the head and uncinate process of the pancreas, with an appearance comparable to the prior examples. Note encasement of the SMA (arrow, *k*).

T2-weighted single-shot SS-ETSE (*l*), immediate postgadolinium T1-weighted SGE (*m*), and 2-min postgadolinium fat-suppressed T1-weighted SGE (*n, o*) images in a fourth patient. A large 4-cm tumor is present in the head of the pancreas that results in obstruction of the pancreatic duct (arrow, *l, m*).

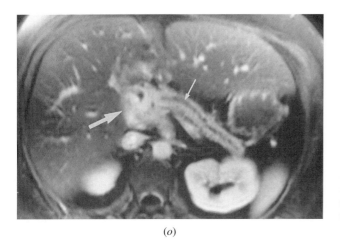

(*o*)

FIG. 4.17 (*Continued*) The tumor is markedly low in signal intensity on the immediate postgadolinium image (short arrows, *m*), and encasement of the SMA is shown (thin arrow, *m*). Adjacent duodenum is thick walled, which is consistent with invasion (curved arrow, *m*). The tumor shows diminished central enhancement on the interstitial-phase fat-suppressed T1-weighted SGE image (arrows, *n*). Small periaortic lymph nodes are identified (long arrow, *n*). Tumor extension into the porta hepatis is present (large arrow, *o*).

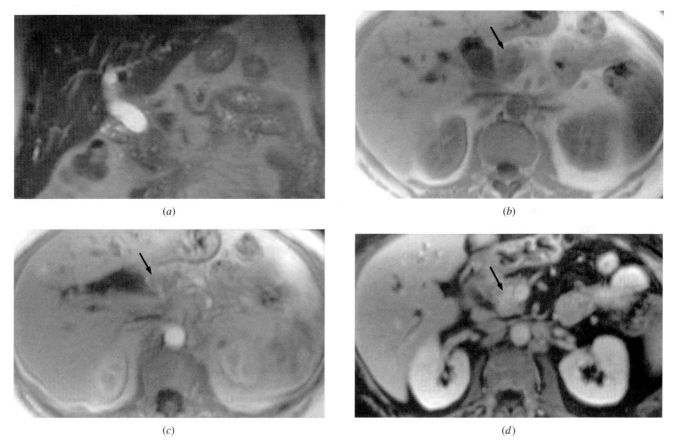

(*a*)   (*b*)

(*c*)   (*d*)

FIG. 4.18 **Infiltrative pancreatic cancer arising in the upper head and neck.** Coronal T2-weighted SS-ETSE (*a*), T1-weighted SGE (*b*), immediate postgadolinium T1-weighted SGE (*c*), and 90-s postgadolinium fat-suppressed SGE (*d*) images. A 3-cm poorly differentiated infiltrative adenocarcinoma is present in the pancreatic head, which causes high-grade obstruction of the CBD. The tumor is ill defined on all imaging sequences (arrow, *b, c*) and demonstrates late increased enhancement (arrow, *d*). These are features of an infiltrative desmoplastic neoplasm.

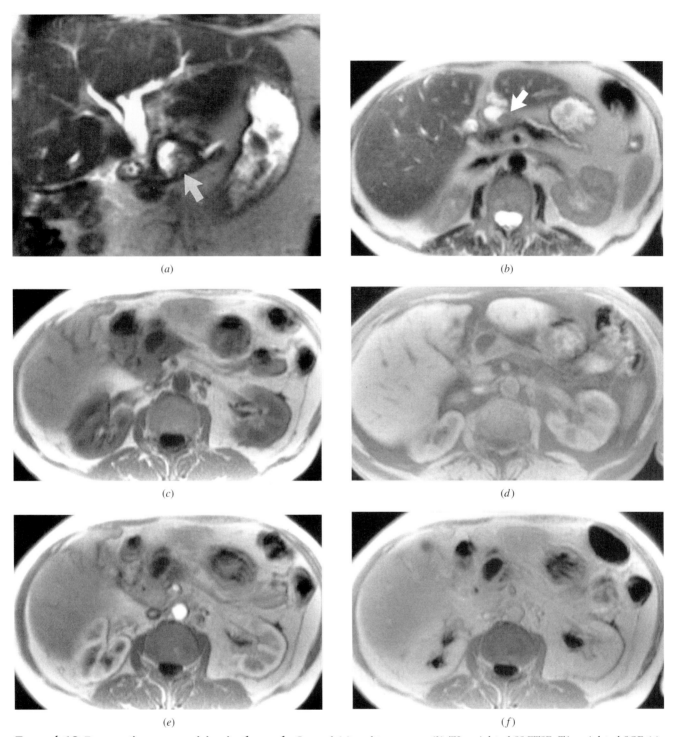

(a)

(b)

(c)

(d)

(e)

(f)

F I G . 4.19 Pancreatic cancer arising in the neck. Coronal (*a*) and transverse (*b*) T2-weighted SS-ETSE, T1-weighted SGE (*c*), T1-weighted fat-suppressed SGE (*d*), and immediate (*e*) and 45-s (*f*) postgadolinium T1-weighted SGE images in a patient with a pancreatic adenocarcinoma arising in the neck of the pancreas. There is a heterogeneous mass in the pancreatic neck, which contains a cystic component (arrow, *a*). The body and tail of the pancreas are atrophic with dilatation of the main pancreatic duct. The biliary tree is markedly dilated (*a*).

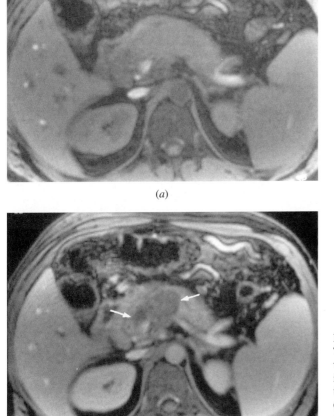
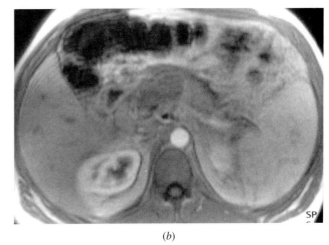

(a)

(b)

(c)

F I G . 4.20 Pancreatic cancer arising in the neck and body. T1-weighted fat-suppressed SGE (*a*), immediate postgadolinium T1-weighted SGE (*b*), and 90-s postgadolinium fat-suppressed SGE (*c*) images. On the noncontrast T1-weighted image, the body and tail of the pancreas are expanded with no definition of a mass. The tumor (arrow, *c*) can be better delineated on gadolinium-enhanced images (*b, c*) because of lesser enhancement of the tumor in relation to the pancreatic parenchyma.

duct. With chronic inflammation of the pancreas, there is progressive fibrosis and glandular atrophy and the proteinaceous fluid of the gland diminishes [34, 37]. In these cases, depiction of cancer is poor on noncontrast T1-weighted fat-suppressed images [34, 35]. However, immediate postgadolinium SGE images are able to define the size and extent of cancers that obstruct the pancreatic duct [34, 35]. Demonstration of a rim, of increased enhancement often thin, surrounding the tumor which represents pancreatic tissue, is commonly observed in pancreatic cancer, particularly those arising in the head. This is an important imaging feature, which helps to establish the focal nature of the disease process. These tumors appear as low-signal intensity mass lesions in a background of slightly greater enhancing chronically inflamed pancreas. Tumors are usually large when they cause changes of surrounding chronic pancreatitis, and in this setting, diagnosis is not problematic. In carcinomas involving the tail, uninvolved pancreatic parenchyma, proximal to the tumor, usually is intact and high in signal intensity on T1-weighted fat-suppressed images (fig. 4.22). This differs from the circumstance of carcinoma within the pancreatic head and reflects the fact that chronic pancreatitis occurs distal to where tumor obstructs the main pancre-

atic duct. An additional imaging feature, which assists in the distinction between carcinoma and chronic pancreatitis, is effacement of the fine, lobular contours of the gland by carcinoma. In the setting of chronic pancreatitis, although the gland may be shrunken and atrophic appearing, background pancreatic architecture is usually preserved. On immediate postgadolinium images, pancreatic carcinoma has diminished signal intensity without well-defined internal structure but with a mild heterogeneous morphology. In contrast, pancreatic enlargement due to subacute or chronic pancreatitis most often shows continuity of the background pancreatic architecture, which has a lobular, feathery or marbled appearance.

In general, pancreatic carcinoma usually appears as a focal mass that is readily detected and characterized on immediate postgadolinium images. In these instances, the tumor is relatively well demarcated from adjacent uninvolved pancreas, which shows greater enhancement. Pancreatic cancer may occasionally be infiltrative in morphology with poorly defined margins (fig. 4.23). In this setting, tumors will be ill defined and decreased in enhancement on immediate postgadolinium images and show slightly increased enhancement on 2-min postgadolinium fat-suppressed SGE images. This appearance

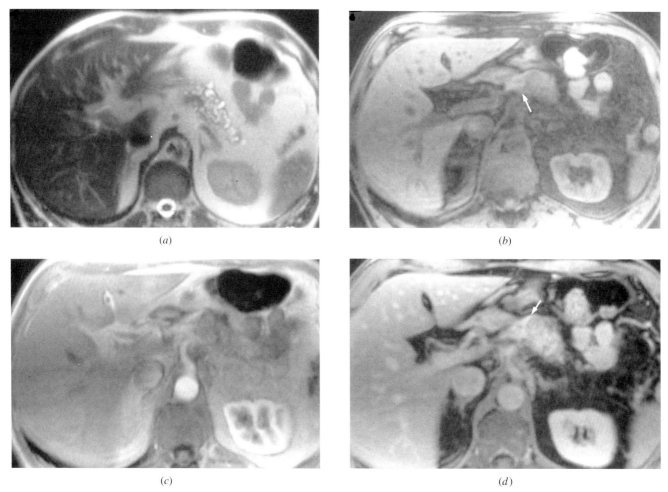

(a)   (b)

(c)   (d)

FIG. 4.21 Pancreatic cancer arising from the body. T2-weighted SS-ETSE (*a*), T1-weighted fat-suppressed SGE (*b*), immediate postgadolinium T1-weighted SGE (*c*), and 90-s postgadolinium fat-suppressed SGE (*d*) images. There is a 3-cm tumor arising in the midpancreatic body. A sharp transition is apparent between proximal normal pancreas and tumor (arrow, *b*), which causes distal chronic pancreatitis on T1-weighted fat-suppressed images (*b*) and the postcontrast images (*c, d*). A claw sign is appreciated (arrow, *d*), reflecting that the mass arises from the pancreas. Dilated ectatic pancreatic duct side branches are present in the distal body and tail, which enhances less than the normal parenchyma.

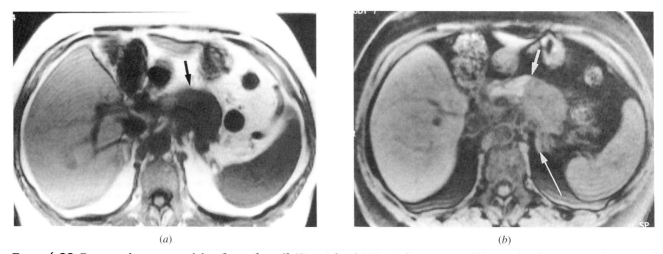

(a)   (b)

FIG. 4.22 Pancreatic cancer arising from the tail. T1-weighted SGE (*a*), fat-suppressed T1-weighted SGE (*b*), and interstitial-phase gadolinium-enhanced T1-weighted SGE (*c*) images. A large pancreatic tail cancer is present that has encased the splenic vein.

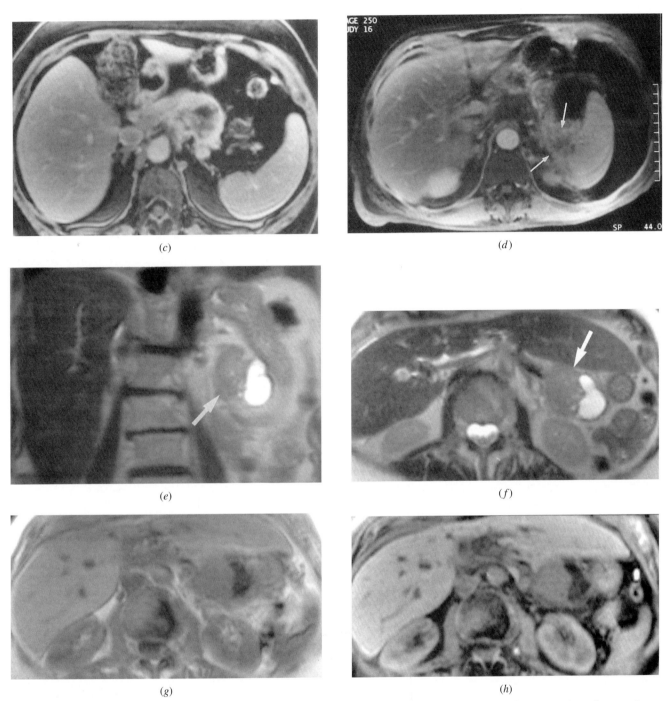

(c)

(d)

(e)

(f)

(g)

(h)

FIG. 4.22 (*Continued*) The tumor is low in signal intensity on the T1-weighted image (arrow, *a*). Demarcation of tumor from uninvolved pancreas (arrow, *b*) is clearly shown on the precontrast T1-weighted fat-suppressed image (*b*). The left adrenal is involved (long arrow, *b*). Heterogeneous enhancement with central low signal intensity is apparent on the interstitial-phase image (*c*).

Interstitial-phase gadolinium-enhanced T1-weighted SGE image (*d*) in a second patient demonstrates a pancreatic tail cancer (arrows, *d*) that invades the splenic hilum.

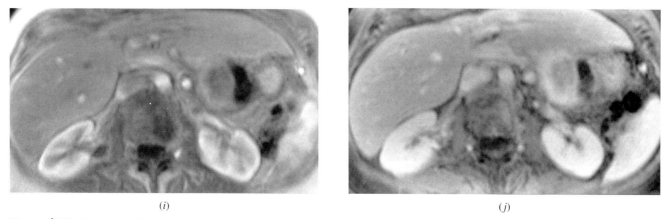

(i)   *(j)*

F I G . **4.22** (*Continued*) Coronal (*e*) and transverse (*f*) T2-weighted SS-ETSE, T1-weighted SGE (*g*), T1-weighted fat-suppressed SGE (*h*), immediate postgadolinium T1-weighted SGE (*i*), and 90-s postgadolinium fat-suppressed SGE (*j*) images in a third patient. A 5-cm cancer (arrow, *e, f*) arises from the tail of the pancreas and contains a cystic component. The tumor displaces the lesser gastric curvature laterally, best appreciated on the coronal image (*e*).

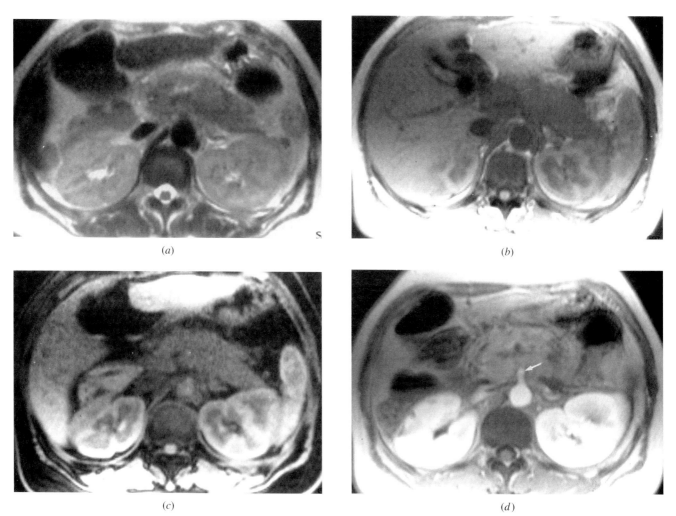

(a)   *(b)*

(c)   *(d)*

F I G . **4.23 Diffuse pancreatic adenocarcinoma.** T2-weighted echo-train spin-echo (*a*), T1-weighted SGE (*b*), T1-weighted fat-suppressed SGE (*c*), immediate postgadolinium T1-weighted SGE (*d*), and 90-s postgadolinium fat-suppressed SGE (*e, f*) images.

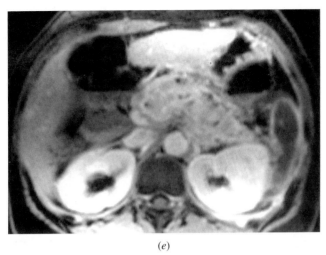

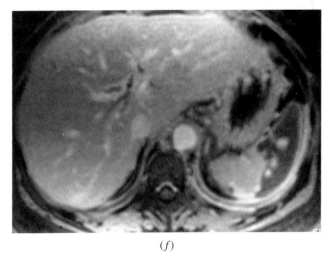

(e)   (f)

F I G . 4.23 (*Continued*) The pancreas is diffusely enlarged and hypointense on T2- (*a*) and T1-weighted (*b*) images, with diminished and heterogeneous enhancement on early (*d*) and late (*e*) gadolinium-enhanced images. The tumor encases the superior mesenteric artery (arrow, *d*) and occludes the superior mesenteric vein and splenic vein. Extensive infarction of the spleen (*f*) reflects the vascular occlusion of splenic vessels.

is commonly observed in pancreatic cancer that has been treated with chemotherapy and radiation therapy (see below) but may also, albeit uncommonly, be seen at initial presentation. Features that may aid in the distinction from chronic pancreatitis are the relatively short history of clinical findings such as abdominal pain and jaundice, and the high-grade ductal obstruction despite ostensibly small-volume disease.

Regarding tumor staging, local extension of cancer and lymphovascular involvement may be evaluated on nonsuppressed T1-weighted images (figs. 4.24 and 4.25) [38, 39]. Low-signal intensity tumor is well shown in a background of high-signal intensity fat. Gadolinium-enhanced fat-suppressed SGE image acquired in the interstitial phase of enhancement (1–10 min after contrast)

demonstrates intermediate-signal intensity tumor tissue extension into low-signal intensity suppressed fat. In comparison, noncontrast T1-weighted fat-suppressed images generally show minimal signal intensitydifference between tumor, which is low in signal intensity, and suppressed background fat [34]. When tumor involves the body or tail of the pancreas, invasion of adjacent organs, such as the left adrenal gland, is well shown on a combination of sequences including nonsuppressed T1-weighted images and interstitial-phase gadolinium-enhanced fat-suppressed T1-weighted images (figs. 4.26 and 4.27).

Vascular encasement by the tumor may be shown using a variety of sequences. T1-weighted spin-echo imaging has been reported to be superior to dynamic

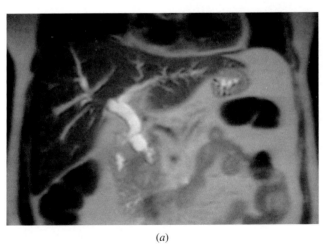

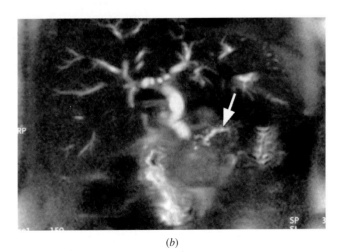

(a)   (b)

F I G . 4.24 Staging pancreatic cancer—vessel involvement. Coronal T2-weighted SS-ETSE (*a*), angled coronal MRCP (*b*), immediate postgadolinium T1-weighted SGE (*c*), and 90-s postgadolinium fat-suppressed SGE (*d*) images. A 5-cm tumor arises from the pancreatic head and obstructs the CBD and pancreatic duct (arrow, *b*), which is well shown on the MRCP image (*b*). The interstitial-phase gadolinium-enhanced image (*d*) shows a nonocclusive thrombus in the superior mesenteric vein (arrow, *d*) and tumor stranding around both superior mesenteric vessels.

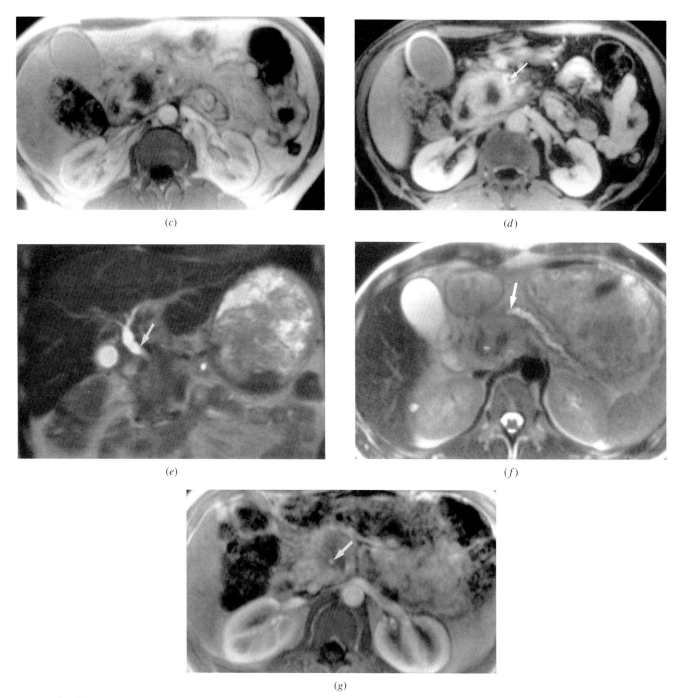

(c)

(d)

(e)

(f)

(g)

FIG. 4.24 (*Continued*) Coronal (*e*) and transverse (*f*) T2-weighted SS-ETSE and immediate postgadolinium T1-weighted SGE (*g*) images in a second patient with pancreatic head adenocarcinoma. Note atrophy of the pancreatic body and tail with dilatation of main pancreatic duct. Ductal dilatations of the CBD (arrow, *e*) and pancreatic duct (arrow, *f*) are best shown on single shot T2-weighted images (including MRCP). The tumor is best shown on immediate postgadolinium images (*g*). Encased superior mesenteric artery is shown (arrow, *g*)

contrast-enhanced CT imaging for the determination of vascular encasement [38]; however, this MR approach may not yield consistent results. Vascular patency may be evaluated by either a flow-sensitive gradient-echo technique [40] or dynamic gadolinium-enhanced SGE (fig. 4.24) [40, 41]. In our experience gadolinium-enhanced SGE generates reproducible, consistently good image quality. Immediate postgadolinium SGE images are useful for evaluating arterial patency and immediate and 45-s postgadolinium SGE images for evaluating venous patency.

When approaches by CT and MRI are compared, interstitial-phase gadolinium-enhanced fat-suppressed images best delineate peritoneal metastases [42, 43]. MR

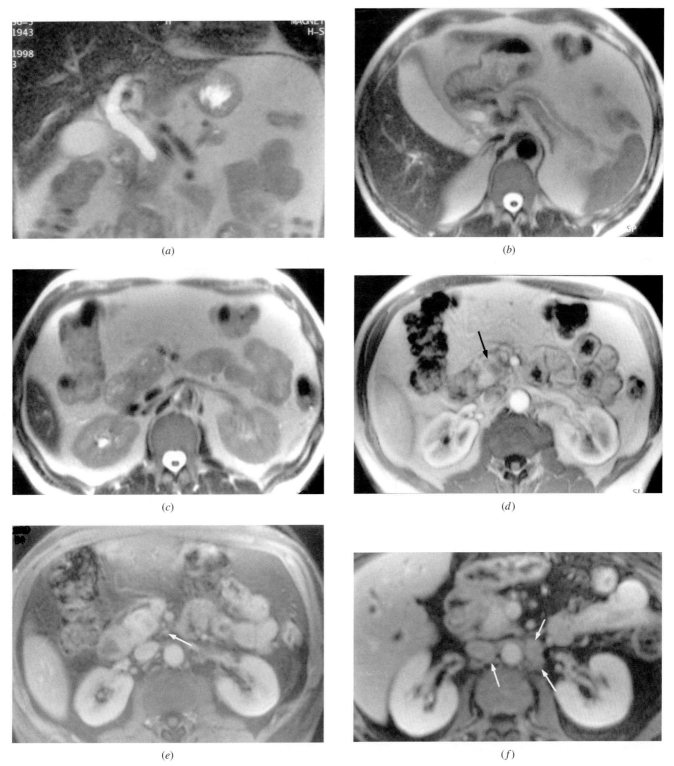

F I G . 4.25 Staging pancreatic cancer—lymph nodes. Coronal (*a*) and transverse (*b, c*) T2-weighted SS-ETSE, immediate post-gadolinium T1-weighted SGE (*d*), and 90-s postgadolinium fat-suppressed SGE (*e*) images in a patient with pancreatic ductal adeno-carcinoma (arrow, *d*) arising from the head. The CBD is markedly dilated (*a*), with mild dilatation of the pancreatic duct (*b*). Tumors are generally not well seen on T2 (*c*). Optimal tumor demonstration is on immediate postgadolinium images (*d*). Small regional nodes (arrow, *e*) are best seen on interstitial-phase gadolinium-enhanced fat-suppressed SGE images (*e*).

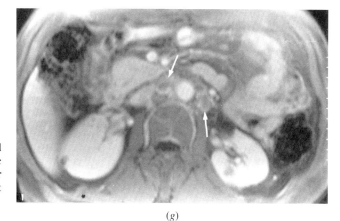

(g)

FIG. 4.25 (*Continued*) Interstitial-phase gadolinium-enhanced fat-suppressed SGE images (*f*, *g*) in two other patients demonstrate malignant retroperitoneal lymph nodes (arrows, *f*, *g*). In the latter patient (*g*) the lymph nodes have low-signal centers consistent with central necrosis.

does not perform well at local staging if this technique is not employed [44]. Peritoneal metastases appear moderately high signal in a dark background of suppressed fat and are very conspicuous even if peritoneal disease is of thin volume and relatively linear (fig. 4.28). Demonstration of focal thickening or nodules increases the likelihood that peritoneal abnormalities represent a malignant process.

Lymph nodes are well shown on T2-weighted fat-suppressed images and interstitial-phase gadolinium-enhanced fat-suppressed T1-weighted images. Lymph nodes are moderately high in signal intensity in a background of low-signal intensity suppressed fat using both of these techniques (figs. 4.25 and 4.29). T2-weighted fat-suppressed imaging is particularly useful for the demonstration of lymph nodes in close approximation to the liver because of the signal intensity difference

between moderately high-signal intensity nodes and moderately low-signal intensity liver. Both lymph nodes and liver appear moderately enhanced on interstitial-phase gadolinium-enhanced fat suppressed SGE images. To detect lymph nodes adjacent to liver it is useful to identify suspicious foci of high signal on the T2-weighted fat-suppressed images and confirm that they have the rounded morphology of lymph nodes on the gadolinium-enhanced fat-suppressed T1-weighted sequences. On nonsuppressed T1-weighted images, lymph nodes are conspicuous as low-signal intensity focal masses in a background of high-signal intensity fat [39]. Liver metastases from pancreatic cancers are generally irregular in shape, are low in signal intensity on conventional or fat-suppressed T1-weighted images and minimally hyperintense on T2-weighted images, and demonstrate irregular rim enhancement on immediate

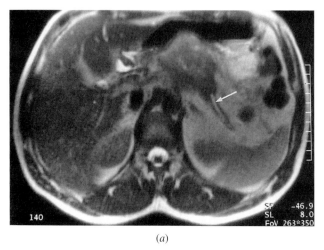

(a)

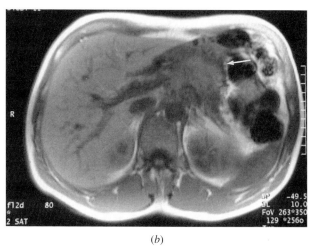

(b)

FIG. 4.26 Staging pancreatic cancer—stomach invasion and splenic vein thrombosis. T2-weighted SS-ETSE (*a*), T1-weighted SGE (*b*), immediate postgadolinium T1-weighted SGE (*c*), interstitial-phase gadolinium-enhanced T1-weighted fat-suppressed SGE (*d*, *e*), and coronal interstitial-phase gadolinium-enhanced T1-weighted fat-suppressed SGE (*f*) images. A large cancer is present arising from the body of the pancreas (arrow, *b*) that invades the posterior wall of the stomach. Atrophy of the pancreatic tail with ductal dilatation (arrow, *a*) is well shown on the single-shot T2-weighted image (*a*). Heterogeneous minimal enhancement of the tumor is present on the immediate postgadolinium T1-weighted SGE image (*c*).

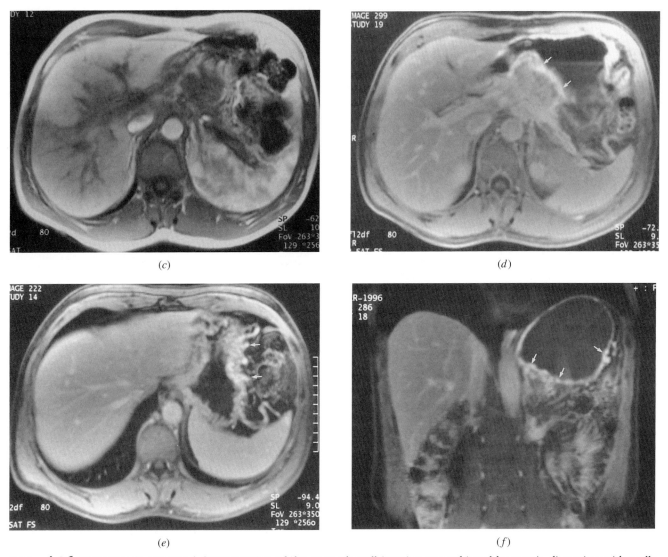

(c)

(d)

(e)

(f)

F I G . 4.26 (*Continued*) Improved demonstration of the stomach wall invasion was achieved by gastric distension with orally administered water on the interstitial-phase fat-suppressed T1-weighted SGE image (small arrows, *d*). Multiple varices along the greater curvature of the stomach are present due to thrombosis of the splenic vein. Varices are well shown on gadolinium-enhanced T1-weighted fat-suppressed T1-weighted SGE images as high-signal intensity tubular structures (arrows, *e*, *f*).

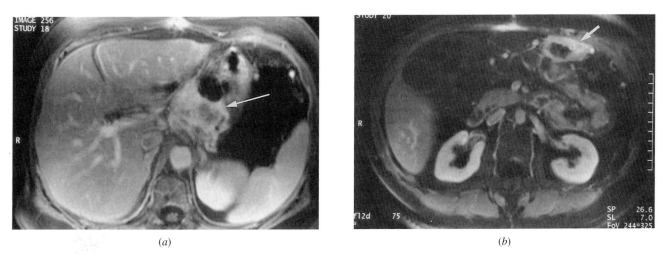

(a)

(b)

F I G . 4.27 Staging pancreatic cancer—extension along the transverse mesocolon. Interstitial-phase gadolinium-enhanced fat-suppressed T1-weighted SGE images (*a–c*). A large cancer arises from the body of the pancreas (arrow, *a*) that is adherent to the posterior wall of the stomach.

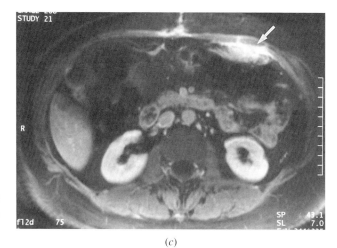

(c)

FIG. 4.27 *(Continued)* Tumor extends inferiorly along the transverse mesocolon to involve the transverse colon (arrow, *b*), greater omentum, and adjacent peritoneum (arrow, *c*).

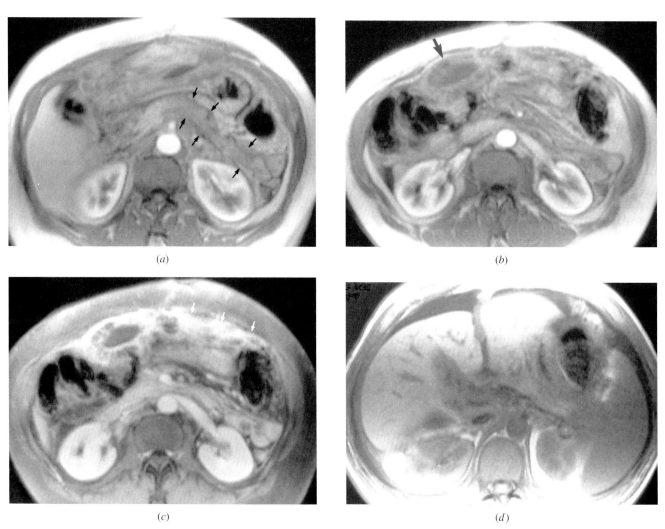

(a)

(b)

(c)

(d)

FIG. 4.28 Staging pancreatic cancer—peritoneal metastasis. Immediate postgadolinium SGE (*a*, *b*) and 90-s postgadolinium fat-suppressed SGE (*c*) images. There is normal enhancement of the pancreatic head and neck with an abrupt transition showing hypo-enhancement of the body and tail of the pancreas (arrows, *a*). A focal mass is not present, and this is consistent with diffusely infiltrative pancreatic cancer. A large peritoneum-based mass (arrow, *b*) along the anterior abdominal wall is present, which has a multiloculated appearance with peripheral enhancement. There is adjacent peritoneal and omental (arrows, *c*) enhancement. These findings are consistent with diffusely infiltrative pancreatic adenocarcinoma with peritoneal metastasis.

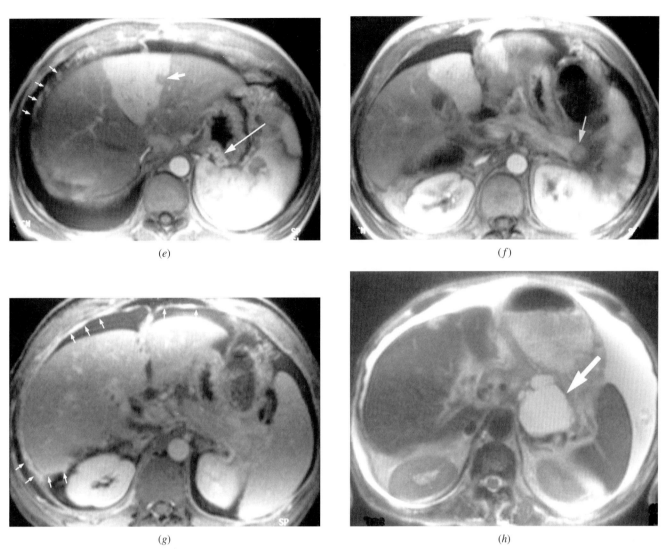

(e) *(f)*

(g) *(h)*

FIG. 4.28 (*Continued*) T1-weighted SGE (*d*), immediate postgadolinium T1-weighted SGE (*e, f*), and 90-s postgadolinium fat-suppressed SGE (*g*) images at the level of the pancreatic body and tail in a second patient. A 2-cm cancer arises from the pancreatic tail (arrow, *f*), which is best shown on the immediate postgadolinium image (*f*). Wedge-shaped transient hyperenhancement of *segment 4* of the liver on the immediate postgadolinium images is present. Perilesional enhancement is commonly observed with pancreatic cancer liver metastases. A small defect is present in the hyperenhanced liver, which may represent a metastasis (small arrow, *e*). Diminished enhancement centrally in the spleen and a gastric wall varix (long arrow, *e*) reflect splenic vein thrombosis. Ascites and extensive peritoneal metastases are present (very small arrows, *e, g*), which are most conspicuous on the interstitial-phase gadolinium-enhanced fat-suppressed SGE images (*g*).

T2-weighted fat suppressed SS-ETSE (*h*) and 90-s postgadolinium fat-suppressed T1-weighted SGE (*i*) images in a third patient who has pancreatic cancer with liver and peritoneal metastases. A 6-cm cystic mass is present in the lesser arc (arrow, *h*). Multiple varices are identified surrounding the cystic lesion (*i*). Ascites is appreciated on both T2 (*h*) and postgadolinium fat-suppressed T1-weighted images (*i*). Extensive thickening and enhancement of the peritoneum (small arrows, *i*) is only appreciated on the fat-suppressed gadolinium-enhanced images (*i*). A 1.5-cm subcapsular metastasis is identified in *segment 4* (curved arrow, *i*).

postcontrast SGE images (figs. 4.29–4.31). The low-signal intensity centers of metastatic lesions reflect the desmoplastic nature of the primary cancer [1]. The low fluid content and hypovascular nature of these metastases permits the distinction between these lesions and cysts and hemangiomas, respectively, even when lesions are <1 cm in diameter. Transient, ill-defined, increased perilesional hepatic parenchyma enhancement may be observed on immediate postgadolinium images. A similar appearance is observed even more commonly for colon cancer metastases. Perilesional enhancement is more typically wedge shaped with pancreatic cancer liver metastases than with colon cancer liver metastases and may have a dramatic appearance. This unique profile of perilesional enhancement may represent effects of neovascularization with increased

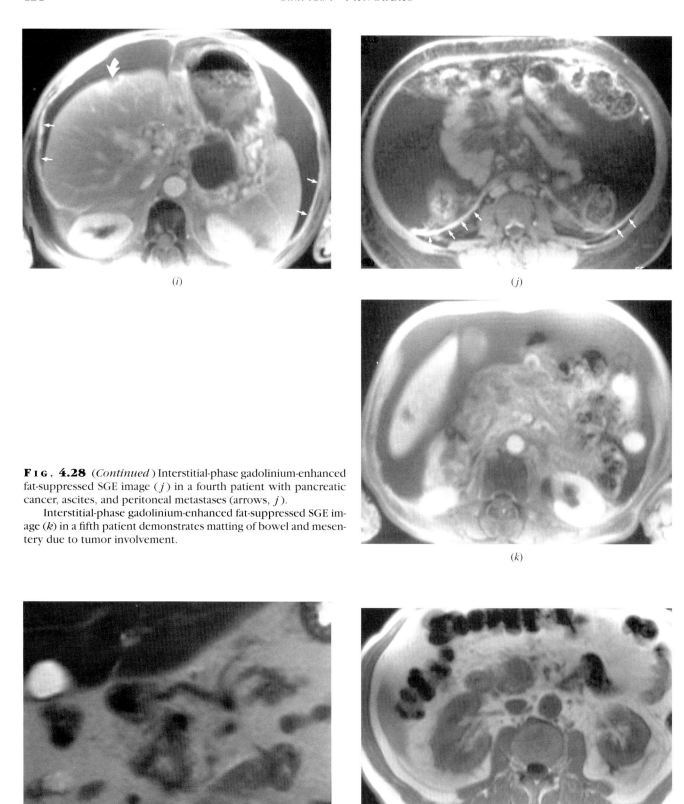

F I G . **4.28** (*Continued*) Interstitial-phase gadolinium-enhanced fat-suppressed SGE image (*j*) in a fourth patient with pancreatic cancer, ascites, and peritoneal metastases (arrows, *j*).

Interstitial-phase gadolinium-enhanced fat-suppressed SGE image (*k*) in a fifth patient demonstrates matting of bowel and mesentery due to tumor involvement.

F I G . **4.29 Staging pancreatic cancer—lymphadenopathy and liver metastases.** Coronal T2-weighted echo-train spin-echo (*a*), T1-weighted SGE (*b*), T1-weighted fat-suppressed SGE (*c*), immediate postgadolinium T1 SGE (*d*, *e*), and 90-s postgadolinium T1-weighted fat-suppressed SGE (*f*, *g*) images. There is a 3-cm pancreatic head cancer (arrow, *d*), which is clearly shown on the immediate postgadolinium image (*d*) as a hypoenhancing mass with demarcated borders and adjacent greater-enhancing pancreatic parenchyma.

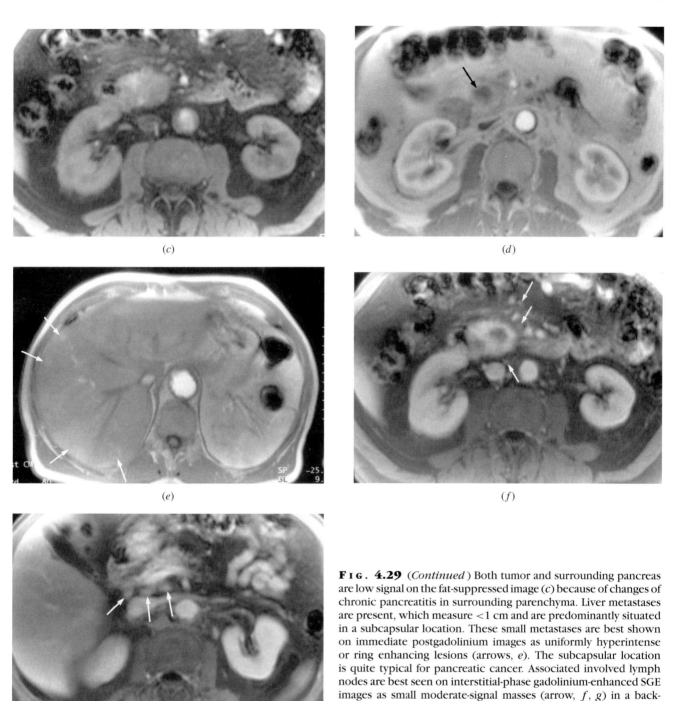

(c)

(d)

(e)

(f)

(g)

F I G . 4.29 (*Continued*) Both tumor and surrounding pancreas are low signal on the fat-suppressed image (*c*) because of changes of chronic pancreatitis in surrounding parenchyma. Liver metastases are present, which measure <1 cm and are predominantly situated in a subcapsular location. These small metastases are best shown on immediate postgadolinium images as uniformly hyperintense or ring enhancing lesions (arrows, *e*). The subcapsular location is quite typical for pancreatic cancer. Associated involved lymph nodes are best seen on interstitial-phase gadolinium-enhanced SGE images as small moderate-signal masses (arrow, *f*, *g*) in a background of suppressed fat. Pancreatic cancer has a propensity to involve nodes without resulting in increased size.

capillary permeability and hypercoagulable state with thrombus formation causing ischemia or tumor embolus. Concomitant liver metastases in the setting of prominent wedge-shaped enhancement abnormalities are commonly small, hypervascular, and subcapsular in location. The pathophysiologic explanation for this pattern of metastases is currently under investigation.

Optimal utilization of MRI in the investigation of pancreatic carcinoma occurs in the following circumstances; 1) detection of small, non-contour-deforming tumors (due to the high contrast resolution of precontrast T1-weighted fat-suppressed imaging and immediate postgadolinium SGE images), 2) determination of tumor location for imaging-guided biopsy, 3) evaluation of

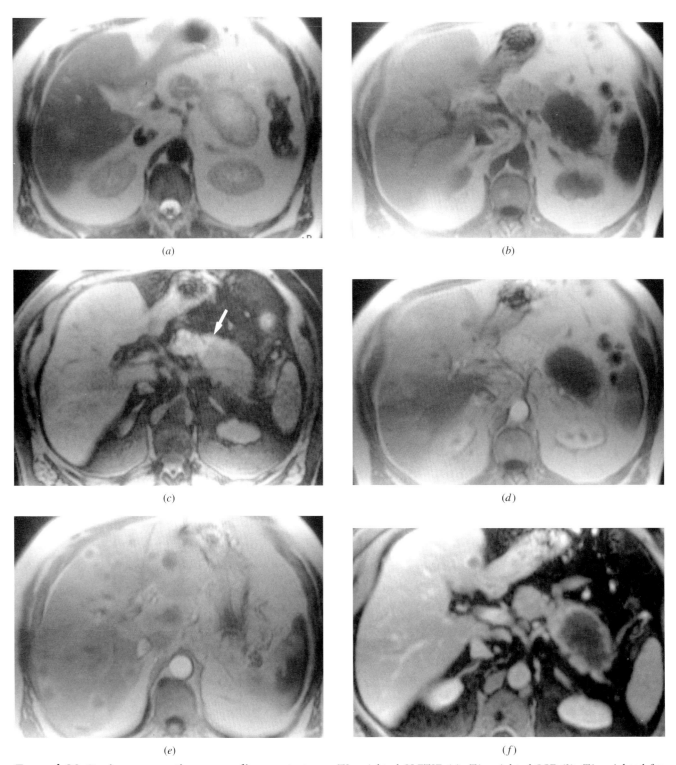

(a)

(b)

(c)

(d)

(e)

(f)

F I G . 4.30 Staging pancreatic cancer—liver metastases. T2-weighted SS-ETSE (*a*), T1-weighted SGE (*b*), T1-weighted fat-suppressed SGE (*c*), immediate postgadolinium T1-weighted SGE (*d*, *e*), and 90-s postgadolinium fat-suppressed SGE (*f*) images. A 4 × 5-cm tumor arises in the pancreatic tail. Note the shape demarcation of normal pancreas (arrow, *c*) proximal to the large pancreatic cancer. There are multiple liver metastases that are mildly hyperintense on T2 (*a*) and mildly low signal on T1, reflecting a low fluid content. Liver metastases are best seen as ring-enhancing lesions on immediate postgadolinium images (*d*, *e*) with ring-enhancing metastases involving both lobes. Pancreatic cancer most commonly metastasizes to the liver.

Immediate postgadolinium SGE image (*g*) in a second patient demonstrates a 1-cm ring-enhancing metastasis (arrow, *g*).

Immediate postgadolinium SGE image (*h*) in a third patient demonstrates a large hypovascular tumor arising from the tail of the tail of the pancreas (arrow, *h*).

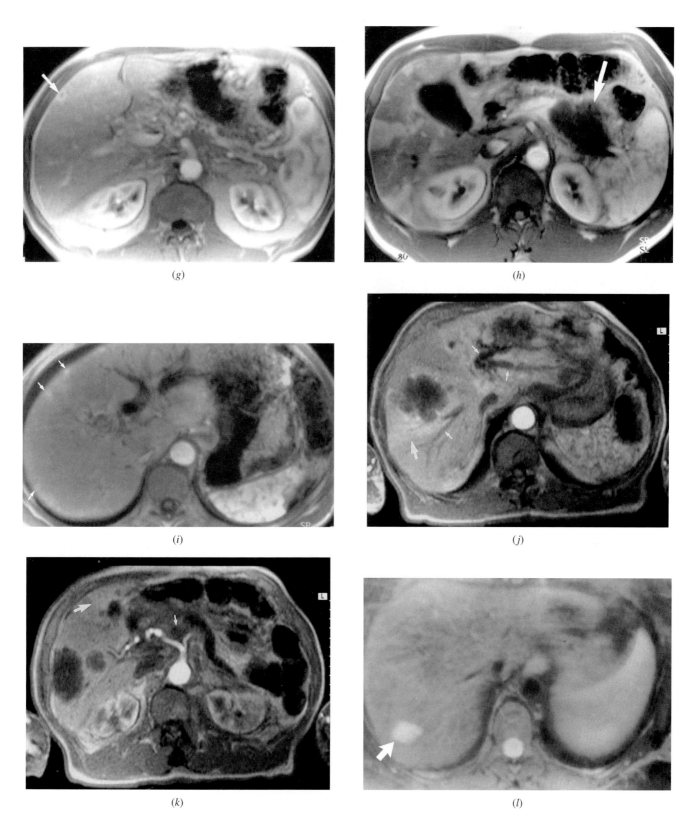

(g)

(h)

(i)

(j)

(k)

(l)

F I G . 4.30 (*Continued*) Note the beak sign with the proximal pancreatic parenchyma. Multiple hyperenhancing liver metastases are present, the majority <1 cm in size. Wedge-shaped areas of transient increased perilesional enhancement are appreciated surrounding several lesions. Perilesional enhancement is not uncommon in pancreatic ductal adenocarcinoma. The most commonly observed metastases with perilesional enhancement are colon adenocarcinoma.

Immediate postgadolinium T1-weighted SGE image (*i*) in a fourth patient. Multiple hyperenhancing <1-cm subcapsular liver metastases (arrow, *i*) are present that were not identifiable on other sequences.

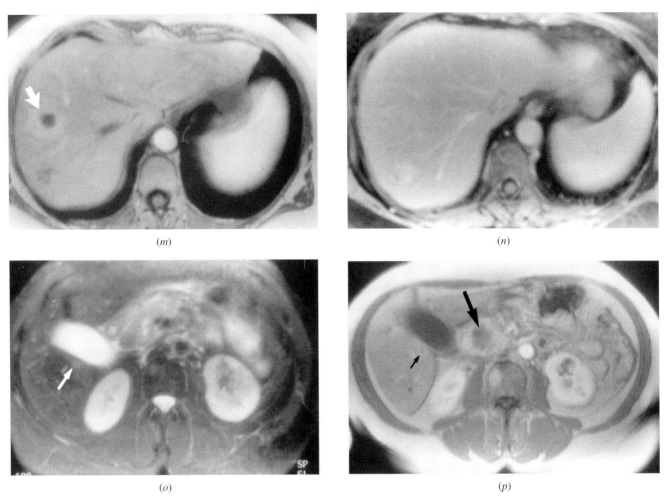

(m)

(n)

(o)

(p)

FIG. 4.30 (*Continued*) Immediate postgadolinium T1-weighted SGE images (*j, k*) in a fifth patient. Multiple irregular hepatic metastases with rim enhancement are present. Ill-defined perilesional enhancement (arrow, *j, k*) is apparent surrounding several metastases. Substantial intrahepatic bile duct dilatation is also identified (small arrows, *j*) secondary to CBD obstruction by the pancreatic head cancer. Low-signal intensity tissue (small arrows, *k*) surrounds the celiac axis, a finding consistent with tumor involvement.

Breathing-averaged T2-weighted ETSE (*l*), immediate postgadolinium SGE (*m*), and 90-s postgadolinium T1-weighted fat-suppressed SGE (*n*) images in a sixth patient who has liver metastases and a hemangioma. Hemangiomas and metastases can usually be readily distinguished. The hemangioma (arrow, *l*) is high signal on T2 (*l*) and demonstrates peripheral nodules on the immediate postgadolinium image (*m*) with relatively uniform hyperintense enhancement on delayed images (*n*). In contrast, the 3-cm metastasis is nearly invisible on T2 (*l*) and late postgadolinium images (*n*), with intense ring enhancement (arrow, *m*) on immediate postgadolinium image (*n*). This constellation of findings is virtually pathognomonic on T2-weighted and postgadolinium images for a liver metastasis coexistent with a hemangioma.

Breathing averaged T2-weighted echo-train spin-echo (*o*) and immediate postgadolinium SGE (*p*) images in a seventh patient. The pancreatic tumor is not well seen on T2, but clearly shown as a hypoenhancing mass (arrow, *p*) on the immediate postgadolinium image (*p*). A <1-cm ring-enhancing lesion (small arrow, *p*) is apparent in a subcapsular location adjacent to the gallbladder in *segment V*. On the T2-weighted image (*o*) the lesion is only mildly hyperintense, consistent with minimal fluid content, characteristic of pancreatic ductal adenocarcinoma metastases.

vascular involvement by tumor, 4) determination and characterization of associated liver lesions, and 5) evaluation of patients with diminished renal function or iodine contrast allergy. MRI may be particularly valuable in patients who have an enlarged pancreatic head with no definition of a mass on CT images. Surgery remains the main therapeutic treatment of patients with pancreatic cancer [27, 45]; therefore, earlier detection of potentially curable disease may result in improved patient survival. Benassai et al. [45] recently reported

on the factors associated with improvement in the 5-year actuarial survival for patients undergoing pancreaticoduodenectomy. Five-year survival was greater for node-negative than for node-positive patients (41.7% vs. 7.8%, *P* < 0.001) and for smaller (<3 cm) than for larger tumors (33.3% vs. 8.8%, *P* < 0.006). The 5-year survival for patients with negative surgical margins was 23.3%, whereas no patients with positive surgical margins survived at 13 months (*P* < 0.001).

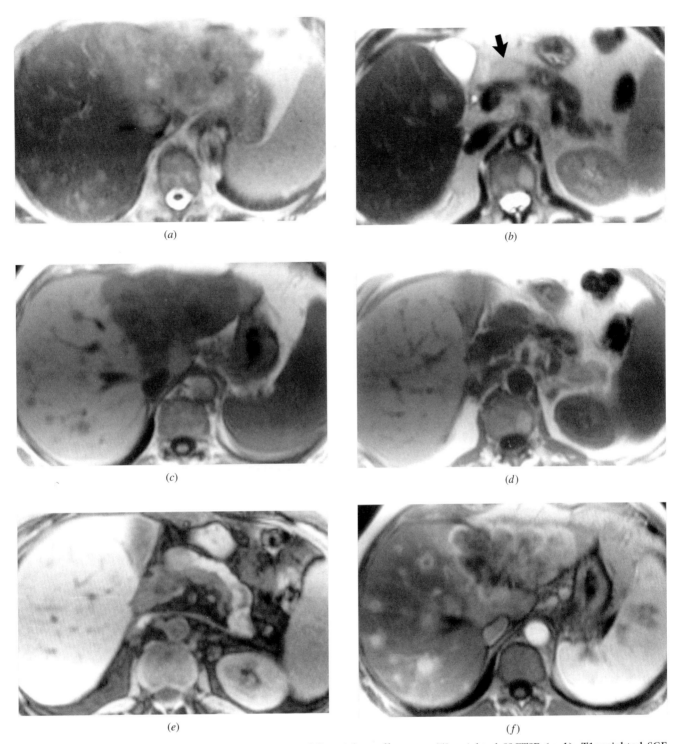

F I G . 4.31 Poorly differentiated carcinoma resembling islet cell tumor. T2-weighted SS-ETSE (*a*, *b*), T1-weighted SGE (*c*, *d*), T1-weighted fat-suppressed SGE (*e*), immediate postgadolinium T1-weighted SGE (*f*, *g*), and 90-s postgadolinium fat-suppressed SGE (*h*, *i*) images. There is a 3-cm tumor (arrow, *b*) arising in the pancreatic neck, which is moderately hyperintense on T2 (*b*) and moderately hypointense on T1 (*d*, *e*), enhances in a uniform intense fashion immediately after gadolinium administration (arrow, *g*), and retains contrast on interstitial-phase images (*i*).

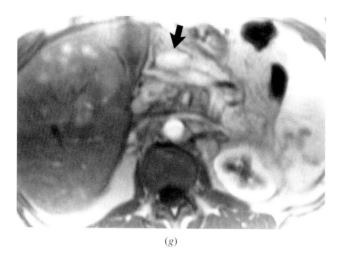

(g)

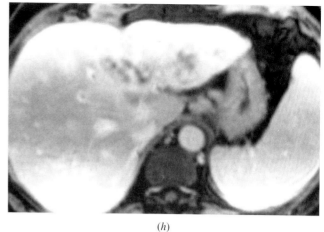

(h)

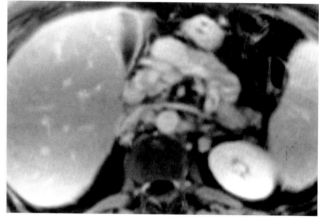

(i)

FIG. 4.31 (*Continued*) There are multiple liver metastases that
are moderately hyperintense on T2 (*a*) and moderately hypointense
on T1 (*c*) and show uniform or ring enhancement on immediate
postgadolinium images (*f*), mimicking an islet cell tumor.

Poorly Differentiated Carcinoma

Rarely, malignant pancreatic cancers may not be clas-
sifiable because of to poorly differentiated or anaplastic
cytology. These cancers may have an appearance similar
to islet cell tumors, with tumors appearing high signal on
T2-weighted images and extensive hypervascular liver
metastases (fig. 4.31). The spectrum of appearance for
poorly differentiated carcinoma has not been elucidated.

Chemotherapy/Radiation Therapy-Treated Pancreatic Ductal Adenocarcinoma

After chemotherapy and radiation therapy, morphologic
and pathophysiologic changes occur in the tumor, in
the pancreas, and in surrounding fatty tissues. In approximately 50% of cases a decrease in the size of tumor and surrounding fibrosis can be demonstrated on
MR images that correlate with clinical response. However, in a sizable proportion of cases, the interface is
indistinct between tumor margin and surrounding background pancreatic tissue. In these instances, evaluation
of tumor dimensions is extremely difficult. In addition,

in some cases, posttreatment studies may show features
suggestive of acute or chronic pancreatitis. On imaging, both processes may demonstrate an increase in
abnormal pancreatic tissue even though the tumor itself has decreased in size. Assessment of treatment response is challenging (fig. 4.32). Further investigation is
necessary to determine positive findings of response to
therapy.

Islet Cell Tumors

Islet cell tumors are a subgroup of gastrointestinal neuroendocrine tumors that occur within the endocrine pancreas. These tumors are rare in comparison with tumors
arising from the exocrine portion. Islet cell tumors are
uncommon, with a reported incidence of less than
1 per 100,000 [46]. Tumors may be nonfunctioning, or,
more commonly, they may present with an endocrine
abnormality resulting from the secretion of hormones
[46]. Histopathologically, only a generic diagnosis of islet
cell tumor can be made with routine staining methods.
However, islet cell tumors are primarily identified by
the peptide they contain, and the tumor itself is named

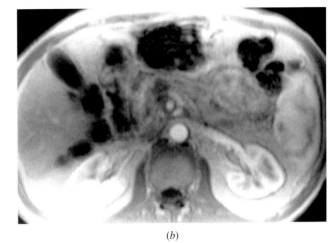

(a)

(b)

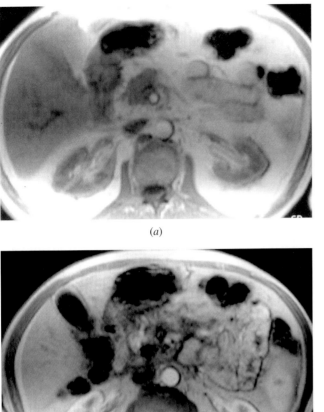

(c)

F I G . 4.32 Pancreatic cancer undergoing chemotherapy and radiation treatment—images from 3 consecutive studies in a patient undergoing chemotherapy and radiation treatment. Immediate postgadolinium SGE images from pretherapy (a), to 3 months (b) and 5 months (c) after initiation of treatment. Pancreatic cancer is initially well defined (arrow, a). After the commencement of treatment, both tumor and pancreas become less defined (b, c).

after the dominant hormone it secretes (e.g., an insulin-secreting tumor is termed an insulinoma). Only the results of special immunohistochemical techniques, such as fluorescence-labeled antibody specific for a peptide, will permit the designation of a specific islet tumor such as insulinoma, gastrinoma, etc. A certain proportion of islet cell tumors will secrete no identifiable substance and remain uncategorized after special immunohistochemical procedures. The most common pancreatic islet cell tumors are insulinomas and gastrinomas, followed in frequency of diagnosis by glucagonomas and VIPomas [47]. In our experience, the majority of clinically or immunohistochemically verified pancreatic neuroendocrine tumors are gastrinomas [48]. Hormonally functional tumors tend to present when they are small because of symptoms related to the hormones secreted by the tumors. Nonfunctional tumors account for at least 15–20% of islet cell tumors and tend to present with symptoms due to large tumor mass or metastatic disease [49]. One cannot diagnose malignancy on the basis of the histologic appearance of islet cell tumors. Instead, malignancy is determined by the presence of metastasis or local invasion beyond the substance of the

pancreas. Insulinomas are most commonly benign tumors; gastrinomas are malignant in approximately 60% of cases, and almost all other types, including nonfunctioning tumors, are malignant in the great majority of cases. The liver is the most common organ for metastatic spread. There is also a particular propensity for splenic metastases.

In the MRI investigation for islet cell tumors, precontrast T1-weighted fat-suppressed images, immediate postgadolinium SGE images, and T2-weighted fat-suppressed images or breath-hold T2-weighted images are useful [1, 50–53]. Because many MR techniques independently demonstrate islet cell tumors well, MR is particularly well suited for the investigation of these tumors. Tumors are low in signal intensity on T1-weighted fat-suppressed images, demonstrate homogeneous, ring, or diffuse heterogeneous enhancement on immediate postgadolinium SGE, and are high in signal intensity on T2-weighted fat-suppressed images [48]. In rare instances, islet cell tumors may be very desmoplastic, appear low in signal intensity on T2-weighted images, and demonstrate negligible contrast enhancement. In these cases, the tumors may mimic the appearance of pancreatic ductal adenocarcinoma. Large, noninsulinoma, islet cell tumors may contain regions of necrosis [54].

Features that distinguish the majority of islet cell tumors from ductal adenocarcinomas include high signal intensity on T2-weighted images, increased homogeneous enhancement on immediate postgadolinium images, and hypervascular liver metastases [52]. Because islet cell tumors rarely obstruct the pancreatic duct, T1-weighted fat-suppressed images most often show high signal intensity of background pancreas rendering clear depiction of low-signal intensity tumors in the majority of cases [51, 52]; however, exceptions may occur (figs. 4.33–4.35). Lack of pancreatic ductal obstruction and vascular encasement by tumor are features generally absent in islet cell tumors that differentiate these tumors from pancreatic ductal adenocarcinoma. In contrast to the frequent occurrence of thrombosis in pancreatic ductal adenocarcinoma, thrombosis is rare in the setting of islet cell tumors. Unlike thrombus in ductal adenocarcinoma, which is usually blood thrombus, thrombus in islet cell tumors have a greater propensity to be tumor

thrombus (fig. 4.36) [55]. Peritoneal metastasis and/or regional lymph node enlargement, characteristic features of pancreatic ductal adenocarcinoma, are generally not present in islet cell tumors.

Islet Cell Tumors, Untyped or Uncategorized

Islet cell tumors do not receive a specific designation when special immunohistochemical stains or serum assays are negative. Tumors are generally large at presentation because they are clinically silent. The imaging appearance of these tumors resembles glucagonomas and somatostatinomas (figs. 4.33–4.36)

Gastrinomas (G cell Tumors)

The Zollinger-Ellison syndrome is defined by the clinical triad of pancreatic islet cell gastrinoma, gastric hypersecretion, and recalcitrant peptic ulcer disease. Ulcers located in the postbulbar region of the duodenum or in the jejunum, particularly if multiple, suggest the diagnosis of a gastrinoma. Esophagitis is ocasionally observed in these patients.

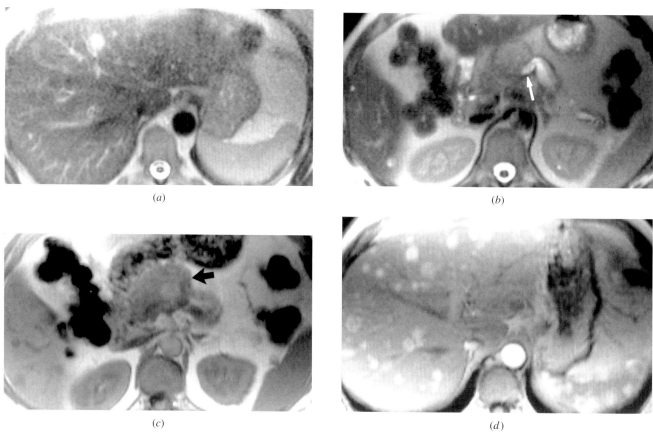

(a)   (b)

(c)   (d)

F I G . 4.33 Nonfunctioning islet cell tumor with pancreatic ductal obstruction. T2-weighted SS-ETSE (*a*, *b*), T1-weighted SGE (*c*), immediate (*d*, *e*) and 45-s (*f*) postgadolinium T1-weighted SGE, and 90-s postgadolinium fat-suppressed SGE (*g*) images. There is a 5-cm lobulated tumor (arrow, *c*) arising from the neck/proximal body of the pancreas. The tumor is mildly hyperintense on T2 (*b*) and mildly hypointense on T1 (*c*) and shows diffuse moderately intense enhancement on immediate postgadolinium SGE (*e*) with moderate washout on interstitial-phase images (*g*).

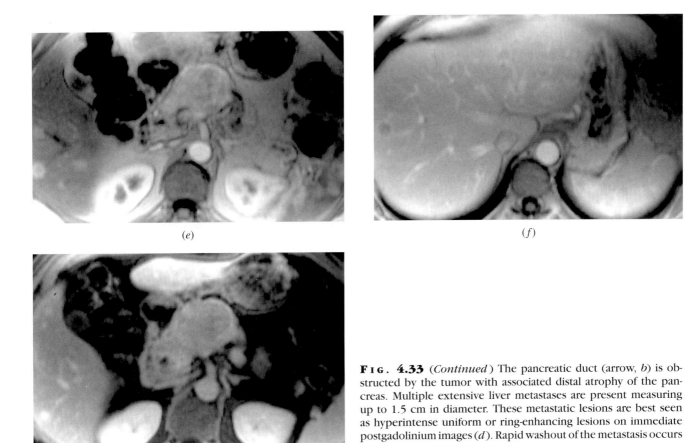

(e)

(f)

(g)

F I G . 4.33 (*Continued*) The pancreatic duct (arrow, *b*) is obstructed by the tumor with associated distal atrophy of the pancreas. Multiple extensive liver metastases are present measuring up to 1.5 cm in diameter. These metastatic lesions are best seen as hyperintense uniform or ring-enhancing lesions on immediate postgadolinium images (*d*). Rapid washout of the metastasis occurs by 45 after injection (*f*).

(a)

(b)

F I G . 4.34 Nonfunctioning well-differentiated neuroendocrine carcinoma. T2-weighted SS-ETSE (*a*), T1-weighted SGE (*b*), T1-weighted fat-suppressed SGE (*c*), immediate postgadolinium T1-weighted SGE (*d*), and 90-s postgadolinium fat-suppressed SGE (*e*) images.

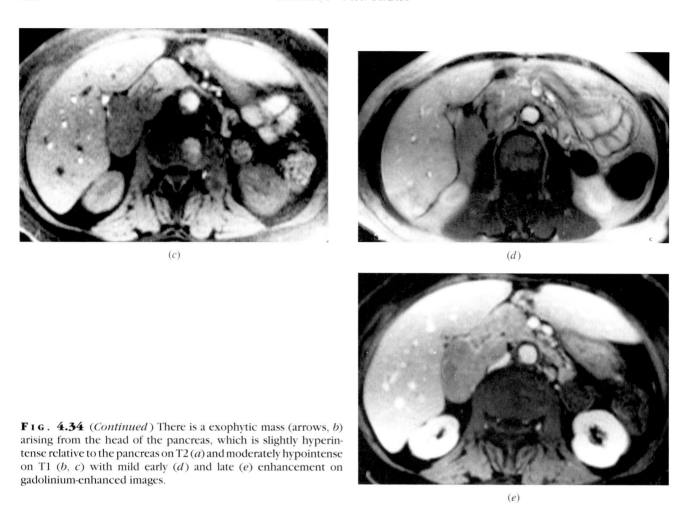

(c)

(d)

(e)

FIG. 4.34 (*Continued*) There is a exophytic mass (arrows, *b*) arising from the head of the pancreas, which is slightly hyperintense relative to the pancreas on T2 (*a*) and moderately hypointense on T1 (*b*, *c*) with mild early (*d*) and late (*e*) enhancement on gadolinium-enhanced images.

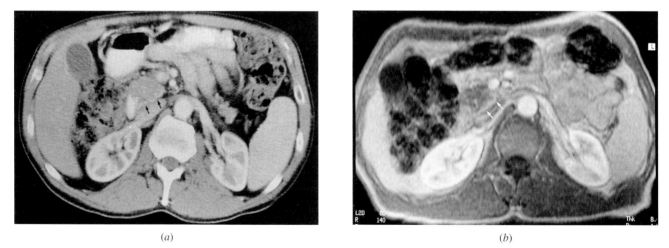

(a)

(b)

FIG. 4.35 **Hypovascular nonfunctioning islet cell tumor with liver metastases.** Spiral CT (*a*) and immediate postgadolinium T1-weighted SGE (*b*) images. Low-attenuation/signal intensity tumor is well shown in the head of the pancreas on both spiral CT (*a*) and MR (*b*) images. A thin rim of greater-enhancing normal pancreas is noted posterior to the tumor (small arrows, *a*, *b*). On a higher tomographic section, an ill-defined low-density lesion is noted in the liver on spiral CT image (arrow, *c*) that was considered indeterminate. On the T2-weighted fat-suppressed spin-echo image (*d*), the liver lesion is noted to be low in signal intensity (arrow, *d*), which is not consistent with cyst or hemangioma and is compatible with a hypovascular metastasis.

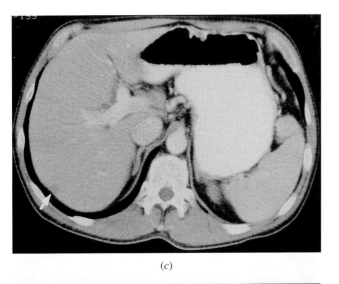

(c)

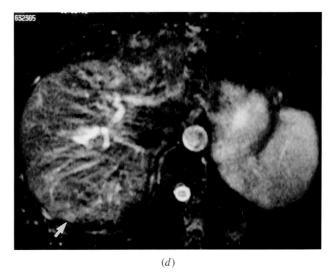

(d)

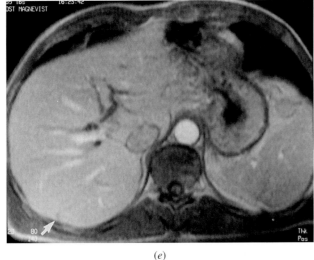

(e)

FIG. 4.35 (*Continued*) On the 45-s postgadolinium T1-weighted SGE images (*e*), the lesion enhances in a diminished fashion with faint peripheral rim enhancement (arrow, *e*) consistent with a hypovascular metastasis. A cyst would appear nearly signal void, which would be comparable in appearance to the dilated biliary ducts on the postgadolinium image (*e*). The hypovascular nature of this primary tumor is uncommon for islet cell tumors.

Gastrinomas occur most frequently in a region including the pancreatic head, duodenum, stomach, and lymph nodes in a territory termed the gastrinoma triangle [32]. The anatomic boundaries of the triangle are the porta hepatis as the superior point of the triangle and the second and third parts of the duodenum forming the base. Although gastrinomas are usually solitary, multiple gastrinomas may occur, especially in the setting of multiple endocrine neoplasias, type 1. In this setting, patients have multiple pancreatic and duodenal islet cell tumors [44, 50, 56].

Gastrinomas are not as frequently hypervascular as insulinomas. Mean size at presentation is 4 cm [54]. CT imaging is able to detect gastrinomas reliably when the tumors measure >3 cm in diameter but performs less well in the detection of smaller tumors [57]. Conventional spin-echo MRI also has been limited in the detection of gastrinomas [58, 59]. However, MRI, using current techniques, is very effective at detecting tumors <1 cm in diameter.

Gastrinomas are low in signal intensity on T1-weighted fat-suppressed images and high in signal intensity on T2-weighted fat-suppressed images, demonstrating peripheral ringlike enhancement on immediate postgadolinium SGE images (fig. 4.36). These imaging features are observed in the primary lesion and in hepatic metastases. Central low signal intensity on postgadolinium images reflects central hypovascularity. Occasionally, lesions will be cystic. The enhancing rim of the primary tumor varies substantially in thickness, with the thickness of the rim reflecting the degree of hypervascularity of the tumor. If the enhancing rim is thin, it may appear nearly imperceptible because of similar enhancement of the surrounding pancreatic parenchyma. Gastrinomas may occur outside the pancreas, and fat-suppressed T2-weighted images are particularly effective at detecting these high-signal intensity tumors in the background of suppressed fat (figs. 4.37 and 4.38). Multiple gastrinomas may be scattered throughout the pancreas and frequently are small. T2-weighted

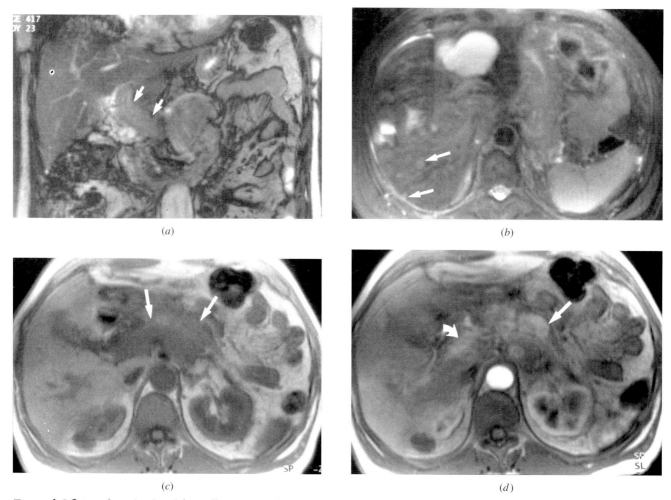

(a)   *(b)*

(c)   *(d)*

F I G . 4.36 Nonfunctioning islet cell tumor with tumor thrombus. Coronal gradient refocused flow-sensitive gradient-echo (*a*), T2-weighted fat-suppressed SS-ETSE (*b*), T1-weighted SGE (*c*), and immediate postgadolinium T1-weighted SGE (*d*) images in a second patient. A 8 × 5-cm mass arises in the pancreatic body (arrow, *c*). Expansile tumor thrombus (arrows, *a*) extending into the intrahepatic portal vein is appreciated on the coronal flow-sensitive gradient-echo image (*a*). Liver cysts and metastases are present with the <1-cm liver metastases (arrows, *b*) best shown on the T2-weighted image (*b*). The primary tumor exhibits diffuse moderately intense heterogeneous enhancement (arrow, *d*), and enhancement of the tumor thrombus is also appreciated (curved arrow, *d*).

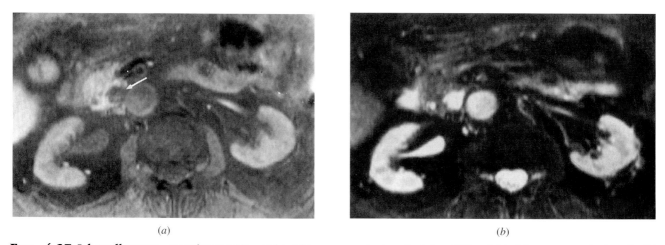

(a)   *(b)*

F I G . 4.37 Islet cell tumor—gastrinoma. T1-weighted fat-suppressed spin-echo (*a*) and T2-weighted fat-suppressed spin-echo (*b*) images. Islet cell tumors (arrow, *a*) are usually low in signal intensity in a background of high-signal intensity pancreas on T1-weighted

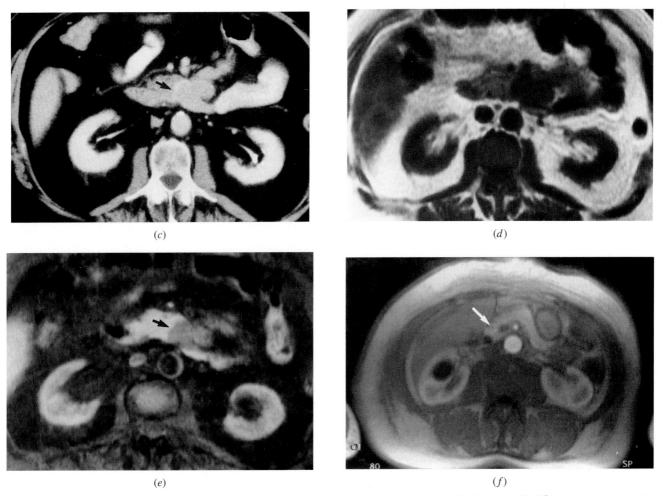

(c)

(d)

(e)

(f)

F I G . 4.37 (*Continued*) fat-suppressed images (*a*) and high in signal intensity on T2-weighted images (*b*). The uncinate process is a common location for gastrinomas, because it is located in the "gastrinoma triangle."

Dynamic contrast-enhanced CT (*c*), T1-weighted SGE (*d*), and T1-weighted fat-suppressed spin-echo (*e*) images in a second patient. A 2-cm gastrinoma is present arising from the uncinate process of the pancreas (*c–e*). The tumor is most conspicuous on the T1-weighted fat-suppressed spin-echo image with a "beak" sign apparent (arrow, *e*) and was not identified on the CT examination prospectively. An enhancing rim (arrow, *c*) is apparent on the CT image.

Immediate postgadolinium SGE image (*f*) in a third patient demonstrates a 8-mm ring-enhancing tumor (arrow, *f*) in the neck of the pancreas diagnostic for a gastrinoma on the appropriate clinical setting. Gastrinomas most commonly possess uniform ring enhancement in both the primary tumor and liver metastases. This patient had two recent CT examinations that were both negative for gastrinoma.

breathing-independent single-shot echo-train spin-echo may be effective at demonstrating even small tumors, because they are high signal intensity and are clearly depicted as the imaged tissue is stationary; in contrast, breathing-averaged T2-weighted sequences may result in image blurring, which may mask the presence of small tumors (fig. 4.39).

Gastrointestinal imaging findings that may be observed in gastrinomas include enlargement of the rugal folds of gastric mucosa (hypertrophic gastropathy) and intense mucosal enhancement on early postgadolinium SGE images (fig. 4.40), increased esophageal enhancement, and abnormal enhancement or and/thickness of

proximal small bowel (fig. 4.38). These features are reflective of the inflammatory changes of peptic ulcer disease and gastric hyperplasia due to the effects of gastrin.

In general, islet cell tumor metastases to the liver are well shown on MR images. Gastrinoma metastases frequently are relatively uniform in size and shape [52]. These metastases are generally hypervascular and possess uniform, intense rim enhancement on immediate postgadolinium SGE images. Less commonly, a varied population of metastases may be present. Metastases may have such an external vascularity that enhancement may appear nearly diffuse heterogeneous on immediate postgadolinium images. In this case, the tumors may

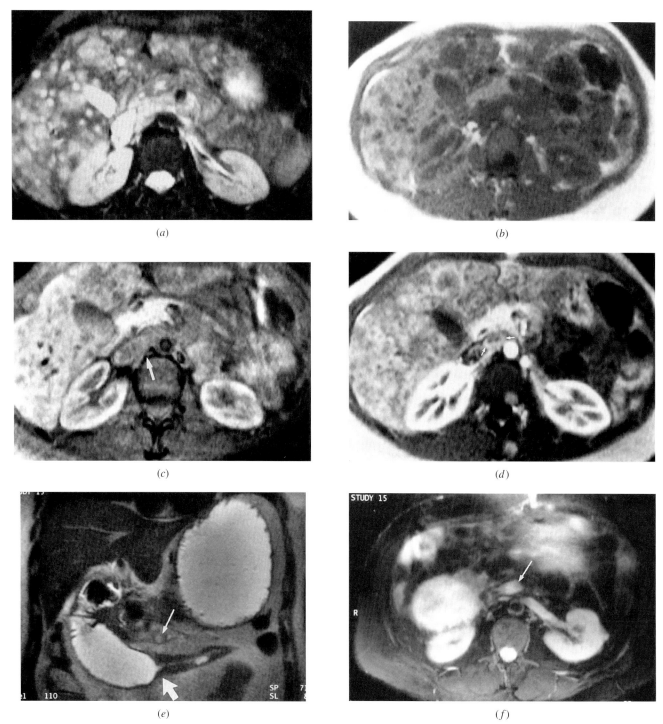

(a)   *(b)*

(c)   *(d)*

(e)   *(f)*

F I G . 4.38 Extrapancreatic gastrinoma. T2-weighted fat-suppressed spin-echo (*a*), T1-weighted SGE (*b*), T1-weighted fat-suppressed spin-echo (*c*), and immediate postgadolinium T1-weighted SGE (*d*) images. On the T2-weighted fat-suppressed image (*a*), multiple high-signal intensity foci are present throughout the primary tumor, located posterior to the head of the pancreas with an identical appearance to the well-defined high-signal intensity liver metastases. T1-weighted images (*b, c*) demonstrate the extra-pancreatic gastrinoma multiple <1.5-cm liver metastases that possess similar low signal intensity. The primary tumor (arrow, *c*) is more clearly visible on the T1-weighted fat-suppressed image (*c*) because of the good signal difference between pancreas and tumor. On the immediate postgadolinium image (*d*), multiple ring-enhancing lesions are apparent in both the primary tumor (arrow, *d*) and the liver metastases.

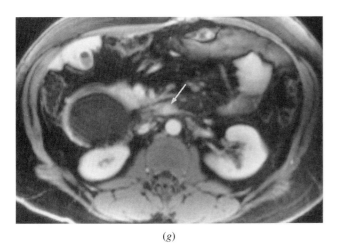

(g)

FIG. 4.38 (*Continued*) Coronal SS-ETSE (*e*), fat-suppressed breathing-averaged ETSE (*f*), and 90-s postgadolinium fat-suppressed T1-weighted SGE (*g*) images in a second patient demonstrate a gastrinoma (arrow, *e–g*) superior to the fourth portion of the duodenum. The mass is uniformly high in signal intensity on T2-weighted (*e, f*) and interstitial-phase gadolinium-enhanced T1-weighted (*g*) images. Stricturing of the fourth part of the duodenum (large arrow, *e*) reflects peptic ulcer disease in Zollinger-Ellison syndrome. Two prior CT imaging examinations were reported as negative.

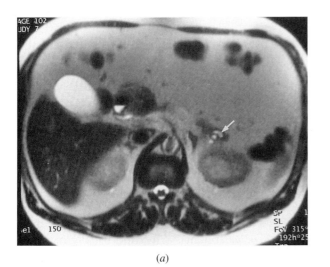

(a)

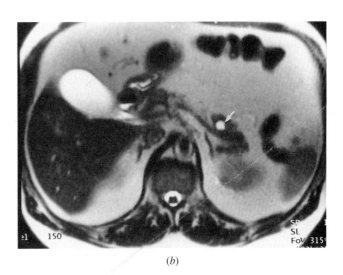

(b)

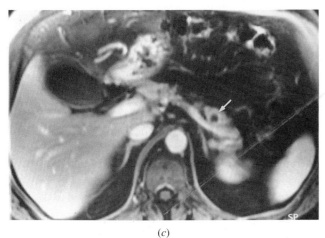

(c)

FIG. 4.39 Multiple gastrinomas. T2-weighted SS-ETSE (*a, b*) and interstitial-phase gadolinium-enhanced fat-suppressed T1-weighted SGE (*c*) images demonstrate multiple high-signal intensity gastrinomas <1 cm in the tail of the pancreas. The absence of breathing artifact on the SS-ETSE images has resulted in good resolution of the small tumors (arrows, *a, b*). Ring enhancement is apparent on the largest 8-mm tumor (arrow, *c*).

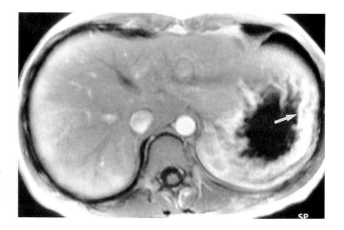

F I G . 4.40 Gastric wall hyperplasia. Immediate postgadolinium T1-weighted SGE image demonstrates intense enhancement of the prominent gastric rugal folds (arrow) in a patient with gastrinoma.

exhibit a spoke-wheel pattern, which appears as intense enhancement with thin radial bonds of diminished enhancement. Unlike pancreatic ductal cancer liver metastases, ill-defined perilesional enhancement is not observed for gastrinoma metastases, despite the substantial hepatic arterial blood supply of these tumors. Typically, lesions are very high in signal intensity on T2-weighted fat-suppressed images and have well-defined margins. This T2-weighted appearance may be confused with hemangiomas, which are also moderately high signal intensity and well defined. Islet cell liver metastases are differentiated from hemangiomas by their enhancement patterns. Islet cell metastases have uniform ring enhancement on immediate postgadolinium images that fades with time [37], whereas hemangiomas have discontinuous peripheral nodular enhancement on immediate postgadolinium images with centripetal progression of enhancement. (For a discussion on hemangiomas, see Chapter 2, *Liver.*) These appearances are better shown on MR than CT images because of the higher sensitivity of MRI to contrast enhancement, faster delivery of a compact bolus of intravenous contrast, and greater imaging temporal resolution [37]. The peripheral enhancing rim may be thin or thick, resulting in differences in the degree of vascularity. Occasionally, thick rim enhancement may have a peripheral-based spoke-wheel enhancement. Centripetal enhancement of gastrinoma metastases may occur on serial postgadolinium images. Peripheral washout is commonly observed for hypervascular gastrinoma metastases (fig. 4.41).

Insulinomas

In the realm of islet cell tumors, insulinomas are common and are frequently functionally active. Tumors present to clinical attention when they are small (<2 cm) because of the severity of the symptomatology [54]. Patients present with signs and symptoms of hypoglycemia. Insulinomas are usually richly vascular. Angiography has been reported as superior to CT imaging in detecting these tumors because of their small size and increased

vascularity [60]. In our experience, MRI may be superior to angiography for the detection of these tumors.

Insulinomas are low in signal intensity on T1-weighted images and high in signal intensity on T2-weighted images. Insulinomas are well shown on T1-weighted fat-suppressed images (fig. 4.42) [51]. Small insulinomas typically enhance homogeneously on immediate postgadolinium SGE images (fig. 4.43) [52]. Larger tumors, which measure >2 cm in diameter, often show ring enhancement. Liver metastases from insulinomas typically have peripheral ringlike enhancement, although small metastases tend to enhance homogeneously. Enhancement of small metastases frequently occurs transiently in the capillary phase of enhancement and fades on images acquired at 1 min after injection.

Glucagonoma, Somatostatinoma, VIPoma, and ACTHoma

These islet cell tumors are considerably rarer than insulinomas or gastrinomas. They are usually malignant, with liver metastases present at the time of diagnosis [46, 53, 54, 61–64]. Glucagonoma and somatostatinoma are large and heterogeneous on MR images [61–64]. They are usually low in signal intensity on T1-weighted fat-suppressed images and high in signal intensity on T2-weighted fat-suppressed images, enhancing heterogeneously on immediate postgadolinium images (fig. 4.44) [53]. Liver metastases are generally heterogeneous in size and shape, unlike gastrinoma metastases, which are typically uniform [52]. Metastases possess irregular peripheral rims of intense enhancement on immediate postgadolinium SGE images (fig. 4.44). Hypervascular liver metastases are best shown on immediate postgadolinium SGE images, which are superior to spiral CT images for this determination [53]. Splenic metastases may occur (fig. 4.44).

ACTHoma may present with a large heterogeneous enhancing primary tumor and small hypervascular liver metastases (fig. 4.45). Their appearance may resemble glucagonomas and somatostatinomas.

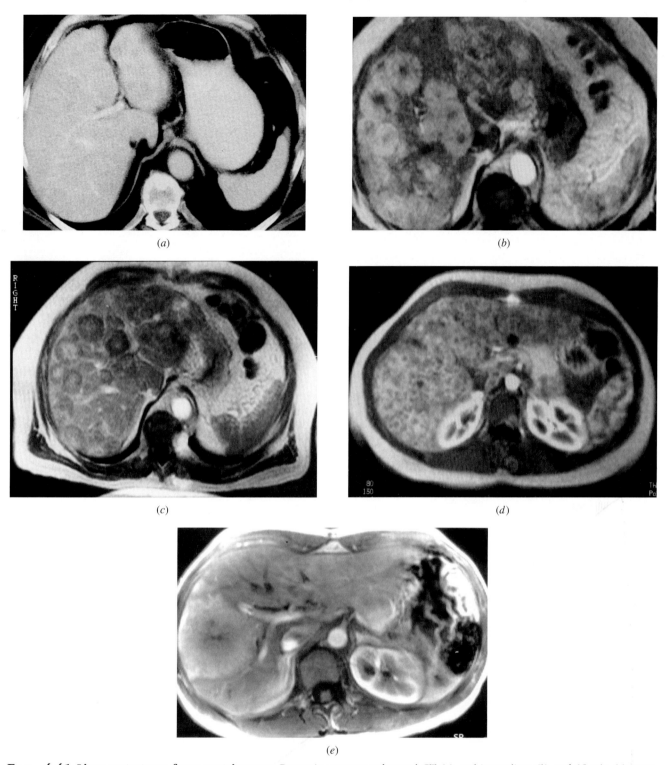

(a)

(b)

(c)

(d)

(e)

F I G . 4.41 Liver metastases from gastrinomas. Dynamic contrast-enhanced CT (*a*) and immediate (*b*) and 10-min (*c*) post-gadolinium T1-weighted SGE images. Metastases are poorly visualized on the CT image (*a*). On the immediate postgadolinium T1-weighted SGE image (*b*), multiple metastases of similar size are identified with uniform intense rim enhancement. Peripheral washout is well shown on the 10-min postcontrast image (*c*).

Immediate postgadolinium SGE images (*d*) in a second patient show extensive <1.5-cm liver metastases throughout the liver with uniform ring enhancement.

Immediate postgadolinium SGE image (*e*) in a third patient show an unusual pattern for gastrinoma liver metastases with varying sized lesions with intense, almost uniform enhancement of a 5-cm metastasis. Often these large hypervascular islet cell metastases that enhance nearly uniformly on immediate postgadolinium images possess a radiating spoke-wheel pattern of bands of lesser-enhancing stroma.

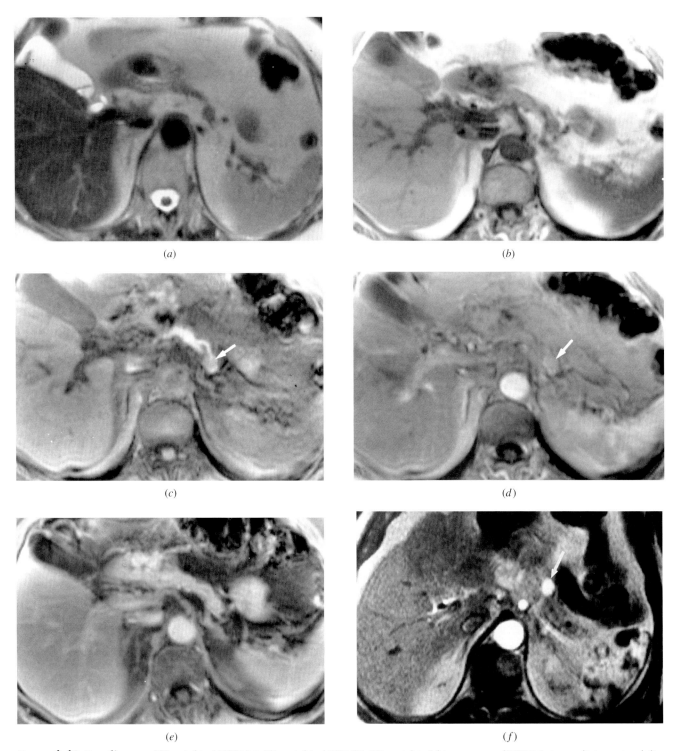

F I G . 4.42 Insulinoma. T2-weighted ETSE (*a*), T1-weighted SGE (*b*), T1-weighted fat-suppressed SGE (*c*), immediate postgadolinium T1-weighted SGE (*d*), and 90-s postgadolinium fat-suppressed SGE (*e*) images. A 1-cm tumor (arrow, *c*) arising in the superior aspect of the midbody of the pancreas is isointense on T2- (*a*) and T1-weighted (*b*) images and low signal on T1-weighted fat-suppressed image (*c*) and enhances intensely and homogeneously (arrow, *d*) on the immediate postgadolinium image. The lesion fades to isointensity with background pancreas (*e*).

Immediate postgadolinium T1 SGE image (*f*) demonstrates a 1.2-cm uniformly enhancing insulinoma (arrow) arising from the body of the pancreas.

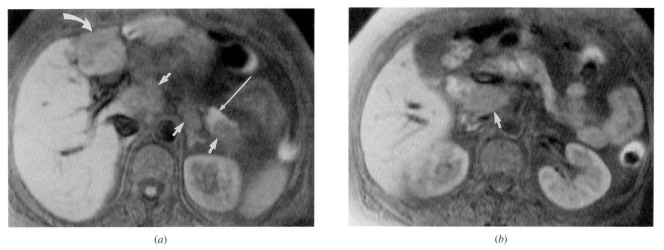

(a)   (b)

F I G . 4.43 Multiple malignant insulinomas. T1-weighted fat-suppressed spin-echo images (*a*, *b*). Multiple low-signal intensity insulinomas (arrows, *a*, *b*) ranging in diameter from 1 to 5 cm are present throughout the pancreas. Intervening pancreatic tissue is noted to be normal in signal intensity (long arrow, *a*). Liver metastases are also present (curved arrow, *a*). Multiple insulinomas are uncommon, occurring in <10% of all cases of B cell tumors.

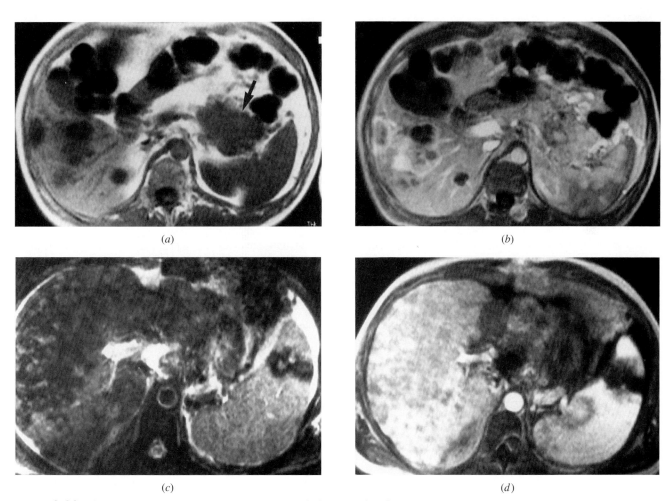

(a)   (b)

(c)   (d)

F I G . 4.44 Glucagonoma and somatostatinoma with liver and spleen metastases. T1-weighted SGE (*a*) and immediate postgadolinium T1-weighted SGE (*b*) images. A 6-cm tumor (arrow, *a*) arises from the tail of the pancreas (*a*). Multiple liver metastases are present, which are low in signal intensity on the precontrast T1-weighted image (*a*). On the immediate postgadolinium T1-weighted SGE image (*b*), the primary tumor enhances heterogeneously. Intense ring enhancement is present in many of the liver metastases, reflecting hypervascularity. Note that the liver metastases are variable in size and shape.

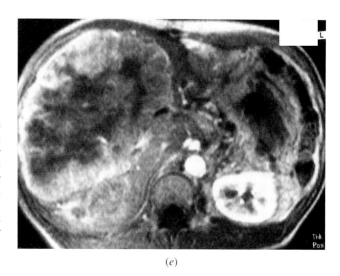

(e)

FIG. 4.44 (*Continued*) T2-weighted fat-suppressed SS-ETSE (*c*) and immediate postgadolinium T1-weighted SGE (*d*) images. On the T2-weighted image (*c*), multiple small, high-signal intensity liver metastases and a large, low-signal intensity splenic metastasis are present. On the immediate postgadolinium image (*d*), the liver metastases enhance intensely and the splenic metastasis is low in signal intensity.

Immediate postgadolinium T1-weighted SGE image (*e*) in a second patient with somatostatinoma demonstrates a 14-cm liver metastasis with intense, irregular rim enhancement.

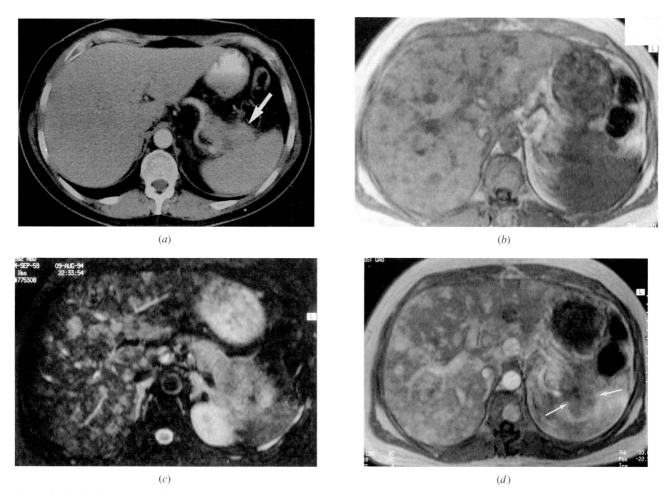

(a)   (b)

(c)   (d)

FIG. 4.45 ACTHoma. Spiral CT (*a*), T1-weighted SGE (*b*), T2-weighted fat-suppressed ETSE (*c*), and immediate postgadolinium T1-weighed SGE (*d*) images. A 4-cm ACTHoma is present in the tail of the pancreas (arrow, *a*). Direct extension of the primary tumor into the spleen is most clearly shown on the immediate postgadolinium T1-weighted SGE image (arrows, *d*). Multiple liver metastases are present, which are poorly seen on the spiral CT image (*a*) but are well shown on the MR images (*b–d*). Liver metastases are most conspicuous on the immediate postgadolinium T1-weighted SGE image (*d*). (Reproduced with permission from Kelekis NL, Semelka RC, Molina PL, Doerr ME: ACTH-secreting islet cell tumor: Appearances on dynamic gadolinium-enhanced MRI. *Magn Reson Imaging* 13: 641–644, 1995.)

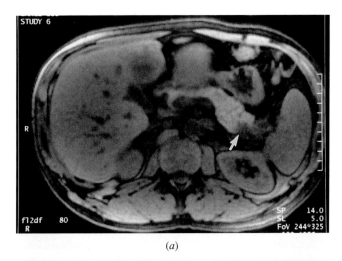

(a)

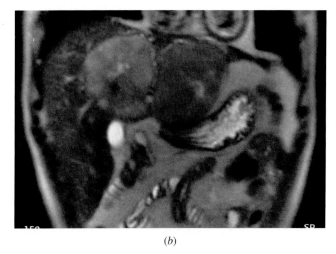

(b)

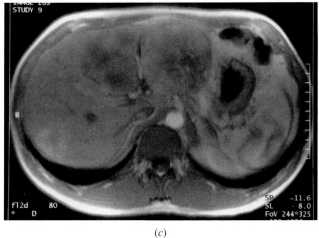

(c)

F I G . 4.46 VIPoma. T1-weighted fat-suppressed SGE (*a*), coronal T2-weighted SS-ETSE (*b*), and immediate postgadolinium T1-weighted SGE (*c*) images in a patient with VIPoma. A 1.5-cm tumor arises from the tail of the pancreas (arrow, *a*) that appears low in signal intensity on the T1-weighted image. Multiple metastases are present that are moderately low signal intensity on the T1-weighted image (*a*) and moderately high signal intensity on the T2-weighted image (*b*) and enhance in a moderately intense peripheral spoke-wheel type radial fashion on the immediate postgadolinium T1-weighted SGE image (*c*).

VIPoma may have a characteristic appearance of a small primary tumor despite large and extensive liver metastases (fig. 4.46). Prior case reports have described ostensibly primary VIPoma of the liver without visualization of a pancreatic primary. The possibility exists that the primary pancreatic tumor may have been minuscule and escaped detection.

Carcinoid Tumors

Rarely, carcinoid tumors may originate in the pancreas. Pancreatic carcinoids arise from the cells of the gastroenteropancreatic neuroendocrine system [48]. Carcinoid tumors are generally large at presentation, with coexistent liver metastases. Focal and diffuse involvements of the pancreas have been observed. Tumors are generally mildly hypointense on T1 and moderately hyperintense on T2 and show diffuse heterogeneous enhancement on immediate postgadolinium images (fig. 4.47) [48]. Liver metastases are variable in size and often exhibit intense enhancement, similar to glucagonoma and somatostatinoma liver metastases.

CYSTIC PANCREATIC NEOPLASMS

In general, this group of pancreatic tumors arises from the exocrine component of the gland and is much less common than solid exocrine carcinomas. Although secondary cystic change can be seen in most types of pancreatic neoplasms, cystic pancreatic neoplasms are characterized by their consistently present cystic configuration.

Serous Cystadenoma (Microcystic Serous Cystadenoma)

Serous cystadenoma is a benign neoplasm characterized by numerous, tiny, serous, fluid-filled cysts [65]. This tumor frequently occurs in older patients and has an increased association with von Hippel-Lindau disease [25, 65]. The tumor is well demarcated and occasionally contains a central scar. Tumors range in size from 1 to 12 cm with an average diameter at presentation of 5 cm. The lesion may exhibit either a smooth or a

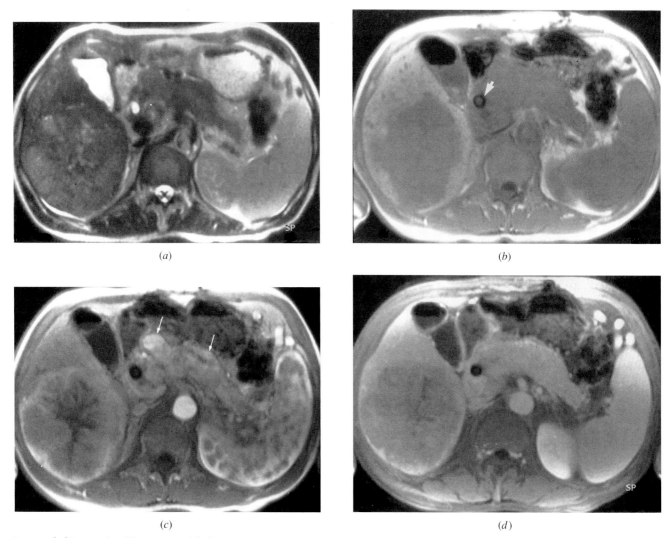

(a)   (b)

(c)   (d)

FIG. 4.47 Carcinoid tumor with liver metastases. T2-weighted echo-train spin-echo (*a*), T1-weighted SGE (*b*), immediate postgadolinium T1-weighted SGE (*c*), and 90-s postgadolinium fat-suppressed SGE (*d*) images in a patient with a carcinoid tumor with diffuse involvement of the pancreas and hypervascular liver metastasis. The pancreas is diffusely enlarged with irregular contour and enhances heterogeneously on the immediate postgadolinium image (arrows, *c*). The metastatic liver lesion shows a radial enhancement on gadolinium-enhanced images (*c, d*) Note a biliary stent in the CBD (arrow, *b*).

nodular contour. On cut surface, small, closely packed cysts are filled with clear, watery (serous) fluid and separated by fine, fibrous septa, creating a honeycomb appearance. On MR images the tumors are well defined and do not demonstrate invasion of fat or adjacent organs [66]. On T2-weighted images, the small cysts and intervening septations may be well shown as a cluster of small grapelike high-signal intensity cysts. This appearance is more clearly shown on breath-hold or breathing-independent sequences such as single-shot echo-train spin-echo, because the thin septations blur using longer-duration non-breath-hold sequence (fig. 4.48). Cystic pancreatic masses that contain cysts measuring <1 cm in diameter most likely represent microcystic cystadenoma. Uncommonly, serous cystadenomas may be macrocystic (cysts measuring from 1 to 8 cm) oligo- or unilocu-

lar (fig. 4.49). Macrocystic or unilocular serous cystadenomas exhibit distinctly different macroscopic features from microcystic lesions and may pose diagnostic difficulties for both radiologist and pathologist. A CT study evaluating these tumors misinterpreted all five cases to be mucinous cystic neoplasms or pseudocysts. Microcystic and macrocystic serous tumors represent morphologic variants of the same benign pancreatic neoplasm, namely serous cystadenoma [66, 67]. Relatively thin uniform septations and absence of infiltration of adjacent organs and structures are features that distinguish serous cystadenoma from serous cystadenocarcinoma. Tumor septations usually enhance minimally with gadolinium on early and late postcontrast images, although moderate enhancement on early postcontrast images may occur. Delayed enhancement of the central scar may

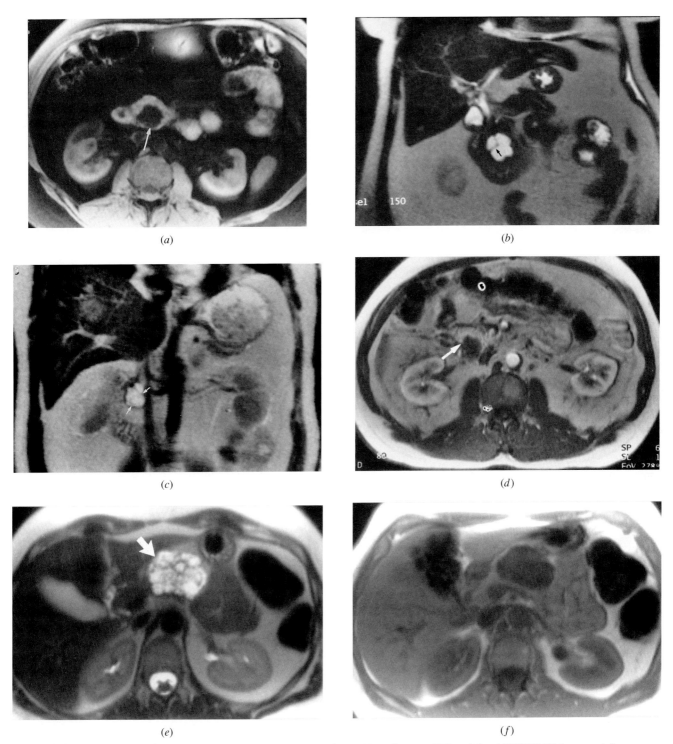

F I G . 4.48 Serous cystadenoma. T1-weighted fat-suppressed SGE (*a*) and coronal T2-weighted SS-ETSE (*b*) images. A 3-cm mass lesion is present in the head of the pancreas. The lesion is well defined and low in signal intensity (arrow, *a*) in a background of high-signal intensity pancreas on the fat-suppressed T1-weighted SGE image (*a*). On the breathing-independent T2-weighted image (*b*), definition of fine septations (small arrow, *b*) within the cystic mass shows that the cysts are microcysts measuring <1 cm in diameter. The serous cystadenoma is high in signal intensity on the T2-weighted image because of the high fluid content.

Coronal T2-weighted ETSE (*c*) and immediate postgadolinium T1-weighted SGE (*d*) images in a second patient demonstrate a 3-cm serous cystadenoma in the head of the pancreas. Fine septations are apparent on the T2-weighted image (arrows, *c*), and the tumor is sharply demarcated from normal-enhancing pancreas on the immediate postgadolinium image (arrow, *d*).

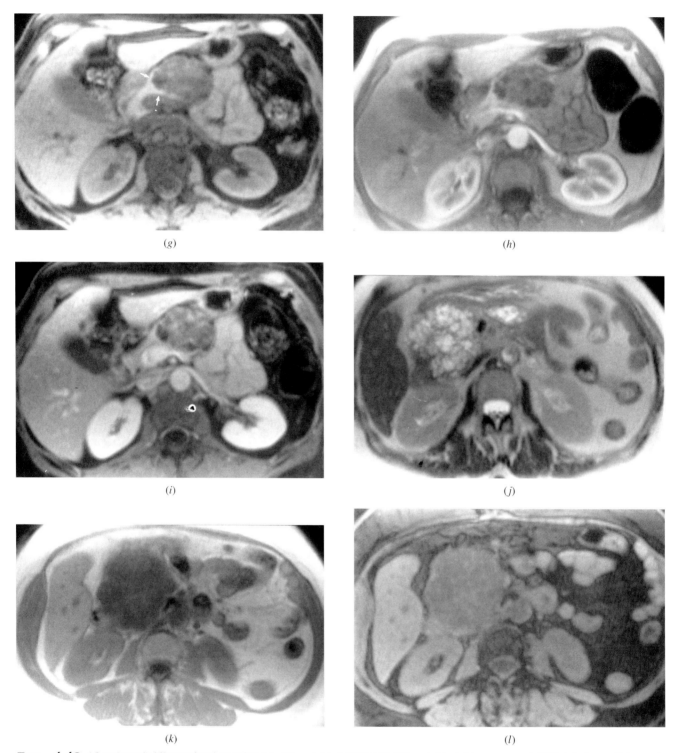

(g)

(h)

(i)

(j)

(k)

(l)

F IG . 4.48 (*Continued*) T2-weighted SS-ETSE (*e*), T1-weighted SGE (*f*), T1-weighted fat-suppressed SGE (*g*), immediate post-gadolinium T1-weighted SGE (*h*), and 90-s postgadolinium fat-suppressed SGE (*i*) images in a third patient. There is a 6-cm multicystic mass (arrows, *e*) arising in the pancreatic body with thin septations creating <2-cm cysts. The single-shot T2-weighted sequence performs very well at defining the septations in cystic masses. A "beak sign" is demonstrated in the pancreas (arrow, *g*) best shown on the noncontrast T1-weighted fat-suppressed (*g*) and immediate postgadolinium SGE (*h*) images, confirming that the mass originates from this organ. The septations enhance minimally on immediate postgadolinium images (*h*) with progressive enhancement on late images (*i*).

T2-weighted ETSE (*j*), T1-weighted fat-suppressed SGE (*k*), immediate postgadolinium T1-weighted SGE (*l*), and 90-s postgadolinium fat-suppressed SGE (*m*) images in a fourth patient.

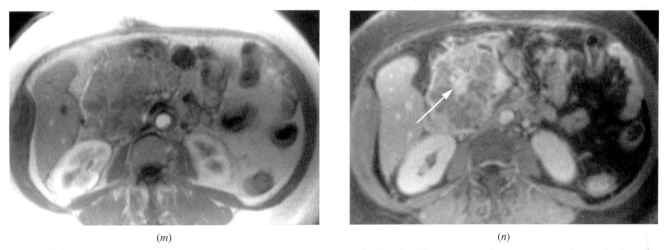

(m)   *(n)*

F I G . 4.48 (*Continued*) An 8-cm serous cystadenoma is present in the head of the pancreas, best shown on the single-shot T2-weighted sequence. There is a central scar, typical for serous cystadenoma, which enhances on late images (arrow), consistent with fibrosis.

Serous cystadenomas occur predominantly in women as seen in these cases. The importance of the MR study is to differentiate this benign entity from mucinous cystadenomas that are potentially malignant.

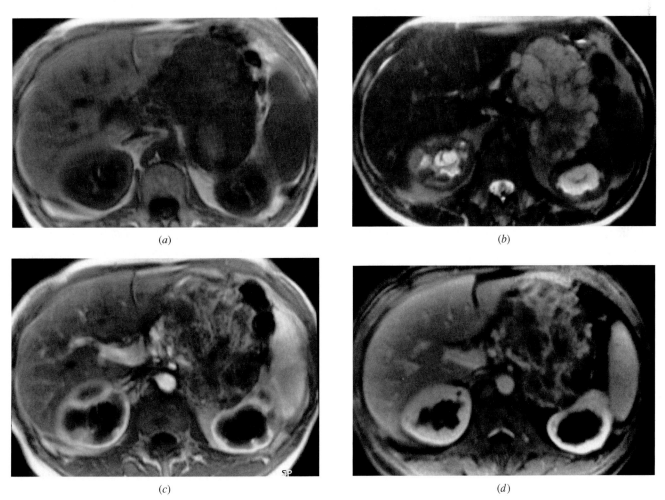

(c)   *(d)*

F I G . 4.49 Macrocystic serous cystadenoma. T1-weighted SGE (*a*), T2-weighted SS-ETSE (*b*), immediate postgadolinium T1-wighted SGE (*c*), and 90-s postgadolinium fat-suppressed SGE (*d*) images. A 10-cm mass arises from the tail of the pancreas. The tumor is mildly hypointense with regions of hyperintensity on precontrast T1-weighted images (*a*). Multiple septations are present throughout the mass, well shown on the breathing-independent T2-weighted image (*b*). Some of the cysts measure >2 cm. Moderately intense enhancement of the septations is present on immediate (*c*) and 90-s (*d*) postcontrast images.

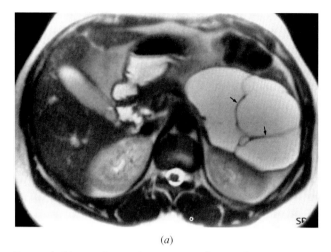
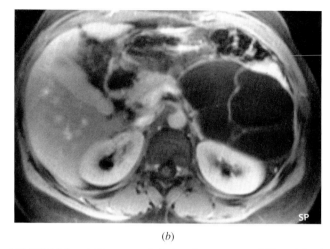

(a)   (b)

FIG. 4.50 Mucinous (macrocystic) cystadenoma. T2-weighted SS-ETSE (a) and 90-s postgadolinium fat-suppressed T1-weighed SGE (b) images. A well-defined cystic mass arises from the body and tail of the pancreas that is low in signal intensity on the T1-weighted image (not shown) and high in signal intensity on the T2-weighted image (a) and demonstrates enhancement of septations on the postgadolinium T1-weighted SGE image (b). No evidence of tumor nodules, invasion of adjacent tissue, or liver metastases is appreciated. The uniform thickness of the septations is clearly defined on the breathing-independent SS-ETSE image (arrows, a). Mucinous cystadenoma is potentially a low-grade malignant neoplasm.

occasionally be observed [1] and is more typical of large tumors. Delayed enhancement of the central scar on postgadolinium images is apparent in larger tumors, and this enhancement pattern is typical for fibrous tissue in general. The central scar may represent compressed contiguous cyst walls of centrally located cysts.

Serous Cystadenocarcinoma (Microcystic Serous Cystadenocarcinoma)

This malignant pancreatic tumor is extremely rare. Distinction from benign serous cystadenoma is difficult on histologic grounds alone and may only be established by the presence of metastatic disease or local invasion.

Mucinous Cystadenoma/Cystadenocarcinoma (Macrocystic Cystadenoma/Cystadenocarcinoma)

Mucinous cystic neoplasms of the pancreas are characterized by the formation of large unilocular or multilocular cysts filled with abundant, thick gelatinous mucin. Histopathologically these tumors are divided into benign (mucinous cystadenoma), borderline, and malignant (mucinous cystadenocarcinoma). However, at many institutions, all cases of mucinous cystic neoplasms are interpreted as mucinous cystadenocarcinomas of low-grade malignant potential to reinforce the need for complete surgical resection and close clinical follow-up [65, 66, 68–70]. Mucinous cystic neoplasms occur more frequently in females (6 to 1) and approximately 50% occur in patients between the ages of 40 and 60 years [71]. These tumors usually are located in the body and

tail of the pancreas. They may be large (mean diameter of 10 cm), multiloculated, and encapsulated [69, 70]. There is a great propensity for invasion of local organs and tissues.

On gadolinium-enhanced T1-weighted fat-suppressed images, large, irregular cystic spaces separated by thick septa are demonstrated [1]. Mucinous cystadenomas are well circumscribed, and they show no evidence of metastases or invasion of adjacent tissues (fig. 4.50). Mucinous cystadenomas described pathologically as having borderline malignant potential may be very large but may not show imaging or gross evidence of metastases or local invasion (figs. 4.51 and 4.52). Histopathologically, these tumors show moderate epithelial dysplasia. Mucinous cystadenocarcinoma may be very locally aggressive malignancies with extensive invasion of adjacent tissues and organs (fig. 4.53). However, absence of demonstration of tumor invasion into surrounding tissue does not exclude malignancy. The higher inherent soft tissue contrast of MRI compared to CT imaging results in superior differentiation between microcystic and macrocystic adenomas because of sharp definition of cysts that permits evaluation of cyst size and margins [69]. Breathing-independent T2-weighted images are particularly effective at defining the cysts.

Mucin produced by these tumors may result in high signal intensity on T1- and T2-weighted images of the primary tumor and liver metastases. Liver metastases are generally hypervascular and have intense ring enhancement on immediate postgadolinium images. Metastases are commonly cystic and may contain mucin, which results in mixed low and high signal intensity on T1- and T2-weighted images (fig. 4.54).

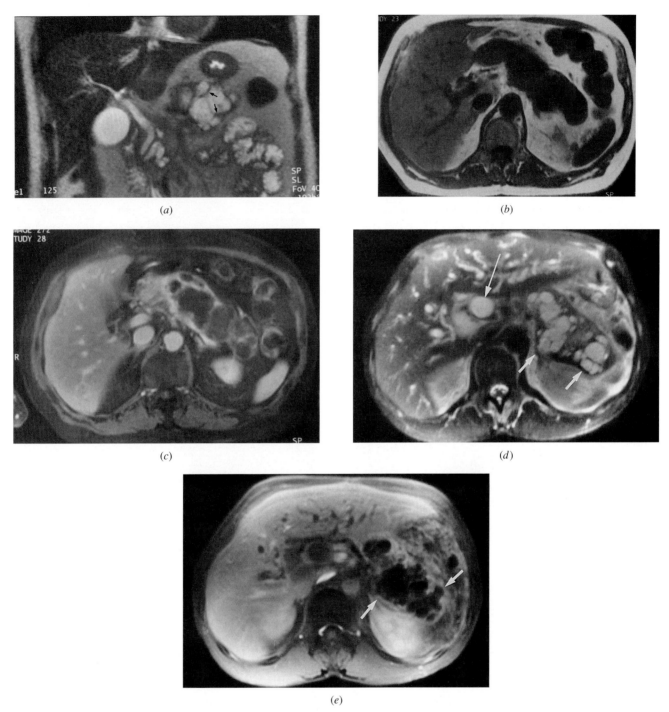

(a)

(b)

(c)

(d)

(e)

F I G . 4.51 Mucinous cystadenoma with carcinoma in situ. Coronal T2-weighted SS-ETSE (*a*), T1-weighted SGE (*b*), and 90-s postgadolinium fat-suppressed SGE (*c*) images. A multicystic mass involves the entire body and tail of the pancreas (*a–c*). Septations are well defined on the breathing-independent T2-weighted image (arrows, *a*). The moderate irregularity of the septations and the extent of tumor are features compatible with malignant changes.

T2-weighted SS-ETSE (*d*) and 90-s postgadolinium fat-suppressed T1-weighted SGE (*e*) images in a second patient demonstrate a mucinous cystadenocarcinoma in the body and tail (arrows, *d*, *e*). Dilatation of the CBD (long arrow, *d*) and intrahepatic biliary tree are also present.

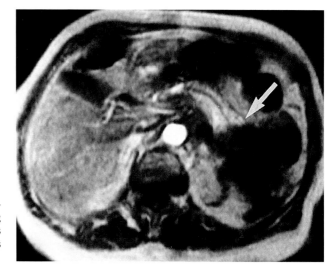

F I G . 4.52 Mucinous cystadenocarcinoma. Immediate post-gadolinium T1-weighted SGE image demonstrates a tumor arising from the tail of the pancreas (arrow) that contains thick septations and multiple large cysts. The tumor is locally aggressive and invades into the splenic hilum (not shown).

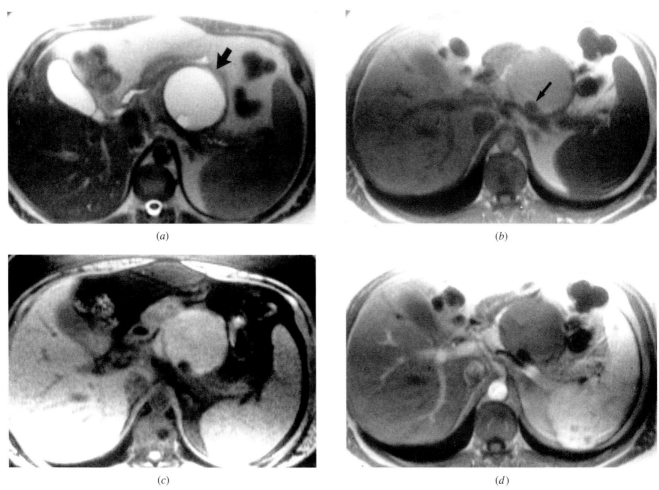

(a)

(b)

(c)

(d)

F I G . 4.53 Mucinous cystadenocarcinoma. T2-weighted ETSE (*a*), T1-weighted SGE (*b*), T1-weighted fat-suppressed SGE (*c*), immediate postgadolinium T1-weighted SGE (*d*), and 90-s postgadolinium fat-suppressed SGE (*e*) images. There is a large cystic mass (arrow, *a*) arising from the pancreatic body, which has a thickened and slightly irregular wall, which demonstrates increased enhancement (arrow, *e*) on interstitial-phase gadolinium-enhanced fat-suppressed images.

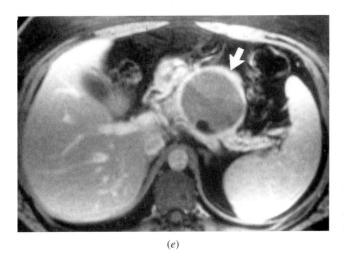

(e)

F I G . 4.53 (*Continued*) The cyst is high in signal on T1-weighted images (*b*, *c*), reflecting the presence of high protein content from mucin. The cyst contains a smaller cystic structure (arrow, *b*).

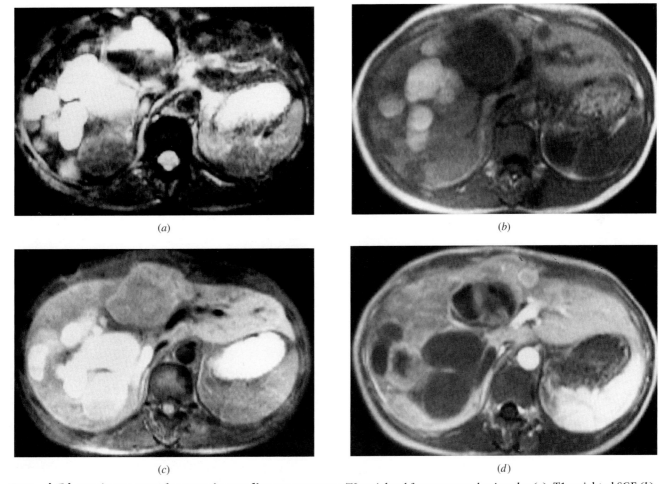

(a)

(b)

(c)

(d)

F I G . 4.54 Mucinous cystadenocarcinoma liver metastases. T2-weighted fat-suppressed spin-echo (*a*), T1-weighted SGE (*b*), T1-weighted fat-suppressed spin-echo (*c*), and immediate postgadolinium T1-weighted SGE (*d*) images. Multiple metastases are present throughout the liver that are mixed low and high signal intensity on T1-weighted (*b*, *c*) and T2-weighted (*a*) images. This appearance is consistent with the presence of mucin in these tumors. On the immediate postgadolinium image (*d*), enhancement of the walls of the cysts is appreciated.

Intraductal Papillary Mucinous Tumors (Duct-Ectatic Mucin-Producing Tumor)

Intraductal papillary mucinous tumors arise in the pancreatic duct epithelium and in general, have a low potential for malignancy. Dysplastic lining epithelium proliferates and forms papillary projections that protrude into and expand the main pancreatic duct or side branch ducts. Duct obstruction is secondary to tenacious plugs of mucin, elaborated by the epithelium, or ductal compression by cystic masses [72]. Clinically, these tumors may result in large volumes of mucin production, which can be appreciated by direct inspection at ERCP investigation. Intraductal papillary mucinous tumors may be classified into main duct and side branch duct types.

Main pancreatic duct involvement presents as diffuse ductal dilatation, copious mucin production, and papillary growth and is typically associated with malignancy [73]. Tumors arising in the main duct exhibit a greatly expanded main pancreatic duct on T2-weighted images or MRCP images (fig. 4.55). Irregular enhancing tissue along the ductal epithelium is appreciated on post gadolinium images, confirming that underlying tumor is the cause of the ductal dilatation. Intraductal papillary mucinous tumors involving predominantly side branch ducts appear as oval-shaped cystic masses in proximity to the main pancreatic duct. These benign tumors appear as localized cystic parenchymal lesions. The majority of side branch intraductal papillary mucinous tumors are located in the head of the pancreas. MRCP images are

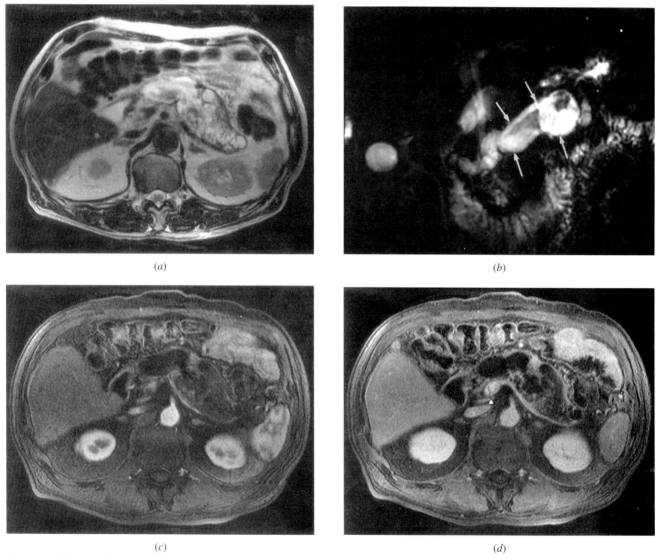

(a)

(b)

(c)

(d)

F I G . 4.55 Intraductal papillary mucin secreting tumor—main duct type. T2-weighted echo-train spin-echo (a), thick-slab MRCP (b), immediate postgadolinium fat-suppressed SGE (c), and interstitial-phase gadolinium-enhanced fat-suppressed SGE (d) images. There is massive dilatation of the entire main pancreatic duct (arrows, b), which is well shown on the T2-weighted sequence (a) and MRCP (b). Enhancing tumor stroma is appreciated on the postcontrast images (c, d), with progressive enhancement on the later interstitial-phase images (d). (Courtesy of Masayuki Kanematsu, M.D., Gifu University School of Medicine, Japan.)

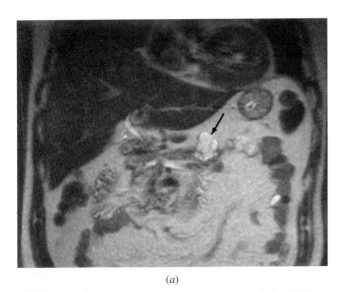

(a)

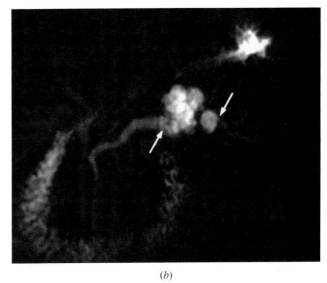

(b)

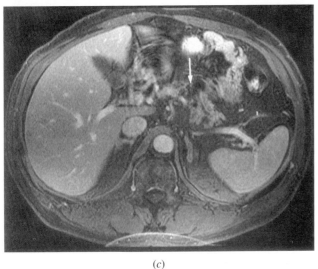

(c)

F I G . 4.56 Intraductal papillary mucin-secreting tumor-side branch type. Coronal T2-weighted SS-ETSE (*a*), thick-section MRCP (*b*), and interstitial-phase gadolinium-enhanced fat-suppressed SGE (*c*) images in a patient with branch-type intraductal mucin-producing papillary neoplasm. There are clusters of multiple small cysts (arrow, *a*) in the pancreatic body, which exhibit communication with the main pancreatic duct. Communication with the main duct is well shown on the MRCP image. No apparent tumor stroma (arrow, *c*) is appreciated on postgadolinium images. Branch duct type tumor usually shows cystic parenchymal lesions and tends to be less aggressive than the main ductal type. (Courtesy of Masayuki Kanematsu, M.D., Gifu University School of Medicine, Japan.)

able to show communication of the cystic tumor with the main pancreatic duct in a number of cases (fig. 4.56) [68, 74–77].

Solid and Papillary Epithelial Neoplasm (Papillary Cystic Neoplasm)

These tumors are generally considered benign neoplasms with occasional examples exhibiting low-grade malignant potential. Solid and papillary epithelial neoplasms occur most frequently in women between 20 and 30 years of age [78]. The gross appearance of tumors is characterized by an encapsulated mass, which on cut surface reveals areas of hemorrhage, necrosis, and cystic spaces. The capsule and inner portion of tumor may contain calcifications. MRI findings of solid and papillary epithelial neoplasms are highly suggestive in the appropriate clinical setting. When seen in a young female patient, a large, well-encapsulated mass, which

demonstrates focal calcification and regions of hemorrhagic degeneration (as evidenced by fluid debris levels or signal intensities on MR images paralleling those of blood products) is virtually diagnostic [79]. A report describing the MRI appearance of solid and papillary epithelial neoplasms found that all tumors were well-demarcated lesions that contained central high signal intensity on T1-weighted images [78]. This central high signal intensity represented hemorrhagic necrosis. The presence of overt hemorrhage may be related to tumor size because smaller tumors may appear heterogeneous but not overtly hemorrhagic (fig. 4.57).

OTHER TUMORS

Lymphoma

Non-Hodgkin lymphoma may involve peripancreatic lymph nodes or may directly invade the pancreas [80].

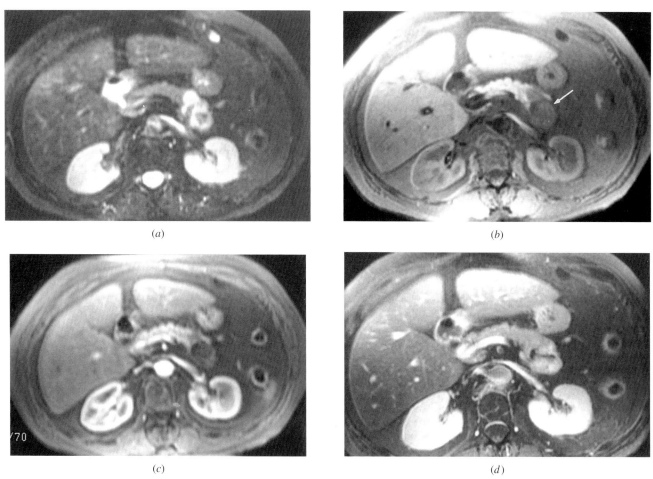

(a)   (b)

(c)   (d)

FIG. 4.57 Solid and papillary epithelial neoplasm. T2-weighted fat-suppressed spin-echo (*a*), T1-weighted fat-suppressed SGE (*b*), immediate postgadolinium T1-weighted fat-suppressed SGE (*c*), and 90-s postgadolinium fat-suppressed SGE (*d*) images. A 4-cm tumor mass arises from the tail of the pancreas that is low in signal intensity on the T1-weighted image (arrow, *b*) and heterogeneous on the T2-weighted image (*a*), enhances negligibly on the immediate postgadolinium T1-weighted SGE image (*c*), and shows heterogeneous enhancement on the interstitial-phase image (*d*). This rare low-grade malignant tumor is more frequent in young females and is typically located in the tail of the pancreas. MRI may be useful in these lesions by showing cystic degeneration and hemorrhagic necrosis, which are characteristic of this entity. (Courtesy of Caroline Reinhold, MD, Dept. of Radiology, McGill University.)

Intermediate-signal intensity peripancreatic lymph nodes are distinguished from high-signal intensity normal pancreas on T1-weighted fat-suppressed images. Invasion of the pancreas is shown by loss of the normal high signal intensity of the pancreas on T1-weighted fat-suppressed images (fig. 4.58).

Burkitt lymphoma has a particular propensity to involve organs and structures within the abdominal cavity, including bowel, gallbladder, peritoneum, and pancreas (fig. 4.58).

Metastases

Involvement of the pancreas by metastatic tumor may be the result of spread by any of the usual routes; direct invasion by the extension of cancers from neighboring organs is common, particularly in carcinoma of the stomach or transverse colon. Hematogenous metastases may occur with carcinomas of the lung, breast, and kidney and malignant melanoma.

The MRI appearance of renal cell carcinoma metastatic to the pancreas has been described as diffuse micronodular, multifocal, and solitary metastatic deposits [81]. Metastases are low in signal intensity on T1-weighted images and high in signal intensity on T2-weighted images. Small metastases (<1 cm in diameter) enhance uniformly on immediate postgadolinium SGE images, and larger metastases enhance in a ring fashion (fig. 4.59). This appearance is analogous to the appearance of hypervascular metastases to the liver and reflects the pathophysiology of parasitization of host blood supply by metastatic disease. Renal cancer metastases resemble the appearance of islet cell tumors. Clinical history of renal cancer, even if remote, is essential to obtain to establish the correct diagnosis.

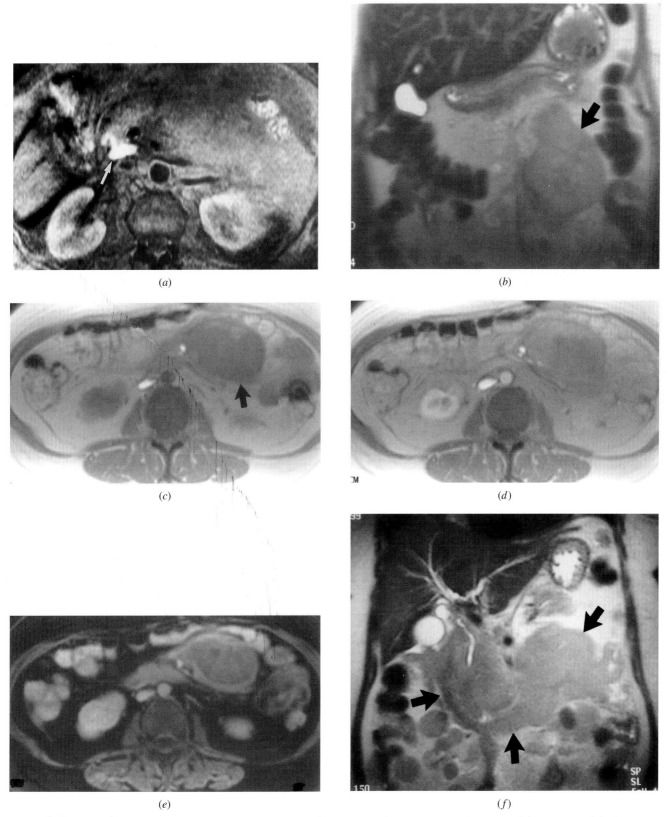

(a)

(b)

(c)

(d)

(e)

(f)

FIG. 4.58 Lymphoma. T1-weighted fat-suppressed spin-echo image (*a*) demonstrates replacement of the majority of the pancreas with intermediate-signal ill-defined lymphomatous tissue. The ventral portion of the pancreatic head is spared (arrow, *a*). (Reproduced with permission from Semelka RC, Shoenut JP, Kroeker MA, Micflikier AB. The Pancreas. In: Semelka RC, Shoenut JP. *MRI of the Abdomen with CT Correlation.* New York: Raven Press, p. 59–76, 1993.)

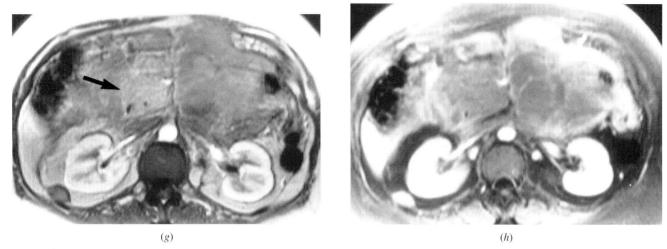

(g)   *(h)*

F I G . 4.58 *(Continued)* Coronal T2-weighted SS-ETSE (*b*), T1-weighted SGE (*c*), immediate postgadolinium T1-weighted SGE (*d*), and 90-s postgadolinium fat-suppressed SGE (*e*) images in a second patient, who has Burkitt lymphoma. A 10-cm mass (arrow, *b*, *c*) involves the pancreatic body and tail, which is mildly hypointense in signal intensity on both T1-(*c*) and T2-weighted (*b*) images and enhances minimally on early (*d*) and late (*e*) postgadolinium images.

Coronal T2-weighted SS-ETSE (*f*), immediate postgadolinium SGE (*g*), and 90-s postgadolinium fat-suppressed SGE (*h*) images in a third patient who has non-Hodgkin lymphoma. A large mass is present in the mesentery, which involves the pancreas as well. Mild enhancement of the mesenteric tumor and tumor involving the pancreatic head (arrow, *g*) is present on early (*g*) and late (*h*) postgadolinium images. As these cases illustrate, lymphoma typically exhibits mild enhancement on early and late postcontrast images.

Metastasis of other primary tumors generally appears as focal pancreatic masses that are mildly hypointense on T1-weighted images, moderately hypointense on T1-weighted fat-suppressed images, and mildly hyperintense on T2-weighted images. Metastases often enhance in a ring fashion (Figs. 4.60 and 4.61), as in the case with liver metastases, and their extent of enhancement generally varies with the angiogenic properties of the primary neoplasms. Ductal obstruction is uncommon, even with larger tumors, which aids the distinction from pancreatic ductal adenocarcinoma. The lack of ductal obstruction, which explains the clear visibility of metastases on

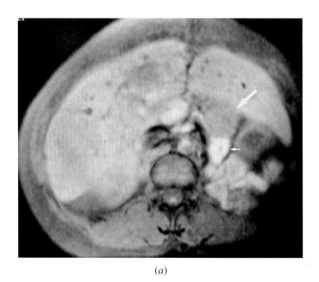
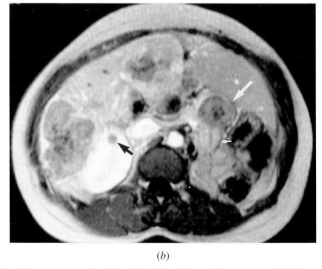

(a)   *(b)*

F I G . 4.59 Pancreatic metastases from renal cancer. T1-weighted fat-suppressed spin-echo (*a*) and immediate postgadolinium T1-weighted SGE (*b*) images demonstrate a 3-cm mass in the distal body of the pancreas (arrow, *a*, *b*). The uninvolved tail of the pancreas has a normal high signal intensity (small arrow, *a*, *b*). Multiple liver metastases are present that demonstrate predominant rim enhancement on the immediate postgadolinium image (*b*). Multiple renal cancers are present (black arrow, *b*).

T1-weighted SGE (*c*) and interstitial-phase gadolinium-enhanced T1-weighted fat-suppressed spin-echo (*d*) images of the body of the pancreas and immediate postgadolinium T1-weighted SGE image (*e*) in a second patient.

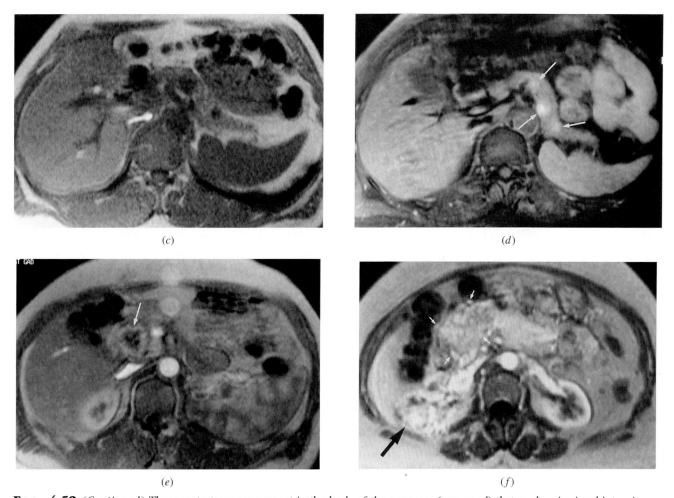

(c) (d)

(e) (f)

F I G . 4.59 (*Continued*) Three metastases are present in the body of the pancreas (arrows, *d*) that are low in signal intensity on the precontrast T1-weighted SGE image (*c*) and enhance uniformly and with moderate intensity on the interstitial-phase gadolinium-enhanced image (*d*). A larger 3-cm metastasis is present in the head of the pancreas that demonstrates rim enhancement on the immediate postgadolinium image (arrow, *e*).

Immediate postgadolinium T1-weighted SGE image (*f*) in a third patient demonstrates multiple micronodular metastases to the pancreas <5 mm, which enhance uniformly and intensely on the immediate postgadolinium image (small arrows, *f*). The renal cancer is also shown (arrow, *f*). (Reproduced with permission from Kelekis NL, Semelka RC, Siegelman ES: MRI of pancreatic metastasis from renal cell cancer. *J Comput Assist Tomogr* 20: 249–253, 1996.)

Renal cell cancer is among the most common metastatic lesions to the pancreas.

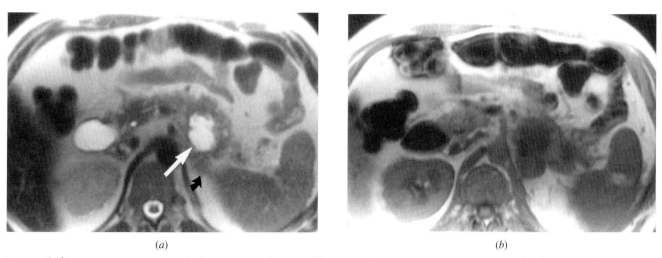

(a) (b)

F I G . 4.60 Pancreatic metastasis from transitional cell cancer. T2-weighted ETSE (*a*), T1-weighted SGE (*b*), T1-weighted fat-suppressed SGE (*c*), immediate postgadolinium T1-weighted SGE (*d*), and 90-s postgadolinium fat-suppressed SGE (*e*) images in a patient with recurrent transitional cell cancer, originally from the left kidney.

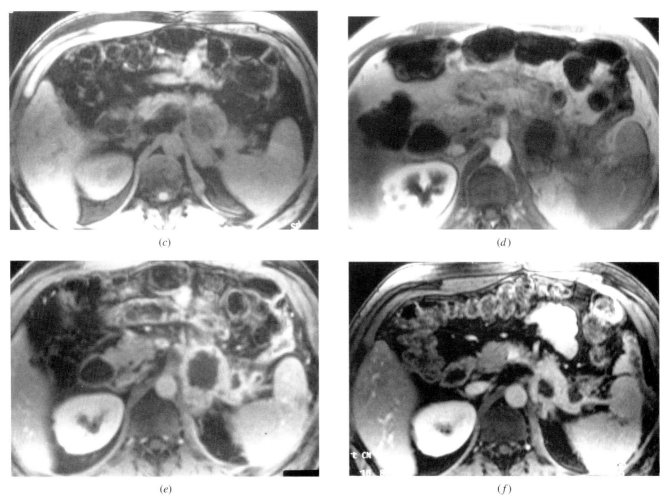

(c)

(d)

(e)

(f)

F I G . 4.60 (*Continued*) There is a cystic mass (arrow, *a*) that involves the pancreatic tail and the left adrenal gland (curved arrow, *a*). A thick enhancing rim is demonstrated on the interstitial-phase gadolinium-enhanced fat-suppressed image.

Interstitial-phase gadolinium-enhanced fat-suppressed SGE image (*f*) obtained after a course of chemotherapy demonstrates substantial decrease in size of the cystic mass.

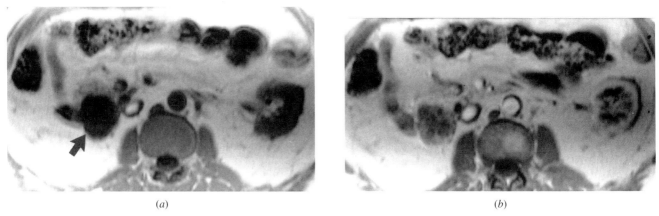

(a)

(b)

F I G . 4.61 Pancreatic metastasis from colon cancer. T1-weighted SGE (*a*), immediate postgadolinium T1-weighted SGE (*b*), and 90-s postgadolinium fat-suppressed SGE (*c*) images in a patient with colon cancer with liver metastases (not shown). There is a 3.5-cm lobulated mass (arrow, *a*) in the pancreatic head.

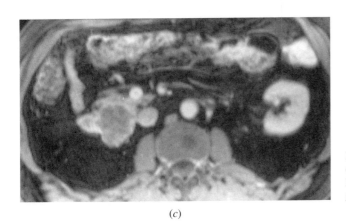

(c)

F I G . 4.61 (*Continued*) The tumor appears hyperintense on T2 (not shown) and hypointense on T1-weighted image (*a*) and shows heterogeneous mild enhancement on early (*b*) and late (*c*) post-gadolinium images.

noncontrast T1-weighted fat-suppressed images. Chronic pancreatitis secondary to ductal obstruction is not present, and therefore background pancreas is moderately high signal intensity, creating sharp contrast with hypointense tumors.

Melanoma metastases may be high in signal intensity on T1-weighted images because of the paramagnetic properties of melanin pigment (fig. 4.62) [1]. Metastatic deposits tend to be focal, well-defined masses (figs. 4.63–4.65).

INFLAMMATORY DISEASES

Pancreatitis

Pancreatitis may occur secondary to chronic alcoholism, gallstones, hypercalcemia, hyperlipoproteinemia, blunt abdominal trauma, penetrating peptic ulcer disease, viral infections (most frequently Epstein-Barr), and certain

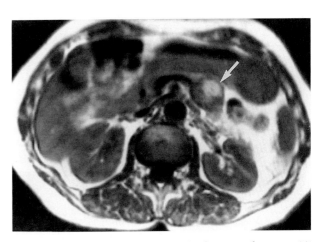

F I G . 4.62 Pancreatic metastasis from melanoma. T1-SGE image demonstrates a high-signal intensity mass in the tail of the pancreas (arrow). The high signal intensity of the mass is due to the paramagnetic effect of melanin. (Reproduced with permission from Semelka RC, Ascher SM: MRI of the pancreas—state of the art. *Radiology* 188: 593–602, 1993.)

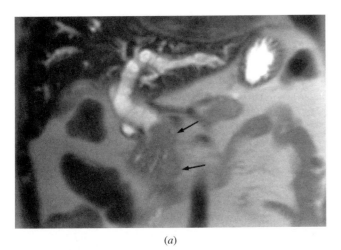

(a)

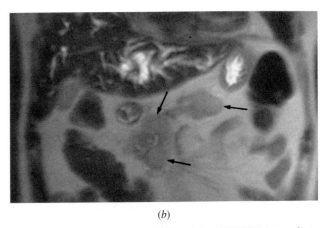

(b)

F I G . 4.63 Pancreatic metastasis from small cell lung cancer. Coronal (*a*, *b*) and transverse (*c*) T2-weighted SS-ETSE, immediate postgadolinium T1-weighed SGE (*d*), and 90-s postgadolinium fat-suppressed SGE (*e*, *f*) images. Multiple masses (arrows, *a*, *b*) are present throughout the pancreas that are mildly hyperintense on T2 (*a–c*) and enhance minimally on early (*d*) and late (*e*, *f*) postgadolinium images.

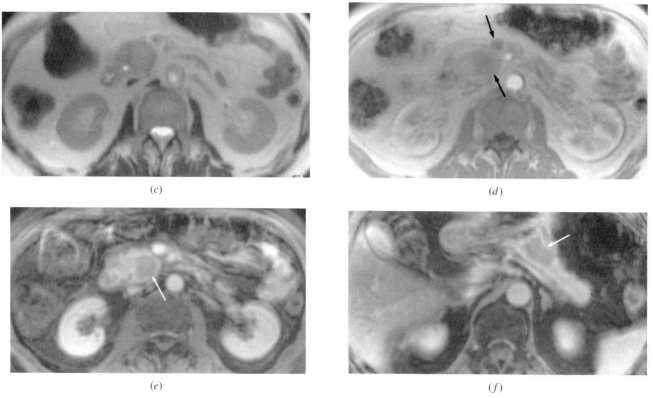

(c)

(d)

(e)

(f)

F I G . 4.63 (*Continued*) Lung cancer is among the most common primary tumors that metastasize to the pancreas.

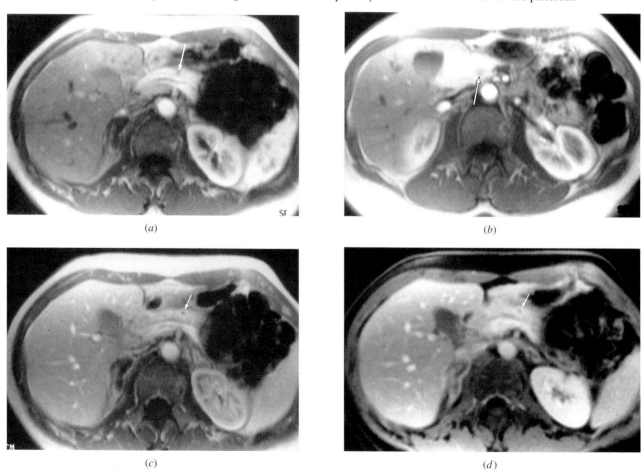

(a)

(b)

(c)

(d)

F I G . 4.64 Pancreatic metastasis from breast cancer. Immediate postgadolinium T1-weighted SGE (*a, b*), 45-s postgadolinium SGE (*c*), and interstitial-phase gadolinium-enhanced SGE (*d*) images demonstrate multiple <1-cm hypointense metastases (arrow, *a, b*) in the pancreatic head and body. Note ring enhancement of the metastases on the post contrast images (arrows, *c, d*).

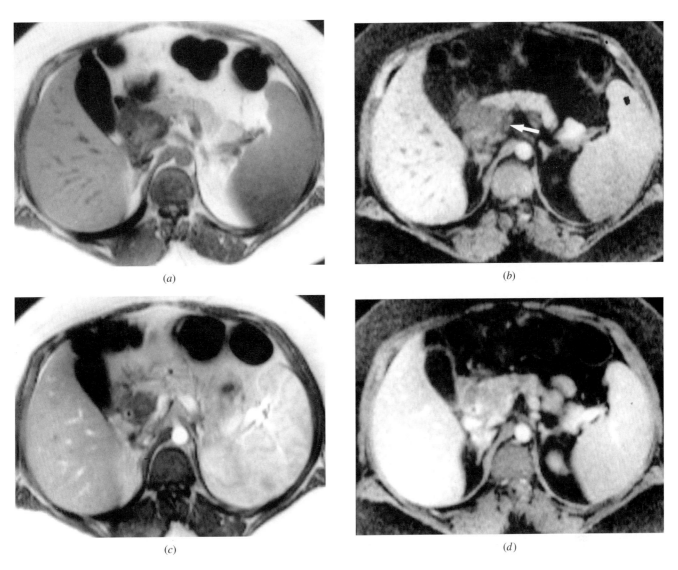

(a)

(b)

(c)

(d)

F I G . 4.65 Pancreatic metastasis from Merkel cell cancer. T1-weighted SGE (*a*), T1-weighted fat-suppressed SGE (*b*), immediate postgadolinium T1-weighted SGE (*c*), and 90-s postgadolinium fat-suppressed SGE (*d*) images in a patient with pancreatic metastasis (arrow, *b*) from a primary neuroendocrine cancer of the skin (Merkel cell carcinoma). There is a well-defined 6-cm mass in the head of the pancreas that is hypointense on T1-weighted images (*a, b*) and enhances minimally on early (*c*) postcontrast images, with progressive enhancement on late images (*d*). Distant metastasis occurs in one-third of patients with Merkel cell cancers.

drugs [82]. Predisposition may also be inherited as an autosomal dominant trait [83].

Acute Pancreatitis

Acute pancreatitis is defined as an acute inflammatory condition typically presenting with abdominal pain and associated with elevations in pancreatic enzymes (particularly amylase and lipase). Acute pancreatitis arises in the majority of cases from alcoholism or cholelithiasis [82]. Alcohol-related acute pancreatitis most frequently results in acute recurrent pancreatitis, whereas gallstone-related pancreatitis typically results in a single attack (fig. 4.66). The passage of biliary sludge may also cause acute pancreatitis [84]. At least 95% of patients with acute pancreatitis experience severe midepigastric pain that ra-

diates to the back. Nausea and vomiting occur in 75–85% of patients, and fever occurs in approximately 50%.

Acute pancreatitis results from the exudation of fluid containing activated proteolytic enzymes into the interstitium of the pancreas and leakage of this fluid into surrounding tissue. Trypsin is suspected to be the primary enzyme involved in the coagulative necrosis. Pathologically, acute pancreatitis is characterized by a spectrum of morphologic features, which may be patchy or diffuse. In mild cases, edema predominates, producing so-called edematous or interstitial pancreatitis. There is scattered peripancreatic fat necrosis without parenchymal or acinar necrosis. In severe cases, extensive pancreatic and peripancreatic fat necrosis, parenchymal necrosis, and hemorrhage occur. In its most devastating form, severe acute pancreatitis may produce an organ that resembles oily mud, where degenerative tissue, fat, and hemorrhage congeal [85].

The signal intensity features of the pancreas in uncomplicated mild acute pancreatitis resemble those of normal pancreatic tissue. The pancreas is high in signal intensity on precontrast T1-weighted fat-suppressed images and enhances in a normal uniform fashion on immediate postgadolinium images reflecting a normal capillary blush (fig. 4.67). The diagnosis of acute pancreatitis on MR images relies on the presence of morphologic and/or signal intensity changes [1]. The acutely inflamed pancreas shows either focal or diffuse enlargement, which may be subtle. Peripancreatic fluid is well shown on noncontrast or immediate postgadolinium SGE images and appears as low-signal intensity strands of fluid or fluid collections in a background of high-signal intensity fat. Breathing-independent single-shot T2-weighted images employing fat suppression are also effective at showing small-volume high-signal fluid in a background of intermediate- to low-signal pancreas and low-signal fat. MRI is sensitive for the detection of subtle changes of acute pancreatitis, particularly minor peripancreatic inflammatory changes. CT imaging examinations appear normal in 15–30% of patients with clinical features of acute pancreatitis [86]. The sensitivity of MRI may exceed that of CT imaging, suggesting a role for MRI in the evaluation of patients with suspected acute pancreatitis and negative CT imaging examination. As the extent of pancreatitis becomes more severe, the pancreas develops a heterogeneous appearance on precontrast T1-weighted fat-suppressed images and enhances in a more heterogeneous, diminished fashion on immediate postgadolinium images (fig. 4.68).

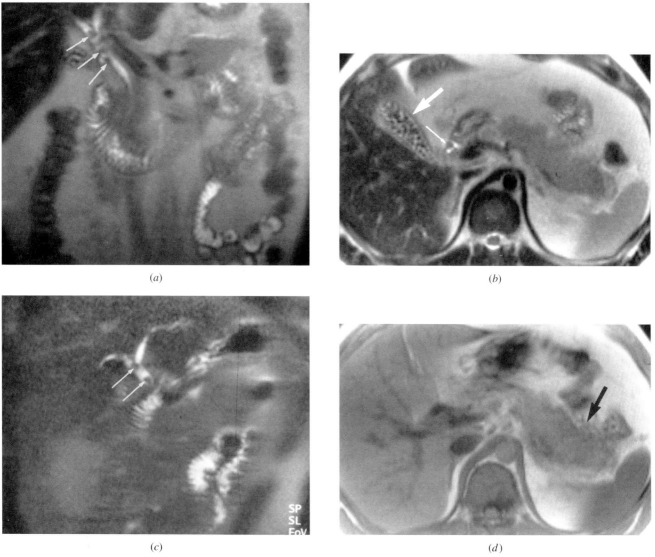

(a)

(b)

(c)

(d)

F I G . 4.66 Mild acute gallstone pancreatitis. Coronal (*a*) and transverse (*b*) T2-weighted ETSE, MRCP (*c*), T1-weighted SGE (*d*), and immediate postgadolinium T1-weighted SGE (*e*) images.

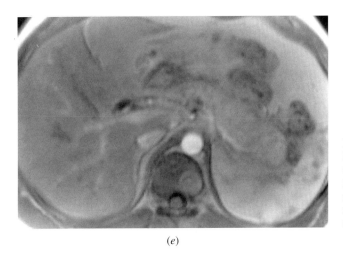

(e)

F I G . 4.66 (*Continued*) Three stones are seen in the mildly dilated CHD and CBD (arrows, *a*, *b*, *c*), and multiple small stones are present in the gallbladder (large arrow, *b*). The pancreas is enlarged slightly and diffusely (arrow, *d*) with ill-defined margins and a minimal volume of surrounding fluid. Passage of calculi through the biliary tree is a common cause of single episodes of acute pancreatitis, which, as in this case, is generally of mild severity.

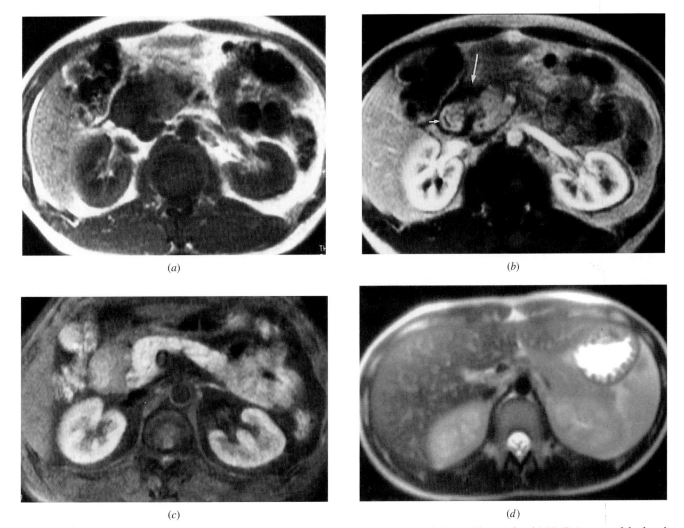

(a) (b)

(c) (d)

F I G . 4.67 Mild acute pancreatitis. T1-weighted SGE (*a*) and immediate postgadolinium T1-weighted SGE (*b*) images of the head of the pancreas and T1-weighted fat-suppressed spin-echo image (*c*) of the body of the pancreas. On the precontrast T1-weighted image (*a*), ill-defined low-signal intensity reticular strands surround a slightly enlarged pancreatic head, a finding consistent with peripancreatic fluid. On the immediate postgadolinium image (*b*), signal-void fluid (arrow, *b*) surrounds the head of the pancreas and duodenum (small arrow, *b*). The body of the pancreas is normal and high in signal intensity on the T1-weighted fat-suppressed image (*c*), reflecting a normal content of aqueous protein in the pancreatic acini consistent with mild pancreatitis. (Reproduced with permission from Semelka RC, Shoenut JP, Kroeker MA, Micflikier AB: The pancreas. In: Semelka RC, Shoenut JP. *MRI of the Abdomen with CT Correlation*. New York: Raven Press, p. 59–76, 1993.)

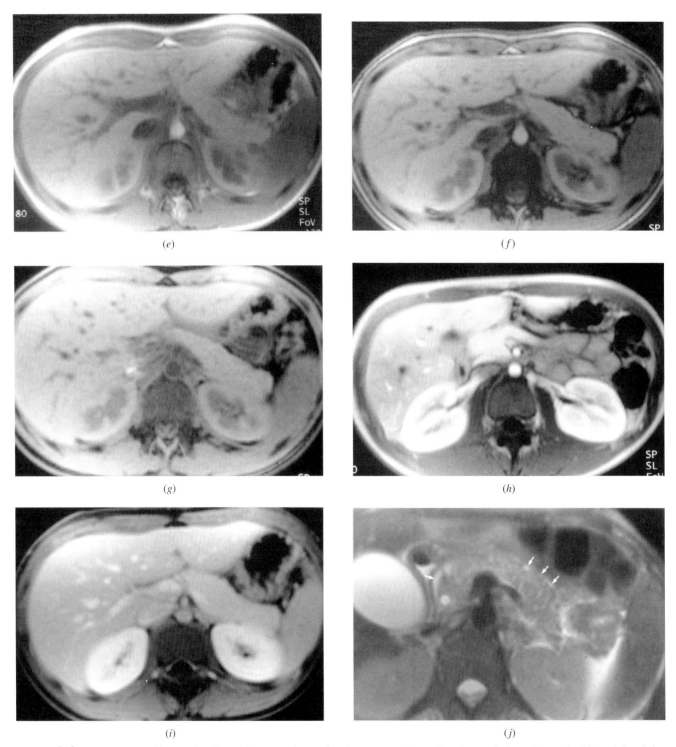

(e)   (f)

(g)   (h)

(i)   (j)

FIG. 4.67 (*Continued*) T2-weighted SS-ETSE (*d*), T1-weighted SGE (*e*), T1-weighted out-of-phase SGE (*f*), T1-weighted fat-suppressed SGE (*g*), immediate postgadolinium SGE (*h*), and 90-s postgadolinium fat-suppressed SGE (*i*) images in a second patient. The pancreas is minimally and diffusely enlarged with subtle loss of lobulated contour. The pancreas is normal in signal on noncontrast T1-weighted fat-suppressed images (*g*) and enhances normally on immediate postgadolinium images (*h*). The appearance is essentially that of normal pancreas, but clinical history and mildly elevated serum amylase were diagnostic for an episode of pancreatitis.

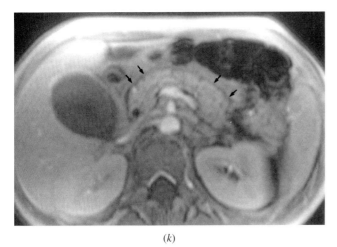

(*k*)

FIG. 4.67 (*Continued*) T2-weighted fat-suppressed SS-ETSE (*j*) and early postgadolinium single-shot magnetization-prepared gradient-echo (*k*) images demonstrate mild diffuse enhancement of the pancreas and a thin film of peripancreatic fluid surrounding the pancreas (small arrows, *j*, *k*) and throughout the interstices of the marbled pancreatic parenchyma. Fat-suppressed breathing-independent single-shot T2-weighted sequences are very effective at showing small volumes of fluid, as surrounding fat and pancreas are both low signal and only fluid will be high signal (*j*). This case is also noteworthy in that image quality is reasonable despite the fact that the patient was very ill and a noncooperative MR imaging protocol was employed, which uses only breathing-independent single-shot images.

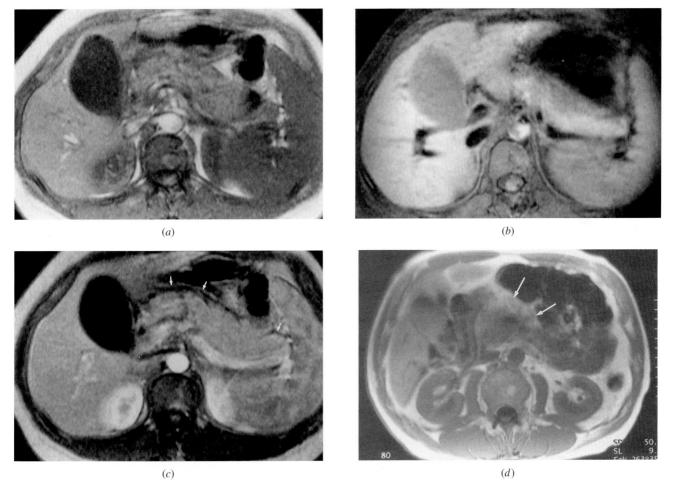

(*a*)

(*b*)

(*c*)

(*d*)

FIG. 4.68 Moderately severe acute pancreatitis. T1-weighted SGE (*a*), T1-weighted fat-suppressed spin-echo (*b*), and immediate postgadolinium T1-weighted SGE (*c*) images. The pancreas is diffusely enlarged (*a*–*c*). The signal intensity of the pancreas is heterogeneous on the T1-weighted fat-suppressed image (*b*), which suggests a decrease in the proteinaceous fluid content within the acini of the pancreas. Signal-void fluid is shown surrounding the body and tail of the pancreas on the immediate postgadolinium image (arrows, *c*). The intensity of pancreatic enhancement is less than normal for pancreas on the capillary-phase image (*c*).

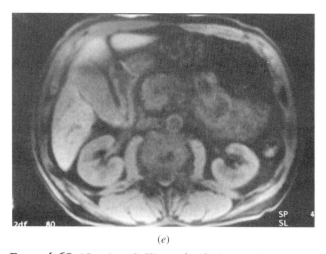

(e)

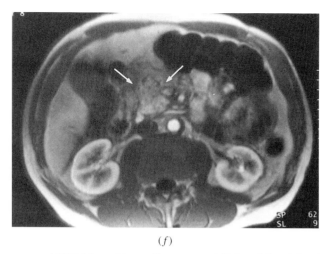

(f)

F I G . 4.68 (*Continued*) T1-weighted SGE (*d*), T1-weighted fat-suppressed SGE (*e*), and immediate postgadolinium T1-weighted SGE (*f*) images in a second patient. Peripancreatic fluid is well shown as low-signal intensity stranding in the high-signal intensity fat on the T1-weighted SGE image (arrows, *d*). The anterior portion of the head of the pancreas is lower in signal intensity on the precontrast fat-suppressed image (*e*) and enhances less (arrows, *f*) on immediate postgadolinium images (*f*), reflecting more severe changes of pancreatitis. Relative sparing of either anterior or posterior portions of the head of the pancreas is not uncommon because of separate pancreatic ductal systems. Despite the focal nature of the diminished enhancement of the dorsal head of the pancreas, there is lobular architecture similar to that of the ventral pancreatic head. A pancreatic neoplasm would not exhibit lobular architecture.

Percentage of pancreatic necrosis has been considered an important prognostic indicator in patients with acute pancreatitis [87, 88]. Dynamic gadolinium-enhanced SGE images may be useful for this determination because MRI is very sensitive in detecting the presence or absence of gadolinium enhancement. Saifuddin et al. [89] described comparable results for dynamic contrast-enhanced CT images and immediate postgadolinium SGE images for determining the presence of pancreatic necrosis. Complications of acute pancreatitis such as hemorrhage (fig. 4.69), pseudocyst formation (fig. 4.70), or abscess are clearly shown on MRI. Hemorrhagic fluid collections are high in signal intensity on T1-weighted fat-suppressed images, and depiction of hemorrhage is superior on MR images compared to CT images. Simple pseudocysts are low in signal intensity or signal void in a background of normal-signal intensity pancreatic tissue on both SGE and T1-weighted

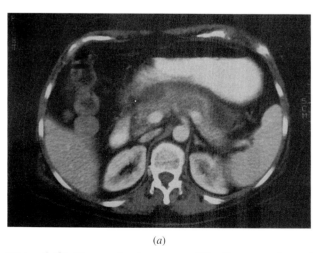

(a)

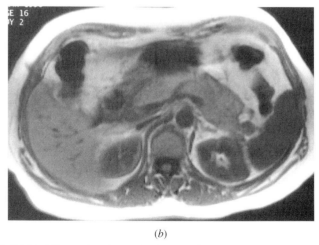

(b)

F I G . 4.69 Hemorrhagic pancreatitis. Contrast-enhanced spiral CT (*a*), T1-weighted SGE (*b*), T1-weighted fat-suppressed SGE (*c*), T2-weighted SS-ETSE (*d*), and immediate postgadolinium T1-weighted SGE (*e*) images. The CT image demonstrates an enlarged pancreas with free fluid along its anterior margin, findings consistent with acute pancreatitis. On the T1-weighted SGE image (*b*), the fluid collections are noted to be hyperintense, which is accentuated on the fat-suppressed image (arrows, *c*).

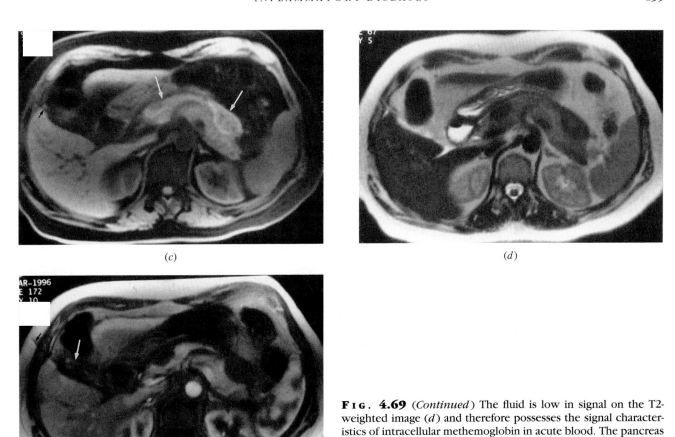

(c)

(d)

(e)

F I G . 4.69 (*Continued*) The fluid is low in signal on the T2-weighted image (*d*) and therefore possesses the signal characteristics of intracellular methemoglobin in acute blood. The pancreas enhances relatively uniformly on the immediate postgadolinium image, reflecting the absence of pancreatic necrosis (*e*). A collapsed acutely inflamed gallbladder (arrow, *e*) is present, in which a cholecystostomy catheter was placed (small arrow, *c, e*).

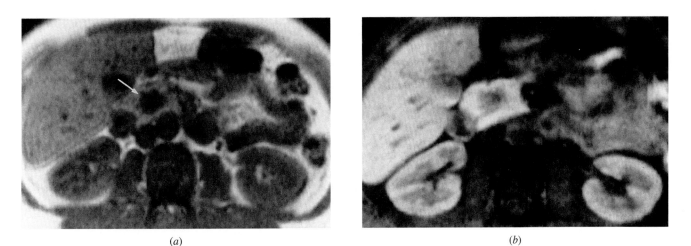

(a)

(b)

F I G . 4.70 Pseudocyst in acute pancreatitis. T1-weighted SGE (*a*), T1-weighted fat-suppressed spin-echo (*b*), and immediate postgadolinium T1-weighted SGE (*c*) images. A low-signal intensity pseudocyst (arrow, *a*) is present in the head of the pancreas (*a–c*). The pancreas has normal high signal intensity on the T1-weighted fat-suppressed image (*b*), and there is normal uniform enhancement of the pancreas on the immediate postgadolinium image (*c*). These imaging features are consistent with a pseudocyst in the setting of acute pancreatitis because the background pancreas has normal signal intensity features. The lesion did not change in size and shape on delayed images, excluding a poorly vascularized tumor.

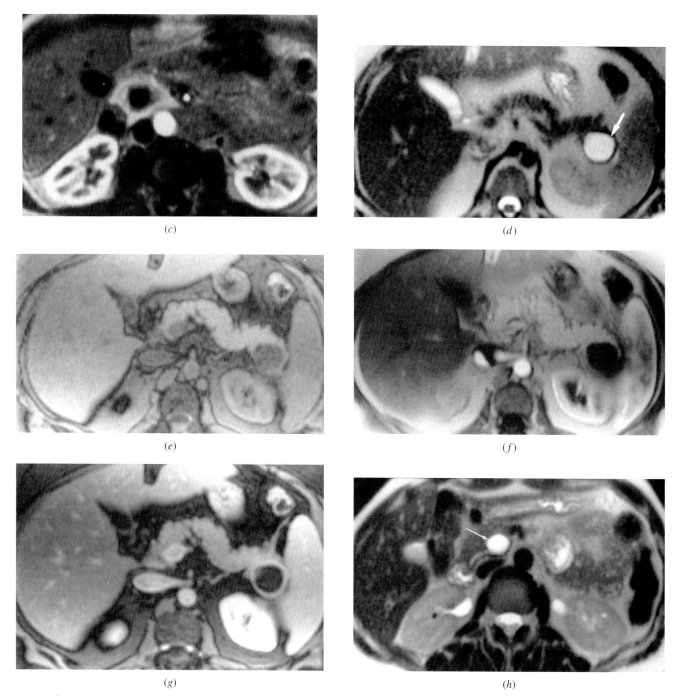

(c)

(d)

(e)

(f)

(g)

(h)

F I G . 4.70 (*Continued*) T2-weighted SS-ETSE (*d*), T1-weighted fat-suppressed SGE (*e*), immediate postgadolinium T1-weighted SGE (*f*), and 90-s postgadolinium fat-suppressed SGE (*g*) images in a second patient. A 3-cm pseudocyst (arrow, *d*) arises in the pancreatic tail. The pancreas is normal in signal on noncontrast T1-weighted fat-suppressed images (*e*) and enhances normally on early (*f*) and late (*g*) images, consistent with no substantial parenchymal disease. There is progressive enhancement of the wall of the pseudocyst (*g*), which is typically for fibrous tissue. The pancreas and liver are hypointense on T2-weighted images (*d*) secondary to iron deposition from multiple blood transfusion.

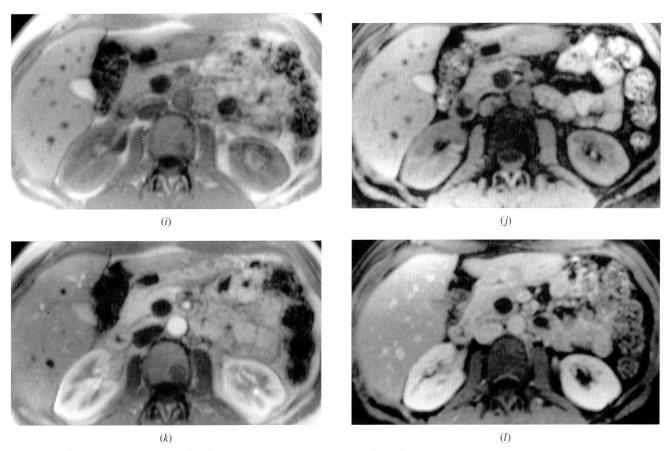

(i)   *(j)*

(k)   *(l)*

FIG. 4.70 (*Continued*) T2-weighted SS-ETSE (*h*), T1-weighted SGE (*i*), T1-weighted fat-suppressed SGE (*j*), immediate postgadolinium T1-weighted SGE (*k*), and 90-s postgadolinium fat-suppressed SGE (*l*) images demonstrate a 2-cm pseudocyst (arrow, *h*) in the uncinate process of the pancreas. The normal signal intensity of the pancreas, especially on noncontrast T1-weighted fat-suppressed (*j*) and immediate postgadolinium SGE (*k*) images, shows that background pancreas is not substantially diseased.

fat-suppressed images (figs. 4.71 and 4.72). Extrapancreatic pseudocysts are well shown on breath-hold SGE images because of high contrast with high-signal intensity fat.

Image acquisition in multiple planes permits determination of pseudocyst location in relation to various organs and structures. Simple pseudocysts are relatively homogeneous and high in signal intensity on T2-weighted images. Pseudocysts complicated by necrotic debris, hemorrhage, or infection are heterogeneous in signal intensity on T2-weighted images [89]. Proteinaceous fluid tends to layer in a gradation of concentration with low-signal intensity concentrated proteinaceous material in the dependent portion of the cyst. Necrotic material may appear as irregularly shaped regions of low signal intensity in the pseudocyst [90]. This information may provide both therapeutic and prognostic information because pseudocysts that contain necrotic material may not respond to simple percutaneous drainage and thus may require open debridement. Breathing-independent T2-weighted sequences may be of particular value in evaluating these pseudocyst collections, as

many patients are very debilitated and unable to cooperate with breath-holding instructions.

Chronic Pancreatitis

Chronic pancreatitis is defined pathologically by continuous or relapsing inflammation of the organ leading to irreversible morphologic injury and typically leading to impairment of function. Chronic pancreatitis is acquired either as a disease process distinct from acute pancreatitis or as a complication of repeated attacks of acute pancreatitis. There is a strong association between alcoholism and development of chronic pancreatitis [91, 92]. Obstruction of the pancreatic duct from various causes, including pancreatic ductal cancer, results in chronic pancreatitis [92]. Acute pancreatitis secondary to gallstone disease rarely results in chronic pancreatitis.

Chronic pancreatitis is associated with decreased endocrine as well as exocrine function [91, 92]. Patients with chronic pancreatitis have an increased risk of developing pancreatic cancer [93]. An analysis of patients with chronic pancreatitis imaged on dynamic contrast-enhanced CT images showed the following features: 66%

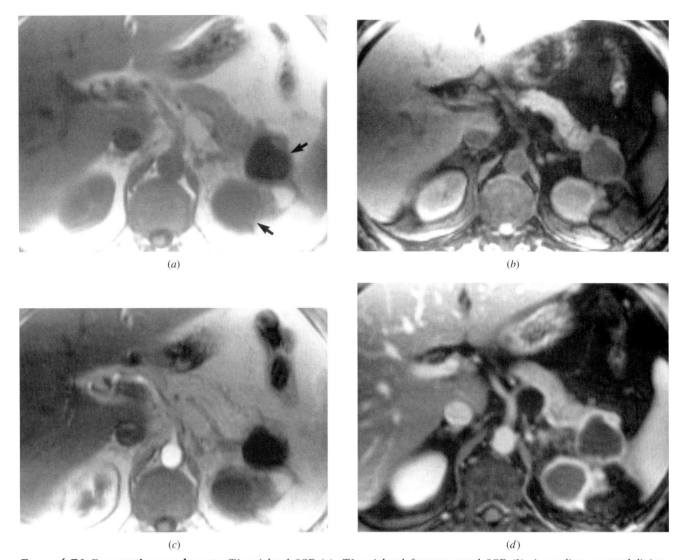

(a)

(b)

(c)

(d)

FIG. 4.71 Pancreatic pseudocysts. T1-weighted SGE (*a*), T1-weighted fat-suppressed SGE (*b*), immediate postgadolinium T1-weighted SGE (*c*) and 90-s postgadolinium T1-weighted fat-suppressed SGE (*d*) images. There is a pseudocyst in the tail of the pancreas and a second one adjacent in the upper pole of the left kidney (arrows, *a*). Late enhancement of the pseudocyst walls is appreciated (*d*).

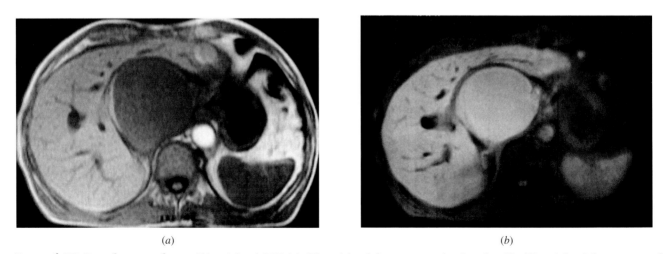

(a)

(b)

FIG. 4.72 Pseudocysts—large. T1-weighted SGE (*a*), T1-weighted fat-suppressed spin-echo (*b*), T2-weighted fat-suppressed SS-ETSE (*c*), and immediate postgadolinium T1-weighted SGE (*d*) images obtained superior to the pancreas, T1-weighted fat-suppressed spin-echo (*e*) and gadolinium-enhanced T1-weighted fat-suppressed spin-echo (*f*) images at the level of the body of the pancreas, coronal gadolinium-enhanced T1-weighted SGE images from midhepatic (*g*) and more anterior (*h*) locations, and sagittal-plane (*i*) T1-weighted SGE images.

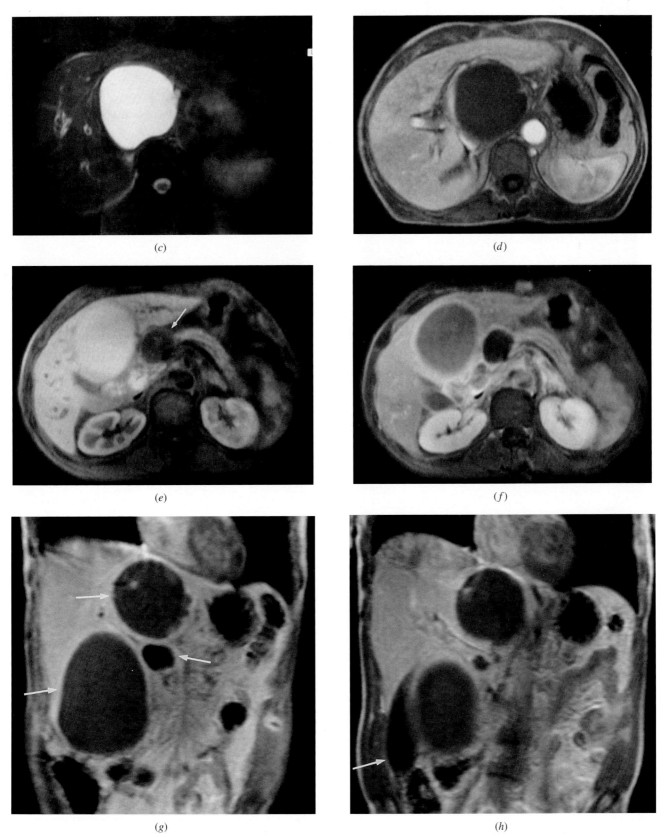

F I G . 4.72 (*Continued*) An 8-cm pseudocyst is present in the region of the porta hepatis that is mildly high in signal intensity on T1-weighted images (*a, b*) and high in signal intensity on the T2-weighted image (*c*).The mild, high signal intensity on T1-weighted images is more conspicuous with fat suppression (*b*) and consistent with dilute blood or protein. The homogeneous signal intensity on T2-weighted images suggests that the fluid, although proteinaceous, is not complicated by infection or cellular debris. A 3-cm pseudocyst (arrow, *e*) is identified within the body of the pancreas (*e, f*).

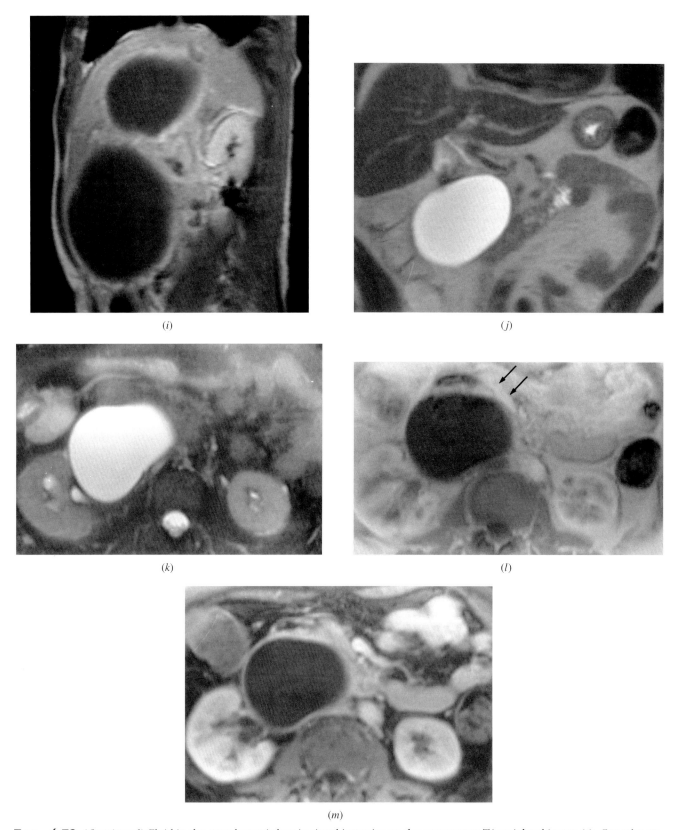

(i)

(j)

(k)

(l)

(m)

F i g . 4.72 (*Continued*) Fluid in the pseudocyst is low in signal intensity on the precontrast T1-weighted image (*e*). Capsular enhancement of the pseudocysts is shown on the fat-suppressed gadolinium-enhanced image (*f*). Coronal plane gadolinium-enhanced T1-weighted SGE images (*g, h*) demonstrate the relationship of the pseudocysts to surrounding structures. Three pseudocysts (arrows, *g*) are shown in the coronal plane (*g*). Gallbladder (arrow, *h*) is displaced laterally by the large pseudocyst in the porta hepatis. The sagittal plane image (*i*) demonstrates the anteroposterior orientation of the pseudocysts to other structures.

Coronal SS-ETSE (*j*), transverse fat-suppressed SS-ETSE (*k*), immediate postgadolinium T1-weighted SGE (*l*), and 90-s postgadolinium fat-suppressed SGE (*m*) images in a second patient. A large, 8 × 7 cm, pancreatic pseudocyst is situated between the right kidney and second portion of the duodenum. The pancreatic head is displaced anteriorly (arrows, *l*).

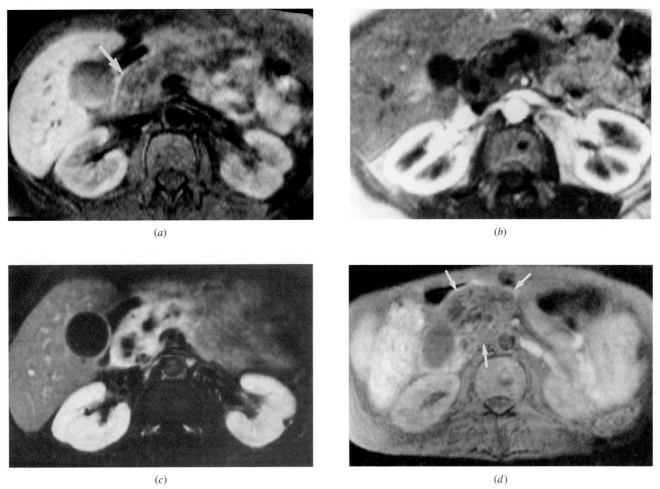

(a)   *(b)*

(c)   *(d)*

F I G . 4.73 Chronic pancreatitis with focal enlargement of the head of the pancreas. T1-weighted fat-suppressed spin-echo (*a*), immediate postgadolinium T1-weighted SGE (*b*), and gadolinium-enhanced T1-weighted fat-suppressed spin-echo (*c*) images. The head of the pancreas is enlarged (arrow, *a*). The pancreas is diffusely low in signal intensity on the precontrast T1-weighted fat-suppressed image (*a*). The pancreas shows diffuse diminished enhancement on the immediate postgadolinium image (*b*). The lack of definition of a focal mass lesion on the immediate postgadolinium image is the most important observation that excludes tumor. On the interstitial-phase gadolinium-enhanced image (*c*), signal-void foci are identified that represent cysts, pseudocysts, dilated pancreatic duct, and calcifications.

had dilation of the main pancreatic duct, 54% had parenchymal atrophy, 50% had pancreatic calcifications, 34% had pseudocysts, 32% had focal pancreatic enlargement, 29% had biliary ductal dilatation, and 16% had densities in peripancreatic fat or fascia. No abnormalities were present in 7% of patients [94]. Calcification, which is the pathognomonic feature of chronic pancreatitis on CT images, is a late phenomenon following development of fibrosis and is observed in only half of these patients. CT imaging is not sensitive for detecting the early changes of fibrosis in chronic pancreatitis. Focal chronic pancreatitis may be difficult to distinguish from adenocarcinoma in the head of the pancreas because both entities may cause focal enlargement (fig. 4.73), obstruction of the common bile duct and pancreatic duct (figs. 4.74), atrophy of the tail of the pancreas, and obliteration of the fat plane around the superior mesenteric artery (SMA)

[95–97]. Unlike the situation with pancreatic cancer in which the pancreatic duct is dilated on the basis of mechanical obstruction alone; in chronic pancreatitis ductal dilatation is more tortuous and irregular, and side branch dilatation occurs more commonly (fig. 4.75).

MRI may perform better than CT imaging at detecting changes of chronic pancreatitis in that MRI detects not only morphologic findings but also the presence of fibrosis. Fibrosis is shown by diminished signal intensity on noncontrast T1-weighted fat-suppressed images and diminished heterogeneous enhancement on immediate postgadolinium SGE images [98]. Low signal intensity on T1-weighted fat-suppressed images reflects loss of the aqueous protein in the acini of the pancreas. Diminished enhancement on capillary-phase images reflects disruption of the normal capillary bed and increased chronic inflammation and fibrous tissue. A study that

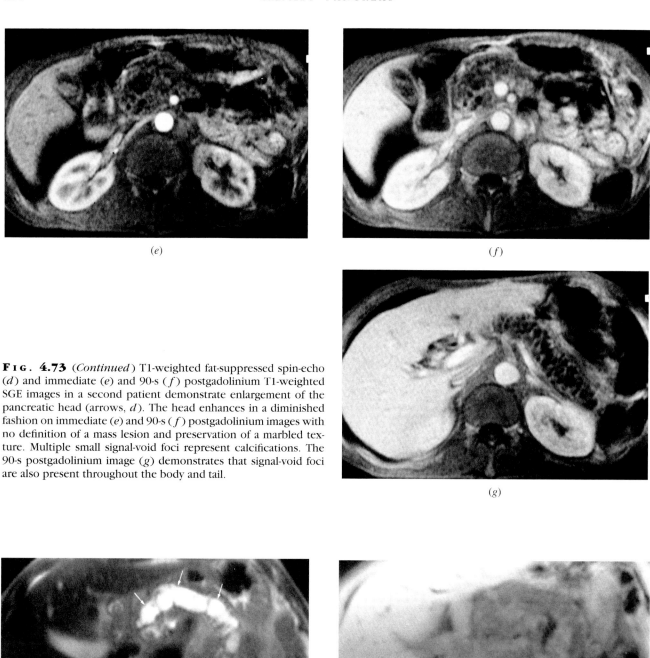

(e)

(f)

(g)

FIG. 4.73 *(Continued)* T1-weighted fat-suppressed spin-echo (*d*) and immediate (*e*) and 90-s (*f*) postgadolinium T1-weighted SGE images in a second patient demonstrate enlargement of the pancreatic head (arrows, *d*). The head enhances in a diminished fashion on immediate (*e*) and 90-s (*f*) postgadolinium images with no definition of a mass lesion and preservation of a marbled texture. Multiple small signal-void foci represent calcifications. The 90-s postgadolinium image (*g*) demonstrates that signal-void foci are also present throughout the body and tail.

(a)

(b)

FIG. 4.74 Chronic pancreatitis with moderate to severe pancreatic duct dilatation. T2-weighted SS-ETSE (*a*), T1-weighted fat-suppressed SGE (*b*), immediate postgadolinium T1-weighted SGE (*c*), and 90-s postgadolinium fat-suppressed SGE (*d*) images in a patient with hereditary pancreatitis and recurrent bouts of pancreatitis. The pancreatic ductal is very dilated (arrows, *a*). The pancreatic parenchyma is atrophic and is low signal on noncontrast T1-weighted fat-suppressed SGE (*b*). The thin rim of atrophic pancreas enhances minimally on immediate postgadolinium image (*c*) and shows late enhancement (arrows, *d*) consistent with changes of fibrosis. The pancreas is atrophic for the patient age (18 years old), and it shows heterogeneous signal intensity on T1-weighted images (*b*) with diminished enhancement on postgadolinium images (*d*). The pancreatic duct is slightly prominent.

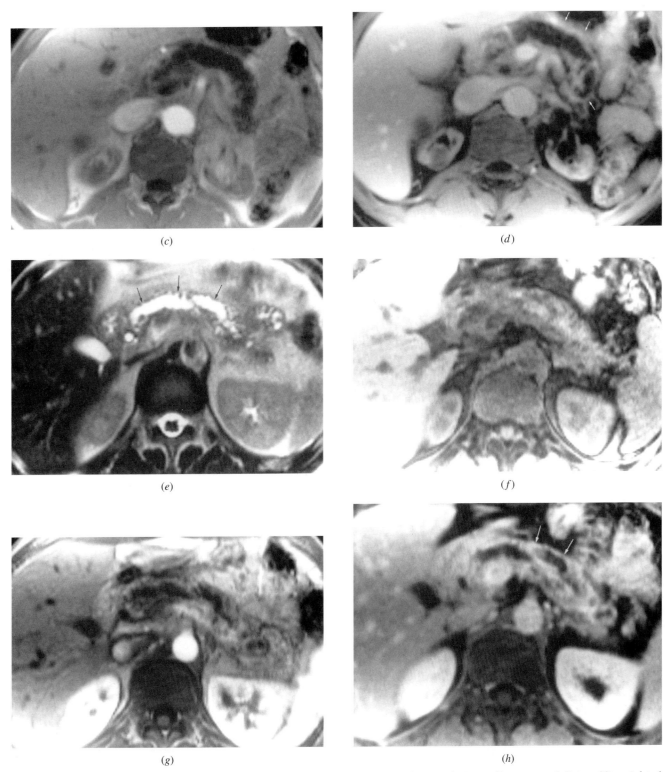

FIG. 4.74 (*Continued*) T2-weighted SS-ETSE (*e*), T1-weighted fat-suppressed SGE (*f*), immediate postgadolinium T1-weighted SGE (*g*), and 90-s postgadolinium fat-suppressed SGE (*h*) images on a second patient demonstrates similar findings. Note moderately severe dilatation of the pancreatic duct (arrows, *e*) and late enhancement of atrophic pancreatic parenchyma (arrows, *h*).

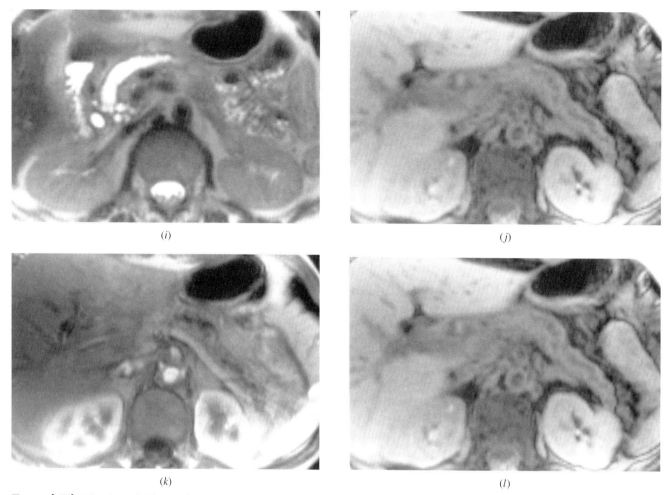

(i)   (j)

(k)   (l)

F I G . 4.74 (*Continued*) T2-weighted SS-ETSE (*i*), T1-weighted fat-suppressed SGE (*j*), immediate postgadolinium fat-suppressed SGE (*k*), and 90-s postgadolinium fat-suppressed SGE (*l*) images in a third patient show the same findings of moderately severe pancreatic ductal dilatation with parenchymal signal intensity changes of chronic pancreatitis.

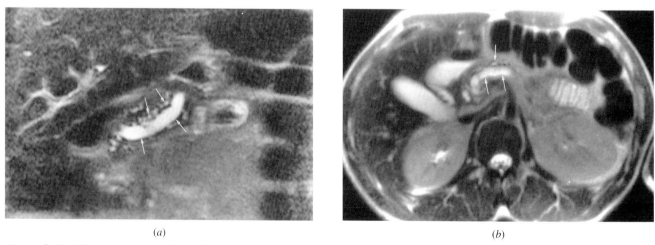

(a)   (b)

F I G . 4.75 Chronic pancreatitis with main pancreatic and side branch ductal dilatation. Coronal MRCP (*a*) and transverse T2-weighted SS-ETSE (*b*), T1-weighted fat-suppressed SGE (*c*), immediate postgadolinium T1-weighted SGE (*d*), and 90-s postgadolinium fat-suppressed SGE (*e*) images. The main pancreatic duct and its side branches are markedly dilated, which is best seen on MRCP and single shot T2-weighted images (arrows, *a, b*).

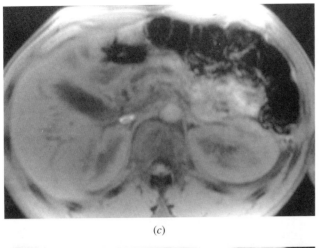

(c)

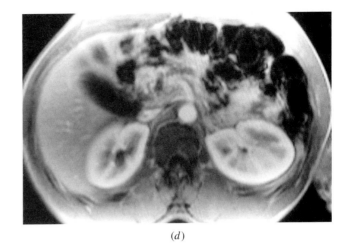

(d)

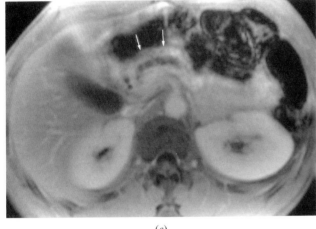

(e)

F I G. 4.75 (*Continued*) Parenchymal changes of chronic pancreatitis are present including low signal on noncontrast T1-weighted fat-suppressed images (*c*) and minimal heterogeneous early enhancement (*d*) with late progressive parenchymal enhancement (arrows, *e*). The presence of dilated ectatic side branches is a feature more consistent with chronic pancreatitis than pancreatic ductal adenocarcinoma, with the latter entity more typically causing dilatation of the main pancreatic duct without side branch ectasia.

described MRI findings in 13 patients with chronic calcifying pancreatitis and 9 patients with acute recurrent pancreatitis demonstrated differences between these groups on T1-weighted fat-suppressed images and immediate postgadolinium SGE images. All patients with pancreatic calcifications on CT examination had a diminished-signal intensity pancreas on T1-weighted fat-suppressed images and an abnormally low percentage of contrast enhancements on immediate postgadolinium SGE images (fig. 4.76). Patients with acute recurrent pancreatitis had signal intensity features of the pancreas comparable to those of normal pancreas. Focal enlargement of the head of the pancreas with chronic pancreatitis may be difficult to distinguish from cancer on CT images. MR images permit the distinction between these two entities (fig. 4.73). Both chronic pancreatitis and carcinoma show signal intensity of the enlarged region of pancreas on noncontrast T1-weighted fat-suppressed and T2-weighted images. On immediate postgadolinium images, focal pancreatitis shows heterogeneous enhancement with the presence of moderately signal-void cysts and calcifications without evidence of well-defined,

minimally enhancing mass lesion. Demonstration of a definable, circumscribed mass lesion is most often diagnostic for tumor. In chronic pancreatitis, the focally enlarged portion of pancreas usually shows preservation of a glandular, feathery, or marbled texture similar to that of remaining pancreas. In contrast, in pancreatic cancer, the focally enlarged portion of pancreas loses its usual anatomic detail. Diffuse low signal intensity of the entire pancreas, including the area of focal enlargement, on T1-weighted fat-suppressed and immediate postgadolinium SGE images is typical for chronic pancreatitis. In the setting of pancreatic cancer, the enhancement of the tumor is markedly less than adjacent pancreatic parenchyma. Rarely, chronic pancreatitis may involve only the focally enlarged portion of pancreas, with the reminder of the pancreas having no inflammatory changes. In these cases, the focus of chronic pancreatitis can simulate the appearance of pancreatic ductal adenocarcinoma (fig. 4.77). In these rare cases, diagnosis can only be established by surgical resection and histopathologic examination confirming the absence of malignancy.

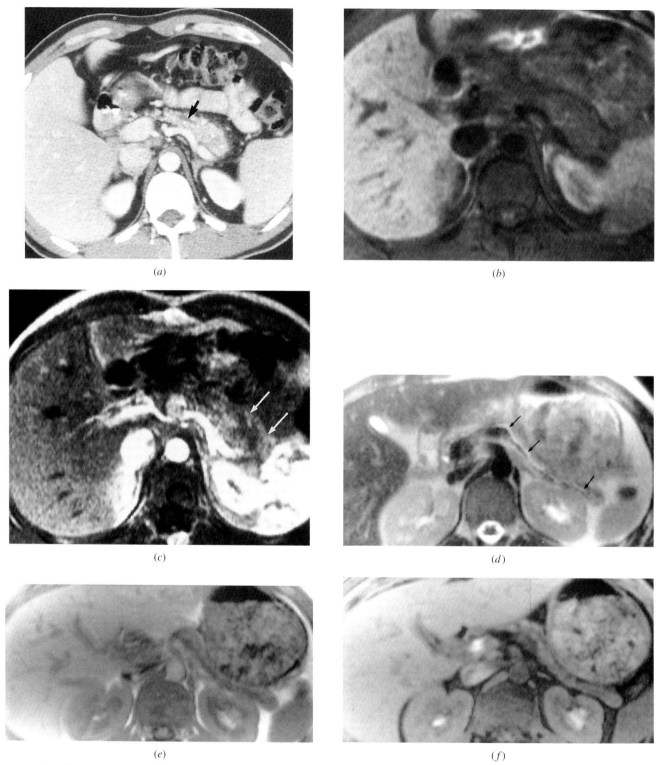

(a)

(b)

(c)

(d)

(e)

(f)

FIG. 4.76 Chronic pancreatitis. Contrast-enhanced CT (*a*) T1-weighted fat-suppressed spin-echo (*b*) and immediate postgadolinium T1-weighted SGE (*c*) images. The CT image demonstrates pancreatic calcifications, which is diagnostic for chronic pancreatitis. Mild pancreatic ductal dilatation (arrow, *a*) and mild pancreatic enlargement are also present. The pancreas is low in signal intensity on the T1-weighted fat-suppressed image, which is consistent with loss of aqueous protein in the acini. The immediate postgadolinium T1-weighted SGE image demonstrates heterogeneous diminished enhancement of the pancreas (arrows, *c*), reflecting replacement of the normal capillary bed with lesser vascularized fibrotic tissue. (Reproduced with permission from Semelka RC, Kroeker MA, Shoenut JP, Kroeker R, Yaffe CS, Micflikier AB: Pancreatic disease: Prospective comparison of CT, ERCP, and 1.5 T MR imaging with dynamic gadolinium enhancement and fat suppression. *Radiology* 181: 785–791, 1991.)

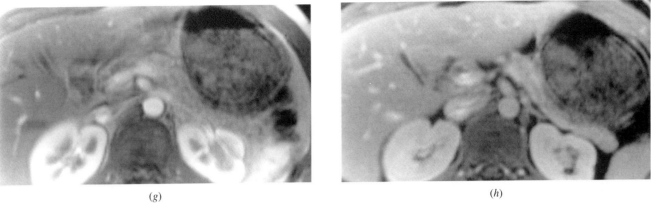

(g)   (h)

F I G . 4.76 (*Continued*) T2-weighted SS-ETSE (*d*), T1-weighted SGE (*e*), noncontrast T1-weighted fat-suppressed SGE (*f*), immediate postgadolinium T1-weighted SGE (*g*) and 90-s postgadolinium fat-suppressed SGE (*h*) images in a second patient. Moderate dilatation of the pancreatic duct is present (arrows, *d*). There is moderate atrophy of the pancreatic parenchyma which is low signal on T1-weighted fat-suppressed SGE (*f*) and demonstrates minimal enhancement on immediate postgadolinium images (*g*) with progressive enhancement on 90-s postcontrast images (*h*). These are classic features for chronic pancreatitis.

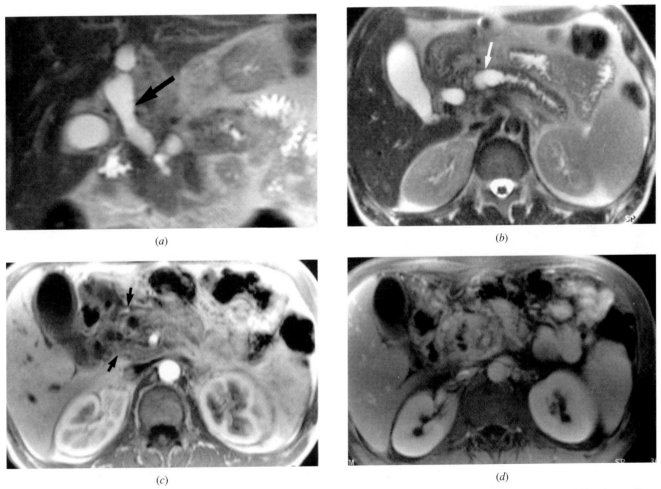

(a)   (b)

(c)   (d)

F I G . 4.77 Chronic pancreatitis simulating pancreatic cancer. Coronal (*a*) and transverse (*b*) T2-weighted SS-ETSE, immediate postgadolinium T1-weighted SGE (*c*), and 90-s postgadolinium fat-suppressed SGE (*d*) images. The CBD (arrow, *a*) and pancreatic (arrow, *b*) ducts are severely dilated, with atrophy of the pancreatic body (*b*) creating the double duct sign. On early (*c*) and late (*d*) postgadolinium images, no demarcated pancreatic mass is observed in the head of the pancreas. Instead, the enlarged pancreas shows a marbled texture (arrows, *c*) comparable in appearance to the remainder of the pancreas.

Recurrent bouts of acute pancreatitis superimposed on the chronic disease typify the usual clinical course of these patients. Acute on chronic pancreatitis is well shown on MR images (fig. 4.78, 4.79, 4.80). Pancreatic pseudocysts occur with an incidence of 10% in patients with chronic pancreatitis [92], often as a sequence of episodes of acute inflammation. Small pseudocysts

and cysts are well shown on gadolinium-enhanced T1-weighted fat-suppressed images as nearly signal-void oval structures (fig. 4.81). Pseudocysts are generally high in signal intensity on T2-weighted images, but signal intensity varies considerably depending on the presence of blood, protein, infection, and debris (fig 4.82).

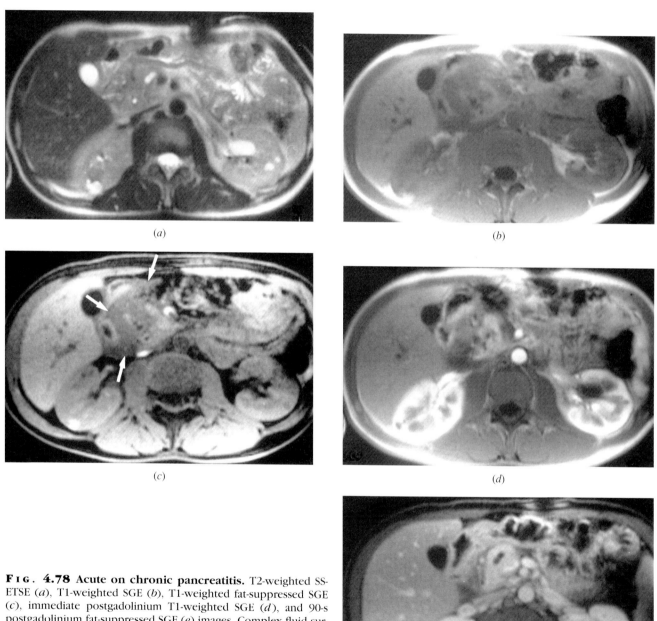

(a)

(b)

(c)

(d)

(e)

FIG. 4.78 Acute on chronic pancreatitis. T2-weighted SS-ETSE (*a*), T1-weighted SGE (*b*), T1-weighted fat-suppressed SGE (*c*), immediate postgadolinium T1-weighted SGE (*d*), and 90-s postgadolinium fat-suppressed SGE (*e*) images. Complex fluid surrounds the pancreas, predominantly located between the head and the second portion of duodenum (arrows, *c*). The pancreatic head is enlarged and shows decreased signal on noncontrast T1-weighted fat-suppressed SGE (*c*) and heterogeneous and reduced enhancement on immediate postgadolinium images (*d*), which is characteristic of chronic pancreatitis.

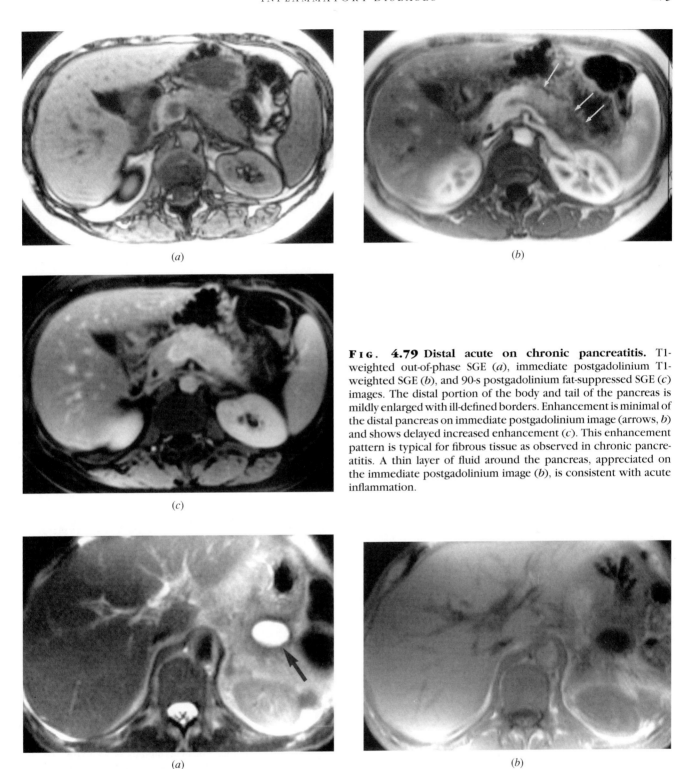

FIG. 4.79 Distal acute on chronic pancreatitis. T1-weighted out-of-phase SGE (*a*), immediate postgadolinium T1-weighted SGE (*b*), and 90-s postgadolinium fat-suppressed SGE (*c*) images. The distal portion of the body and tail of the pancreas is mildly enlarged with ill-defined borders. Enhancement is minimal of the distal pancreas on immediate postgadolinium image (arrows, *b*) and shows delayed increased enhancement (*c*). This enhancement pattern is typical for fibrous tissue as observed in chronic pancreatitis. A thin layer of fluid around the pancreas, appreciated on the immediate postgadolinium image (*b*), is consistent with acute inflammation.

FIG. 4.80 Acute on chronic pancreatitis with pseudocyst formation. T2-weighted SS-ETSE (*a*), T1-weighted SGE (*b*), T1-weighted fat-suppressed SGE (*c, d*), immediate postgadolinium T1-weighted SGE (*e, f*), and 90-s postgadolinium fat-suppressed SGE (*g*) images. There is a pseudocyst (arrow, *a*) in the pancreatic tail, which has a thickened wall that exhibits progressive late enhancement (arrow, *g*). The pancreatic head and neck region (arrows, *d*) are enlarged (*d, f*) and exhibit low signal on noncontrast fat-suppressed images (*d*) and diminished heterogeneous enhancement on immediate postgadolinium SGE images (*f*) consistent with focal acute on diffuse chronic pancreatitis. Note that renal corticomedullary difference is diminished on the noncontrast T1-weighted fat-suppressed image consistent with decreased renal function (*d*).

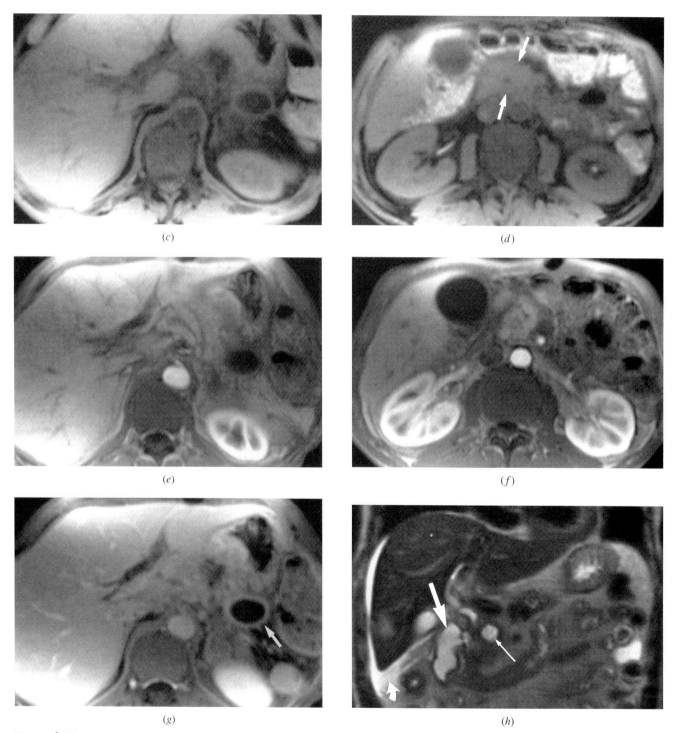

(c)

(d)

(e)

(f)

(g)

(h)

FIG. 4.80 (*Continued*) Coronal (*h*) and transverse (*i, j*) T2-weighted SS-ETSE, immediate postgadolinium T1-weighted SGE (*k*), and 90-s postgadolinium fat-suppressed SGE (*l*) images in a second patient. There is mild pancreatic duct dilatation and irregularity (arrow, *i*), which is commonly observed in chronic pancreatitis (*i*). A 2-cm pseudocyst is present in the posterior aspect of the pancreatic head (small arrow, *h, j*), and an irregular 4-cm pseudocyst (large arrow, *h, j*) adjacent to the second portion of the duodenum. A small volume of ascites is present (curved arrow, *h*). Note an incidental hemangioma on the liver that is high signal on T2 (curved arrow, *j*) and peripheral nodular enhancement with enlargement and coalescence of the nodules (*k, l*).

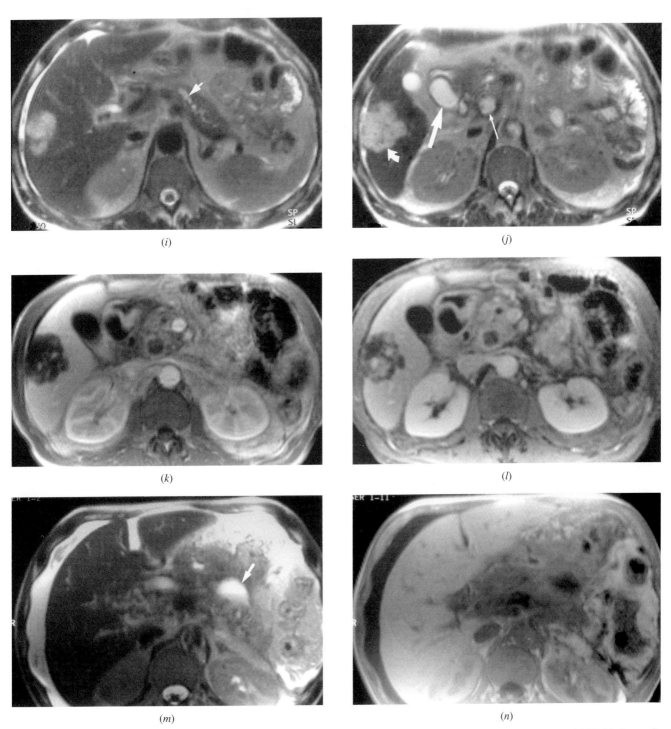

FIG. 4.80 (*Continued*) T2-weighted echo-train spin-echo (*m*), T1-weighted SGE (*n*), T1-weighted fat-suppressed SGE (*o*), immediate postgadolinium T1 SGE (*p*), and 90-s postgadolinium T1-weighted fat-suppressed SGE (*q*) images in a third patient. The pancreas is enlarged and ill-defined with blurring of the adjacent fat. The pancreas is low signal (arrows, *o*) on noncontrast T1-weighted fat-suppressed images (*o*) and on immediate postgadolinium SGE images (*q*) consistent with chronic pancreatitis. The pancreatic parenchyma shows progressive enhancement on late gadolinium-enhanced images (*q*), which is also a feature of chronic pancreatitis. There is a thick-walled pseudocyst anterior to the distal body of the pancreas, which contains a fluid-fluid level (arrow, *m*) on T2 (*m*). Multiple varices (small arrows, *q*) observed on the interstitial-phase gadolinium-enhanced image (*q*) reflect thrombosis of the splenic vein from longstanding severe chronic pancreatitis.

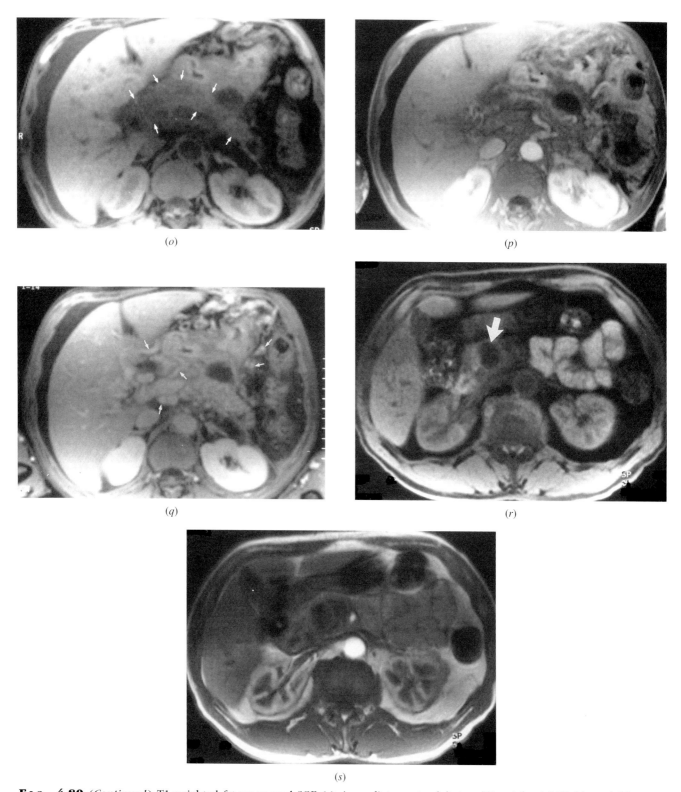

(o)

(p)

(q)

(r)

(s)

FIG. 4.80 (*Continued*) T1-weighted fat-suppressed SGE (*r*), immediate postgadolinium T1-weighted SGE (*s*), and 90-s post-gadolinium fat-suppressed SGE (*t*) images in a fourth patient. A pseudocyst is present in the head of the pancreas (arrow, *r*). Note the decreased signal on the noncontrast T1-weighted fat-suppressed SGE image (*r*), and minimal heterogeneous enhancement on the immediate postgadolinium SGE image (*s*) with progressive enhancement on the parenchyma (*t*), which are imaging features of chronic pancreatitis. Compare this appearance to the pseudocyst in the pancreatic head of patients with acute pancreatitis (fig. 4.70).

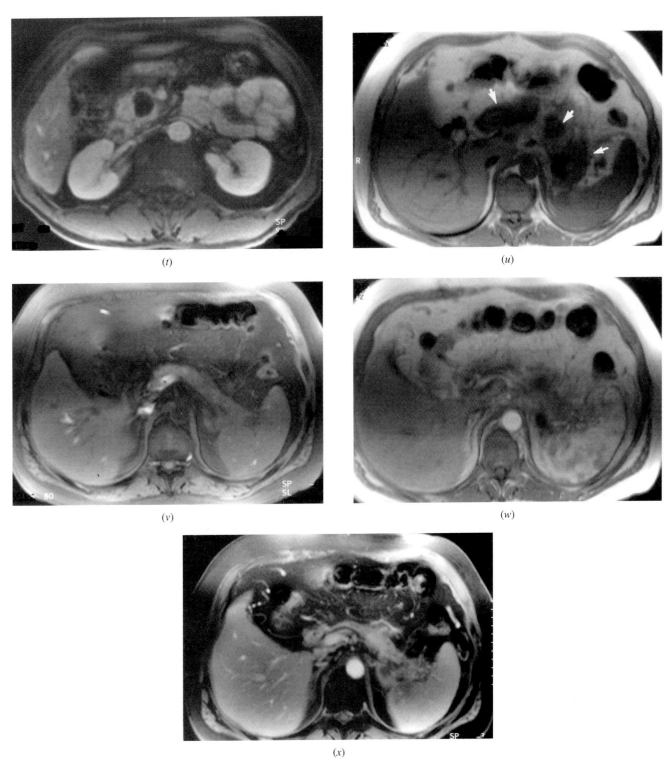

F I G. 4.80 (*Continued*) T1-weighted SGE (*u*), T1-weighted fat-suppressed SGE (*v*), immediate postgadolinium SGE (*w*), and 90-s postgadolinium fat-suppressed SGE (*x*) images in a fifth patient. Multiple pseudocysts (arrows, *u*) and peripancreatic fluid strands from acute inflammation present superimposed on chronic pancreatitis. The peripancreatic fluid strands are more clearly shown on the non-fat-suppressed images (*u, w*) than on the fat-suppressed images (*v, x*), because of the excellent contrast between low-signal fluid and high-signal background fat. Background chronic pancreatitis is shown as low signal of a small pancreas on noncontrast T1-weighted fat-suppressed image (*v*) and minimal early enhancement of the pancreas (*w*) with progressive enhancement on late images (*x*).

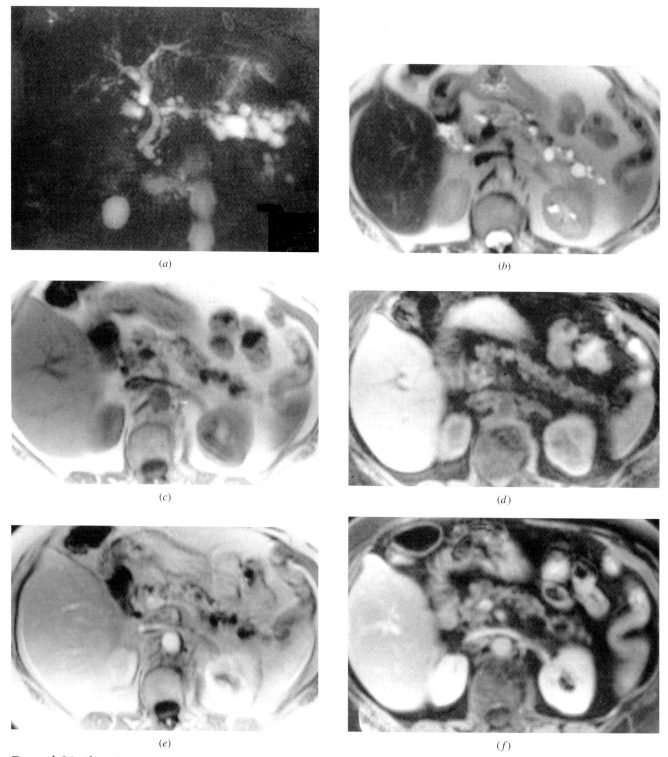

F I G .   4.81 Chronic pancreatitis with multiple small pseudocysts. MRCP (*a*), T2-weighted SS-ETSE (*b*), T1-weighted SGE (*c*), T1-weighted fat-suppressed SGE (*d*), immediate postgadolinium T1-weighted SGE (*e*), and 90-s postgadolinium fat-suppressed SGE (*f*) images. Multiple small pseudocysts are present throughout the atrophic background pancreatic parenchyma and appear hyperintense on T2-weighted images (*a, b*) and hypointense on T1-weighted images (*c, d*) and show lack of enhancement on early (*e*) and late (*f*) postgadolinium images, consistent with pseudocysts.

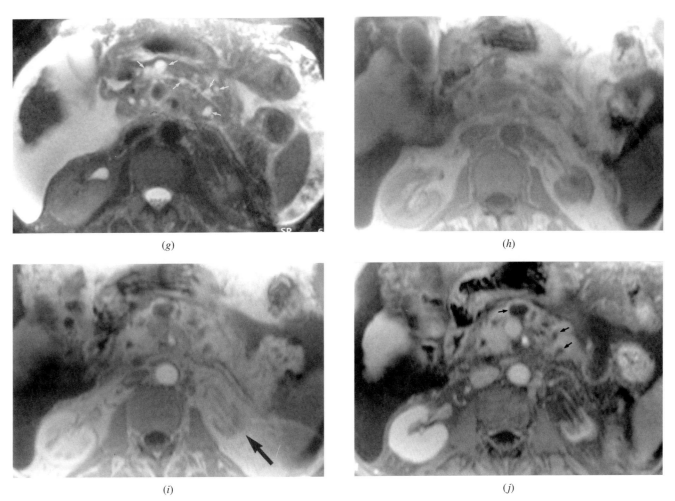

(g)

(h)

(i)

(j)

FIG. 4.81 (*Continued*) T2-weighted SS-ETSE (*g*), T1-weighted SGE (*h*), immediate postgadolinium T1-weighted SGE (*i*), and 90-s postgadolinium fat-suppressed SGE (*j*) images in a second patient with alcoholic pancreatitis. There are numerous cysts (arrows, *g, j*) scattered throughout the pancreas, and the pancreatic parenchyma enhances poorly on postgadolinium images. There is a large volume of ascites secondary to liver cirrhosis. Note also ischemic nephropathy of the left kidney (arrow, *i*) from main renal artery disease.

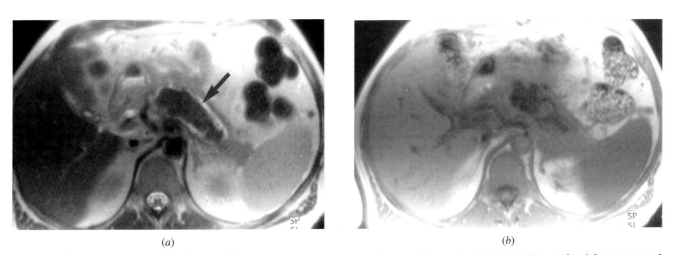

(a)

(b)

FIG. 4.82 Hemorrhagic pseudocyst. T2-weighted echo-train spin-echo (*a*), T1-weighted SGE (*b*), T1-weighted fat-suppressed SGE (*c*), immediate postgadolinium T1-weighted SGE (*d*), and 90-s postgadolinium T1-weighted fat-suppressed SGE (*e*) images.

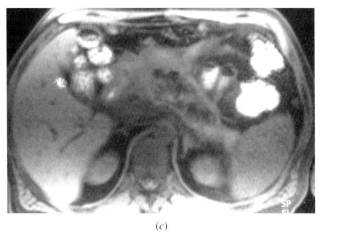

(c)

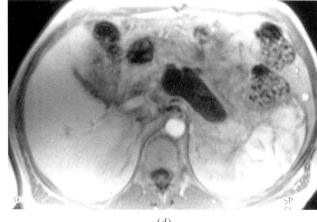

(d)

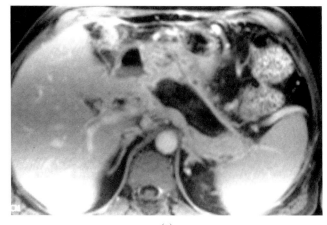

(e)

Fig. 4.82 (*Continued*) There is a tubule-shaped fluid collection (arrow, *a*) within the pancreas that has heterogeneous signal intensity on T1-(*b, c*) and T2-weighted (*a*) images compatible with hemorrhage. The pancreas is enlarged and has a blurred contour.

Chronic Autoimmune Pancreatitis

Most patients presenting with chronic pancreatitis will have alcohol-related disease. In approximately 30% of patients the nature and course of chronic pancreatitis is unclear, and these cases may be labeled idiopathic. A subgroup of these cases have been associated with autoimmune disorders such as Sjögrens syndrome, primary biliary cirrhosis, and primary sclerosing cholangitis [99, 100]. Histopathologic examination in cases of chronic nonalcoholic pancreatitis, including associated autoimmune disorders, shows periductal chronic inflammation and fibrosis. This process may result in obstruction or destruction of ducts [101]. Recent studies underscore the importance of diagnosing cases of suspected autoimmune-related chronic pancreatitis because these disorders may have a salutary response to steroid therapy [102]. Recent studies have described the MR appearance of autoimmune chronic pancreatitis characterized by enlarged pancreas with decreased signal intensity on T1-weighted images, high signal intensity on T2-weighted images, and delayed enhancement of the pancreatic parenchyma after the gadolinium administration. Additional findings that may be observed in autoimmune pancreatitis include 1) capsulelike rim sur-

rounding the diseased parenchyma that is hypointense on T2-weighted images and demonstrates delayed enhancement after gadolinium administration [99], 2) absence of parenchymal atrophy, 3) ductal dilatation proximal to the site of stenosis, 4) absence of extrapancreatic fluid, and 5) clear demarcation of the lesion [100].

Inflammatory Conditions and Infections of the Pancreas

A variety of bacterial, granulomatous, viral, and parasitic diseases may rarely affect the pancreas. Inflammatory diseases may appear as ill-defined focal masses that show irregular infiltration of pancreatic tissue (fig. 4.83). Differentiation between malignant and inflammatory diseases may not, however, reliably be made on imaging studies. Pancreatitis may also arise as a reactions to drugs (fig 4.84) or toxins.

TRAUMA

Traumatic injury of the pancreas may result in a spectrum of abnormalities (fig. 4.85) from mild contusion to

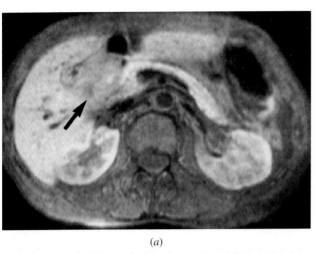

(a)

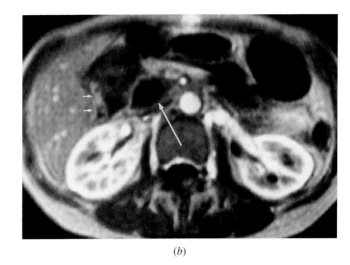

(b)

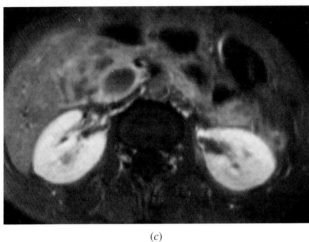

(c)

FIG. 4.83 Necrotizing granulomatous pancreatitis. T1-weighted fat-suppressed spin-echo (*a*), immediate postgadolinium T1-weighted SGE (*b*), and gadolinium-enhanced T1-weighted fat-suppressed spin-echo (*c*) images. A heterogeneous low-signal intensity mass is present, arising from the lateral aspect of the head of the pancreas (arrow, *a*). The remainder of the pancreas is normal and moderately high in signal intensity on T1-weighted fat-suppressed spin-echo images (*a*). The lesion enhances in a heterogeneous minimal fashion on immediate postgadolinium T1-weighted SGE images (*b*). The duodenum (small arrows, *b*) is displaced laterally by the mass. The mass contains a cystic component (thin arrow, *b*). Heterogeneous enhancement of the mass is also present on the interstitial-phase gadolinium-enhanced T1-weighted fat-suppressed image (*c*).

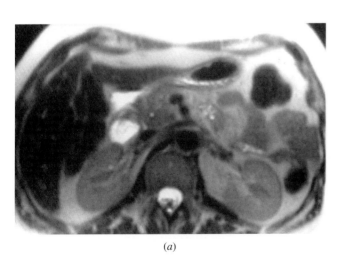

(a)

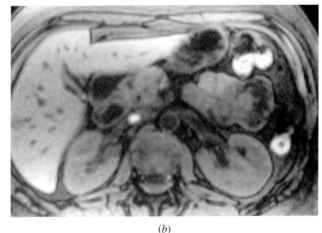

(b)

FIG. 4.84 Chemotherapy-induced pancreatitis. T2-weighted ETSE (*a*), T1-weighted fat-suppressed SGE (*b*), immediate post-gadolinium T1-weighted SGE (*c*), and 90-s postgadolinium fat-suppressed SGE (*d*) images.

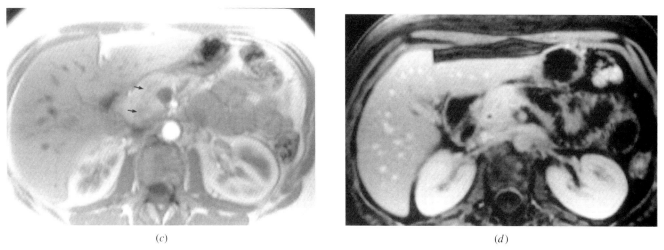

(c)   *(d)*

F I G . 4.84 *(Continued)* In this patient, undergoing chemotherapy for breast cancer, there is a heterogeneous low-signal region in the head of the pancreas on the noncontrast T1-weighted fat-suppressed image (*b*) that also shows heterogeneous decreased enhancement (arrows, *c*) on the immediate postgadolinium SGE image (*c*) consistent with pancreatitis secondary to chemotherapy toxicity.

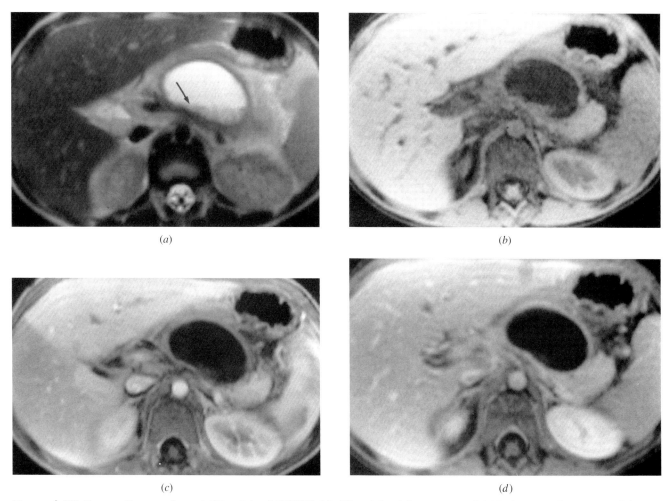

(a)   *(b)*

(c)   *(d)*

F I G . 4.85 Traumatic pseudocyst. T2-weighted SS-ETSE (*a*), T1-weighted fat-suppressed SGE (*b*), immediate postgadolinium T1-weighted SGE (*c*), and 90-s postgadolinium fat-suppressed SGE (*d*) images in a patient with a history of recent abdominal trauma.

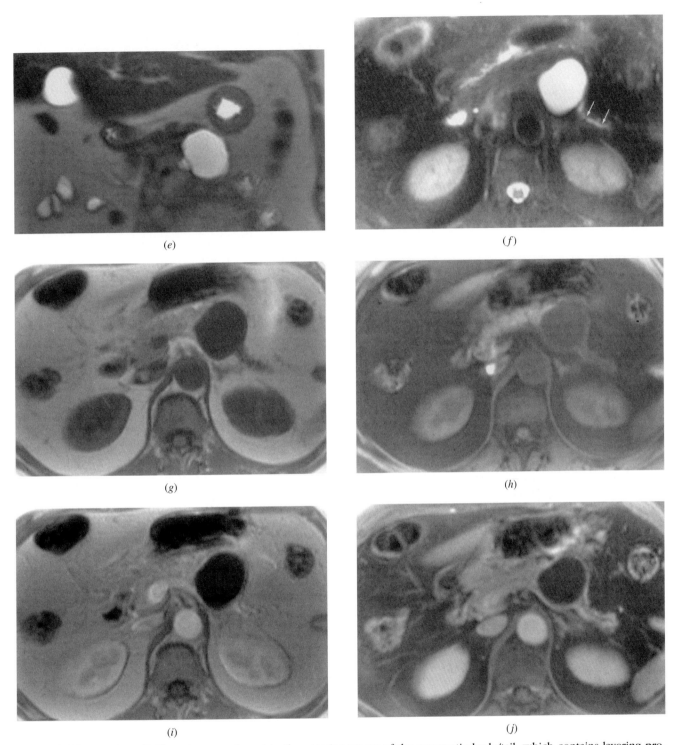

(e)

(f)

(g)

(h)

(i)

(j)

F I G . 4.85 (*Continued*) There is a pseudocyst in the anterior aspect of the pancreatic body/tail, which contains layering protein/hemoglobin in the dependent portion of the cyst, best appreciated on the T2-weighted image (arrow, *a*). Note transient increased enhancement of the left lobe of the liver on the immediate postgadolinium image (*c*), which reflects compromise of the left portal vein.

Coronal (*e*) and transverse (*f*) T2-weighted SS-ETSE, T1-weighted SGE (*g*), T1-weighted fat-suppressed SGE (*h*), immediate postgadolinium SGE (*i*), and 90-s postgadolinium SGE (*j*) images in a second patient. There is a 4-cm pseudocyst transversing the pancreas at the junction of the body and tail. The pancreas proximal to the traumatic pseudocyst appears normal. Distal to the pseudocyst, the tail shows ductal dilatation (arrows, *f*) and atrophy consistent with changes of long-term ductal obstruction and resultant chronic pancreatitis, in this patient with a remote history of abdominal trauma.

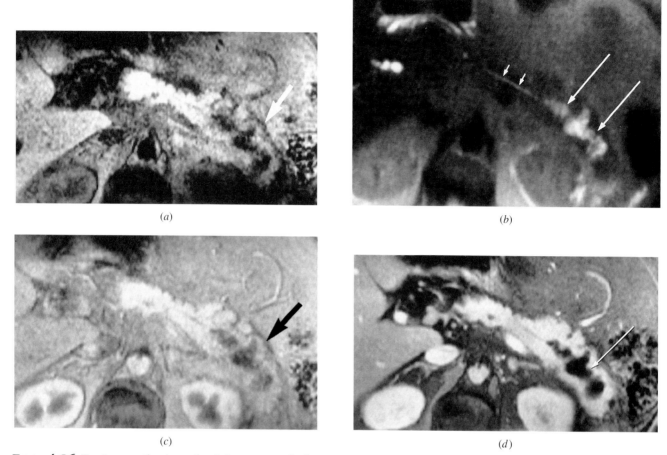

FIG. 4.86 Posttraumatic stenosis of the pancreatic duct. Fat-suppressed T1-weighted SGE (*a*), T2-weighted SS-ETSE (*b*), and immediate (*c*) and 90-s postgadolinium fat-suppressed T1 SGE (*d*) images in a patient who had undergone abdominal trauma 6 years earlier. A transition is noted in the body of the pancreas between normal-appearing proximal pancreas and abnormal-appearing distal pancreas containing an irregularly dilated pancreatic duct. On the precontrast, fat-suppressed image (*a*), the distal pancreas (arrow, *a*) is noted to be low in signal intensity, consistent with changes of chronic pancreatitis. On the SS-ETSE image (*b*) a transition is well shown between normal-caliber pancreatic duct (small arrows, *b*) and abnormally expanded distal pancreatic duct (long arrows, *b*). The distal pancreas is noted to enhance minimally on the immediate postgadolinium image (arrow, *c*). Enhancement of the pancreas is more uniform on the interstitial phase image (*d*), with clear definition of the irregularly dilated pancreatic duct (long arrow, *d*). (Courtesy of Susan M. Ascher, MD, Dept. of Radiology, Georgetown University Medical Center.)

laceration and transection. Stenosis of the pancreatic duct with distal ductal dilatation may be observed as a sequel of trauma. A combination of tissue imaging sequences and MR pancreatography can facilitate this diagnosis by the demonstration of ductal dilatation and changes of chronic pancreatitis of the pancreas distal to the stenosis (fig. 4.86).

PANCREATIC TRANSPLANTS

Dynamic gadolinium-enhanced MRI has been employed to assess rejection of pancreatic transplants [103–106]. In one study, enhancement in six normal grafts was $98 \pm 23\%$ within the first minute compared to $42 \pm 20\%$ in six dysfunctional grafts [98]. MR angiography also has

been employed to detect acute vascular compromise, with high sensitivity and specificity (fig. 4.87) [103]. Complications such as venous thrombosis are well shown on gadolinium-enhanced SGE or 3D gradient-echo imaging (fig. 4.88) [106].

FUTURE DIRECTIONS

The role of new contrast agents, such as manganese (Mn)-DPDP, to evaluate disease of the pancreas is currently under investigation. Normal pancreas enhances with Mn-DPDP, and most focal lesions do not. The degree of enhancement is less than with gadolinium, but the duration of enhancement is longer (fig. 4.89) [107]. New tissue-specific pancreatic agents are also under

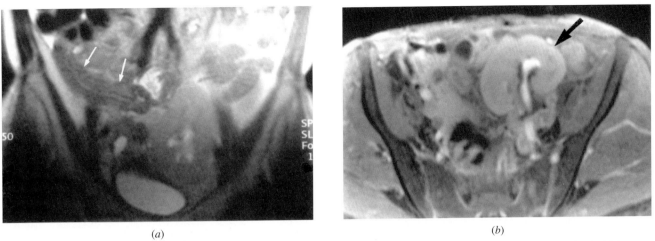

FIG. 4.87 Normal pancreatic transplant. Coronal T2-weighted ETSE (*a*) and 90-s postgadolinium fat-suppressed SGE (*b*) images in a patient status postpancreas and renal transplant. The transplanted pancreas is normal in signal intensity and is located in the right lower quadrant (arrows, *a*). The transplanted kidney is in the left lower quadrant (arrow, *b*).

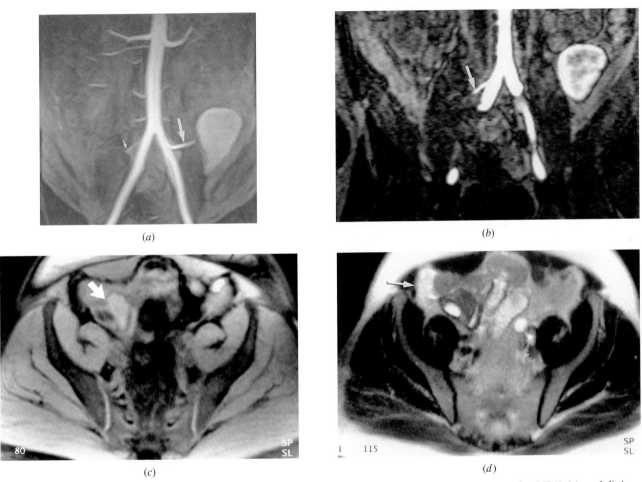

FIG. 4.88 Pancreatic transplant with arterial thrombosis. Coronal MIP reconstructed MR angiography (MRA) (*a*), gadolinium-enhanced 2-mm 3D gradient-echo source image (*b*), T1-weighted fat-suppressed SGE (*c*), and T2-weighted SS-ETSE (*d*) images. The MIP reconstructed MRA image demonstrates a normal artery (arrow, *a*) feeding the renal transplant in the left pelvis and an occluded artery (small arrow, *a*) feeding the pancreas transplant in the right pelvis. To establish the diagnosis of occlusion, examination of the source images is essential; occlusion is confirmed on the source image (arrow, *b*) as abrupt termination of the contrast-enhanced vascular lumen. The transplant is identified in the right side of the pelvis on T1-weighted (arrow, *c*) and T2-weighted (*d*) images. Inflammatory fluid (arrow, *d*) is noted adjacent to the pancreas transplant.

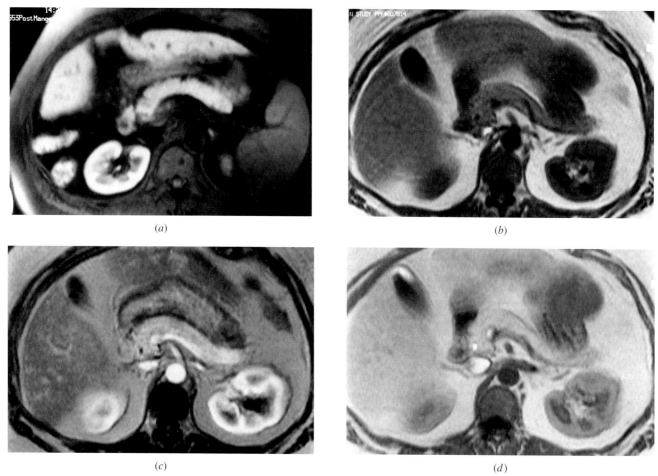

(a)

(b)

(c)

(d)

FIG. 4.89 Manganese (Mn)-DPDP-enhanced pancreas. Mn-DPDP-enhanced T1-weighted fat-suppressed SE image (*a*) demonstrates uniform enhancement of the pancreas. Intense renal cortical enhancement is also identified. T1-weighted SGE (*b*), immediate postgadolinium T1-weighted SGE (*c*), and Mn-DPDP-enhanced T1-weighted SGE (*d*) images in a second patient demonstrate that the pancreas enhances greater with gadolinium than with Mn-DPDP. The pancreas is higher in signal intensity relative to background fat on the gadolinium-enhanced image (*c*) and lower than background fat on the Mn-DPDP-enhanced image (*d*).

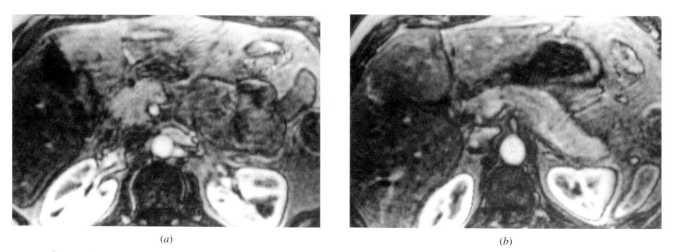

(a)

(b)

FIG. 4.90 Thin section 3D imaging of the pancreas. Transverse gadolinium-enhanced 2-mm 3D gradient-echo source images (*a, b*) and coronal 3D reconstructed MIP of these source images (*c*) of a normal pancreas.

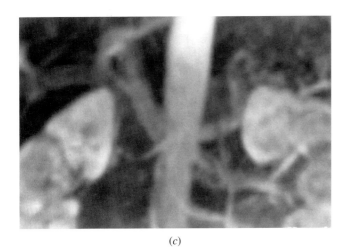

(c)

FIG. 4.90 (*Continued*) The 3D acquisition permits thin-section acquisition which can than be reconstructed into an MRA projection.

development [108]. Gradient-echo sequences that are 3D acquisition combined with gadolinium enhancement allow for thin-section data acquisition of the pancreas, with sections measuring 2 mm in thickness. This may improve detection of small tumors and may allow improved demonstration of vascular involvement by 3D reconstruction into an angiographic projection (fig. 4.90).

CONCLUSION

MRI is a valuable tool in the assessment of the full spectrum of pancreatic diseases. MRI techniques are sensitive for the evaluation of pancreatic disorders in the following settings: 1) T1-weighted fat-suppressed and dynamic gadolinium-enhanced SGE imaging for the detection of chronic pancreatitis, ductal adenocarcinoma, and islet cell tumors; 2) T2-weighted fat-suppressed imaging and T2-weighted breath-hold imaging for the detection of islet cell tumors; and 3) precontrast breath-hold SGE imaging for the detection of acute pancreatitis. Relatively specific morphologic and signal intensity features permit characterization of acute pancreatitis, chronic pancreatitis, ductal adenocarcinoma, insulinoma, gastrinoma, glucagonoma, microcystic cystadenoma, macrocystic cystadenoma, and solid and papillary epithelial neoplasm. MRI is effective as a problem-solving modality, because it is able to distinguish chronic pancreatitis from normal pancreas and chronic pancreatitis with focal enlargement from pancreatic cancer in the majority of cases.

MRI studies should be considered in the following settings: 1) patients with elevated serum creatinine, allergy to iodine contrast, or other contraindications for iodine contrast administration; 2) patients with prior CT imaging who have focal enlargement of the pancreas with no definable mass; 3) patients in whom clinical history is worrisome for malignancy and findings on CT imaging are equivocal or difficult to interpret; and 4) situations requiring distinction between chronic pancreatitis with focal enlargement and pancreatic cancer. Patients with biochemical evidence of islet cell tumors should be examined by MRI as the first-line imaging modality because of the high sensitivity of current MRI techniques for detecting the presence of islet cell tumors and determining the presence of metastatic disease.

REFERENCES

1. Semelka RC, Ascher SM: MRI of the pancreas—state of the art. *Radiology* 188: 593–602, 1993.
2. Winston CB, Mitchell DG, Outwater EK, Ehrlich SM: Pancreatic signal intensity on T1-weighted fat saturation MR images: Clinical correlation. *J Magn Reson Imaging* 5: 267–271, 1995.
3. Mitchell DG, Vinitski S, Saponaro S, Tasciyan T, Burk DL Jr, Rifkin MD: Liver and pancreas: Improved spin-echo T1 contrast by shorter echo time and fat suppression at 1.5 T. *Radiology* 178: 67–71, 1991.
4. Semelka RC, Kroeker MA, Shoenut JP, Kroeker R, Yaffe CS, Micflikier AB: Pancreatic disease: Prospective comparison of CT, ERCP, and 1.5 T MR imaging with dynamic gadolinium enhancement and fat suppression. *Radiology* 181: 785–791, 1991.
5. Takehara Y, Ichijo K, Tooyama N, et al.: Breath-hold MR cholangiopancreatography with a long-echo-time fast spin-echo sequence and a surface coil in chronic pancreatitis. *Radiology* 192: 73–78, 1994.
6. Bret PM, Reinhold C, Taourel P, Guibaud L, Atri M, Barkun AN: Pancreas divisum: Evaluation with MR cholangiopancreatography. *Radiology* 199: 99–103, 1996.
7. Soto JA, Barish MA, Yucel EK, et al.: Pancreatic duct: MR cholangiopancreatography with a three-dimensional fast spin-echo technique. *Radiology* 196: 459–464, 1995.
8. Semelka RC, Simm FC, Recht M, Deimling M, Lenz G, Laub GA: MRI of the pancreas at high field strength—a comparison of six sequences. *J Comput Assist Tomogr* 15(6): 966–971, 1991.
9. Mitchell DG, Winston CB, Outwater EK, Ehrlich SM: Delineation of pancreas with MR imaging: Multiobserver comparison of five pulse sequences. *J Magn Reson Imag* 5: 193–199, 1995.
10. Fulcher AS, Turner MA: MR pancreatography: A useful tool for evaluationg pancreatic disorders. *Radiographics* 19: 5–24, 1999.
11. Catalano C, Pavone P, Laghi A, Panebianco V, Scipioni A: Pancreatic adenocarcinoma: combination of MR imaging, MR

angiography and MR cholangiopancreatography for the diagnosis and assessment of respectability. *Eur Radiol* 8: 428–434, 1998.

12. Cruikshank AH, Benbow EW: *Pathology of the Pancreas* (2nd edition). London: Springer, p. 30, 1995.

13. Delhaye M, Engelholm, Cremer M: Pancreas divisum: Congenital anatomic variant or anomaly. Contribution of endoscopic retrograde dorsal pancreatography. *Gastroenterology* 89: 951–958, 1985.

14. Delhaye M, Cremer M: Clinical significance of pancreas divisum. *Acta Gastroenterol Bel* 55:306–313, 1992.

15. Rosai J: *Ackerman's Surgical Pathology* (8th edition). New York: Mosby, p. 1004, 1996.

16. Quest L, Lombard M: Pancreas divisum: opinio divisa. *Gut* 47: 317–319, 2000.

17. Deasi MB, Mitchell DG, Munoz SJ: Asymptomatic annular pancreas: Detection by magnetic resonance imaging. *Magn Reson Imaging* 12: 683–685, 1994.

18. Applegate KE, Goske MJ, Pierce G, Murphy D: Situs revisited: Imaging of the heterotaxy syndrome. *Radiographics* 19: 837–852, 1999.

19. Gayer G, Apter S, Jonas T, Amitai M, Zissin R, Sella T, Weiss P, Hetz M: Polysplenia syndrome detected in adulthood: Report of sight cases and review of the literature. *Abdom Imaging* 24: 178–184, 1999.

20. Tham RTOTA, Heyerman HGM, Falke THM, et al.: Cystic fibrosis: MR imaging of the pancreas. *Radiology* 179: 183–186, 1991.

21. Ferroi F, Bova D, Campodonico F, et al.: Cystic fibrosis: MR assessment of pancreatic damage. *Radiology* 198: 875–879, 1996.

22. King LF, Scurr ED, Murugan N: Hepatobiliary and pancreatic manifestation of cystic fibrosis: MR imaging appearances. *Radiographics* 20: 767–777, 2000.

23. Siegelman ES, Mitchell DG, Outwater E, Munoz SJ, Rubin R: Idiopathic hemochromatosis: MR imaging findings in cirrhotic and precirrhotic patients. *Radiology* 188: 637–641, 1993.

24. Siegelman ES, Mitchell DG, Semelka RC: Abdominal iron deposition: Metabolism, MR findings, and clinical importance. *Radiology* 199: 13–22, 1996.

25. Hough DM, Stephens DH, Johnson CD, Binkovitz LA: Pancreatic lesions in von Hippel-Lindau disease: Prevalence, clinical significance, and CT findings. *Am J Roentgenol* 162: 1091–1094, 1994.

26. Boring CC, Squires TS, Tong T: Cancer statistics, 1991. *CA Cancer J Clin* 41: 19–51, 1991.

27. Warshaw AL, Fernandez-del Castillo C: Pancreatic carcinoma. *N Engl J Med* 326: 455–465, 1992.

28. Moossa AR: Pancreatic cancer: Approach to diagnosis, selection for surgery and choice of operation. *Cancer* 50: 2689–2698, 1982.

29. Clark LR, Jaffe MH, Choyke PL, Grant EG, Zeman RK: Pancreatic imaging. *Radiol Clin N Am* 23: 489–501, 1985.

30. Rosai J: *Ackerman's Surgical Pathology* (8th edition). New York: Mosby, p. 976, 1966.

31. Baron RL, Stanley RJ, Lee JKT, Koehler RE, Levitt RG: Computed tomographic features of biliary obstruction. *Am J Roentgenol* 140: 1173–1178, 1983.

32. Wittenberg J, Simeone JF, Ferrucci JT Jr, Mueller PR, van Sonnenberg E, Neff CC: Non-focal enlargement in pancreatic carcinoma. *Radiology* 144: 131–135, 1982.

33. Megibow AJ, Bosniak MA, Ambos MA, Beranbaum ER: Thickening of the celiac axis and/or superior mesenteric artery: A sign of pancreatic carcinoma on computed tomography. *Radiology* 141: 449–453, 1981.

34. Gabata T, Matsui O, Kadoya M, et al.: Small pancreatic adenocarcinomas: Efficacy of MR imaging with fat suppression and gadolinium enhancement. *Radiology* 193: 683–688, 1994.

35. Semelka RC, Kelekis NL, Molina PL, Scharp T, Calvo B: Pancreatic masses with inconclusive findings on spiral CR. Is there a role for MRI? *J Magn Reson Imaging* 6: 585–588, 1996.

36. Steiner E, Stark DD, Hahn PF, et al.: Imaging of pancreatic neoplasms: Comparison of MR and CT. *Am J Roentgenol* 152: 487–491, 1989.

37. Sarles H, Sahel J: Pathology of chronic calcifying pancreatitis. *Am J Gastroenterol* 66: 117–139, 1976.

38. Vellet AD, Romano W, Bach DB, Passi RB, Taves DH, Munk PL: Adenocarcinoma of the pancreatic ducts: Comparative evaluation with CT and MR imaging at 1.5 T. *Radiology* 183: 87–95, 1992.

39. Pavone P, Occhiato R, Michelini O, et al.: Magnetic resonance imaging of pancreatic carcinoma. *Eur Radiol* 1: 124–130, 1991.

40. Patt R, Zeman RK, Nauta R, Ascher SM, Wooley P, Silverman P: Vascular encasement by pancreatobiliary neoplasms: Assessment with dynamic CT, spin-echo MR imaging, and gradient-echo MR imaging. *Radiology* 181(P): 259, 1991.

41. McFarland EG, Kaufman JA, Saini S, et al.: Preoperative staging of cancer of the pancreas: Value of MR angiography versus conventional angiography in detecting portal venous invasion. *Am J Roentgenol* 166: 37–43, 1996.

42. Low RN, Semelka RC, Worawattanakul S, Alzate GD: Extrahepatic abdominal imaging in patients with malignancy: comparison of MR imaging and helical CT in 164 patients. *J Magn Reson Imag* 12: 269–277, 2000.

43. Low RN, Semalka RC, Worawattanakul S, Alzate GD, Siget JS: Extrahepatic abdominal imaging in patients with malignancy: Comparison of MR imaging and helical CT, with subsequent surgical correlation. *Radiology.* 210: 625–632, 1999.

44. Nishiharu T, Yamashita Y, Abe Y, Mitsuzaki K, Tsuchigame T, Nakayama Y, Takahashi M: Local extension of pancreatic carcinoma: Assessment with thin-section helical CT versus with breath-hold fast MR imaging—ROC analysis. *Radiology* 212: 445–452, 1999.

45. Benassai G, Mastrorilli M, Quarto G, Cappiello A, Giani U, Forestieri P: Factors influencing survival after resection for ductal adenocarcinoma of the head of the pancreas. *J Surg Oncol* 73: 212–218, 2000.

46. Mozell E, Stenzel P, Woltering EA, Ro-sch J, O'Dorisio TM: Functional endocrine tumors of the pancreas: Clinical presentation, diagnosis, and treatment. *Curr Probl Surg* 27: 304–385, 1990.

47. Beger HG, Warshal AL: *The Pancreas* (1st edition). London: Blackwell Science, p. 1183, 1998.

48. Semelka RC, Custodio CM, Balci C, Woosley JT: Neuroendocrine tumors of the pancreas: Spectrum of appearances on MRI. *Magn Res Imaging* 11: 141–148, 2000.

49. Thompson NW, Eckhauser FE, Vinik AI, Lloyd RV, Fiddian-Green RD, Strodel WE: Cystic neuroendocrine neoplasms of the pancreas and liver. *Ann Surg* 199: 158–164, 1984.

50. Mitchell DG, Cruvella M, Eschelman DJ, Miettinen MM, Vernick JJ: MRI of pancreatic gastrinomas. *J Comput Assist Tomogr* 16: 583–585, 1992.

51. Kraus BB, Ros PR: Insulinoma: Diagnosis with fat-suppressed MR imaging. *Am J Roentgenol* 162: 69–70, 1994.

52. Semelka RC, Cummings M, Shoenut JP, Yaffe CS, Kroeker MA, Greenberg HM: Islet cell tumors: A comparison of detection by dynamic contrast-enhanced CT and MR imaging with dynamic gadolinium enhancement and fat suppression. *Radiology* 186: 799–802, 1993.

53. Kelekis NL, Semelka RC, Molina PL, Doerr ME: ACTH-secreting islet cell tumor: Appearances on dynamic gadolinium-enhanced MRI. *Magn Reson Imaging* 13: 641–644, 1995.

54. Buetow PC, Parrino TV, Buck JL, et al.: Islet cell tumors of the pancreas: Pathologic-imaging correlation among size, necrosis and

cysts, calcification, malignant behavior, and functional status. *Am J Roentgenol* 165: 1175–1179, 1995.

55. Smith TM, Semelka RC, Noone TC, Balci C, Woosley JT: Islet cell tumor of the pancreas associated with tumor thrombus in the portal vein. *Magn Reson Imaging* 17 (7): 1093–1096, 1999.

56. Pipeleers-Marichal M, Donow C Heitz PU, Kloppel G: Pathologic aspects pf gastrinomas in patients with Zollinger-Ellison syndrome with and without multiple endocrine neoplasia type I. *World J Surg;* 17: 481–488, 1993.

57. Wank SA, Doppman JL, Miller DL, et al.: Prospective study of the ability of computed axial tomography to localize gastrinomas in patients with Zollinger-Ellison syndrome. *Gastroenterology* 92: 905–912, 1987.

58. Frucht H, Doppman JL, Norten JA, et al.: Gastrinomas comparison of MR imaging with CT, angiography, and US. *Radiology* 171: 713–717, 1989.

59. Muller MF, Meyenberger C, Bertschinger P, Schaer R, Marincek B: Pancreatic tumors: Evaluation with endoscopic US, CT, and MR imaging. *Radiology* 190: 745–751, 1994.

60. Galiber AK, Reading CC, Charboneau JW, et al.: Localization of pancreatic insulinoma: Comparison of pre- and intraoperative US with CT and angiography. *Radiology* 166: 405–408, 1988.

61. Tjon A, Tham RTO, Jansen JBMJ, Falke THM, et al.: MR, CT, and ultrasound findings of metastatic vipoma in pancreas. *J Comput Assist Tomogr* 13(1): 142–144, 1989.

62. Carlson B, Johnson CD, Stephens DH, Ward EM, Kvois LK: MRI of pancreatic islet cell carcinoma. *J Comput Assist Tomogr* 17: 735–740, 1993.

63. Tjon A, Tham RTO, Jansen JBMJ, Falke THM, Lamers CBMW: Imaging features of somatostatinoma: MR, CT, US, and angiography. *J Comp Assist Tomogr* 18: 427–431, 1994.

64. Doppman JL, Nieman LK, Cutler GB Jr, et al.: Adrenocorticotripic hormone-secreting islet cell tumors: Are they always malignant? *Radiology* 190: 59–64, 1994.

65. Ros PR, Hamrick-Turner JE, Chiechi MV, Ross LH., Gallego P, Burton SS: Cystic masses of the pancreas. *Radiographics* 12: 673–686, 1992.

66. Lewandrowski K, Warshaw A, Compton C: Macrocystic serous cystadenoma of the pancreas: A morphologic variant differing from microcystic adenoma. *Hum Pathol* 23: 871–875, 1992.

67. Lewandrowski K, Warshaw A, Compton C: Macrocystic serous cystadenoma of the pancreas: a morphologic variant differing from microcystic adenoma. *Hum Pathol* 23: 871–875, 1992.

68. Buetow PC, Rao P, Thompson LDR: From the archives of the AFIP. Mucinous cystic neoplasm of the pancreas: Radiologic-pathologic correlation. *Radiographics* 18: 433–449, 1998.

69. Minami M, Itai Y, Ohtomo K, Yoshida H, Yoshikawa K, Iio M: Cystic neoplasms of the pancreas: Comparison of MR imaging with CT. *Radiology* 171: 53–56, 1989.

70. Friedman AC, Liechtenstein JE, Dachman AH: Cystic neoplasms of the pancreas: Radiological-pathological correlation. *Radiology* 149: 45–50, 1983.

71. Compagno J, Oertel JE: Mucinous cystic neoplasms of the pancreas with overt and latent malignancy (cystadenocarcinoma and cystadenoma): A clinicopathologic study of 41 cases. *Am J Clin Pathol* 69: 573–580, 1978.

72. Silas AM, Morrin MM, Raptopoulos V, Krogan MT: Intradictal papillary mucinous tumor of the pancreas. *Am J Roentgenol* Jan, 176 (1): 179–185, 2001.

73. Traverso LM, Peralta EA, Ryan JA, Kozarek RA: Intraductal neoplasm of the pancreas. *Am J Surg* 175: 426–432, 1998.

74. Procacci C, Megibow AJ, Carbognin G, Guarise A, Spoto E: Intraductal papillary mucinous tumor of the pancreas: a pictorial essay. *Radiographics* 19: 1447–1463, 1999.

75. Koito K, Namieno T, Ichimura T, Yama N, Hareyama M: Mucin-producing pancreatic tumors: comparison of MR cholangiopancreatography with endoscopy retrograde cholangiopancreatography. *Radiology.* 208: 231–237, 1998.

76. Onaya H, Itai Y, Niitsu M, Chiba Y, Michishita N, Saida Y: Ductectatic mucinous cyst neoplasm of pancreas: evaluation with MR cholangiopancreatography. *Am J Roentgenol* 171: 171–177, 1998.

77. Irie H, Honda H, Aibe H, Kuroiwa T, Yoshimizu K: MR cholangiopancreatography differentiation of benign and malignant intraductal mucin-producing tumors of the pancreas. *Am J Roentgenol* 174: 1403–1408, 2000.

78. Ohtomo K, Furai S, Oneone M, Okada Y, Kusano S, Uchiyama G: Solid and papillary epithelial neoplasm of the pancreas: MR imaging and pathologic correlation. *Radiology* 184: 567–570, 1992.

79. Buetow PC, Buck JL: Solid and papillary epithelial neoplasm of the pancreas: imaging-pathologic correlation in 56 cases. *Radiology* 199: 707–771, 1996.

80. Zeman RK, Schiebler M, Clark LR, et al.: The clinical and imaging spectrum of pancreaticoduodenal lymph node enlargement. *Am J Roentgenol* 144: 1223–1227, 1985.

81. Kelekis NL, Semelka RC, Siegelman ES: MRI of pancreatic metastases from renal cancer. *J Comput Assist Tomogr* 20: 249–253, 1996.

82. Steinberg W, Tenner S: Acute pancreatitis. *N Engl J Med* 330: 1198–1210, 1994.

83. Kattwinkel J, Lapey A, DiSant'Agnese PA, Edwards WA, Jufty MP: Hereditary pancreatitis: Three new kindreds and a critical review of the literature. *Pediatrics* 51: 5–69, 1973.

84. Lee SP, Nicholls JF, Park HZ: Biliary sludge as a cause of acute pancreatitis. *N Engl J Med* 326: 589–593, 1992.

85. Shearman DJ, Finlayson N: *Diseases of the Gastrointestinal Tract and Liver.* New York: Churchill Livingstone, p. 1253, 1997.

86. Balthazar E: CT diagnosis and staging of acute pancreatitis. *Radiol Clin N Am* 27: 19–37, 1989.

87. Balthazar EJ, Robinson DL, Megibow AJ, Ranson JHC: Acute pancreatitis: Value of CT in establishing prognosis. *Radiology* 174: 331–336, 1990.

88. Johnson CD, Stephens DH, Sarr MG: CT of acute pancreatitis: Correlation between lack of contrast enhancement and pancreatic necrosis. *Am J Roentgenol* 156: 93–95, 1991.

89. Saifuddin A, Ward J, Ridgway J, Chalriners AG: Comparison of MR and CT scanning in severe acute pancreatitis: initial experiences. *Clin Radiol* 48: 111–116, 1993.

90. Morgan DE, Baron TH, Smith JK, Robbin ML, Kenney PJ: Pancreatic fluid collections prior to intervention: evaluation with MR imaging compared with CT and US. *Radiology* 203: 773–778, 1997.

91. Bank S: Chronic pancreatitis: clinical features and medical management. *Am J Gastroenterol* 81: 153–167, 1986.

92. Steer ML, Waxman I, Freedman S: Chronic pancreatitis. *N Engl J Med* 332: 1482–1490, 1995.

93. Lowenfels AB, Maisonneuve P, Cavallini G, et al.: Pancreatitis and the risk of pancreatic cancer. *N Engl J Med* 328: 1433–1437, 1993.

94. Luetmer PH, Stephens DH, Ward EM: Chronic pancreatitis reassessment with current CT. *Radiology* 171: 353–357, 1989.

95. Aranha GV, Prinz RA, Freeark RJ, Greenlee HB: The spectrum of biliary tract obstruction from chronic pancreatitis. *Arch Surg* 119: 595–600, 1984.

96. Lammer J, Herlinger H, Zalaudek G, Hofler H: Pseudotumorous pancreatitis. *Gastrointest Radiol* 10: 59–67, 1985.

97. Sostre CF, Flournoy JG, Bova JG, Goldstein HM, Schenker S: Pancreatic phlegmon: Clinical features and course. *Dig Dis Sci* 30: 918–927, 1985.

98. Semelka RC, Shoenut JP, Kroeker MA, Micflikier AB: Chronic pancreatitis: MR imaging features before and after administration of

gadopentetate dimeglumine. *J Magn Reson Imaging* 3: 79–82, 1993.

99. Irie H, Honda H, Baba S, Kuroiwa T, Yoshimitsu K: Autoimmune pancreatitis: CT and MR characteristics. *Am J Roentgenol* 170: 1323–1327, 1998.

100. Van Hoe L, Gryspeerdt S, Ectors N, Steenbergen WV: Nonalcoholic duct-destructive chronic pancreatitis: imaging findings. *Am J Roentgenol* 170: 643–647, 1998.

101. Ectors N, Maillet B, Aerts R, Geboes K, Donner A: Non-alcoholic duct destructive chronic pancreatitis. *Gut* 41: 263–268, 1997.

102. Ito T, Nakano I, Koyanagi S, Miyahara T, Migita Y, Ogoshi K: Autoimmune pancreatitis as a new clinical entity. Three cases of autoimmune pancreatitis with effective steroids therapy. *Dig Dis Sci* 42(7): 1458–1468, 1997.

103. del Pilar Fernandez M, Bernardino ME, Neylan JF, Olson RA: Diagnosis of pancreatic transplant dysfunction: Value of gadopentatate dimeglumine-enhanced MR imaging. *Am J Roentgenol* 156: 1171–1176, 1991.

104. Krebs TL, Daly B, Wong JJ, Chow CC, Bartlett ST: Vascular complications of pancreatic transplantation: MR evaluation. *Radiology* 196: 793–798, 1995.

105. Krebs TL, Daly B, Cheong JJWY, Carroll K, Barlett ST: Acute pancreatic transplant rejection: evaluation with dynamic contrast-enhanced MR imaging compared with histopathologic analysis. *Radiology* 210: 437–442, 1999.

106. Eubank WB, Schmiedl UP, Levy AE, Marsh CL: Venous thrombosis and occlusion after pancreas transplantation: evaluation with breath-hold gadolinium-enhanced three-dimensional MR imaging. *Am J Roentgenol* 175: 381–385, 2000.

107. Kettritz U, Warshauer DM, Brown ED, Schlund JF, Eisenberg LB, Semelka RC: Enhancement of the normal pancreas: Comparison of manganese-DPDP and gadolinium chelate. *Eur Radiol* 6: 14–18, 1996.

108. Reiner P, Weissleder R, Shen T, Knoefel WT, Brady TJ: Pancreatic receptors: Initial feasibility studies with a targeted contrast agent for MR imaging. *Radiology* 193: 527–531, 1994.

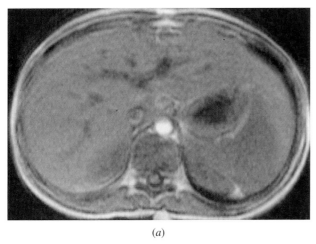

(a)

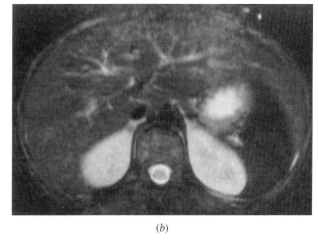

(b)

F I G . 5.2 Iron deposition in the spleen. T1-weighted SGE (a) and T2-weighted fat-suppressed spin-echo (b) images. Signal intensity of the spleen is only slightly lower than normal on the T1-weighted image (a), which is consistent with mild iron deposition in the RES. Signal intensity of the spleen is noted to be nearly signal void on the T2-weighted image (b), with low signal intensity also noted of liver and bone marrow due to iron deposition in the RES in these organs.

termed arciform. This pattern has been observed in all normal spleens in nondiseased patients and in some spleens of patients with inflammatory or neoplastic disease (fig. 5.3). The second most common pattern (16% of patients) is homogeneous high signal intensity enhancement (fig. 5.4). This has been observed in patients with inflammatory or neoplastic diseases, hepatic focal fatty infiltration, or hepatic enzyme abnormalities. A nonspecific immune response may be responsible for this pattern of enhancement. This appearance may represent the conversion of a mixture of slow and fast channels to only fast channels, reflecting a mechanism to increase transit of immune system cells. The third pattern is uniform low signal intensity (5% of patients) (fig. 5.5) this was found in all patients who had undergone multiple recent blood transfusions. The T2-shortening effects from

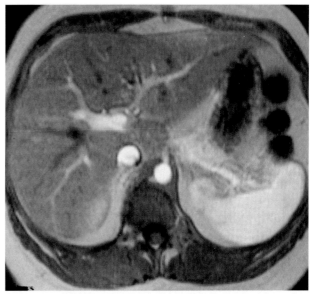

F I G . 5.4 Homogeneous intense splenic enhancement. The spleen is noted to enhance intensely and uniformly in the capillary phase of enhancement. Contrast in hepatic arteries and portal veins and no contrast in hepatic veins demonstrate that the image was acquired in the capillary phase of enhancement.

hemosiderin deposition in the RES supersede the T1-shortening effects of gadolinium [5–6].

Superparamagnetic iron oxide particles are selectively taken up by the RES and have been used to evaluate the spleen. These particles diminish the signal intensity of the normal spleen on T2-weighted sequences, whereas tumors remain unchanged in signal characteristics [7–9]. Superparamagnetic iron oxide crystals embedded in a starch matrix [magnetic starch microspheres (MSM); Nycomed Imaging, Oslo, Norway] have been studied in animal models and have been shown to increase conspicuity of both focal and diffuse splenic lesions [9]. Normal spleen diminishes in

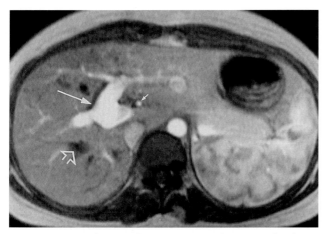

F I G . 5.3 Arciform enhancement in the normal spleen. Note the serpiginous, tubular bands of low signal intensity throughout the splenic parenchyma. Contrast identified in portal vein (long arrow), hepatic arteries (short arrow), and lack of contrast in hepatic veins (hollow arrow) defines the capillary or hepatic arterial dominant phase of enhancement.

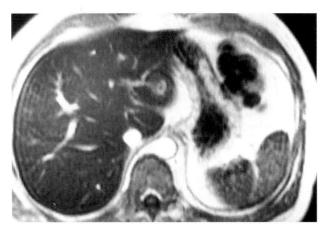

FIG. 5.5 Homogeneous low-signal intensity splenic enhancement. The spleen is low in signal intensity on immediate postgadolinium images because of the predominant T2-shortening effects of iron in the spleen.

signal on T2-weighted or T2*-weighted images, whereas focal or diffuse disease retains signal, which renders disease conspicuous by being relatively high in signal intensity.

In the neonate and until the infant is approximately 8 months old, the spleen signal intensity is isointense to the liver on T1-weighted images and varies from iso- to hypointense relative to the liver on T2-weighted images (fig. 5.6). As the reticuloendothelial system matures, the spleen displays a hypointense signal relative to the liver on T1-weighted images, with a gradual increase in the spleen signal relative to the liver on T2-weighted images, approaching the normal appearance of the adult spleen [10].

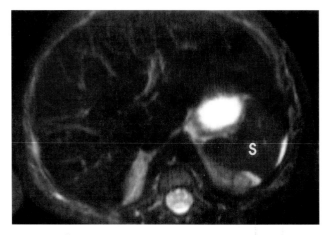

FIG. 5.6 Normal spleen in a 1-month-old patient. T2-weighted fat-suppressed spin-echo image. Normal spleen (S) is low signal intensity, comparable to liver on T2-weighted image.

Normal Variants and Congenital Disease

Accessory spleens
Accessory spleens, or "spleniculi," are common and may occur in up to 40% of individuals [12,13]. They are clinically important insofar as they must be differentiated from other mass lesions. In patients with hypersplenism, identification of accessory spleens is critical before splenectomy to avoid accessory spleen hypertrophy and recurrence [12,13]. Accessory spleens parallel the signal intensity of the spleen on all MRI sequences, including their enhancement on immediate postgadolinium images (fig. 5.7). Spleniculi may also be confidently characterized in the patient who has undergone repeated blood transfusions because they will be nearly signal void on T2- or T2*-weighted sequences because of iron deposition within the RES of the splenules. This effect also may be achieved with the use of iron oxide particles [14].

Asplenia
Asplenia syndrome, right isomerism, or Ivemark syndrome is a congenital syndrome characterized by absence of the spleen associated with thoracoabdominal abnormalities (fig. 5.8). The majority of patients die in infancy with few surviving longer than 1 year. The mortality in the first year of life approaches 80% because of complex and severe cardiovascular anomalies and a compromised immune system. In cardiac MRI studies in which cardiovascular anomalies raise the possibility of asplenia, a limited abdominal MRI should be performed at the same time to evaluate abdominal situs inversus and associated abnormalities, abdominal vessels, and the presence of the spleen, because asplenic patients are at risk of sepsis [15].

Polysplenia
Polysplenia syndrome is a congenital syndrome characterized by multiple small splenic masses and left isomerism. The splenic masses vary from 2 to 16 in number and are distributed along the greater curvature of the stomach (fig 5.9). Other associated abnormalities include cardiopulmonary anomalies, malrotation of the intestinal tract, absence of the hepatic segment of the inferior vena cava with azygous or hemiazygous continuation, and a short pancreas. Polysplenia has also been associated with polycystic kidney disease. In comparison with asplenia, polysplenia has a lower mortality, and serious cardiac malformations are less common. MRI can demonstrate the situs inversus, abdominal vessels, and the number of spleens together with such complications as splenic hemorrhages or infarcts [15].

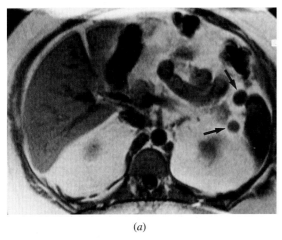

(a)

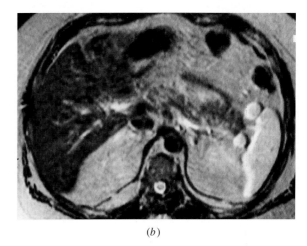

(b)

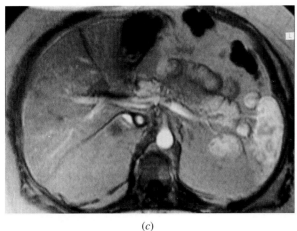

(c)

Fig. 5.7 Splenules. T1-weighted SGE (a), T2-weighted spin echo (b), and immediate postgadolinium SGE (c) images. Two splenules are identified (arrows, a) that parallel the signal intensity of the spleen. They are low in signal intensity on T1-weighted images (a) and high in signal intensity on T2-weighted images (b) and enhance intensely on immediate postgadolinium image (c). The splenules show heterogeneous enhancement on immediate postcontrast images, which suggests that they have architecture similar to that of the spleen.

Gaucher Disease

Gaucher disease is a multisystem hereditary disease caused by deficient glucocerebrosidase activity. Glucocerebroside, a glycolipid, accumulates in the mononuclear phagocytic cells of organs [16]. The abdominal manifestations of Gaucher disease in a population of 46 patients have been described using conventional spin-echo technique [16]. All patients had hepatosplenomegaly. Splenic nodules of variable signal intensity were present in 14 patients (30%). Fifteen patients

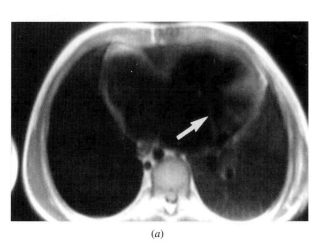

(a)

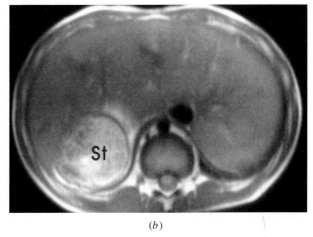

(b)

Fig. 5.8 Asplenia. T2 black blood single-shot echo-train spin-echo images (a, b) at the level of the heart (a) and liver (b) and coronal source MRA (c) images.

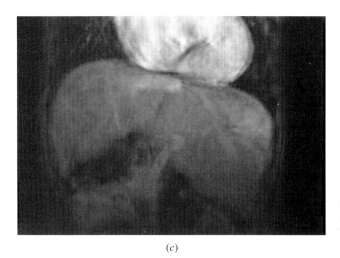

(c)

F I G. 5.8 (*Continued*) Eight-month-old patient with endocardial cushion defect, common AV valve (arrow, *a*), and situs inversus, with the stomach (St, *b*) on the right side. No spleen is present.

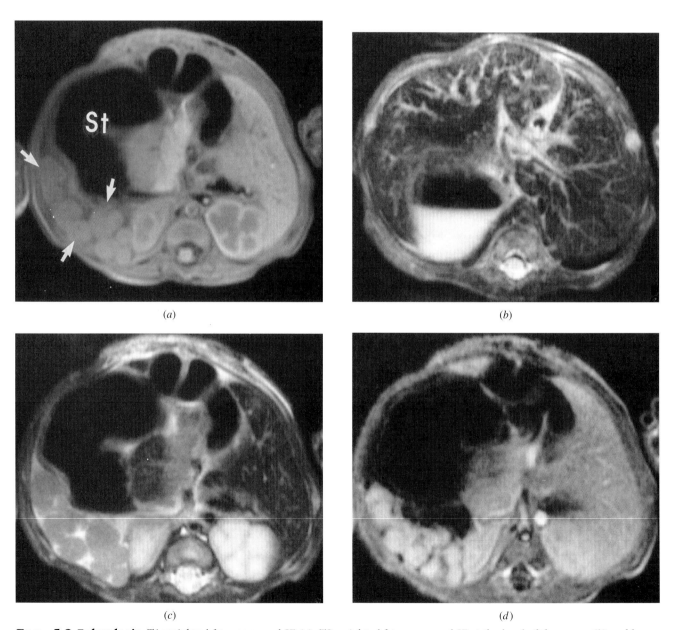

(a)

(b)

(c)

(d)

F I G. 5.9 Polysplenia. T1-weighted fat-suppressed SE (*a*), T2-weighted fat-suppressed SE at the level of the upper (*b*) and lower (*c*) liver, immediate postgadolinium T1-weighted snap-shot gradient-echo (*d*) and 2-min postgadolinium T1-weighted fat-suppressed spin-echo (*e*) images. Situs inversus is present in this 3-month-old patient (*a, b*), with the liver in the left upper abdomen and stomach (St, *a*) in the right upper abdomen.

496

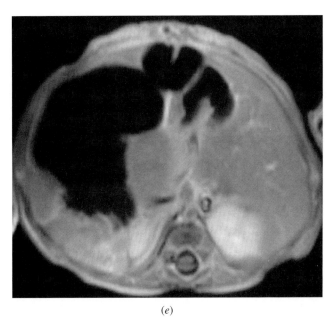

(e)

FIG. 5.9 (*Continued*) Multiple small spleens are noted along the greater curvature of the stomach (arrows, *a*), which are moderately low signal on T1 (*a*) and moderately high signal on T2 (*c*) and demonstrate early intense enhancement (*d*) with fading on delayed postgadolinium images (*e*), consistent with the MR imaging appearance of multiple spleens.

(33%) had splenic infarcts with or without associated subcapsular fluid collections, and four patients (9%) had both infarcts and nodules. Focal areas of abnormal signal intensity were noted in the livers of nine patients (20%).

Sickle Cell Disease

The manifestations of sickle cell anemia vary and depend on whether the patient is homozygous or heterozygous for the hemoglobinopathy. In patients with homozygous disease, the spleen is nearly signal void because of the sequela of iron deposition from blood transfusions coupled with microscopic perivascular and parenchymal calcifications [17]. This decrease in signal intensity was found to be diffuse in most patients with signal-void foci due to calcifications and/or foci of greater iron deposition (fig. 5.10*a*). Hyperintense focal lesions on proton density images may occur and are believed to represent infarcts (fig. 5.10*b–d*).

MASS LESIONS

The appearance of common splenic lesions on T1-weighted, T2-weighted, and early and late postgadolinium images is presented in Table 5.1.

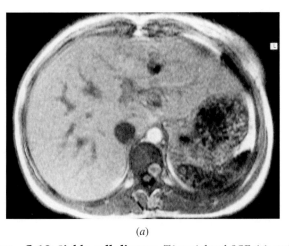

(a)

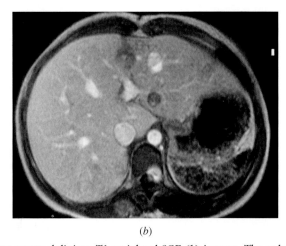

(b)

FIG. 5.10 Sickle-cell disease. T1 weighted SGE (*a*) and immediate postgadolinium T1 weighted SGE (*b*) images. The spleen is noted to be small and low in signal intensity on all MR images (*a, b*). On the precontrast T1-weighted SGE image (*a*), multiple 1-cm signal-void foci are noted in the small low-signal intensity spleen. These foci are better demarcated after contrast administration (*b*) because of enhancement, although minimal, of surrounding splenic parenchyma.

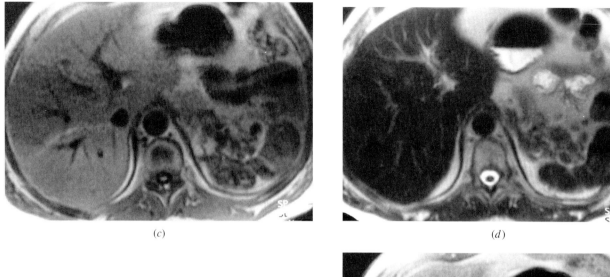

(c)   (d)

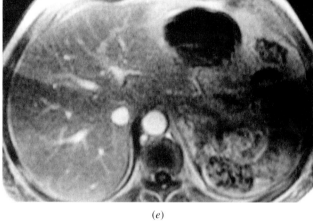

FIG. 5.10 (*Continued*) T1-weighted SGE (*c*), T2-weighted echo-train spin echo (*d*), and immediate postgadolinium T1-weighted SGE (*e*) images in a second patient. The spleen is small and irregular with extensive low-signal iron deposition, regions of scarring, and infarction.

(e)

Table 5.1 Pattern Recognition: Most Common Splenic Lesions

	T1	T2	Early Gd	Late Gd	Other Features
Cyst	↓–Ø	↑↑	None	None	Well defined
Hamartoma	Ø	Ø–↑	Heterogeneous intense	Homogeneous isointense	Usually >4 cm and arise from the medial surface of the midspleen
Hemangioma	↓–Ø	↑	Peripheral nodules or homogeneous	Centripetal enhancement; retain contrast	Usually <2 cm. Lesion more commonly enhances homogeneously on immediate post-Gd images compared with liver hemangiomas, reflecting their small size. Peripheral nodules are not as clearly defined as liver hemangiomas
Metastases	↓–Ø	Ø–↑	Focal lesions with minimal enhancement	Isointense	Metastases commonly become isointense by 1 min post-Gd.
Lymphoma— Focal	↓–Ø	↓–↑	Focal lesions with minimal enhancement	Isointense	Other sites of nodal disease. Lymphomatous lesions commonly become isointense by 1 min post-Gd.
Lymphoma— Diffuse	↓–Ø	↓–↑	Irregular regions with minimal enhancement	Isointense	Other sites of nodal disease. Lymphomatous lesions commonly become isointense by 1 min post-Gd.

Keys: ↓↓: moderately to markedly decreased; ↓: mildly decreased; Ø: isointense; ↑: mildly increased; ↑↑: moderately to markedly increased.

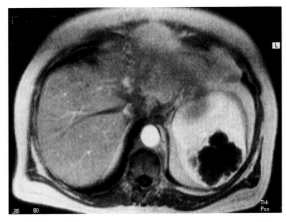

FIG. 5.11 Epidermoid cyst. Immediate postgadolinium T1-weighted SGE image demonstrates a signal-void cystic lesion with peripheral septations.

Benign Masses

Cysts

Cysts are the most common of the benign splenic lesions. Three types of nonneoplastic cysts exist: posttraumatic or pseudocyst, epidermoid cysts, and hydatid cysts [18]. Most splenic cysts are posttraumatic in origin. They are not lined by epithelium and thus are pseudocysts. Epidermoid cysts are true cysts discovered in childhood or early adulthood that may have trabeculations or septations in their walls with occasional peripheral calcification [18,19] (fig. 5.11). Hydatids, or echinococcal cysts, are rare. They are characterized by extensive wall calcification. The MRI features of cysts include sharp lesion margination, low signal intensity on T1-weighted images, and very high signal intensity on T2-weighted images. Cysts complicated by proteinaceous fluid or hemorrhage may have regions of high signal intensity on T1-weighted images, regions of mixed signal intensity on T2-weighted images, or both. Cysts do not enhance on postgadolinium images. Pseudocysts may be complicated by hemorrhage particularly early in their evolution and thus may contain foci of high signal intensity on precontrast T1-weighted images (fig. 5.12).

Hemangiomas

Hemangiomas are the most common of the benign splenic neoplasms [20, 21]. Lesions may be single or multiple. Splenic hemangiomas are mildly low to isointense on T1-weighted images and mildly to moderately hyperintense on T2-weighted images, similar to hepatic hemangiomas. Hemangiomas are minimally hypointense to isointense with background spleen on T1-weighted images because of the relatively low signal intensity of spleen on these images and minimally hyperintense relative to spleen on T2-weighted images because of the moderately high signal intensity of spleen on T2-weighted images. Three patterns of contrast enhancement are observed: 1) immediate homogeneous enhancement with persistent enhancement on delayed images, 2) peripheral enhancement with progression to uniform enhancement on delayed images (fig. 5.13), and 3) peripheral enhancement with centripetal progression but persistent lack of enhancement of central scar. These patterns are similar to those observed for hepatic hemangiomas. However, unlike hepatic hemangiomas, splenic hemangiomas generally do not demonstrate well-defined nodules on early postgadolinium images. This may, in part, reflect the blood supply from

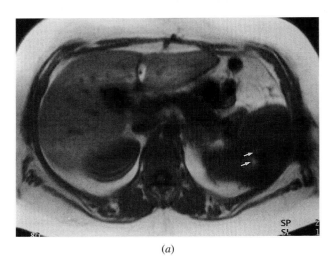

(a)

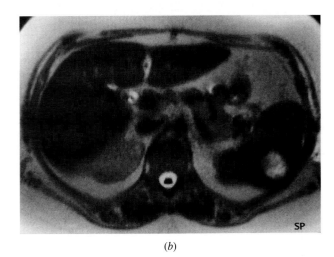

(b)

FIG. 5.12 Pseudocyst. T1-weighted SGE (*a*), T2-weighted single-shot echo-train spin-echo (*b*), and 90-s gadolinium-enhanced fat-suppressed SGE (*c*) images. High-signal intensity foci are identified in the cyst on the precontrast SGE image (arrows, *a*), a finding consistent with hemorrhage. Slight heterogeneity of the cyst on the T2-weighted image (*b*) also reflects the presence of blood degradation products. The cyst is sharply demarcated after gadolinium administration (*c*). The foci of blood remain high in signal intensity on postgadolinium images.

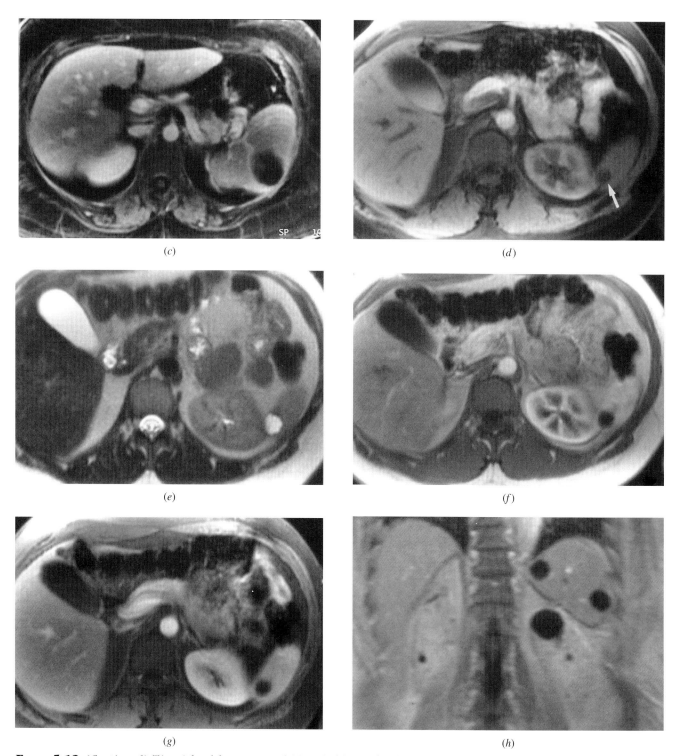

(c)

(d)

(e)

(f)

(g)

(h)

FIG. 5.12 (*Continued*) T1-weighted fat-suppressed SGE (*d*), T2-weighted single-shot echo-train spin-echo (*e*), immediate post-gadolinium T1-weighted SGE (*f*), and 90-s gadolinium-enhanced T1-weighted fat-suppressed SGE (*g*) images in a second patient. The pseudocyst is low signal on T1 (arrow, *d*), high signal on T2 (*e*), and does not enhance on early (*f*) or late (*g*) postgadolinium images.

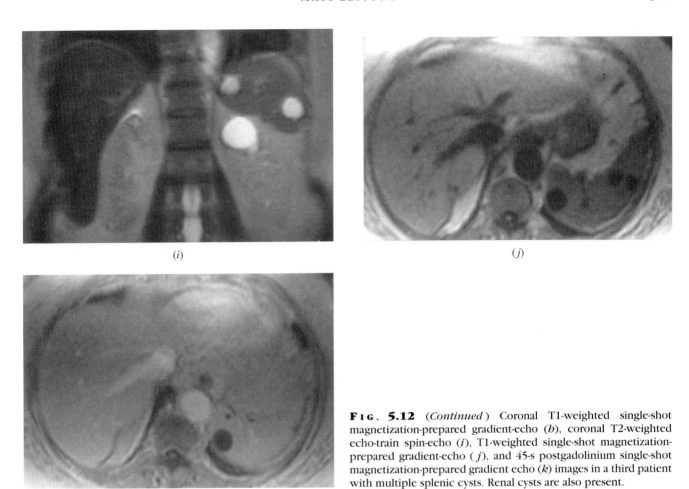

(i)

(j)

(k)

FIG. 5.12 (*Continued*) Coronal T1-weighted single-shot magnetization-prepared gradient-echo (*h*), coronal T2-weighted echo-train spin-echo (*i*), T1-weighted single-shot magnetization-prepared gradient-echo (*j*), and 45-s postgadolinium single-shot magnetization-prepared gradient echo (*k*) images in a third patient with multiple splenic cysts. Renal cysts are also present.

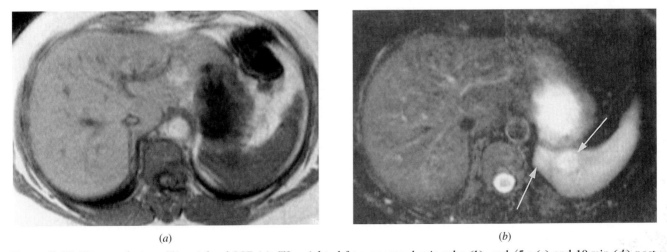

(a)

(b)

FIG. 5.13 Hemangiomas. T1-weighted SGE (*a*), T2-weighted fat-suppressed spin-echo (*b*), and 45-s (*c*) and 10-min (*d*) postgadolinium SGE images. Two small, <1.5 cm, hemangiomas are present that are minimally hypointense on T1-weighted images (*a*) and moderately hyperintense on T2-weighted images (arrows, *b*). Peripheral nodules are present on early postgadolinium images (*c*), and enhancement progresses to uniform high signal intensity by 10 min (*d*).

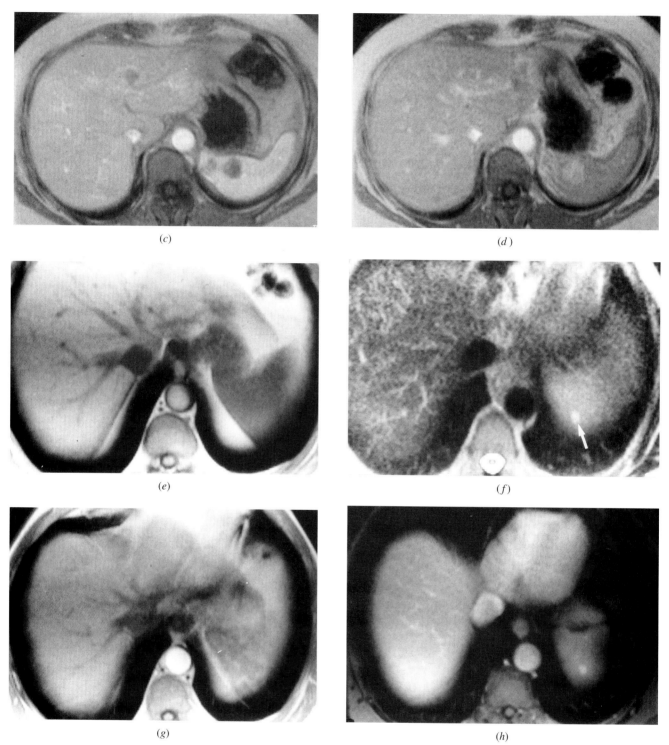

(c)

(d)

(e)

(f)

(g)

(h)

FIG. 5.13 (*Continued*) T1-weighted SGE (*e*), T2 fat-suppressed spin-echo (*f*), immediate postgadolinium T1 SGE (*g*), and 90-s postgadolinium T1-fat-suppressed SGE (*h*) images in a second patient. The small hemangioma in the superior aspect of the spleen is isointense on T1, moderately hyperintense on T2 (arrow, *f*) and shows early uniform enhancement (*g*) that persists on the late postgadolinium image (*h*). The hemangioma is better demonstrated on the later postgadolinium image as background splenic enhancement has diminished and is uniform. Early uniform enhancement is common in <1.5-cm hemangiomas.

T1-weighted SGE (*i*), T2-weighted fat-suppressed spin echo (*j*), immediate postgadolinium T1-weighted SGE (*k*), and 90-s postgadolinium T1-weighted fat-suppressed SGE (*l*) images in a third patient.

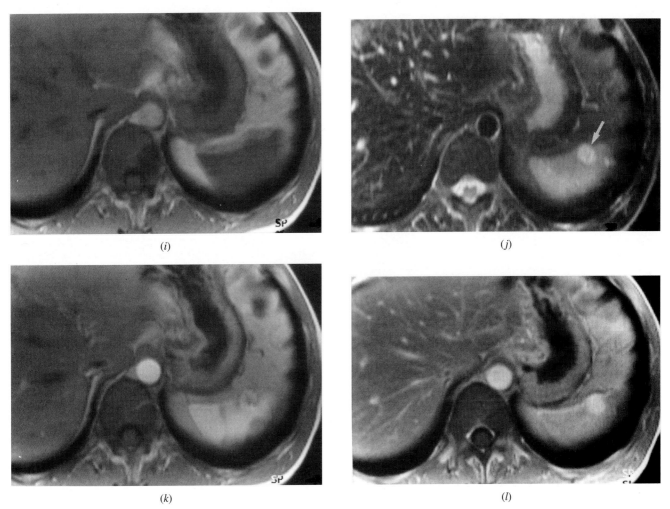

(i) (j)

(k) (l)

F I G . 5.13 (*Continued*) The lesion is isointense on T1 (*i*) and moderately hyperintense on the T2-weighted image (arrow, *j*). Note centripetal (*k, l*) progressive enhancement of the hemangioma resembling the pattern of a hepatic hemangioma.

the background organ. Uniform high signal on immediate postgadolinium SGE images is a common appearance for small (<1.5 cm) hemangiomas, as it is with hepatic hemangiomas. Rarely, hemangiomas with a very large central scar can appear hypointense on T2-weighted images, reflecting the lower fluid content of the central scar (fig. 5.14). These may be termed sclerosing hemangiomas.

Hamartomas

Hamartomas are rare and composed of structurally disorganized mature splenic red pulp elements. The lesions tend to be single, spherical, and predominantly solid. They are most likely to occur in the midportion of the spleen, arising from the anterior or posterior aspect of the medial surface. These tumors are mildly low to isointense on T1-weighted images and moderately high in signal intensity on T2-weighted images [21–23]. They frequently are moderately heterogeneous in part because of the presence of cystic spaces of varying size. If the

composition of fibrous tissue is substantial, hamartomas may have regions of low signal intensity on T2-weighted images [23]. They enhance on immediate postgadolinium SGE images in an intense diffuse heterogeneous fashion [21, 23] (fig. 5.15). Diffuse enhancement on immediate postgadolinium images is generally observed in tumors that are native to the organ in which they occur. Lesion size and enhancement pattern may mimic a more aggressive lesion. Lesions may also resemble normal splenic parenchyma (fig. 5.15). Enhancement becomes homogeneous on more delayed images with signal intensity slightly greater than in background spleen. The early diffuse heterogeneous enhancement permits distinction from hemangioma [21].

Lymphangiomas

Lymphangiomas are composed of collections of small and cystically dilated lymphatic channels. Splenic lymphangiomatosis is rare and usually appears as a subcapsular multiloculated mass with increased signal intensity

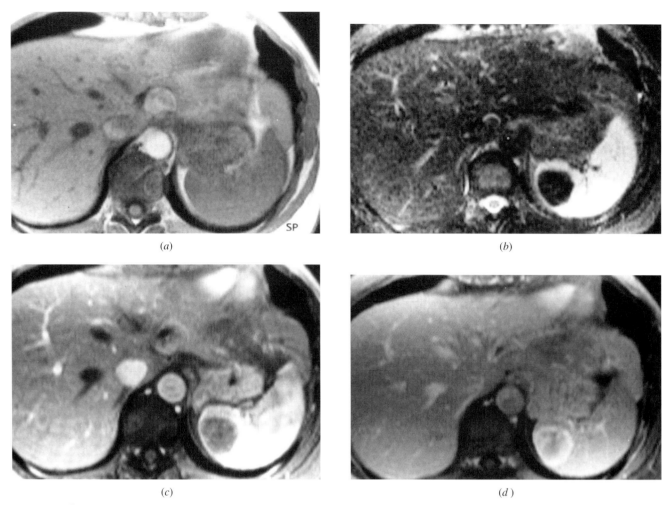

(a)

(b)

(c)

(d)

FIG. 5.14 Sclerosing hemangioma. T1-weighted SGE (*a*), T2-weighted fat-suppressed spin-echo (*b*), immediate postgadolinium T1-weighted SGE (*c*), and 90-s postgadolinium T1-weighted fat-suppressed SGE (*d*) images. A 3-cm hemangioma is isointense to the spleen on T1- (*a*) and markedly hypointense on the T2-weighted image (*b*). Peripheral nodules of enhancement are present on the early postgadolinium image (*c*), with moderate progressive enhancement on the delayed postgadolinium (*d*) images. The combination of hypointensity on T2 with only moderate progression of nodular enhancement on postcontrast T1-weighted images is consistent with a sclerosing hemangioma. (courtesy of Bert te Strake M.D., Manukau Radiology Institute Ltd., Auckland, New Zealand).

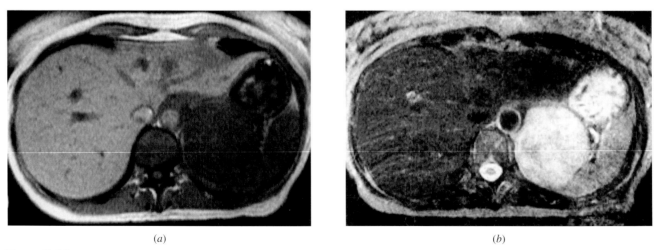

(a)

(b)

FIG. 5.15 Hamartoma. T1-weighted SGE (*a*), T2-weighted fat-suppressed single-shot echo-train spin-echo (*b*), immediate post-gadolinium T1-weighted SGE (*c*), 5-min postgadolinium T1-weighted fat-suppressed spin-echo (*d*), and 10-min postgadolinium SGE (*e*) images.

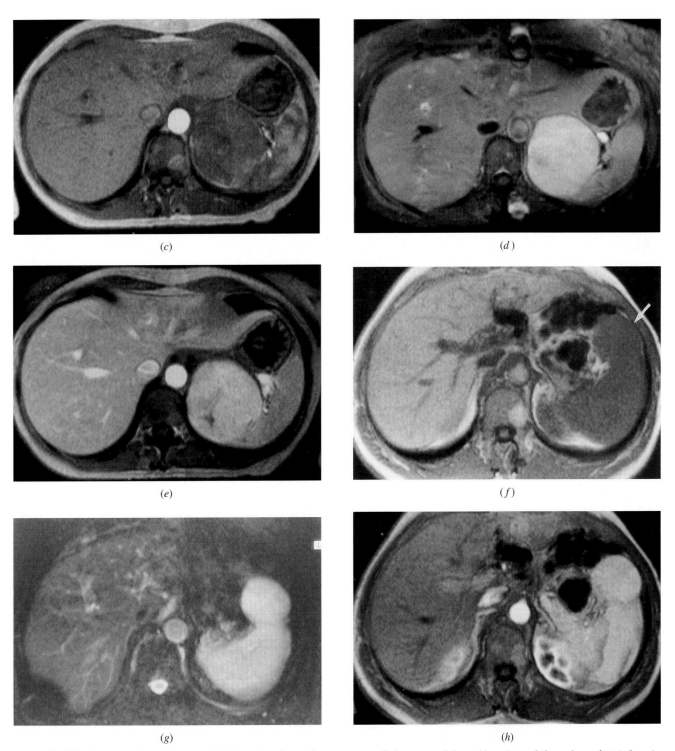

(c)

(d)

(e)

(f)

(g)

(h)

FIG. 5.15 (*Continued*) A 7-cm mass lesion arises from the posteromedial aspect of the midportion of the spleen that is low in signal intensity on the T1-weighted image (*a*), moderately high in signal intensity on the T2-weighted image (*b*), and demonstrates diffuse heterogeneous enhancement on the immediate postgadolinium SGE image (*c*). On more delayed images (*d*, *e*) enhancement becomes more homogeneous and is greater than that of background spleen.

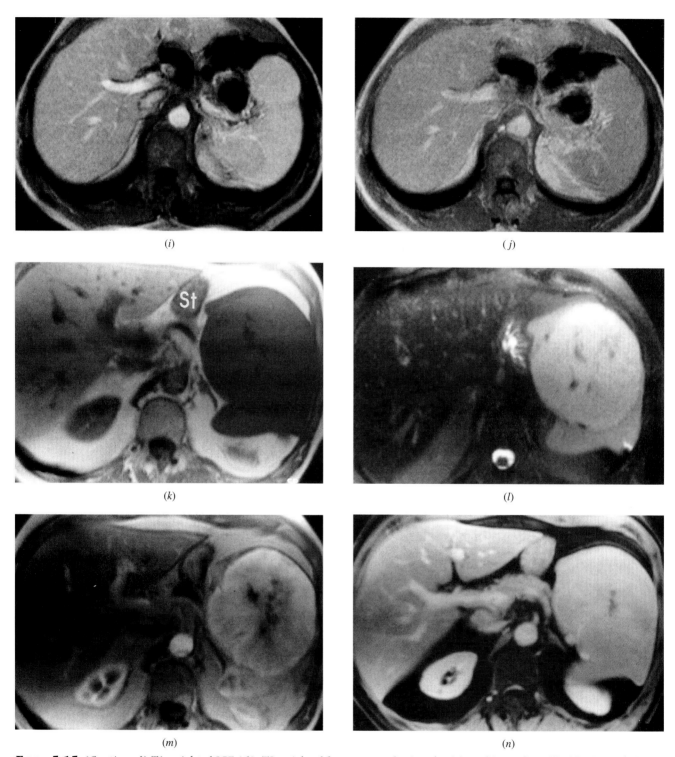

(i)

(j)

(k)

(l)

(m)

(n)

F I G . 5.15 (*Continued*) T1-weighted SGE (*f*), T2-weighted fat-suppressed spin-echo (*g*), and immediate (*h*), 90-s (*i*), and 10-min (*j*) postgadolinium images in a second patient. A 4-cm hamartoma arises from the anterior aspect of the midportion of the spleen (arrow, *f*). The signal intensity of the hamartoma is very similar to that of background spleen on all imaging sequences. A cleavage plane from spleen is noted on the T2-weighted image (*g*). On the immediate postgadolinium image (*h*) the tumor has intense, uniform enhancement, which is different from the arciform enhancement of the normal splenic parenchyma.

T1-weighted SGE (*k*), T2-weighted fat-suppressed echo-train spin-echo (*l*), immediate postgadolinium T1-weighted SGE (*m*), and 90-s gadolinium-enhanced T1-weighted fat-suppressed SGE (*n*) images in a third patient. A large hamartoma in the anterior aspect of the spleen displaces the stomach (St, *m*) medially. The mass is near isointense to the spleen on all sequences. It shows intense heterogeneous enhancement on the immediate postgadolinium image, similar to the intensity of spleen but with a differing pattern.

on T2 weighted images and enhancing septa on late-phase gadolinium-enhanced imaging [24].

Malignant Masses

Lymphoma and Other Hematologic Malignancies

Hodgkin and non-Hodgkin lymphomas often involve the spleen [25–27]. Lymphomatous deposits in the spleen frequently parallel the signal intensity of splenic parenchyma on T1- and T2-weighted images. Therefore, conventional unenhanced spin-echo MRI has had only limited success in imaging lymphomatous involvement of the spleen [26]. Immediate postgadolinium SGE images, however, surpass CT images for the evaluation of lymphoma [4]. This is explained by the higher sensitivity of MRI for gadolinium and its ability to acquire images of the entire spleen in a rapid fashion after a compact bolus of contrast.

Splenic involvement may have various appearances on immediate postgadolinium images. Diffuse involvement may appear as large, irregularly enhancing regions of high and low signal intensity (fig. 5.16), in contrast to the uniform bands that characterize normal arciform enhancement. Multifocal disease is also common, appearing as focal low-signal intensity mass of lesions scattered throughout the spleen [4]. Focal lesions may occur in a background of arciform-enhancing spleen or in a background of uniformly enhancing spleen. Focal lymphomatous involvement with persistent arciform enhancement is more typical of Hodgkin than non-Hodgkin lymphoma. Focal involvement appears as spherical lesions in distinction to the wavy tubular pattern of arciform enhancement of uninvolved spleen. Focal lymphomatous deposits may be low in signal intensity compared with background spleen on

T2-weighted images (fig. 5.17), which is a feature distinguishing lymphomas from metastases, which are rarely low in signal intensity and usually isointense to hyperintense. Although splenomegaly is most often present, lymphoma may involve normal-sized spleens (fig. 5.18). Lymphoma also may appear as a large mass involving spleen and contiguous organs such as stomach, adrenal, or kidney. Bulky lymphadenopathy is frequently, but not invariably, present. It is critical to acquire SGE images within the first 30 s after contrast administration because foci of lymphoma equilibrate early, becoming isointense with normal splenic tissue within 2 min and frequently earlier [2, 4]. A rare appearance is that of a solitary mass involving the spleen, which may also show moderately intense diffuse heterogeneous enhancement on immediate postgadolinium SGE images (fig. 5.19). This appearance may mimic that of splenic hamartomas, although the intensity of contrast enhancement is less. The presence of symptoms and signs of systemic disease may suggest the diagnosis of lymphoma.

Superparamagnetic particles also improve the accuracy of diagnosing splenic lymphoma [9, 10]. These particles are selectively taken up by the RES cells and cause a decrease in signal intensity. By contrast, malignant cells do not take up superparamagnetic particles. Therefore, splenic lymphoma remains hyperintense compared to the normal spleen, improving tumor-spleen contrast [9, 10].

Chronic lymphocytic leukemia frequently involves the spleen and may result in massive splenomegaly. Focal deposits are more infiltrative and less well defined than lymphoma. Deposits are well shown after gadolinium administration and appear as irregular hypointense masses on early postcontrast images (fig. 5.20). Malignancies related to leukemia, such as angioimmunoblastic

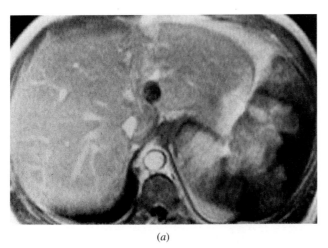

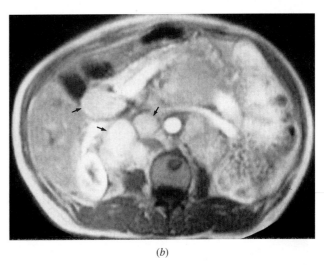

(a)   (b)

F I G . 5.16 Diffuse infiltration with lymphoma. Immediate postgadolinium T1-weighted SGE image (*a*) demonstrates irregular regions of high and low signal intensity in the spleen in this patient with non-Hodgkin lymphoma. Irregular enhancement is observed in the setting of diffuse infiltration.

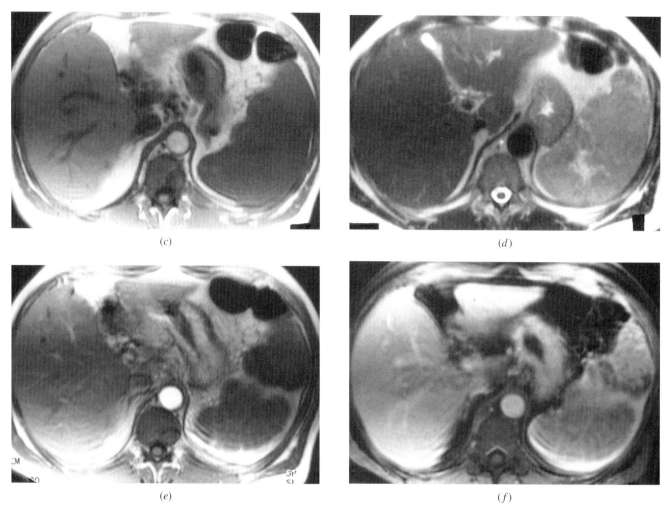

(c)

(d)

(e)

(f)

FIG. 5.16 (*Continued*) Immediate postgadolinium SGE image (*b*) in a second patient with non-Hodgkin lymphoma demonstrates irregular enhancement of the spleen consistent with diffuse infiltration. Enhancing lymph nodes (arrows, *b*) are also noted.

T1-weighted SGE (*c*), T2-weighted echo-train spin-echo (*d*), immediate postgadolinium T1-weighted SGE (*e*), and 90-s post-gadolinium T1-weighted fat-suppressed SGE (*f*) images in a third patient with B cell lymphoma infiltrating the spleen. The spleen is homogeneous in signal intensity on T1 (*c*) and is heterogeneous on the T2-weighted image (*d*). Diffuse heterogeneous enhancement with large irregular foci of decreased enhancement is appreciated on the immediate postgadolinium image (*e*) that persists on the late image (*f*).

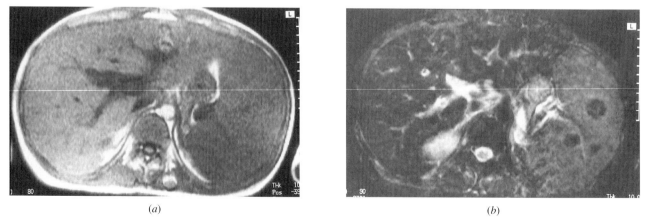

(a)

(b)

FIG. 5.17 Non-Hodgkin lymphoma with multifocal splenic involvement. T1-weighted SGE (*a*), T2-weighted fat-suppressed spin-echo (*b*), and immediate (*c*) and 2-min (*d*) postgadolinium SGE images.

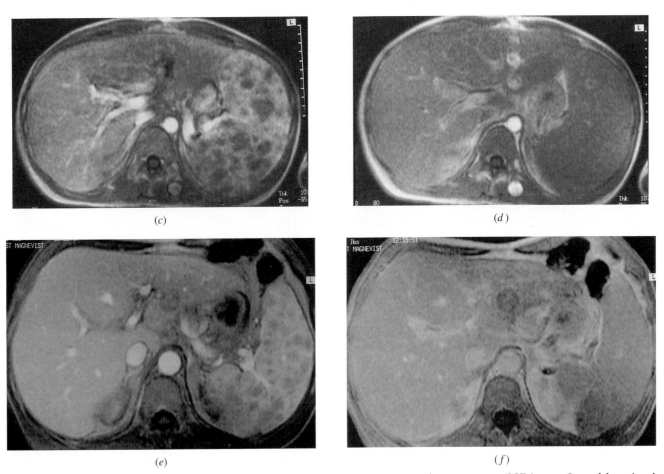

(c)

(d)

(e)

(f)

FIG. 5.17 (*Continued*) Splenomegaly is present. Lesions are not apparent on the precontrast SGE image. Several low-signal intensity focal mass lesions are identified on T2-weighted images, an appearance that is not uncommon for lymphoma but rare for other malignant tumors. Multiple focal masses are most clearly demonstrated on immediate postgadolinium images (*c*). Lymphomatous foci become isointense with background spleen by 2-min after contrast (*d*).

Immediate (*e*) and 90-s (*f*) postgadolinium SGE images in a second patient. Multiple low-signal intensity masses are identified on the immediate postgadolinium image (*e*). Lesions become isointense with background spleen by 90-s.

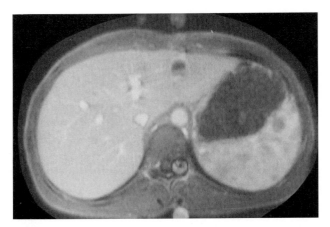

FIG. 5.18 Hodgkin lymphoma. Immediate postgadolinium image demonstrates multiple low-signal intensity masses within a normal-sized spleen. Rounded lesions are present in a background of arciform-enhancing spleen.

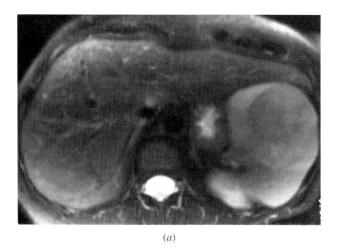

(a)

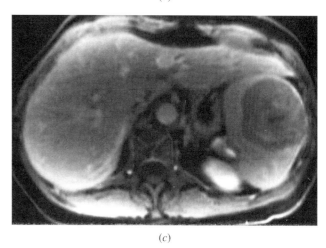

(b)

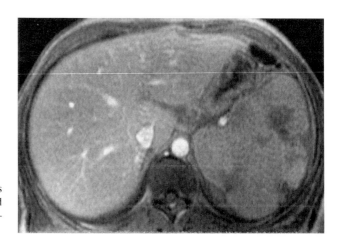

(c)

FIG. 5.19 Splenic lymphoma presenting as a solitary mass. T2-weighted fat-suppressed echo-train spin-echo (*a*), immediate postgadolinium T1-weighted SGE (*b*), and 90-s postgadolinium fat-suppressed SGE (*c*) images. A 6-cm solitary mass arises from the spleen that is mildly heterogeneous and hyperintense on the T2-weighted image (*a*). The mass enhances moderately in a diffuse heterogeneous fashion on the immediate postgadolinium image (arrow, *b*) with slightly increased signal intensity by 90 s after contrast (*c*). The appearance resembles a hamartoma, with diffuse heterogeneous enhancement. Substantially less enhancement is present of this lymphomatous mass than is typically seen with a hamartoma. The patient presented with systemic symptoms, which is a picture in keeping with lymphoma and not hamartoma. The patient did not have retroperitoneal adenopathy, which is another uncommon feature of splenic lymphoma.

lymphadenopathy with dysproteinemia, have a similar appearance, with irregular regions of low signal intensity within the spleen on immediate postgadolinium images (fig. 5.21). Lymphadenopathy is frequently present.

Chemotherapy-treated lymphomatous deposits in the spleen can appear as fibrotic nodules that are low signal intensity on T1-weighted and T2-weighted images and demonstrate negligible enhancement on early and late postgadolinium images (fig. 5.22). These imaging features may be correlated clinically with a favorable response to therapy.

Metastases

Although tumors may invade the spleen from contiguous viscera, true tumor metastasis to the spleen is rare, usually occurring only in the setting of disseminated

FIG. 5.20 Chronic lymphocytic leukemia. The spleen is noted to be massively enlarged and contains irregularly marginated focal low-signal intensity masses on the 45-s postgadolinium T1-weighted SGE image.

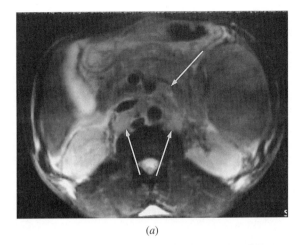

(a)

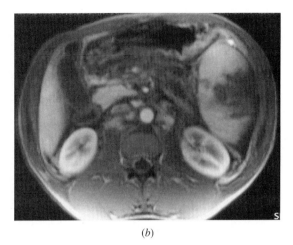

(b)

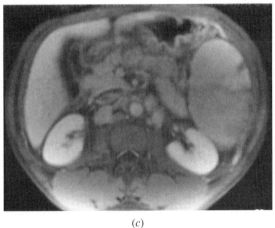

(c)

FIG. 5.21 Angioimmunoblastic lymphadenopathy with dysproteinemia. T2-weighted fat-suppressed spin-echo (a), immediate postgadolinium T1-weighted SGE (b), and 90-s postgadolinium fat-suppressed SGE (c) images. The spleen is noted to be markedly enlarged. Lymphadenopathy is moderately high in signal intensity on T2-weighted images and is rendered conspicuous because of the suppression of fat signal intensity (arrows, a). Mild enhancement of lymph nodes is noted on immediate postgadolinium SGE (b). Lymph nodes enhance more intensely in the interstitial phase and are more clearly defined by the suppression of fat signal intensity (c). Splenic involvement is demonstrated by irregular, poorly marginated, large regions of diminished enhancement on the immediate postgadolinium image (b). Enhancement of the spleen is more uniform by 90 s after contrast (c), and signal intensity is mildly heterogeneous on the T2-weighted image (a).

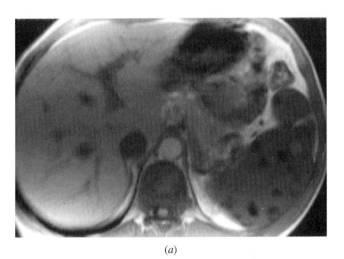

(a)

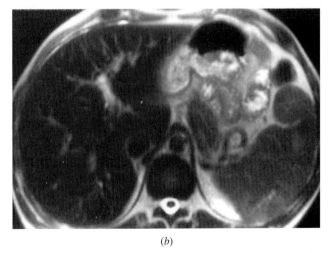

(b)

FIG. 5.22 Chemotherapy-treated splenic lymphoma. T1-weighted SGE (a), T2-weighted single-shot echo-train spin-echo (b), immediate postgadolinium T1-weighted SGE (c), and 90-s postgadolinium T1-weighted fat-suppressed SGE (d) images. Foci of treated lymphoma are hypointense on T1 (a), and hypo to isointense on T2 (b) and demonstrate negligible enhancement on early (c) and late (d) postgadolinium images. The low signal on T2 reflects a diminished fluid content, and fibrous changes result in the diminished enhancement.

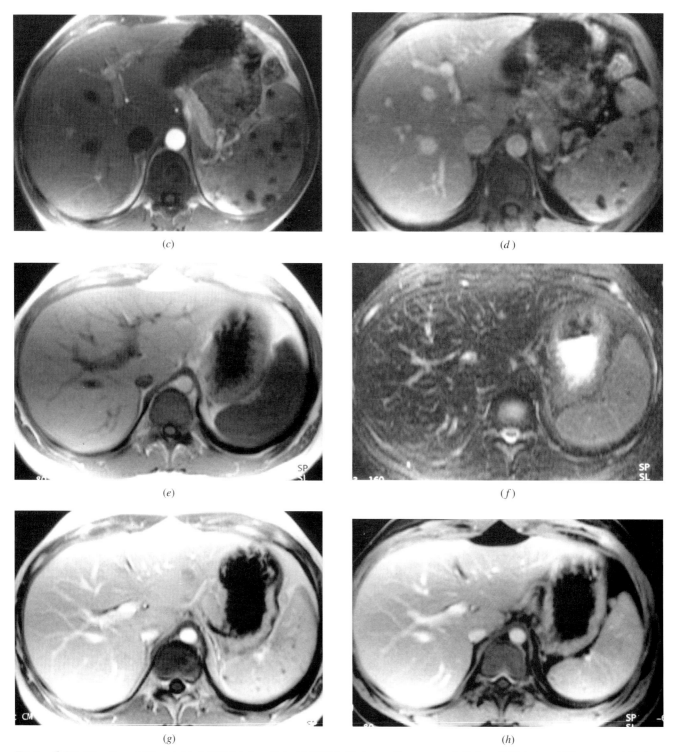

(c)

(d)

(e)

(f)

(g)

(h)

F IG . 5.22 (*Continue*) T1-weighted SGE (*e*), breath-hold STIR (*f*), immediate postgadolinium SGE (*g*) and 90-s postgadolinium SGE (*h*) in a second patient with Hodgkin lymphoma receiving chemotherapy. There are multiple small hypointense lesions on T1- (*e*) and T2- (*f*) weighted images, which shows peripheral or diffuse enhancement after contrast administration (*g, h*) reflecting the different stages of the fibrotic process. These lesions remained stable in appearance in follow-up MRI exams (not shown).

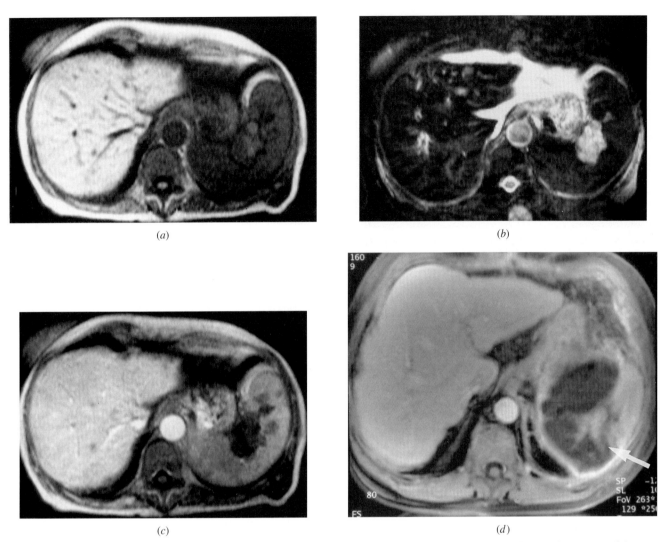

F I G . 5.23 Splenic metastases. T1-weighted SGE (*a*), T2-weighted fat-suppressed spin-echo (*b*), and immediate postgadolinium T1-weighted SGE (*c*) images in a woman with endometrial cancer. Metastases are noted throughout the spleen that are mixed hypointense and isointense on the T1-weighted image (*a*), mixed isointense and hyperintense on the T2-weighted image (*b*), and low in signal intensity on the immediate postgadolinium image (*c*). Note that metastases are best shown on the immediate postgadolinium image. The largest metastasis is distinctly demonstrated on the T2-weighted image (*b*). The smaller lesions are poorly shown, despite the presence of iron deposition. Ascites is also present and is low in signal intensity on pre- and postcontrast T1-weighted images and high in signal intensity on the T2-weighted image.

Transverse 90-s postgadolinium fat-suppressed SGE image (*d*) in a second patient demonstrates an expansile destructive lesion (arrow, *d*) in the posterior aspect of the spleen associated with a large subcapsular fluid collection.

disease in the terminal stage. Breast cancer, lung cancer, and melanoma are the most common primary tumors [28]. The most generally accepted theory to account for the relative scarcity of splenic metastasis is based on the absence of afferent lymphatic channels within the spleen [29]. Metastases tend to be in the form of nodules or aggregates of tumor, and they are particularly prone to disrupt the normal splenic architecture. Splenic metastases often are occult on conventional spin-echo imaging [27]. One notable exception is melanoma, because its paramagnetic properties may result in a mixed population of high- and low-signal intensity lesions on both T1-and T2-weighted images. Lesion detection is improved by acquiring immediate postgadolinium SGE images [3] (fig. 5.23). Metastases are lower in signal intensity than normal splenic tissue on these images. Images must be acquired within the first 30 s after gadolinium administration because metastases rapidly equilibrate with splenic parenchyma. Image acquisition with superparamagnetic iron oxide particles renders metastases higher in signal intensity than normal spleen [7, 9]. An attractive feature of iron oxide particles is that the imaging window is longer (60 min) than for gadolinium (<1 min) [7–9].

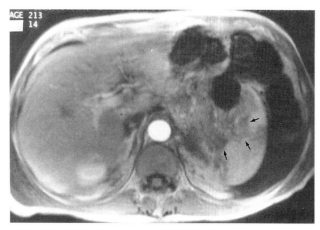

F I G . 5.24 Direct tumor invasion. Immediate postgadolinium T1-weighted SGE image demonstrates invasion of the splenic hilum by a large infiltrative pancreatic ductal adenocarcinoma (arrows).

Direct Tumor Invasion

Direct tumor invasion is most commonly observed with pancreatic cancers including ductal adenocarcinoma, islet cell tumor, and macrocystic cystadenocarcinoma (fig. 5.24). Direct extension from tumors of gastric, colonic, renal and adrenal origins, in a decreasing order of frequency, is also observed. Lymphoma has a particular propensity to involve the spleen in continuity with other organs.

Angiosarcoma

Angiosarcoma is rare but represents the most common primary nonlymphoid malignant tumor of the spleen. Tumors may be single or multiple and demonstrate an aggressive growth pattern. Rupture is not uncommon, and hemorrhage is a frequent finding. Angiosarcomas commonly demonstrate a variety of signal intensities on T1-weighted images because of the varying ages of blood products [30]. Tumors are usually highly vascular and enhance intensely with gadolinium [30].

MISCELLANEOUS

Splenomegaly

Splenomegaly may be observed in a number of disease states including venous congestion (portal hypertension), leukemia, lymphoma, metastases, and various infections. In North America, the most common cause of splenomegaly is secondary to portal hypertension. On immediate postgadolinium images demonstration of arciform or uniform high-signal intensity enhancement is consistent with portal hypertension and excludes the presence of malignant disease (fig. 5.25).

Infection

Viral infection may result in splenomegaly. The three most common viruses to involve the spleen are Epstein-Barr, varicella, and cytomegalovirus. Nonviral infectious agents that involve the spleen in patients with normal immune status include histoplasmosis, tuberculosis, and echinococcosis [31]. These infectious agents are observed in immunocompromised patients with an even greater frequency (fig. 5.26). In the immunocompromised patient, the most common hepatosplenic infection is fungal infection with *Candida albicans* and *Cryptococcus* [32, 33]. Patients with acute myelogenous leukemia are at particular risk for developing this fungal infection. Multiorgan involvement is common. The gastrointestinal tract is almost invariably involved, and although esophageal disease is well shown on MR images, involvement of the intestines is frequently not visible. Esophageal candidiasis is common and rarely associated with hepatosplenic candidiasis, whereas small intestine candidiasis is more frequently associated with this infection. Lesions are most commonly observed in the spleen and liver, whereas renal disease is somewhat uncommon. MR images can demonstrate lesions in the acute phase, subacute treated phase, and chronic healed phase [32, 34]. Lesions in each of these phases have distinctive MRI appearances. These varying appearances are more distinct for liver lesions. (For an in-depth discussion, see Chapter 2, *Liver.*) Acute lesions are generally more apparent in the spleen than in the liver, whereas the reverse is true for subacute-treated and chronic-healed lesions. In the acute phase, hepatosplenic candidiasis results in small (<1 cm), well-defined abscesses in the spleen and liver. They are well shown on T2-weighted fat-suppressed images as high-signal intensity rounded foci (fig. 5.27). Lesions also may be visible on postgadolinium images, but they usually are not visualized on precontrast SGE images. MRI has been shown to be superior to contrast-enhanced CT imaging for the detection of fungal microabscesses [32]. MRI should be used routinely in the investigation of hepatosplenic candidiasis because patient survival depends on swift pharmacologic intervention with antifungal agents.

Bacterial and fungal abscesses are rare in the spleen. Abscesses appear slightly hypo- to isointense on T1-weighted images and heterogeneous and mildly to moderately hyperintense on T2-weighted images. These lesions show intense mural enhancement on early gadolinium-enhanced images. This pattern persists on later postgadolinium images, accompanied by the presence of periabscess increased enhancement of surrounding tissue on immediate postgadolinium images (fig. 5.28).

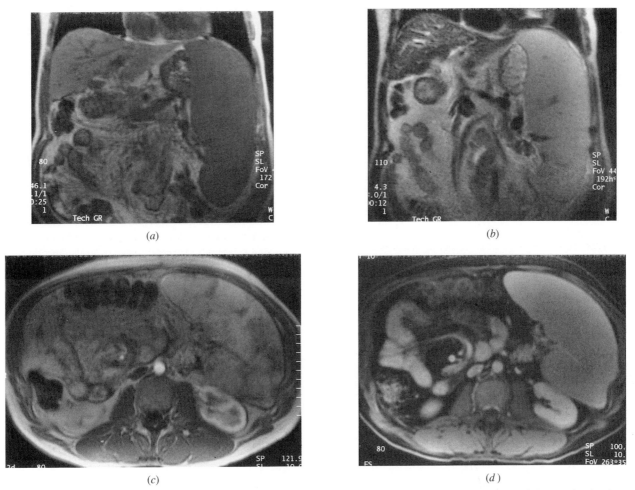

(a)

(b)

(c)

(d)

FIG. 5.25 Splenomegaly secondary to portal hypertension. Coronal T1-weighted SGE (*a*), coronal T2-weighted echo-train spin-echo (*b*), immediate postgadolinium T1-weighted SGE (*c*), and 90-s postgadolinium fat-suppressed SGE (*d*) images. Massive splenomegaly is demonstrated on all MR images. No focal lesions are present on precontrast T1 (*a*) or T2-weighted (*b*) images. The presence of arciform enhancement on the immediate postgadolinium SGE image (*c*) excludes the presence of malignant disease. At 90 s, the spleen becomes homogeneous in signal (*d*).

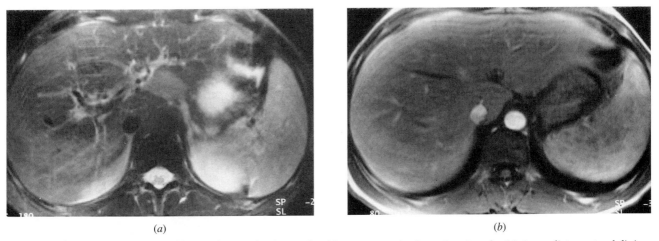

(a)

(b)

FIG. 5.26 Hepatosplenorenal histoplasmosis. T2-weighted fat-suppressed echo-train spin-echo (*a*), immediate postgadolinium T1-weighted SGE (*b*), and 90-s postgadolinium fat-suppressed SGE (*c*) images in a patient with human immunodeficiency virus (HIV) infection. Multiple lesions <1 cm are demonstrated in the liver, spleen, and kidneys.

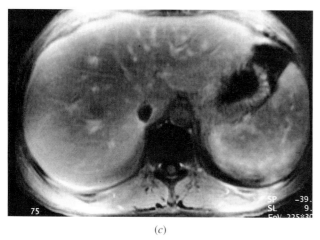

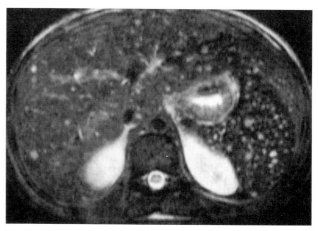

(c)

FIG. 5.26 (*Continued*) Lesions are poorly visualized on T2-weighted images and appear as small minimally hyperintense lesions (*a*). On immediate postgadolinium image lesions appear low in signal intensity (*b*). By 90 s after gadolinium, lesions enhance more than background tissue (arrows, *c*)

FIG. 5.27 Hepatosplenic candidiasis. T2-weighted fat-suppressed echo-train spin-echo image demonstrates multiple, well-defined, high-signal intensity candidiasis abscesses <1 cm in the liver and spleen.

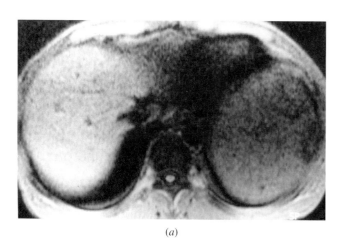

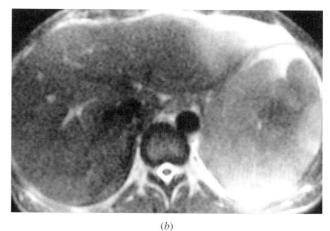

(a)

(b)

FIG. 5.28 Cryptococcal abscess. T1-weighted magnetization-prepared gradient-echo (*a*), T2 fat-suppressed single-shot echo-train spin-echo (*b*), and coronal 3-min postgadolinium T1-weighted magnetization-prepared gradient-echo (*c*) images in an immunocompromised patient with AIDS and generalized cryptococcal infection. The abscess appears mildly hypointense on T1 (*a*) and mildly hyperintense on T2 (*b*), with subtle signal difference compared to spleen. Lack of enhancement and peripheral ring enhancement (arrow, *c*) are present on the post-gadolinium image (*c*), which are features of bacterial and some fungal abscesses.

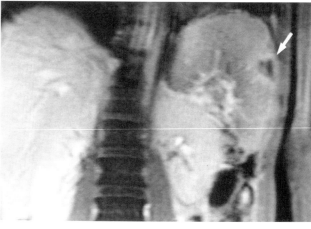

(c)

Sarcoidosis

Lesions of sarcoidosis are small (<1 cm) and hypovascular. Because of their hypovascularity, the lesions are low in signal intensity on T1- and T2-weighted images and enhance on gadolinium-enhanced images in a minimal and delayed fashion [35] (fig. 5.29). Low signal intensity on T2-weighted images is a feature that distinguishes these lesions from acute infective lesions.

Gamna-Gandy Bodies

Foci of iron deposition occur commonly in patients with cirrhosis and portal hypertension due to microhemorrhages in the splenic parenchyma. On occasion, such foci are observed in patients receiving blood transfusions [36, 37]. Lesions vary in size but are generally <1 cm.

Lesions appear signal void on all pulse sequences [36, 37] (fig. 5.30). Susceptibility artifact is demonstrated on gradient-echo images as blooming artifact, and this artifact is pathognomonic for this entity. An imaging feature that is helpful to distinguish Gamna-Gandy bodies from fibrotic nodules is that Gamna-Gandy bodies appear smaller on shorter TE sequences because of a diminution of susceptibility artifact (e.g., smaller on TE = 2 ms sequence compared to TE = 4 ms sequence) whereas the size of fibrotic nodules is unchanged on shorter TE sequences.

Trauma

The spleen is the most commonly ruptured abdominal organ in the setting of trauma. Injury to the spleen may take several forms: subcapsular hematoma, contusion,

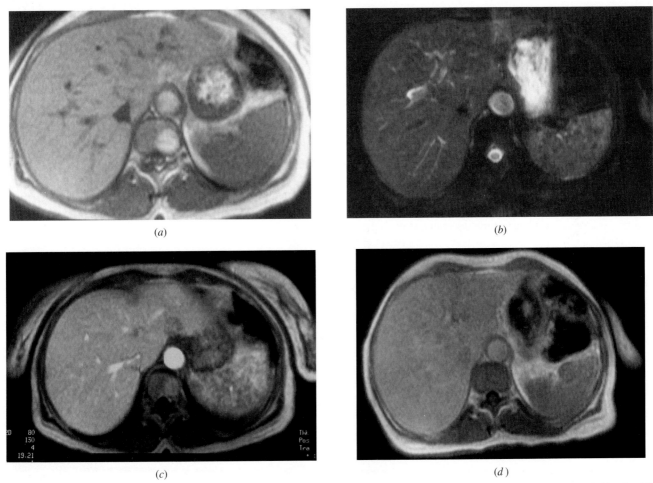

(a)   *(b)*

(c)   *(d)*

F I G . 5.29 Sarcoidosis. T1-weighted SGE (*a*), T2-weighted fat-suppressed spin-echo (*b*), and immediate (*c*) and 10-min (*d*) postgadolinium T1-weighted SGE images. Multiple sarcoidosis granulomas, <1 cm, are present in the spleen. Lesions are mildly hypointense to isointense on T1-weighted images (*a*), moderately hypointense on T2-weighted images (*b*), and hypointense on immediate postgadolinium images (*c*), gradually enhancing to near-isointensity on delayed postgadolinium images (*d*). Hypointensity on T2-weighted images distinguish these lesions from those of infectious etiologies (Reproduced with permission from Warshauer DM, Semelka RC, Ascher SM, Nodular sarcoidosis of the liver and spleen: appearance on MR images. J Magn Reson Imaging 4: 553–557, 1994.

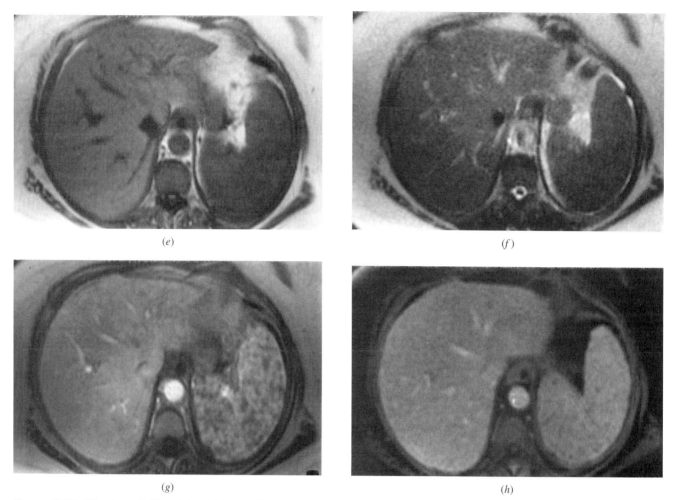

(e)

(f)

(g)

(h)

FIG. 5.29 (*Continued*) T1-weighted SGE (*e*), T2-weighted single-shot echo-train spin echo (*f*), immediate postgadolinium T1 single-shot magnetization-prepared gradient-echo (*g*) and 90-s postgadolinium T1-weighted fat-suppressed spin-echo (*h*) images in a second patient. The imaging features are comparable to the above described patient.

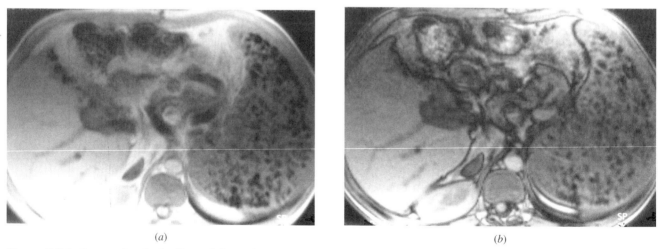

(a)

(b)

FIG. 5.30 Gamna-Gandy bodies of the spleen. T1-weighted SGE (*a*), T1-weighted out-of-phase SGE (*b*), T2-weighted fat-suppressed single-shot echo-train spin-echo (*c*), immediate postgadolinium T1-weighted SGE (*d*), and 90-s postgadolinium T1-weighted fat-suppressed SGE (*e*) images. Gamna-Gandy bodies are typically multiple and <1 cm in diameter.

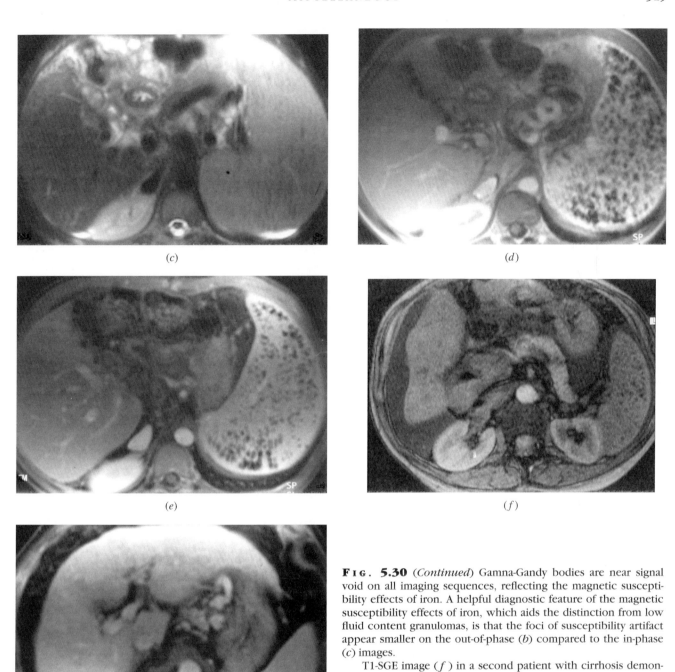

(c)

(d)

(e)

(f)

(g)

F I G . 5.30 (*Continued*) Gamna-Gandy bodies are near signal void on all imaging sequences, reflecting the magnetic susceptibility effects of iron. A helpful diagnostic feature of the magnetic susceptibility effects of iron, which aids the distinction from low fluid content granulomas, is that the foci of susceptibility artifact appear smaller on the out-of-phase (*b*) compared to the in-phase (*c*) images.

T1-SGE image (*f*) in a second patient with cirrhosis demonstrates multiple <5-mm Gamna-Gandy bodies.

Ninety-second postgadolinium fat-suppressed SGE image (*g*) in a third patient shows a solitary Gamna-Gandy body (arrow, *g*). Note large varices along the lesser curve of the stomach, accentuated with the use of fat suppression.

laceration, and devascularization/infarct. Subcapsular or intraparenchymal hematoma secondary to contusion or laceration demonstrates a time course of changes in signal intensity due to the paramagnetic properties of the degradation products of hemoglobin (fig. 5.31). Subacute hemorrhage is particularly conspicuous because of its distinctive high signal intensity on T1- and T2-weighted images (fig. 5.32). Traumatic injury of the spleen, especially devascularization, is well shown on immediate postgadolinium SGE images. Areas of devascularization are nearly signal void compared to the high signal intensity of enhancement vascularized tissue.

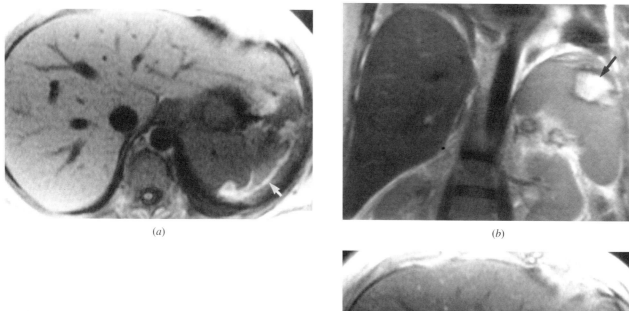

(a)

(b)

F I G . 5.31 Splenic laceration with subcapsular hematoma. T1-weighted single-shot magnetization-prepared gradient-echo (*a*), coronal T2-weighted single-shot echo-train spin-echo (*b*), and immediate postgadolinium single-shot magnetization-prepared gradient-echo (*c*) images. Subcapsular blood (arrow, *a*) is appreciated as high-signal fluid on the precontrast T1-weighted image (*a*). The laceration is isointense on T1 (*a*) and high signal on T2 (arrow, *b*) and demonstrates lack of enhancement (arrow, *c*) on the postgadolinium image (*c*).

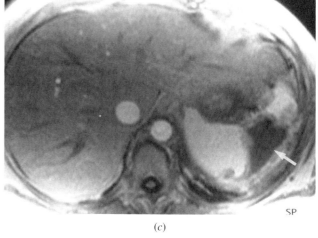

(c)

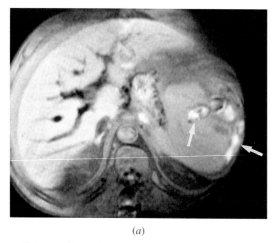

(a)

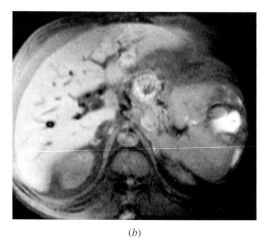

(b)

F I G . 5.32 Splenic laceration. T1-weighted fat-suppressed spin-echo images from adjacent cranial (*a*) and caudal (*b*) transverse sections. Mixed, predominantly high-signal intensity fluid is present in an intraparenchymal and subcapsular location (arrows, *a*) in the spleen, which represents subacute blood.

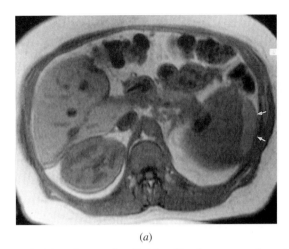 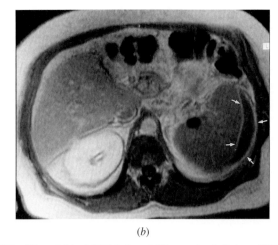

(a)   (b)

F I G . 5.33 Subcapsular fluid collection secondary to pancreatitis. T1-weighted SGE (*a*) and 90-s postgadolinium SGE (*b*) images. A subcapsular fluid collection is present that is slightly high in signal intensity on the T1-weighted image, a finding consistent with the presence of blood or protein (arrows, *a*). Enhancement of the capsule and surface of the spleen on the postgadolinium image (arrows, *b*) confirms the subcapsular location of the fluid collection.

Subcapsular Fluid Collections

Multiple causes for subcapsular fluid collections exist, the most common being sequela to trauma. Enhancement of the capsule and surface of the spleen may be observed on postgadolinium images, which confirms the location of these fluid collections (fig. 5.33).

Splenosis

Splenosis is the term used for ectopic tissue resulting from splenic injury. The most common appearance of splenosis on magnetic resonance imaging is solid, well-circumscribed nodules in the abdominal cavity, with signal intensity similar to the normal spleen (fig. 5.34).

Infarcts

Splenic infarcts are a common occurrence in the setting of obstruction of the splenic artery or one of its branches. The most common cause is cardiac emboli, but local thrombosis, vasculitis and splenic torsion are also described. Infarcts appear as peripheral wedge-shaped, round, or linear defects that are most clearly defined on 1- to 5-min postgadolinium images as low-signal intensity wedge-shaped regions (fig. 5.35). The splenic

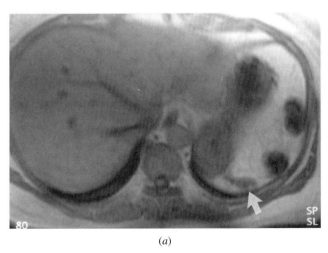 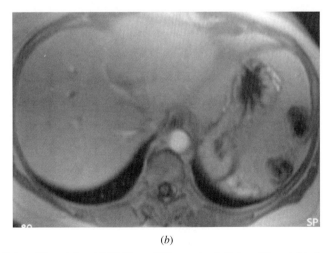

(a)   (b)

F I G . 5.34 Splenosis. T1-weighted SGE (*a*), immediate postgadolinium T1-weighted SGE (*b*), and 90-s postgadolinium T1-weighted fat-suppressed SGE (*c*) images. A small elongated mass is present in the left upper abdominal quadrant in a patient with prior splenectomy. The mass is slightly hypointense to the liver on the T1-weighted image (arrow, *a*), with intense enhancement on the immediate postgadolinium image (*b*) and persistent enhancement on the delayed postgadolinium image (*c*).

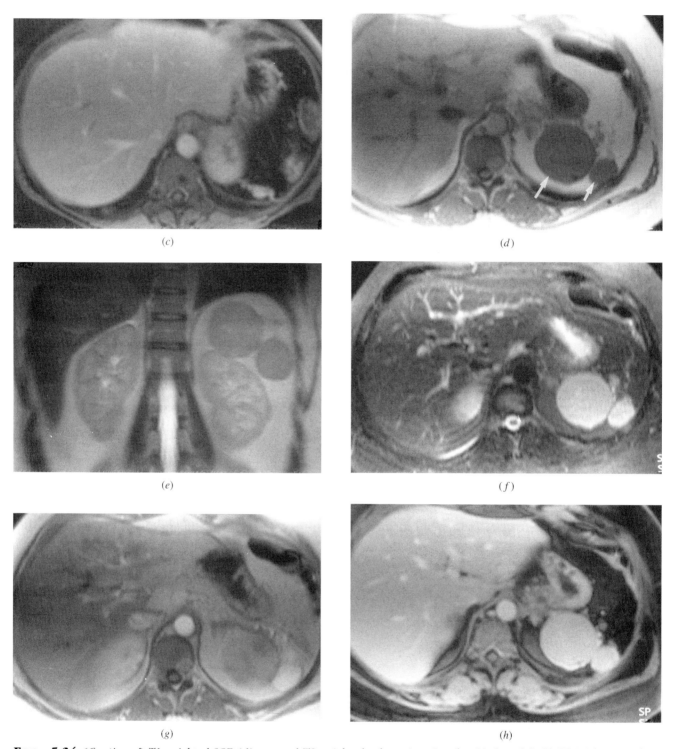

FIG. 5.34 (*Continued*) T1-weighted SGE (*d*), coronal T2-weighted echo-train spin-echo (*e*), breath-hold STIR (*f*), immediate postgadolinium T1-weighted SGE (*g*), and 90-s postgadolinium T1-weighted fat-suppressed SGE (*h*) images in a second patient with prior splenectomy. Two splenules are present in the left upper abdomen (arrows, *d*). The masses have an appearance similar to normal spleen, with mild hypointensity on T1 (*d*), moderate hyperintensity on T2 (*e*), and early heterogeneous enhancement (*g*), which becomes more homogeneous on delayed images (*h*). Note that the enhancement of the larger mass is less than that of the smaller mass, presumably reflecting a smaller feeding arterial supply.

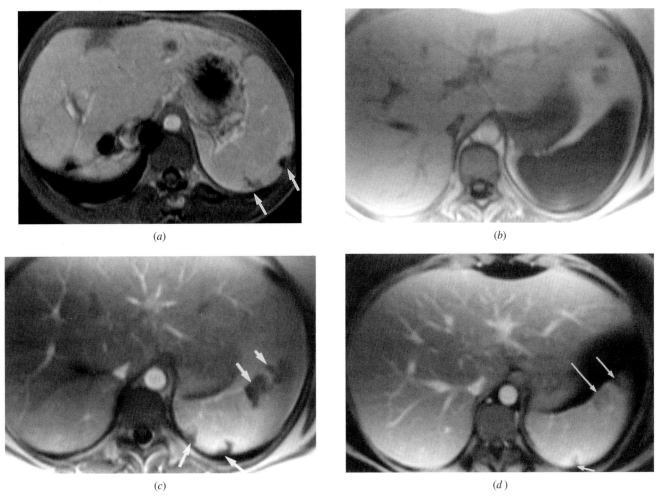

FIG. 5.35 Splenic infarct. One minute postgadolinium T1-weighted SGE image (*a*). Peripheral wedge-shaped defects are noted in the spleen (arrows, *a*) secondary to infarcts.

T1-weighted SGE (*b*), immediate postgadolinium T1-weighted SGE (*c*) and 90-s postgadolinium T1-weighted fat-suppressed SGE (*d*) images in a second patient. An ill-defined posterior subcapsular hyperintensity is present on the T1-weighted image (*b*). Infarct regions are best seen on post gadolinium images (*c*, *d*), and appear as well-defined wedge-shaped defects (arrows, *c* and *d*). Peripheral linear enhancement of the capsule may also be appreciated. Note that some of the regions that have no enhancement on the immediate postgadolinium images show delayed enhancement. These are consistent with areas of ischemia.

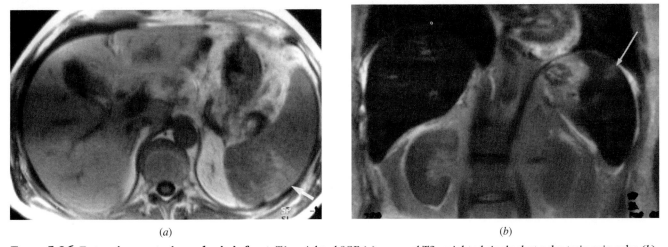

FIG. 5.36 Extensive posterior splenic infarct. T1-weighted SGE (*a*), coronal T2-weighted single-shot echo-train spin-echo (*b*), immediate (*c*) and 45-s postgadolinium T1-weighted SGE (*d*), and 90-s postgadolinium T1-weighted fat-suppressed SGE (*e*) images.

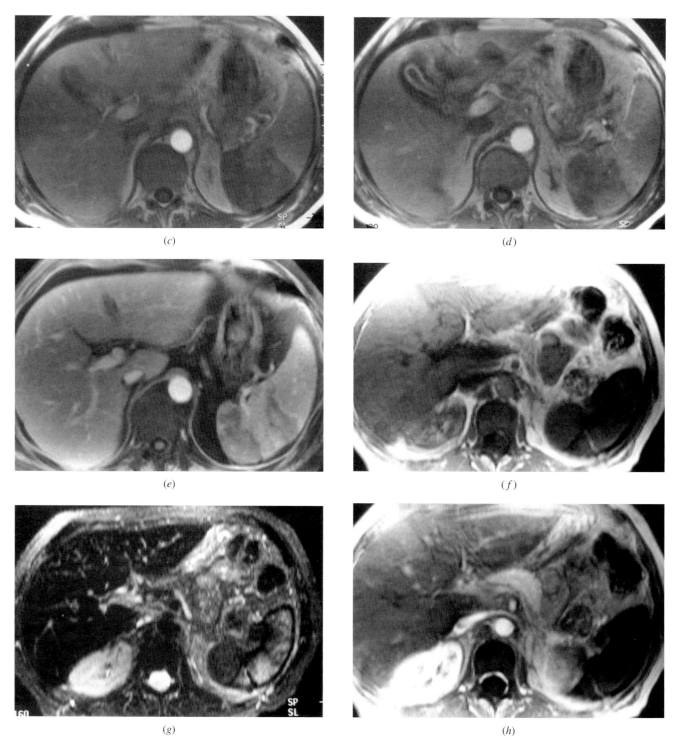

(c)

(d)

(e)

(f)

(g)

(h)

F I G . 5.36 (*Continued*) The splenic infarcts appear heterogeneous and mildly high signal on T1-weighted (arrow, *a*) and heterogeneous and moderately high signal on T2-weighted (arrow, *b*) images. On the immediate (*c*), 45-second (*d*) and 90-s (*e*) postgadolinium images there is heterogeneous lack of enhancement of the regions of infarction.

T1-weighted SGE (*f*), breath-hold STIR (*g*), immediate postgadolinium SGE (*h*) and 90-s postgadolinium fat-suppressed SGE (*i*) image in a second patient with splenic infarcts. The large anterior splenic infarct is heterogeneous on T1 (*f*) and T2 (*g*) weighted images.

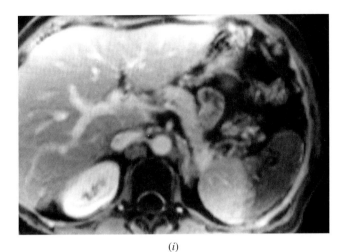

(*i*)

F i g . 5.36 (*Continued*) Lack of enhancement on early (*h*) and late (*i*) postgadolinium images most clearly demonstrates that this region has undergone infarction. Lack of enhancement is more apparent on the later postcontrast image.

capsule is commonly observed as a thin peripheral, enhancing linear structure. Massive splenic infarcts may appear as diffuse low-signal intensity regions on T1-weighted images that are inhomogeneous and high signal on T2-weighted images. Lack of enhancement on early and late postgadolinium images of wedge-shaped regions is the most diagnostic feature (fig. 5.36).

CONCLUSION

MRI is a valuable tool in the evaluation of the spleen and surpasses CT imaging in many clinical settings. One of the major indications for MRI is the investigation of hepatosplenic candidiasis. Other circumstances in which MRI may be of value include the detection of malignant lesions (metastases or lymphoma), infections, and the characterization of lesions such as hemangiomas or hamartomas. MRI should be considered in patients with elevated serum creatinine or those with allergy to iodinated contrast material for the investigation of possible splenic disease. MRI is useful in the further investigation of patients with a CT diagnosis of splenomegaly to determine whether underlying tumor infiltration is present. The future of superparamagnetic iron oxide particles for evaluating the spleen will depend on their efficacy, cost, and patient tolerance, as well as their performance compared with dynamic gadolinium-enhanced MRI.

REFERENCES

1. Mirowitz SA, Brown JJ, Lee JKT, Heiken JP: Dynamic gadolinium-enhanced MR imaging of the normal spleen: Normal enhancement patterns and evaluation of splenic lesions. *Radiology* 179: 681–686, 1991.

2. Mirowitz SA, Gutierrez E, Lee JKT, Brown JJ, et al.: Normal abdominal enhancement patterns with dynamic gadolinium-enhanced MR imaging. *Radiology* 180: 637–640, 1991.

3. Semelka RC, Shoenut JP, Lawrence PH, Greenberg HM, Madden TP, Kroeker MA: Spleen: Dynamic enhancement patterns on gradient-echo MR images enhanced with gadopentetate dimeglumine. *Radiology*, 185: 479–482, 1992.

4. Hamed MM, Hamm B, Ibrahim ME, Taupitz M, et al.: Dynamic MR imaging of the abdomen with gadopentate dimeglumine: Normal enhancement patterns of liver, spleen, stomach, and pancreas. *Am J Roentgenol* 158: 303–307, 1992.

5. Siegelman ES, Mitchell DG, Rubin R, et al.: Parenchymal versus reticuloendothelial iron overload in the liver: Distinction with MR imaging. *Radiology* 179: 361–366, 1991.

6. Siegelman ES, Mitchel DG, Semelka RC: Abdominal iron deposition: Metabolism, MR findings, and clinical importance. *Radiology* 199: 13–22, 1996.

7. Weissleder R, Hahn PF, Stark DD, Elizondo G, et al.: Superparamagnetic iron oxide: Enhanced detection of focal splenic tumors with MR imaging. *Radiology* 169: 399–403, 1988.

8. Weissleder R, Elizondo G, Stark DD, Hahn PF, et al.: The diagnosis of splenic lymphoma by MR imaging: Value of superparamagnetic iron oxide. *Am J Roentgenol* 152: 175–180, 1989.

9. Kreft BP, Tanimoto A, Leffler S, Finn JP, Oksendal AN, Stark DD: Contrast-enhanced MR imaging of diffuse and focal splenic disease with use of magnetic starch micropheres. *J Magn Reson Imaging* 4: 373–379, 1994.

10. Paterson A, Frush DP, Donnelly LF, Foss JN, O'Hara SM, Bisset GS 3rd: A pattern-oriented approach to splenic imaging in infants and children. *Radiographics* 19(6): 1465–85, 1999.

11. Ambriz P, Munoz R, Quintanar E, Sigler L, et al.: Accessory spleen compromising response to splenectomy for idiopathic thrombocytopenic purpura. *Radiology* 155: 793–796, 1985.

12. Beahrs JR, Stephens DH: Enlarged accessory spleens: CT appearance in post splenectomy patients. *Am J Roentgenol* 141: 483–486, 1981.

13. Storm BL, Abbitt PL, Allen DA, Ros PR: Splenosis: Superparamagnetic iron oxide-enhanced MR imaging. *Am J Roentgenol* 159: 333–335, 1992.

14. Applegate KE, Goske MJ, Pierce G, Murphy D: Situs revisited: Imaging of the heterotaxy syndrome. *Radiographics* 19: 837–852, 1999.

15. Vito F, Federico A: Association of splenic syndromes with renal cystic disease. *Hum Pathol* 20: 496,1989

16. Hill SC, Damaska BM, Ling A, Patterson K, et al.: Gaucher disease: Abdominal MR imaging findings in 46 patients. *Radiology* 184: 561–566, 1992.

17. Adler DD, Glazer GM, Aisen AM: MRI of the spleen: Normal appearance and findings in sickle-cell anemia. *Am J Roentgenol* 147: 843–845, 1986.

18. Urrutia M, Mergo PJ, Ros LH, Torres GM, Ros PR: Cystic masses of the spleen: Radiologic-pathologic correlation. *Radiographics* 16: 107–129, 1996.

19. Shirkhoda A, Freeman J, Armin AR, Cacciarelli AA, Morden R: Imaging features of splenic epidermoid cyst with pathologic correlation. *Abdom Imaging* 20: 449–451, 1995.

20. Disler DG, Chew FS: Splenic hemangioma. *Am J Roentgenol* 157: 44, 1991.

21. Ramani M, Reinhold C, Semelka RC, Siegelman ES, Liang L, Ascher SM, Brown JJ, Eisen RN, Bret PM: Splenic hemangiomas and hamartomas: MR imaging characteristics of 28 lesions. *Radiology* 202: 166–172, 1997.

22. Ohtomo K, Fukuda H, Mori K, Minami M, et al.: CT and MR appearances of splenic hamartoma. *J Comput Assist Tomogr*, 16: 425–428, 1992.

23. Pinto PO, Avidago P, Garcia H, Aves FC, Marques C: Splenic hamartoma: A case report. *Eur Radiol* 5: 93–95, 1995.

24. Ito K, Mitchell DG, Honjo K, Fujita T, et al.: MR imaging of acquired abnormalities of the spleen. *Am J Roentgenol* 168: 697–702, 1997.

25. Bragg DG, Colby TV, Ward JH: New concepts in the non-Hodgkin lymphoma: Radiologic implications. *Radiology* 159: 289–304, 1986.

26. Castellino RA: Hodgkin disease: Practical concepts for the diagnostic radiologist. *Radiology* 159: 305–310, 1986.

27. Hahn PF, Weissleder R, Stark DD, et al.: MR imaging of focal splenic tumors. *Am J Roentgenol* 150: 823–827, 1988.

28. Klein B, Stein M, Kuten A, et al.: Splenomegaly and solitary spleen metastases in solid tumors. *Cancer* 60: 100;1987

29. Drinkr CK, Yoffey JM: *Lymphatics, Lymph and Lymphoid Tissue*, Cambridge: Harvard University Press, p. 23, 1941

30. Rabushka LS, Kawashima A, Fishman EK: Imaging of the spleen: CT with supplemental MR examination. *Radiographics* 14: 307–332, 1994.

31. Senturk H, Kocer N, Papila C, Uras C, Dogusoy G: Primary macronodular hepatosplenic tuberculosis: Two cases with US, CT, and MR findings. *Eur Radiol* 5: 451–455, 1995.

32. Semelka RC, Shoenut JP, Greenberg HM, Bow EJ: Detection of acute and treated lesions of hepatosplenic candidiasis: Comparison of dynamic contrast-enhanced CT and MR imaging. *J Magn Reson Imaging* 2: 341–345, 1992.

33. Cho J-S, Kim EE, Varma DGK, Wallace S: MR imaging of hepatosplenic candidiasis superimposed on hemochromatosis. *J Comput Assist Tomgr* 14: 774–776, 1990.

34. Kelekis N, Semelka RC, Burdeny DA: Dark ring sign: Finding in patients with fungal liver lesions undergoing treatment with antifungal antibiotics. *Magn Reson Imaging* 14: 615–618, 1996.

35. Warshauer DM, Semelka RC, Ascher SM: Nodular sarcoidosis of the liver and spleen: Appearance on MR images. *J Magn Reson Imaging* 4: 553–557, 1994.

36. Sagoh T, Hoh K, Togashi K, et al.: Gamna-Gandy bodies of the spleen: Evaluation with MR imaging. *Radiology* 172: 685–687, 1989.

37. Minami M, Itai Y, Ohtomo K, et al.: Siderotic nodules in the spleen: MR imaging of portal hypertension. *Radiology* 172: 681–684, 1989.

GASTROINTESTINAL TRACT

RICHARD C. SEMELKA, M.D., MONICA S. PEDRO, M.D.,
DIANE ARMAO, M.D., HANI B. MARCOS, M.D.
AND SUSAN M. ASCHER, M.D.

I hav finally kum to the konklusion,
that a good reliable sett ov bowels
iz wurth more tu a man, than enny
quantity ov brains.

Josh Billings
(early American aphorism)

Breath-hold SGE sequences, fat-suppressed T1-weighted sequences, and single-shot echo-train T2-weighted sequences, combined with intravenous gadolinium chelates, have resulted in consistent image quality of the gastrointestinal tract. These techniques arrest bowel motion, remove competing high signal of intra-abdominal fat, expand the dynamic range of abdominal tissue signal intensities, decrease susceptibility artifacts, and distinguish between intraluminal bowel contents and bowel wall [1]. Currently, the role of oral contrast agents remains uncertain. Direct multiplanar imaging has achieved an important role in distinguishing the bowel, which shows tubular configuration in at least one of two planes, from masses, which do not. Current applications of gastrointestinal MRI include 1) distinguishing type and severity of inflammatory bowel disease (IBD) [1–6]; 2) identifying enteric abscesses and fistulae [7, 8]; 3) preoperative staging of malignant neoplasms, especially rectal carcinoma [5, 9, 10]; and 4) dif-

ferentiating postoperative and radiation therapy changes from recurrent carcinoma [11–16].

THE ESOPHAGUS

Normal Anatomy

The organization of tissues within the esophageal wall follows the general scheme of the entire digestive tract, namely (from lumen outward), the mucosa with an epithelial lining, submucosa, muscularis externa (propria) with an inner circular and outer longitudinal muscle layer, and, below the level of the diaphragm, mesothelium-lined serosa instead of adventitia. Except for that portion of the esophagus in the peritoneal cavity, the rest is covered by a layer of loose connective tissue, or adventitia, which blends into surrounding tissue. The lack of a serosal surface explains the rapid spread of esophageal cancer into adjacent mediastinal fat. The esophagus lies posterior to the trachea in the neck. As it enters the thoracic inlet, the esophagus courses toward the left to reside in the posterior mediastinum. The esophagus then enters the abdomen via the diaphragmatic esophageal hiatus and lies immediately anterior

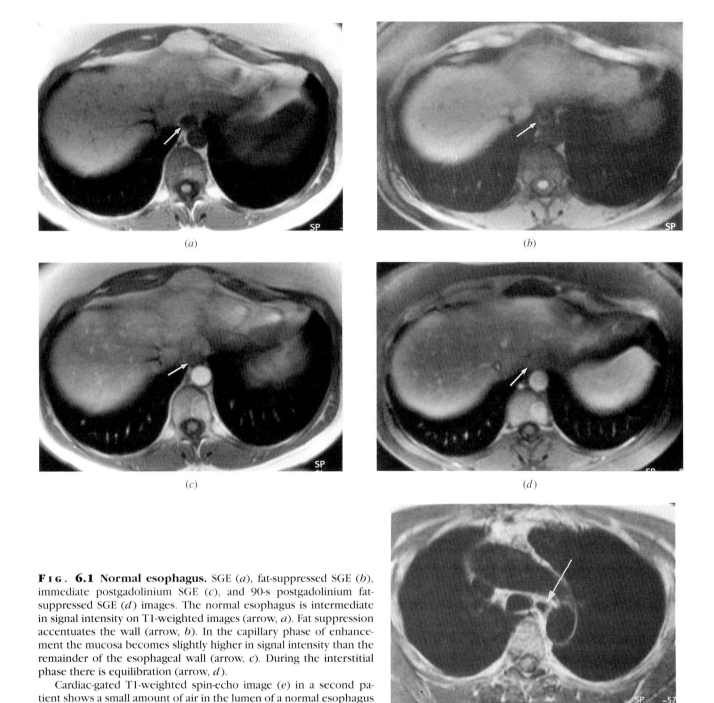

FIG. 6.1 Normal esophagus. SGE (*a*), fat-suppressed SGE (*b*), immediate postgadolinium SGE (*c*), and 90-s postgadolinium fat-suppressed SGE (*d*) images. The normal esophagus is intermediate in signal intensity on T1-weighted images (arrow, *a*). Fat suppression accentuates the wall (arrow, *b*). In the capillary phase of enhancement the mucosa becomes slightly higher in signal intensity than the remainder of the esophageal wall (arrow, *c*). During the interstitial phase there is equilibration (arrow, *d*).

Cardiac-gated T1-weighted spin-echo image (*e*) in a second patient shows a small amount of air in the lumen of a normal esophagus (arrow, *e*).

to the aorta. The normal esophageal wall thickness is 3 mm. On cross-sectional images the esophagus tends to be collapsed, although a small amount of air in the lumen is not abnormal.

MRI Technique

Techniques that have been used for MRI of the esophagus include fat saturation, gadolinium enhancement, and cardiac gating (fig. 6.1). The difficulty with T1-weighted ECG-gated fat-suppressed spin-echo imaging is that the sequence is lengthy and the image quality is inconsistent because of the combination of phase artifacts from breathing, patient motion, and cardiac pulsation. The esophagus, therefore, of all bowel segments, suffers the most from image artifacts and uniquely experiences artifacts from cardiac pulsation resulting in severe artifacts on SGE sequences, which form an important component

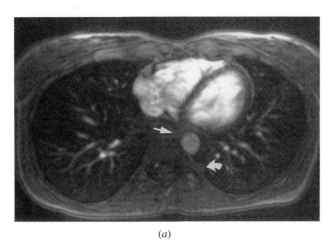
(a)

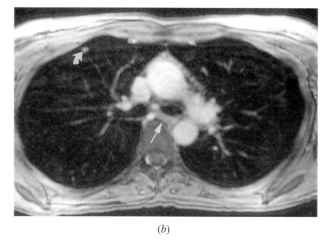
(b)

F I G . 6.2 Normal esophagus. Transverse gadolinium-enhanced 3D gradient-echo (*a* and *b*) images in two different patients. On the gadolinium-enhanced 3D images the esophagus is well shown (short arrow, *a*, *b*) and is free of cardiac motion artifact. Note also a subtle pleural-based density along the posterior left hemithorax in *a* (curved arrow, *a*) and pulmonary metastasis in *b* (curved arrow, *b*).

of imaging protocols of other bowel segments. As such, until the present time, MRI has not achieved a role for imaging the esophagus. The lack of a role for MR imaging of the esophagus may now be changing, because it has recently been observed that gadolinium-enhanced 3D gradient echo (also termed VIBE) results in minimal artifact in the thorax and consistent display of the esophagus (fig. 6.2). This sequence has the further important feature of being short duration.

Congenital Lesions

Duplication Cysts

Gastrointestinal duplication cysts may occur throughout the alimentary tube. The cysts occur in or adjacent to the wall of a portion of the gastrointestinal tract, and, although they are lined by epithelium, it may not be of the same histologic type as that of the involved segment. Duplication cysts usually are discovered in childhood or infancy secondary to mass effect and/or infection resulting from intestinal stasis combined with bowel communication [17]. Patients may also present later in life with peptic ulcers or pancreatitis if the cysts contain gastric or pancreatic epithelium, respectively. In the esophagus they tend to be small, ovoid, fluid-filled structures in the lower one-third of the esophagus located posteriorly in a periesophageal location or within the esophageal wall. Cysts have variable signal intensity on T1-weighted images, depending on the concentration of mucin or protein within them. Duplication cysts are generally high in signal intensity on T2-weighted images [18]. The cyst wall enhances after intravenous gadolinium administration, whereas the fluid-filled lumen does not enhance and may appear near signal void. Relatively intense cyst wall enhancement may reflect the presence of gastric mucosa or inflammatory changes.

Mass Lesions

Benign Masses

Leiomyomas. Leiomyomas are the most common benign tumors of the esophagus. These tumors are composed of smooth muscle and arise from the muscularis externa. They most frequently occur in the distal esophagus and may be single or multiple [19, 20]. Esophageal leiomyomas appear as small, oval masses that may be pedunculated on MRI images. They are often close to isointensity with surrounding bowel wall on T1- and T2-weighted images; however, with gadolinium, leiomyomas will enhance in a uniform fashion and to a greater degree than adjacent bowel wall in the interstitial phase of enhancement. (fig. 6.3).

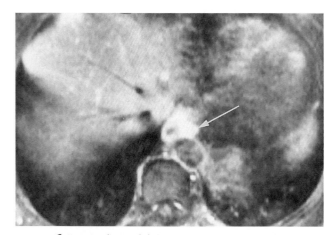

F I G . 6.3 Esophageal leiomyoma. Gadolinium-enhanced T1-weighted fat-suppressed spin-echo image shows a 2-cm leiomyoma (arrow) arising from the lateral aspect of the distal esophagus. Leiomyomas are the most common benign tumors of the esophagus. (Reprinted with permission from Shoenut JP, Semelka RC, Silverman R, Yaffe CS, Mickflikier AB: The gastrointestinal tract. In Semelka RC, Shoenut JP (eds.), *MRI of the Abdomen with CT Correlation*. New York: Raven Press, p. 119–143, 1993.)

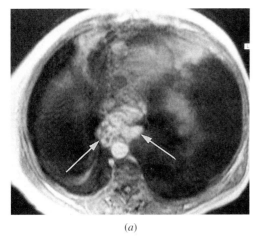
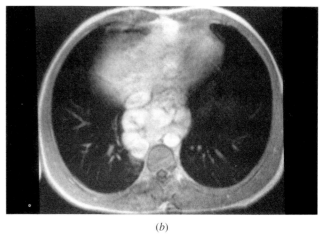

(a)   (b)

F I G . 6.4 Esophageal varices. Transverse 45-s postgadolinium SGE image (*a*) in a patient with portal hypertension. Enhancing serpiginous tubular structures (arrows) in the lower esophagus represent varices.

Transverse gadolinium-enhanced T1-weighted SGE (*b*) image in a second patient with congenital hepatic fibrosis demonstrates massive esophageal varices.

Varices. Varices, or tortuous, dilated submucosal veins, develop in the setting of portal hypertension or splenic vein thrombosis. They occur along the lower esophagus, the stomach, and other locations with portosystemic communications. Varices can be demonstrated as signal-void tubular structures on spin-echo images, high-signal intensity structures on 2D time-of-flight (TOF) MR angiography (MRA), or enhancing serpiginous structures on dynamic 2D or 3D gadolinium-enhanced SGE or fat-suppressed SGE images (fig. 6.4). The most consistent display of varices in bowel is on gadolinium-enhanced fat-suppressed SGE images acquired 2 min after gadolinium administration, although esophageal varices may benefit from imaging with gadolinium-enhanced 3D gradient echo.

Malignant Masses

Before 1975, squamous cell carcinoma accounted for 95% of all cases of esophagus cancer. Since that time there has been a marked increase in the incidence of adenocarcinomas among esophagus cancers. At the present time, the overall relative incidence of squamous cell carcinoma and adenocarcinoma is about equal in the United States [21].

The etiology of squamous cell carcinoma is unknown, but there is an association with alcohol consumption and tobacco use [22]. It occurs more commonly in males (3 to 1) and African-Americans [23]. Primary adenocarcinoma of the esophagus may arise de novo in Barrett esophagus, or it may arise in the stomach and cross the gastroesophageal junction to involve the distal esophagus and simulate achalasia [24]. It is more common in Caucasian males. Tumors that commonly metastasize to the esophagus include breast and lung carcinoma and melanoma. Gadolinium-enhanced fat-

suppressed SGE technique delineates primary tumors of the distal esophagus, whereas cardiac gating is useful to image midesophageal cancers posterior to the heart (fig. 6.5) [25]. Squamous cell cancers (see fig. 6.5) and adenocarcinomas (fig. 6.6) appear similar on MR images. Predisposing factors or tumor location may aid in making this distinction. The success of MRI in staging esophageal cancer has been inconsistent, reflecting the variable image quality of breathing-averaged, cardiac-gated sequences [26, 27]. At present, there is no reported series describing the use of gadolinium-enhanced 3D gradient echo in the evaluation of esophageal cancers. This may prove to be the most consistent MR technique to investigate these tumors. The combined use of fat suppression and intravenous gadolinium may facilitate identification of mediastinal involvement. The presence of multiple (>5) paraesophageal normal-sized lymph nodes is worrisome for tumor involvement; however, accurate determination awaits the use of contrast agents that can define the presence of tumor in normal-sized lymph nodes. A comprehensive exam for staging patients with esophageal carcinoma should include a metastatic survey of the liver.

Metastases to the esophagus may appear indistinguishable from a primary esophageal tumor, and clinical history helps to establish the diagnosis (fig. 6.7).

Inflammatory and Infectious Disorders

Reflux Esophagitis

Gastroesophageal reflux is defined as the retrograde flow of gastric and sometimes duodenal contents into the esophagus. In general, reflux esophagitis refers to esophageal inflammation resulting from gastroesophageal reflux. Reflux esophagitis may result from several

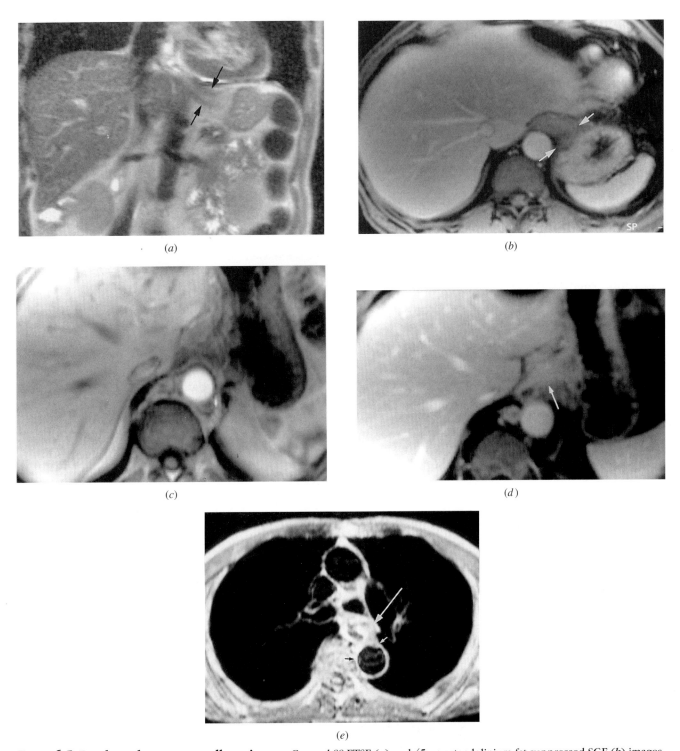

F I G . 6.5 Esophageal squamous cell carcinoma. Coronal SS-ETSE (*a*) and 45-s postgadolinium fat-suppressed SGE (*b*) images. Increased thickness of the distal esophagus is present on the precontrast image (arrows, *a*). The squamous cell carcinoma of the distal esophagus is clearly defined, and tumor is shown to extend to the gastroesophageal junction (arrows, *b*). Lack of extension into the stomach is well shown by demonstration of normal-enhancing higher-signal gastric mucosa.

Transverse immediate postgadolinium T1-weighted SGE (*c*) and interstitial-phase gadolinium-enhanced fat-suppressed SGE (*d*) images in a second patient demonstrate a mass lesion centered in the region of the gastroesophageal junction (arrow, *d*) consistent with distal esophageal squamous cell carcinoma.

Gadolinium-enhanced gated T1-weighted spin-echo image (*e*) in a third patient with squamous cell carcinoma of the midesophagus. A 2-cm cancer (arrow, *e*) is present that shows heterogeneous extension into the aortic wall (small arrows, *e*).

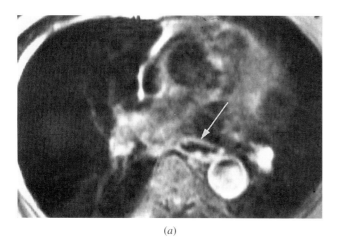

(a)

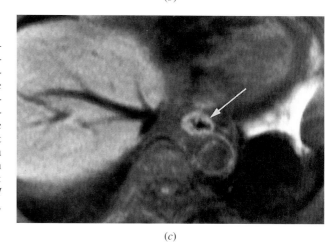

(b)

FIG. 6.6 Esophageal adenocarcinoma. Gadolinium-enhanced T1-weighted fat-suppressed (*a, b*) and T1-weighted fat-suppressed (*c*) spin-echo images in a patient with esophageal adenocarcinoma. Above the tumor at the level of the midthorax, the esophagus has a normal-appearing thin wall (arrow, *a*). More inferiorly at the level of the mitral valve, a 2.5-cm tumor (long arrow, *b*) is identified in the esophagus. Note the interface of the tumor with the descending aorta (*a, b*) is less than 90° (short arrow, *b*). Below the tumor, the esophagus once again has a normal thin wall (arrow, *c*). (Reprinted with permission from Shoenut JP, Semelka RC, Silverman R, Yaffe CS, Mickflikier AB: The gastrointestinal tract. In Semelka RC, Shoenut JP (eds.), *MRI of the Abdomen with CT Correlation*. New York: Raven Press, p. 119–143, 1993.)

(c)

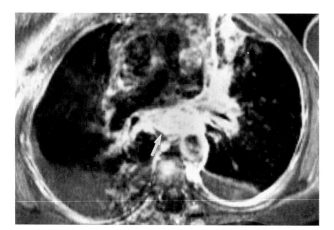

FIG. 6.7 Esophageal metastases. Gadolinium-enhanced T1-weighted fat-suppressed image in a woman with metastatic breast carcinoma. Enhancing tumor (arrow) encases the esophagus and extends along the left hilum and left mediastinum and invades the chest wall. (Reprinted with permission from Shoenut JP, Semelka RC, Silverman R, Yaffe CS, Mickflikier AB: The gastrointestinal tract. In Semelka RC, Shoenut JP (eds.), *MRI of the Abdomen with CT Correlation*. New York: Raven Press, p. 119–143, 1993.)

disease entities and/or their treatments: hiatal hernia, achalasia, and scleroderma. Gastroesophageal reflux is common in the setting of hiatal hernia. (For a more complete discussion of hiatal hernia, see Chapter 7, *Peritoneal Cavity*.) Achalasia is a primary esophageal disorder, which results in failure of relaxation of the lower esophageal sphincter (LES) coupled with nonperistaltic esophageal contractions. Balloon dilation of the LES is the mainstay of treatment and may lead to reflux esophagitis. Scleroderma involvement of the esophagus results in a patulous gastroesophageal junction with substantial reflux of gastric contents. In all of these conditions, MRI demonstrates a thickened esophageal wall, and, after the administration of gadolinium, the inflamed wall shows marked enhancement (fig. 6.8).

Radiation Esophagitis

Patients undergoing radiation therapy to the thorax are at risk of developing radiation damage to the esophagus. In the early period, 4–6 weeks after treatment, mucosal edema may be seen. Approximately 6–8 months after treatment, strictures may begin to develop.

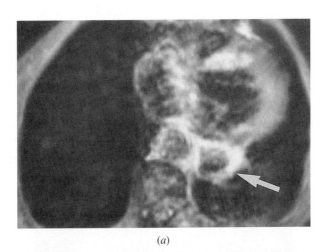

(a)

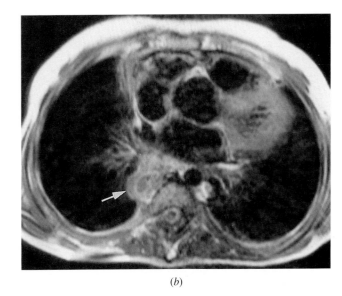

(b)

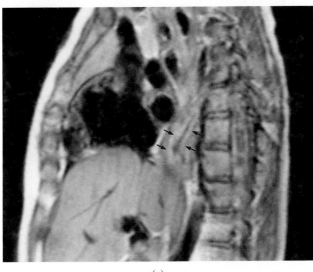

(c)

F I G . 6.8 Reflux esophagitis. Gadolinium-enhanced T1-weighted fat-suppressed spin-echo (a), gadolinium-enhanced gated transverse (b), and sagittal (c) T1-weighted spin-echo images in two different patients (a) and (b, c) with reflux esophagitis. In a patient with achalasia (a), balloon dilation for achalasia predisposes to reflux esophagitis. The esophagus appears dilated, and the wall is thickened with increased mural enhancement. The esophagus in a second patient with reflux esophagitis due to hiatal hernia shows increased thickness of the esophageal wall (arrow, b) and increased signal intensity of the mucosa. The superior extent of inflamed mucosa (small arrows, c) is well shown on the sagittal image (c).

Corrosive Esophagitis

Ingestion of caustic material such as strong alkaline or acidic agents or very hot liquids may cause esophagitis. Damage to tissue is most severe after ingestion of strongly alkaline agents. These substances cause a liquefactive necrosis that penetrates the entire esophageal wall rapidly. Acute changes include edema and ulceration. Stricture formation occurs later, and there is a strong association between corrosive stricture and the development of carcinoma.

Infectious Disease

Esophageal infection by *Candida albicans*, cytomegalovirus (CMV), and herpes simplex virus (HSV) is observed with increasing frequency. This reflects the large numbers of immunocompromised patients. Bone marrow transplant, chemotherapy, acquired immunodeficiency syndrome (AIDS), administration of exoge-nous steroids, and blood dyscrasias predispose to infection by *Candida albicans* a fungus that may occur normally in the esophagus. Infection is diffuse, with white-colored plaques coating the mucosa. The mucosa becomes friable, and ulceration results. MRI demonstrates a high-signal intensity thickened esophageal wall on T2-weighted images. Hyperemia and capillary leakage account for the marked enhancement after intravenous gadolinium injection (fig. 6.9).

THE STOMACH

Normal Anatomy

The stomach serves two important functions: It is a reservoir for ingested food and a mixer for their mechanical and chemical breakdown. Although the stomach is typically J-shaped and resides in the posterior aspect

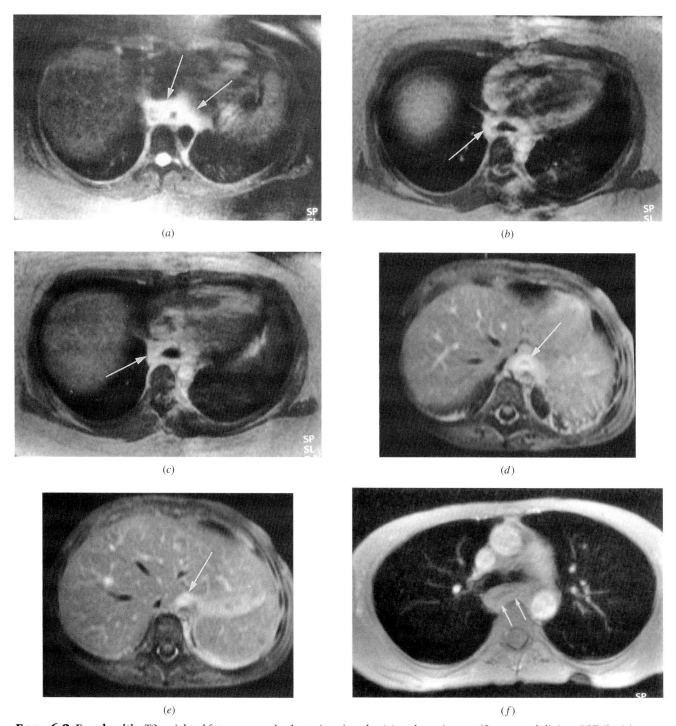

F I G . 6.9 Esophagitis. T2-weighted fat-suppressed echo-train spin-echo (*a*) and contiguous 45-s postgadolinium SGE (*b*, *c*) images in a patient with AIDS and esophageal candidiasis. The high signal intensity on the T2-weighted images reflects both the fungal plaques that coat the esophagus as well as the underlying inflamed wall (arrows, *a*). After contrast, the thickened esophageal wall enhances (arrow, *b*, *c*).

Gadolinium-enhanced T1-weighted fat-suppressed spin-echo images (*d*, *e*) in a second immunocompromised patient with acute myelogenous leukemia on chemotherapy. Capillary leakage associated with inflammation leads to marked mucosal enhancement (arrow, *d*, *e*) in this patient with *Candida albicans* esophageal invasion.

Transverse gadolinium-enhanced SGE (*f*) image in a third patient who has AIDS and dysphagia shows diffuse esophageal wall thickening (arrows, *f*) consistent with inflammatory changes.

of the left upper quadrant, its position varies with degree of distension and body habitus. Gross inspection shows four anatomic regions: cardia, fundus, body, and antrum. The antrum ends at the pylorus, from the Greek "pylorus" or gatekeeper, a narrow channel that connects the stomach to the duodenum. The stomach's curved morphology also gives rise to a greater (caudal) and a lesser (cephalic) curvature in addition to anterior and posterior walls. Four distinct layers comprise the stomach wall: mucosa, submucosa, muscularis, and serosa. Subdivisions exist within each layer. The mucosa is composed of distinct populations of endocrine and exocrine cells. The muscularis externa has three different muscle groups: inner oblique, middle circular, and outer longitudinal.

MRI Technique

Imaging the stomach achieves best results with distension and hypotonia. MRI examinations of the stomach may benefit from administering water in an approximate volume of 1 liter and intravenous glucagon, with 0.5 mg given immediately before the start of the examination and 0.5 mg before the administration of gadolinium [28]. A recommended imaging protocol includes 1) T1-weighted fat-suppressed SGE imaging before and after intravenous gadolinium, 2) unenhanced T1-weighted SGE imaging, and 3) T2-weighted single-shot echo-train spin-echo [e.g., half-Fourier single-shot turbo spin-echo (HASTE) imaging; fig. 6.10]. Gastric mucosa enhances more intensely than other bowel mucosa after intravenous gadolinium [29]. This observation may be helpful for the detection of gastric mucosa-lined duplication cyst or Meckel diverticulum.

Congenital Lesions

Congenital lesions, except for hypertrophic pyloric stenosis, are rare in the stomach.

Gastric Duplication Cysts

Gastric duplication cysts account for <4% of duplications of the gastrointestinal tract. They occur along the greater curvature and are more common in females. Occasionally, gastric duplication cysts calcify, and in 15% the cysts communicate with the gastric lumen. Although gastric duplication cysts are uncommon, they are important to recognize because 35% of these patients will have other congenital anomalies [30].

Congenital Heterotopias

Congenital heterotopias result from cellular entrapment during the morphogenic movements throughout embryogenesis. Pancreatic rests occur throughout the alimentary tract but are most common along the greater curvature or posterior antral wall of the stomach. Heterotopic pancreas usually appears as a solitary, submucosal globoid mass with a central nipplelike structure representing ductal openings into the gastric lumen [31].

Congenital Diverticula

Congenital diverticula may also be demonstrated in the stomach (fig. 6.11) [28]. Gastric diverticula are rare, and >75% of them occur in a juxtacardiac position high on the posterior wall of the stomach, approximately 2 cm below the esophagogastric junction and 3 cm from the lesser curvature of the stomach. [32]. Congenital diverticula are characterized as solitary, well-defined, oval or pear-shaped pouches that communicate with the gastric

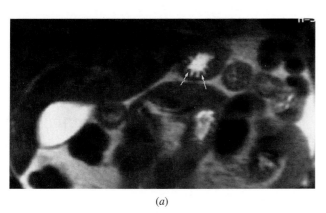

(a)

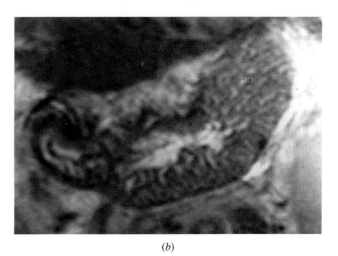

(b)

F I G . 6.10 Normal Stomach. Coronal T2-weighted SS-ETSE (*a* and *b*), coronal (*c*), and transverse (*d*) interstitial-phase gadolinium-enhanced fat-suppressed SGE images in four different patients with a normal stomach. T2-weighted SS-ETSE is well suited for imaging the rugal folds (arrows, *a*). After intravenous contrast the stomach wall shows marked enhancement (arrow, *c*, *d*). The normal gastroesophageal junction (arrowhead, *c*) is frequently well defined by imaging in transverse and coronal planes. Optimal stomach ("s," *d*) distention was obtained after ingestion of a negative oral contrast agent.

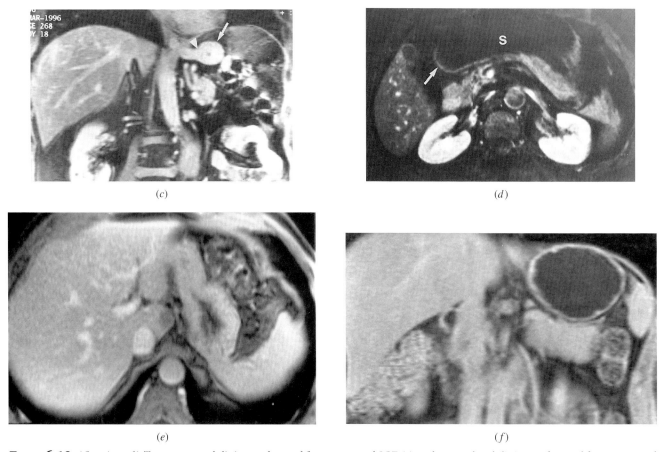

(c)

(d)

(e)

(f)

F i g . 6.10 (*Continued*) Transverse gadolinium-enhanced fat-suppressed SGE (*e*) and coronal gadolinium-enhanced fat-suppressed SGE (*f*) images in a another patient before and after water ingestion. Optimal gastric distention can also be achieved with water.

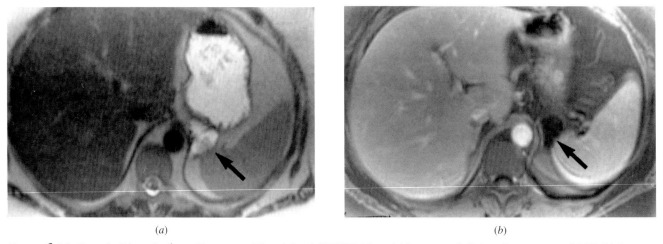

(a)

(b)

F i g . 6.11 Gastric Diverticulum. Transverse T2-weighted SS-ETSE (*a*) and 90-s postgadolinium fat-suppressed SGE (*b*) images. A small cystic thin-walled mass (arrow, *a*) is shown, which is high signal intensity and intimately related to the posterior aspect of cardiac portion of the stomach. On the 90-s postgadolinium image (*b*) the diverticulum appears signal void with a thin enhancing wall (arrow, *b*). (Reprinted with permission from Marcos HB, Semelka RC: Stomach diseases: MR evaluation using combined T2-weighted single-shot echo train spin-echo and gadolinium-enhanced spoiled gradient-echo sequences. *J Magn Reson Imaging* 10: 950–960, 1999.)

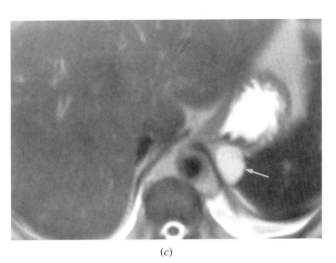
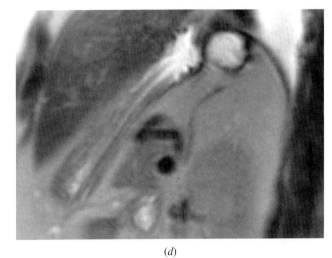

(c)   (d)

F ɪ ɢ . 6.11 (*Continued*) Transverse (*c*) and sagittal (*d*) T2-weighted SS-ETSE in a second patient. A small posterior gastric diverticulum (arrow, *c*) is seen in the fundus of the stomach.

lumen via a narrow or broad-based opening [33]. The clinical presentation depends on location, size, type of mucosa of the diverticulum, and presence or absence of communication with the stomach.

Mass Lesions

Benign Masses

Polyps. Gastric polyps may be hyperplastic, adenomatous, or hamartomatous. They may be isolated findings or associated with a polyposis syndrome. Eighty to ninety percent of gastric polyps are hyperplastic and benign, whereas approximately 10 percent are adenomatous. Hyperplastic polyps are nonneoplastic lesions that result from an exaggerated regenerative response to injury, namely, ulcers, gastroenterostomy stomas, or a background of chronic gastritis. In contrast to hyperplastic polyps, adenomatous polyps are true neoplasms, morphologically similar to those seen in the colon. Microscopic features show close-packed glandular structures lined by neoplastic cells with cytologic atypia. Approximately one-third of adenomatous polyps contain a focus of adenocarcinoma [34]. Malignant potential is related to size, with up to 46% of adenomas >2 cm containing carcinoma [35]. Both hyperplastic and adenomatous polyps are found in patients with chronic atrophic gastritis and Gardner and familial polyposis syndromes, conditions associated with an increased incidence of malignancy. (For a more complete discussion on polyposis syndromes, see the section on the large intestine later in this chapter.) Although most polyps are asymptomatic, anemia related to chronic blood loss, iron deficiency, or malabsorption of vitamin B12 may be present. Hamartomatous gastric polyps refer to lesions produced by excessive, disorganized overgrowth of ma-

ture normal cells and tissues indigenous to the stomach. Hamartomatous polyps may be an isolated finding or can occur in patients with Peutz-Jeghers syndrome. Although both isolated hamartomatous polyps and those associated with Peutz-Jeghers syndrome are benign lesions, patients with Peutz-Jeghers syndrome have an increased risk of developing carcinomas of the gastrointestinal tract, pancreas, breast, lung, ovary, and uterus.

Benign polyps are generally isointense with the gastric wall on unenhanced MR images. Adequate distension of the stomach is mandatory to distinguish a polyp from a prominent rugal fold. Benign polyp enhancement is usually isointense to slightly hyperintense compared with normal gastric mucosa on early postgadolinium images and mildly hyperintense on 2-min postgadolinium images, reflecting retention of contrast in the interstitial space (fig. 6.12). In polyps complicated by invasive adenocarcinoma, more heterogeneous gadolinium enhancement and disruption of the underlying gastric wall may be observed.

Leiomyomas. Leiomyomas are the most common benign nonepithelial tumors of the stomach. They arise from the smooth muscle of the gastric wall. They may grow inward toward the lumen and mimic a polyp or extend to the serosa and present as an exophytic mass. When large, the overlying gastric mucosa may ulcerate, leading to gastrointestinal bleeding. Other mesenchymal gastric wall elements may give rise to benign neoplasms: fibromas, hemangiomas, lipomas, and neurogenic tumors. Except for lipomas, these mesenchymal tumors are indistinguishable from each other on MRI. Similar to fatty lesions elsewhere in the body, lipomas will be high in signal intensity on T1-weighted images and decrease in signal intensity on fat-suppressed images.

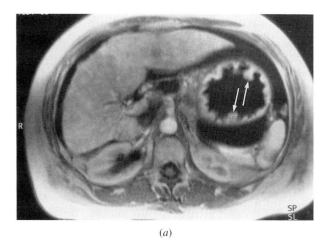

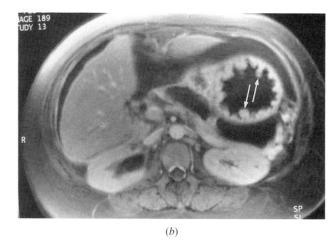

(a)   *(b)*

FIG. 6.12 Gastric polyps. Immediate postgadolinium SGE (*a*) and 90-s postgadolinium fat-suppressed SGE (*b*) images in a patient with Gardner syndrome demonstrate multiple enhancing gastric polyps (arrows, *a, b*). The polyps possess intense enhancement.

Varices. Portal hypertension and splenic vein thrombosis lead to gastric varices. Varices restricted to the short gastric veins along the greater curvature of the stomach should raise the suspicion of splenic vein thrombosis (fig. 6.13).

Bezoar. The word bezoar derives from the Arabic "bazahr" or "badzeahr," meaning antidote. Bezoars were valued for their medicinal qualities and were thought to be imbued with magical powers and to be effective antidotes for poisoning [36].

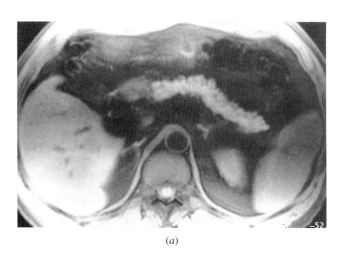

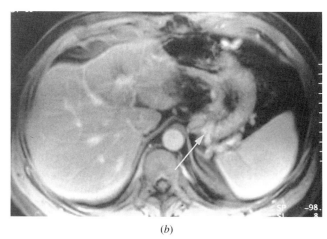

(a)   *(b)*

FIG. 6.13 Gastric varices. Fat-suppressed SGE (*a*) and 90-s post-gadolinium fat-suppressed SGE (*b*) images. No splenic vein is identified posterior to the pancreas (*a*). After intravenous gadolinium administration (*b*), gastric varices enhance. These veins are part of the portosystemic circulation that are recruited to provide alternative venous channels in the presence of splenic vein thrombosis. A prominent varix is identified in the gastric wall (arrow, *b*).

Transverse interstitial-phase gadolinium-enhanced fat-suppressed SGE image (*c*) in a second patient with hepatic cirrhosis. Large-caliber varices (arrow, *b*) are seen within the posterior wall stomach, immediately distal to the GE junction.

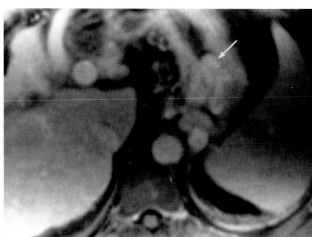

(c)

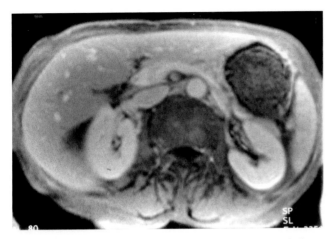

F I G . 6.14 Gastric bezoar. Transverse interstitial-phase gadolinium-enhanced fat-suppressed SGE image. The stomach is distended and filled with debris, which demonstrates a rounded configuration that represents a bezoar.

The term bezoar is used to refer to an intragastric mass composed of accumulated ingested material. It may be composed of hair (trichobezoar), fruit or vegetable products (phytobezoar), or concretions such as resins, asphalt, or other material. Factors that predispose to bezoar development include psychiatric illness, lack of teeth, previous vagotomy or gastric surgery, and diseases such as diabetes and muscular dystrophies. Altered gastric motility or anatomy that causes retention of material in the stomach underlies most of the risk factors (fig. 6.14).

Malignant Masses

Carcinoma is the most important and the most common tumor of the stomach. Most gastric carcinomas are adenocarcinomas [37].

Adenocarcinoma. The incidence of gastric adenocarcinoma is on the decline. At present, 22,800 Americans are diagnosed with gastric cancer each year [38]. Males are affected twice as often as females. Predisposing conditions include atrophic gastritis, pernicious anemia, adenomatous polyps, dietary nitrates, and Japanese heritage [39, 40]. The tumors show a predilection for the lesser curvature of the antropyloric region. Grossly, adenocarcinomas of the stomach can be divided generally into three forms: 1) exophytic or polypoid, projecting into the lumen; 2) ulcerated, with a shallow or deeply erosive crater; and 3) diffusely infiltrative. The last-named form of adenocarcinoma creates a rigid, thickened "leather" stomach wall termed linitis plastica carcinoma. Gastric cancer may spread hematogenously to the liver and lung, contiguously to adjacent organs, lymphatically to regional and remote lymph nodes, and/or intraperitoneally to the abdominal lining, mesentery, and

Table 6.1 TNM Staging for Cancer of the Stomach

T—Primary tumor

Tx	Primary tumor cannot be assessed
T0	No evidence of primary tumor
Tis	Preinvasive carcinoma (carcinoma in situ)
T1	Tumor limited to the mucosa or mucosa and submucosa regardless of extent and location
T2	Tumor with deep infiltration occupying not more than one-half of one region
T3	Tumor with deep infiltration occupying more than one-half but not more than of one region
T4	Tumor with deep infiltration occupying more than one-half but not more than one region or extending to neighboring structures

N—Regional lymph nodes

Nx	Regional lymph nodes cannot be assessed
N0	No evidence of regional lymph node metastasis
N1	Metastasis in lymph node(s) within 3 cm of the primary tumor along the greater or lesser curvatures
N2	Evidence of lymph node metastasis more than 3 cm from the primary tumor including those along the left gastric, splenic, celliac, and common hepatic arteries
N3	Evidence of involvement of the para-aortic and hepatodu-odenal lymph nodes and/or other intra-abdominal lymph nodes

M—Metastases

Mx	Distant metastases cannot be assessed
M0	No distant metastases
M1	Distant metastases

serosa. The overall prognosis is poor. A TNM system is used for staging (Table 6.1).

Early in the disease, symptoms are vague and include dyspepsia, anorexia, and weight loss. Later, vomiting and hematemesis may occur in association with a palpable epigastric mass and anemia. The goals of MRI in patients with gastric cancer is to demonstrate the primary tumor, assess the depth of invasion, and detect extragastric disease. Adequate distension is necessary for surveying the gastric wall. On T1-weighted sequences, gastric adenocarcinoma is isointense to normal stomach and may be apparent as focal wall thickening. On T2-weighted images, tumors usually are slightly higher in signal intensity than adjacent normal stomach [41].

An important observation on gadolinium-enhancement MRI images is that collapsed normal gastric wall enhances identically to the remainder of the wall on early and late postgadolinium images (fig. 6.15), whereas tumors show more heterogeneous enhancement that may be decreased or increased relative to the gastric wall on early, late, or both sets of images [28].

Tumors that originate in the cardia (fig. 6.16), body (fig. 6.17), antrum (fig. 6.18), and pylorus (fig. 6.19) are

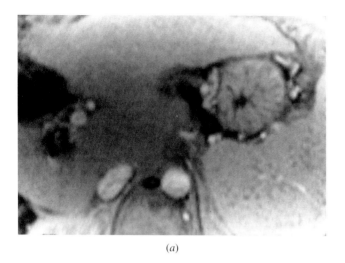

(a)

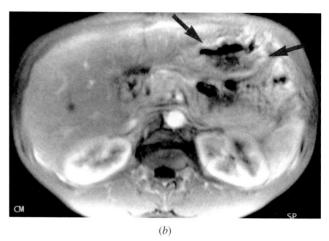

(b)

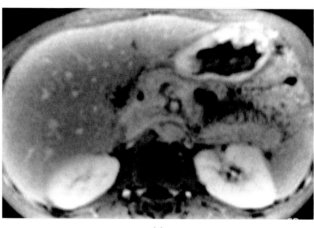

(c)

F I G . 6.15 Comparison between normal collapsed gastric wall and tumor. Transverse interstitial-phase gadolinium-enhanced fat-suppressed SGE (*a*) image in a normal patient. Note that the stomach is collapsed and the gastric wall enhancement is homogeneous. Note the symmetric radial fold pattern of the gastric rugae in the collapsed stomach.

Transverse immediate postgadolinium (*b*) and interstitial-phase gadolinium-enhanced fat-suppressed SGE (*c*) images in a second patient with gastric cancer show diffuse gastric wall thickening and heterogeneous enhancement of the gastric wall. (Reprinted with permission from Marcos HB, Semelka RC: Stomach diseases: MR evaluation using combined T2-weighted single-shot echo train spin-echo and gadolinium-enhanced spoiled gradient-echo sequences. *J Magn Reson Imaging* 10: 950–960, 1999.)

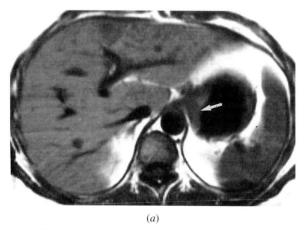

(a)

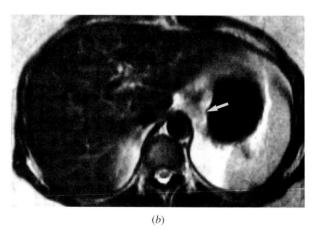

(b)

F I G . 6.16 Gastric adenocarcinoma, cardia. T1-weighted (*a*), T2-weighted (*b*), and gadolinium-enhanced Interstitial-phase T1-weighted fat-suppressed spin-echo (*c*, *d*) images in a patient with gastric cancer. The stomach has been distended with negative oral contrast agent. The gastric adenocarcinoma causes wall thickening medially, which is intermediate in signal intensity on the T1-weighted image (arrow, *a*) and heterogeneous and slightly hyperintense on the T2-weighted image (arrow, *b*). After intravenous gadolinium administration, the tumor (open arrows, *c*, *d*) enhances more than the normal stomach. The distal esophagus is also abnormally thickened with increased enhancement (arrowheads, *d*), which is consistent with spread across the gastroesophageal junction.

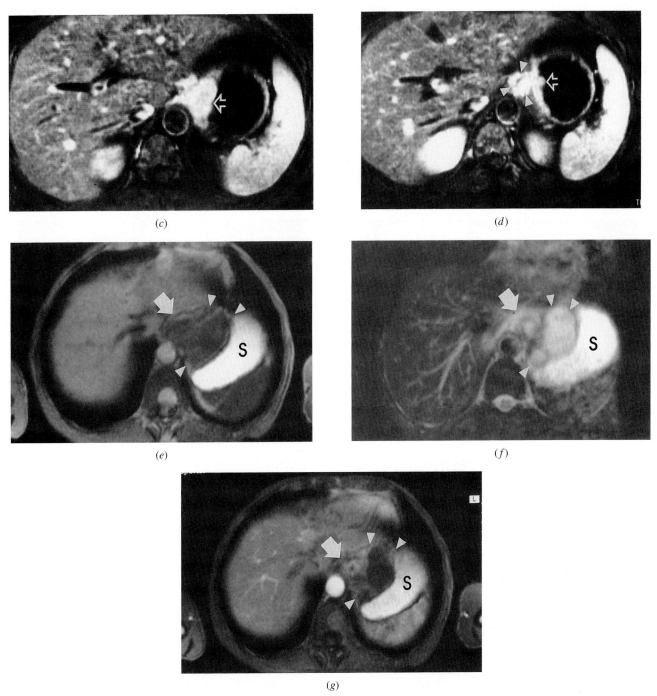

(c)   *(d)*

(e)   *(f)*

(g)

FIG. 6.16 *(Continued)* SGE (*e*), T2-weighted fat-suppressed echo-train spin-echo (*f*), and immediate postgadolinium SGE (*g*) images in a second patient. The stomach ("S," *e, f, g*) has been distended with a positive oral contrast agent. A large tumor in the cardia of the stomach (arrowheads, *e, f, g*) causes mass effect upon the lumen. The cancer is low in signal intensity on the T1-weighted image (*e*), heterogeneous and high in signal intensity on the T2-weighted image (*f*), and enhances heterogeneously after intravenous contrast (*g*). Note that the tumor also involves the distal esophagus (large arrow, *e, f, g*).

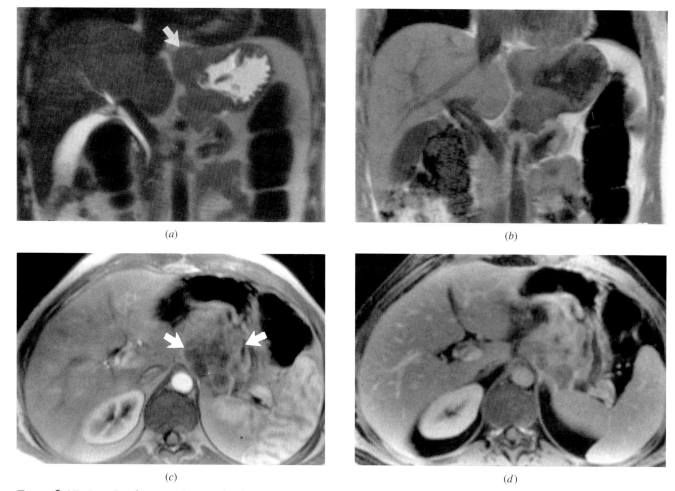

F I G . 6.17 Gastric adenocarcinoma, body. Coronal T2-weighted SS-ETSE (*a*), coronal precontrast SGE (*b*), transverse immediate postgadolinium SGE (*c*), and transverse 2-min postgadolinium fat-suppressed SGE (*d*) images. A circumferential low-signal intensity mass is demonstrated in the body of the stomach. The high-signal intensity fluid contents of the stomach permit good deliniation of the low-signal intensity mass on the T2-weighted SS-ETSE image (arrow, *a*). The mass is isointense to the stomach wall on precontrast T1-weighted image (*b*). On immediate postgadolinium images, the tumor (arrows, *c*) shows mild heterogeneous enhancement. On 2-min postgadolinium image (*d*), the tumor continues to enhance but to a lesser extent and heterogeneously compared to the remainder of the gastric wall. Note the intense enhancement of the normal renal cortex, which is greater than the enhancement of gastric wall or tumor. (Reprinted with permission from Marcos HB, Semelka RC: Stomach diseases: MR evaluation using combined T2-weighted single-shot echo train spin-echo and gadolinium-enhanced spoiled gradient-echo sequences. *J Magn Reson Imaging* 10: 950–960, 1999.)

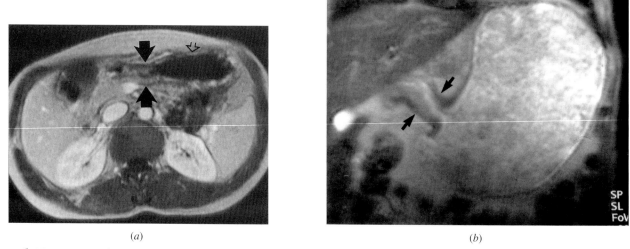

F I G . 6.18 Gastric adenocarcinoma, antrum. Transverse 45-s postgadolinium SGE image (*a*) demonstrates thickening and increased enhancement of the antrum secondary to gastric carcinoma (solid arrows, *a*). The remaining normal stomach has a thin wall (open arrow, *a*).

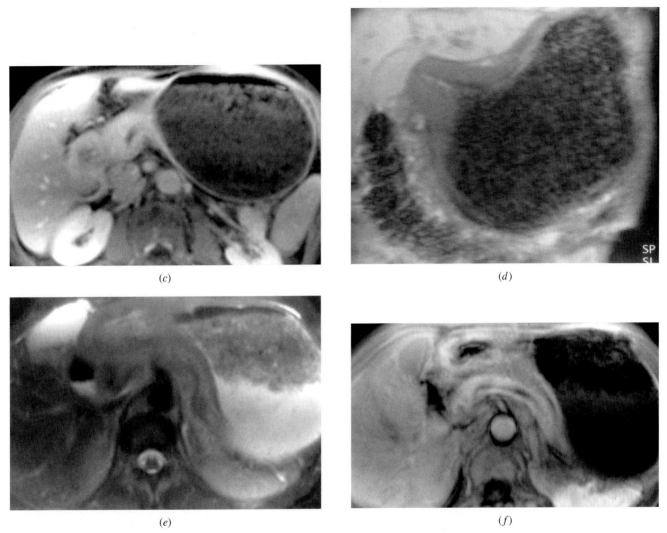

(c)

(d)

(e)

(f)

FIG. 6.18 (*Continued*) Coronal SS-ETSE (*b*) and transverse interstitial phase gadolinium-enhanced SGE (*c*) images in a second patient with antral tumor demonstrate a large, distended, debris-filled stomach secondary to gastric outlet obstuction. Note the substantial thickening (arrows, *b*) and increased enhancement with gadolinium (*c*) of the antrum.

Coronal (*d*) and transverse (*e*) T2-weighted SS-ETSE and transverse interstitial-phase gadolinium-enhanced fat-suppressed SGE (*f*) images in a third patient also show circumferential thickening and increased enhancement of the gastric antrum, with marked distension of the stomach.

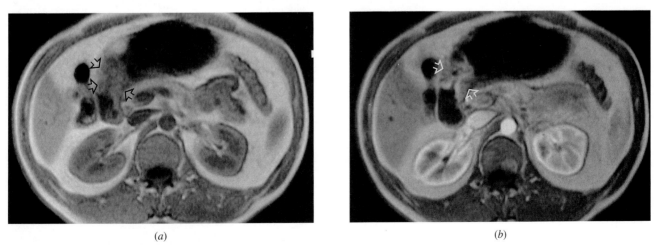

(a)

(b)

FIG. 6.19 **Gastric adenocarcinoma, pylorus.** SGE (*a*), 1-s (*b*) and 45-s (*c*) postgadolinium SGE, and interstitial-phase gadolinium-enhanced T1-weighted fat-suppressed spin-echo (*d*) images.

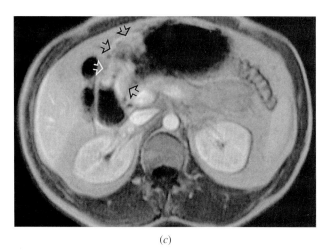

(c)

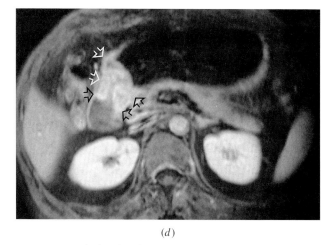

(d)

F I G . 6.19 (*Continued*) A circumferential pyloric channel adenocarcinoma with duodenal extension (arrows, *a–d*) is present. The tumor enhances heterogeneously (*b*) and increases in signal intensity on the 3-min interstitial-phase image (*d*). This reflects accumulation of contrast in the interstitial space of the tumor.

all well shown. Diffusely infiltrative carcinoma (linitis plastica carcinoma) tends to be lower in signal intensity than normal adjacent stomach on T2-weighted images because of its desmoplastic nature. Linitis plastica carcinoma enhances only modestly after intravenous contrast (fig. 6.20). In contradistinction, the other morpho-

logic types of gastric carcinoma enhance more intensely with intravenous gadolinium. Gadolinium-enhanced fat-suppressed SGE imaging aids in identification of transmural spread including peritoneal disease (fig. 6.21) and tumor involvement of lymph nodes. In vitro work with resected gastric cancer specimens at high field strength

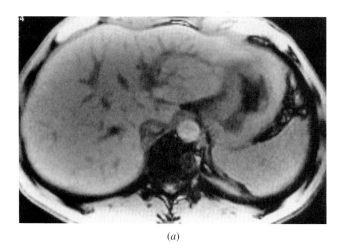

(a)

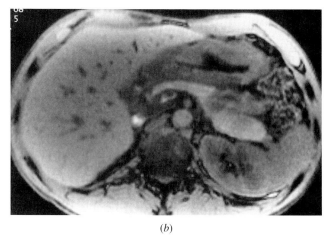

(b)

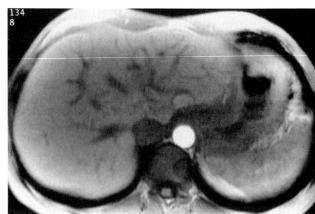

(c)

F I G . 6.20 Gastric adenocarcinoma, linitis plastica. Fat-suppressed SGE (*a, b*) and immediate postgadolinium SGE (*c*) images. Diffuse relatively homogeneous gastric wall thickening is present (*a, b*). Minimal enhancement is appreciated on the immediate postgadolinium SGE image (*c*).

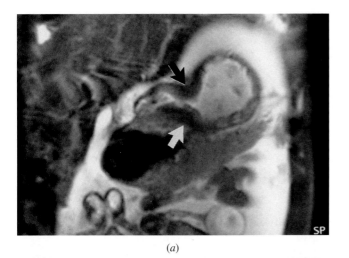

(a)

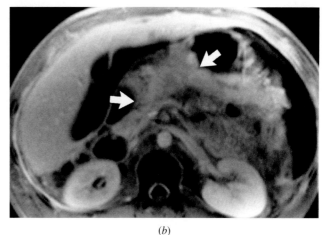

(b)

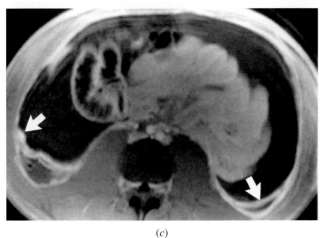

(c)

F I G . 6.21 Gastric adenocarcinoma with extensive carcinomatosis. Coronal T2-weighted SS-ETSE (*a*) and transverse 2-min postgadolinium fat-suppressed SGE images at more superior (*b*) and inferior (*c*) tomographic levels. Diffuse thickening of a low-signal intensity gastric wall is appreciated (arrows, *a*). Ascites is shown as high-signal intensity intraperitoneal fluid on the T2-weighted image (*a*). The gastric tumor (arrows, *b*) is mildly enhanced on the 2-min postgadolinium image (*b*) compared with gastric wall. At a lower tomographic level (*c*), intense peritoneal enhancement (arrows, *c*) with nodules is shown, representing peritoneal metastases. (Reprinted with permission from Marcos HB, Semelka RC: Stomach diseases: MR evaluation using combined T2-weighted single-shot echo train spin-echo and gadolinium-enhanced spoiled gradient-echo sequences. *J Magn Reson Imaging* 10: 950–960, 1999.)

has demonstrated mucosal, submucosal, and muscle invasion [41].

Metastases enhance conspicuously against a background of low-signal intensity fat. Detection of hepatic involvement is facilitated by T2-weighted fat-suppressed sequences and dynamic gadolinium-enhanced SGE techniques. This combined approach is superior to conventional CT imaging [42].

Marcos and Semelka reported on the detection and staging of gastric carcinoma [28]. In five of eight patients, focal, asymmetric gastric wall thickening or mass, consistent with gastric adenocarcinoma, was well demonstrated on MR evaluation. Failure of detection was related to small tumor size (<1–2 cm), lack of gastric distension, tumor enhancement similar to stomach wall, and tumoral isointensity on T2-weighted images. Staging accuracy was good, reflecting the adequate display of tumor and tumor extent on gadolinium-enhanced fat-suppressed SGE images.

Gastrointestinal Stromal Tumors (GIST). Gastrointestinal mesenchymal neoplasms can be divided into two broad categories, those that represent clear-cut diagnostic entities (such as leiomyomas and lipomas) and those that are difficult to classify into any specific cell lineage, that is, ultrastructural or immunohistochemical studies are not able to determine the histogenesis of the neoplastic cell population. The latter group of tumors falls into the category of gastrointestinal stromal tumors (GISTs). Although rare, GISTs most commonly occur in the stomach. All symptomatic GISTs are potentially malignant. These tumors are divided pathologically into lesions of 1) uncertain malignant potential, 2) low-grade malignant GIST, and 3) high-grade GIST. Grossly, these tumors differ from adenocarcinoma and lymphoma in that they often have a large exophytic component. Liquefactive necrosis and intratumoral hemorrhage are common. Spread is via direct extension and hematogenous metastases. High-grade GISTs are heterogeneous and high in signal on T2-weighted and gadolinium-enhanced fat-suppressed SGE images because of their increased vascularity (figs. 6.22–6.25). During the capillary phase of imaging, they show marked enhancement that persists throughout the interstitial phase. Hasegawa et al. reported that high-grade tumors have ill-defined tissue planes with adjacent tissues and organs, reflecting

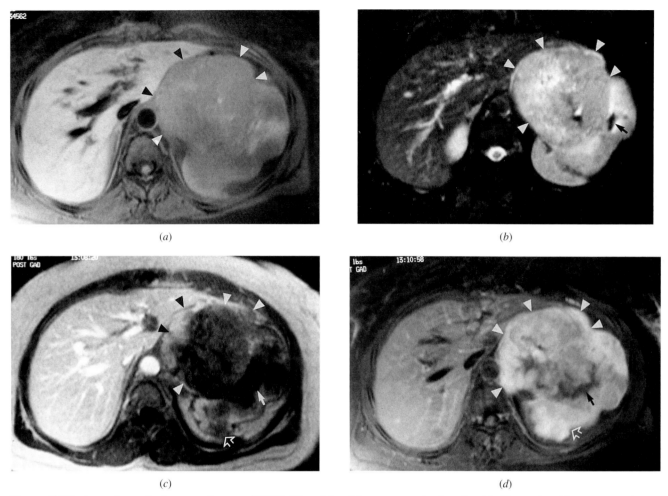

F I G . 6.22 Gastrointestinal stromal tumor (GIST). T1-weighted fat-suppressed spin-echo (*a*), T2-weighted fat-suppressed spin-echo (*b*), 45-s postgadolinium SGE (*c*), and gadolinium-enhanced fat-suppressed spin-echo (*d*) images. A large exophytic GIST arises from the lesser curvature (arrowheads, *a, b, c, d*) and is contiguous with the spleen. The tumor is heterogeneous and high in signal intensity on the T2-weighted image (*b*) and enhances intensely (*c, d*). Enhancing tumor extends adjacent to the spleen (open arrow, *c, d*). Signal-void areas within the tumor are consistent with necrosis. Air within the gastric lumen is also signal void (solid arrow, *b, c, d*).

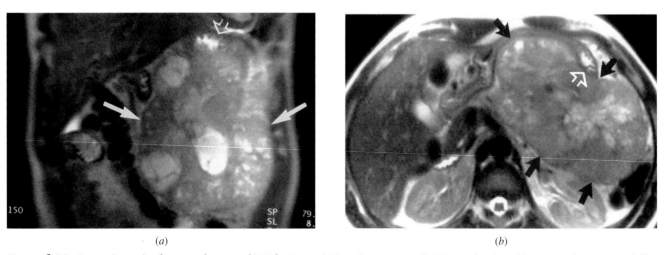

F I G . 6.23 Gastrointestinal stromal tumor (GIST). Coronal (*a*) and transverse (*b*) T2-weighted SS-ETSE, immediate postgadolinium SGE (*c*), and 90-s postgadolinium fat-suppressed SGE (*d*) images. A large multilobulated tumor (arrows, *a, b*) measuring 18 × 16 × 13 cm is shown arising from the gastric wall (open arrow, *a, b*). Multiple internal foci of high signal intensity are seen, representing areas of hemorrhage and necrosis.

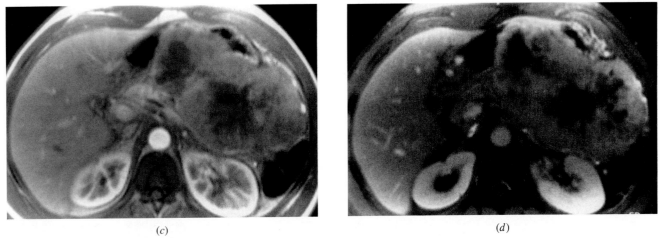

(c) *(d)*

F I G . 6.23 (*Continued*) On the immediate postgadolinium images (*c*), the tumor enhances heterogeneously and is mildly hyper-intense. On the 90-s fat-suppressed SGE image (*d*), increased heterogeneous enhancement of the mass is shown, which contains nonenhancing areas of necrosis and hemorrhage. (Reprinted with permission from Marcos HB, Semelka RC: Stomach diseases: MR evaluation using combined T2-weighted single-shot echo train spin-echo and gadolinium-enhanced spoiled gradient-echo sequences. *J Magn Reson Imaging* 10: 950–960, 1999.)

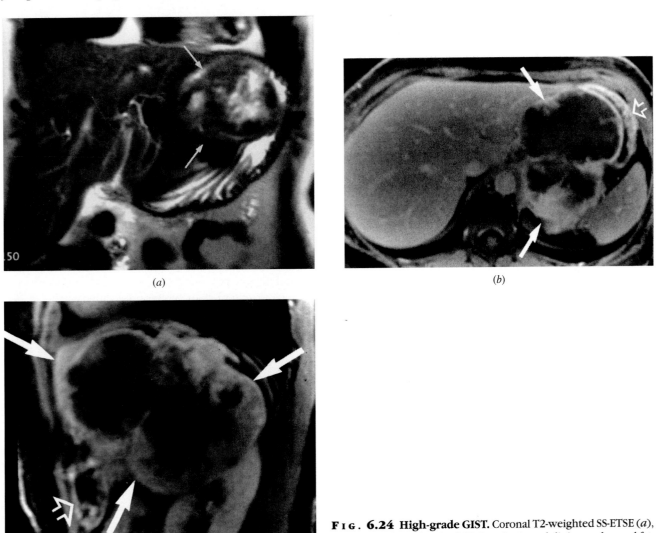

(a) *(b)*

(c)

F I G . 6.24 High-grade GIST. Coronal T2-weighted SS-ETSE (*a*), transverse (*b*), and sagittal (*c*) 2- to 3-min gadolinium-enhanced fat-suppressed SGE images. A large, heterogeneous tumor (arrow, *a–c*) arises from the gastric fundus and body. The lesion has ill-defined margins that correspond to high-grade cellular features seen at histopathologic examination. The stomach (open arrow, *b, c*) is compressed and deviated by the mass.

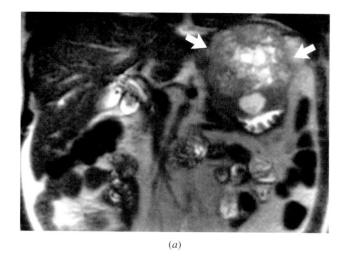

(a)

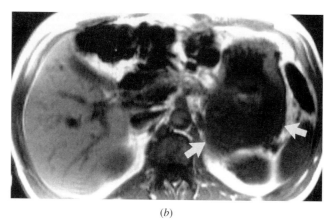

(b)

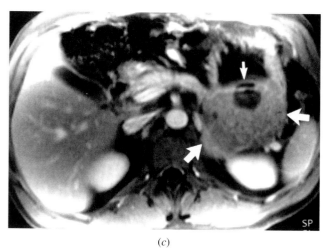

(c)

F I G . 6.25 Intermediate- to high-grade GIST. Coronal T2-weighted SS-ETSE (*a*), SGE (*b*), and 90-s gadolinium-enhanced fat-suppressed SGE (*c*) images. A large mass is seen (arrows, *a–c*) arising from the posterosuperior aspect of the gastric fundus. The tumor has heterogeneous signal intensity, contains hemorrhagic foci, and demonstrates moderate signal intensity. The mass has a long interface with the left hemidiaphragm and surrounding organs, but there is no evidence of deep invasion. A dominant necrotic focus is evident that represents an ulcer crater (small arrow, *c*).

invasion, whereas low-grade tumors have well-defined planes, reflecting less aggressive tumor behavior [43]. The necrotic portions of the tumor remain signal void on postcontrast images. Dynamic gadolinium-enhanced T1-weighted imaging also detects hepatic metastases.

The hypervascular lesions show early ring or uniform enhancement, which rapidly becomes isointense with normal hepatic parenchyma. Low-grade tumors enhance to a lesser extent than higher-grade tumors (fig. 6.26). GIST of the stomach may be submucosal, intramural, or

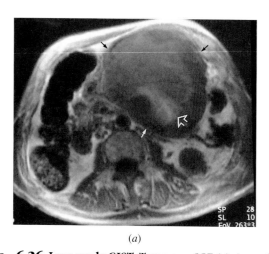

(a)

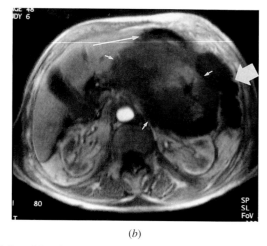

(b)

F I G . 6.26 Low-grade GIST. Transverse SGE (*a*), immediate postgadolinium SGE (*b*), and 90-s postgadolinium fat-suppressed SGE (*c, d*) images in a low-grade GIST (short arrows, *a–d*).

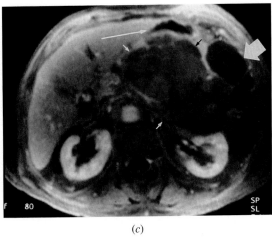

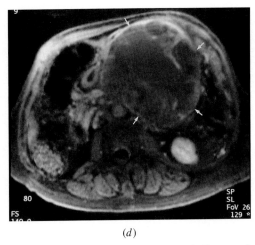

(c)   (d)

F I G . 6.26 On the precontrast image, high signal within the tumor represents hemorrhage (open arrow, *a*). Low-grade GIST enhance minimally after intravenous contrast. The tumor causes mass effect on the remaining stomach (long arrow, *b*, *c*) and the adjacent colon (large arrow, *b*, *c*).

subserosal; subserosal lesions may be predominantly exophytic, and their origin from the gastric wall may not be apparent on radiologic evaluation [44]. In the Hasegawa series, the gastric origin of the tumor was uncertain in three of nine cases because of the large exophytic component, relatively small gastric pedicle, and absence of mucosal invasion. It is therefore prudent to consider the possibility of GIST for any large tumor with central necrosis and hemorrhage that may appear radiologically to only abut the stomach.

Kaposi Sarcoma. Kaposi sarcoma most commonly occurs in immunocompromised patients, usually AIDS patients or recipients of organ transplantation. Grossly, the lesions of gastrointestinal tract Kaposi sarcoma consist of solitary, but frequently multiple, submucosal nodules. Microscopically, tumor is characterized by proliferation of spindled cells admixed with numerous vascular channels and red blood cell extravasation. Although approximately 50% of patients with AIDS-related Kaposi sarcoma will have gastrointestinal lesions at autopsy, most patients are asymptomatic. In rare instances, gastrointestinal Kaposi sarcoma may cause obstruction, intussusception, or hemorrhage. The stomach is the most common site of gut involvement, but lesions may occur throughout the gastrointestinal tract. Kaposi sarcoma should be considered in an AIDS patient who has gastrointestinal lesions in concert with bulky retroperitoneal lymphadenopathy, hepatic and splenic lesions, and infiltration of the psoas or abdominal wall [45].

Lymphoma. Primary gastric lymphoma is rare. Hodgkin and non-Hodgkin lymphomas (NHL) are more commonly observed in the context of disseminated disease. Approximately 50% of gastrointestinal NHL arise in the stomach, 40% in the small intestine, and 10% in

the colon [46]. Infiltration of the gastric wall by tumor cells results in diffuse mural thickening [47, 48]. Non-Hodgkin lymphoma often preserves gastric distensibility, whereas Hodgkin lymphoma mimics diffusely infiltrating form of primary gastric adenocarcinoma (linitis plastica): a desmoplastic reaction predominates, leading to a noncompliant aperistaltic viscus. Diffuse gastric wall thickening is best seen on single-shot echo-train spin-echo and gadolinium-enhanced fat-suppressed SGE images (fig. 6.27). Involved regional lymph nodes also can be identified with these techniques.

Carcinoid. These tumors were first described by Obendorfer in 1907 as "karzinoide" (resembling carcinoma), because, despite their malignant potential, tumors exhibited slow growth patterns and were slow to metastasize. Carcinoids are best characterized as well-differentiated neuroendocrine neoplasms that occur most commonly in the appendix and small intestine (see discussion under small intestine). Gastric carcinoids are divided into two basic clinicopathologic categories, depending on whether they arise in the presence or absence of chronic atrophic gastritis [49].

Gastrin is secreted in a normal physiologic state by G cells in the gastric antrum. Secretion rates are normally controlled by gastric acid levels (mainly hydrochloric acid secretion by parietal cells in the fundus). When hydrochloric acid levels decrease, as occurs in the setting of chronic atrophic gastritis, increased secretion by G cells causes hypergastrinemia. Gastrin acts as a trophic factor to neuroendocrine-like cells in the fundic mucosa, resulting in hyperplasia progressing to carcinoid tumors. These tumors arise in situations of hypergastrinemia in such conditions as chronic autoimmune atrophic gastritis (pernicious anemia), chronic atrophic gastritis associated with *Helicobacter pylori* infection, and prolonged

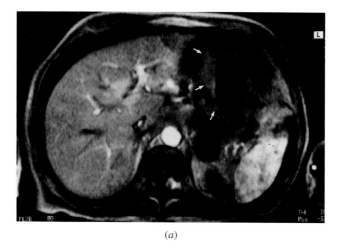

(a)

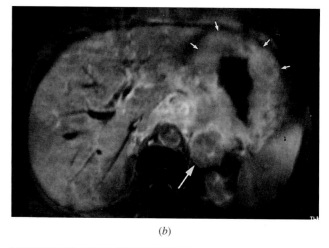

(b)

FIG. 6.27 Non-Hodgkin lymphoma of the stomach. Immediate postgadolinium SGE (*a*) and gadolinium-enhanced T1-weighted fat-suppressed spin-echo (*b*, *c*) images. There is diffuse circumferential lymphomatous infiltration of the stomach wall (short arrows, *a*, *b*, *c*). Lymphoma extends to the left adrenal gland (long arrow, *b*). At a lower tomographic section, prominent retroperitoneal lymphadenopathy is present (arrow, *c*), which is commonly observed in the setting of gastric lymphoma.

(c)

iatrogenic acid suppression with proton pump inhibitors (such as omeprazole) [50]. Hypergastrinemia may also occur in patients with Zollinger-Ellison syndrome and multiple endocrine neoplasia (MEN) type I. Gastric carcinoid tumors associated with chronic atrophic gastritis tend to occur in the fundus and are multiple, limited to the mucosa and submucosa. Lesions are rarely malignant and regress when gastrin levels are decreased, usually after antrectomy (gastrin-producing cells reside predominantly in the antrum). This situation is in sharp contrast to gastric carcinoid tumors that arise sporadically in a normogastrinemic state. Sporadic gastric carcinoid tumors arise anywhere in the stomach and may be small (<2 cm diameter) submucosal nodules or large tumors that invade deeply and promote prominent fibrosis in surrounding tissues. Sporadic gastric carcinoids should be regarded as malignant neoplasms and be completely surgically resected.

On MR images, carcinoid tumors are near-isointense on T1 and mildly hyperintense and heterogeneous on T2 and often show increased enhancement on early and later postgadolinium images (fig. 6.28).

Metastases. Metastatic involvement of the stomach is uncommon. Gastric metastatic lesions are generally submucosal. Tumors of neighboring organs, such as esophagus, pancreas, and transverse colon, may involve the stomach by direct extension. Specifically, colon carcinoma arising in the transverse colon invades the stomach via the gastrocolic ligament, whereas pancreatic carcinoma invades the posterior wall of the gastric body and antrum via the transverse mesocolon.

Carcinomas of lung and breast and melanoma are the most common primary malignancies that result in hematogenous gastric metastases (fig. 6.29). Breast cancer metastases are noteworthy in that submucosal involvement with diffuse thickening of gastric wall may be indistinguishable from diffusely infiltrative gastric adenocarcinoma (linitis plastica).

Inflammatory and Infectious Disorders

Gastric Ulceration

Ulcers are defined pathologically as localized, destructive lesions involving full-thickness mucosa. Ulcer craters

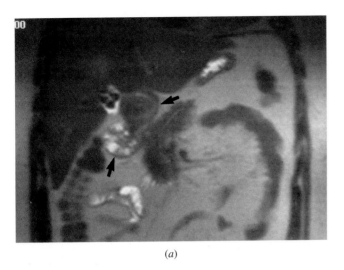

(a)

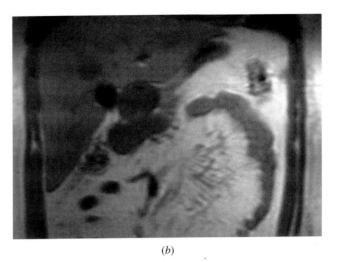

(b)

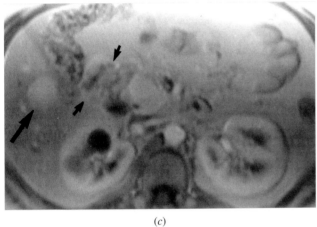

(c)

FIG. 6.28 Gastric carcinoid. Coronal T2-weighted SS-ETSE (a), coronal SGE (b), and transverse immediate postgadolinium SGE (c) images. This primary carcinoid tumor of the stomach appears as a mass in the wall of the antrum that invades the duodenum and pancreas. The tumor is mixed solid with cystic spaces (arrows, a) on T2 and isointense on T1 (b) and enhances heterogeneously after contrast administration (arrows, c). There are also hepatic metastases that are moderately hyperintense on T2-weighted image and hypointense on precontrast SGE image (b) and show homogeneous early enhancement (large arrow, c). A simple cyst is also seen in the right kidney.

may extend into submucosa or deeper aspects of the gut wall. The two most important factors involved in the etiology of chronic peptic ulcer disease are the amount of gastric acid and the mucosal resistance. An almost invariable feature of gastric ulcer disease is evidence of diffuse inflammation of surrounding mucosa, indicative of chronic antral gastritis that is mainly caused by *H. pylori* infection. In some cases, gastritis may result from repeated exposure to toxic substances including alcohol, drugs, and bile salts. Approximately 10% of patients have ulcers in both the antrum and duodenum [51].

Benign gastric ulcers most commonly occur along the lesser curvature in the region of the border zone between the corpus and antral mucosa.

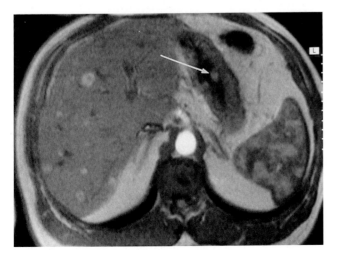

FIG. 6.29 Melanoma metastasis to the stomach. Immediate postgadolinium SGE image in a patient with metastatic melanoma. Malignant melanoma metastasizes hematogenously, and in this patient multiple liver metastases and a gastric metastasis (long arrow) are identified. The metastases are high in signal on this T1-weighted image because of the paramagnetic properties of melanin.

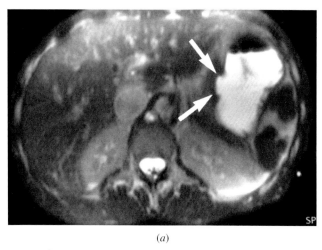
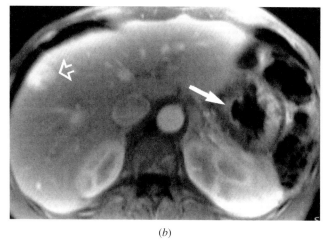

(a)   (b)

F I G . 6.30 Gastric ulcer. Transverse T2-weighted SS-ETSE (a) and transverse 1-min postgadolinium SGE (b) images. The high signal intensity of gastric contents (orally administered water) deliniates the ulcer crater (arrows, a), on the mucosal surface of the lesser curvature. On the 1-min postgadolinium SGE image (b), the ulcer shows mildly increased enhancement (arrow, b). A 2-cm hemangioma is incidentally noted as an intensely enhancing mass lesion in the liver on the 1-min postgadolinium image (open arrow, b). (Reprinted with permission from Marcos HB, Semelka RC: Stomach diseases: MR evaluation using combined T2-weighted single-shot echo train spin-echo and gadolinium-enhanced spoiled gradient-echo sequences. *J Magn Reson Imaging* 10: 950–960, 1999.)

Marcos and Semelka reported on the MR appearance of gastric ulcers [28]. Gastric inflammatory disease in general results in increased mural enhancement on both early and late gadolinium images. Ulcer craters may be demonstrated both on single-shot echo-train spin-echo and on gadolinium enhancement fat-suppressed SGE images (fig. 6.30).

Gastritis

Gastritis is defined as inflammation of the gastric mucosa. Inflammation may be acute, consisting predominantly of neutrophils, or chronic with a preponderance of lymphocytes or plasma cells. Acute gastritis is usually transient in nature and may be associated with a variety of factors including heavy use of drugs, especially NSAIDs, excessive alcohol consumption, smoking, and severe stress (e.g., trauma, burns, surgery). Severe acute gastritis is often characterized pathologically by the presence of erosions and hemorrhage. The term "erosion" denotes the loss of superficial epithelium, in contrast to ulcers, which involve the full-thickness mucosa.

Chronic gastritis is characterized by the presence of chronic inflammation leading to mucosal atrophy and abnormal changes in the epithelium (fig. 6.31). Erosions generally do not occur in this setting. The major etiologies of chronic gastritis include immunologic (pernicious anemia), chronic infection, especially with *Helicobacter*

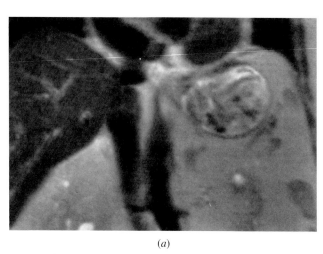
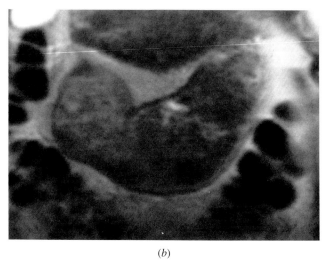

(a)   (b)

F I G . 6.31 Atrophic gastritis. Coronal T2-weighted SS-ETSE image (a). The gastric wall is noted to be thin and featureless, consistent with atrophy of the gastric rugae.

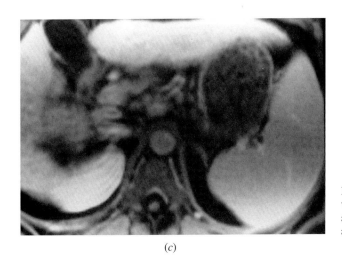

(c)

FIG. 6.31 Coronal T2-weighted SS-ETSE image (*b*) and transverse interstitial-phase fat-suppressed postgadolinium SGE (*c*) images in a second patient show similar features of gastric wall atrophy.

pylori and toxic, as in alcohol consumption and cigarette smoking.

Both acute and chronic gastritis may occur in patients receiving high-dose radiation therapy. A chronic ulcer may develop months to several years after radiation exposure. Gastric inflammation, fibrosis, and stricture formation may lead to outlet obstruction (fig. 6.32) [52].

Hypertrophic Rugal Folds

Localized or diffuse thickening and gross enlargement of rugal folds ("cerebriform") may result from discrete hyperplasia of one of the epithelial mucosal components, inflammatory diseases, or tumors, most notably lymphoma or carcinoma. Causes of diffuse mucosal hypertrophy include hyperplasia of the parietal cells in Zollinger-Ellison syndrome (fig. 6.33) or of surface

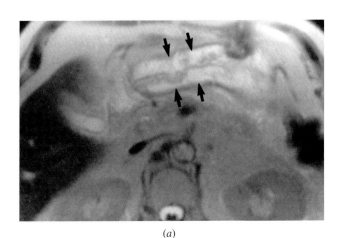

(a)

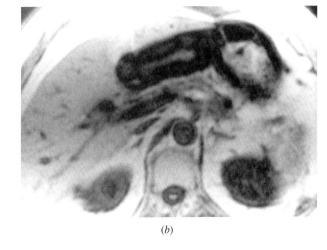

(b)

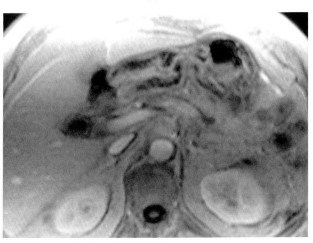

(c)

FIG. 6.32 Radiation gastritis. Transverse T2-weighted SS-ETSE (*a*), SGE (*b*), and 90-s postgadolinium fat-suppressed SGE (*c*) images is a patient after radiation therapy for pancreatic cancer. There is a marked wall thickening of the stomach with submucosal edema. Note the high signal of the thickened submucosal on the T2-weighted image (arrows, *a*) reflecting edema. After contrast administration, mucosal enhancement is noted.

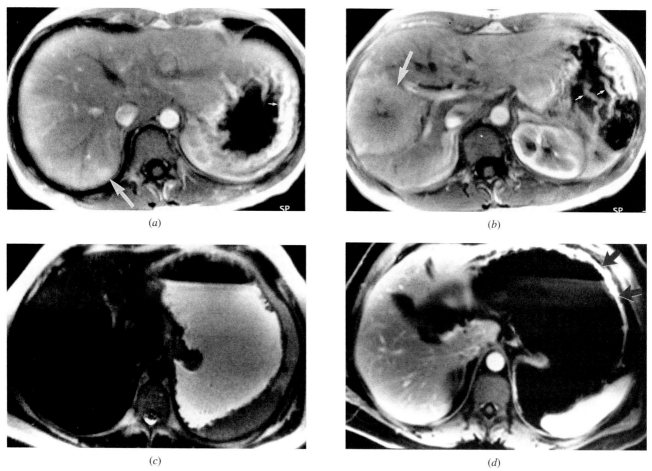

(a)   *(b)*

(c)   *(d)*

F I G . 6.33 Zollinger-Ellison syndrome. Immediate postgadolinium SGE images (*a*, *b*). Intense enhancement and increased thickness of gastric rugae are appreciated (small arrows, *a*, *b*). Hypervascular liver metastases are also present (large arrow, *a*, *b*).
    Transverse T2-weighted SS-ETSE (*c*) and transverse 90-s fat-suppressed postgadolinium SGE (*d*) images in a second patient. There is a marked distension of the stomach and duodenum, and the anterior gastric wall is thickened. On the 90-s postgadolinium fat-suppressed SGE image (*d*), the gastric wall shows intense enhancement (arrows, *b*). (Reprinted with permission from Marcos HB, Semelka RC: Stomach diseases: MR Evaluation using combined T2-weighted single-shot echo train spin-echo and gadolinium-enhanced spoiled gradient-echo sequences. *J Magn Reson Imaging* 10: 950–960, 1999.)

foveolar mucous cells in Menetrier disease. Types of specific inflammatory conditions that may cause rugal enlargement, often localized to the antrum, include infections such as tuberculosis and syphilis, chronic granulomatous diseases, and sarcoidosis [53].
    The use of the single-shot echo-train spin-echo technique coupled with adequate distension permits detection of rugal thickening. The hyperemia and capillary leakage that accompany inflammation are highlighted on T1-weighted fat-suppressed SGE images: the inflamed tissue demonstrates early marked enhancement, which persists as the contrast pools in the interstitium. The inflammatory nature of some of these gastric diseases is best shown on gadolinium-enhanced images.

The Postoperative Stomach

A spectrum of surgical procedures involves the stomach. These procedures may be categorized as drainage with

or without partial gastric resection, antireflux operations, gastroplasty, resection, and feeding gastrostomy. Familiarity with the exact surgical procedure performed aids radiologic investigation. The single-shot T2-weighted technique allows visualization of the anatomic changes after surgery, such as bowel anastomoses (fig. 6.34). Evaluation of inflammatory changes is accomplished with gadolinium-enhanced images.

THE SMALL INTESTINE

Normal Anatomy

The small bowel measures approximately 20–22 feet from the ligament of Treitz to the ileocecal valve. On gross inspection the lining of the small intestine shows a series of permanent circular folds, plicae circulares. Each fold is covered by mucosa and contains a core of

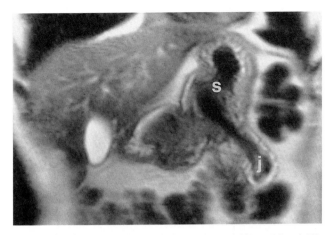

F I G . 6.34 Gastrojejunostomy. Coronal T2-weighted T2-weighted SS-ETSE image shows the side-to-end anastomosis of the stomach (s) to the jejunum (j) in this patient status postgastrointestinal bypass surgery.

submucosa. Plicae circulares increase the surface area and act as partial barriers that attenuate the forward flow of intraluminal contents, thus increasing the time of contact with absorptive surfaces. The duodenum is in continuation with the pylorus. It extends in a C shape to curve around the pancreatic head to end at the duodenal-jejunal flexure. The duodenum is divided into four parts: bulb, descending, horizontal, and ascending segments. The bulb is the only intraperitoneal portion of the duodenum and is the most mobile. The second portion is in close proximity to the head of the pancreas, and both the pancreatic and common bile duct enter its postero-medial aspect. The mesenteric small intestine begins at the jejunum. The jejunum occupies the superior and left abdomen, whereas the ileum occupies the inferior and right abdomen. Their mesenteric attachment gives rise to two distinct borders, the concave or mesenteric border and the convex or antimesenteric border. In addition to differences in location, the ileum has a narrower lumen with fewer mucosal folds and a greater number of mesenteric arcades. Normal bowel wall thickness should not exceed 3–4 mm.

MRI Technique

Previously, MRI had a limited role in assessing the small bowel because of poor intrinsic contrast resolution and motion artifacts caused by peristalsis. The combination of breathing-independent single-shot echo-train spin-echo images and pre- and postgadolinium fat-suppressed SGE images is an effective approach for imaging the bowel (fig. 6.35). As a routine, patients should fast for at least 5 h before the exam to decrease bowel motion and peristalsis with the resulting blurring artifact. Ingested water coupled with the single-shot echo-train spin-echo technique provides high-quality images of the small bowel (fig. 6.35). Images of the upper and midabdomen should be obtained in the axial and coronal planes to distinguish bowel, which will show tubular-shaped configuration in at least one plane, from masses, which will not. Unenhanced SGE images with and without fat suppression followed by gadolinium-enhanced T1-weighted fat-suppressed SGE images are necessary for a comprehensive exam. Normal bowel on unenhanced images has a

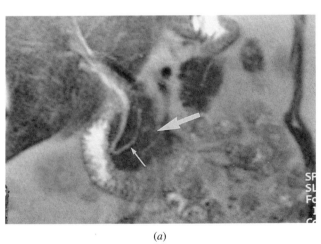

(a)

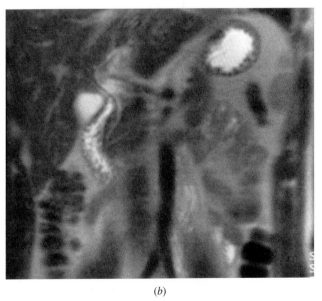

(b)

F I G . 6.35 Normal bowel. Coronal T2-weighted SS-ETSE (a–e) in five different patients. The valvulae conniventes of the C loop of the duodenum (a–c) and of multiple loops of jejunum and ileum are well shown as low-signal intensity bands on the T2-weighted images and stand out in relief against the high-signal intensity intraluminal contents and moderately high-signal intensity fat. Normal head of pancreas (large arrow, a), and pancreatic duct (thin arrow, a) are demonstrated.

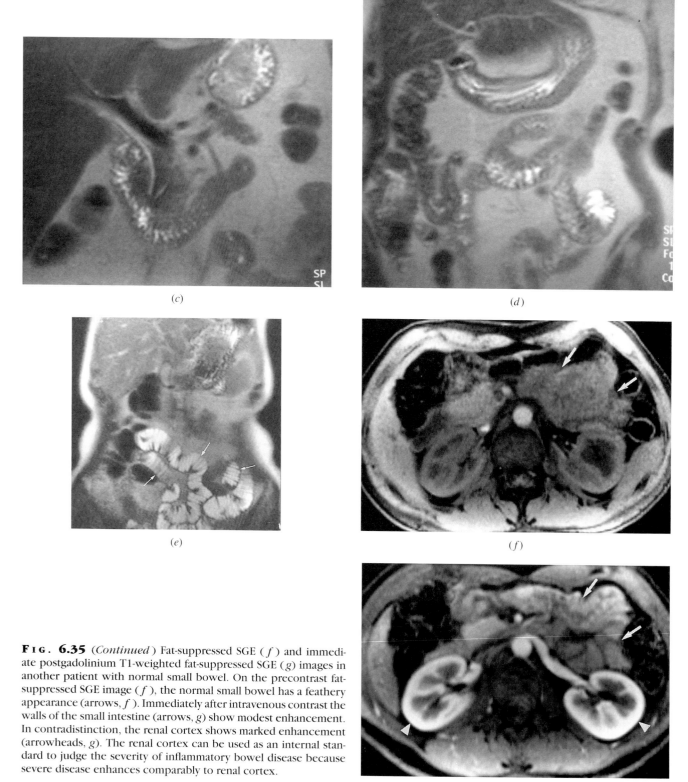

Fig. 6.35 (*Continued*) Fat-suppressed SGE (*f*) and immediate postgadolinium T1-weighted fat-suppressed SGE (*g*) images in another patient with normal small bowel. On the precontrast fat-suppressed SGE image (*f*), the normal small bowel has a feathery appearance (arrows, *f*). Immediately after intravenous contrast the walls of the small intestine (arrows, *g*) show modest enhancement. In contradistinction, the renal cortex shows marked enhancement (arrowheads, *g*). The renal cortex can be used as an internal standard to judge the severity of inflammatory bowel disease because severe disease enhances comparably to renal cortex.

feathery appearance because of the plicae circulares and after intravenous gadolinium enhances in a moderate and uniform fashion [54] (see fig. 6.35). Small bowel enhances less than the gastric wall (see fig. 6.35) and pancreas. The lesser enhancement of small bowel compared to pancreas generally allows clear distinction between these two organs on immediate postgadolinium images. The administration of intravenous gadolinium permits evaluation of the bowel wall and assessment of lymphadenopathy, associated peritoneal disease, and accompanying fistula, if present.

Recent studies have described small bowel follow-through and small bowel enema performed as MR studies. The technique involves administering a large volume of fluid (water is often sufficient) by mouth or enteric tube and acquiring thick-section (5–8 cm) single-shot echo-train spin-echo images with strong T2 weighting to obtain images that resemble fluoroscopic small bowel images (fig. 6.36).

Congenital Lesions

Rotational Abnormalities

Intestinal malrotations or nonrotations result from disordered or interrupted embryonic intestinal counterclockwise rotations around the axis of the superior mesenteric artery. In rotational abnormalities, the normal rotations and fixations are either incomplete or occur out of sequence [55]. The most common form, nonrotation, is readily apparent on tomographic images, demonstrated by the lack of normal passage of the third and fourth parts of the duodenum from right to left of midline. The other types of malrotation occur less frequently and include incomplete rotation, reversed rotation, and anomalous fixation or fusion of the mesenteries. Marcos et al. [56] has shown that rotational abnormalities can be well visualized on snap-shot echo-train spin-echo images (fig. 6.37).

Diverticulum

A diverticulum is defined as a mucosal outpouching emanating from the alimentary tract that communicates with the gut lumen. Congenital diverticula usually contain all three layers with a complete muscularis externa in the outpouching; in contrast, acquired diverticula lack a muscularis externa. Diverticula of the jejunum and ileum involve the mesenteric side of the bowel. In the small intestine muscular wall, points at which mesenteric vessels and nerves enter provide potential sites of weakness where mucosa may herniate into the mesentery.

Small bowel diverticula occur most commonly in the duodenum. Multiple small bowel diverticula may

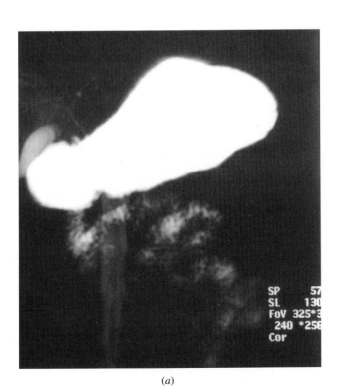

(a)

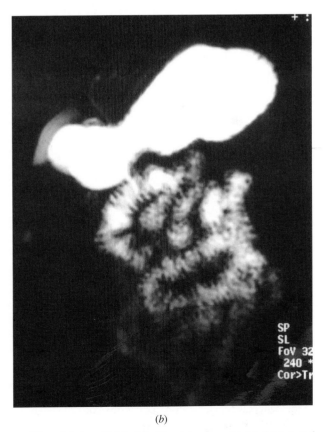

(b)

F I G . 6.36 Small bowel follow-through. SS-ETSE images with strong T2 weighting. Thick slab (6 cm) images obtained 5 (a) and 20 (b) min after ingestion of a large volume of water resemble fluoroscopic small bowel images.

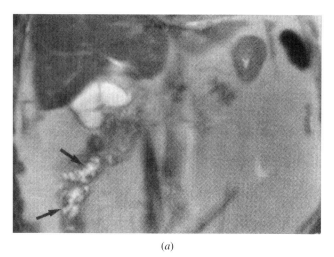

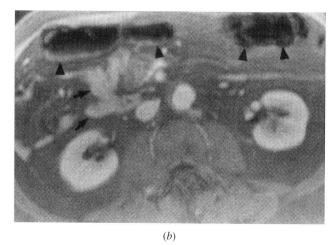

(a)   (b)

F I G . 6.37 Rotational abnormalities of small bowel. Coronal T2-weighted SS-ETSE (a) and transverse 90 s postgadolinium fat-suppressed SGE images. Coronal T2 (a) demonstrates that small bowel is predominantly located in the right side of the abdomen (arrows). The 90-s postgadolinium fat-suppressed SGE image demonstrates that the third and fourth portions of the duodenum are located to the right of midline (arrows, b). Note that the large bowel is in a normal location (arrowheads). (Reprinted with permission from Marcos HB, Semelka RC, Noone TC, Woosley JT, Lee JKT: MRI of normal and abnormal duodenum using half-Fourier single-shot RARE and gadolinium-enhanced spoiled gradient-echo sequences. *Magn Reson Imaging* 17: 869–880, 1999.

be associated with intestinal bacterial overgrowth and resultant metabolic complications. Diverticula may be demonstrated on MR images as air or air fluid-containing structures that arise from the bowel (fig. 6.38). Change in size of the diverticulum may be observed between sequences in an MRI examination reflecting contraction and expansion. Single-shot echo-train spin echo is effective at demonstrating this entity. The absence of appreciable susceptibility artifact from air in the diverticula using this technique allows clear delineation of diverticula and their origin from bowel [56].

Meckel Diverticulum

Meckel diverticulum is a remnant of the omphalomesenteric duct (vitelline duct). Normally, this duct is obliterated by the fifth week of gestation. Meckel diverticulum is common with a prevalence of about 2% in the general population. It occurs within 25 cm of the ileocecal valve along the antimesenteric border. Most patients with Meckel diverticulum are asymptomatic. If the diverticulum contains acid-secreting epithelium of gastric mucosa, ulceration and bleeding may result. Intussusception and inflammation may also occur, irrespective

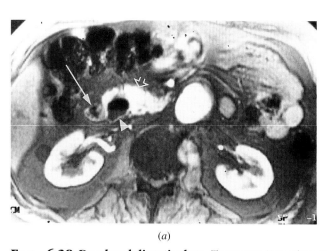

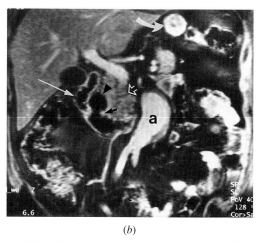

(a)   (b)

F I G . 6.38 Duodenal diverticulum. Transverse immediate (a), and coronal 90-s (b) postgadolinium fat-suppressed SGE images. An air- and fluid-containing diverticulum (arrowhead, a, b) is interposed between the duodenum (long arrow, a, b) and the head of the pancreas (open arrow, a, b). On the coronal image, a neck (short arrow, b) connecting the diverticulum to the duodenum is well shown, which confirms that the lesion represents a diverticulum and not a cystic mass in the head of the pancreas. Duodenal diverticula are common and usually incidental findings. The normal gastric wall (curved arrow, b) enhances more intensely than normal small bowel. An abdominal aortic aneurysm ("a", b) is also present.

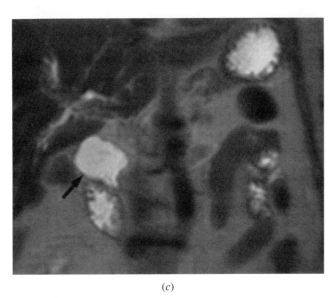

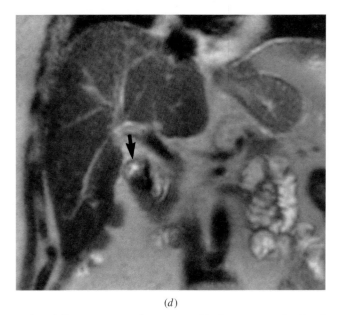

(c)   (d)

F I G . 6.38 (*Continued*) Coronal T2-weighted SS-ETSE (*c, d*) in two other different patients demonstrate fluid-containing duodenal diverticula (arrow, *c, d*).

of the type of mucosa present. The mainstay of diagnosis has been 99m Tc-pertechnetate scintigraphy and enteroclysis. MRI, like scintigraphy, exploits the presence of gastric mucosa in making the diagnosis. Because gastric mucosa enhances more than any other segment of bowel, a gastric-lined Meckel diverticulum will demonstrate marked enhancement on immediate (capillary phase) and interstitial-phase postgadolinium images (fig. 6.39) [57, 58].

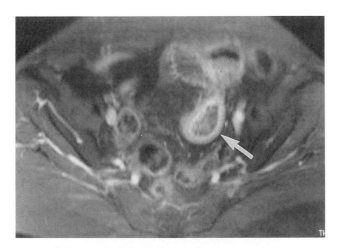

F I G . 6.39 Meckel diverticulum. Gadolinium-enhanced T1-weighted fat-suppressed spin-echo image in a patient with lower gastrointestinal bleeding. A teardrop-shaped Meckel diverticulum (arrow) extends from a loop of mildly dilated ileum. The inner wall of the diverticulum enhances to a greater extent than adjacent small bowel and colon. This allows detection of the diverticulum, and the degree of enhancement is consistent with the presence of gastric mucosa.

Atresia and Stenosis

Intestinal atresia results in complete absence of a portion of bowel or closure by an occluding mucosal diaphragm, whereas congenital stenosis implies a narrowing of an intestinal segment by fibrosis or stricture. Both may cause intestinal obstruction. Duodenal atresia represents the most common gastrointestinal atresia; jejunal and ileal atresia are rare and occur with equal frequency.

Approximately 25% of cases will have associated congenital anomalies including malrotation of the gut and Meckel diverticulum. Although the precise etiology of congenital atresia and stenosis is not known, lesions appear to arise from developmental failure, intrauterine vascular accidents, or intussusceptions occurring after the intestine has developed. Barium studies are the most common means of diagnosis, although T2-weighted single-shot echo-train spin-echo images can highlight the atretic/stenotic segment and proximal dilatation (fig. 6.40).

Choledochocele

Choledochocele is a congenital anomaly characterized by cystic dilation of the distal common bile duct in the region of the papilla. Clinically, it may be associated with abdominal pain, bleeding, jaundice, and pancreatitis. The diverticulum can contain calculi. On imaging examinations, these may appear as polypoid masses indistinguishable from papillary edema or carcinoma. When large enough, they can protrude into the duodenum and even occlude it. MR cholangiopancreatography (MRCP) (see Chapter 3, *Gallbladder and Biliary System*) and single-shot echo-train spin-echo images facilitate establishing the correct diagnosis (fig. 6.41).

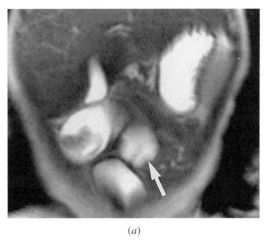 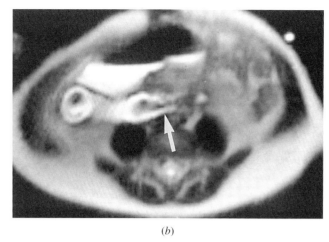

(a)   (b)

F I G . 6.40 Congenital stenosis, duodenum. Coronal (*a*) and transverse (*b*) T2-weighted SS-ETSE images. The coronal image demonstrates dilation of the third part of the duodenum (arrow, *a*). The duodenum is noted to narrow (arrow, *b*) at the crossing of the superior mesenteric artery on the transverse image (*b*).

Mass Lesions

Benign and malignant small intestinal tumors are uncommon. Adenomas, leiomyomas, and lipomas constitute the three most common primary benign small intestinal tumors [59]. In general, benign tumors occur less commonly in the duodenum and increase in frequency as one reaches the ileum.

Benign Masses

Polyps. The term "polyp" is a clinical term for any tumorous mass that projects above the surrounding normal mucosa. Hamartomatous, hyperplastic, and inflammatory polyps are benign, nonneoplastic lesions; adenomatous polyps are true neoplastic tumors containing dysplastic epithelium and are precursors of carcinoma.

Polyps are infrequently symptomatic and are usually incidental findings at autopsy. Clinically evident polyps present with pain, obstruction, or bleeding. Polyps are the most common lead points for intussusception in adults. Except in hereditary polyposis syndrome, adenomatous polyps of the small intestine are rare, with <0.05% of all intestinal adenomas arising in the small intestine [60]. Overall, the frequency of cancer in adenomas ranges from 45% to 63% [61]. Multiple adenomas predominate in the setting of Gardner and familial polyposis syndromes. Small bowel hamartomas occur commonly in Peutz-Jeghers syndrome and rarely in juvenile polyposis syndromes.

Similar to polyps elsewhere in the gastrointestinal tract, small bowel polyps appear as enhancing masses on gadolinium-enhanced fat-suppressed SGE images

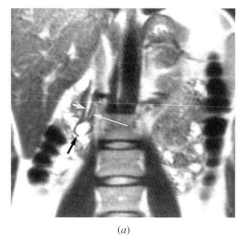 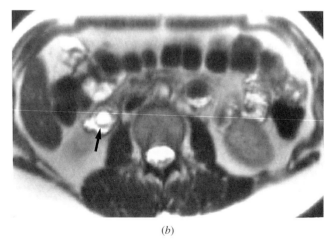

(a)   (b)

F I G . 6.41 Choledochocele. Coronal (*a*) and transverse (*b*) T2-weighted SS-ETSE images in a patient with recurrent bouts of pancreatitis. A high-signal intensity choledochocele (black arrow, *a*, *b*) protrudes into the duodenum. The SS-ETSE image clearly defines the cystic nature of the lesion, which excludes an ampullary tumor, and demonstrates the relationship to the common bile duct (small arrow, *a*) and the pancreatic duct (long arrow, *a*). (Courtesy of Susan M Ascher, MD, Dept Radiology, Georgetown University Medical Center).

(fig. 6.42). On single-shot echo-train spin-echo images polyps appear as rounded low-signal intensity masses. Polyps are termed pedunculated when they are anchored by a slender stalk and sessile when they are attached by a broad base. Although it may not be possible to exclude a focus of carcinoma within the polyp, extraserosal extension of a polyp is compatible with malignant degeneration.

Neurofibromas. Primary neurogenic tumors of the gastrointestinal tract are rare. Pathologically, neurofibromas consist of neoplastic cells arising from the nerve sheath. Gastrointestinal involvement in neurofibromatosis type 1, or von Recklinghausen disease, is well recognized, and solitary or multiple gastrointestinal tumors have been reported in 11–25% of patients with this disease [62, 63].

Neurofibromatosis type 1 predisposes individuals to an increased risk of a variety of gastrointestinal lesions, including neurofibromas, schwanomas, smooth muscle tumors, and neuroendocrine tumors of the duodenum and ampullary region [62]. The detection of these tumors by MRI depends essentially on their size [64]. They appear as intraluminal masses that enhance to the same extent as bowel wall (fig. 6.43).

Leiomyomas. The frequency of small bowel leiomyoma is comparable to that of adenoma. Leiomyomas are smooth muscle proliferations that usually originate in the submucosa or muscularis externa. Depending on their location, they may protrude into the lumen or produce a mass effect on adjacent bowel. In general, leiomyomas are usually solitary lesions. As leiomyomas enlarge, they may undergo central necrosis and bleeding. On MRI the submucosal lesions may be indistinguishable from polyps. Uniform enhancement greater than that of adjacent bowel is observed on postgadolinium images (fig. 6.44).

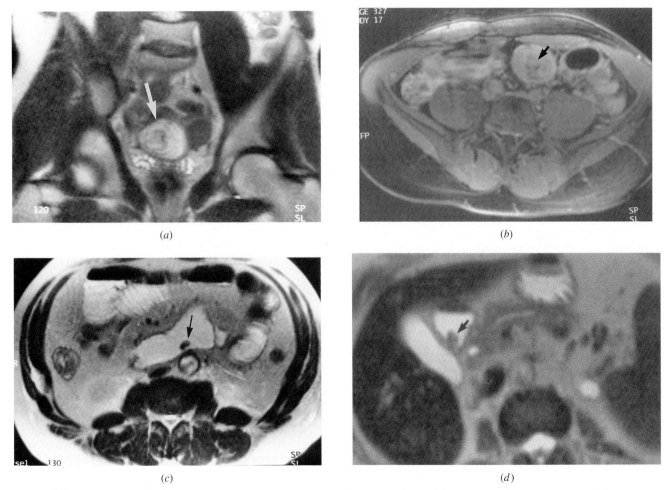

(a)

(b)

(c)

(d)

F I G . 6.42 Small bowel polyps. T2-weighted SS-ETSE (*a*) and gadolinium-enhanced fat-suppressed SGE (*b*) images of a hamartoma in Peutz-Jeghers syndrome. A bowel-within-bowel appearance (arrow, *a*) is identified on the T2-weighted image (*a*) in the proximal jejunum because of intussusception. The intussusception is caused by a hamartomatous polyp that has acted as a lead point. The hamartoma is shown as a 1-cm uniformly enhancing mass (arrow, *b*) on the gadolinium-enhanced fat-suppressed SGE image (*b*).

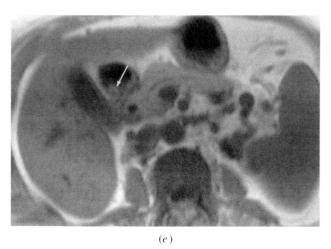

(e)

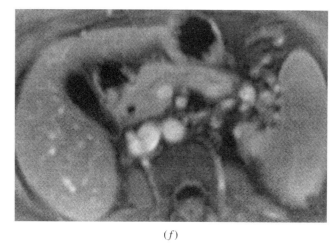

(f)

F I G . 6.42 (*Continued*) T2-weighted image (*c*) in a second patient demonstrates a 1-cm polyp (arrow, *c*) within a slightly dilated loop of duodenum.

T2-weighted SS-ETSE (*d*), SGE (*e*), and 90-s postgadolinium fat-suppressed SGE (*f*) images in a third patient. T2 image shows a low-signal intensity mass (arrow, *d*), measuring 1.5 cm located in the descending portion of the duodenum. Note that the high signal intensity of intraluminal fluid within the duodenum clearly deliniates the polyp, which appears moderately low in signal intensity. Comparing precontrast (*e*) and postgadolinium (*f*) images, enhancement of the polyp is demonstrated, showing it to remain comparable in signal to the duodenal wall, reflecting the tissue nature of the polyp. (Reprinted with permission from Marcos HB, Semelka RC, Noone TC, Woosley JT, Lee JKT: MRI of normal and abnormal duodenum using half-Fourier single-shot RARE and gadolinium-enhanced spoiled gradient-echo sequences. *Magn Reson Imaging* 17: 869–880, 1999.)

Lipomas. Lipomas are mature adipose tissue proliferations that arise in the submucosa and occur predominantly in the duodenum and ileum. Similar to leiomyomas, they may ulcerate and bleed. Lipomas are high in signal intensity on T1-weighted images and will have signal intensity comparable to intra-abdominal fat on T2-weighted images. On T1-weighted fat-suppressed images these lesions will show a characteristic loss of signal intensity.

Varices. Duodenal varices may be seen in isolation or in conjunction with portal vein obstruction. SGE or

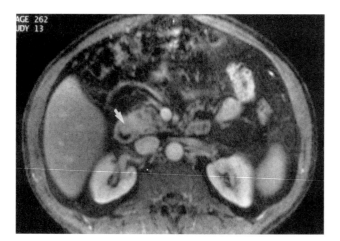

F I G . 6.43 Neurofibroma of duodenum. Transverse 90-s postgadolinium fat-suppressed SGE image in a patient with type 1 neurofibromatosis. A 1-cm intraluminal mass (arrow) arises in the second part of duodenum. This mass enhances to the same extent as the duodenal wall, reflecting the tissue composition of the neurofibroma. The patient expired, and at autopsy multiple cutaneous and gastrointestinal neurofibromas were found. (Reprinted with permission from Semelka RC, Marcos HB: Polyposis syndromes of the gastrointestinal tract. *J Magn Reson Imaging* 11: 51–55, 2000.)

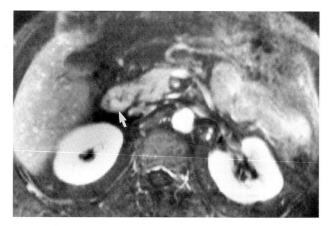

F I G . 6.44 Duodenal leiomyoma. Gadolinium-enhanced T1-weighted fat-suppressed spin-echo image shows a uniformly enhancing mass (arrow) protruding into the duodenum. When intraluminal, leiomyomas are indistinguishable from polyps. (Reprinted with permission from Shoenut JP, Semelka RC, Silverman R, Yaffe CS, Mickflikier AB: The gastrointestinal tract. In Semelka RC, Shoenut JP (eds.). *MRI of the Abdomen with CT Correlation.* New York: Raven Press, p. 119–143, 1993.)

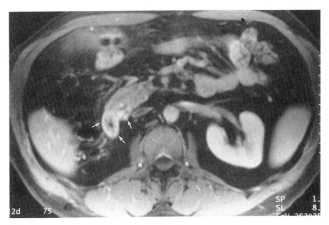

FIG. 6.45 Periduodenal and duodenal varices. Transverse 90-s postgadolinium fat-suppressed SGE image in a patient with splenic vein thrombosis. Periduodenal and duodenal varices are clearly shown as thin enhancing tubular structures adjacent to and within the wall of the duodenum. Venous blood is rerouted to periduodenal and duodenal varices as one of the collateral pathways in the setting of splenic vein thrombosis.

fat-suppressed SGE images obtained between 30 and 90s after gadolinium administration demonstrate the varices as thin tubular structures within the bowel wall (fig. 6.45).

Malignant Masses

Adenocarcinomas. Small bowel tumors account for only 1% of all gastrointestinal malignancies, and one-half are adenocarcinomas [26]. The most common site for small bowel adenocarcinoma is the duodenum. This tumor frequently occurs in close proximity to the ampulla and as a result may cause obstructive jaundice [65]. Other symptoms, regardless of location, include intestinal obstruction, chronic blood loss, or both. Patients

usually are asymptomatic early in the course of their disease; as a result, presentation is often late with advanced disease [26]. The combined use of T2-weighted single-shot echo-train spin-echo and gadolinium-enhanced fat-suppressed SGE imaging has resulted in reproducible high image quality for the evaluation of small bowel neoplasms [66].

Duodenal neoplasms are particularly well shown because of the relatively fixed position of the duodenum in the anterior pararenal space. The most consistent MR imaging feature that permits their detection is that tumors enhance in a heterogeneous moderate fashion on interstitial-phase gadolinium-enhanced images (fig. 6.46). T2-weighted single-shot echo-train spin-echo images provide information about the tumor itself, and can also be performed as an MRCP study to evaluate the biliary tree. Immediate postgadolinium SGE images may be used to survey the liver for metastatic disease, whereas 2-min postgadolinium fat-suppressed SGE images may be obtained to determine the presence of lymphadenopathy and intraperitoneal spread.

Gastrointestinal Stromal Tumor (GIST). Although the stomach is the principal site for approximately two-thirds of all gut stromal tumors (see description above), the small intestine contains about 25% of the tumors. As in the stomach, these may be large and ulcerating. Gadolinium-enhanced SGE or fat-suppressed SGE images demonstrate heterogeneous and substantial enhancement of the primary tumor (fig. 6.47). Local or intraperitoneal recurrence is not uncommon after surgical resection (fig. 6.48). MRI using immediate postgadolinium SGE is particularly effective at detecting liver metastases because these tend to be hypervascular and often are small.

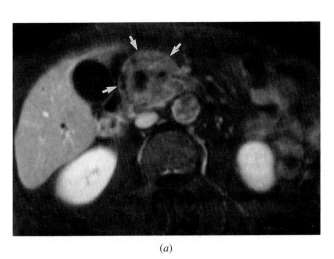

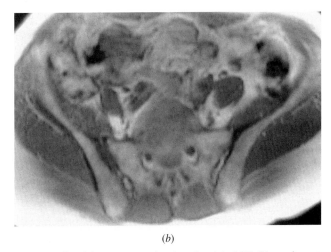

(a)   (b)

FIG. 6.46 Small bowel adenocarcinoma. Gadolinium-enhanced T1-weighted fat-suppressed spin-echo (*a*), SGE (*b*), and postgadolinium T1-weighted fat-suppressed spin-echo (*c*) images in two different patients (*a*) and (*b*, *c*) with small bowel adenocarcinoma. In the first patient (*a*), the size and extent of a large duodenal tumor (arrows, *a*) are well shown on the gadolinium-enhanced fat-suppressed image.

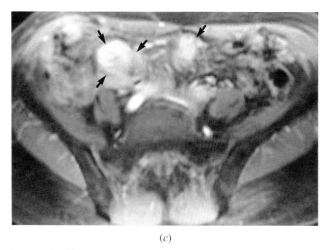

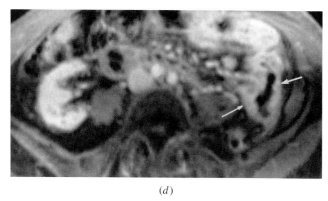

(c)

(d)

FIG. 6.46 (*Continued*) In the second patient (*b, c*), the neoplasm is difficult to identify on the precontrast SGE image (*b*) because it is isointense with background bowel. On the gadolinium-enhanced fat-suppressed SGE image (*c*), the distal jejunal tumors are conspicuous (arrows, *c*) because they are higher in signal intensity and heterogeneous compared with background bowel.

Transverse 90-s postgadolinium fat-suppressed SGE image (*d*) in another patient with adenocarcinoma of the jejunum. Irregular thickening and enhancement of a segment of proximal jejunum is apparent (arrows, *d*).

Lymphoma. Throughout the small intestine and colon are nodules of lymphoid tissue within the mucosa and submucosa. Primary gastrointestinal non-Hodgkin lymphomas are most commonly of the B cell type, and appear to arise from B cells of mucosa-associated lymphoid tissue (MALT) (fig. 6.49). In the small intestine, the terminal ileum is the most common site affected, which reflects the relatively greater amount of lymphoid tissue present in this segment compared with the duodenum and jejunum [67]. Gastrointestinal lymphomas comprise 1–2% of all gastrointestinal malignancies and can assume different gross appearances: 1) diffusely infiltrating lesions that often produce full-thickness mural thickening with effacement of overlying mucosal folds, 2) polypoid lesions that protude into the lumen, and 3) large, exo-

phytic, fungating masses that are prone to ulceration and fistula formation.

The small intestine is involved in up to 50% of patients with widespread primary nodal non-Hodgkin lymphoma. The MRI features of small intestine lymphoma include moderately enhancing thickened loops of bowel and large tumor masses that invade the bowel but usually do not result in obstruction (fig. 6.50). The presence of splenic lesions and mesenteric and retroperitoneal lymphadenopathy supports the diagnosis.

Carcinoid. Carcinoids are the most common primary neoplasm of the small bowel. Tumors are well-differentiated neuroendocrine neoplasms that occur primarily in the distal ileum, in which location they are

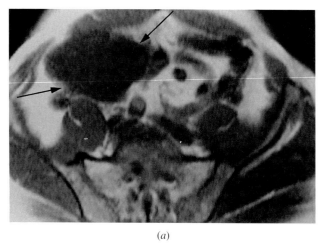

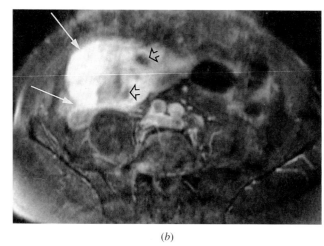

(a)

(b)

FIG. 6.47 **Gastrointestinal stromal tumor (GIST).** SGE (*a*) and gadolinium-enhanced T1-weighted fat-suppressed spin-echo (*b*) images. A large exophytic mass (arrows, *a*) arises from the ileum. Lack of proximal bowel obstruction is consistent with its eccentric origin. The tumor's large size coupled with intense enhancement (arrows, *b*) and regions of necrosis (open arrows, *b*) are typical features of GIST.

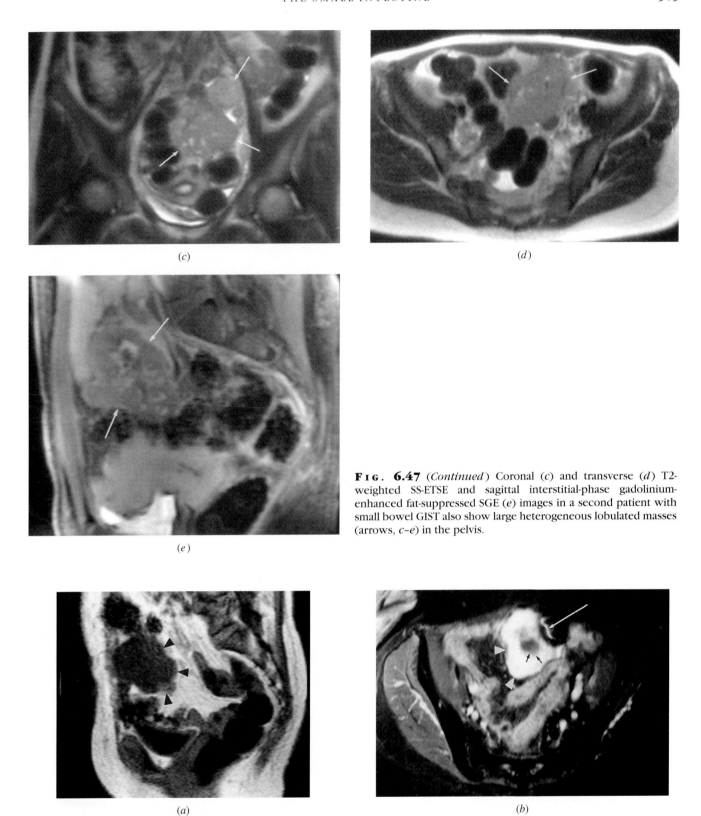

(c)

(d)

(e)

FIG. 6.47 (*Continued*) Coronal (*c*) and transverse (*d*) T2-weighted SS-ETSE and sagittal interstitial-phase gadolinium-enhanced fat-suppressed SGE (*e*) images in a second patient with small bowel GIST also show large heterogeneous lobulated masses (arrows, *c–e*) in the pelvis.

(a)

(b)

FIG. 6.48 Recurrent GIST. Sagittal SGE (*a*) and gadolinium-enhanced T1-weighted fat-suppressed spin-echo (*b, c*) images in a patient with previous surgical resection for GIST. Recurrent GIST exhibits features similar to those of the primary tumor: large size, exophytic growth, hypervascularity, and central necrosis. The eccentric location of the tumor (arrowheads, *a–c*) is seen on all imaging planes.

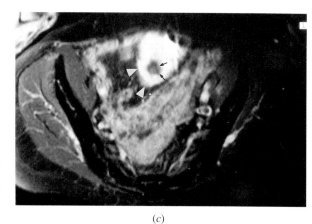

(c)

FIG. 6.48 (*Continued*) Marked enhancement after intravenous contrast reflects hypervascularity. Necrosis often accompanies these large tumors (short arrows, *b*, *c*). Note the susceptibility artifact (long arrow, *b*) associated with surgical clips from prior resection.

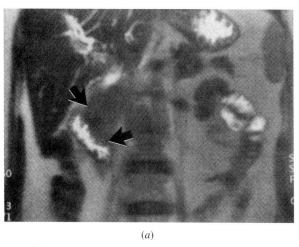

(a)

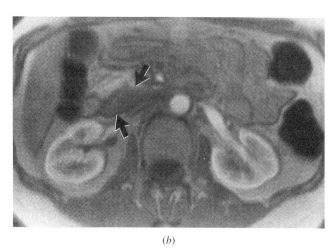

(b)

FIG. 6.49 **Duodenal MALToma.** Coronal T2-weighted SS-ETSE (*a*) and immediate postgadolinium fat-suppressed SGE (*b*) images. T2-weighted image demonstrates irregular thickening of the superior aspect of the duodenal wall caused by a paraduodenal mass (arrows, *a*). postgadolinium image shows a mass that is interposed between the third portion of the duodenum and the head of the pancreas. This mass shows mild heterogeneous enhancement compared to duodenal wall and pancreas, which permits a good distinction between mass and pancreas. Low-grade lyphoma (MALToma type) was proven by endoscopic biopsy. (Reprinted with permission from Marcos HB, Semelka RC, Noone TC, Woosley JT, Lee JKT: MRI of normal and abnormal duodenum using half-Fourier single-shot RARE and gadolinium-enhanced spoiled gradient-echo sequences. *Magn Reson Imaging* 17: 869–880, 1999.)

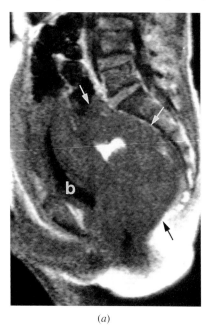

(a)

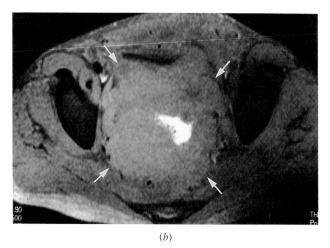

(b)

FIG. 6.50 **Small intestine lymphoma.** Sagittal SGE (*a*), T1-weighted fat-suppressed spin-echo (*b*), sagittal 45-s post- gadolinium SGE (*c*), and gadolinium-enhanced T1-weighted fat-suppressed spin-echo (*d*) images in a patient with diffuse lymphomatous infiltration of the distal jejunum and ileum.

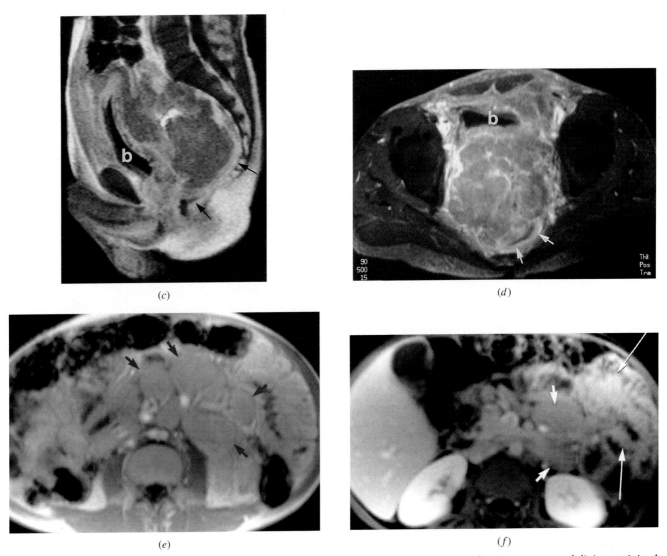

(c)

(d)

(e)

(f)

FIG. 6.50 (*Continued*) A large pelvic mass (arrows, *a, b*) is seen on precontrast images. After intravenous gadolinium, minimal enhancement of the mass is present on early postgadolinium images (*c*), and heterogeneous, slightly greater enhancement is present on the interstitial-phase image (*d*). Minimal enhancement on early postgadolinium images with slight increase and minimal heterogeneous enhancement on more delayed images are common imaging findings for lymphoma in general. The relationship of the mass to adjacent structures can be assessed by imaging in multiple planes. The rectum (arrows, *c, d*) is displaced and compressed by the tumor. Despite extensive disease, there is no proximal small bowel obstruction, a characteristic finding with small intestine lymphoma. High signal intensity within the pelvic mass is consistent with hemorrhage. Bladder = "b," a, c.

Transverse gadolinium-enhanced SGE (*e*) and interstitial-phase gadolinium-enhanced fat-suppressed SGE (*f*) images in a second patient with non-Hodgkin lymphoma. Bulky mesenteric lymphadenopathy (small arrows, *e, f*) is observed as well as thickening of small bowel loops (long arrows, *f*).

almost always malignant. Men and women are affected with equal frequency. Most patients present with tumor-related symptoms of bleeding and bowel obstruction or intussusception. Particular to ileal carcinoids are regional mesenteric metastases and vascular sclerosis. The primary tumor may be quite small, with the accompanying lymphadenopathy and desmoplastic reaction in the root of the mesentery presenting as the only visible manifestation of disease. However, when large enough, the primary tumor causes asymmetric bowel wall thickening and enhances heterogeneously, usually moderate in intensity after intravenous gadolinium (fig. 6.51). The char-

acteristic desmoplastic changes in the mesentery and retroperitoneum that occur in response to the secretion of serotonin and tryptophan are low in signal on both T1- and T2-weighted images and show negligible enhancement after contrast. Liver metastases are responsible for the "carcinoid syndrome," which is characterized by vasomotor instability, intestinal hypomotility, and bronchoconstriction [68]. Liver metastases are often hypervascular and high in signal intensity on T2-weighted images, possessing intense ring or uniform enhancement on immediate postgadolinium SGE images. In the recent series by Bader et al. [69] 98% of liver metastases

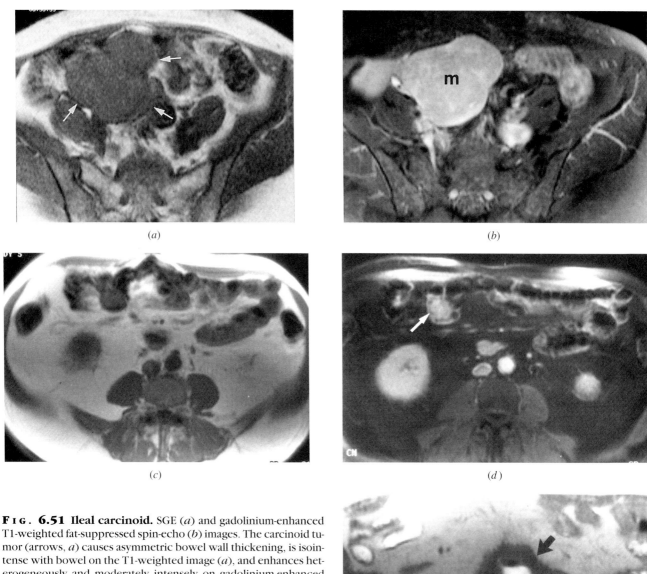

(a)

(b)

(c)

(d)

(e)

F I G . 6.51 Ileal carcinoid. SGE (*a*) and gadolinium-enhanced T1-weighted fat-suppressed spin-echo (*b*) images. The carcinoid tumor (arrows, *a*) causes asymmetric bowel wall thickening, is isointense with bowel on the T1-weighted image (*a*), and enhances heterogeneously and moderately intensely on gadolinium-enhanced interstitial-phase images (*b*).

Transverse SGE (*c*) and and interstitial-phase gadolinium-enhanced fat-suppressed SGE (*d*) images in a second patient with ileal carcinoid demonstrate a nodular mass originating from the bowel loop that is isointense on transverse precontrast T1-weighted image and enhances moderately and heterogeneously on the delayed image (arrow, *d*).

Transverse T2-weighted SS-ETSE (*e*) in a third patient shows irregular circunferential thickening small bowel consistent with carcinoid tumor.

were hypervascular. Occasionally, carcinoid liver metastases are hypovascular and appear nearly isointense with liver on T2-weighted images and demonstrate faint ring enhancement on immediate postgadolinium SGE images.

Metastases. Tumors arising in the mesentery, pancreas, stomach, or colon may involve the small intestine through contiguous extension (fig. 6.52). Metastases to small intestine from melanoma and carcinomas of

the lung, testes, adrenal, ovary, stomach, large intestine, uterus, cervix, liver, and kidney have been reported. Of these malignancies, ovarian tumors are the most common cause of disseminated serosal implants.

On gadolinium-enhanced fat-suppressed SGE images, metastases are moderately high in signal intensity in contrast to the low signal intensity of intra-abdominal fat. Malignant peritoneal tissue enhances moderately to substantially on interstitial-phase gadolinium-enhanced images and appears as nodular or irregularly thickened

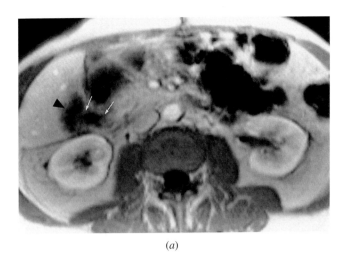 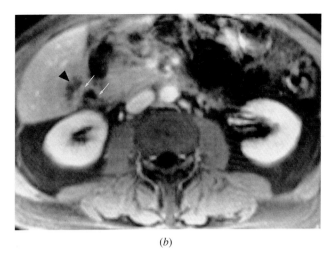

(a)   (b)

F I G . 6.52 Colon cancer liver metastasis with invasion of the duodenum. Immediate postgadolinium SGE (*a*) and 90-s postgadolinium fat-suppressed SGE (*b*) images in a patient with colon cancer metastasis to liver and duodenum. A peripheral hepatic metastasis (arrowhead, *a*, *b*) transgresses the liver capsule to directly invade the adjacent duodenum (arrows, *a*, *b*).

peritoneal or serosal tissue (fig. 6.53). Gadolinium-enhanced fat-suppressed imaging has been shown to be more sensitive than CT imaging in detecting small tumor nodules [70, 71]. Metastatic spread of carcinomas from distal sites such as breast and lung occur, and lesions often lodge on the antimesenteric border of the small bowel. These lesions may be visualized as intramural masses (fig. 6.54). Metastatic tumor may create large submucosal masses and serve as lead points for intussusception.

Inflammatory, Infectious, and Diffuse Disorders

Inflammatory Bowel Disease

Crohn disease and ulcerative colitis are the most common forms of chronic idiopathic inflammatory bowel disease (IBD). MRI findings correlate well with clinical evaluation, endoscopy, and histologic findings. It is a robust technique capable of diagnosing type, evaluating severity, and monitoring response to treatment in patients with IBD [1-4].

Crohn Disease. In North America Crohn disease is the most common inflammatory condition to affect the small bowel. The incidence is greatest in the second and third decades of life, and Crohn's disease is most prevalent in urban-dwelling women. There is evidence for familial associations in Crohn disease, and there is an increased incidence in Jews. The etiology is unknown, but is likely multifactorial including genetic, immunologic, and infectious influences [72]. Crohn disease usually presents in young adults, but can occur in any age group including children and the elderly. Symptoms

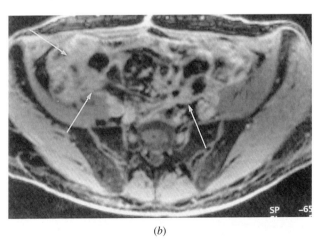

(a)   (b)

F I G . 6.53 Ovarian carcinoma metastases to the peritoneal and serosal surfaces. Transverse 512-resolution T2-weighted echo-train spin-echo (*a*) and 90-s postgadolinium fat-suppressed SGE (*b*) images highlight the improvement in disease detection afforded by breath-hold gadolinium-enhanced fat-suppressed SGE. On the high-resolution T2-weighted image, bowel motion degrades image quality; no metastatic disease can be identified. On the gadolinium-enhanced fat-suppressed SGE image (*b*), the acquisition during suspended respiration avoids breathing artifact and minimizes bowel motion. Enhancement of irregularly thickened tissue along the peritoneum and serosal surface of bowel (arrows, *b*) is consistent with widespread metastatic disease.

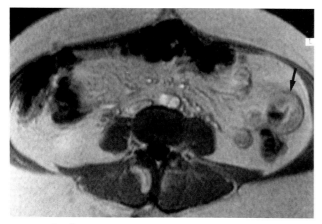

F I G . 6.54 Hematogenous metastases. Transverse 45-s postgadolinium SGE image demonstrates an eccentric mural tumor in the midjejunum (arrow). This tumor was a hematogenous metastasis from uterine leiomyosarcoma.

include watery diarrhea, crampy abdominal pain, weight loss, and fever. Patients with longstanding Crohn disease have a well-documented increased incidence of cancer (approximately 3% of patients) of the gastrointestinal tract, usually involving the colon or ileum. Although any part of the gastrointestinal tract, from the mouth to the anus, may become involved with Crohn disease, it classically involves the terminal ileum, often in association with disease in the right colon. Involvement of the terminal ileum occurs in approximately 70% of patients, with combined terminal ileal and cecal disease present in 40% of the total and isolated terminal ileal involvement in the remaining 30%. Five percent of patients will manifest Crohn disease in the duodenum or jejunum. Twenty to thirty percent will have isolated colon involve-

ment [73]. Crohn disease is characterized pathologically by sharply defined areas showing transmural involvement by chronic inflammation, fibrosis, and noncaseating granulomas.

Sometimes several well-demarcated lesions are separated by normal bowel, producing what are termed "skip lesions." This particular pattern is not found in ulcerative colitis, which produces instead a confluent or continuous region of inflammation. Prominent lymph follicles, lymphangiectasia, and submucosal edema are also noted. Grossly, at the beginning stages of Crohn disease, the mucosa may show only small, hyperemic ("aphtoid") ulcerations. In time, the ulcers extend transmurally, often beyond the intestinal serosa, to become sinus tracts or fistulae. With the evolution of the disease, the bowel wall becomes thickened and inflexible, secondary to fibrosis. In addition, strictures, abscesses, and lymphoid hyperplasia may complicate the disease. The mesenteric changes include inflammatory stranding, a reflection of dilated vasa rectae and sinus tracts, reactive lymphadenopathy, and abundant ("creeping") fat. Patients are usually treated medically. Surgery is reserved for complicated cases, but anastomotic recurrence is common.

Changes of Crohn disease are well shown on MRI. Severe disease is characterized by wall thickness more than 1 cm, length of involvement more than 15 cm, and mural enhancement more than 100% (fig. 6.55). Mild disease results in subtle findings that may only be appreciated on gadolinium-enhanced fat-suppressed images (fig. 6.56). Multiplanar imaging provides comprehensive information on disease extent and complications. T2-weighted single-shot echo-train spin-echo and gadolinium-enhanced T1-weighted fat-suppressed SGE

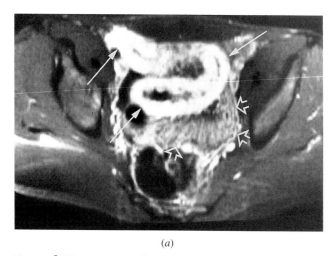

(a)

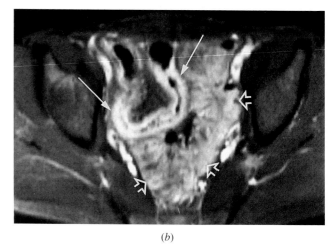

(b)

F I G . 6.55 Severe Crohn disease. Gadolinium-enhanced T1-weighted fat-suppressed spin-echo images (*a–c*) in 3 patients with severe Crohn disease. A thickened loop of substantially enhancing ileum (arrows, *a*) and associated mesenteric inflammation (open arrows, *a*) are characteristic findings for Crohn disease.

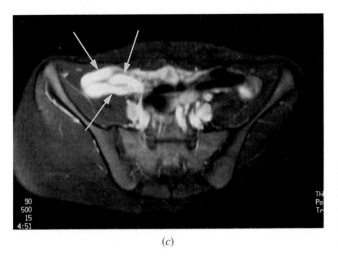

(c)

FIG. 6.55 (*Continued*) In the second patient (*b*), similar findings of a thickened, intensely enhancing loop of ileum (arrows, *b*) with associated mesenteric inflammation (open arrow, *b*) are identified. In the third patient (*c*), multiple thickened loops of intensely enhancing ileum are present (arrows, *c*).

images demonstrate characteristic findings: transmural involvement, skip lesions, and mesenteric inflammatory changes (figs. 6.57–6.59).

Marcos and Semelka evaluated the capability of single-shot echo-train spin-echo and gadolinium-enhanced T1 SGE images for evaluating bowel changes and complications of Crohn disease [74]. The results of this study showed that single-shot echo-train spin-echo image is a very effective technique to demonstrate dilated obstructed bowel, whereas gadolinium-enhanced fat-suppressed SGE is useful in demonstrating inflammatory changes in bowel. Both techniques were effective in showing wall thickening and abscess formation.

Good correlation has been reported between MRI findings and disease activity [2, 4, 5]. These results are in contrast to barium studies, which have limited correlation with symptomatology or response to therapy. Moreover, the potential harm of radiation exposure from serial barium examinations in pregnant women and patients of reproductive age is not inconsequential [73]. MRI may be the modality of choice for evaluation of Crohn disease in patients with contraindication to barium examinations or CT imaging (fig. 6.60).

The MRI criteria of mild, moderate, and severe disease has been described and is a function of wall thickness, length of diseased segment, and percentage of mural contrast enhancement (Table 6.2). The extent of mural enhancement may also be determined by comparison of bowel enhancement on gadolinium-enhanced fat-suppressed SGE with that of the renal parenchyma

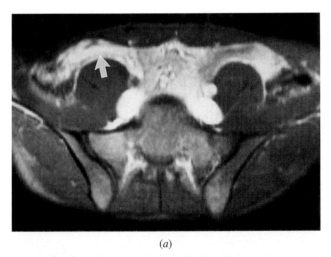

(a)

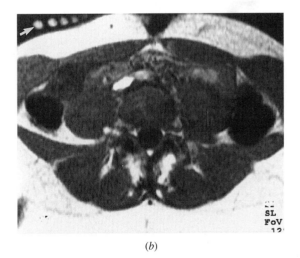

(b)

FIG. 6.56 Mild to moderate Crohn disease. Transverse gadolinium-enhanced T1-weighted fat-suppressed image (*a*) demonstrates moderate inflammatory disease of the terminal ileum (arrow, *a*), which has a wall thickness of 5 mm, <10 cm of diseased bowel, and moderate wall enhancement.

SGE (*b*) and gadolinium-enhanced T1-weighted fat-suppressed spin-echo (*c*) images in a second patient with mild Crohn disease. The unenhanced image (*b*) appears unremarkable. On the gadolinium-enhanced image, transmural enhancement is apparent with wall thickness of 5 mm, length of involved segment of <10 cm, and moderate mural enhancement.

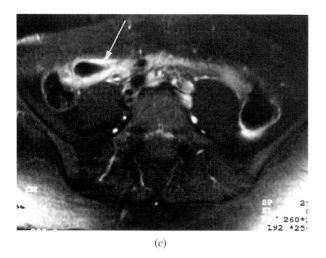

(c)

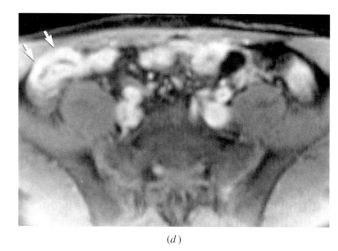

(d)

FIG. 6.56 (*Continued*) This constellation of imaging findings is consistent with mild disease. Assessment of severity of disease must be determined on the nondependent bowel wall (arrow, *c*) after intravenous contrast administration. Lipid beads (small arrow, *b*) demarcate the area of patient tenderness.

Transverse (*d*) and sagittal (*e*) interstitial-phase gadolinium-enhanced fat-suppressed SGE images in a third patient show segmental wall thickening and abnormal enhancement of the distal ileum (arrows, *d*, *e*).

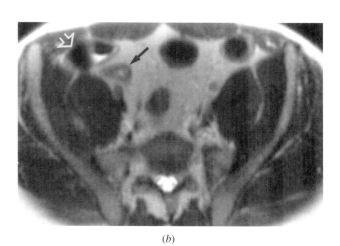

(e)

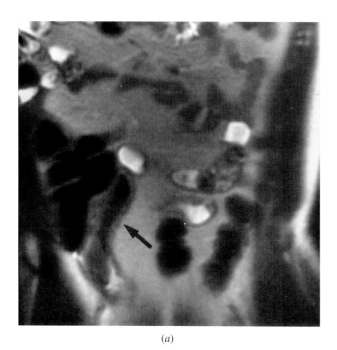

(a)

(b)

FIG. 6.57 **Moderate Crohn disease.** Coronal (*a*) and transverse (*b*) T2-weighted SS-ETSE and 2-min fat-suppressed SGE (*c*) images.

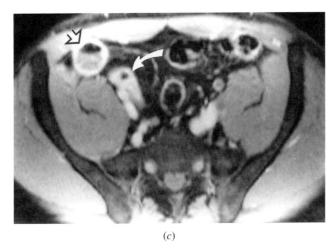

(c)

F I G . 6.57 (*Continued*) The distal terminal ileum (arrow, *a*, *b*) shows increased wall thickness, whereas the ascending colon (open arrow, *b*) demonstrates normal wall thickness. On the 2-min fat-suppressed SGE image (*c*), moderate enhancement of the thickened distal terminal ileum (curved arrow, c) and ascending colon (open arrow, c) are present, reflecting moderate severity of the disease. Note that the ascending colon has a normal wall thickness associated with moderately increased enhancement because of Crohn disease involvement. (Reprinted with permission from Marcos HB, Semelka RC: Evaluation of Crohn's disease using half-Fourier RARE and gadolinium-enhanced SGE sequences: Initial results. *Magn Reson Imaging* 18: 263–268, 2000.)

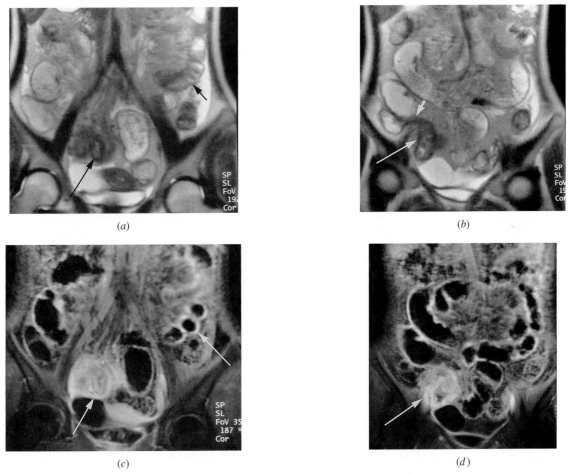

(a)   (b)

(c)   (d)

F I G . 6.58 Severe Crohn disease. Coronal SS-ETSE (*a*, *b*), coronal (*c*, *d*), and transverse (*e*, *f*) 2- to 3-min postgadolinium fat-suppressed SGE images in a patient with severe disease. Coronal T2-weighted images from midabdominal plane (*a*) and 2 cm more anterior (*b*) demonstrate thickened loops of distal small bowel (long arrows, *a*, *b*). The terminal ileum is well shown at its entry into the cecum (small arrow, *b*). Coronal gadolinium-enhanced fat-suppressed SGE images acquired from similar tomographic sections, respectively, demonstrate substantial enhancement of the thickened loops of bowel and surrounding tissues. An enhancing fistulous tract (arrow, *d*) is apparent close to the ileocecal valve. Transverse gadolinium-enhanced images demonstrate intense enhancement of multiple loops of bowel, including loops with wall thickness of 4 mm (arrows, *e*). On the more inferior tomographic section, narrowing of distal ileum is apparent (long arrows, *f*), which accounts for the mild dilation of more proximal loops (arrows, *e*).

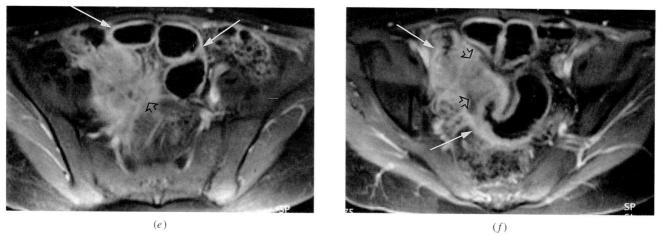

(e)   (f)

F I G . 6.58 (*Continued*) Inflammatory mesenteric changes are evident (hollow arrows, *e, f*). Normal-appearing proximal jejunum (small arrow, *a*) is appreciated on the T2-weighted image.

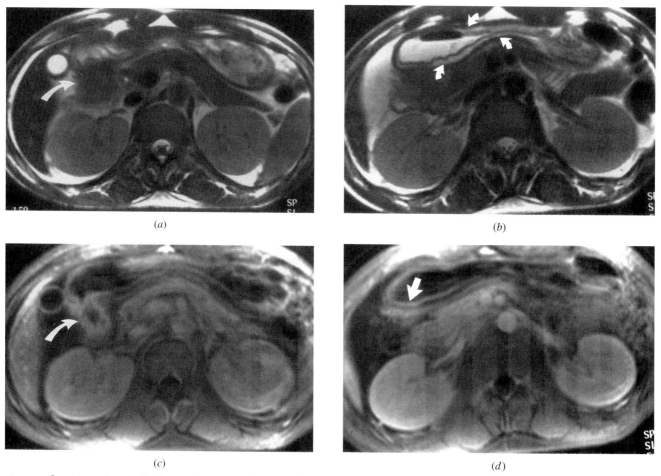

(a)   (b)

(c)   (d)

F I G . 6.59 Duodenal Crohn disease and gastric outlet obstruction. Transverse T2-weighted SS-ETSE (*a, b*) and 2-min postgadolinium fat-suppressed (*c, d*) images. The stomach and proximal duodenum are dilated with a transition point in the second portion of the duodenum. The duodenum at the level of obstruction shows increased wall thickness on the T2-weighted image (curved arrow, *a*). High signal intensity of the submucosa of the antrum and first portion of the duodenum is identified (curved arrows, *b*). The thickened portion of the duodenum demonstrate moderately increased mural enhancement (curved arrow, *c*), with mucosa and serosa layers of the antrum and proximal duodenum demonstrating enhancement reflecting moderate chronic inflammatory changes (arrow, *d*). Low signal intensity of the submucosa on the postgadolinium T1-weighted images (*c, d*) represents submucosal edema and corresponds to high signal intensity on the T2-weighted image. (Reprinted with permission from Marcos HB, Semelka RC: Evaluation of Crohn's disease using half-Fourier RARE and gadolinium-enhanced SGE sequences: Initial results. *Magn Reson Imaging* 18: 263–268, 2000.)

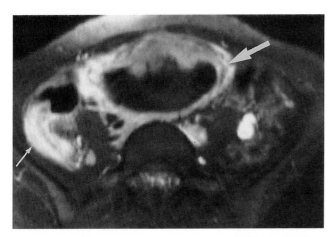

FIG. 6.60 Crohn disease in pregnancy. Gadolinium-enhanced T1-weighted fat-suppressed spin-echo image in a patient in the second trimester of pregnancy. Thickened and intensely enhancing distal ileum is present (arrow). The pregnant uterus is also well shown (large arrow).

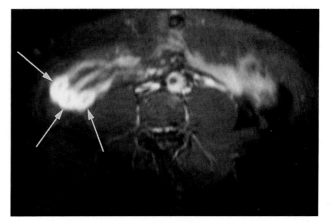

FIG. 6.61 Crohn disease activity assessment. Gadolinium-enhanced T1-weighted fat-suppressed spin-echo image in a patient with active Crohn disease. There is good correlation between clinical indices [CDAI, 185, (active disease 1150); modified IOIBD index, 8 (scale 1–10)] and MRI findings (arrows) of thickened wall, length of diseased segment, and percentage of mural enhancement (MRP, 4664). (Reprinted with permission from Kettritz U, Isaacs K, Warshauer DM, Semelka RC: Crohn's disease: Pilot study comparing MRI of the abdomen with clinical evaluation. *J Clin Gastroenterol* 21: 249–253, 1995.)

[74]. Bowel should not enhance to the same degree as renal cortex on either early capillary-phase images or >1-min interstitial-phase images. Enhancement equivalent or greater than renal cortex is abnormal and most often reflects the presence of inflammatory change.

MRI assessment is made on gadolinium-enhanced T1-weighted fat-suppressed images using the nondependent bowel surface. It is critical that the time point for determining percentage of enhancement is standardized. This establishes reproducible measures of disease activity between studies in the same patient. We have used a time point of 2.5 min after injection. Immediate postgadolinium images reflect significant perivascular inflammation and increased capillary blood flow. Commonly, the inner half of the bowel wall enhances most intensely in this phase of enhancement in severely inflamed bowel. Later interstitial-phase images demonstrate more uniform enhancement in diseased bowel, reflecting capillary leakage and decreased venous removal in transmurally inflamed bowel. A recent pilot study found good correlation between clinical indices to mea-

sure Crohn activity [Crohn Disease Activity Index (CDAI) and modified Index of the International Organization for the Study of Inflammatory Bowel Disease (IOIBD)] and an MRI determinant, the MRI product [wall thickness × length of diseased segment × percentage mural enhancement (MRP)] (fig. 6.61) [4]. This work suggests that MRI may be the best modality for evaluating the severity of Crohn disease. It may provide complementary or confirmatory information to clinical assessment.

MRI also may have a role in the evaluation of acute exacerbations of Crohn disease. Specifically, in patients with longstanding disease, marked enhancement of the mucosa with a substantially thickened wall and minimal enhancements of the outer layer is suggestive of acute-on-chronic involvement (fig. 6.62). Crohn disease may also result in large patulous segments of small bowel that may contain debris due to the presence of chronic distal small bowel obstruction. Patients may be symptomatic from the effects of bacterial overgrowth. On MR images, greatly dilated segments of bowel are shown that contain substantial debris. Single-shot echo-train spin-echo technique is very effective in delineating the extent of dilatation, and gadolinium-enhanced fat-suppressed SGE technique for showing the inflammation (fig. 6.63).

Ulcerative Colitis. Ulcerative colitis is a recurrent acute and chronic ulcero-inflammatory disorder of unknown etiology that affects the large bowel and is discussed below. Small bowel involvement ("backwash ileitis") is the sequela of pancolonic disease. Free reflux of colon contents into the ileum via a patulous,

Table 6.2 Crohn's Disease Severity Criteria

Severity	Contrast Enhancement (%)	Wall Thickness (mm)	Length of Diseased Segment (cm)
Mild*	<50	<5	<5
Moderate	50–100	5–20	variable
Severe	>00	>10	>5**

*Bowel-wall thickening must be at least 4 mm, and one of the other 2 criteria must be satisfied.
**Typically >10 cm of affected bowel.
Reprinted with permission from Ascher SM, Semelka RC: MRI of the gastrointestinal tract. In Higgins CB, Hricak H, Helms CA (eds.). Magnetic Resonance Imaging of the Body. New York: Raven Press, p. 677–700, 1997.

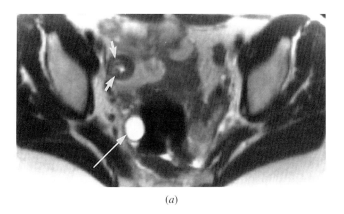

(a)

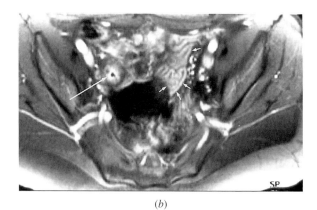

(b)

F I G . 6.62 Acute-on-chronic Crohn disease. T2-weighted SS-ETSE (*a*) and gadolinium-enhanced T1-weighted fat-suppressed spin-echo (*b*) images in a patient with longstanding disease. Increased thickness of distal ileum is present, which demonstrates increased signal intensity in the inner aspect of the wall (short arrows, *a*). Acute exacerbation is characterized by intense mucosal enhancement (long arrow, *b*) with minimal enhancement of the outer wall in substantially thickened bowel. Accompanying hyperemia of the mesentery reflects the active inflammatory process (short arrows, *b*). Incidental note is made of a right adnexal cyst (long arrow, *a*) and free fluid in the pelvis.

Gadolinium-enhanced T1-weighted fat-suppressed spin-echo image (*c*) in a second patient with a long history of Crohn disease. Thickened loops of small bowel with intense enhancement of the inner wall are apparent (arrows, *c*). This appearance is that of acute mucosal exacerbation superimposed on a chronically thickened wall.

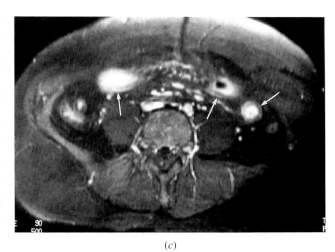

(c)

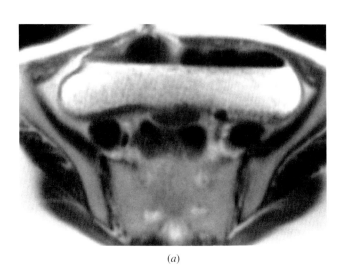

(a)

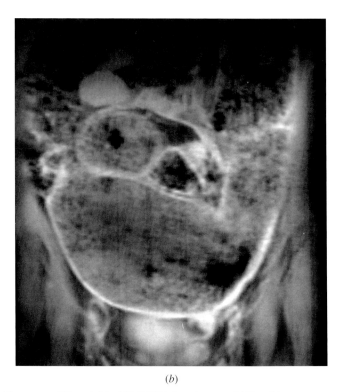

(b)

F I G . 6.63 Crohn disease with dilated stagnant bowel loop. Transverse T2-weighted SS-ETSE (*a*) and coronal (*b*) and transverse (*c*) gadolinium-enhanced interstitial-phase fat-suppressed SGE images.

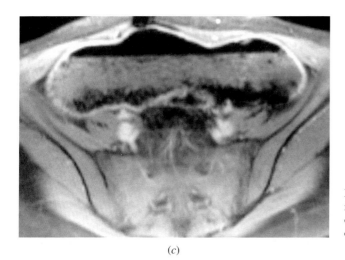

(c)

F I G . 6.63 (*Continued*) An enlarged loop of distal small bowel is present that contains substantial debris. Enlarged stagnant loops of small bowel is a complication of longstanding distal small bowel obstruction as observed in Crohn disease.

incompetent ileocecal valve is believed to be responsible [73]. The lumen of the ileum is moderately dilated, and on MRI the diseased ileal wall is abnormal, showing mild dilatation and moderately increased enhancement with gadolinium, reflective of diffuse inflammation, erosion, and ulcerations (fig. 6.64).

Gluten-Sensitive Enteropathy (Celiac Disease, Celiac Sprue)

Gluten-sensitive enteropathy (GSE) is an immunologically mediated gastrointestinal disease that produces a malabsorption syndrome. GSE likely results from a specific immunologic hyperactivity to a constituent of dietary gluten. The diagnosis is made through jejunal biopsy and is based on the presence of mucosal at-

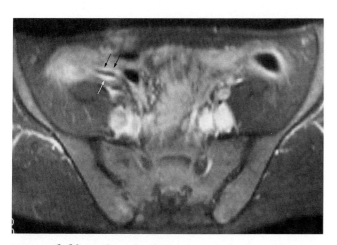

F I G . 6.64 Backwash ileitis. Gadolinium-enhanced T1-weighted fat-suppressed spin-echo image in a patient with ulcerative colitis. Pancolonic involvement with ulcerative colitis results in a patulous ileocecal valve. Reflux of colon contents into the ileum causes inflammatory changes (arrows). (Reprinted with permission from Shoenut JP, Semelka RC, Silverman R, Yaffe CS, Mickflikier AB: The gastrointestinal tract. In Semelka RC, Shoenut JP (eds). *MRI of the Abdomen with CT Correlation*. New York: Raven Press, p. 119–143, 1993.)

rophy with blunting or complete loss of the villi and inflammation within the mucosa of the small intestine. T2-weighted single-shot echo-train spin-echo technique may demonstrate an abnormal mucosal fold pattern of the small bowel, associated with an increase of intraluminal fluid (fig. 6.65) [56].

Scleroderma

Scleroderma, or progressive systemic sclerosis, is a connective tissue disease that often involves the GI tract. There is a patchy destruction of the muscularis propria in the small intestine, mainly involving the duodenum and jejunum. There is also degeneration of both circular and longitudinal muscle layers and replacement by collagen tissue [75]. Dilatation is the most common finding in imaging studies (fig. 6.66), and sacculation with formation of pseudodiverticula also may develop.

Pouchitis

A continent ileostomy ("pouch") is often fashioned for patients after total colectomy. The creation of an ileal pouch changes the usual function of this part of the small intestine from absorption to fecal storage. With fecal storage, stasis and bacterial overgrowth may occur. The most common long-term complication of an ileal resevoir is inflammation known as "pouchitis." This condition is more common in patients with Crohn disease [76] MRI features of which include an enhancing and thickened pouch wall and inflammatory stranding of the "peripouch" fat (fig. 6.67).

Fistula

A fistula is defined as an abnormal passage or communication, generally between two internal organs or leading from an organ to the surface of the body. In the setting of small bowel pathology, fistulae result from compromise in the integrity of the visceral wall and may be sequelae of infection, inflammation, neoplasia, radiation therapy, and ischemia (embolic, thrombotic, or vasoconstrictive).

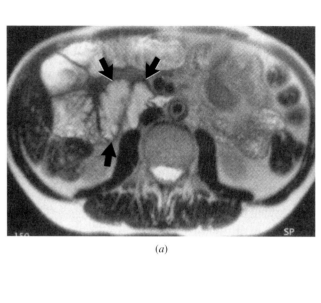

(a)

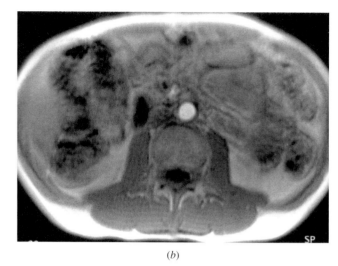

(b)

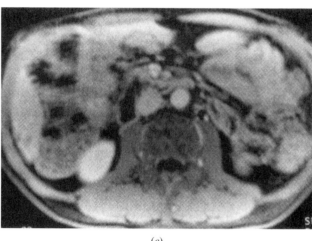

(c)

FIG. 6.65 Gluten-sensitive enteropathy. T2-weighted SS-ETSE (*a*), immediate postgadolinium SGE (*b*), and 90-s post-gadolinium fat-suppressed SGE (*c*) images. T2-weighted image demonstrates an abnormally prominent mucosal pattern in the duodenum associated with an increase in intraluminal fluid (short arrows, *a*). The duodenal mucosa enhances normally, which reflects a lack of vascular changes related to the disease process. Upper gastrointestinal endoscopy with biopsy was performed, and histopathologic examination established the diagnosis of gluten-sensitive enteropathy. (Reprinted with permission from Marcos HB, Semelka RC, Noone TC, Woosley JT, Lee JKT: MRI of normal and abnormal duodenum using half-Fourier single-shot RARE and gadolinium-enhanced spoiled gradient-echo sequences. *Magn Reson Imaging* 17: 869–880, 1999.)

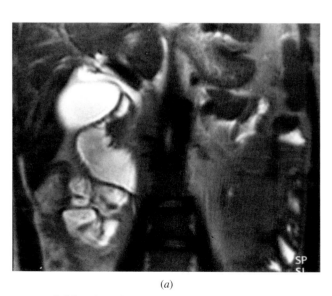

(a)

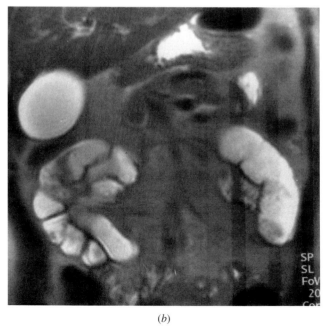

(b)

FIG. 6.66 Scleroderma. Coronal (*a*, *b*) and transverse (*c*) T2-weighted SS-ETSE images show dilatation of the duodenum and multiple small bowel loops without evidence of obstruction.

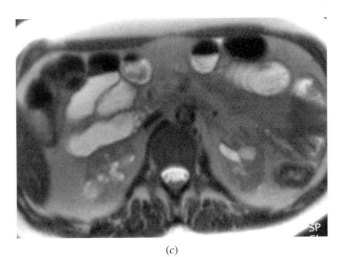

(c)

FIG. 6.66 (*Continued*).

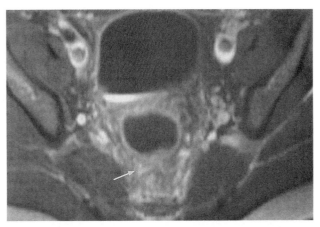

FIG. 6.67 Pouchitis. Gadolinium-enhanced T1-weighted fat-suppressed spin-echo image demonstrates slight thickening of the pouch with stranding in the surrounding fat (arrow).

MRI's good contrast and spatial resolution, in conjunction with direct image acquisition in any plane, makes it a very effective modality in the workup of fistulae. The appearance of a fistula will depend on its contents, the degree of inflammation, and the type of sequence employed. Fluid-filled tracts are high in signal intensity on T2-weighted sequences, whereas gas-filled tracts are signal void. Fat suppression combined with intravenous gadolinium highlights the enhancing fistulous tracts amid the surrounding low-signal intensity intraabdominal fat. Focal discontinuity of the involved organ

at the site of tract penetration is diagnostic (fig. 6.68) [7, 8].

Infectious Enteritis

Active inflammation may be caused by a variety of bacterial, protozoal, fungal, or viral pathogens. *Yersinia enterocolitica* infection may cause acute gastroenteritis, terminal ileitis, mesenteric lymphadenitis, and colitis [77]. *Yersinia ileitis* and *Yersinia enterocolitis* may mimic appendicitis and Crohn disease, respectively. *Campylobacter jejuni* may produce diarrhea, severe

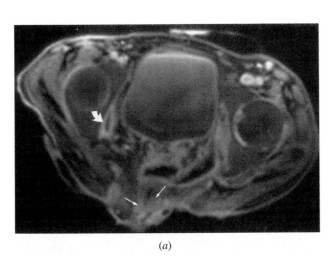

(a)

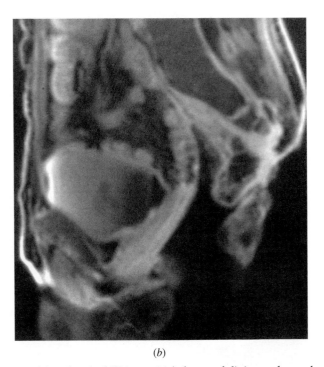

(b)

FIG. 6.68 Pelvic fistulas in a patient with Crohn disease. Transverse (*a*) and sagittal (*b*) interstitial-phase gadolinium-enhanced fat-suppressed SGE images. There is a large decubitus ulcer associated with destruction of the coccyx and lower part of the sacrum. Extensive pelvic cutaneous fistulas appear as enhancing track walls (arrows, *a*). An abscess of the obturator internus muscle is present (curved arrow, *a*).

gastroenteritis, or colitis [78]. *Giardia lamblia* and *Strongyloides stercoralis* are protozoa that typically involve proximal small bowel. The increasing population of immunocompromised patients has led to an increase in occurrence of infectious granulomatous disease of the bowel. Tuberculosis mycobacteria infection involves the terminal ileum. Patients may be symptomatic from the acute inflammatory response, late fibrotic stenosis, or both. *Mycobacterium avium intracellulare* favors the colon and is frequently accompanied by bulky retroperitoneal lymphadenopathy. Cytomegalovirus and *Cryptosporidium parvum* are infections common in AIDS patients. In all of these inflammatory conditions, the MRI findings may be nonspecific, demonstrating bowel wall thickening, increased secretions, and mesenteric edema. Gadolinium- enhanced fat-suppressed SGE imaging demonstrates bowel wall thickening and increased enhancement (fig. 6.69) and detects the presence of abscesses by the identification of encapsulated fluid collections that possess an enhancing rim. Clinical history, coupled with the segment of bowel affected, may suggest the correct diagnosis. For example, in an AIDS patient, small bowel wall thickening and submucosal hemorrhage may be seen in cytomegalovirus infection, whereas focal thickening of the bowel wall and mildly dilated, fluid-filled segments may suggest *Cryptosporidium* infection [45].

Pancreatitis

Small bowel changes also may occur adjacent to an active inflammatory process. Specifically, in patients with pancreatitis, small bowel wall thickening and focal ileus are seen on gadolinium-enhanced SGE images (fig. 6.70). An MRI colon cutoff sign also may be demonstrated.

Drug Toxicity

Inflammatory changes of small bowel may result from a number of etiologies. Chemotherapy toxicity is one example. Diffuse wall thickening and increased enhancement are observed (fig. 6.71), which is typically symmetric and regular in increased wall thickness.

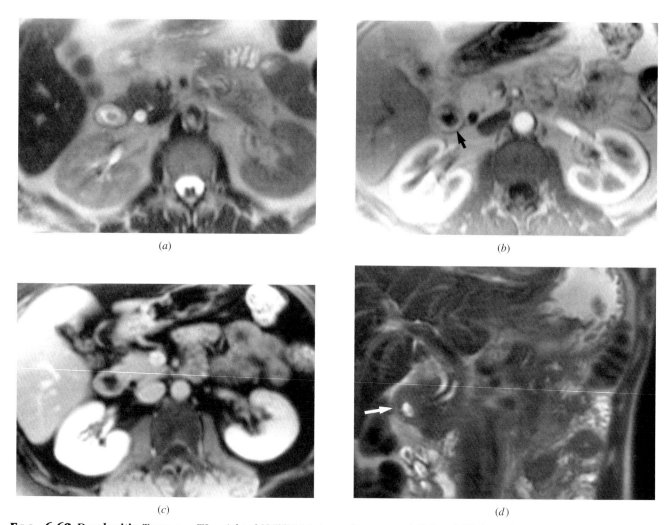

(a)   *(b)*

(c)   *(d)*

F I G . 6.69 Duodenitis. Transverse T2-weighted SS-ETSE (*a*), immediate postgadolinium SGE (*b*), and interstitial-phase gadolinium-enhanced fat-suppressed SGE (*c*) images.

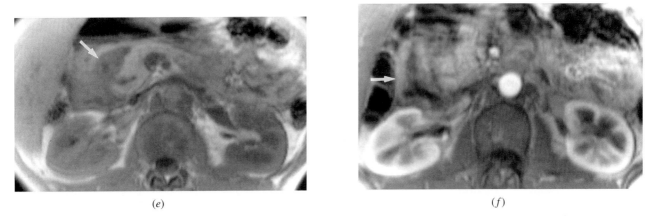

(e)   (f)

F I G . 6.69 (*Continued*) Diffuse wall thickening and enhancement (arrow, *b*), involving the second part of the duodenum are observed in a patient with infectious enteritis.

Coronal T2-weighted SS-ETSE (*d*), transverse SGE (*e*), and immediate postgadolinium T1-weighted SGE (*f*) in a second patient who has eosinophilic enteritis. There is thickening of the the first and second portions of the duodenum (arrows, *d–f*) with duodenal dilatation.

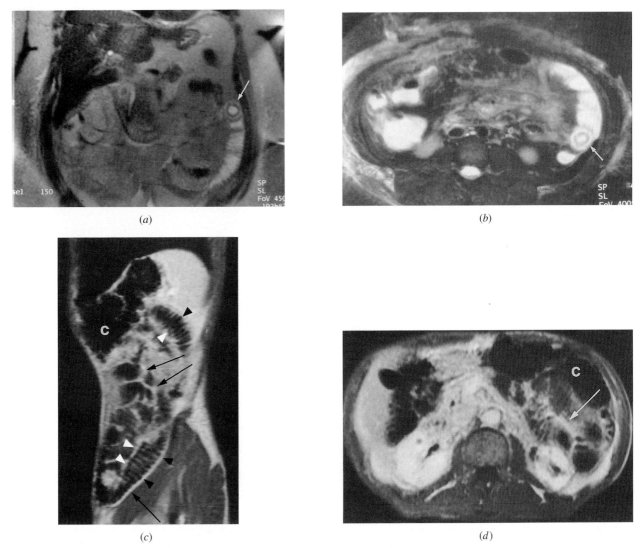

(a)   (b)

(c)   (d)

F I G . 6.70 Small intestine inflammation secondary to pancreatitis. Coronal T2-weighted SS-ETSE (*a*) and T2-weighted fat-suppressed echo-train spin-echo (*b*) images demonstrate circumferential high signal intensity of the wall of the jejunum (arrow, *a*, *b*) secondary to edema caused by inflammatory changes induced by pancreatitis. The outer wall is high in signal intensity, whereas the inner wall is low in signal intensity, reflecting the extrinsic nature of the bowel inflammation.

Sagittal (*c*) and transverse (*d*) interstitial-phase gadolinium-enhanced SGE images in a second patient demonstrate dilation (arrowheads, *c*) of small bowel with increased wall enhancement (arrows, *c*, *d*). The transverse colon ("c", *c*, *d*) shows a transition from normal caliber to narrowed, which is the transverse colon cutoff sign of pancreatitis.

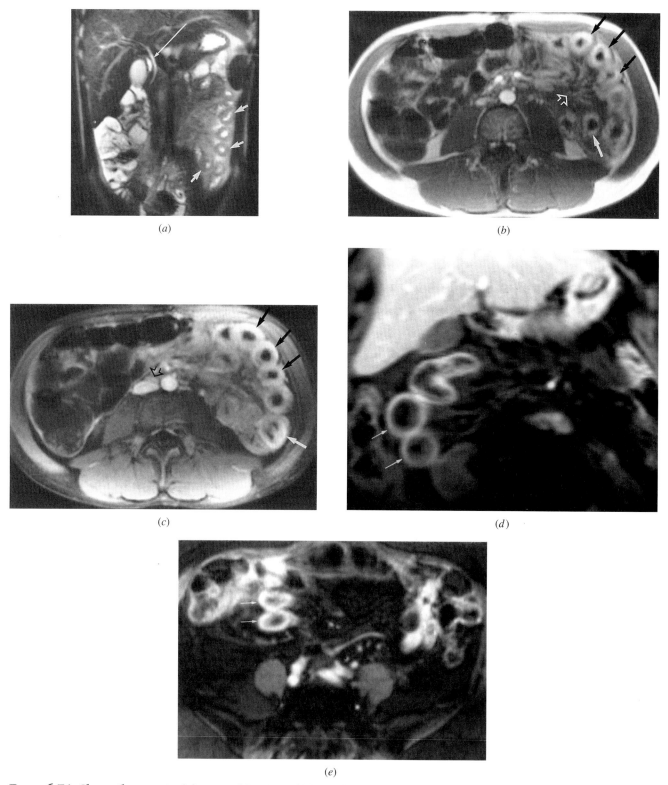

(a)

(b)

(c)

(d)

(e)

F I G . 6.71 Chemotherapy toxicity enteritis. Coronal T2-weighted SS-ETSE (*a*), immediate postgadolinium SGE (*b*), and 90-s postgadolinium fat-suppressed SGE (*c*) images in a patient with chemotherapy toxicity enteritis. Many etiological agents may cause inflammation of the small bowel. The findings are nonspecific and include diffuse circumferential wall thickening (short arrows, *a*), marked bowel wall enhancement (arrows, *b*, *c*), mesenteric infiltration and hyperemia (open arrow, *b*), and lymphadenopathy (open arrow, *c*). Note the normal common bile duct on the T2-weighted image (long arrow, *a*).

Coronal (*d*) and transverse (*e*) interstitial-phase gadolinium-enhanced fat-suppressed SGE images in a second patient, who underwent chemotherapy for ovarian cancer. There is abnormal enhancement of multiple loops of small bowel (arrows, *d*, *e*), consistent with chemotherapy toxicity enteritis.

Radiation Enteritis

In the gastrointestinal tract, the small intestine is the region most sensitive to radiation injury. Radiation therapy for malignant disease may cause an enteritis with tumor doses greater than 45 Gy. The majority of cases are secondary to treatment for female genital tract malignancy. The distal jejunum and ileum are the most common sites affected. Acute injury to the small intestine occurs within hours to days after radiation therapy. Although some damage to the intestinal wall is a regular occurrence, lesions are variable in severity. Microscopic inspection may show sloughed villi with mucosal hemorrhage, edema, focal necrosis, and inflammation. Early postradiotherapy complications include ulceration, necrosis, bleeding, perforation, and abscess formation. The development of chronic radiation enteritis is variable, developing months to years after the radiation event. Chronic radiation enteritis is a progressive disease resulting from underlying vascular damage. Vascular injury includes fibrosis and hyalinization of blood vessel walls leading to obliterative endarteritis within the intestinal wall and mesentery. Progression of the vascular pathology causes ischemia. Normal tissue is replaced by parenchymal atrophy and progressive fibrosis. Complications of chronic radiation enteritis include strictures, fistulae, bowel fixation, and angulation. Varying degrees of small bowel obstruction may result. Gadolinium-enhanced fat-suppressed SGE imaging is the most effective technique for detecting the diffuse early ischemic and inflammatory changes of radiation enteritis as well as the more focal late fibrotic sequelae. Changes caused by radiation effect are reflected in diffuse symmetric bowel wall thickening and enhancement of multiple loops of small bowel in the same region of the abdomen. Radiation effect can be readily distinguished from recurrent tumor, which demonstrates irregular, nodular bowel wall thickening (fig. 6.72).

Ischemia and Hemorrhage

Ischemia and hemorrhage may occur in tandem or as isolated events. Ischemia, regardless of etiology, leads to wall edema secondary to capillary leakage (fig. 6.73). If ischemia is prolonged, infarction can result. The MRI findings parallel the severity of blood flow compromise. Early changes include mural thickening and increased enhancement on late postcontrast images (fig. 6.74). Increased enhancement on immediate postgadolinium images reflects leaky capillaries. Necrotic bowel manifests MRI findings consistent with hemorrhage, and in severe cases, portal venous gas may be observed (see fig. 6.74). Vascular compromise or thrombosis may be well shown on early (>1 min) postgadolinium images (fig. 6.75) and MRA images. Bowel wall hemorrhage from trauma or ischemia may be diagnosed by high signal intensity within the submucosa on both T1- and T2-weighted sequences because of the presence of extracellular methemoglobin. Noncontrast T1-weighted fat-suppressed images are the most sensitive for the detection of subacute blood (fig. 6.76).

Hypoproteinemia

Hypoproteinemia may arise from a number of causes, the most common of which are cirrhosis and malnourishment. In the setting of cirrhosis, hypoproteinemia has been postulated as the primary cause of intestinal wall edema of the large and small bowel. It is generally thought that edema is diffuse and results from changes in oncotic pressure [79]. Generalized bowel wall thickening is present, which is best appreciated in the jejunum. Unlike inflammatory conditions, enhancement on gadolinium-enhanced images is negligible (fig. 6.77).

Intussusception

Intussusception is a form of intestinal obstruction characterized by the telescoping of one intestinal segment into another. Predisposing factors include masses and motility disorders [80]. Transient asymptomatic intussusceptions are not uncommon imaging findings, but multiple nonobstructing intussusceptions suggest an underlying bowel disorder such as sprue. The invaginating bowel segment is referred to as the intussusceptum, and the bowel segment into which the prolapse has occurred is referred to as intussuscipiens. Intussusception is clearly demonstrated on T2-weighted single-shot echo-train spin-echo images because of the sharp anatomic detail of this sequence. In the setting of intussusception, fluid in dilated bowel provides excellent intrinsic contrast for the bowel-within-bowel appearance (fig. 6.78).

Graft-versus-Host Disease

Graft-versus-host disease (GVHD) is an immunologic disorder that occurs in any situation in which immunologically competent donor cells are transplanted into an immunologically incompetent recipient. GVHD most commonly follows bone marrow or organ transplantation. The acute form involves the gastric antrum, small bowel, and colon and occurs within days (7–100) in recipients. Histologically, acute GVHD shows loss of normal intestinal mucosal architecture with ulceration, mucosal denudation, and submucosal edema. On MR images there is diffuse bowel wall thickening with increased enhancement of the inner wall layers (fig. 6.79). The chronic form of GVHD disease may follow the acute form or occur insidiously and is usually associated with esophageal involvement. Microscopic examination of the esophagus shows a sloughed and hyperemic mucosa. This desquamative esophagitis may lead to webs and strictures.

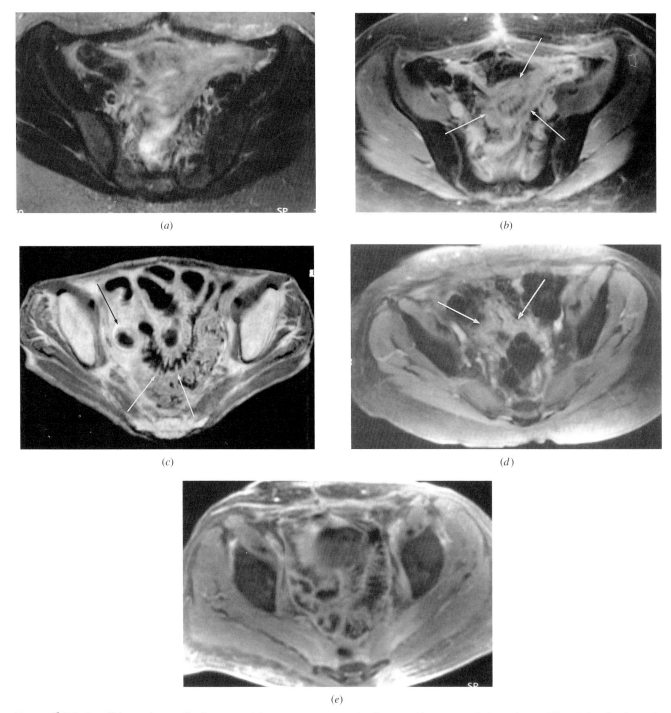

(a)

(b)

(c)

(d)

(e)

F I G . 6.72 Small intestine radiation enteritis versus metastatic disease. Transverse 512-resolution T2-weighted echo-train spin-echo (*a*), 90-s postgadolinium fat-suppressed SGE (*b*), and 90-s postgadolinium SGE (*c*) images in two patients (*a*, *b*) and (*c*) with radiation enteritis, respectively. In the first patient, the T2-weighted echo-train spin-echo image (*a*) is degraded by blurring artifact secondary to peristalsis. Breath-hold technique coupled with gadolinium-enhanced fat-suppressed imaging at the same level highlights postradiation therapy changes of the small bowel: diffuse, symmetric wall thickening with increased enhancement (arrows, *b*). Similar changes are noted in the second patient after radiation therapy (arrows, *c*).

Transverse 90-s postgadolinium fat-suppressed SGE image (*d*) in a third patient, who has recurrent ovarian cancer, demonstrates irregular focal thickening of small bowel. Note the difference between the symmetric and uniform bowel thickening associated with radiation changes (*b*, *c*) and the more focal and asymmetric changes produced by metastatic disease to the small bowel (arrows, *d*).

Transverse gadolinium-enhanced interstitial-phase fat-suppressed SGE (*e*) image in a fourth patient, after radiation therapy for colon cancer, shows circumferential small bowel thickening.

THE LARGE INTESTINE

Normal Anatomy

The large bowel measures approximately 4.5 ft in length and is divided into the appendix, cecum, ascending colon, transverse colon, descending colon, sigmoid colon, rectum, and anal canal. Its main functions include absorption of water and electrolytes, storage of fecal matter, and mucus secretion.

The cecum lies below the level of the ileocecal valve. Although the cecum is in the right iliac fossa, it possesses a mesentery and sometimes is freely mobile. This mobility predisposes the cecum to volvulus formation. The ascending and descending colon are retroperitoneal and located in the anterior pararenal space. The transverse colon is located anteriorly in the peritoneal cavity suspended by the transverse mesocolon, which originates from the peritoneal covering of the anterior surface of the pancreas. The gastrocolic ligament connects the superior surface of the transverse colon to the greater curvature of the stomach. The sigmoid colon is intraperitoneal and suspended by a mesentery, whereas the rectum is retroperitoneal and relatively fixed. The frontal and lateral surfaces of the rectum are covered with peritoneum, which is then reflected anteriorly, forming the rectovaginal recess in females and the rectovesical recess in males. Below the coccyx, the rectum traverses the levator ani muscles to become the anal canal.

Colonic microstructure consists of four layers: mucosa, submucosa, muscularis externa, and serosa. The bowel wall is usually less than 4 mm thick. The muscularis consists of an inner circular and an outer

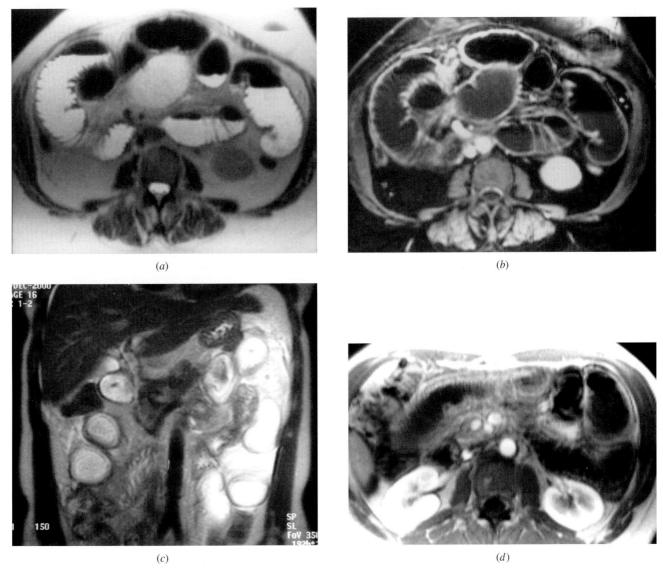

(a)

(b)

(c)

(d)

F I G . 6.73 Small bowel ischemia. T2-weighted SS-ETSE (a) and interstitial-phase gadolinium-enhanced fat-suppressed SGE (b) images in a patient with encarcerated hernia. Multiple dilated enhancing loops of small bowel with increased mural enhancement are observed. Air-fluid levels are identified on T2-weighted image (a).

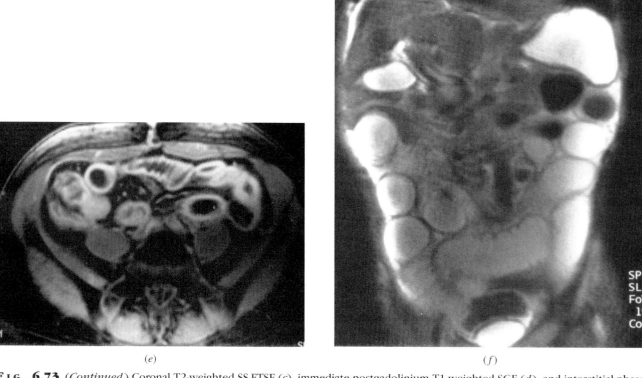

(e)   (f)

F I G . 6.73 (*Continued*) Coronal T2-weighted SS-ETSE (*c*), immediate postgadolinium T1-weighted SGE (*d*), and interstitial-phase gadolinium-enhanced fat-suppressed SGE (*e*) images in a second patient, who underwent radiotherapy for cervix cancer. Small bowel dilatation with increased thickness and enhancement is present. Operative finding were consistent with multiple adhesions and bowel ischemia.

Coronal T2-weighted SS-ETSE (*f*) image in a third patient shows diffuse, markedly dilated small bowel loops.

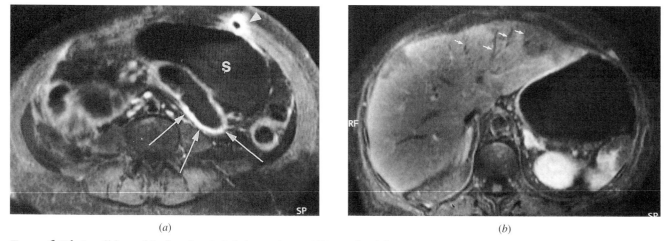

(a)   (b)

F I G . 6.74 Small bowel ischemia. Gadolinium-enhanced T1-weighted fat-suppressed spin-echo images (*a, b*). The patient had undergone previous small bowel resection. Increased enhancement of a loop of proximal small bowel (arrows, *a*) is present. The stomach ("s," *a*) also contains regions of increased mural enhancement. Increased enhancement results from leaky capillaries in ischemic bowel disease. Portal venous gas (small arrows, *b*) is an ominous finding suggesting bowel necrosis. Susceptibility artifact (arrowhead, *a*) is noted within the anterior abdominal wall.

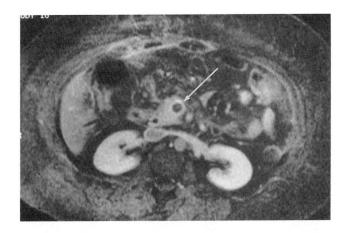

FIG. 6.75 Superior mesenteric vein (SMV) thrombosis. Transverse 90-s postgadolinium fat-suppressed SGE image demonstrates signal void thrombus in the SMV with increased enhancement of the SMV wall (arrow), which was caused by infection associated with thrombosis.

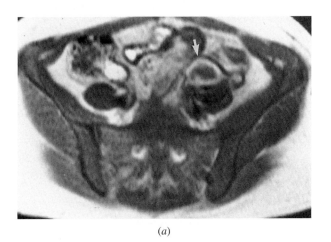

(a)

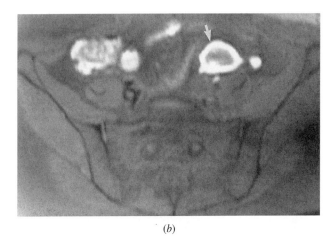

(b)

FIG. 6.76 Submucosal hemorrhage. SGE (*a*) and T1-weighted fat-suppressed spin-echo (*b*) images in a woman status posthysterectomy who had undergone vigorous intraoperative bowel retraction. Increased signal intensity in the bowel wall on the SGE image (arrow, *a*) becomes more conspicuous after fat suppression (arrow, *b*). (Reprinted with permission from Shoenut JP, Semelka RC, Silverman R, Yaffe CS, Mickflikier AB: The gastrointestinal tract. In Semelka RC, Shoenut JP (eds.). *MRI of the Abdomen with CT Correlation.* New York: Raven Press, p. 119–143, 1993.)

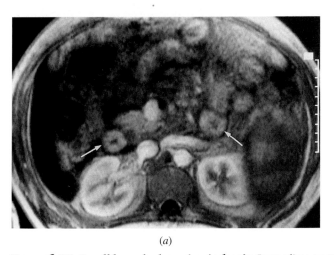

(a)

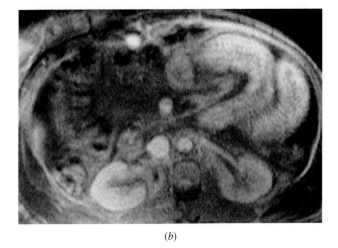

(b)

FIG. 6.77 Small bowel edema in cirrhosis. Immediate postgadolinium SGE (*a*), 90-s postgadolinium SGE (*b*), and T2-weighted single-shot echo train spin echo (*c*) images in 3 patients with cirrhosis.

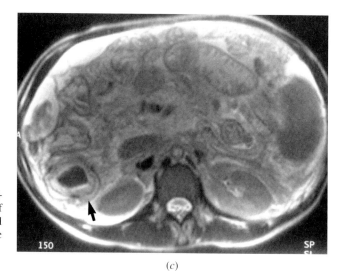

(c)

F I G . 6.77 (*Continued*) Ascites and diffuse thickening of multiple loops of small bowel (arrows, *a*) are present. Third spacing of fluid secondary to hypoproteinemia accounts for the bowel wall thickening. High-signal submucosal edema is well shown on the single-shot T2-weighted image (arrow, *c*).

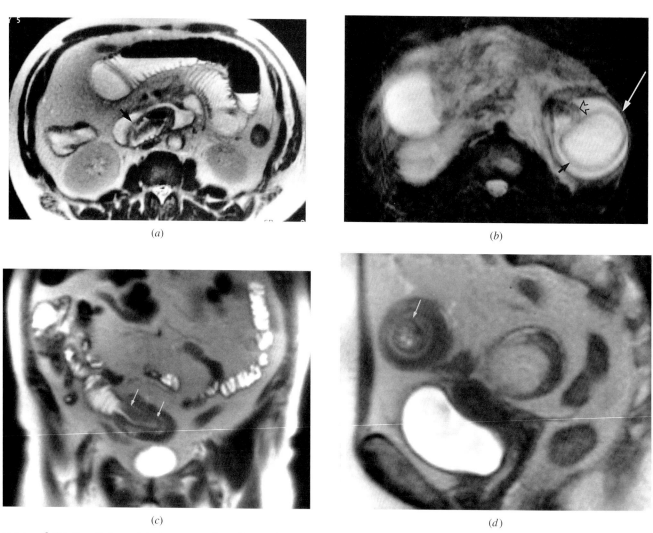

(a)

(b)

(c)

(d)

F I G . 6.78 Small bowel intussusception. T2-weighted SS-ETSE (*a*) and T2-weighted fat-suppressed echo-train spin-echo (*b*) images in 2 patients. In the first patient, the T2-weighted image (*a*) provides clear definition of the bowel-within-bowel appearance (arrow, *a*) of intussusception. In the second patient (*b*), respiratory and bowel motion degrades the majority of the peritoneal cavity. However, the dilated, relatively fixed, hypotonic loop of the intussuscipiens (long arrow, *b*) is relatively well shown.

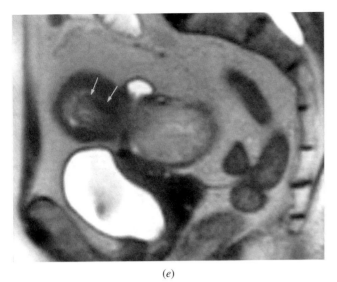

(e)

F I G. 6.78 (*Continued*) The intussusceptum (short arrows, *a*) is clearly shown, and its mesentery (hollow arrow, *b*) is also appreciated. In this second patient adequate visualization of the intussusception occurred in this non-breath-hold study because of the hypotonicity of the involved bowel segments.

Coronal (*c*) and sagittal (*d*, *e*) T2-weighted SS-ETSE images in a third patient. The bowel-within-bowel appearance (arrows, (*c–e*) is clearly demonstrated. (Courtesy of N. Cem Balci, Florence Nightingale Hospital, Istanbul, Turkey).

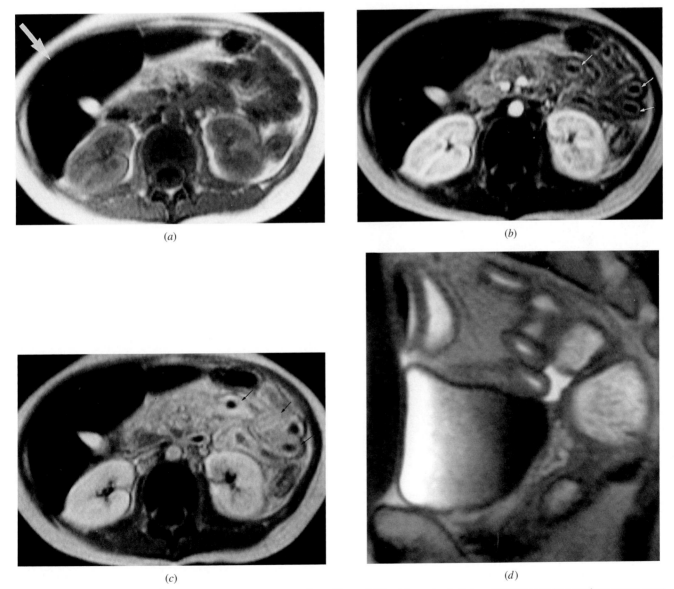

(a)

(b)

(c)

(d)

F I G. 6.79 Graft-versus-host disease. SGE (*a*), immediate (*b*), and 90-s (*c*) postgadolinium SGE images in a patient status post bone marrow transplant. Unenhanced images suggest thickening of multiple loops of small bowel.

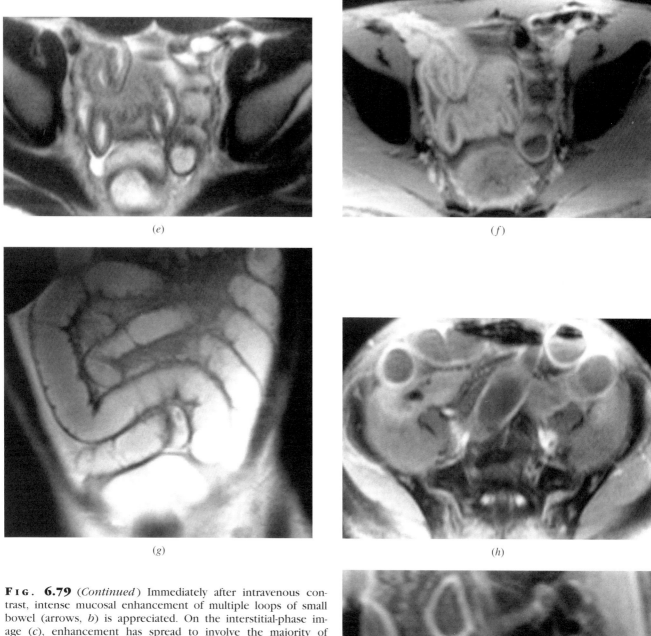

(e)

(f)

(g)

(h)

FIG. 6.79 (*Continued*) Immediately after intravenous contrast, intense mucosal enhancement of multiple loops of small bowel (arrows, *b*) is appreciated. On the interstitial-phase image (*c*), enhancement has spread to involve the majority of the wall (arrows, *c*). This enhancement pattern reflects hyperemia and capillary leakage, respectively. The decreased signal intensity of the liver (arrow, *a*) is consistent with iron overload secondary to multiple blood transfusions. (Reprinted with permission from Ascher SM, Semelka RC: MRI of the gastrointestinal tract. In Higgins CB, Hricak H, Helms CA (eds.), *Magnetic Resonance Imaging of the Body*. New York: Raven Press, p. 677–700, 1997.)

Sagittal (*d*) and transverse (*e*) T2-weighted SS-ETSE and transverse interstitial-phase gadolinium-enhanced fat-suppressed SGE (*f*) images in a second patient after bone marrow transplant. There is marked and diffuse wall thickening and increased mural enhancement of multiple bowel loops.

Coronal T2-weighted SS-ETSE (*g*), transverse (*h*), and sagittal (*i*) interstitial-phase gadolinium-enhanced fat-suppressed SGE images in a third patient after bone marrow transplant for acute lymphocytic leukemia. There are dilated, fluid-filled small bowel loops associated with diffuse enhancement of the bowel wall.

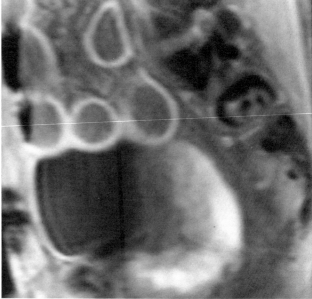

(i)

longitudinal layer. Thickened muscular bundles of the outer muscle layer form the taeniae coli. Because the taeniae are shorter in length than the colonic wall itself, taeniae coli gather the wall into sacculations or haustra. Colonic luminal diameter is greatest in the cecum and gradually decreases distally to the level of the rectal ampulla, where the caliber again increases.

MRI Technique

The technique and considerations for studying the large bowel parallel those for the small bowel. Fasting at least 4–6 h before imaging is recommended to reduce peristalsis. Blurring artifact from bowel motion decreases image quality of long-acquisition time T2-weighted conventional and fast spin-echo techniques. T2-weighted single-shot echo-train spin-echo technique overcomes this limitation and should be performed in the axial

and coronal planes for imaging colonic disease, with the sagittal plane reserved for imaging the rectum. Gadolinium-enhanced fat-suppressed SGE imaging is an important sequence for imaging the colon, as with all other segments of intra-abdominal bowel. Normal colon is thin-walled, has haustrations, and enhances minimally with gadolinium (fig. 6.80).

The rectum deserves special mention. Unlike the remaining large intestine, the relatively fixed position of the rectum benefits from high-resolution (512 matrix) T2-weighted echo-train spin-echo imaging. This technique is particularly useful for the evaluation of rectal carcinoma, in assessing the extent of bowel wall involvement by tumor, determining the relationship of tumors to adjacent structures, and distinguishing tumor recurrence from fibrosis. Endorectal MRI also may be used to study the rectum. The endoluminal surface coil optimizes spatial resolution and demonstrates the rectal wall layers,

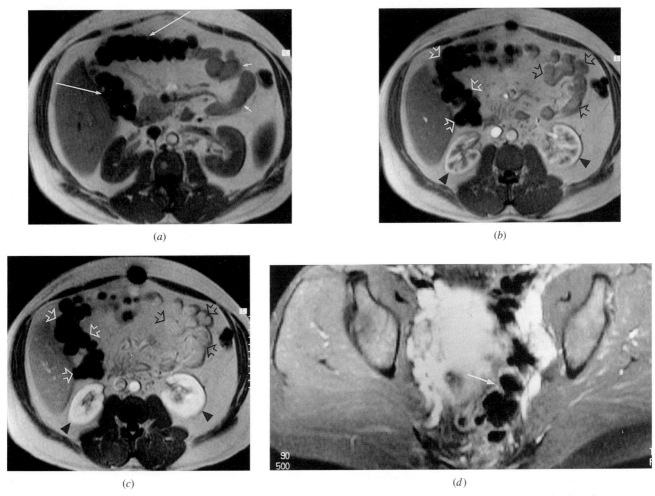

(a) (b) (c) (d)

F I G . 6.80 Normal large bowel. SGE (*a*), immediate (*b*), and 90-s (*c*) postgadolinium SGE images. Air-filled colon (long arrows, *a*) and normal small bowel (short arrows, *a*) are seen on the precontrast T1-weighted image (*a*). After intravenous gadolinium administration, the walls of the large and small bowel (open arrows, *b, c*) enhance less than adjacent renal parenchyma (arrowheads, *b, c*) on capillary-phase (*b*) and interstitial-phase (*c*) images. Gadolinium-enhanced T1-weighted fat-suppressed spin-echo image (*d*) in another subject demonstrates a normal-appearing sigmoid colon that shows minimal mural enhancement, thin wall, and haustrations (arrow, *d*).

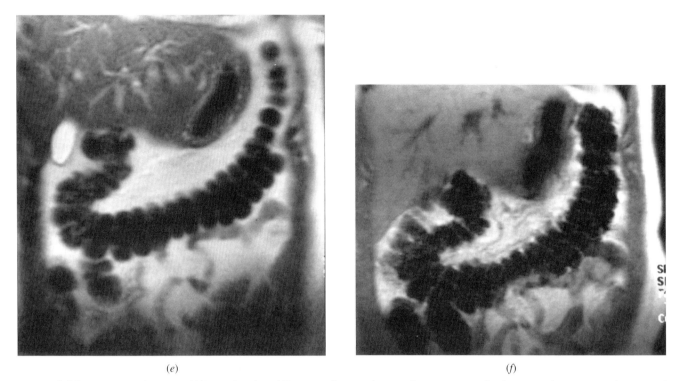

(e)   (f)

F I G . 6.80 (*Continued*) Coronal T2-weighted SS-ETSE (*e*) and coronal SGE (*f*) images in a third patient demonstrate the normal transverse colon with multiple haustrations.

anal sphincter complex, and disease processes [9, 10, 81, 82]. The use of intraluminal contrast to distend the colon may improve detection of mucosal abnormalities [83].

The layers of the rectal wall can be visualized on gadolinium-enhanced T1-weighted fat-suppressed images, high-resolution T2-weighted images, and endorectal coil T2-weighted images (see fig. 6.80). The transition between the rectum and the anal canal can be deter-

mined by the observation that the rectum contains intraluminal air and the anal canal is collapsed (fig. 6.81). MR colonography is a relatively recent technique that involves distending the colon with fluid and obtaining coronal thick-slab (5–8 cm) T2-weighted single-shot echo-train spin echo to generate images that resemble fluoroscopic barium enemas. Water serves well as an intraluminal contrast agent.

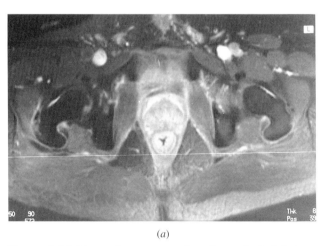

(a)

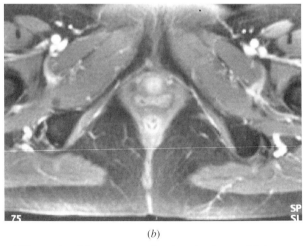

(b)

F I G . 6.81 Normal rectum and anal canal. Gadolinium-enhanced T1-weighted fat-suppressed spin-echo image (*a*) in a man highlight the different layers of the rectum (from inner layer to outer layer): high-signal intensity mucosa, low-signal intensity muscularis mucosa and lamina propria, high-signal intensity submucosa, and low-signal intensity muscularis propria. The rectum contains air within the lumen.

Gadolinium-enhanced T1-weighted fat-suppressed spin-echo image (*b*) in a woman demonstrates the same enhancement features of the anal canal. Note that the anal canal is collapsed and does not contain air.

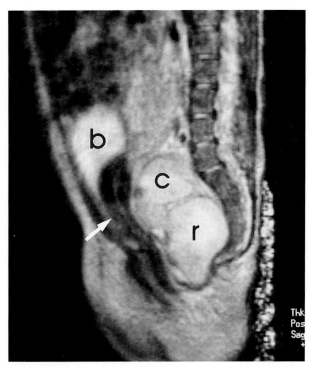

F I G. 6.82 Colonic duplication. T2-weighted spin-echo image in a patient with colonic duplication. The uterus (arrow) and bladder (b) are anteriorly displaced by two fluid-filled viscous structures that represent the rectum (r) and the duplication cyst (c).

Congenital Anomalies

Malrotation

Nonrotation, the most common rotational abnormality, is discussed above. In this condition the large bowel will occupy the left side of the abdomen.

Duplication

Colonic duplications represent a congenital longitudinal division of the developing gut. Grossly, two intestinal

lumens are identified. The abnormalities may be limited to a single segment of large bowel, or they can involve the entire colon (fig. 6.82). Symptoms will depend on whether or not there is communication of the duplication with the remainder of the colon. Patients with right colon duplication are at risk for intussusception.

Anorectal Anomalies

Most cases of anorectal anomalies occur in association with other congenital malformations. MRI has been successful in evaluating these patients because it directly demonstrates the rectal pouch and sphincter muscles in multiple planes. This permits exact determination of the location and developmental status of the sphincter muscles as well as identification of associated anomalies of the kidneys and spine. MRI is also valuable for post-operative assessment of the neorectum and sphincteric muscles (figs. 6.83 and 6.84) [84].

Mass Lesions

Benign Masses

Polyps and Polyposis Syndromes. Adenomas are the most common form of colorectal polyp. Colonic adenomatous polyps are the most common large bowel neoplasm. All adenomatous polyps arise as the result of epithelial proliferative dysplasia or deranged development (fig. 6.85). In this regard, adenomas are the precursor lesion for colorectal adenocarcinoma. Three basic patterns of adenomatous polyps are discerned pathologically: tubular, tubulovillous, and villous. Villous adenomas are characterized by a neoplastic growth composed of fine fingerlets or villi that project from the muscularis mucosae to the outer tip of the adenoma and show a propensity for the rectum and rectosigmoid area. Villous architecture tends to be found more frequently in larger adenomas and is associated with a higher risk of malignancy (fig. 6.86) [85]. Multiple colonic adenomas

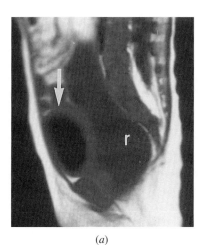

(a)

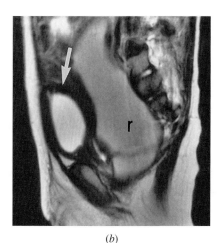

(b)

F I G. 6.83 Surgical repair of persistent cloaca. Sagittal T1-weighted spin-echo (a), sagittal T2-weighted echo-train spin-echo (b), and transverse T2-weighted echo-train spin-echo (c) images.

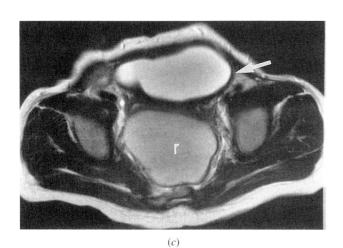

(c)

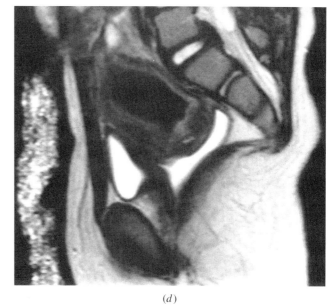

(d)

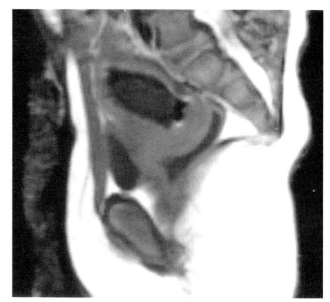

(e)

FIG. 6.83 (*Continued*) A capacious neorectum ("r," *a, b, c*) is present. The bladder (large arrow, *a–c*) is thick walled and anteriorly displaced. Absence of the vagina is noted.

Sagittal T2-weighted SS-ETSE (*d*) and T1-weighted SGE (*e*) images in a second patient with cloacal anomaly who had undergone multiple surgeries. The levator ani complex is diminutive in size, and distal sacral segments are absent. There is a fluid-filled structure situated posterior to the uterus that represents the anal canal and rectum.

are seen in association with familial adenomatous polyposis or Gardner syndromes, whereas multiple colonic hamartomas may be seen in Peutz-Jeghers syndrome or juvenile polyposis syndromes.

A number of polyposis syndromes have been described. The most common are familial adenomatous polyposis, Gardner, and Peutz-Jeghers syndromes and the juvenile polyposis syndromes. Familial adenomatous polyposis syndrome is an autosomal dominant disorder characterized by numerous adenomas affecting primarily the colon and the rectum. Familial adenomatous polyposis represents a prototype of a hereditary precancerous syndrome because the risk of malignant transformation to colorectal carcinoma approaches 100% [86]. Patients with familial adenomatous polypo-

sis syndrome have an increased risk of developing periampullary duodenal carcinoma. Gardner syndrome is an autosomal dominant condition with diffuse adenomatous polyps, bony abnormalities (osteomas), and soft tissue tumors. Presently regarded as a variation of familial adenomatous polyposis syndrome, Gardner syndrome confers the same risk of progression to colon adenocarcinoma. Peutz-Jeghers syndrome is an autosomal dominant disorder characterized clinically by skin and mucosal pigmented macules and gastrointestinal hamartomas. The hamartomas favor the small bowel in 95% of cases, with colonic and stomach involvement in up to 25%. Although the hamartomatous polyps themselves do not have malignant potential, patients with this syndrome have an increased incidence of both benign and

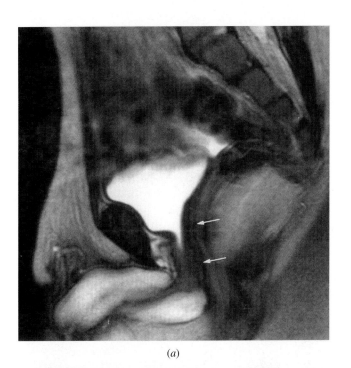

(a)

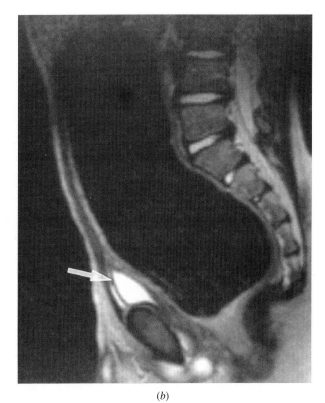

(b)

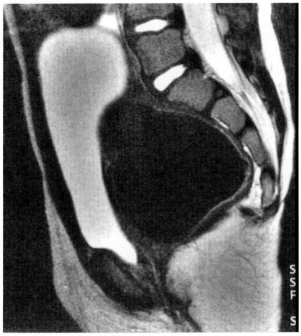

(c)

FIG. 6.84 Reconstructed imperforate anus. Sagittal T2-weighted SS-ETSE (a) image in a one-year-old boy shows that the anal canal (arrows, a) is situated in an anterior location, just posterior to the prostate. The levator ani muscle is intact.

Sagittal T2-weighted echo-train spin-echo images in a second (b) and a third (c) patient demonstrate a markedly dilated air-filled rectum, compressing and displacing the bladder anterosuperiorly (arrow, b).

malignant tumors arising in many organs. Up to 3% of patients with Peutz-Jeghers syndrome will develop adenocarcinoma of the stomach or duodenum, and 5% of women will have ovarian cysts or tumors. There are three distinct syndromes associated with juvenile polyps of the alimentary tract: juvenile polyposis, gastrointestinal juvenile polyposis, and the Cronkhite-Canada syndromes. Hamartomas are common to all three syndromes [87, 88].

Gadolinium-enhanced fat-suppressed SGE images can demonstrate polyps, whether they occur in isolation or in association with a polyposis syndrome. Semelka and Marcos reported on the MR appearance of polyposis syndromes [64]. In that series, polyps were

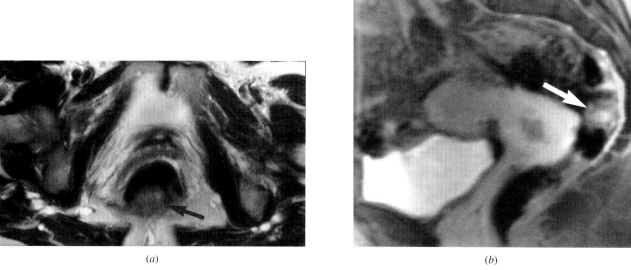

(a) (b)

F I G . 6.85 Adenomatous polyp of rectum. Transverse T2-weigthed echo train spin-echo (a) and sagittal interstitial-phase gadolinium-enhanced fat-suppressed SGE (b) images. There is a 1.6-cm polypoid mass (arrows, a, b) arising from the posterior wall of the rectum, without evidence of extension beyond the rectal wall.

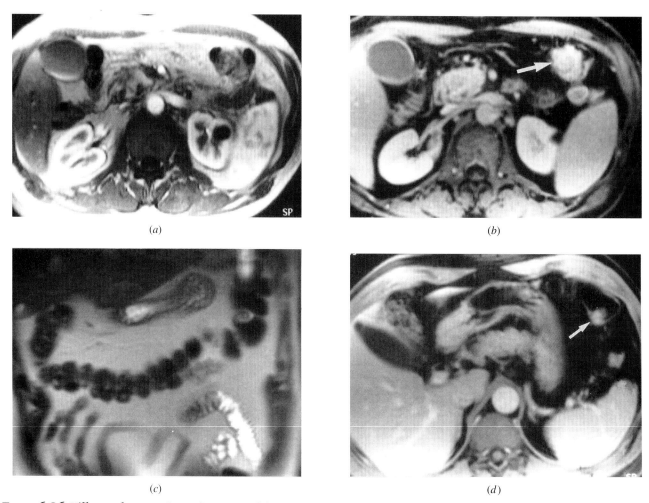

(a) (b)

(c) (d)

F I G . 6.86 Villous adenoma. Immediate-postgadolinium SGE (a) and interstitial-phase gadolinium-enhanced fat-suppressed SGE (b) images. A polypoid mass is seen within the distal transverse colon. The mass enhances minimally on immediate postgadolinium images (a) and in a moderately intense fashion with mild heterogeneity on 2-min postgadolinium images (arrow, b).

Coronal T2-weighted SS-ETSE (c) and transverse interstitial-phase gadolinium- enhanced fat-suppressed SGE (d) images in a second patient with villous adenoma of transverse colon (arrow, d) demonstrates a similar appearance to the previous patient. Most tumors show moderately intense enhancement with mild heterogeneity on 2-min postgadolinium interstitial-phase images, reflecting a larger and more irregular interstitial space than adjacent normal bowel.

well seen using a combination of gadolinium-enhanced fat-suppressed SGE images and T2-weighted single-shot echo-train spin-echo images. The importance of demonstrating polyp enhancement comparing precontrast and postcontrast fat-suppressed SGE images was emphasized, because this observation permitted distinction between polyps and colon contents. Polyps smaller than 1 cm in familial polyposis syndrome were not commonly observed. The most common appearance is an enhancing sessile or pedunculated mass arising from the bowel wall and protruding into the lumen (fig. 6.87). If frond-like polyp morphology or enhancement is observed, the possibility of a villous adenoma should be raised. Similarly, extension beyond the bowel wall signifies malignant degeneration.

Lipomas. Lipomas are the second most common benign neoplasm of the large bowel. They usually originate in the submucosa. Most are asymptomatic, although changes in bowel habits, bleeding, or both have been reported in patients with large lesions. The most common locations for colonic lipomas are the cecum, ascending colon, and sigmoid colon. The MRI appearance of lipomas with T1-weighted and fat-suppressed T1-weighted sequences is pathognomonic: high in signal intensity on T1-weighted images and diminished in signal intensity on fat-suppressed T1-weighted images (fig. 6.88) [89]. Additional use of out-of-phase SGE may demonstrate fat-water black ring phase cancellation surrounding the polyp (fig. 6.89). Lipomas may also act as lead point for intussusceptions (fig. 6.90).

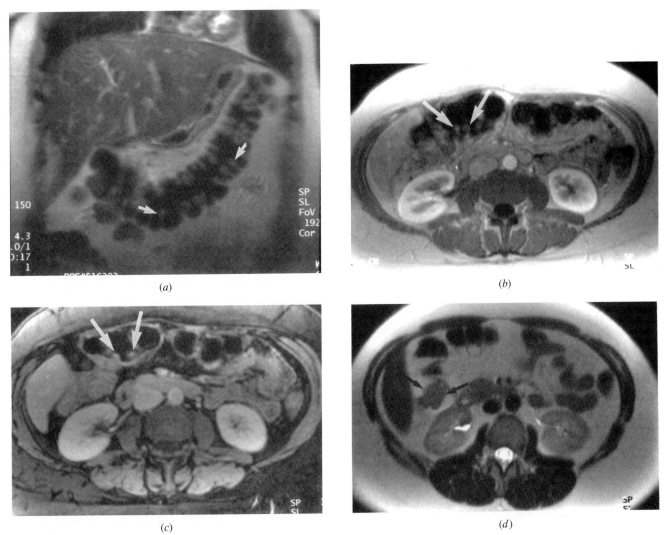

(a)

(b)

(c)

(d)

F I G. 6.87 Familial adenomatous polyposis syndrome. Coronal T2-weighted SS-ETSE (*a*), immediate postgadolinium SGE (*b*), and interstitial-phase gadolinium-enhanced fat-suppressed SGE (*c*) images. Numerous polyps are seen measuring <1 cm in diameter in the transverse colon (arrows, *a*). The signal void of the air in the colon provides good contrast from the soft tissue polyps on the T2-weighted image (*a*). The polyps are mildly enhanced (arrows, *b*) on the immediate postgadolinium image (*b*). Polyps demonstrate persistent enhancement on interstitial-phase images (arrows, *c*). This patient underwent total colectomy, which demonstrated numerous adenomatous polyps.

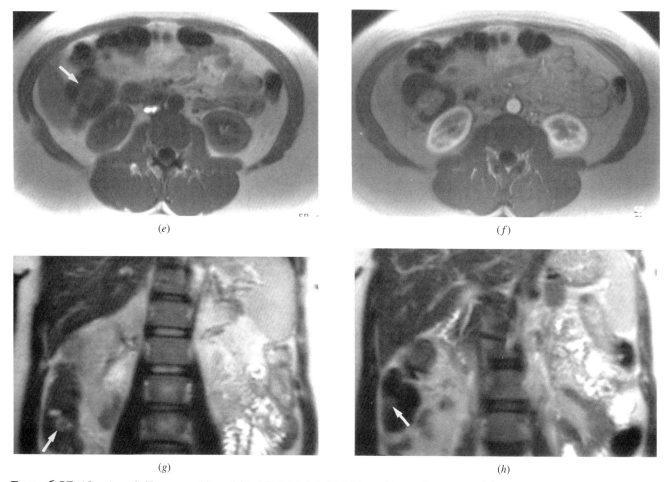

(e)

(f)

(g)

(h)

F I G . 6.87 (*Continued*) Transverse T2-weighted SS-ETSE (*d*), SGE (*e*), and immediate postgadolinium SGE (*f*) images in another patient with familial polyposis syndrome. A 2.5-cm polyp is present that arises in the ascending colon. The high signal intensity of the fluid contents of the colon permits good delineation of the low signal intensity of the polyp on the SS-ETSE image (arrows, *d*). The polyp is isointense to the bowel wall on the precontrast T1-weighted image (arrow, *e*). On the early postgadolinium image, the polyp shows mild heterogeneous enhancement comparable to the bowel wall. Note the intense enhancement of the normal renal cortex, which is greater than the enhancement of the bowel wall or the polyp. This patient underwent sigmoidoscopy with biopsy followed by total colectomy (Reprinted with permission from Semelka RC, Marcos HB: Polyposis syndromes of the gastrointestinal tract. *J Magn Reson Imaging* 11: 51–55, 2000.)

Coronal SS-ETSE (*g*, *h*) images in a third patient with familial adenomatous polyposis demonstrate polypoid lesions in the cecum (arrow, *g*, *h*).

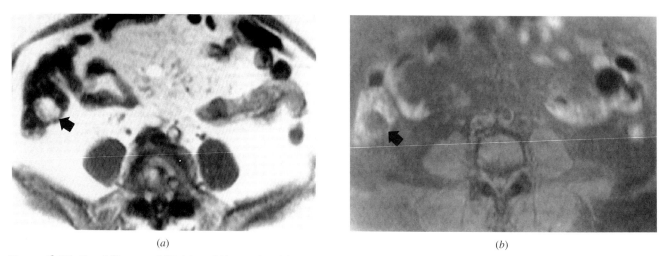

(a)

(b)

F I G . 6.88 Cecal lipoma. SGE (*a*) and T1-weighted fat-suppressed spin-echo (*b*) images. A mass in the cecum is high in signal intensity on the T1-weighted image (arrow, *a*) and diminishes in signal intensity on the fat-suppressed image (arrow, *b*). These imaging characteristics are pathognomonic for a fat containing tumor. The cecum is a common location for large bowel lipomas. (Reprinted with permission from Shoenut JP, Semelka RC, Silverman R, Yaffe CS, Mickflikier AB: Magnetic Resonance imaging evaluation of the local extent of colorectal mass lesions. *J Clin Gastroenterol* 17: 248–253, 1993.)

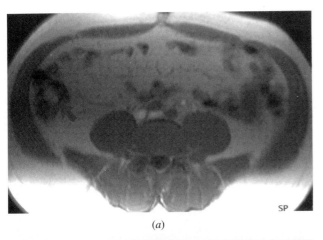

(a)

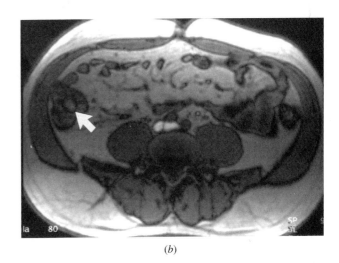

(b)

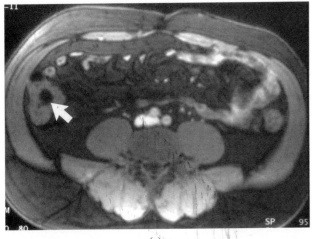

(c)

F I G . 6.89 Cecal lipoma. Precontrast SGE (*a*), precontrast out-of-phase SGE (*b*), and 90 s postgadolinium fat-suppressed SGE (*c*) images. A 2-cm mass in the cecum is high in signal intensity in the precontrast SGE image (arrow, *a*) and demonstrates a phase cancellation artifact in the out-of-phase SGE image (arrow, *b*). Markedly diminished signal intensity of the mass is noted on postcontrast fat-suppressed SGE image (arrow, *c*). (Reprinted with permission from Chung JJ, Semelka RC , Martin DR, Marcos HB: Colon diseases: MR evaluation using combined T2-weighted single-shot echo train spin-echo and gadolinium-enhanced spoiled gradient-echo sequences. *J Magn Reson Imaging* 12: 297–305, 2000.)

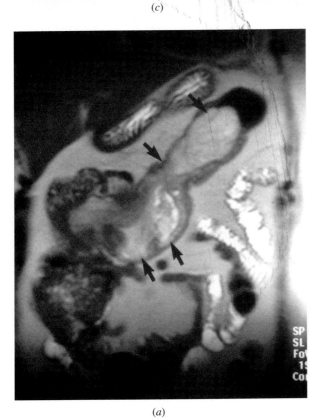

(a)

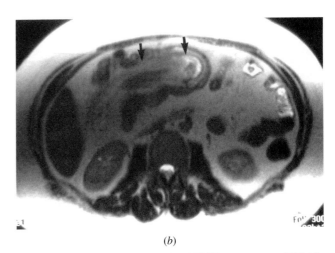

(b)

F I G . 6.90 Colonic lipoma as a lead point for intussusception. Coronal (*a*) and transverse (*b*) SS-ETSE, precontrast SGE (*c*), and 90-s postgadolinium fat-suppressed SGE (*d, e*) images.

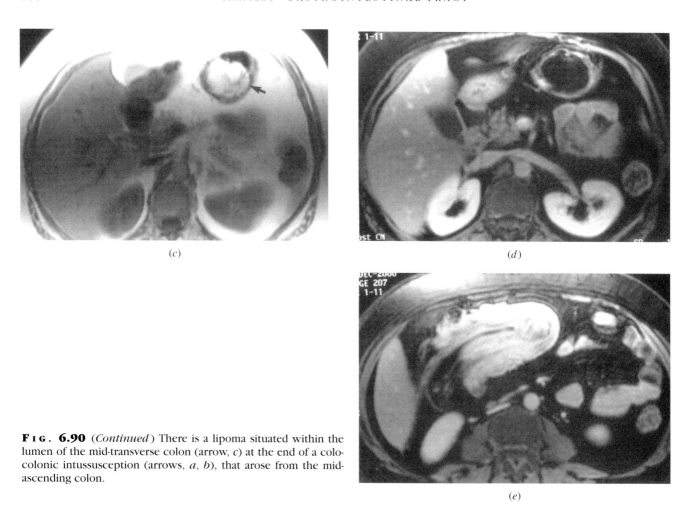

(c)

(d)

(e)

F I G . 6.90 (*Continued*) There is a lipoma situated within the lumen of the mid-transverse colon (arrow, *c*) at the end of a colo-colonic intussusception (arrows, *a*, *b*), that arose from the mid-ascending colon.

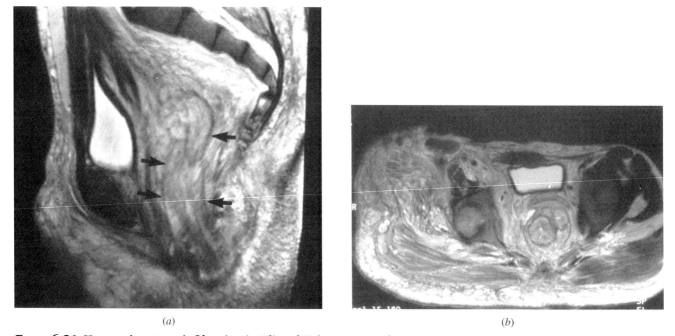

(a)

(b)

F I G . 6.91 **Hemangiomatous infiltration in Klippel-Trénaunay syndrome.** Sagittal (*a*) and transverse (*b*) T2-weighted ETSE and transverse SGE (*c*) in a patient with Klippel-Trénaunay syndrome.

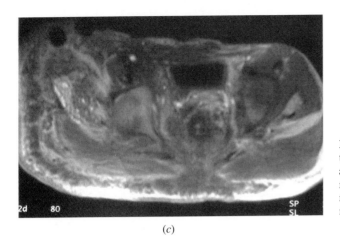

(c)

F I G . 6.91 (*Continued*) The intrapelvic fat is extensively infiltrated with hemangiomatous tissue. The wall of the rectum and anal canal are noted to be expanded (arrows, *a*) because of hemangiomatous infiltration. Note also the extensive infiltrative hemangiomas involving the soft tissues of the pelvis and right gluteal region, which are expanded.

Other Mesenchymal Neoplasms. Leiomyomas, hemangiomas (fig. 6.91), and neurofibromas are all rare.

Mucocele. A mucocele is defined as dilatation of the appendiceal lumen resulting from mucus accumulation associated with luminal obstruction. Mucoceles are frequently asymptomatic unless they become secondarily infected or rupture. Pathologically it is important to distinguish between nonneoplastic lesions (retention) mucoceles and neoplastic mucoceles. Nonneoplastic lesions show an inflamed mucosa or hyperplastic epithelium. Neoplastic mucoceles are best classified as mucinous cystadenoma or mucinous cystadenocarcinoma. In mucinous cystoadenocarcinoma, spread of malignant cells beyond the appendix in the form of peritoneal implants is frequently present. Pseudomyxoma peritonei, with the findings of adenocarcinomatous cells, distinguishes this malignant process from simple mucinous spillage, which may occur with rupture of a retention mucocele or cystadenoma. Because of the possibility of

an underlying malignancy and the risk of rupture, mucoceles should be prophylactically removed. T2-weighted single-shot echo-train spin-echo images show a high-signal intensity tubular structure in the region of the appendix. Mucoceles have a higher signal intensity than simple fluid on T1-weighted sequences owing to their protein content. In uncomplicated cases, the wall of the mucocele is thin and enhances minimally after intravenous gadolinium administration (fig. 6.92).

Varices. Rectal varices develop in patients with portal hypertension. The incidence of hemorrhoids is not increased in these patients [90].

Malignant Masses

Adenocarcinoma. Adenocarcinoma of the colon is the most common gastrointestinal tract malignancy and the second most common visceral cancer in North America. The estimated incidence in the United States is 138,000 new cases per year and the 5-year survival is 50–60% [38]. The incidence of adenocarcinoma

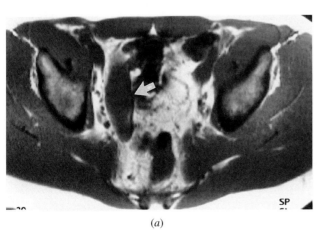

(a)

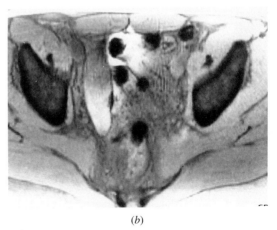

(b)

F I G . 6.92 Mucocele of the appendix. SGE (*a*), fat-suppressed SGE (*b*), SS-ETSE (*c*), sagittal SS-ETSE (*d*), and immediate post-gadolinium fat-suppressed SGE (*e*) images. An oblong-shaped mucocele of the appendix is present (arrow, *a*) that contains high-signal intensity material in the dependent portion of the cyst on the T1-weighted image (*a*), which is accentuated with the application of fat suppression (*b*). The mucocele is high in signal intensity on the T2-weighted image, with slight heterogeneity in the dependent portion (*c*).

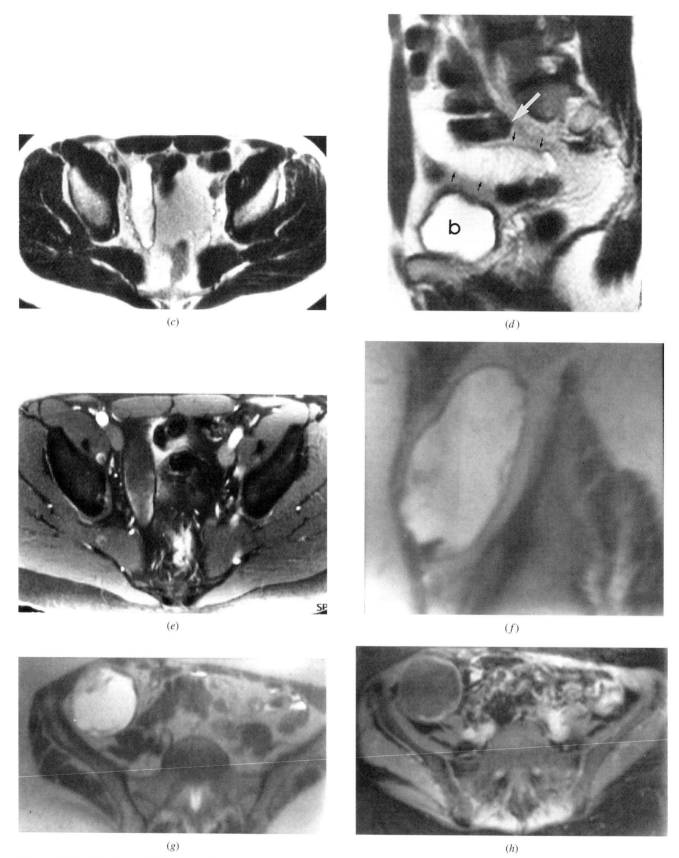

(c)

(d)

(e)

(f)

(g)

(h)

F I G . 6.92 (*Continued*) The sagittal plane image (*d*) shows the orientation of the mucocele (small arrows, *d*) to the base of the cecum (arrow, *d*) and the relationship to the bladder ("b," *d*). No appreciable enhancement of the mucocele wall is noted on the postgadolinium image (*e*), which excludes the diagnosis of abscess.

Sagittal (*f*) and transverse (*g*) SS-ETSE and interstitial-phase gadolinium-enhanced SGE (*h*) images in a second patient show a large cystic mass in the lower right quadrant of the abdomen extending into the pelvic inlet. Note the presence of septations and a thin rim enhancement.

Table 6.3 TNM Staging for Cancer of the Colon

T—Primary Tumor

Tx	Primary tumor cannot be assessed
T0	No evidence of primary tumor
Tis	Preinvasive carcinoma (carcinoma in situ)
T1	Tumor limited to the mucosa or mucosa and sub-mucosa
T2	Tumor with extension to muscle or muscle and serosa
T3	Tumor with extension beyond the colon to immediately contiguous structures
T3a	Tumor without fistula formation
T3b	Tumor with fistula formation
T4	Tumor with deep infiltration occupying more than one-half but not more than one region or extending to neighboring structures

N—Regional lymph nodes

Nx	Regional lymph nodes cannot be assessed
N0	No evidence of regional lymph node metastasis
N1	Evidence of regional lymph node involvement
N2, N3	*Not applicable*
N4	Evidence of involvement of juxta-regional lymph nodes

M—Metastases

Mx	Distant metastases cannot be assessed
M0	No distant metastases
M1	Distant metastases

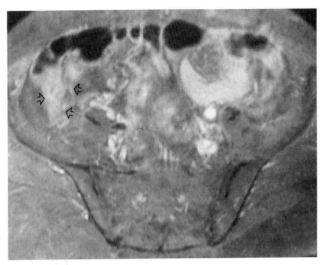

F I G . 6.93 Appendiceal adenocarcinoma. Gadolinium-enhanced T1-weighted fat-suppressed spin-echo image demonstrates heterogeneous enhancing infiltrative tumor arising from the appendix (open arrows).

of the colon increases with advancing age. Sporadic cancers are increased in first-degree family relatives of patients with known colorectal carcinoma. Other conditions that predispose to the development of colon cancer include familial adenomatous polyposis, Gardner syndrome, Lynch syndrome, ulcerative colitis, Crohn's colitis, and previous ureterosigmoidostomies. Cancers occur most often in the rectosigmoid colon, but right-sided cancers are reported to occur in increasing frequency [91]. Tumors may be polypoid, circumferential ("apple core"), or plaquelike. Symptoms reflect tumor location and morphology, with most patients reporting a combination of change in bowel habits, bleeding, pain, and weight loss. A TNM system is used for staging (Table 6.3).

Good correlation is observed between gadolinium-enhanced fat-suppressed MRI techniques and surgical specimens for tumor size, bowel wall involvement, peritumoral extension, and lymph node detection [5]. Malignant lymph nodes are usually not enlarged in gastrointestinal adenocarcinoma. However, the presence of more than five lymph nodes that measure smaller than 1 cm in a regional distribution related to the tumor correlates well with tumor involvement. All segments of the colon and the appendix are well shown on MR images. The combination of T2-weighted single-shot echo train spin-echo and gadolinium-enhanced fat-suppressed SGE images result in the most reproducible image quality for the colon above the rectum (Figs. 6.93–

6.100). Rectal cancers benefit from the combined use of gadolinium-enhanced fat-suppressed SGE and high-resolution T2-weighted echo-train spin-echo images (fig. 6.101). Gadolinium-enhanced fat-suppressed SGE imaging is valuable in demonstrating perirectal tumor extension, regional lymph nodes, and seeding of peritoneal by tumor. This reflects the high-contrast resolution of this technique for detecting enhancing diseased tissue (figs. 6.102 and 6.103). Image acquisition of T2-weighted echo-train spin echo or single-shot echo-train spin echo after the administration of gadolinium is commonly done when abdomen and pelvis studies are combined in one examination. As an additional benefit to a shortened MR

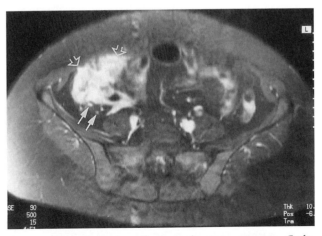

F I G . 6.94 Colonic adenocarcinoma, cecum. Gadolinium-enhanced T1-weighted fat-suppressed spin-echo image demonstrates a large heterogeneous intensely enhancing cecal carcinoma (hollow arrow) that extends to the anterior peritoneal wall. Multiple enhancing lymph nodes <5 mm are identified (arrows), which are malignant.

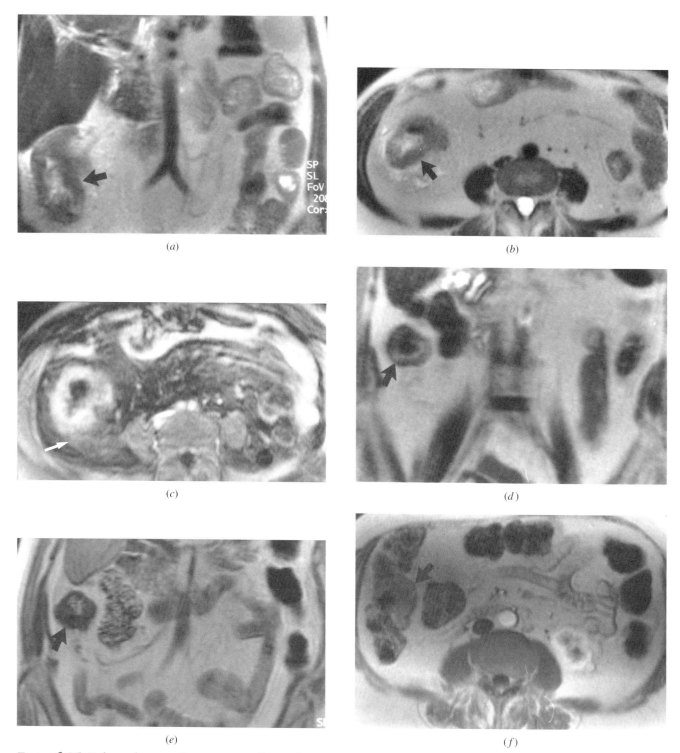

(a)

(b)

(c)

(d)

(e)

(f)

F I G . 6.95 Colon adenocarcinoma, ascending colon. Coronal (*a*) and transverse (*b*) SS-ETSE and 90-s postgadolinium fat-suppressed SGE (*c*) images. Irregularly thickened bowel wall with intermediate signal intensity representing cancer is noted in the ascending colon (arrow, *a, b*). The cancer enhances in a moderate and slightly heterogeneous fashion. Pericolonic fat infiltration is demonstrated in the ascending colon on postcontrast fat-suppressed SGE image as enhancing strands of tissue (arrow, *c*).

Coronal SS-ETSE (*d*), coronal precontrast SGE (*e*), and transverse immediate postcontrast SGE (*f*) images in a second patient also demonstrate an irregular thickening of the ascending colon wall (arrow, *d–f*). There is no evidence of pericolonic fat infiltration with sharp external margins to the tumor.

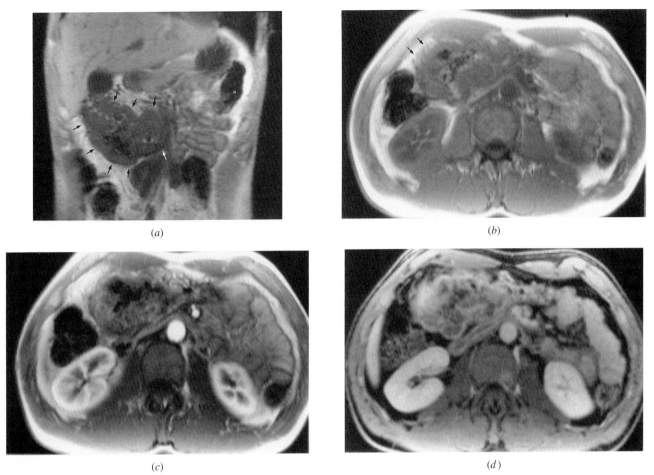

F I G. 6.96 Colon adenocarcinoma, transverse colon. Coronal SGE (*a*), SGE (*b*), immediate postgadolinium SGE (*c*), and 90-s postgadolinium fat-suppressed SGE (*d*) images. A large cancer arises from the transverse colon (small arrows, *a*). The outer margin of the tumor is indistinct (small arrows, *b*), a finding consistent with lymphovascular extension. The tumor is heterogeneous and moderate in signal intensity on capillary-phase (*c*) and interstitial-phase (*d*) images.

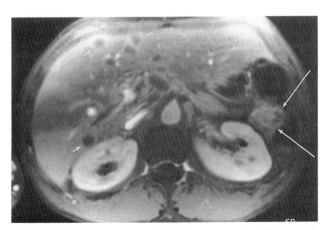

F I G. 6.97 Colon adenocarcinoma, proximal descending colon. Transverse 90-s postgadolinium SGE image demonstrates a heterogeneously enhancing tumor (long arrows) in the proximal descending colon with prominent enhancing strands in the surrounding mesentery consistent with lymphovascular extension. Multiple ring-enhancing liver metastases are apparent (small arrows).

examination, dependent, concentrated gadolinium in the bladder, which is low in signal intensity, may increase the conspicuity of high-signal intensity rectal tumor invasion of the bladder wall (see fig. 6.101).

When feasible, surface torso coils (e.g., phased-array torso coil) should be employed to ensure better definition of perirectal tumor extension [92]. Phased-array torso coils also provide good overall topographic display that improves detection of features such as regional lymph nodes. Endorectal coil imaging permits differentiation of the anatomic layers of the rectal wall on T2-weighted fat-suppressed images [10]. Local staging of rectal carcinoma also benefits from endorectal coil imaging (fig. 6.104) [9, 10].

Recurrence rates for rectosigmoid carcinoma, which are reported to range from 8 to 50%, are a function of the stage of the primary tumor at initial presentation [12]. Tumors tend to recur locally, and curative surgery is feasible. The sagittal imaging plane facilitates MRI detection of recurrent rectal carcinoma. Using T1-weighted,

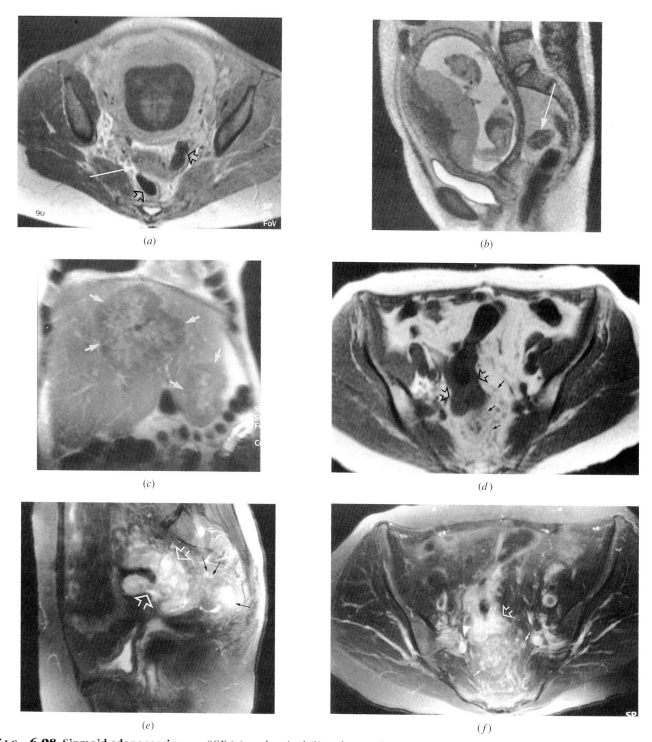

F I G . 6.98 Sigmoid adenocarcinoma. SGE (*a*), and sagittal (*b*) and coronal (*c*) SS-ETSE images in a pregnant patient with colon cancer. The SGE image shows air-filled colon (hollow arrows, *a*) proximal and distal to the 4-cm sigmoid cancer (long arrow, *a*). The SS-ETSE images show the primary tumor (arrow, *b*) and the liver metastases (arrows, *c*). The gravid uterus is well imaged with the single-shot T2-weighted breathing-independent technique (*b*).

SGE (*d*), sagittal T2-weighted fat-suppressed spin-echo (*e*), and gadolinium-enhanced T1-weighted fat-suppressed spin-echo (*f*) images in a second patient with advanced sigmoid adenocarcinoma. The precontrast image demonstrates abnormal thickening of the sigmoid colon (open arrows, *d*) with low-signal intensity strands infiltrating the pericolonic fat (small arrows, *d*). The primary tumor (open arrows, *e*, *f*) and pericolonic extension are well shown as high-signal intensity structures in a low-signal intensity background on both fat-suppressed T2-weighted (*e*) and gadolinium-enhanced T1-weighted fat-suppressed (*f*) images. Multiple small regional malignant lymph nodes are identified (small arrows, *e*, *f*).

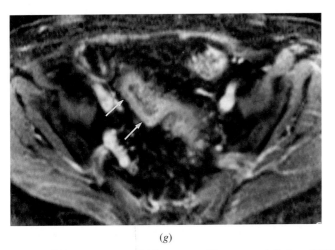

(g)

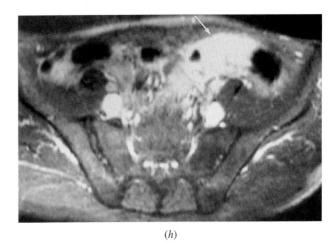

(h)

F I G . 6.98 (*Continued*) Transverse 90-s postgadolinium SGE image (*g*) in a third patient demonstrates a circumferential 4-cm sigmoid colon cancer (arrows, *g*) that does not show lymphovascular extension.

Gadolinium-enhanced T1-weighted fat-suppressed spin-echo image (*b*) in a fourth patient demonstrates an intensely enhancing sigmoid colon cancer (arrow, *b*) involving the anterior peritoneum.

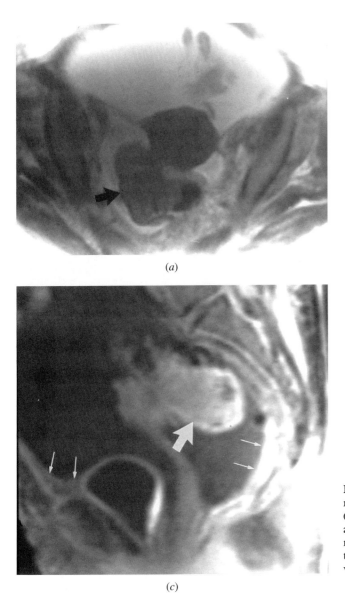

(a)

(c)

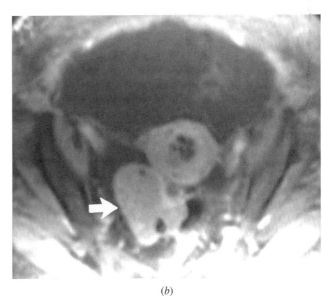

(b)

F I G . 6.99 Sigmoid adenocarcinoma with peritoneal metastases. Transverse SS-ETSE (*a*) and transverse (*b*) and sagittal (*c*) 2- to 3-min postgadolinium fat-suppressed SGE images. There is a soft tissue enhancing mass in the sigmoid colon representing tumor (arrow, *a–c*). Note the increased peritoneal enhancement and thickening (small arrows, *c*) and large volume of ascites, consistent with peritoneal disease.

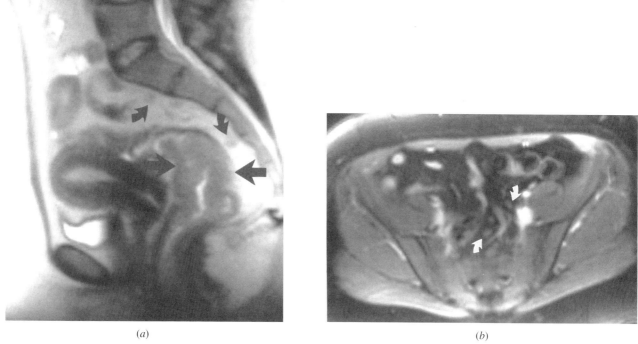

(a)

(b)

F I G . 6.100 Rectosigmoid colon adenocarcinoma. Sagittal SS-ETSE (*a*) and 90-s postgadolinium fat-suppressed SGE (*b*) images. Markedly thickening tumor mass (large arrows, *a*) is noted in the rectosigmoid region on the SS-ETSE images. Multiple regional lymph nodes <1 cm in diameter are well demonstrated in the pelvis (curved arrows *a, b*). Small nodes are best shown on gadolinium-enhanced fat-suppressed SGE images. (Reprinted with permission from Chung JJ, Semelka RC, Martin DR, Marcos HB: Colon diseases: MR evaluation using combined T2-weighted single-shot echo train spin-echo and gadolinium-enhanced spoiled gradient-echo sequences. *J Magn Reson Imaging* 12: 297–305, 2000.)

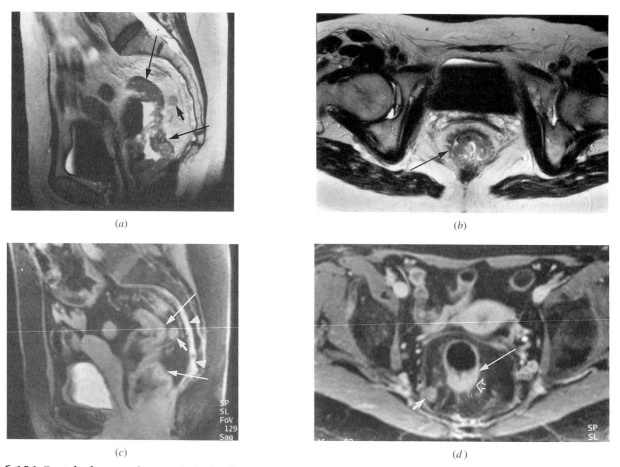

(a)

(b)

(c)

(d)

F I G . 6.101 Rectal adenocarcinoma. Sagittal and transverse postgadolinium high-resolution T2-weighted echo-train spin-echo (*a, b*) and sagittal and transverse postgadolinium fat-suppressed SGE (*c, d*) images in a patient with advanced colon cancer.

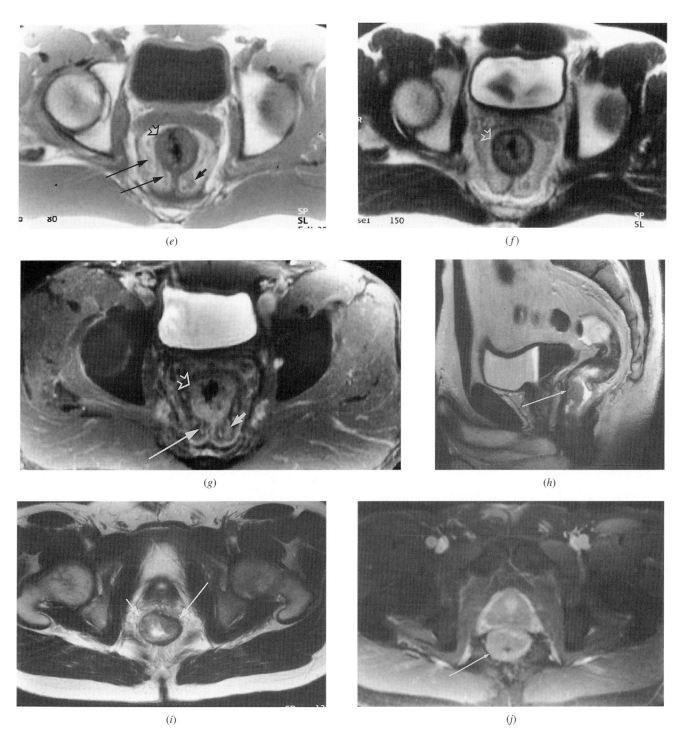

(e)

(f)

(g)

(h)

(i)

(j)

F I G. 6.101 (*Continued*) A large rectal cancer is present (long arrows, *a, c*). The craniocaudal extent of tumor is well shown on sagittal images (*a, c*). The tumor extends inferiorly in the rectum (arrow, *b*) to the anal verge. Lymphovascular extension with involved lymph nodes (small arrows, *a, c, d*) is present. At the superior margin, the tumor is mainly posterior in location (hollow arrow, *d*). The transition from normal colon to tumor (long arrow, *d*) is clearly shown. Presacral spread of tumor is shown as enhancing tissue on the sagittal gadolinium-enhanced fat-suppressed image (arrowheads, *c*).

SGE (*e*), SS-ETSE (*f*), and postgadolinium fat-suppressed SGE (*g*) images in a second patient with rectal adenocarcinoma and similar imaging findings. The rectal tumor (hollow arrows, *e, f, g*), lymphovascular extension (long arrows, *e, g*), and perirectal lymph nodes (short arrow, *e, g*) are well shown.

Sagittal and transverse postgadolinium 512-resolution T2-weighted echo-train spin-echo (*h, i*) and interstitial-phase gadolinium-enhanced fat-suppressed SGE (*j*) images in a third patient. Asymmetric tumor involvement of the rectal wall is apparent on the 512-resolution T2-weighted images (long arrow, *h, i*). Tumor penetrates the full thickness of the right aspect of the rectum (short arrow, *i*). This is shown by interruption of the muscular wall that appears low signal intensity on the T2-weighted image (long arrow, *i*). On the gadolinium-enhanced fat-suppressed SGE image, lower-signal intensity tumor (arrow, *j*) penetrates the full thickness of the higher-signal intensity wall. Postgadolinium T2-weighted imaging is a novel technique for assessing possible bladder invasion. Enhancing tumor is conspicuous against the low signal intensity produced by concentrated gadolinium excreted into the bladder. In this case, the bladder is spared.

609

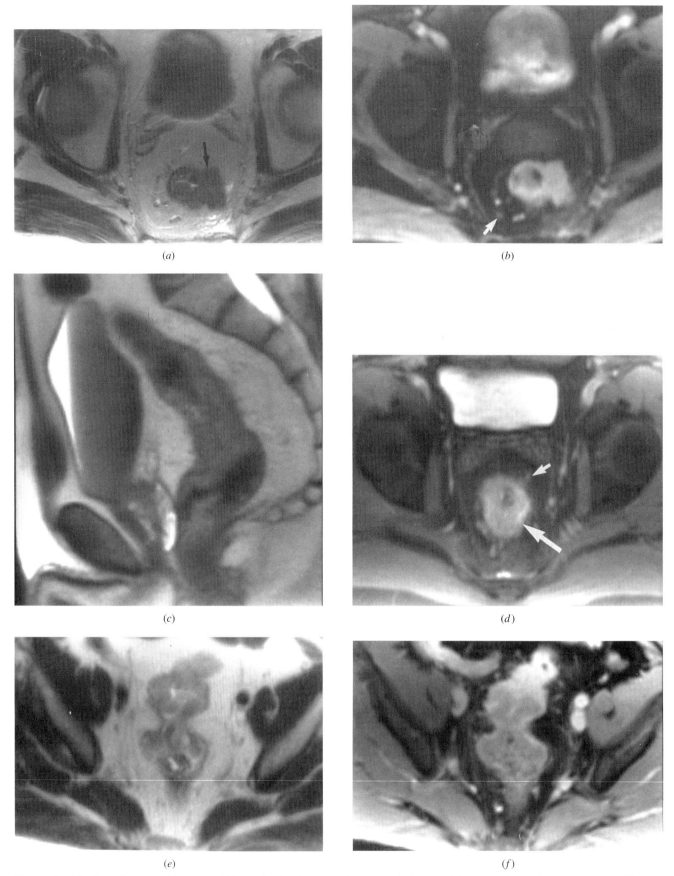

(a)

(b)

(c)

(d)

(e)

(f)

F I G . 6.102 Rectal cancer. Transverse T2-weighted ETSE (*a*) and interstitial-phase gadolinium-enhanced SGE (*b*) images. There is a soft tissue mass involving the wall of rectosigmoid with gross tumor extension through the left aspect of the wall (arrow, *a*). Small regional lymph nodes are also identified (arrow, *b*).

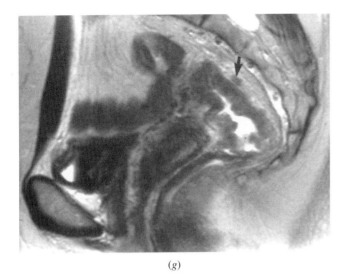

(g)

F I G . 6.102 (*Continued*) Sagittal postgadolinium SS-ETSE (*c*) and interstitial-phase gadolinium-enhanced SGE (*d*) images in a second patient demonstrate circumferential thickening of the rectum with infiltration of perirectal fat (large arrow, *d*). Small regional nodes are present (arrow, *d*).

   Transverse SS-ETSE (*e*) and interstitial-phase gadolinium-enhanced SGE (*f*) images in a third patient also show diffuse thickening of the rectal wall associated with stranding of perirectal fat and small perirectal nodes.

   Sagittal T2-weighted ETSE (*g*) image in a fourth patient demonstrates similar features. Small regional nodes are present (arrow, *g*).

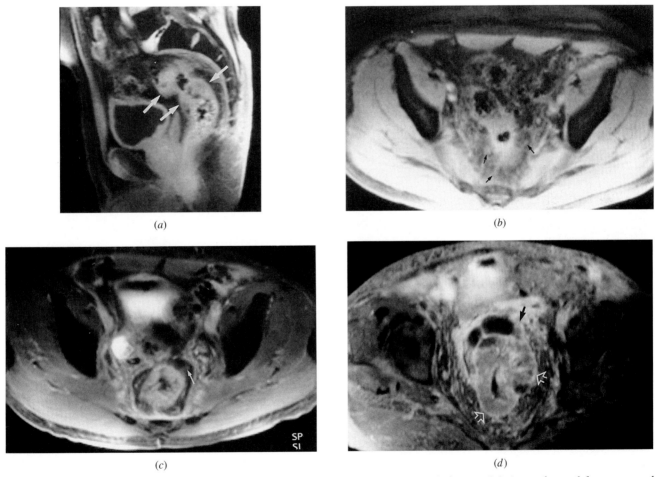

(a)   (b)

(c)   (d)

F I G . 6.103 Rectal adenocarcinoma. Sagittal (*a*) and transverse (*b, c*) interstitial-phase gadolinium-enhanced fat-suppressed SGE images demonstrate a large rectal adenocarcinoma (arrows, *a*) with prominent lymphovascular extension and multiple small malignant lymph nodes (arrows, *b, c*). The sagittal imaging plane (*a*) highlights the inferior and superior extent of the tumor.

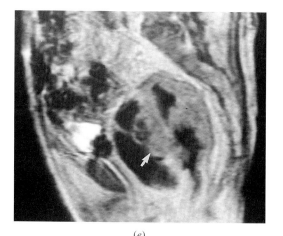

(e)

FIG. 6.103 (*Continued*) Transverse gadolinium-enhanced fat-suppressed SGE (*d*) and sagittal postgadolinium SGE (*e*) images in a second patient demonstrate a large rectal cancer (hollow arrows, *d*) that has prominent lymphovascular invasion. Invasion of adjacent small bowel (arrow, *d*, *e*) is shown.

T2-weighted, and gadolinium-enhanced T1-weighted sequences, one study reported 93.3% accuracy in detecting recurrent disease [12]. Others have shown that MRI is superior to conventional CT imaging and is more specific than transrectal ultrasound for identifying recurrent tumor [11, 13–15]. Specifically, MRI correctly diagnosed recurrent rectal carcinoma in 83.2% of patients versus transrectal ultrasound, which diagnosed recurrence in only 41.6% [16].

Recurrent tumor tends to be low in signal intensity on T1-weighted images and enhances moderately after

intravenous gadolinium (figs. 6.105–6.107) [6, 11, 93]. On T2-weighted images, recurrent tumor usually is moderately high in signal intensity. This may be difficult to appreciate on echo-train spin-echo sequences because the surrounding fat is also moderately high in signal intensity on these sequences (see fig. 6.105). Caution must be exercised in interpreting images in patients with possible recurrent disease on echo-train spin-echo sequences; tumor appears lower in signal intensity compared with its appearance on conventional spin-echo sequences. This reflects the relatively high signal intensity

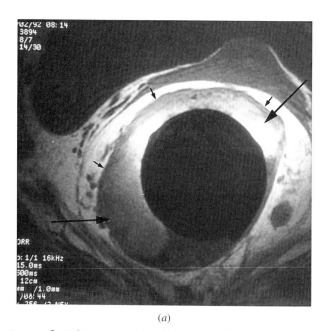

(a)

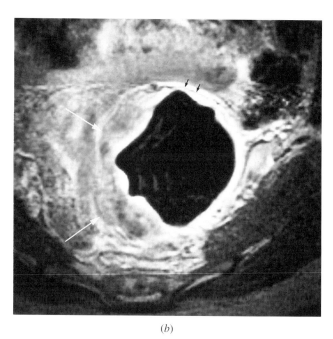

(b)

FIG. 6.104 Endorectal coil imaging of rectal cancer. Gadolinium-enhanced T1-weighted image (*a*) demonstrates a T2 rectal cancer (long arrows, *a*). Preservation of low-signal intensity muscular wall (short arrows, *a*) along the outer margin of the tumor confirms lack of full-thickness involvement.

Gadolinium-enhanced T1-weighted fat-suppressed spin-echo image (*b*) in a second patient with T3 rectal cancer. Heterogeneous moderate enhancing tumor (long arrows, *b*) is noted to extend beyond the confines of muscularis propria (short arrows, *b*). [Courtesy of Rahel A. Kubik Huch].

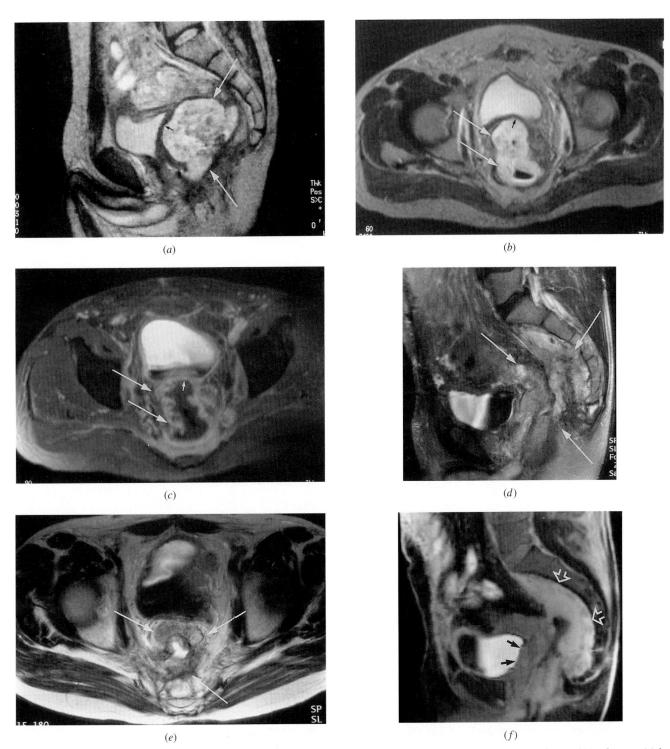

F I G . 6.105 Recurrent rectal adenocarcinoma. Sagittal and transverse T2-weighted echo-train spin-echo (*a, b*) and interstitial-phase gadolinium-enhanced T1-weighted fat-suppressed spin-echo (*c*) images. A large heterogeneous mass occupies the rectal fossa, a finding consistent with recurrence. Recurrent tumors are usually moderately high in signal intensity on T2-weighted images (long arrows, *a, b*) and enhance moderately after intravenous contrast (long arrows, *c*). Central necrosis is well shown on the gadolinium-enhanced T1-weighted fat-suppressed image. The tumor is contiguous with the bladder wall (short arrow, *a–c*), but the low signal intensity of the bladder wall on the T2-weighted images shows that the bladder wall is not invaded.

Sagittal and transverse postgadolinium 512-resolution T2-weighted echo-train spin-echo (*d, e*) and sagittal and transverse interstitial-phase gadolinium-enhanced fat-suppressed SGE (*f, g*) images in a second patient with recurrent rectal tumor. The 512-resolution T2-weighted images show a large heterogeneous tumor in the rectal bed (arrows, *d, e*).

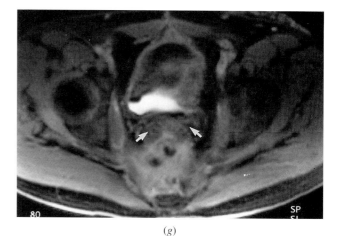

FIG. 6.105 (*Continued*) Low-signal intensity urine reflects concentrated gadolinium dependently. The gadolinium-enhanced fat-suppressed SGE images (*f*, *g*) demonstrate extensive recurrent disease involving the rectal fossa, rectovesical space (arrows *f*, *g*), presacral space (open arrows, *f*), and sciatic foramina.

(*g*)

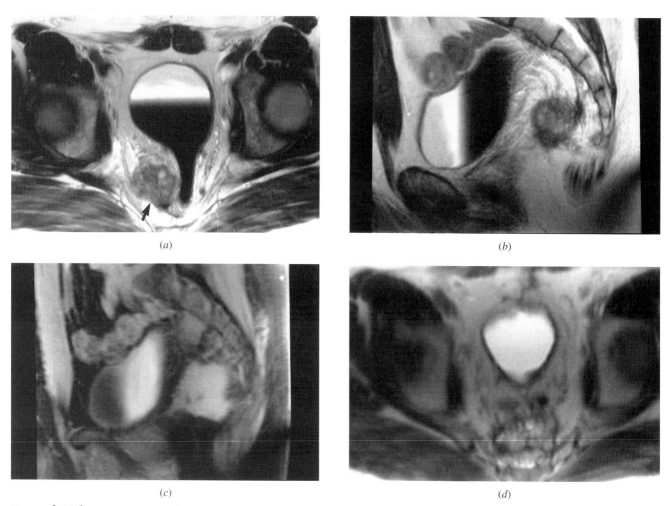

(*a*) (*b*)

(*c*) (*d*)

FIG. 6.106 Recurrent rectal cancer. Transverse (*a*) and sagittal T2-weighted postcontrast SS-ETSE (*b*) and sagittal interstitial-phase gadolinium-enhanced SGE (*c*) images in a patient after abdominoperineal resection (APR) for rectal cancer . There is a 4-cm mass in the right presacral space that is mildly heterogeneous on T2 (arrow, *a*) and heterogeneously enhancing consistent with tumor recurrence. Note the abnormal posterior position of the bladder after APR surgery.

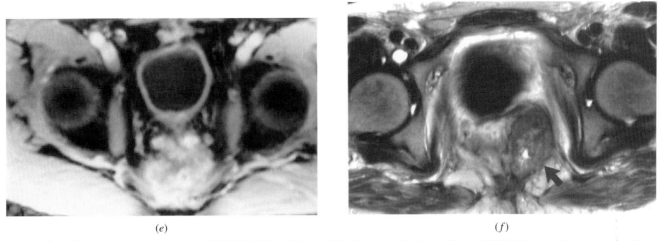

(e)   (f)

F I G . 6.106 (*Continued*) T2-weighted SS-ETSE (*d*) and interstitial-phase gadolinium-enhanced SGE (*e*) images in a second patient demonstrate an irregular presacral mass, which enhances heterogeneously after gadolinium administration.

T2-weighted ETSE (*f*) image in a third patient with tumor recurrence also shows a mass (arrow, *f*) in the presacral space.

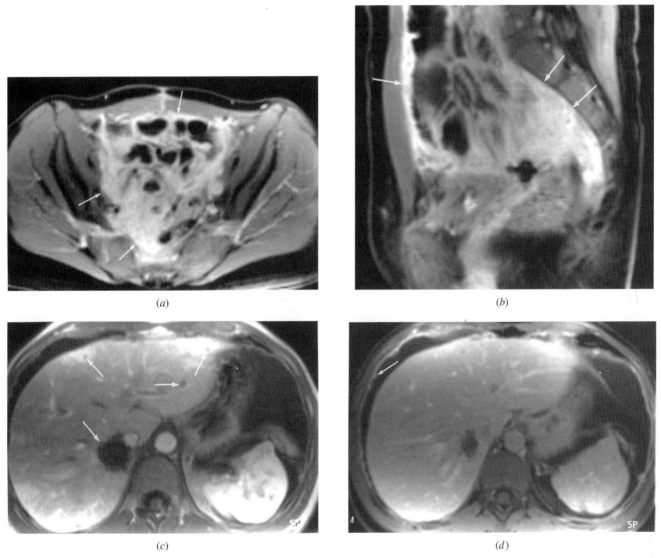

(a)   (b)

(c)   (d)

F I G . 6.107 Colon cancer with peritoneal disease and hepatic metastases. Transverse (*a*) and sagittal (*b*) T2-weighted SS-ETSE, transverse immediate postgadolinium SGE (*c*), and 90-s postgadolinium fat-suppressed SGE (*d*) images demonstrate a large recurrent rectal carcinoma in the presacral space, with extensive local infiltration in the pelvis (arrows, *a*, *b*). Immediate postgadolinium image demonstrates the presence of hepatic metastases (arrows, *c*). The peritoneal involvement in the upper abdomen is well shown on interstitial-phase postcontrast image (arrow, *d*).

615

of fat on echo-train spin-echo sequences. Demonstration of sacral invasion is well shown on T2-weighted fat-suppressed echo-train spin-echo and gadolinium-enhanced T1-weighted fat-suppressed images. Marrow is low in signal intensity on both of these sequences, particularly in the setting of postradiation fatty replacement, which is often present in these patients, and tumor extension is conspicuous because of its high signal intensity (fig. 6.108). In the assessment of sacral involvement, imaging in the sagittal plane is essential for visualizing invasion of the cortex of the sacrum. In selected cases, oblique coronal images (following the angulation of the sacrum) are helpful (see fig. 6.108). Recurrent tumor often has a nodular configuration. Recurrent rectosigmoid cancer and posttreatment (surgical and/or radiation) fibrosis frequently coexist (figs. 6.109 and 6.110).

Postradiation fibrosis in patients more than 1 year after therapy often demonstrates low signal intensity in the surgical bed on T1- and T2-weighted images and may show negligible enhancement after intravenous gadolinium administration (fig. 6.111) [6, 11, 91, 93]. Enhancement of fibrosis with gadolinium, particularly on fat-suppressed images, often persists for 1.5–2 years after therapy, which is longer than the period of time that fibrosis is high in signal intensity on T2-weighted images. Morphologically, fibrosis often has a plaquelike appearance. Unfortunately, the imaging features of postradiation changes, especially in patients receiving doses in excess of 45 Gy, may not always follow a predictable time course and overlap in signal behavior between recurrent tumor and posttreatment fibrosis exists [94]. On echo-train spin-echo images, the high signal intensity of fat admixed with fibrous tissue may simulate recurrence (fig. 6.112). Although the T2-weighted signal intensity of fibrosis usually decreases 1 year after radiation, granulation tissue may show persistent high signal

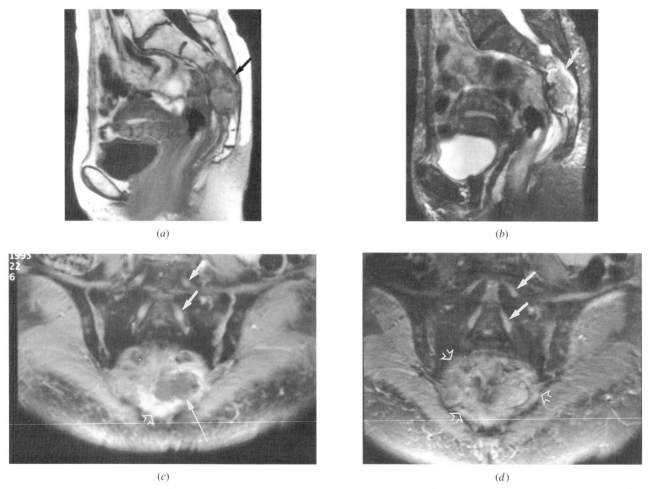

(a)

(b)

(c)

(d)

Fig. 6.108 Recurrent rectal adenocarcinoma invading sacrum. Sagittal T1-weighted SGE (*a*), sagittal 512-resolution T2-weighted fat-suppressed echo-train spin-echo (*b*), and oblique coronal postgadolinium fat-suppressed SGE (*c, d*) images. A large recurrent tumor mass invades the sacrum and is intermediate in signal intensity on the T1-weighted image (arrow, *a*) and heterogeneously high in signal intensity on the T2-weighted image (arrow, *b*). After contrast, the tumor enhances heterogeneously (open arrows, *c, d*) and contains an area of central necrosis (long arrow, *c*). S1 and S2 sacral segments are not involved, and uninvolved S1 and S2 nerve roots are shown (short arrows, *c, d*).

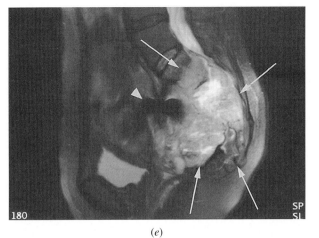

(e)

F I G . 6.108 (*Continued*) Sparing of the upper two sacral segments is a finding on which surgeons once based surgical resection. At surgery the upper margin of the tumor involved S3, sparing the S2 sacral segment.

Sagittal 512-resolution T2-weighted echo-train spin-echo image (*e*) in a second patient demonstrates sacral invasion by a large recurrent rectal adenocarcinoma (arrows, *e*). This tumor involves the entire sacrum and precludes a surgical resection attempt. Surgical clip from prior resection produces a signal-void susceptibility artifact (arrowhead, *e*).

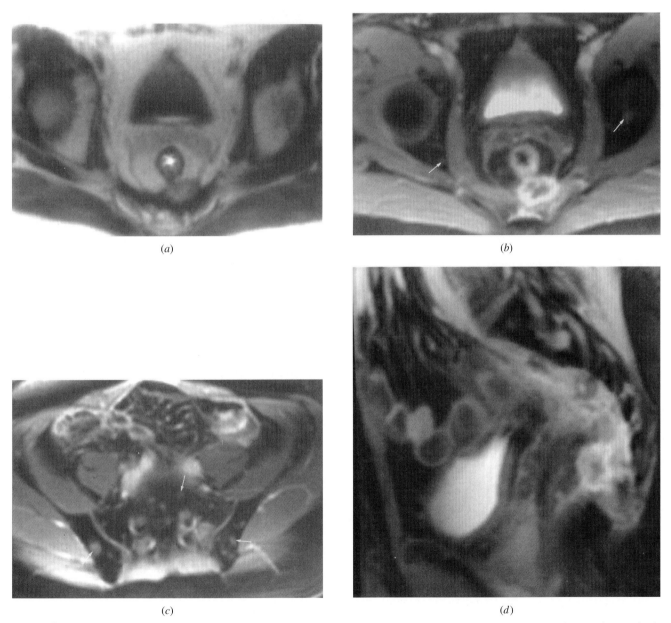

(a)

(b)

(c)

(d)

F I G . 6.109 Recurrent rectal carcinoma with bone metastases. T2-weighted SS-ETSE (*a*) and transverse (*b*, *c*) and sagittal (*d*) interstitial-phase gadolinium-enhanced SGE images. A soft tissue mass is present in the left presacral region. The tumor demonstrates peripheral enhancement. Additionally, there are multiple enhancing lesions within the bone marrow of the sacrum and pelvis (arrows, *b*, *c*), consistent with metastases.

617

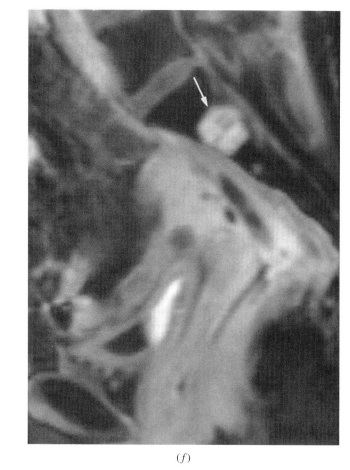

(e)

(f)

F I G . 6.109 (*Continued*) Transverse (*e*) and sagittal (*f*) interstitial-phase gadolinium-enhanced SGE images in a second patient show presacral abnormalities consistent with tumor recurrence associated with radiation changes. Note the presence of metastatic lesions (arrow, *e, f*) within the sacrum and left iliac wing.

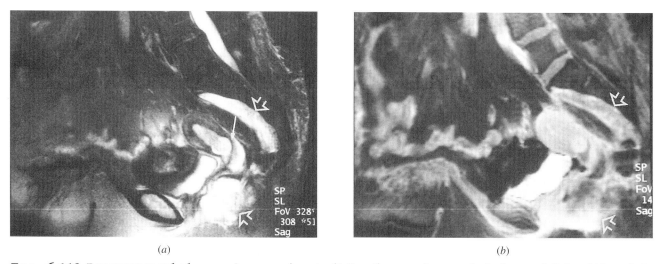

(a)

(b)

F I G . 6.110 Recurrent rectal adenocarcinoma and postradiation therapy changes. Sagittal postgadolinium 512-resolution T2-weighted fat-suppressed echo-train spin-echo (*a*) and sagittal interstitial-phase gadolinium-enhanced fat-suppressed SGE (*b*) images in a woman status postradiotherapy for rectal adenocarcinoma. Recurrent tumor is high in signal intensity on the T2-weighted fat-suppressed image and enhances after gadolinium administration (open arrows, *a, b*). Cervical stenosis (arrow, *a*) secondary to radiation therapy causes widening of the proximal endocervical and endometrial canal.

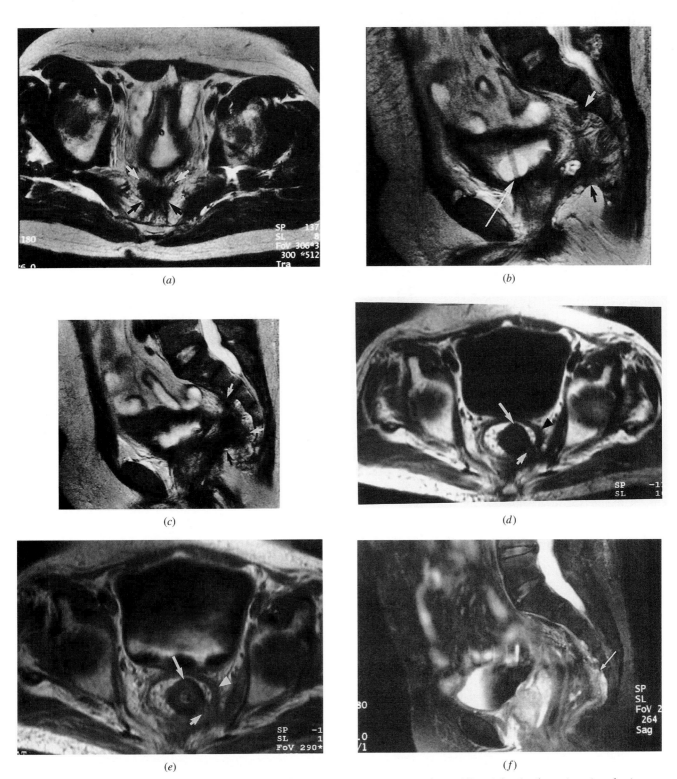

FIG. 6.111 Posttreatment fibrosis. Transverse (*a*) and sagittal (*b, c*) 512-resolution T2-weighted echo-train spin-echo images demonstrate low signal intensity in the surgical bed (arrows, *a–c*) consistent with fibrosis. Fibrosis has a plaquelike morphology, whereas recurrence tends to be more nodular. A Foley catheter is in place (long arrow, *b*).

SGE (*d*) and 4-min postgadolinium SGE (*e*) images in a second patient show thickening of the rectal wall (long arrow, *d, e*) and perirectal tissue (arrowhead, *d, e*). Prominent perirectal strands are also present (short arrow, *d, e*). Negligible enhancement is consistent with perirectal fibrosis. The perirectal halo of fibrotic tissue is a common finding after radiation therapy for rectal cancer.

Sagittal (*f*) and transverse (*g*) 512-resolution T2-weighted fat-suppressed echo-train spin-echo images and interstitial-phase gadolinium-enhanced fat-suppressed SGE (*h*) images in a third patient demonstrate platelike tissue in the presacral space that is low in signal intensity on T2-weighted images (arrow, *f, g*) and does not enhance substantially after gadolinium administration (arrow, *h*).

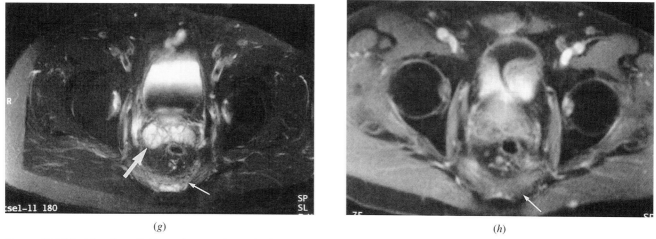

(g)   (h)

F I G . 6.111 (*Continued*) Normal seminal vesicles have a "cluster of grapes" appearance (large arrow, g) on T2-weighted images, which permits distinction from recurrent tumor.

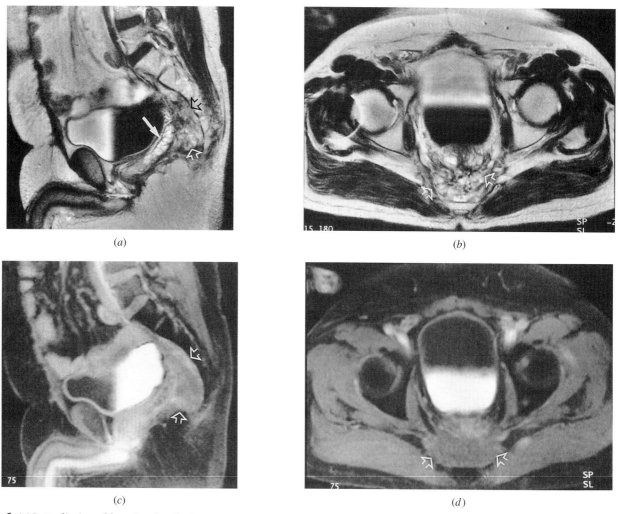

(a)   (b)

(c)   (d)

F I G . 6.112 Radiation fibrosis simulating recurrence. Sagittal (*a*) and transverse (*b*) postgadolinium 512-resolution T2-weighted echo-train spin-echo and sagittal (*c*) and transverse (*d*) interstitial-phase gadolinium-enhanced fat-suppressed SGE images in a patient 1.5 years after treatment for rectal cancer. Heterogeneous, bulky high-signal intensity tissue occupies the rectal fossa (open arrows, *a*, *b*), on the T2-weighted echo-train spin-echo images worrisome for recurrent disease. Other diagnostic possibilities include granulation tissue associated with radiation, inflammation, or infection. The heterogeneity is misleading because it reflects low-signal intensity fibrotic tissue interspersed with high-signal intensity fat. The high signal of fat is a consequence of the echo-train spin-echo technique. Minimal enhancement on the gadolinium-enhanced fat-suppressed SGE is consistent with fibrosis (open arrows, *c*, *d*). The seminal vesicles are distinguished from tissue in the rectal bed by the normal high signal intensity and grapelike morphology on the T2-weighted image (arrow, *a*).

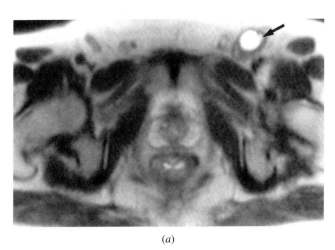
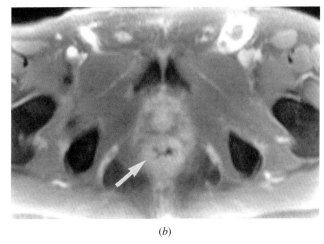

(a)   (b)

F I G . 6.113 Squamous cell carcinoma of anal canal. T2-weighted SS-ETSE (*a*) and interstitial-phase gadolinium-enhanced SGE (*b*) images. There is a diffuse wall thickening of the anal canal associated with stranding in the perianal fat, consistent with cancer (arrow, *b*). Note the necrotic left inguinal lymph node, which contains central high signal on T2 (arrow, *a*) and is centrally low signal with intense peripheral enhancement on postgadolinium fat-suppressed T1-weighted image.

intensity up to 3 years after therapy, particularly if intervening inflammation or infection has developed. Persistent increased signal intensity is most pronounced on gadolinium-enhanced T1-weighted fat-suppressed images. Finally, recurrent tumor may mimic radiation fibrosis when desmoplastic features predominate [6, 11]. Clinical history will often aid radiologic diagnosis: elevation of CEA levels, onset of presacral pain, or both are harbingers of tumor recurrence irrespective of imaging features.

Squamous Cell Carcinoma. Squamous cell cancer occurs in the anal canal, and its imaging characteristics resemble those of adenocarcinoma. Evaluation of local and distant spread is aided by gadolinium-enhanced fat-suppressed SGE images (fig. 6.113).

Lymphoma. Primary non-Hodgkin lymphoma accounts for approximatelly 0.5% of all colorectal malignancies. Primary lymphoma is most often seen in patients with human immunodeficiency virus (HIV) infection or chronic ulcerative colitis [95, 96]. The cecum is the most common site of involvement, followed by the rectosigmoid colon. Secondary involvement of the colon by lymphoma occurs in the setting of widespread disease, especially in the elderly population. The MRI appearance includes isolated or multiple enhancing masses. Alternatively, diffuse nodularity with wall thickening may be seen after intravenous gadolinium administration (fig. 6.114) [47, 48]. Coexistent lymphadenopathy and splenic lesions may aid in the diagnosis.

Carcinoid Tumors. The rectum is a common location for carcinoid tumor (fig. 6.115). A retrospective report of 170 carcinoid tumors found that 94 (55%) were

primary rectal lesions. Larger tumors were associated with metastatic disease and poor survival [97]. The imaging features of carcinoid tumors have been discussed elsewhere. As with other rectal diseases, direct sagittal plane imaging is useful. Liver metastases are best studied with dynamic gadolinium-enhanced SGE technique.

Melanoma. Primary colonic melanoma is rare and carries a poor prognosis [98]. Owing to the paramagnetic effects of melanin, the lesion can have a characteristic high signal intensity on T1-weighted images (fig. 6.116). Tumors may demonstrate ring enhancement after gadolinium administration.

Metastases. The large intestine may be the site of metastasis from a number of tumors including lung and breast carcinoma. The most common mode of secondary colonic involvement is peritoneal seeding [99]. Ovarian carcinoma commonly extends along peritoneal surfaces to involve the large bowel. Prostate or cervical carcinoma may affect the rectum by direct extension. Colorectal involvement is well shown on gadolinium-enhanced fat-suppressed T1-weighted images [70] (fig. 6.117).

Inflammatory and Infectious Disorders

Ulcerative Colitis
Ulcerative colitis is a chronic ulcero-inflammatory disease limited to the large bowel. It has a predictable distribution: disease begins in the rectum and extends proximally in a continuous fashion to involve part or all of the colon. "Skip" lesions, such as occur in Crohn disease, are absent. The incidence of ulcerative colitis is greatest in the second through fourth decades of life. There is a Caucasian, Jewish, and female predominance, and a

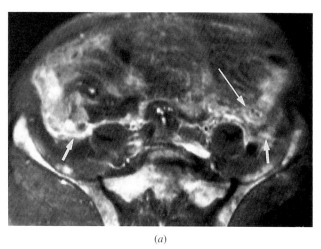

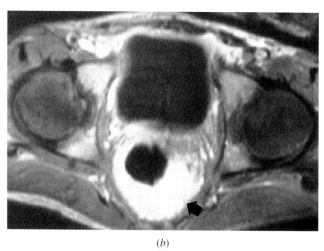

(a)   (b)

F I G . 6.114 Colonic lymphoma. Gadolinium-enhanced T1-weighted fat-suppressed spin-echo images (*a*, *b*) in 2 patients with lymphoma. In the first patient, with Burkitt lymphoma (*a*), there is enhancing soft tissue in both paracolic gutters (arrows, *a*), thickening of the descending colon (long arrow, *a*), and ill-defined stranding in the mesentery. Note the diffuse enhancing bone marrow involvement. The second patient (*b*) has HIV infection and a primary rectal lymphoma (arrow, *b*). HIV patients are at risk for developing primary large bowel lymphoma. (Reprinted with permission from Shoenut JP, Semelka RC, Silverman R, Yaffe CS, Mickflikier AB: The gastrointestinal tract. In Semelka RC, Shoenut JP (eds.), *MRI of the Abdomen with CT Correlation.* New York: Raven Press, p. 119–143, 1993.)

positive family history is reported in up to 25% of cases [100]. The cause is unknown, but similar to Crohn disease, a multifactorial etiology has been postulated. Ulcerative colitis is variable in presentation, but symptoms tend to be indolent with intermittent diarrhea and rectal bleeding. Patients with ulcerative colitis are at risk for

developing toxic megacolon, which may be the presenting feature. Chronic ulcerative colitis is associated with an increased risk of colon cancer.

In contrast to Crohn disease, which affects full-thickness bowel wall, ulcerative colitis is a mucosal disease. In active ulcerative colitis, there are multifocal

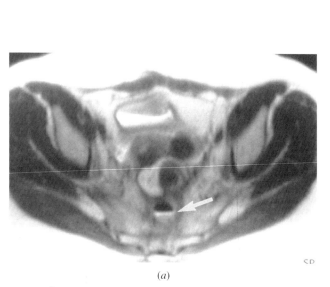

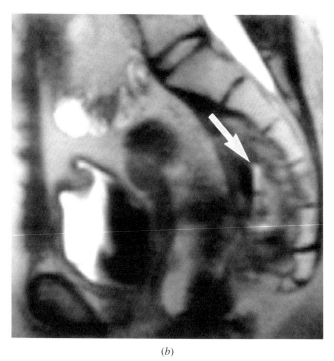

(a)   (b)

F I G . 6.115 Rectal carcinoid recurrence associated with abscess. Transverse (*a*) and sagittal (*b*) postgadolinium T2-weighted SS-ETSE and transverse (*c*) and sagittal (*d*) interstitial-phase gadolinium-enhanced T1-weighted SGE fat-suppressed images.

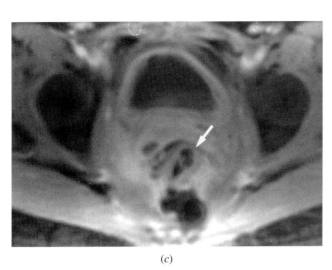

(c)

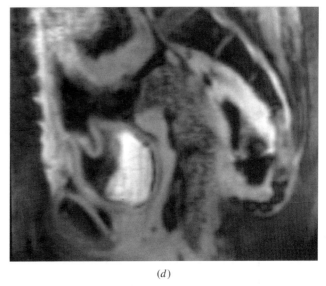

(d)

F i g . 6.115 (*Continued*) There is thickening and enhancement of the rectal wall (arrow, *c*) associated with soft tissue stranding within the pelvis. An air-fluid level is present in the presacral space (arrow, *a, b*), consistent with a small abscess.

full-thickness ulcerations of the mucosa. Adjacent to these sites, edematous, inflammatory tags of mucosa may bulge upward, toward the lumen, as "pseudo-polyps." In longstanding ulcerative colitis, intestinal shortening with loss of haustral folds may occur. This abnormality is ascribed to muscular abnormalities and is most marked in the distal colon and rectum.

The MRI appearance of ulcerative colitis reflects the underlying physiology: 1) rectal involvement progressing in a retrograde fashion to involve a variable amount of colon and (2) submucosal sparing (fig. 6.118). The latter is especially well seen on gadolinium-enhanced

fat-suppressed SGE images showing marked mucosal enhancement and negligible submucosal enhancement. Comparable to other inflammatory processes, the vasa rectae are prominent. The appearance of submucosal sparing is particularly pronounced in longstanding disease because of the combination of submucosal edema and lymphangiectasia [1, 2, 3, 6].

Toxic megacolon is characterized by total or segmental colonic dilatation with loss of its contractile ability. Toxic megacolon usually affects patients with universal colonic involvment ("pancolitis") and, unlike acute exacerbation and chronic indolent ulcerative colitis, is a

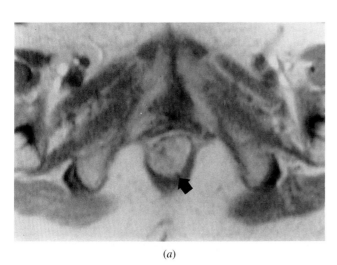

(a)

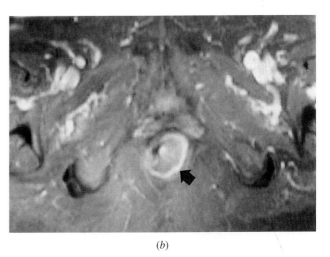

(b)

F i g . 6.116 Anorectal malignant melanoma. SGE (*a*) and gadolinium-enhanced T1-weighted fat-suppressed spin-echo (*b*) images in a patient with melanoma. Melanoma may be bright on T1-weighted sequences (arrow, *a*) because of the paramagnetic properties of melanin. Rim enhancement is apparent after contrast and allows accurate determination of mural extent (arrow, *b*) (Reprinted with permission from Shoenut JP, Semelka RC, Silverman R, Yaffe CS, Mickflikier AB: The gastrointestinal tract. In Semelka RC, Shoenut JP (eds.), *MRI of the Abdomen with CT Correlation.* New York: Raven Press, p. 119–143, 1993.)

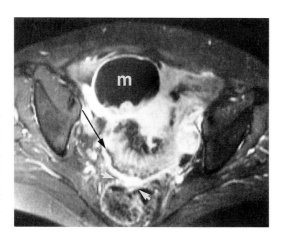

FIG. 6.117 Ovarian carcinoma metastatic to colon. Gadolinium-enhanced T1-weighted fat-suppressed spin-echo image in a patient with metastatic ovarian carcinoma. A complex cystic mass (m) encases the sigmoid colon (long arrow) and invades the rectum (short arrows). Tumor extension is clearly defined as enhancing tissue in a background of suppressed fat. (Reprinted with permission from Shoenut JP, Semelka RC, Silverman R, Yaffe CS, Mickflikier AB: The gastrointestinal tract. In Semelka RC, Shoenut JP (eds.), *MRI of the Abdomen with CT Correlation.* New York: Raven Press, p. 119–143, 1993.)

transmural process. The entire bowel wall enhances after intravenous contrast administration (fig. 6.119). Patients are prostrate with debilitating bloody diarrhea, fever, leukocytosis, and abdominal pain.

Inflammatory bowel disease may be exacerbated during pregnancy. These patients are particularly well suited for MR examination because of the relative safety of the procedure (fig. 6.120).

Crohn Colitis

Isolated colon involvement is noted in approximately one-fourth of cases. When Crohn colitis is limited to the anorectal region, differentiation from ulcerative colitis may be difficult [73]. In rare instances, Crohn colitis also may present with toxic megacolon (fig. 6.121). Crohn colitis is distinguished from ulcerative colitis by the following features: 1) persistence of colonic redundancy and haustrations in pancolonic disease and 2)

transmural enhancement, which at times may show the most intense enhancement in the submucosal layer, a layer that is spared in ulcerative colitis (fig. 6.122). As with ulcerative colitis, submucosal edema may also be present (fig. 6.123).

Diverticulitis

Diverticula occur throughout the colon and tend to be most numerous in the sigmoid colon (fig. 6.124). Inflamed diverticula favor the left colon, whereas hemorrhagic diverticula tend to occur in the right colon. Several studies have shown cross-sectional imaging to be equivalent to, and in some cases superior to, barium enema in the evaluation of diverticulitis (fig. 6.125) [101, 102]. Bowel wall thickening and diverticular abscesses are well seen using a combination of gadolinium-enhanced fat-suppressed T1-weighted SGE images and T2-weighted single-shot echo-train spin-echo images

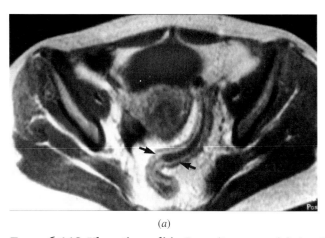

(a)

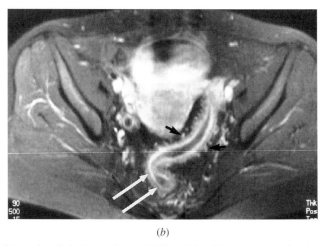

(b)

FIG. 6.118 Ulcerative colitis. Immediate postgadolinium SGE (*a*) and gadolinium-enhanced T1-weighted fat-suppressed spin-echo (*b*) images in a patient with ulcerative colitis. Increased enhancement on the immediate postgadolinium image (*a*) reflects increased capillary blood flow observed in severe disease. On the interstitial-phase image (*b*), there is marked mucosal enhancement with prominent vasa rectae (short arrows, *b*) and submucosal sparing (long arrows, *b*).

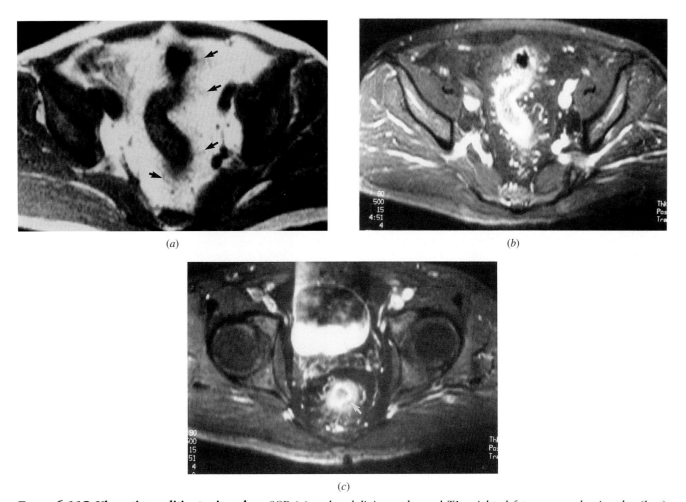

(a)   *(b)*

(c)

F I G. 6.119 Ulcerative colitis, toxic colon. SGE (*a*) and gadolinium-enhanced T1-weighted fat-suppressed spin-echo (*b, c*) images. The precontrast image shows irregular low-signal intensity strands (arrows, *a*) related to a thick-walled sigmoid colon. After contrast there is marked mural enhancement. Enhancement of the pericolonic strands reflects prominent vasa rectae. Submucosal sparing is apparent (arrow, *c*), which is a feature of ulcerative colitis. Note the very intense enhancement of the colon wall, which appears to involve full thickness in the sigmoid colon. This is consistent with patient's presentation of toxic colon.

(figs. 6.126 and 6.127) [103]. Similarly, sinus tracts and fistulas can be identified with this technique. On unenhanced T1-weighted SGE images, inflammatory changes appear as low-signal intensity curvilinear strands located within the high signal intensity of the pericolonic fat. Sinus tracts, fistulas, and abscess walls enhance and are well shown in a background of suppressed fat on gadolinium-enhanced fat-suppressed SGE images. It may be difficult to distinguish a perforated colon cancer from diverticulitis, and the two may coexist (fig. 6.128).

Appendicitis

Diagnostic imaging in cases of appendicitis is typically reserved for unusual presentations. Although CT imaging and ultrasound have surpassed barium enema in the workup of appendicitis [104, 105], MRI has several features that make it an attractive alternative. Specifically, MRI has high contrast-resolution for inflammatory processes and does not involve ionizing radiation. The lat-

ter feature is not inconsequential, because appendicitis is most common in children and young adults of reproductive age. On gadolinium-enhanced T1-weighted fat-suppressed images the inflamed appendix and surrounding tissues show marked enhancement (fig. 6.129). Inflammatory stranding in the surrounding fat is well visualized on unenhanced T1-weighted SGE images. In cases complicated by a periappendiceal abscess, the abscess wall will show enhancement with intravenous contrast administration, whereas the cavity remains signal void (fig. 6.130).

Abscess

Abscess formation may be a complication of gastrointestinal or biliary surgery, diverticulitis, appendicitis, or inflammatory bowel disease (IBD). CT imaging and ultrasound are the mainstays of diagnosis and have the added advantage of ease of percutaneous drainage capabilities. For MRI to compete effectively with these

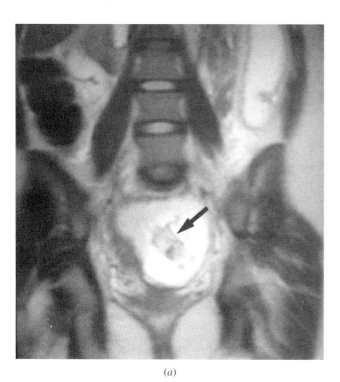

(a)

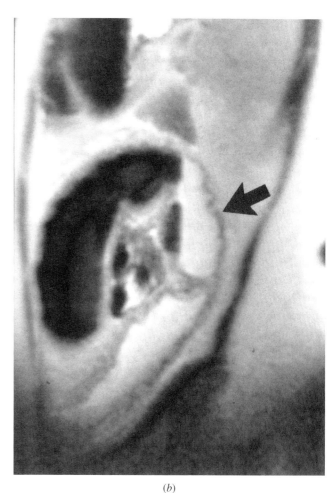

(b)

F I G . 6.120 Ulcerative colitis with acute exacerbation in pregnancy. Coronal (*a*) and sagittal (*b*) T2-weighted SS-ETSE images in a pregnant patient with history of ulcerative colitis. Diffuse irregular circumferential wall thickening of the descending (arrow, *b*) and sigmoid colon is present. Note the fetus (arrow, *a*) in the gestational sac.

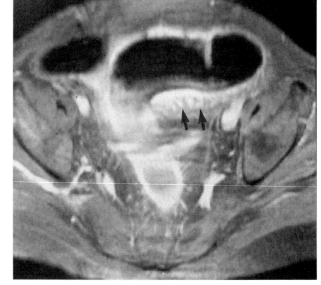

F I G . 6.121 Crohn disease presenting as toxic megacolon. Gadolinium-enhanced T1-weighted fat-suppressed spin-echo image in a patient with toxic megacolon. Dilatation and full-thickness involvement characterize toxic megacolon, a complication of inflammatory bowel disease (IBD). Note the prominent vasa rectae (arrows), a common finding in the setting of bowel inflammation. (Reprinted with permission from Shoenut JP, Semelka RC, Silverman R, Yaffe CS, Mickflikier AB: Magnetic Resonance Imaging in inflammatory bowel disease. *J Clin Gastroenterol* 17: 73–78, 1993.)

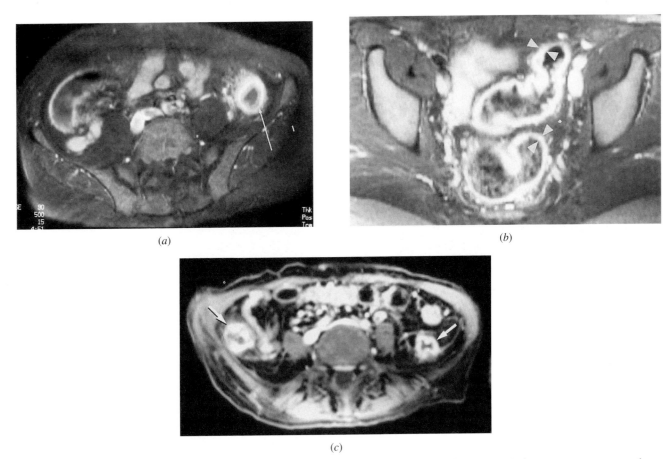

(a)

(b)

(c)

FIG. 6.122 Crohn colitis. Gadolinium-enhanced T1-weighted fat-suppressed spin-echo image (a) demonstrates transmural enhancement with greater enhancement of the submucosa (arrow, a) than the other bowel wall layers, which is diagnostic of Crohn disease and excludes the diagnosis of ulcerative colitis.

In a second patient with Crohn colitis, gadolinium-enhanced T1-weighted fat-suppressed spin-echo image (b) shows full-thickness enhancement of the sigmoid colon (arrowheads, b). The distribution of colon involvement is compatible with ulcerative colitis. However, the colon has remained redundant with persistence of haustrations despite severe disease. These findings combined with transmural enhancement are consistent with Crohn's colitis. Note the enhancing pericolonic inflammation in both patients. (Reprinted with permission from Shoenut JP, Semelka RC, Magro CM, Silverman R, Yaffe CS, Mickflikier AB: Comparison of Magnetic Resonance Imaging and endoscopy in distinguishing the type and severity of inflammatory bowel diseases. *J Clin Gastroenterol* 19: 31–35, 1994.)

Interstitial-phase gadolinium-enhanced T1-weighted SGE (c) image in a third patient with Crohn colitis shows thickening and enhancement of the ascending and descending colon (arrows, c).

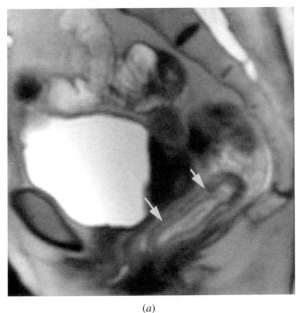

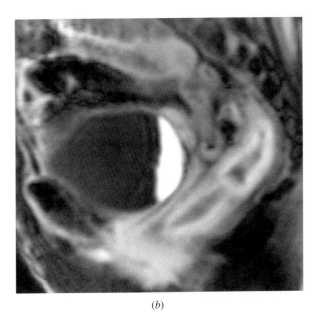

(a)

(b)

FIG. 6.123 Crohn proctitis. Sagittal (a) T2-weighted postgadolinium SS-ETSE and transverse (b) and sagittal (c) interstitial-phase gadolinium-enhanced SGE images.

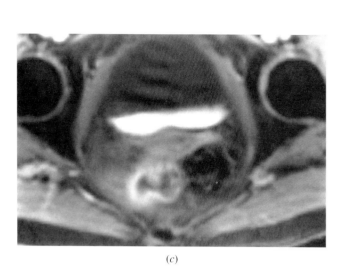

(c)

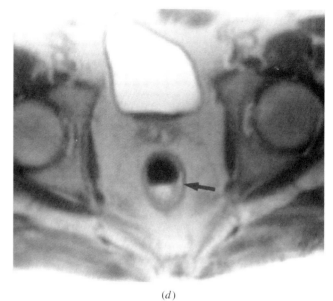

(d)

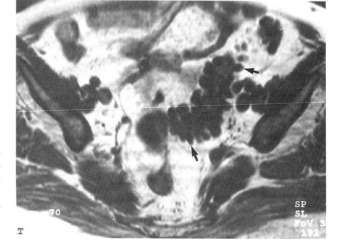

(e)

FIG. 6.123 (*Continued*) Prominent enhancement and thickening of the rectal wall are observed. Submucosal edema is appreciate as a high-signal stripe on the T2-weighted image (arrows, *a*). There is also diffuse perirectal soft tissue enhancement consistent with perirectal inflammatory changes.

Transverse (*d*) and sagital (*e*) T2-weighted SS-ETSE images in a second patient demonstrate thickening of the rectum associated with submucosal edema (arrow, *d*).

FIG. 6.124 **Diverticulosis.** SGE image demonstrates multiple signal-void sacculations arising from the sigmoid colon consistent with diverticulosis. Diverticula are common and often incidental findings. Complications of diverticula include diverticulitis and frank abscess. (Reprinted with permission from Ascher SM, Semelka RC: MRI of the gastrointestinal tract. In: Higgins CB, Hricak H, Helms CA (eds.), *Magnetic Resonance Imaging of the Body*, Raven Press, p. 677–700, 1997.)

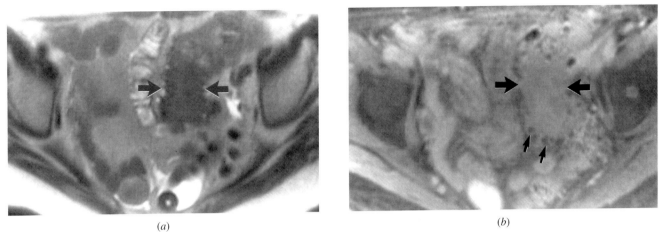

(a)   (b)

F I G . 6.125 Diverticulitis. T2-weighted SS-ETSE (*a*) and 90-s postgadolinium fat-suppressed SGE (*b*) images. Marked concentric wall thickening of an 8-cm segment of sigmoid colon is noted on the T2-weighted SS-ETSE image (arrows, *a*). The thickness of the colon wall measures up to 1 cm. Moderate contrast enhancement and marked wall thickening in the sigmoid colon (large arrows, *b*) are shown with small diverticula (small arrow, *b*) on the postcontrast fat-suppressed SGE image. (Reprinted with permission from Chung JJ, Semelka RC, Martin DR, Marcos HB : Colon diseases: MR evaluation using combined T2-weighted single-shot echo train spin-echo and gadolinium-enhanced spoiled gradient-echo sequences. *J Magn Reson Imaging* 12: 297–305, 2000.)

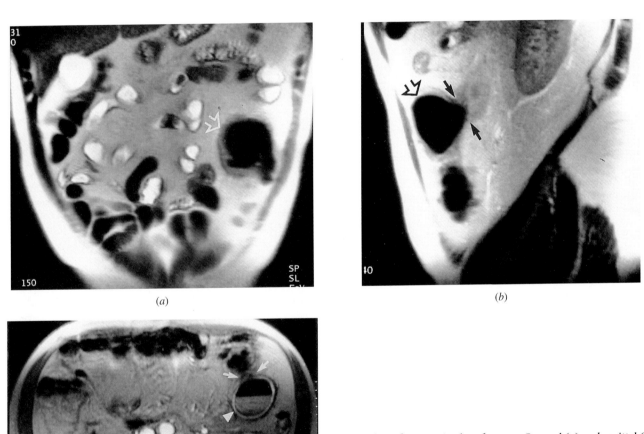

(a)   (b)

F I G . 6.126 Diverticular abscess. Coronal (*a*) and sagittal (*b*) SS-ETSE, and immediate postgadolinium SGE (*c*) images. An air- and fluid-containing collection (open arrow, *a*, *b*) originates from the descending colon (solid arrows, *b*, *c*), a finding consistent with a diverticular abscess. On the immediate postgadolinium image the inner wall of the abscess (arrowhead, *c*) enhances. An airfluid level is apparent on the transverse image (*c*).

(c)

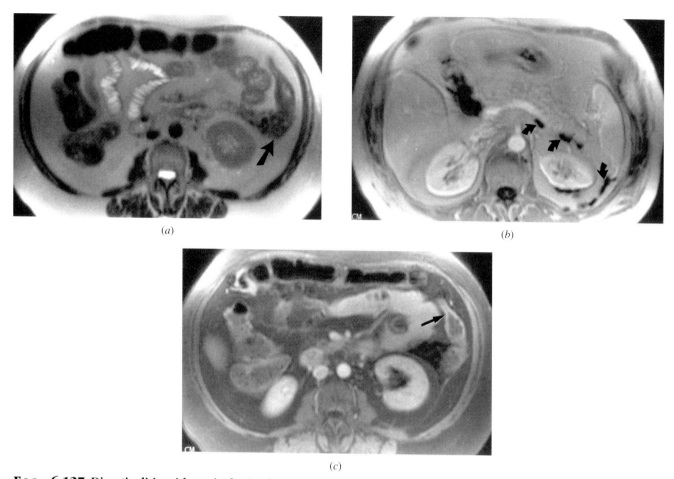

(a)

(b)

(c)

FIG. 6.127 Diverticulitis with pericolonic abscess. T2-weighted SS-ETSE (*a*), immediate postgadolinium SGE (*b*) and 90-s postgadolinium fat-suppressed SGE (*c*) images. An irregularly shaped gas collection is noted in the left anterior pararenal space, posterior to the descending colon, on the T2-weighted image (arrow, *a*). This appears to be in direct communication with a thickened segment of descending colon with an irregular focus of mural discontinuity. Multiple small gas pockets in the left retroperitoneal space are also apparent on the immediate postcontrast SGE image (curved arrows, *b*). The involved descending colon shows marked contrast enhancement (arrow, *c*) with an adjacent gas-containing abscess in the pericolonic fat on the 90-s postgadolinium fat-suppressed SGE image. (Reprinted with permission from Chung JJ, Semelka RC, Martin DR, Marcos HB: Colon diseases: MR evaluation using combined T2-weighted single-shot echo train spin-echo and gadolinium-enhanced spoiled gradient-echo sequences. *J Magn Reson Imaging* 12: 297–305, 2000.)

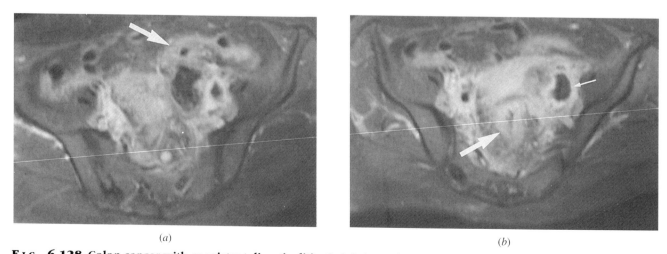

(a)

(b)

FIG. 6.128 Colon cancer with coexistent diverticulitis. Gadolinium-enhanced T1-weighted fat-suppressed spin-echo images (*a*, *b*) demonstrate a heterogeneously enhancing thickened segment of sigmoid colon (large arrow, *a*, *b*) with an adjoining abscess (thin arrow, *b*), features that were considered compatible with diverticulitis. Colon cancer was found in conjunction with diverticulitis at surgery.

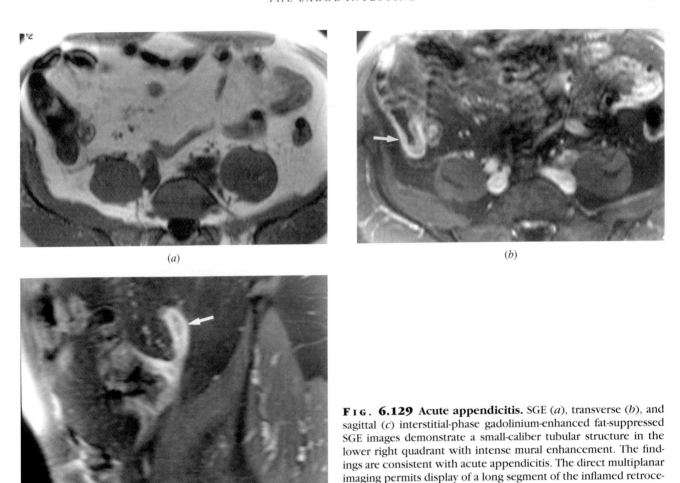

(a)

(b)

(c)

FIG. 6.129 Acute appendicitis. SGE (*a*), transverse (*b*), and sagittal (*c*) interstitial-phase gadolinium-enhanced fat-suppressed SGE images demonstrate a small-caliber tubular structure in the lower right quadrant with intense mural enhancement. The findings are consistent with acute appendicitis. The direct multiplanar imaging permits display of a long segment of the inflamed retrocecal abscess on the sagittal projection (*c*).

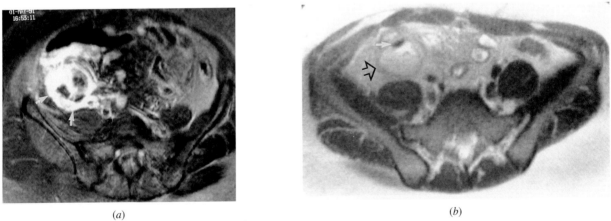

(a)

(b)

FIG. 6.130 Appendiceal abscess. Gadolinium-enhanced T1-weighted fat-suppressed spin-echo image (*a*) demonstrates a low-signal intensity appendiceal abscess with a prominent enhancing rim (arrow, *a*).

SS-ETSE (*b*), transverse (*c, d*), and sagittal (*e*) postgadolinium fat-suppressed SGE images in a second patient. A large multiloculated appendiceal abscess is present (hollow arrow, *b, c, e*).

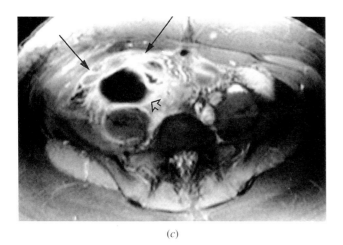

(c)

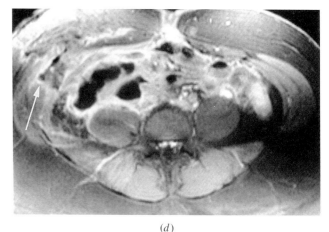

(d)

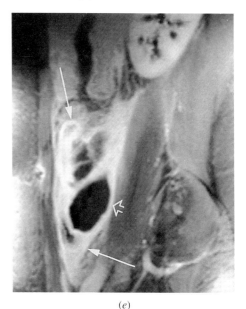

(e)

F I G . 6.130 (*Continued*) Air within the abscess is signal void (arrow, *b*) on the T2-weighted image. After gadolinium administration (*c, d, e*) the abscess rim enhances (open arrow, *c, e*), and extensive enhancement of periabscess tissue is present (long arrows, *c, d, e*).

modalities, automatic table motion, MRI-compatible needle and drainage equipment, and ultrafast imaging techniques must be in common usage.

Noone et al. [106] reported high diagnostic accuracy of MRI in evaluating suspected acute intraperitoneal abscess. In that series, abscesses were visualized as well-defined fluid collections with peripheral rim enhancement on gadolinium-enhanced T1-weighted fat-suppressed images. The presence of signal-void air within the collection confirms the diagnosis (fig. 6.131) [107]. The role of oral or rectal contrast to distinguish bowel from abscess is not firmly established. Most abscesses can be confidently differentiated from bowel with gadolinium-enhanced T1-weighted fat-suppressed SGE and T2-weighted single-shot echo-train spin-echo images acquired in two planes. This approach demonstrates the oval shape of abscesses and permits their distinction from adjacent tubular bowel. Enhancement of periabscess tissues on gadolinium-enhanced T1-

weighted fat-suppressed SGE images confirms the inflammatory nature of the fluid collections (fig. 6.132). The layering effect of low-signal intensity material in the dependent portion of the abscess on T2-weighted images is an important ancillary feature observed in the majority of abscesses [107]. The absence of motion artifact on T2-weighted single-shot echo-train spin echo facilitates identification of the dependent low-signal material in abscesses. The low signal reflects the high protein content of products of infection.

In patients with a contraindication for iodinated intravenous contrast (allergy and/or diminished renal function), MRI should be considered for the evaluation of abscess. MRI is particularly advantageous over CT in patients in whom high-density barium is present in bowel, because the barium creates severe artifacts on CT and may, if anything, improve the image quality in MRI. MRI also may be effective as a method to follow therapeutic interventions (fig. 6.133).

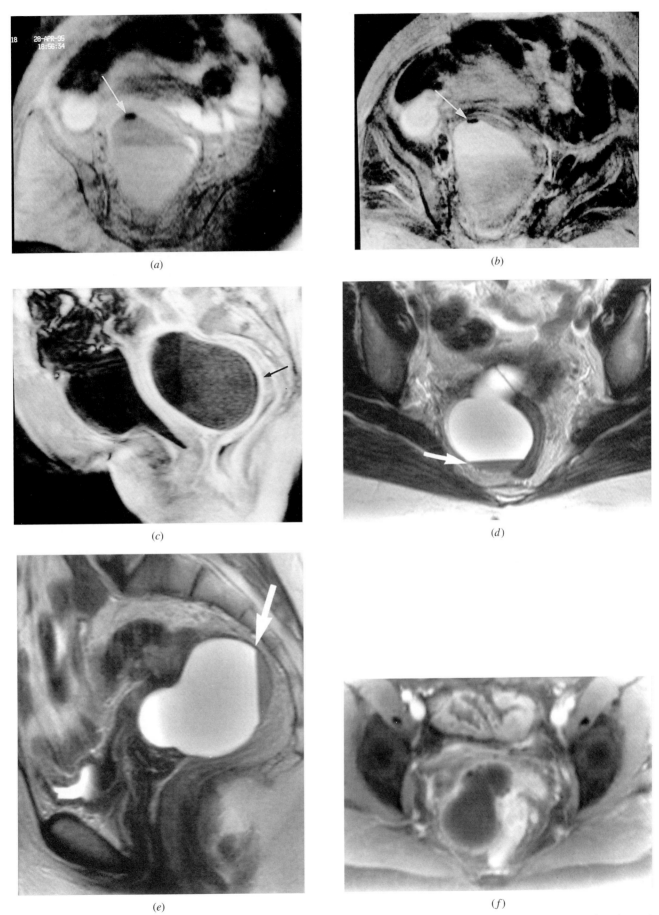

(a)

(b)

(c)

(d)

(e)

(f)

FIG. 6.131 Pouch of Douglas abscess. T1-weighted fat-suppressed spin-echo (*a*), T2-weighted echo-train spin-echo (*b*), and sagittal 45-s postgadolinium SGE (*c*) images.

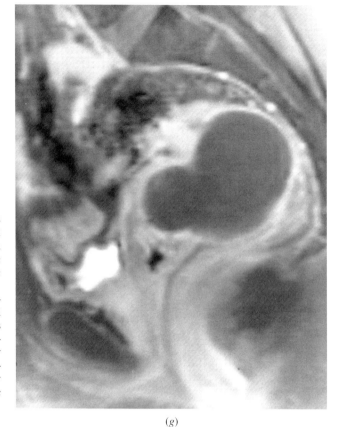

(g)

FIG. 6.131 (*Continued*) An 8-cm pouch of Douglas abscess is present that contains a focus of air that is signal void on T1-weighted (*a*) and T2-weighted (*b*) images (arrow, *a, b*). The abscess has a thick, enhancing rim (arrow, *c*) on the early postgadolinium image (*c*) with increased enhancement of surrounding tissue. Note the layering of debris on all the MR images (*a–c*).

Transverse (*d*) and sagittal (*e*) T2-weighted SS-ETSE and transverse (*f*) and sagittal (*g*) interstitial-phase gadolinium-enhanced fat-suppressed images in a second patient. There is a cystic mass situated in a right perirectal location that exhibits layering of low-signal material (arrow, *a, b*) on T2-weighted images. Moderately intense enhancement is observed of the abscess wall (*c*). The abscess displaces the rectal-sigmoid region to the left. Layering of low signal material on T2-weighted images is a relatively specific feature of abscesses.

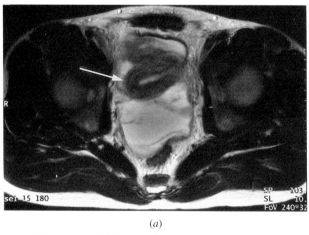

(a)

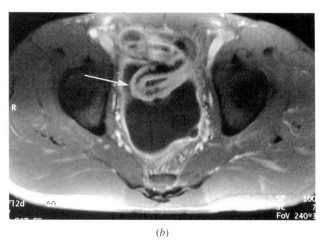

(b)

FIG. 6.132 Midabdominal and pelvic abscesses. Transverse 512-resolution echo-train spin-echo (*a*) and gadolinium-enhanced fat-suppressed SGE (*b*) images through the pelvis and sagittal 512-resolution echo-train spin-echo (*c*) and sagittal gadolinium-enhanced fat-suppressed SGE (*d*) images through the pelvis and midabdomen. An 8-cm, irregular, oval-shaped abscess is present in the recto-vesicle space that demonstrates dependent layering of low-signal intensity debris on the T2-weighted image (*a*) and substantial enhancement of the abscess wall (*b*). Inflammatory thickening of a loop of ileum (arrow, *a*) abutting the abscess is identified. Enhancement of the serosal surface of the bowel is appreciated (arrow, *b*). The sagittal plane images demonstrate the pelvic and the midabdominal abscesses (arrows, *c, d*). Layering of low-signal intensity material in the dependent portion of the pelvic abscess is shown on the T2-weighted image (*c*). Enhancement of the abscess wall and increased enhancement of multiple loops of small bowel are noted on the gadolinium-enhanced fat-suppressed SGE image (*d*).

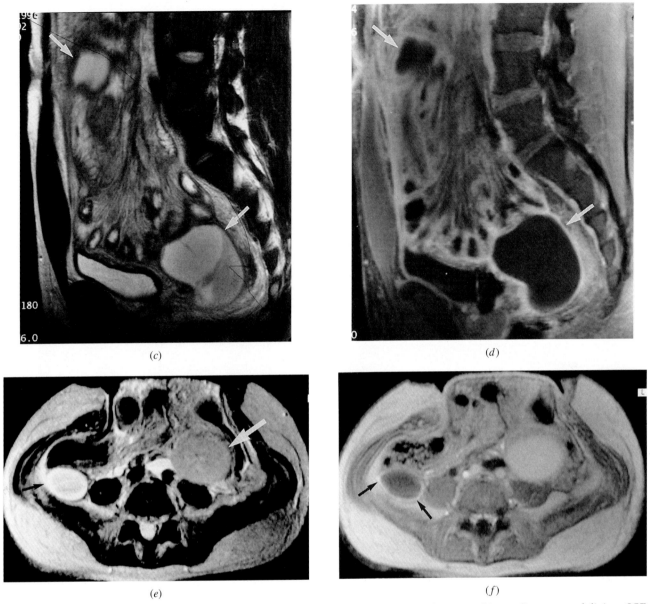

F I G . 6.132 (*Continued*) Transverse 512-resolution T2-weighted echo-train spin-echo (*e*) and immediate postgadolinium SGE (*f*) images in a second patient. This patient with chronic renal failure had undergone multiple abdominal surgical procedures for bowel ischemia and has a large anterior abdominal wall dehiscence with exposed peritoneal lining. A retrocecal abscess collection is present (arrows, *e,f*) that is high in signal intensity on the T2-weighted image and demonstrates ring enhancement on the immediate postgadolinium image. A chronically failed renal transplant is also identifiable (large arrow, *e*).

Colonic Fistulas

MRI is an effective imaging modality for evaluating colonic fistulas [7, 8, 108–110]. In particular, the multiplanar imaging capability of MRI has been shown to be useful for surgical planning for perirectal/perianal fistulas. The relationship of fistulas to the levator ani muscle is well shown on a combination of transverse, coronal, and sagittal plane images. T1-weighted images, T2-weighted images, and gadolinium-enhanced T1-weighted fat-suppressed images all provide good contrast between fistulas and surrounding tissues (fig. 6.134).

Infectious Colitis

Pseudomembranous colitis is defined as an acute colitis characterized pathologically by the formation of an adherent inflammatory "membrane" (pseudomembrane) overlying areas of mucosal damage. This disease occurs in the setting of broad-spectrum antibiotic use. The infectious organism most frequently implicated is *Clostridium difficile* [111]. The severity of the disease varies from mild to life-threatening. MRI shows thickening of the affected large bowel with marked enhancement (fig. 6.135).

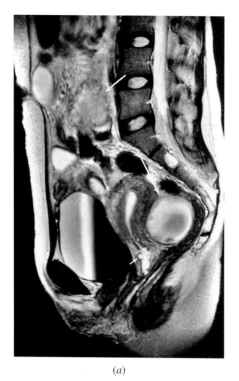

(a)

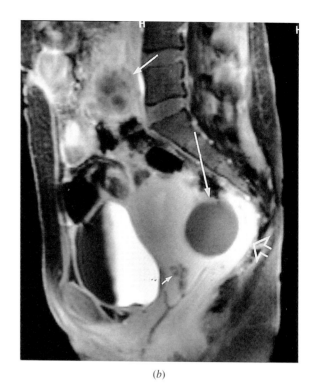

(b)

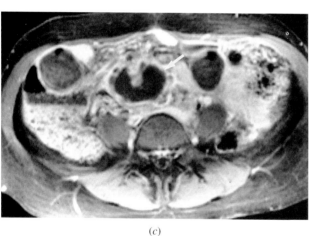

(c)

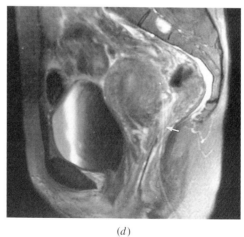

(d)

FIG. 6.133 Pelvic abscess, before and after catheter drainage. Sagittal 512-resolution T2-weighted echo-train spin-echo (*a*) and sagittal (*b*) and transverse (*c*) interstitial-phase gadolinium-enhanced fat-suppressed SGE images. The sagittal images demonstrate a 5-cm abscess in the pouch of Douglas (long arrow, *a*, *b*) and a smaller midabdominal abscess (short arrow, *a*, *b*). On the T2-weighted image, heterogeneous low signal is present in the dependent portion, which is a common finding in abscesses. On the postgadolinium images, substantial enhancement of the abscess wall and the adjacent rectum (hollow arrow, *b*) is present. Multiple Nabothian cysts are present in the cervix (small arrow, *a*, *b*). The transverse gadolinium-enhanced fat-suppressed image through the midabdomen demonstrates a 4-cm abscess (arrow, *c*) with enhancement of the abscess wall and the periabscess tissue.

Sagittal 512-resolution T2-weighted echo-train spin-echo image (*d*) and transverse interstitial-phase gadolinium-enhanced fat-suppressed SGE (*e*) images obtained 1 week after transrectal placement of a drainage catheter demonstrate substantial resolution of the pelvic abscess. The drainage catheter is identified as a signal-void tube (arrow, *d*, *e*). The degree of inflammatory reaction has also substantially diminished, but persistent enhancing tissue around the catheter is visualized (*e*).

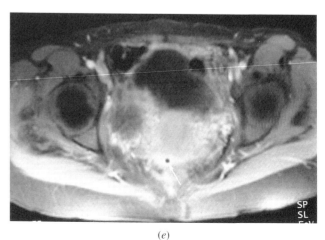

(e)

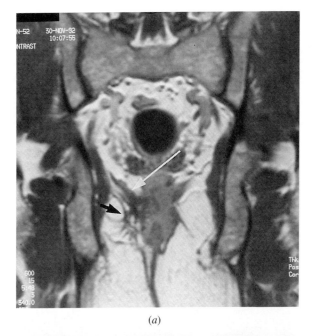

(a)

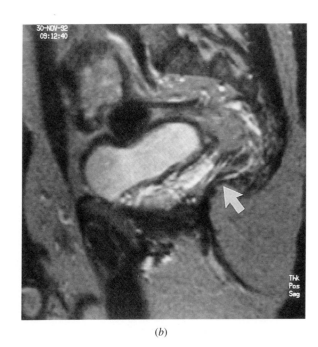

(b)

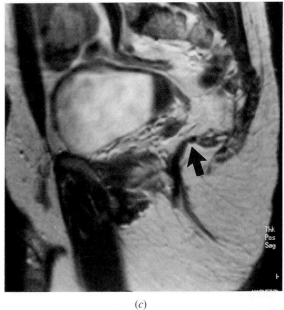

(c)

FIG. 6.134 Perianal fistula. Coronal T1-weighted spin-echo (*a*), sagittal T2-weighted spin-echo (*b*), and gadolinium-enhanced T1-weighted spin-echo (*c*) images. A complex fistula (arrow, *a*) is present in a right perianal location that extends to the levator ani muscle (long arrow, *a*). The fistula is low in signal on T1-weighted (arrow, *a*), T2-weighted (arrow, *b*), and postgadolinium (arrow, *c*) images, reflecting its chronic fibrotic nature.

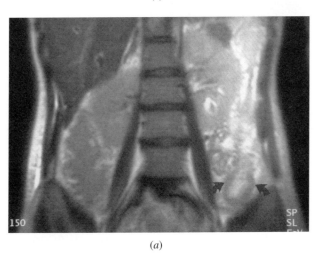

(a)

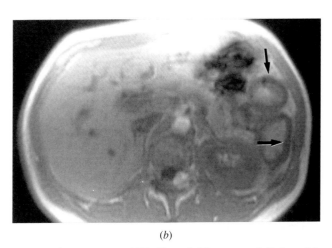

(b)

FIG. 6.135 Pseudomembranous colitis. T2-weighted SS-ETSE (*a*) and precontrast SGE (*b*) and 90-s postgadolinium fat-suppressed SGE (*c*) images. Diffuse bowel wall thickening is noted in the descending colon on the coronal T2-weighted image (arrows, *a*).

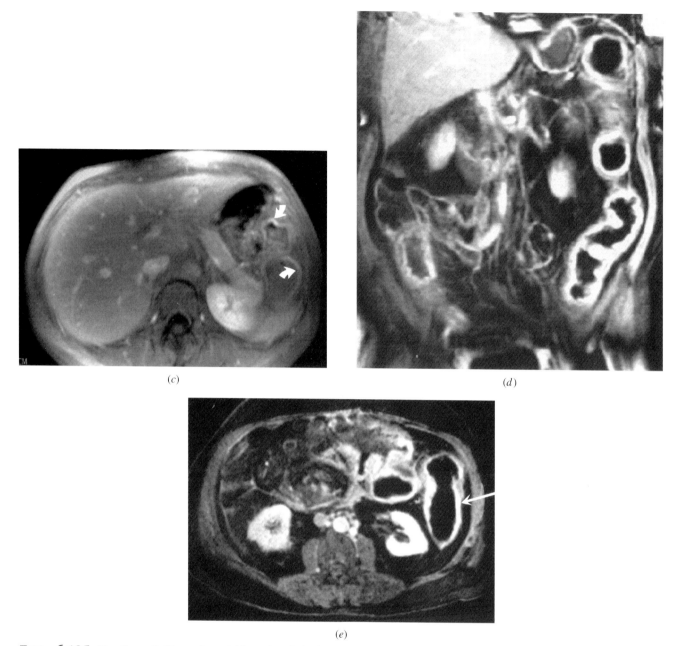

(c)

(d)

(e)

F I G . 6.135 (*Continued*) Circumferential bowel wall thickening is seen in the splenic flexure of the large bowel on precontrast SGE image (arrows, *b*). Moderately increased enhancement and wall thickening of the splenic flexure is noted on the postcontrast fat-suppressed SGE image (arrows, *c*). (Reprinted with permission from Chung JJ, Semelka RC , Martin DR, Marcos HB : Colon diseases: MR evaluation using combined T2-weighted single-shot echo train spin-echo and gadolinium-enhanced spoiled gradient-echo sequences. *J Magn Reson Imaging* 12: 297–305, 2000.)

Coronal (*d*) and transverse (*e*) interstitial-phase gadolinium-enhanced fat-suppressed SGE images in a second patient demonstrate diffuse thickening of the descending colon (arrow, *e*) with intense mural enhancement. (Courtesy of Russel Low, MD, Sharp Clinic, San Diego, CA).

In the past, neutropenic enterocolitis (typhlitis) was a disease affecting predominantly children treated for leukemia. The disorder also affects healthier neutropenic patients with solid tumors and other conditions. The cecum and ascending colon are the segments most commonly affected (fig. 6.136). MRI findings are nonspecific in patients with infectious colitis and generally demon-strate increased wall thickness and enhancement. Other infectious agents that target the colon include *Shigella*, *Salmonella*, *Escherichia coli*, amebiasis, and cholera.

Patients with AIDS are prone to cytomegalovirus colitis. Bowel wall thickening secondary to submucosal hemorrhage is the most characteristic finding. *Mycobac-terium avium intracellulare* also affects the large bowel and produces wall thickening (fig. 6.137) [45]. Patients with AIDS frequently develop proctitis. Opportunistic infection leads to rectal wall thickening and stranding in the perirectal space. Occasionally, frank perirectal abscesses occur. Gadolinium-enhanced T1-weighted fat-suppressed SGE images demonstrate bowel wall thickening with increased enhancement and abscess formation. Unenhanced SGE imaging is effective for show-

ing perirectal stranding, which appears low in signal intensity in a background of high-signal intensity fat.

Radiation Enteritis

The rectum is the most susceptible segment of large bowel to develop radiation enteritis. This finding may be attributed to the large radiation doses used to treat tumors arising in the pelvic area and the relatively fixed

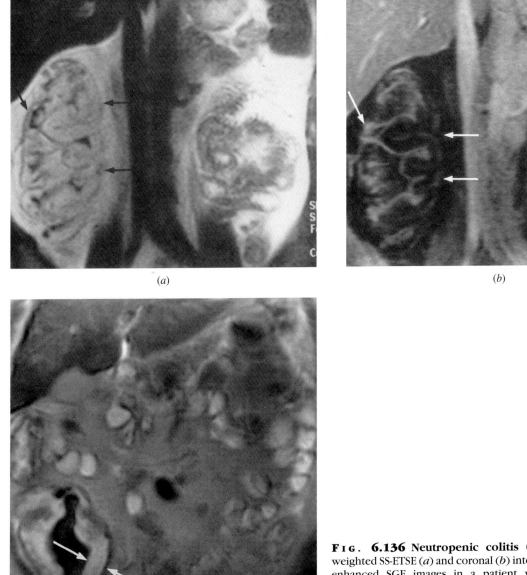

(a)

(b)

(c)

F I G . 6.136 Neutropenic colitis (typhlitis). Coronal T2-weighted SS-ETSE (*a*) and coronal (*b*) interstitial-phase gadolinium-enhanced SGE images in a patient with acute myelogenous leukemia history. There is marked thickening of the ascending colon (arrows, *a*, *b*) consistent with neutropenic colitis. Small bowel thickening and ascites are also present.

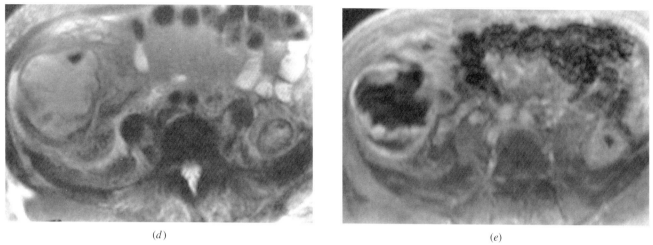

(d)

(e)

FIG. 6.136 *(Continued)* Coronal (*c*) and transverse (*d*) T2-weighted SS-ETSS and transverse interstitial-phase gadolinium-enhanced SGE (*e*) images in a second patient after chemotherapy. The cecum shows dilatation with marked thickening and enhancement of the wall (arrows, *c*).

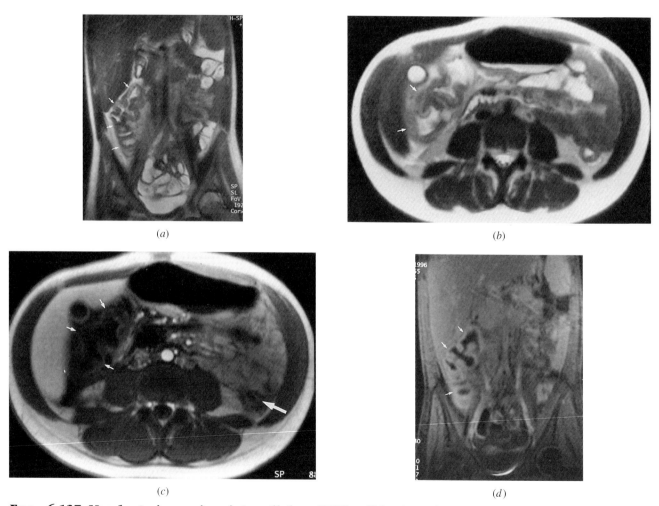

(a)

(b)

(c)

(d)

FIG. 6.137 *Mycobacterium avium intracellulare* **(MAI) colitis.** Coronal (*a*) and transverse (*b*) SS-ETSE, immediate postgadolinium SGE (*c*), and coronal 90-s postgadolinium fat-suppressed SGE (*d*) images in a patient with MAI colitis. SS-ETSE images (*a, b*) demonstrate marked wall thickening of the ascending colon (small arrows, *a, b*) with relative sparing of the descending colon. The mucosal surface enhances on the immediate postgadolinium image (small arrows, *c*), with negligible enhancement of the thickened outer wall. Less severe involvement is also seen of the descending colon (arrow, *c*). Enhancement of the wall increases and becomes more uniform (small arrows, *d*) on interstitial-phase images, reflecting capillary leakage.

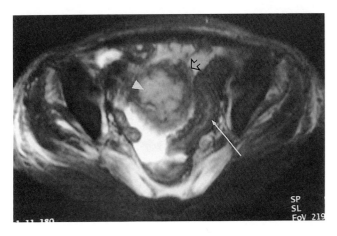

FIG. 6.138 Radiation enteritis. Transverse 512-resolution T2-weighted echo-train spin-echo image in a patient after radiation therapy. The sigmoid colon is thick walled with marked submucosal edema (arrow). The circumferential and symmetric nature of the bowel wall changes are suggestive of radiation enteritis. Note the thick-walled bladder (open arrow) and its heterogeneous contents (arrowhead), findings consistent with hemorrhagic cystitis, another sequela of radiation therapy. Free pelvic fluid is also present.

position of the rectosigmoid colon. Pathologic changes of acute radiation injury include prominent submucosal edema, ulceration, inflammatory polyps, and ischemic changes. Chronic radiation injury may show the histologic features of mucosal atrophy, vascular occlusion, and fibrosis. Late effects of radiation damage are evidenced pathologically by mucosal, submucosal, and muscular fibrosis with stricture formation [112]. In one study, the T1- and T2-weighted MRI features of the rectum in 42 patients status postradiation therapy were graded with respect to wall thickness and signal intensity of the muscular layers and submucosa. A spectrum of tissue changes were seen in the rectum regardless of the time from initiation of therapy. MRI had excellent sensitivity for depicting abnormalities, but specificity was limited [94]. The results of this study emphasize the need for detailed clinical history to ensure optimal MRI. The routine use of gadolinium-enhanced T1-weighted fat-suppressed imaging is effective for evaluating postradiation changes because of the high sensitivity of this technique for inflammatory changes. High-resolution T2-weighted images demonstrate the findings of submucosal edema in acute radiation proctocolitis well (figs. 6.138 and 6.139).

Rectal Surgery

A number of surgical procedures are performed for rectal cancer and other disease processes. Abdominoperineal resection (APR) is performed for tumors that are distal in the rectum, in which a tumor-free distal margin may not be achievable. After APR, more anteriorly positioned pelvic structures reposition more posteriorly, as the bladder, the prostate, and seminal vesicles and uterus. The pelvis is often packed with omental fat to prevent small bowel from filling the potential space when postoperative radiation therapy is contemplated (fig. 6.140).

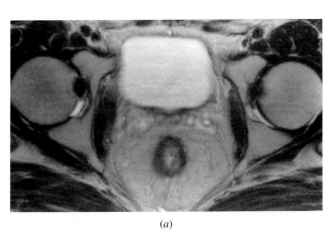

(a)

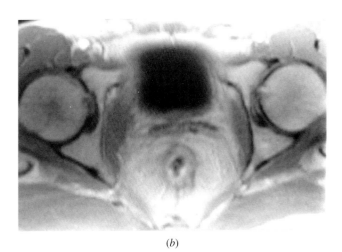

(b)

FIG. 6.139 Radiation proctitis. Transverse T2-weighted ETSE (a), immediate postgadolinium SGE (b), and interstitial-phase gadolinium-enhanced SGE (c) images. The rectal wall is thickened with multiple radiating soft tissue strands (arrow, c) in the perirectal fat. There is intense enhancement of the rectum consistent with radiation-induced inflammation. Abundant perirectal fat is also appreciated. These findings are consistent with postradiation changes.

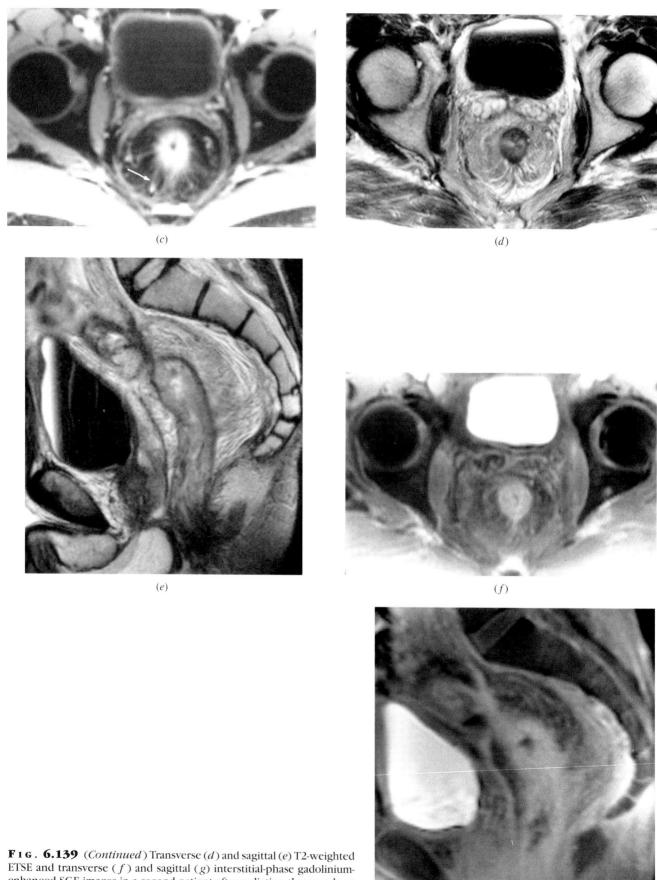

(c)

(d)

(e)

(f)

FIG. 6.139 (*Continued*) Transverse (*d*) and sagittal (*e*) T2-weighted ETSE and transverse (*f*) and sagittal (*g*) interstitial-phase gadolinium-enhanced SGE images in a second patient after radiation therapy show substantial thickening of the rectal wall with extensive linear strands in the enlarged perirectal fat.

(g)

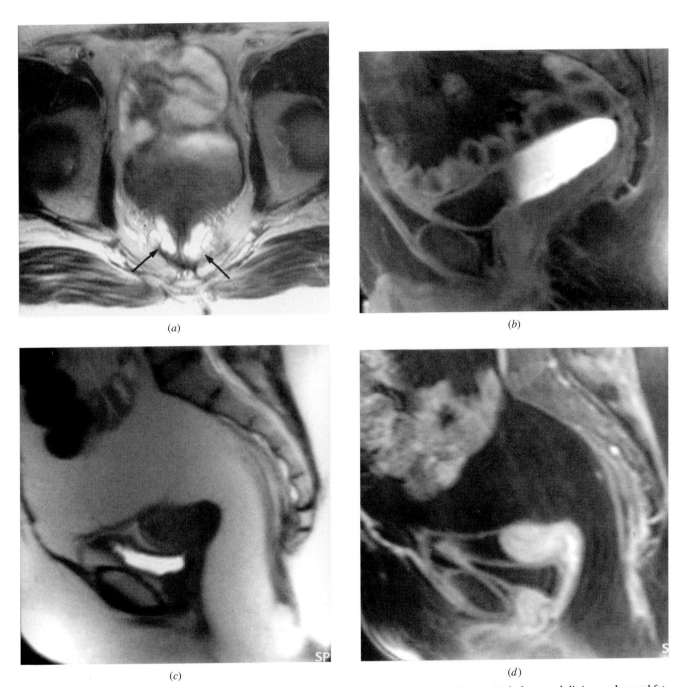

F I G . 6.140 Abdominoperineal resection (APR). T2-weighted ETSE (*a*) and sagittal interstitial-phase gadolinium-enhanced fat-suppressed SGE (*b*) images. The bladder and the seminal vesicles (arrows, *a*) are shifted posteriorly in the pelvis.

Sagittal T2-weighted SS-ETSE (*c*) and sagital interstitial-phase gadolinium-enhanced fat-suppressed SGE (*d*) images in a second patient show increase of pelvic fat consistent with omental packing.

Intraluminal Contrast Agents

The goals of intraluminal contrast agent use are twofold: 1) reliable differentiation of bowel from adjacent structures and 2) better delineation of pathologic processes involving the bowel wall. Oral contrast agents fall into two major categories, positive (signal intensity increasing) and negative (signal intensity decreasing) agents. Positive agents shorten T1-relaxation time, whereas negative agents either shorten T2-relaxation time or rely on

immobile protons to decrease intraluminal signal intensity. Biphasic intraluminal agents are formulated to produce high signal intensity on T1-weighted images and low signal intensity on T2-weighted images [113].

Positive Intraluminal Contrast Agents

Manganese-containing agents, ferric ammonium citrate, and gadolinium-containing agents have been employed as positive intraluminal agents (fig. 6.141). They are all

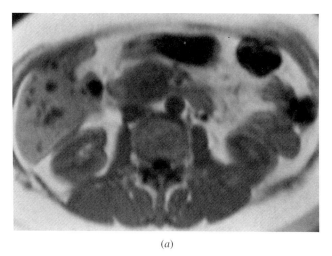 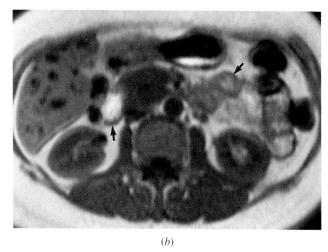

(a)   (b)

F I G . 6.141 Positive oral contrast agent. SGE images before (*a*) and after (*b*) ingestion of ferric ammonium citrate (FAC). Oral contrast causes high signal intensity within the bowel (arrows, *b*). The bowel loops are readily distinguished from the adjacent pancreas after oral contrast administration. Note that FAC not only results in signal intensity change of the bowel lumen but distends it as well.

paramagnetic [114–116]. To date, none of these agents is in routine use. Positive intraluminal agents may be useful to distinguish bowel (which would be rendered as high signal) from encapsulated fluid collections such as abscesses (which would remain low signal). Opacification of fistulous tract could also be demonstrated with these agents. On the other hand, positive intraluminal agents may mask the enhancement of inflammatory bowel wall or bowel masses.

Negative Intraluminal Contrast Agents
Intraluminal contrast agents may result in darkening of the bowel lumen because of lack of mobile protons

(perfluorooctylbromide) (fig. 6.142) [117] or superparamagnetic susceptibility effects (oral magnetic particles) (fig. 6.143) [118]. Because of high cost, perfluorooctylbromide is not available at present. A drawback of oral magnetic particles is occasional disturbing susceptibility artifact on T1-weighted SGE images, particularly in the region of the pancreas. Dilute barium results in a high fluid content of bowel and therefore low signal intensity on T1-weighted images and has achieved routine clinical use by some investigators [119]. Water functions well as a low-signal agent on T1-weighted images in the stomach (by oral administration) and colon (by rectal administration).

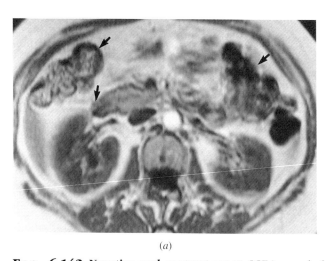 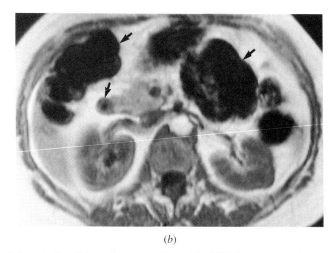

(a)   (b)

F I G . 6.142 Negative oral contrast agent. SGE images before (*a*) and after (*b*) perfluorooctylbromide (PFOB) ingestion, intravenous gadolinium-enhanced SGE image after PFOB ingestion (*c*), and gadolinium-enhanced T1-weighted fat-suppressed spin-echo image after PFOB ingestion (*d*) in 3 patients. In the first patient (*a, b*), bowel contents are heterogeneous before PFOB intake (arrows, *a*), but after ingestion of PFOB, they become nearly signal void (arrows, *b*).

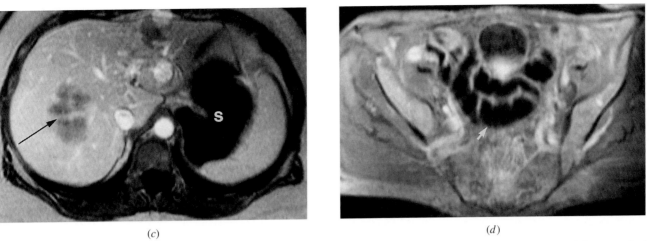

(c)   (d)

F I G . 6.142 (*Continued*) PFOB is signal void in the stomach ("s," *c*) of a woman with hepatic metastases (arrow, *c*) from cervical carcinoma. In a third patient (*d*), distal small bowel is signal void (arrow, *d*) after PFOB administration. Oral agents distend the bowel, which may aid detection of mucosal abnormalities.

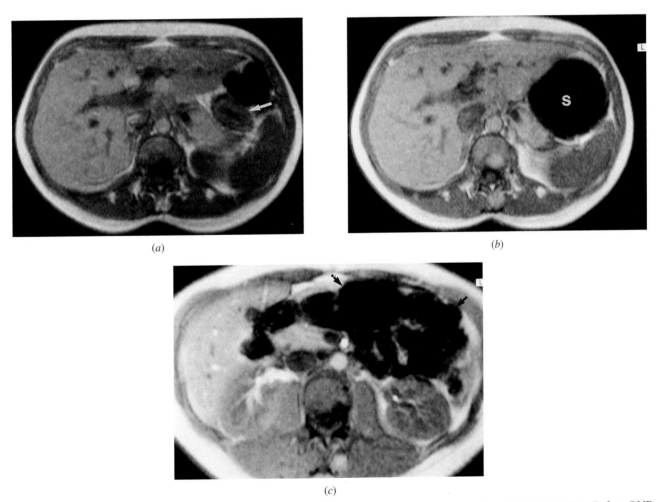

(a)   (b)

(c)

F I G . 6.143 Negative oral contrast agent. SGE before (*a*) and after (*b*, *c*) oral magnetic particle (OMP) ingestion. Before OMP ingestion, the stomach is collapsed with apparent wall thickening. Once distended with oral contrast, the stomach wall is barely perceptible. Similarly, the small and large bowel are distended and marked by OMP (arrows, *c*). Susceptibility artifact is visualized in many of the loops of bowel (*c*).

FUTURE DIRECTIONS

Future directions include the use of oral contrast agents described earlier, new intravenous agents, and new imaging techniques. Regarding intravenous agents, iron oxide particle agents have been used for MR lymphography in experimental models [120]. These agents are taken up by normal lymphoid tissue and hyperplastic lymph nodes, which decrease uniformly in signal intensity on T2-weighted images, whereas nodes involved with malignant disease retain signal intensity. These agents may increase the specificity of detecting malignancy involvement in normal-sized (<1 cm) lymph nodes. Normal-sized malignant lymph nodes are a common occurrence with gastrointestinal malignancies; therefore, improved specificity is of particular value for these tumors. Future imaging directions include real-time, dynamic alimentary track imaging (MRI upper GI), 3D intraluminal display (MRI endoscopy, colonography) and therapeutic interventions (e.g., abscess drainage).

CONCLUSION

Breath-hold scanning techniques as well as reproducible chemically selective excitation-spoiling fat suppression, T2-weighted single-shot echo-train spin echo, and routine usage of intravenous gadolinium have all contributed to the emergence of gastrointestinal MRI. MRI is well established for the investigation of primary or recurrent rectal carcinomas. Current imaging technique renders MRI comparable to CT imaging for the investigation of colonic, small bowel, and gastric malignancies. The superior ability of MRI to evaluate liver metastases may render MRI preferable to CT imaging in the investigation of these malignancies. Inflammatory bowel disease and abscesses are extremely well shown on MR images because of the high sensitivity of gadolinium-enhanced T1-weighted fat-suppressed SGE procedures for the detection of inflammatory enhancement. MRI should be considered in the investigation of these entities in patients with contraindications for iodinated contrast or CT examination. MRI also shows findings of intussusception very well.

REFERENCES

1. Semelka RC, Shoenut JP, Silverman R, Kroeker MA, Yaffe CS, Micflikier AB: Bowel disease: Prospective comparison of CT and 1.5 T pre- and postcontrast MR imaging with T1-weighted fat-suppressed and breath-hold FLASH sequences. *J Magn Reson Imaging* 1: 625–632, 1991.

2. Shoenut JP, Semelka RC, Silverman R, Yaffe CS, Mickflikier AB: Magnetic resonance imaging in inflammatory bowel disease. *J Clin Gastroenterol* 17: 73–78, 1993.

3. Shoenut JP, Semelka RC, Magro CM, Silverman R, Yaffe CS, Mickflikier AB: Comparison of magnetic resonance imaging and endoscopy in distinguishing the type and severity of inflammatory bowel diseases. *J Clin Gastroenterol* 19: 31–35, 1994.

4. Kettritz U, Isaacs K, Warshauer DM, Semelka RC: Crohn's disease: Pilot study comparing MRI of the abdomen with clinical evaluation. *J Clin Gastroenterol* 21: 249–253, 1995.

5. Shoenut JP, Semelka RC, Silverman R, Yaffe CS, Mickflikier AB: Magnetic resonance imaging evaluation of the local extent of colorectal mass lesions. *J Clin Gastroenterol* 17: 248–253, 1993.

6. Shoenut JP, Semelka RC, Silverman R, Yaffe CS, Mickflikier AB: The gastrointestinal tract. In Semelka RC, Shoenut JP (eds.), *MRI of the Abdomen with CT Correlation.* New York: Raven Press, p. 119–143, 1993.

7. Outwater E, Schiebler ML: Pelvic fistulas: Findings on MR images. *Am J Roentgenol* 160: 327–330, 1993.

8. Semelka RC, Hricak H, Kim B, et al.: Pelvic fistulas: Appearances on MR images. *Abdom Imaging* 22: 91–95, 1997.

9. Chan TW, Kressel HY, Milestone B, Tomachefski J, Schnall M, Rosato E, Daly J: Rectal carcinoma: Staging at MR imaging with endorectal surface coil. *Radiology* 181: 461–467, 1991.

10. Schnall MD, Furth EE, Rosato F: Rectal tumor stage: Correlation of endorectal MR imaging and pathologic findings. *Radiology* 190: 709–714, 1994.

11. De Lange EE, Fechner RE, Wanebo HJ: Suspected recurrent rectosigmoid carcinoma after abdominoperineal resection: MR imaging and histopathologic correlation. *Radiology* 170: 323–328, 1989.

12. Balzini L, Ceglia E, D'Ippolito G, et al.: Local recurrence of rectosigmoid cancer: What about the choice of MRI for diagnosis? *Gastrointest Radiol* 15: 338–342, 1990.

13. Gomberg JS, Friedman AC, Radecki PD, Grumbach K, Caroline DF: MRI differentiation of recurrent colorectal carcinoma from postoperative fibrosis. *Gastrointest Radiol* 11: 361–363, 1986.

14. Krestin GP, Steibrich W, Friedman G: Recurrent rectal cancer: Diagnosis with MR versus CT. *Radiology* 168: 307–311, 1988.

15. Pema PJ, Bennett WF, Bova JG, Warman P: CT vs. MRI in diagnosis of recurrent rectosigmoid carcinoma. *J Comput Assist Tomogr* 18: 256–261, 1994.

16. Waizer A, Powsner E, Russo I, et al.: Prospective comparative study of magnetic resonance imaging versus transrectal ultrasound for preoperative staging and follow-up of rectal cancer. *Dis Colon Rectum* 34: 1068–1072, 1991.

17. Macpherson RI: Gastrointestinal tract duplications: Clinical, pathologic, etiologic and radiologic considerations. *Radiographics* 13: 1063–1080, 1993.

18. Rafal RB, Markisz JA: Magnetic resonance imaging of an esophageal duplication cyst. *Am J Gastroenterol* 86: 1809–1811, 1991.

19. American Joint Committee: Clinical staging systems for cancer of the esophagus. *Cancer* 25: 50–57, 1975.

20. Habrey K, Winnfield AL: Multiple leiomyomas of the esophagus. *Am J Dig Dis* 19: 678–680, 1974.

21. Blot, WJ et al.: Continuing climb in rates of esophageal adenocarcinoma: An update. *JAMA* 270(11): 1320, 1993.

22. Winbeck M, Berges W: Oesophageal lesions in the alcoholic. *Clin Gastroenterol* 10: 375–388, 1981.

23. Maram ES, Kurland LT, Ludwig J, Brian DD: Esophageal carcinoma in Olmstead County, Minnesota, 1935–1971. *Mayo Clin Proc* 52: 24–27, 1977.

24. Kahrihas PJ, Kishk SM, Helm JF, Dodds WJ, et al.: Comparison of pseudoachalasia and achalasia. *Am J Med* 82: 439–446, 1987.

25. Templeton PA, Kui M, White CS, Krasna MJ: Use of gadolinium-enhanced MR imaging to evaluate for airway invasion in patients with esophageal carcinoma. *Radiology* 193(P): 311, 1994.

26. Trenker SW, Halvorsen RA, Thompson WM: Neoplasms of the upper gastrointestinal tract. *Radiol Clin N Am* 32: 15–24, 1994.

27. Halvorsen RA, Thompson WM: Primary neoplasms of the hollow organs of the gastrointestinal tract. *Cancer* 67: 188–189, 1991.

28. Marcos H, Semelka RC: Stomach Diseases : MR evaluation using combined T2-weighted single-shot echo train spin echo and gadolinium-enhanced spoiled gradient-echo sequences. *J Magn Reson Imaging* 10: 950–960, 1999.

29. Hamed MM, Hamm B, Ibrahim ME, Taupitz M, Mahfouz AE: Dynamic MR imaging of the abdomen with gadopentetate dimeglumine: Normal enhancement pattern of liver, spleen, stomach, and pancreas. *Am J Roentgenol* 158: 303–307, 1992.

30. Scholz FJ, Vincent ME: The stomach. In: Putnam CE, Ravin CE (eds.), *Textbook of Diagnostic Imaging*. Philadelphia: Saunders, p. 778–807, 1988.

31. Fenoglio-Preiser CM, Noffsinger AE, Stemmermann GN, Lantz PE, Listrom MB, Rilke FO: *Gastrointestinal Pathology*. Philadelphia: Lippincott, p. 156, 1999.

32. Ciftci AO, Tanyel FC, Hicsonmez A: Gastric diverticulum: An uncommon cause of abdominal pain in a 12 year old. *J Pediat Surg* 33: 529–531, 1998.

33. Fenoglio-Preiser CM, Noffsinger AE, Stemmermann GN, Lantz PE, Listrom MB, Rilke FO: *Gastrointestinal Pathology*. Philadelphia: Lippincott, p. 154, 1999.

34. Nakamura T, Nakano G: Histopathological classification and malignant change in gastric polyps. *J Clin Pathol* 38: 754–764, 1985.

35. Eisenberg RL: Single filling defects in the colon. In Eisenberg RL (ed.), *Gastrointestinal Radiology*. Philadelphia: Lippincott, p. 681–710, 1983.

36. Fenoglio-Preiser CM, Noffsinger AE, Stemmermann GN, Lantz PE, Listrom MB, Rilke FO: *Gastrointestinal Pathology*. Philadelphia: Lippincott, p. 232, 1999.

37. Ming SC, Goldman H: *Pathology of the Gastrointestinal Tract*. Philadelphia: Lippincott, p. 608, 1998.

38. Wingo PA, Tong T, Bolden S: Cancer statistics, 1995. *CA Cancer J Clin* 45(1): 8–30, 1995.

39. Haenszel W, Kurihara M: Studies of Japanese migrants. 1. Mortality from Cancer and other disease among Japanese in the United States. *J Natl Cancer Inst* 40: 43–68, 1968.

40. Coggon D, Acheson ED: The geography of Cancer of the stomach. *Br Med Bull* 40: 335–341, 1984.

41. Auh Yh, Lim T-H, Lee DH, Young YK, et al.: In vitro MR imaging of the resected stomach with a 4.7-T super conducting magnet. *Radiology* 191: 129–134, 1994.

42. Semelka RC, Shoenut JP, Kroeker MA, et al.: Focal liver disease: Comparison of dynamic contrast-enhanced CT and T2-weighted fat-suppressed, FLASH, and dynamic gadolinium-enhanced MR imaging at 1.5 T. *Radiology* 184: 687–694, 1992.

43. Hasegawa S, Semelka RC, Noone TC, Woosley JT, Marcos HB, Kenney PJ, Siegelman ES: Gastric stromal sarcomas: Correlation of MR imaging and histopathologic findings in nine patients. *Radiology* 208: 591–595, 1998.

44. Chandrasoma P: *Gastrointestinal Pathology*. Stamford, CT: Appleton & Lange, p, 371, 1999.

45. Jeffrey RB: Abdominal imaging in the immunocompromised patient. *Radiol Clin N Am* 30: 579–596, 1992.

46. Liang R, Todd D, Chan TK, Chiu E, Lie A, Kwong YL, Choy D, Ho FC: Prognostic factors for primary gastrointestinal lymphoma. *Hematol Oncol* 13(3): 153–163, 1995.

47. Chou CK, Chen LT, Sheu RS, Yang CW, et al.: MRI manifestations of gastrointestinal lymphoma. *Abdom Imaging* 19: 495–500, 1994.

48. Chou CK, Chen LT, Sheu RS, Wang ML, et al.: MRI manifestations of gastrointestinal wall thickening. *Abdom Imaging* 19: 389–394, 1994.

49. Fenoglio-Preiser CM, Noffsinger AE, Stemmermann GN, Lantz PE, Listrom MB, Rilke FO: *Gastrointestinal Pathology*. Philadelphia: Lippincott, p. 266, 1999.

50. Der R, Chandrasoma P. Chapter 5. Gastre neoplasms. In: Chandrasoma P: *Gastrointestinal Pathology*. Stamford, CT: Appleton & Lange, pp. 105–144, 1999.

51. Ming SC, Goldman H: *Pathology of the Gastrointestinal Tract*. Philadelphia: Lippincott, p. 563, 1998.

52. Yamada T, Alpers DH: *Textbook of Gastroenterology*. Philadelphia: Lippincott, p. 1302–1305, 1991.

53. Ming SC, Goldman H: *Pathology of the Gastrointestinal Tract*. Philadelphia: Lippincott, p. 583, 1998.

54. Lee JK, Marcos HB, Semelka RC: MR imaging of the small bowel using the HASTE sequence. *Am J Roentgenol* 170: 1457–1463, 1998.

55. Fenoglio-Preiser CM, Noffsinger AE, Stemmermann GN, Lantz PE, Listrom MB, Rilke FO: *Gastrointestinal Pathology*. Philadelphia: Lippincott, p. 309, 1999.

56. Marcos HB, Semelka RC, Noone TC, Woosley JT, Lee KT: MRI of normal and abnormal duodenum using half-fourier single-shot RARE and gadolinium-enhanced spoiled gradient-echo. *Magn Reson Imaging* 17(6): 869–880, 1999.

57. MacKey WC, Dineen P: A fifty year experience with Meckel's diverticulum. *Surg Gynecol Obstet* 156: 56–64, 1983.

58. Chew FS, Zambuto DA: Meckel's diverticulum. *Am J Roentgenol* 159: 982, 1992.

59. Fenoglio-Preiser CM, Noffsinger AE, Stemmermann GN, Lantz PE, Listrom MB, Rilke FO: *Gastrointestinal Pathology*. Philadelphia: Lippincott, p. 458, 1999.

60. Perzin KH, Bridge MY: Adenomas of the small intestine: a clinicopathologic review of 51 cases and a study of their relationship to carcinoma. *Cancer* 48(3): 799–819, 1981.

61. Chappuis CW, Divincenti FC, Cohn I Jr: Villous tumors of the duodenum. *Ann Surg* 209(5): 593–598, 1989.

62. Shekitka KM, Sobin LH: Ganglioneuromas of the gastrointestinal tract. *Am J Surg Pathol* 18(3): 250–257, 1994.

63. Losty P, Hu C, Quinn F, Fitzgerald RJ: Gastointestinal manifestations of neurofibromatosis in childhood. *Pediatr Surg*. 3: 57–58, 1993.

64. Semelka RC, Marcos HB: Polyposis syndromes of the gastrointestinal tract: MR findings. *J Magn Reson Imaging*. 11: 51–55, 2000.

65. Teplick SK, Glick SN, Keller MS: The duodenum. In Putnam CE, Ravin CE (eds.), *Textbook of Diagnostic Imaging*. Philadelphia: Saunders, p. 808–846, 1988.

66. Semelka RC, John G, Kelekis NL, Burdeny DA, Ascher SM: Small bowel neoplastic disease: Demonstration by MRI. *J Magn Reson Imaging*. 6: 855–860, 1996.

67. Al-Mondhiry H: Primary lymphomas of the intestine: East-west contrast. *Am J Hematol* 22: 89–105, 1986.

68. Rubesin SE, Gilchrist AM, Bronner M, Saul SH, et al.: Non-Hodgkin lymphoma of the small intestine. *Radiographics* 10: 985–998, 1990.

69. Bader TR, Semelka RC, Chiu VCY, Armao DM, Woosley JT: MRI of carcinoid tumors: spectrum of appearances in the gastrointestinal tract and liver. J Magn Reson Imaging 14: 261–269, 2001.

70. Semelka RC, Lawrence PH, Shoenut JP, Heywood M, et al.: Primary malignant ovarian disease: Prospective comparison of contrast enhanced CT and pre- and post intravenous Gd-DPTA enhanced fat-suppressed and breath hold MRI with histological correlation. *J Magn Reson Imaging* 3: 99–106, 1993.

71. Low RN, Barone RM, Lacey C, Sigeti JS, Alzate GD, Sebrechts CP: Peritoneal tumor: MR imaging with dilute oral barium and intravenous gadolinium-containing contrast agents compared with unenhanced MR imaging and CT. *Radiology* 204: 513–520, 1997.

72. Brahme F, Linstrom C, Wenckert A: Crohn's disease in a defined population. *Gastroenterology* 69: 342–351, 1975.

73. Goldberg HI, Caruthers B Jr, Nelson JA, Singleton JW: Radiographic findings of the national cooperative Crohn's disease study. *Gastroenterology* 77: 925, 1979.

74. Marcos HB, Semelka RC: Evaluation of Crohn's disease using half-fourier RARE and gadolinium-enhanced SGE sequences initial results. *Magn Reson Imaging* 18: 263–268, 2000.

75. Feeny PC, Stevenson GW: *Margulis and Burhenne's Alimentary Tract Radiology* (5th ed.) St. Louis: Mosby, p. 678–679, 1994.

76. Deutsch AA, McLeod RS, Cullen J, Cohen Z: Results of the pelvic-pouch procedure in patients with Crohn's disease. *Dis Colon Rectum* 34: 475–477, 1991.

77. Gutmann LT: *Yersinia enterocolitica* and *Yersinia pseudotuberculosis*. In Gorbach SI (ed.), *Infectious Diarrhea*. Boston: Blackwell Scientific, p. 65, 1986.

78. Lambert ME, Schofield PF, Ironside AG, Mandal BK: *Campylobacter* colitis. *Br Med J* 1: 857–859, 1979.

79. Guingrich JA, Kuhlman JE: Colonic wall thickening in patients with cirrhosis: CT findings and clinical implications. *Am J Roentgenol* 172: 919–924, 1999.

80. Fenoglio-Preiser CM, Noffsinger AE, Stemmermann GN, Lantz PE, Listrom MB, Rilke FO: *Gastrointestinal Pathology*. Philadelphia: Lippincott, p. 327, 1999.

81. Hussain SM, Stoker J, Lameris JS: Anal sphincter complex: Endoanal MR imaging of normal anatomy. *Radiology* 197: 671–677, 1995.

82. Stoker J, Hussain SM, van Kempen D, Elevelt AJ, Laneris JS: Endoanal coil MR imaging in anal fistulas. *Am J Roentgenol* 166: 360–362, 1996.

83. Okizuka HO, Sugimura K, Ishida T: Preoperative local staging of rectal carcinoma with MR imaging and a rectal balloon. *J Magn Reson Imaging* 3: 329–335, 1993.

84. Sato YS, Pringle KC, Bergman RA, Yuh WT, et al.: Congenital anorectal anomalies: MR imaging. *Radiology* 168: 157–162, 1988.

85. Ma Y, Chandrasoma P. Colorectal polyps and polyposis syndromes, In: Chandrasoma P: *Gastrointestinal Pathology*. Stamford, CT: Appleton & Lange, pp. 313–338, 1999

86. Burt RW, DeSario JA, Cannon-Albright L. Genetics of colon cancer: impact of inheritance on colon cancer risk. Annu Rev Med 46: 371–379, 1995.

87. Eisenberg RL: Multiple filling defects in the colon. In Eisenberg RL (ed.), *Gastrointestinal Radiology*. Philadelphia: Lippincott, p. 711–739, 1983.

88. Eisenberg RL: Solitary filling defects in the jejunum and ileum. In Eisenberg RL (ed.); *Gastrointestinal Radiology*. Philadelphia: Lippincott, p. 492–504, 1983.

89. Younathan CM, Ros PR, Burton SS: MR imaging of colonic lipoma. *J Comput Assist Tomogr* 15: 492–494, 1991.

90. Bernstein WC: What are hemorrhoids and what is their relationship to the portal venous system? *Dis Colon Rectum* 26: 829–834, 1983.

91. Kee F, Wilson RH, Gilliland R, Sloan JM, et al.: Changing site distribution of colorectal Cancer. *Br Med J* 305: 158, 1992.

92. De Lange EE, Gechner RE, Edge SB, Spaulding CA: Preoperative staging of rectal carcinoma with MR imaging: Surgical and histopathologic correlation. *Radiology* 176: 623–628, 1990.

93. Ito K, Kato T, Tadokoro M, et al.: Recurrent rectal Cancer and scar: Differentiation with PET and MR imaging. *Radiology* 182: 549–552, 1992.

94. Sugimura K, Carrington BM, Quivey JM, Hricak H: Postirradiation changes in the pelvis: Assessment with MR imaging. *Radiology* 175: 805–813, 1990.

95. Bartolo D, Goepel JR, Parsons MA: Rectal malignant lymphoma in chronic ulcerative colitis. *Gut* 23: 164–168, 1982.

96. Dragosics B, Bauer P, Radaasziewicz T: Primary gastrointestinal non-Hodgkin's lymphomas. *Cancer* 55: 1060–1073, 1985.

97. Jetmore AB, Ray JE, Gathright BJ, McMullen KM, et al.: Rectal carcinoids: The most frequent carcinoid tumor. *Dis Colon Rectum* 35: 717–725, 1992.

98. Pack GT, Oropeza R: A comparative study of melanoma and epidermoid carcinoma of the anal canal. *Dis Colon Rectum* 10: 161–176, 1967.

99. Fenoglio-Preiser CM, Noffsinger AE, Stemmermann GN, Lantz PE, Listrom MB, Rilke FO: *Gastrointestinal Pathology*. Philadelphia: Lippincott, p. 1050, 1999.

100. Acheson ED: The distribution of ulcerative colitis and regional enteritis in United States veterans with particular reference to the Jewish religion. *Gut* 1: 291–293, 1960.

101. Hulnick DH, Megibow AJ, Balthazar EJ, Naidich DP, Bosniak MA: Computed tomography in the evaluation of diverticulitis. *Radiology*; 152: 491–495, 1984.

102. Cho KC, Morehouse HT, Alterman DD, Thornhill BA: Sigmoid diverticulitis: Diagnostic role of CT—comparison with barium enema studies. *Radiology* 170: 111–115, 1990.

103. Chung JJ, Semelka RC, Martin DR, Marcos HB: Colon diseases: MR evaluation using combined T2-weighted single-shot echo train spin-echo and gadolinium-enhanced spoiled gradient-echo sequences. *J Magn Reson Imaging* 12: 297–305, 2000.

104. Balthazar E, Megibow AJ, Siegal SE, Birnbaum BA: Appendicitis: Prospective evaluation with high-resolution CT. *Radiology* 180: 21–24, 1991.

105. Jeffrey RB, Laing FC, Townsend RR: Acute appendicitis: Sonographic criteria based on 250 cases. *Radiology* 167: 327–329, 1988.

106. Noone TC, Semelka RC, Worawattanakul S, Marcos HB: Intraperitoneal abscesses: Diagnostic accuracy of and appearances at MR imaging. *Radiology* 208: 525–528, 1998.

107. Semelka RC, John G, Kelekis NL, Burdeny DA, Ascher SM: Bowel related abscesses: Demonstration by current MR techniques. *J Magn Reson Imaging* 16: 855–861, 1998.

108. Luniss PJ, Armstrong P, Barker PG, Reznek RH, Phillips RKS: Magnetic resonance imaging of anal fistulae. *Lancet* 340: 394–396, 1992.

109. Barker PG, Luniss PJ, Armstrong P, Reznek RH, Cottam K, Phillips RK: Magnetic resonance imaging of fistula-in-ano: Technique, interpretation and accuracy. *Clin Radiol* 49: 7–13, 1994.

110. Myhr GE, Myrvold HE, Nilsen G, Thoresen JE, Rinck PA: Perianal fistulas: Use of MR imaging for diagnosis. *Radiology* 191: 545–549, 1994.

111. Larson H, Price AB, Honour P: *Clostridium difficile* and the etiology of pseudomembranous colitis. *Lancet* 1: 1063–1066, 1978.

112. Fenoglio-Preiser CM, Noffsinger AE, Stemmermann GN, Lantz PE, Listrom MB, Rilke FO: *Gastrointestinal Pathology*. Philadelphia: Lippincott, p. 819, 1999.

113. Tammo HPR, Davis MA, Ros PR: Intraluminal contrast agents for MR imaging of the abdomen and pelvis. *J Magn Reson Imaging* 4: 291–300, 1994.

114. Bernardino ME, Weinreb JC, Mitchell DG: Fast MR imaging of the bowel with a manganese chloride T1/T2 contrast agent (Abstract). *Radiology* 189(P): 203, 1993.

115. Wesbey GE, Brasch RC, Goldberg HI, Engelstad BL: Dilute oral iron solutions as gastrointestinal contrast agents for magnetic

resonance imaging: Initial clinical experience. *Magn Reson Imaging* 3: 57–66, 1985.

116. Kaminsky S, Laniado M, Gogoll M, et al.: Gadopentetate dimeglumine as a bowel contrast agent: Safety and efficacy. *Radiology* 178: 503–508, 1991.

117. Brown JJ, Duncan JR, Heiken JP, et al.: Perfluorooctylbromide as a gastrointestinal contrast agent for MR imaging: Use with and without glucagon. *Radiology* 181: 455–460, 1991.

118. Rubin DL, Muller HH, Sidhu MK, Young SW, et al.: Liquid oral magnetic particles as a gastrointestinal contrast agent for MR imaging: Efficacy in vivo. *J Magn Reson Imaging* 3: 113–118, 1993.

119. Low RN, Francis IR: MR imaging of the gastrointestinal tract with IV gadolinium and diluted barium oral contrast media compared with unenhanced MR imaging and CT. *Am J Roentgenol* 169: 1051–1059, 1997.

120. Guimaraes R, Clemont O, Bittoun J, Carnot F, Frija G: MR lymphadenopathy with superparamagnetic iron manoparticles in rats: Pathologic basis for contrast enhancement. *Am J Roentgenol* 162: 201–207, 1994.

CHAPTER 7

PERITONEAL CAVITY

MONICA S. PEDRO, M.D., RICHARD C. SEMELKA, M.D.,
DIANE ARMAO, M.D., AND SUSAN M. ASCHER

NORMAL ANATOMY

The peritoneum is the most extensive and complexly arranged of the serous membranes in the human body. Like the serous membranes that line the pericardial and pleural cavities, the peritoneal cavity is lined by a specialized epithelium termed mesothelium.

The peritoneum can be analogized to an empty yet intricately folded sac. The parietal peritoneum lines the abdominal wall, whereas a continuation of the parietal peritoneum is reflected over viscera as the visceral peritoneum. The free surface of the peritoneum is lined by a smooth layer of mesothelium, moistened by a thin film of serous fluid. In the normal state, viscera are able to glide freely against the wall of the abdominal cavity or upon each other without impediment. Loss of this specialized mesothelial surface may lead to the adherence of underlying tissues. In certain conditions, transformation of mesothelial cells into fibroblasts and proliferation of submesothelial connective tissue can lead to macroscopic adhesions between peritoneal surfaces, disrupting intestinal motility or causing complete obstruction [1].

Some abdominal viscera are completely covered by peritoneum and are suspended from the posterior abdominal wall by a thin sheet of peritoneal covered connective tissue that contains a network of blood vessels. These folds of peritoneum are termed mesenteries. Peritoneal ligaments are serous membranes, often serving as neurovascular pedicles, extending between two structures. The apronlike greater omentum extends from the greater curvature of the stomach to lie draped over the coils of the small intestine and is reflected back onto the transverse colon. It forms a protective covering over the abdominal contents. The omentum may limit peritoneal infections because it tends to adhere to areas of infection. In a patient with perforation of the appendix, the omentum may wall off the infection to form an abscess, preventing gereralized peritonitis. The lesser omentum or gastrohepatic ligament joins the lesser curvature of the stomach to the liver. Its medial free edge is termed the hepatoduodenal ligament, which encloses the portal vein, hepatic artery, and common bile duct. The transverse mesocolon is a broad fold of peritoneum connecting the transverse colon to the posterior abdominal wall. Its layers pass from the pancreas to the transverse colon.

Because the parietal and visceral layers of the peritoneum are always in sliding contact, the peritoneal "cavity" is, in fact, best viewed as a potential space. The peritoneal cavity is divided into two regions, a main region, termed the greater sac, and a diverticulum, termed the lesser sac, which is located behind the stomach and the lesser omentum. The opening of the diverticulum, the epiploic foramen, provides communication between the greater and lesser sacs.

The peritoneum has the capacity to exude cells and fluid in response to injury or infection. Certain potential peritoneal spaces or recesses, normally in communication with each other, may be walled off by adhesions and create sites of abnormal fluid collections. The greater sac is further divided by the transverse mesocolon into an upper part, the supramesocolic space, and a lower part, the inframesocolic space. The supramesocolic space is subdivided into right and left peritoneal spaces. The right peritoneal space includes the right perihepatic space and the lesser sac, demarcated anteriorly by the lesser omentum. These spaces communicate via the epiploic foramen, which is bounded by the hepatoduodenal ligament of the lesser omentum. The lesser sac is a potential space that distends in the presence of certain disease processes, especially pancreatitis. The right perihepatic space consists of a subphrenic space and a subhepatic space and is partially divided by the right coronary ligament. The posterior aspect of the right subhepatic space encloses a recess between the liver and kidney called the hepatorenal fossa (Morison pouch). This space commonly accumulates fluid in the setting of diseases affecting gallbladder, second portion of duodenum, liver, or ascending colon. Malignant disease has a tendency to affect the lesser sac in addition to the greater sac. Benign disease, except for pancreatitis, primarily affects the greater sac [2, 3].

The left peritoneal space can be divided into anterior and posterior perihepatic spaces and anterior and posterior subphrenic spaces. The perihepatic spaces tend to be involved with diseases affecting the left lobe of the liver and stomach, whereas the anterior subphrenic space may also be affected by disease involving the splenic flexure. The posterior subphrenic space is most commonly involved in disease of the spleen.

The inframesocolic compartment of the peritoneal cavity is divided into a small right space and a larger infracolic space. The right side is limited inferiorly by the junction of the distal small bowel mesentery with the cecum, whereas the left infracolic space drains into the pelvis.

The paracolic gutters are located lateral to the peritoneal attachment of the ascending and descending colon. The right paracolic gutter is continuous with the right perihepatic space. On the left side, however, the phrenicocolic ligament forms a partial barrier between the paracolic gutter and the left subphrenic space. The pelvis is the most dependent portion of the peritoneal cavity in both the erect and recumbent positions. Therefore, both benign and malignant fluid preferentially pool in this location [4, 5]. The pelvic cavity consists of the lateral paravesical spaces and the midline rectovaginal space (pouch of Douglas or cul de sac) in women, and rectovesical space in men.

The peritoneal reflections are conduits for intraperitoneal fluid, which flows along the path of least resistance. Specifically, flow along the right paracolic gutter and into the pelvis is relatively unimpeded. Greater resistance to flow occurs along the left paracolic gutter, and flow across midline is impeded by the falciform ligament [6].

MRI TECHNIQUE

Techniques that minimize motion and maximize spatial and contrast resolution are well suited for imaging peritoneal disease. The multiplanar capabilities of MRI are also useful. Our standard MRI protocol includes breath-hold T1-weighted SGE, T2-weighted single-shot echo-train spin-echo, and immediate and delayed postgadolinium SGE techniques, with the delayed images acquired with fat suppression. The essential sequence to evaluate peritoneal disease is 2- to 5-min gadolinium-enhanced T1-weighted fat suppressed SGE (fig. 7.1).

For fibrotic processes, the T1-weighted SGE technique maximizes contrast resolution between high-signal intraperitoneal fat and low-signal diseased tissue, whereas, for inflammatory and neoplastic conditions, gadolinium-enhanced T1-weighted fat-suppressed SGE technique is the most sensitive imaging sequence for disease detection. Peritoneal diseases are best studied during the interstitial phase (2–10 min after injection), when leaky capillaries allow contrast to pool in the interstitium. This time course allows for dynamic scanning of a target organ (e.g., the liver) during the capillary phase and a survey of the peritoneum during the interstitial phase. This is particularly advantageous in conditions that simultaneously affect the solid viscera and peritoneum, such as ovarian, colorectal, pancreatic, and gastric carcinoma.

DISEASE ENTITIES

Normal Variants and Congenital Disease

Congenital variation of the peritoneal reflections are rare. They usually are related to malrotation of the bowel or situs anomalies during gestation [7]. Lymphangiomas of the omentum and mesentery are true cysts lined by endothelium. Cystic lymphangioma represents the single most frequent tumor of the omentum in children [8]. Possible pathogenic mechanisms for these lesions include developmental disturbance with abnormality in the lymphatic system or drainage obstruction with secondary

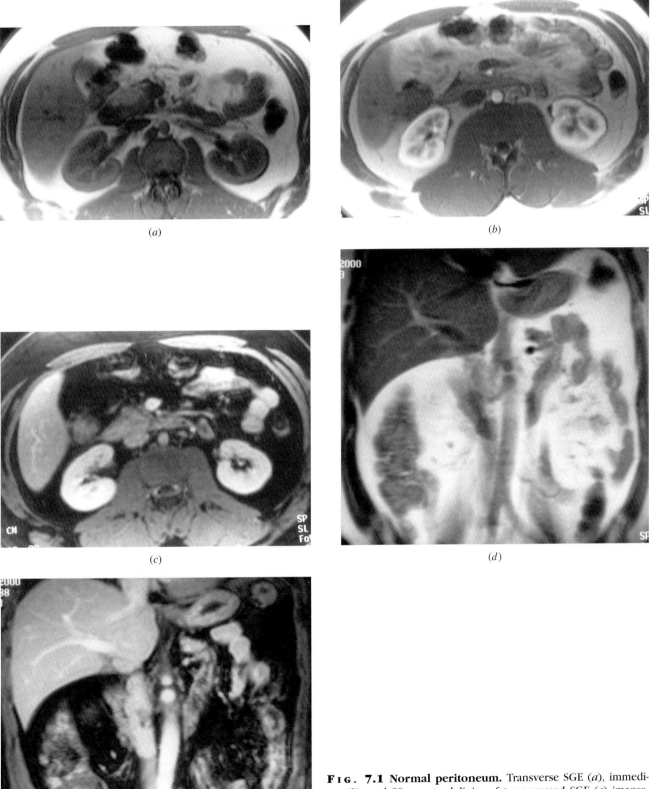

(a)

(b)

(c)

(d)

(e)

FIG. 7.1 Normal peritoneum. Transverse SGE (*a*), immediate (*b*), and 90-s postgadolinium fat-suppressed SGE (*c*) images. The normal peritoneum is faintly appreciable on current MRI techniques. The abdominal fat is uniform and provides good contrast with abdominal organs, using a combination of nonsuppressed (*a, b*) and fat-suppressed (*c*) sequences.

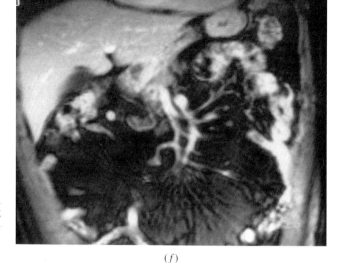

(*f*)

F I G . 7.1 (*Continued*) Coronal T2-weighted SS-ETSE (*d*) and coronal interstitial-phase gadolinium-enhanced fat-suppressed SGE (*e, f*) images in a second patient. Note that bowel, vessels, and the mesentery are well demarcated.

expansion of the lymphatic channels. They usually are multiloculated cysts containing serous or chylous fluid, but may be complicated by hemorrhage. The imaging characteristics reflect the cyst contents in that lymphangiomas with high protein content are high in signal intensity on T1-weighted images [9].

Hernias

Bochdalek hernia
Posterolateral defect of the diaphragm is a common congenital diaphragm abnormality. Defective formation and/or fusion of the pleuroperitoneal membrane results in herniation of abdominal contents into the thoracic cavity. This defect, usually unilateral and on the left side, consists of a large opening (refered to as the foramen of Bochdalek) in the posterior aspect of the diaphragm

[10]. The discontinuity of the diaphragm may be shown by MRI in multiple planes (fig. 7.2).

Hiatus hernia
Partial congenital herniation of the stomach through an enlarged esophageal hiatus is rare. Most hiatal hernias are acquired lesions occurring during adult life. Esophageal hernias are divided into two types, sliding (axial) and paraesophageal. Paraesophageal hiatal hernias are characterized by herniation of all or part of the stomach into the thorax immediately adjacent and to the left of an undisplaced gastroesophageal junction. In contrast, sliding hiatal hernias are characterized by displacement of the upper stomach and gastroesophageal junction upward into the thorax. Sliding hernias result from weakened or torn phrenoesophageal membranes, resulting in a gastroesophageal junction that is above the esophageal hiatus of the diaphragm (fig. 7.3).

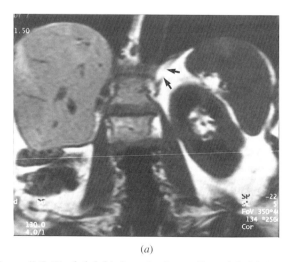

(*a*)

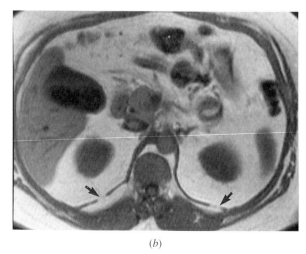

(*b*)

F I G . 7.2 Bochdalek's hernia. Coronal breath-hold T1-weighted SGE image (*a*) shows the discontinuity of the posterior diaphragm (arrows). The rent in the diaphragm allows fat and/or viscera to migrate superiorly into the chest.

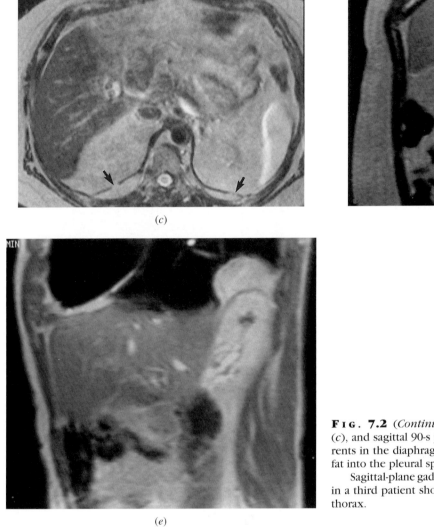

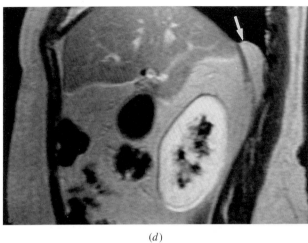

(c)

(d)

F I G . 7.2 (*Continued*) SGE (*b*), T2-weighted spin-echo (T2-SE) (*c*), and sagittal 90-s postgadolinium SGE (*d*) images demonstrate rents in the diaphragm bilaterally (arrows, *b*, *c*) and herniation of fat into the pleural space (arrow, *d*).

Sagittal-plane gadolinium-enhanced T1-weighted SGE (*e*) image in a third patient shows the herniation of kidney and fat into the thorax.

(e)

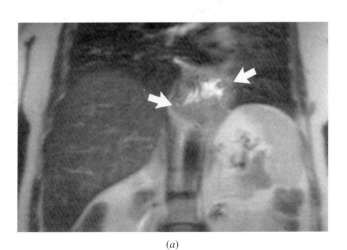

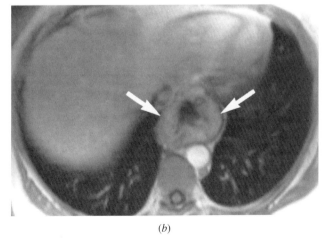

(a)

(b)

F I G . 7.3 Hiatus hernia. Coronal T2-weighted SS-ETSE (*a*) and transverse immediate postgadolinium SGE (*b*) images. The coronal T2-weighted image demonstrates extension of the stomach (arrows, *a*) above the diaphragm. On the transverse postgadolinium image the extent of gastric wall enhancement of the herniated part of the stomach (arrows, *b*) is comparable to the remainder of the stomach.

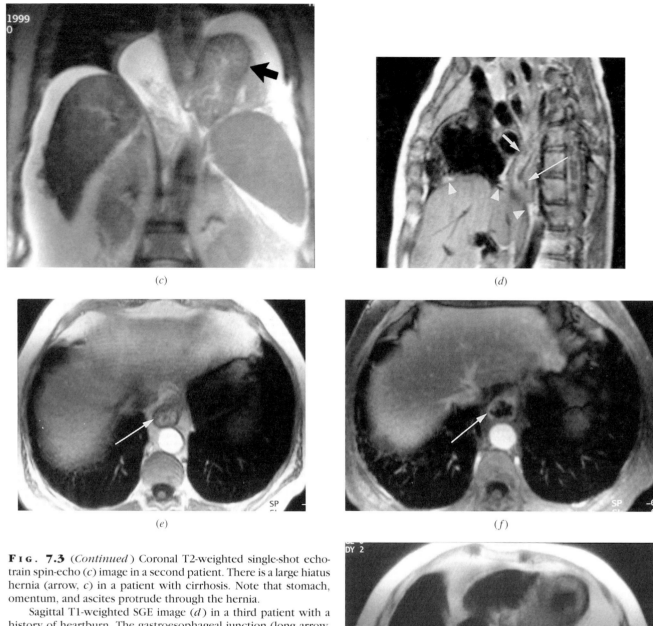

(c)

(d)

(e)

(f)

FIG. 7.3 (*Continued*) Coronal T2-weighted single-shot echo-train spin-echo (*c*) image in a second patient. There is a large hiatus hernia (arrow, *c*) in a patient with cirrhosis. Note that stomach, omentum, and ascites protrude through the hernia.

Sagittal T1-weighted SGE image (*d*) in a third patient with a history of heartburn. The gastroesophageal junction (long arrow, *d*) is above the diaphragm (arrowheads, *d*), which is diagnostic of a hiatal hernia. Thickening of the esophageal wall (short arrow, *d*) is consistent with reflux esophagitis.

Immediate postgadolinium SGE (*e*), and 90-s post-gadolinium SGE imaging (*f*) in a fourth patient demonstrate stomach in the lower mediastinum (arrows, *e*, *f*). Gastric rugae are well shown on the gadolinium-enhanced fat-suppressed image (*f*).

T2-weighted SS-ETSE image (*g*) in a fifth patient shows a large hiatal hernia with surrounding herniated fat.

(g)

Abdominal Wall Hernias

MR images acquired as breath-hold or single-shot techniques identify abdominal wall hernias. This may be helpful in obese patients where physical exam is hampered. Single-shot echo-train spin-echo (SS-ETSE) is particularly effective at demonstrating hernias and, in addition, experiences negligible magnetic susceptibility artifact, which improves visualization of bowel wall in the setting of dilated air-filled loops of bowel.

- **Inguinal hernia:** Inguinal hernias result from a persistent processus vaginalis, which is that portion of the abdominal peritoneum that enters the deep, or internal, inguinal ring. At birth, the patent processus

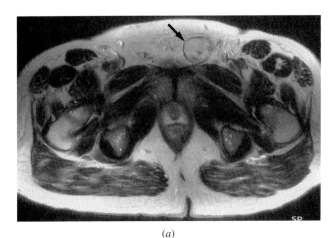

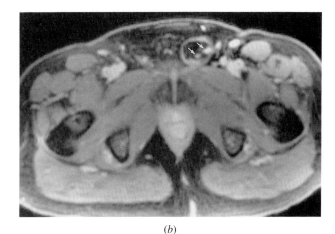

(a)   (b)

F I G . 7.4 Inguinal hernia. Transverse 512-resolution T2-weighted echo-train spin-echo (*a*) and interstitial-phase gadolinium-enhanced fat-suppressed SGE (*b*) images in a patient with inguinal hernia. Expansion of the left inguinal canal (arrow, *a*) is well shown on the T2-weighted image (*a*), which contains high-signal intensity tissue with an appearance identical to surrounding fat. Fat within the expanded inguinal canal diminishes in signal intensity on the fat-suppressed image, and enhancing testicular vessels are well seen (arrows, *b*).

vaginalis communicates with the peritoneal cavity; it normally closes during infancy. If, however, the processus remains patent, abdominal viscera may protrude into it, forming an inguinal hernia [11] (fig. 7.4).

- ***Spigelian hernia*** is a rare hernia of the anterior abdominal wall caused by a defect in the aponeurosis between the transversus abdominis and the rectus abdominis muscle. The peritoneal sac herniates through the rent in the aponeurosis and dissects laterally (fig. 7.5).
- ***Paraumbilical hernia:*** This hernia arises near the umbilicus and protrudes through the linea alba (fig. 7.6). Although they may be congenital, paraum-

bilical hernias are more common in obese and multiparous women; diastasis of the recti abdomini is the common underlying factor [11].

MASS LESIONS

Benign Masses

Cysts

Mesenteric cysts most commonly occur in the small bowel mesentery. Their etiology is not well understood. Although most mesenteric cysts are incidental findings, they can be symptomatic. They may produce chronic

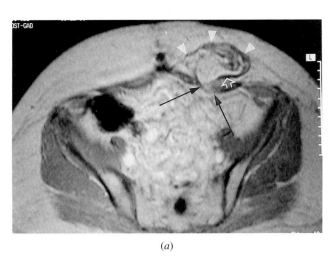

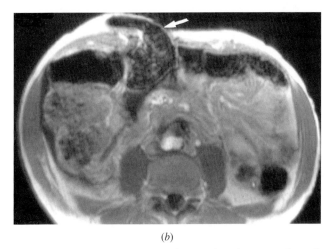

(a)   (b)

F I G . 7.5 Spigelian hernia. Gadolinium-enhanced T1-weighted SGE image (*a*) in a patient with spigelian hernia. A bowel-containing hernia sac (arrowheads, *a*) protrudes through a defect in the aponeurosis between the transversus and rectus muscles (solid arrows, *a*). The lateral margin of the hernia sac is the intact external oblique muscle and fascia (open arrow, *a*).

Transverse immediate postgadolinium T1-weighted SGE image (*b*) in a second patient. A spigelian hernia with protrusion of bowel contents (arrow, *b*) is noted in the right anterior abdomen.

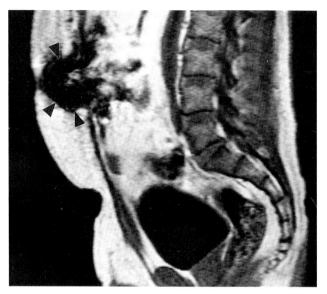

FIG. 7.6 Paraumbilical hernia. Sagittal T1-weighted SGE image shows signal void air-containing bowel (arrowheads) in the subcutaneous tissues in a patient with a paraumbilical hernia.

or acute pain if complicated by rupture, hemorrhage, torsion, or bowel obstruction. The cysts tend to be singular and thin walled and may contain septae. Different types of mesenteric cysts may be lined by a diversity of cell types including endothelium, mesothelium, and fallopian tube-like epithelium. Their fluid contents may be serous, resembling plasma, or chylous, displaying a white, milky consistency. In complicated cases, blood and/or other proteinaceous fluid predominates [12, 13]. The MRI appearance reflects the cyst contents. Simple cysts will be round, well marginated, low in signal intensity on T1-weighted images, and high in signal intensity on T2-weighted images (fig. 7.7). Cysts complicated by protein or hemorrhage will have higher signal intensity on T1-weighted images and/or heterogeneous signal intensity on T2-weighted images. After contrast administration, the cyst wall and septae, if present, will enhance (see fig. 7.7).

Pseudocysts in the peritoneal cavity lack an epithelial or mesothelial lining. As localized collections of fluid,

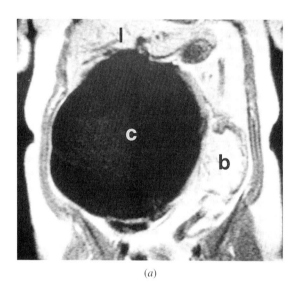

(a)

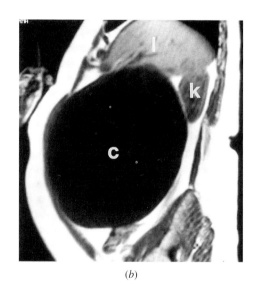

(b)

FIG. 7.7 Mesenteric cyst. Coronal T1-weighted magnetization-prepared single-shot gradient-echo (a), sagittal T1-weighted SGE (b), and immediate postgadolinium fat-suppressed SGE (c) images. A large septated cystic mass ("c," a, b) arising from the small bowel mesentery causes mass effect upon the adjacent bowel ("b," a, c), left kidney ("k," b, c) and liver ("l," a, b). Cysts that are low in signal intensity on T1-weighted images (a, b) and high in signal intensity on T2-weighted images (not shown) are consistent with serous fluid. Immediately after intravenous gadolinium administration (capillary phase) the septae traversing the cyst enhance (arrowheads, c). These imaging characteristics are consistent with an uncomplicated mesenteric cyst.

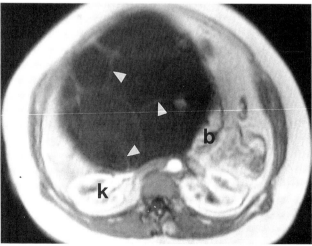

(c)

peritoneal pseudocysts may occur secondary to inflammatory processes such as pancreatitis, perforated ulcerative colitis or appendicitis. Pseudocysts may be a rare complication of ventriculo-peritoneal shunt or indwelling peritoneal catheters [14]. In uncomplicated cases, they are low in signal intensity on T1-weighted images and very high in signal intensity on T2-weighted images. Contrast-enhanced T1-weighted images surpass CT imaging and ultrasound by showing that the lesions are encapsulated and contain complex fluid and septations and by defining the relationship of the pseudocyst to other organs and tissues by direct multiplanar imaging [15]. These findings are more apparent on gadolinium-enhanced fat-suppressed images.

Lipomas and Mesenteric Lipomatosis

Lipomas are benign tumors that rarely involve the peritoneal cavity. Their imaging features parallel those of lipomas elsewhere in the body and are comparable to those of surrounding fat. These lesions are high in signal intensity on nonsuppressed T1-weighted images. Because fat signal varies considerably on T2-weighted images depending on the sequence employed, comparison of the signal intensity of the lesion should be made to that of adjacent fat. T1-weighted fat-suppressed SGE images will show loss of the tumor's signal intensity in comparison to non-fat-suppressed images, thereby definitively characterizing their fatty nature.

On occasion, excessive proliferation of benign fat may occur within the mesentery, producing a mass effect on adjacent structures simulating malignancy. This benign process may be idiopathic or associated with corticosteroid therapy, Cushing syndrome or obesity [16, 17]. MRI is helpful in identifying diffuse or focal prominence of mesenteric fat and excluding the presence of nonfatty soft tissue masses. The signal characteristics of this entity mimic those of benign lipomas [16] with the signal intensity of the tissue identical to fat on all sequences.

Endometriosis

Endometriosis is defined as the presence of endometrial glands or stroma in abnormal locations outside of the uterus. The three imaging hallmarks of endometriosis are pelvic peritoneal endometrial implants, ovarian endometriomas (endometriotic cysts), and adhesions. The most common peritoneal sites of involvement are, in decreasing order of frequency, the ovaries, uterine ligaments, cul de sac and pelvic peritoneum reflected over the uterus, fallopian tubes, rectosigmoid region, and bladder. Rare extraperitoneal sites include the lungs and the central nervous system [18]. The pathogenesis of endometriosis remains controversial. It likely is related to induction and/or transplantation of endometrial cells into the abdominal cavity [19]. Endometriomas have vari-

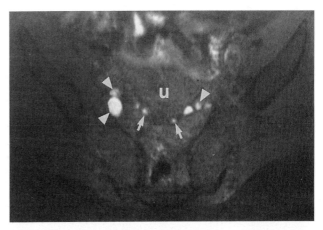

F I G . 7.8 Endometriosis. T1-weighted fat-suppressed spin-echo image demonstrates high-signal intensity foci of ovarian endometriomas (arrowheads) and smaller endometriosis implants adherent to the uterine serosa (arrows). T1-weighted fat-suppressed spin-echo or SGE technique is the most sensitive and specific sequence for detecting the blood product-laden deposits of endometriosis. (Reprinted with permission from Ascher SM, Agrawal R, Bis KG, Brown E, et al: Endometriosis: Appearance and detection with conventional, fat-suppressed, and contrast-enhanced fat-suppressed spin-echo techniques. *J Magn Reson Imaging* **5**: 251–257, 1995.)

able signal intensity but are commonly high in signal intensity on T1-weighted images and heterogeneously high in signal intensity on T2-weighted images [20]. Protein and blood breakdown products tend to demonstrate a gradation of signal intensity on T2-weighted images, which has been termed shading [20]. Noncontrast T1-weighted fat-suppressed imaging is the most sensitive MRI technique for identifying endometriomas (fig. 7.8) [21]. Unfortunately, detecting small, <1 cm, peritoneal endometriosis implants remains problematic [22], although contrast-enhanced fat-suppressed imaging has met with mixed results.

Desmoid Tumor (Aggressive Fibromatosis)

Desmoid tumor is a rare gastrointestinal mesenchymal tumor whose biologic behavior lies in the interface between exuberant fibroproliferations and low-grade fibrosarcoma. Diffuse mesenteric fibromatosis may arise in the postsurgical abdomen or spontaneously [23]. Desmoid tumors are locally invasive lesions that lack the ability to metastasize but tend to recur after incomplete surgical excision [24]. Intra-abdominal desmoid tumors occur in the mesentery or the pelvic wall. These tumors may occur sporadically or in association with Gardner syndrome or familial adenomatous polyposis [25].

Grossly, desmoid tumors vary in size, from 1 to 15 cm in greater diameter. In general, they are unicentric, infiltrative lesions with poorly defined borders (fig. 7.9). Discrete, well-circumscribed tumors also occur (fig. 7.9). Longstanding tumors are low in signal intensity on T1-

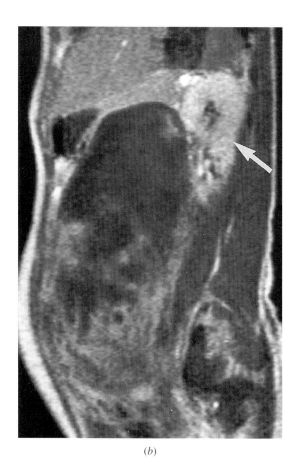

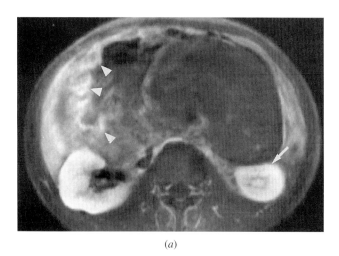

(a)

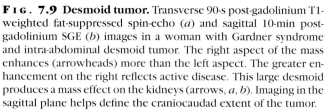

(b)

F I G . 7.9 Desmoid tumor. Transverse 90-s post-gadolinium T1-weighted fat-suppressed spin-echo (*a*) and sagittal 10-min post-gadolinium SGE (*b*) images in a woman with Gardner syndrome and intra-abdominal desmoid tumor. The right aspect of the mass enhances (arrowheads) more than the left aspect. The greater enhancement on the right reflects active disease. This large desmoid produces a mass effect on the kidneys (arrows, *a, b*). Imaging in the sagittal plane helps define the craniocaudad extent of the tumor.

Transverse interstitial phase gadolinium-enhanced T1-weighted fat-suppressed spin-echo image (*c*) in a second woman with Gardner syndrome and intra-abdominal desmoid tumor. The desmoid tumor ("*d*," *c*) exhibits minimal enhancement, confirming its fibrous nature. Thin mural enhancement is apparent (arrow, *c*). On the basis of this image alone, the tumor could be mistaken for a cyst. T2-weighted images distinguish the two: a desmoid tumor remains low in signal intensity, whereas a cyst is high signal intensity.

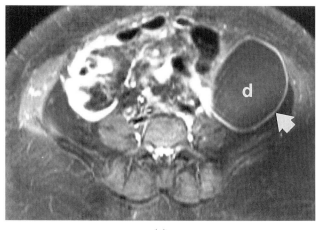

(c)

and T2-weighted images and enhance only minimally after intravenous gadolinium chelate (see fig. 7.9). In the acute phase, tumors may have regions of high signal intensity on T2-weighted images that also show heterogeneous increased enhancement (see fig. 7.9).

Malignant Masses

Diffuse Malignant Mesothelioma

The term mesothelioma is generally used for a malignant tumor derived from mesothelial cells that line serous membranes (e.g., peritoneum, pleura).

Diffuse malignant mesothelioma of the peritoneum is much less common than its counterpart involving the pleura. Heavy exposure to asbestos is an important risk factor. Diffuse malignant peritoneal mesotheliomas have also been described as a late complication of abdominal pelvic therapeutic radiation and after protracted recurrent peritonitis [26]. In the beginning stages of disease, nodules or plaques of tumor may stud the peritoneal surfaces. In time, these lesions become confluent, encasing viscera and mesenteries in a thick mat of tumor. As peritoneal malignant mesothelioma spreads along serosal surfaces, it may invade underlying tissue, especially the

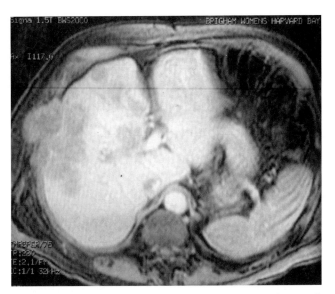

FIG. 7.10 Mesothelioma. Transverse interstitial-phase gadolinium-enhanced fat-suppressed SGE image in a patient with peritoneal mesothelioma demonstrates a large lobulated hypointense mass in the right upper abdomen with invasion of the liver and abdominal wall. Note also the presence of extensive liver metastases. (Courtesy of Gregory Sica, M.D., Brigham and Women's Hospital, Boston, MA)

wall of the intestine, and adjacent organs such as the liver (fig. 7.10). Peritoneal mesothelioma may be accompanied by intraperitoneal adhesions with dense fibrosis and shortening of the mesentery. Such a desmoplastic response within the mesentery is signified by rigid encasement of vessels and adjacent bowel, creating a stellate appearance on imaging [27–29]. The MRI appearance of mesothelioma is nonspecific, but a solid peritoneal mass seen in the setting of pre-existent pleural disease should suggest the correct diagnosis.

Primary Serous Papillary Carcinoma of the Peritoneum

Peritoneal serous papillary carcinoma (PSPC) is a tumor that is often widely distributed over the peritoneal surfaces and is histopathologically indistinguishable from ovarian papillary serous carcinoma. However, in PSPC, the ovaries may be no longer present (e.g., after ovariectomy), appear normal, or show only minimal surface involvement by tumor. Imaging findings of PSPC include ascites and focal or diffuse peritoneal nodules. Nevertheless, these imaging features are nonspecific, and similar appearances are observed for metastatic peritoneal carcinomatosis or malignant mesothelioma [30] (fig. 7.11).

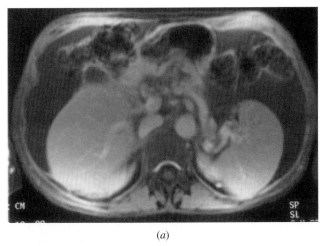

(a)

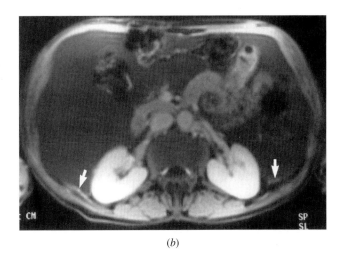

(b)

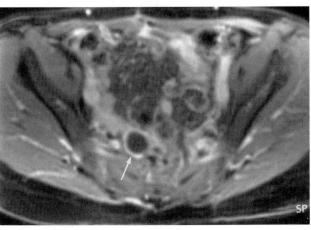

(c)

FIG. 7.11 Primary peritoneal papillary carcinoma of the peritoneum. Transverse 90-s gadolinium-enhanced fat-suppressed SGE (a, b) of the abdomen and 5-to 6-min transverse (c) and sagittal (d) gadolinium-enhanced fat-suppressed SGE images of the pelvis. Thin-volume diffuse peritoneal thickening with layering in the paracolic gutters (arrows, b) is noted in the abdomen. In the pelvis, a 2-cm cystic structure (arrow, c) is noted in the right pelvis.

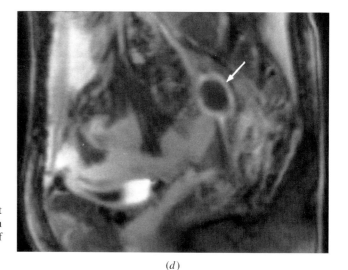

(d)

FIG. 7.11 (*Continued*) The sagittal projection confirms that the lesion is a cystic implant (arrow, *d*) by its oval configuration in both planes, unlike bowel, which would appear tubular in one of the projections.

Metastases

Metastatic tumors that involve the peritoneum most commonly arise from the female genital tract, particularly the ovary, followed by colon, stomach, and pancreas [31, 32]. The gross appearance of metastases ranges from single, well-defined nodules to diffuse peritoneal thickening. Dissemination occurs by several routes: contiguous spread, intraperitoneal seeding, hematogenous spread, and lymphatic dissemination [5, 33].

Contiguous spread. Primary tumors that are highly invasive may involve adjacent viscera by contiguous extension [31, 34, 35]. This process of direct extension is facilitated by the ligaments that interconnect the various organs.

Intraperitoneal Seeding. Seeding of body cavities and surfaces may occur whenever a malignant tumor invades a natural cavity and gains entrance into an "open field." The peritoneal cavity is most frequently involved in this pathway of spread [36].

The most commonly affected areas are the rectovesical/rectovaginal fossa, sigmoid mesocolon, right paracolic gutter, and the small bowel mesentery near the ileocecal valve [5, 37]. Peritoneal seeding is particularly characteristic of ovarian carcinoma when peritoneal surfaces become coated with a heavy glaze of tumor. Other malignancies that commonly spread in this manner include colon, stomach, and pancreatic carcinoma. Gadolinium-enhanced T1-weighted fat-suppressed imaging is essential for demonstrating intraperitoneal seeding. Both patterns of peritoneal involvement, whether focal metastatic nodules or confluent thickening of peritoneal surfaces, stand out as high signal against the low signal intensity of the suppressed intraperitoneal fat (figs. 7.12–7.22) [31, 38].

Breathing-independent T2-weighted single-shot echo-train spin-echo imaging is a useful complementary sequence to gadolinium-enhanced T1-weighted fat-suppressed sequence for detecting peritoneal metastases (figs 7.18 and 7.19). In recent large series, gadolinium-enhanced T1-weighted fat-suppressed SGE was shown to be superior to spiral CT for the detection of peritoneal disease [39], confirming findings in earlier studies [38, 40]. Orally and/or rectally administered contrast may improve delineation of bowel [41, 42], with water or enteric CT contrast having been used successfully. Intraluminal air should not be used at 1.5 T, because of susceptibility effects that may obscure both normal and diseased tissue on gradient echo sequences. Peritoneal metastases along the liver capsule are also well shown on T2-weighted fat-suppressed echo-train spin-echo images because both the fat and liver are relatively low in signal intensity, rendering moderately high-signal intensity peritoneal metastases conspicuous. Because breathing artifact is less problematic in the pelvis, peritoneal metastases also may be well shown with echo-train spin-echo imaging. The sagittal plane is particularly effective at showing implants along the bladder surface (fig. 7.22).

Peritoneal and serosal-based metastases must be distinguished from radiation changes, particularly in patients with gynecological malignancies. Multifocal lesions of peritoneal metastases, regardless of the primary tumor of origin, appear as moderately enhancing masses with slight internal heterogeneity. They lack the round, oval, or tubular contours of bowel and the uniform enhancement of bowel wall with the associated lack of enhancement of the internal dot or stripe of bowel lumen.

Omental metastases frequently coexist in patients with peritoneal metastases. Four imaging patterns of omental involvement have been described: rounded, cakelike, ill defined, and stellate [28, 43]. Regardless

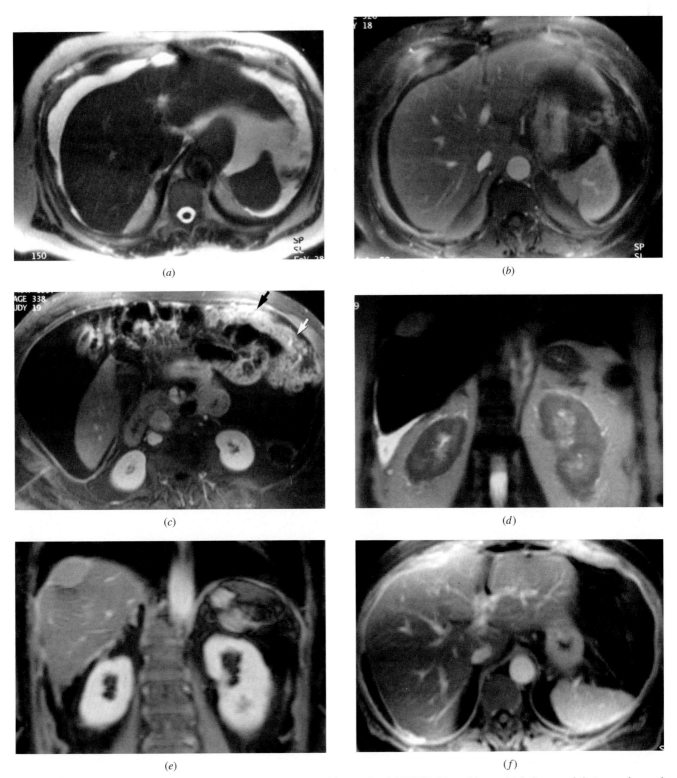

(a) (b)

(c) (d)

(e) (f)

F I G . 7.12 Peritoneal metastases from ovarian cancer. T2-weighted SS-ETSE (a) and interstitial-phase gadolinium-enhanced fat-suppressed SGE (b, c) images in a patient with a history of ovarian cancer. There is a large volume of ascites associated with diffuse thickening and enhancement of peritoneal surfaces on interstitial phase gadolinium-enhanced images. Omental metastases (arrows, c) are also appreciated.

Coronal T2-weighted SS-ETSE (d), coronal (e), and transverse (f) interstitial-phase gadolinium-enhanced fat-suppressed SGE images in a second patient. Diffuse and irregular thickening and enhancement of the peritoneum are observed throughout the abdomen. There is nodular thickening and enhancement of the liver capsule and the diaphragm. The coronal projection facilitates detection of diaphragm-based metastases. A large subcapsular metastases is present in the dome of the liver.

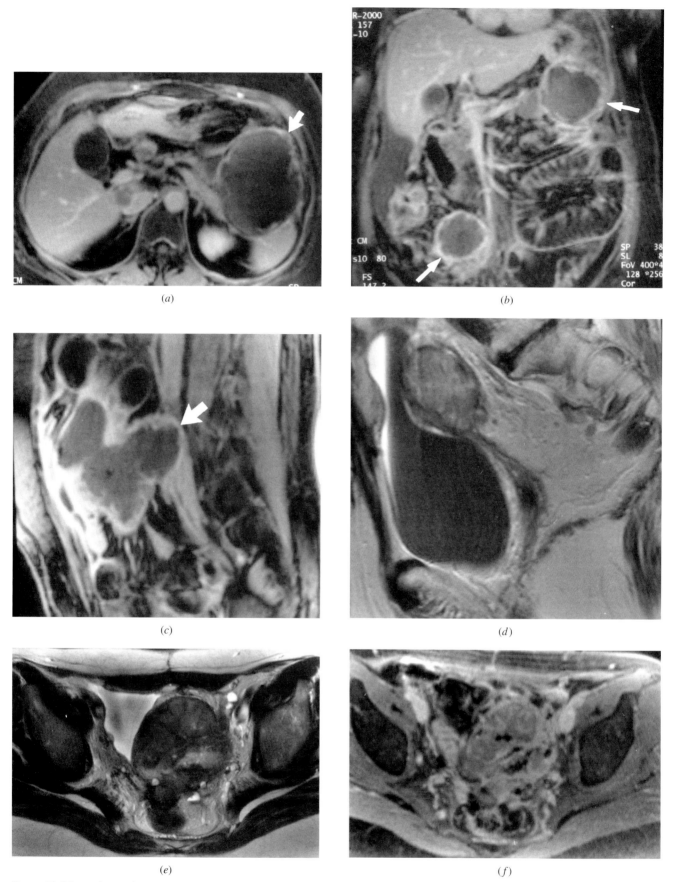

FIG. 7.13 Peritoneal Metastases from Ovarian Cancer. Transverse (*a*), coronal (*b*), and sagittal (*c*) interstitial-phase gadolinium-enhanced fat-suppressed SGE images. There is diffuse enhancement of the peritoneal and serosal surfaces, with multiple peritoneal and serosal-based cystic masses (arrows, *a-c*) throughout the abdomen, consistent with metastases.

664

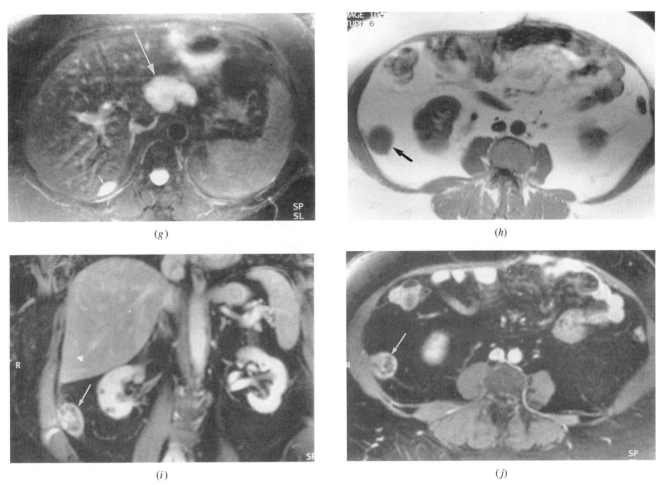

(g)

(h)

(i)

(j)

F I G . 7.13 (*Continued*) Sagittal (*d*) and transverse (*e*) T2-weighted echo train spin-echo and interstitial-phase gadolinium-enhanced fat-suppressed SGE (*f*) images in a second patient with ovarian cancer demonstrate the presence of a large metastatic heterogeneous mass in the pelvis that compresses the bladder.

T2-weighted fat-suppressed echo-train spin-echo (*g*) and SGE (*h*) images of the liver, and coronal (*i*) and transverse (*j*) interstitial-phase gadolinium-enhanced fat-suppressed SGE images of the midabdomen. A lobulated 4-cm peritoneal implant along the gastro-hepatic ligament is moderately high in signal intensity on T2 (arrow, *g*) and contrasts well with moderately low-signal intensity liver. A subcapsular liver metastasis is also present (small arrow, *g*) that demonstrates a characteristic biconvex lens shape indicating its subcapsular location. Noncontrast SGE image shows a 2-cm low-signal intensity peritoneal metastasis (arrow, *h*) that contrasts well with high-signal intensity fat. Gadolinium-enhanced fat-suppressed SGE images demonstrate heterogenous speckled enhancement of the mass (arrow, *i, j*).

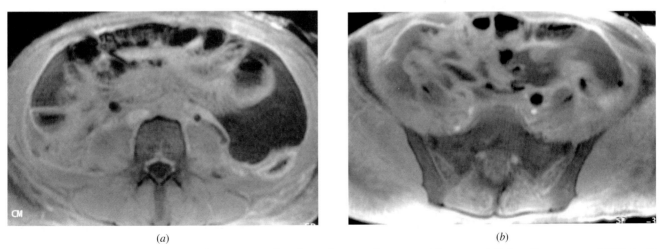

(a)

(b)

F I G . 7.14 Peritoneal metastases from appendiceal carcinoma. Transverse 90-s postgadolinium fat-suppressed SGE (*a, b*) images in a patient with appendiceal carcinoma. A large volume of ascites is present within the abdomen and pelvis. Extensive serosal and peritoneal enhancement is noted associated with thickening of small bowel loops.

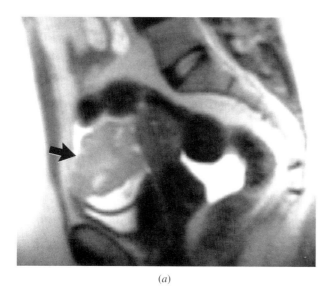

(a)

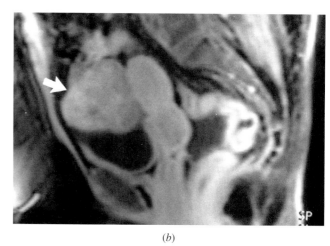

(b)

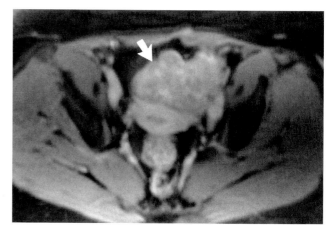

(c)

FIG. 7.15 Peritoneal metastases from colon cancer. Sagittal T2-weighted SS-ETSE (*a*), and sagittal (*b*) and transverse (*c*) interstitial-phase gadolinium-enhanced fat-suppressed SGE images in a patient with colon cancer. There is a large heterogeneous metastasis (arrow, *a–c*) in the pelvis, anterior to the uterus and superior to the bladder, surrounded by fluid.

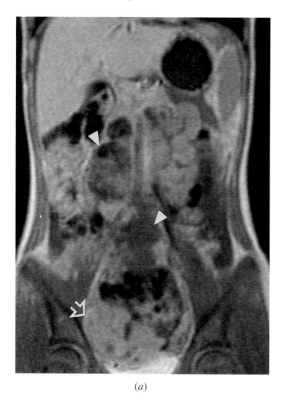

(a)

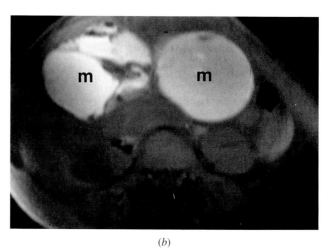

(b)

FIG. 7.16 Metastatic immature teratoma. Coronal T1-weighted magnetization-prepared gradient echo (*a*), transverse T1-weighted fat-suppressed spin-echo (*b*), and transverse gadolinium-enhanced T1-weighted fat-suppressed SGE (*c*) images in a patient

666

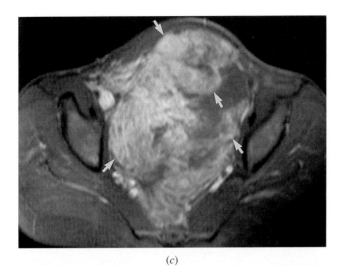

(c)

F I G . 7.16 (*Continued*) with metastatic immature teratoma. The primary tumor (open arrow, *a*) originates in the ovary and has spread to the peritoneal cavity (arrowheads, *a*). The unenhanced fat-suppressed image highlights the nonlipomatous metastases ("*m*," *b*). After gadolinium administration, extensive metastases along peritoneal and serosal surfaces are appreciated (arrows, *c*).

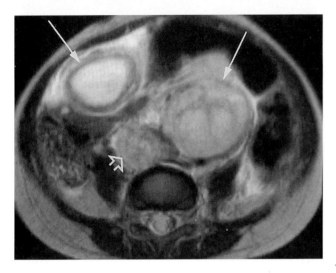

F I G . 7.17 Metastatic yolk sac tumor. Transverse 512-resolution T2-weighted echo-train spin-echo image in a patient with metastatic yolk sac tumor. Ovarian yolk sac tumors spread to the peritoneum (solid arrows), omentum, and retroperitoneal lymph nodes (open arrow).

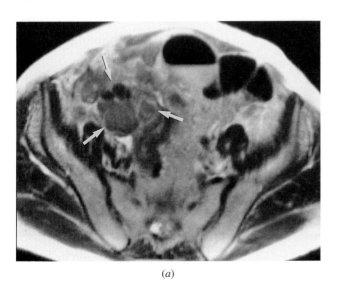

(a)

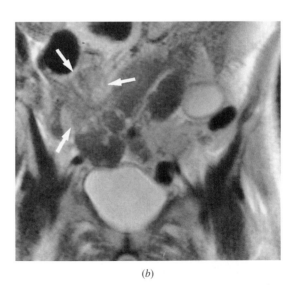

(b)

F I G . 7.18 Metastatic pancreatic cancer. Transverse (*a*) and coronal (*b*) T2-weighted single-shot echo-train spin-echo and interstitial-phase gadolinium-enhanced T1-weighted fat-suppressed SGE (*c*) images in a patient with metastatic pancreatic adeno-carcinoma. The T2-weighted images show a mass in the right lower quadrant (arrows, *a*, *b*). After intravenous contrast the serosal and peritoneal metastases enhance (long arrows, *c*). Incidental note is made of an enhancing bone metastasis in the left ilium (short arrow, *c*).

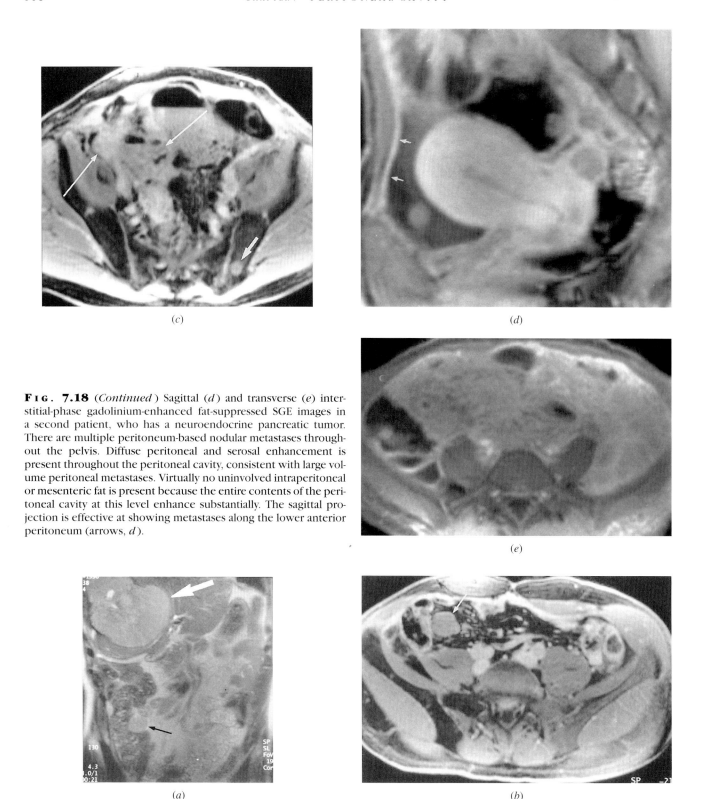

(c)

(d)

F I G . 7.18 (*Continued*) Sagittal (*d*) and transverse (*e*) interstitial-phase gadolinium-enhanced fat-suppressed SGE images in a second patient, who has a neuroendocrine pancreatic tumor. There are multiple peritoneum-based nodular metastases throughout the pelvis. Diffuse peritoneal and serosal enhancement is present throughout the peritoneal cavity, consistent with large volume peritoneal metastases. Virtually no uninvolved intraperitoneal or mesenteric fat is present because the entire contents of the peritoneal cavity at this level enhance substantially. The sagittal projection is effective at showing metastases along the lower anterior peritoneum (arrows, *d*).

(e)

(a)

(b)

F I G . 7.19 Peritoneal metastases from sarcomas. Coronal SS-ETSE (*a*) and interstitial-phase gadolinium-enhanced T1-weighted fat-suppressed SGE (*b*, *c*) images in a patient with synovial sarcoma. The coronal T2-weighted image demonstrates a large subcapsular liver metastasis (large arrow, *a*) and a 2-cm peritoneal metastasis (small arrow, *a*) medial to the ascending colon. The gadolinium-enhanced fat-suppressed image demonstrates moderate uniform enhancement of this metastatic deposit (arrow, *b*). On a transverse section through the pelvis, a 6-mm moderately enhancing metastatic deposit is well shown (arrow, *c*).

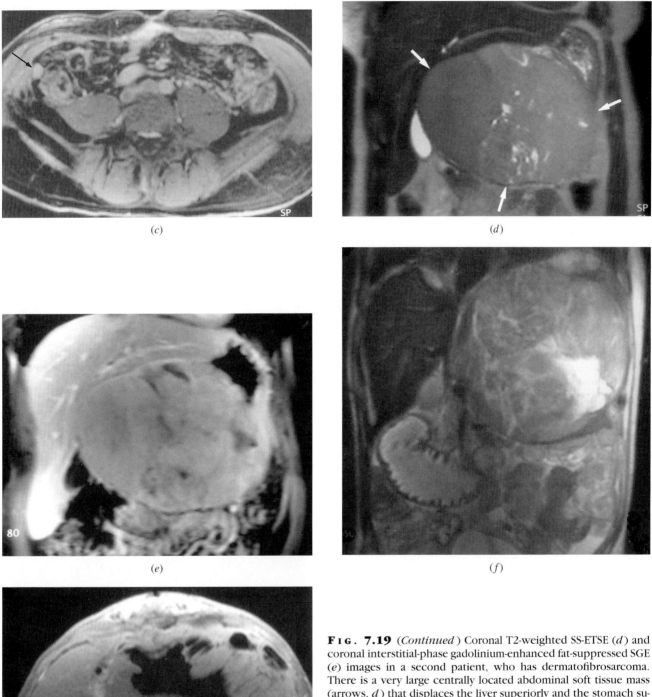

(c)

(d)

(e)

(f)

(g)

FIG. 7.19 (*Continued*) Coronal T2-weighted SS-ETSE (*d*) and coronal interstitial-phase gadolinium-enhanced fat-suppressed SGE (*e*) images in a second patient, who has dermatofibrosarcoma. There is a very large centrally located abdominal soft tissue mass (arrows, *d*) that displaces the liver superiorly and the stomach superiorly and laterally. This mass is mildly hyperintense with small high-signal foci on the T2-weighted image (*d*) and has heterogeneous enhancement on the postgadolinium image (*e*).

Coronal T2-weighted SS-ETSE (*f*) and gadolinium-enhanced magnetization-prepared gradient-echo (*g*) images in a third patient, who has metatatic osteosarcoma. There is a large heterogeneous mass in the left upper quadrant that has central necrosis. Multiple peritoneal metastases are also present (arrows, *g*).

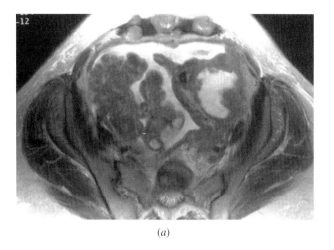

(a)

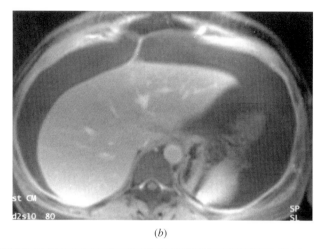

(b)

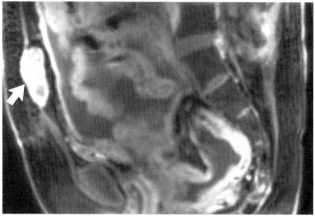

(c)

FIG. 7.20 Extensive peritoneal disease in a patient with leiomyosarcoma. Transverse T2-weighted ETSE (*a*) and transverse (*b*) and sagittal (*c*) interstitial-phase gadolinium-enhanced fat-suppressed SGE images. A large volume of ascites is present. There is thickening and enhancement of the peritoneal surfaces consistent with metastatic disease. Multiple metastatic deposits are present within the anterior abdominal wall (arrow, *c*).

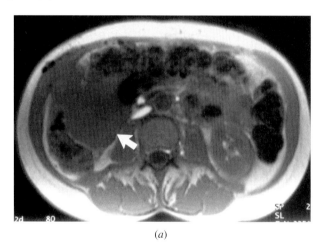

(a)

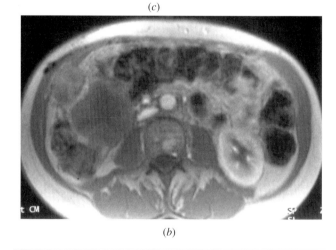

(b)

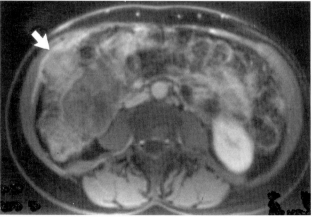

(c)

FIG. 7.21 Peritoneal metastatic masses from hepatocellular carcinoma. SGE (*a*), immediate postgadolinium SGE (*b*) and interstitial-phase gadolinium-enhanced fat-suppressed SGE (*c*) images in a patient with hepatocellular carcinoma. There are two large metastasis in the right abdomen. The larger mass is applied to the medial aspect of the right colon (arrow, *a*), and the other abuts and extends into the abdominal wall (arrow, *c*). These lesions show mild and heterogeneous enhancement after gadolinium administration.

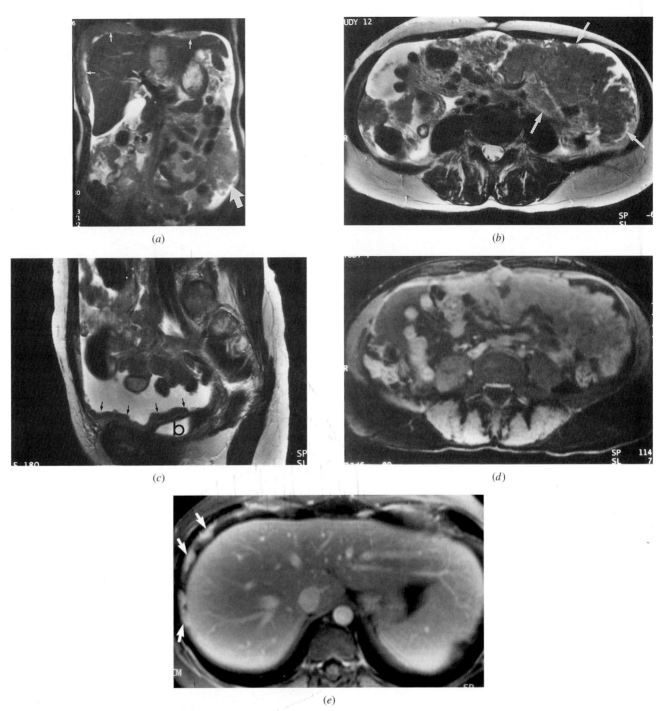

(a) *(b)*

(c) *(d)*

(e)

F I G . 7.22 Peritoneal metastases from nonovary gynecological malignancies. Coronal T2-weighted SS-ETSE (*a*), transverse (*b*) and sagittal (*c*) 512-resolution T2-weighted echo-train spin-echo, and interstitial-phase gadolinium-enhanced SGE (*d*) images in a patient with fallopian tube carcinoma. Extensive peritoneal-based metastases are present that appear intermediate in signal intensity on T2-weighted images (*a–c*). The coronal image demonstrates an irregular layer of metastatic deposit measuring up to 2 cm in thickness along the diaphragmatic surface and the liver capsule (small arrows, *a*). Bulky peritoneal metastases are present in the left lower abdomen (large arrow, *a*) and in the pelvis. The transverse high-resolution T2-weighted image demonstrates extensive bulky peritoneal metastases (arrows, *b*). Peritoneal seeding along the peritoneal reflection over the bladder ("*b*," *c*) is well shown on the sagittal plane image (small arrows, *c*). Heterogeneous and moderate enhancement of the metastases is shown on the gadolinium-enhanced fat-suppressed SGE image obtained at the midabdomen level (*d*).

Interstitial-phase gadolinium-enhanced fat-suppressed SGE image (*e*) in a second patient, who has endometrial stromal sarcoma, demonstrates extensive peritoneal involvement including multiple peritoneal nodules (arrows, *e*).

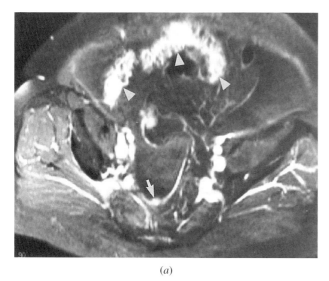

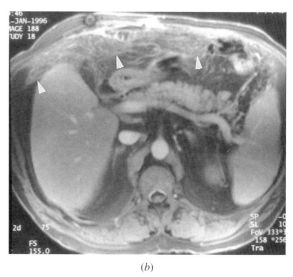

(a)   (b)

F I G . 7.23 Omental metastases. Transverse gadolinium-enhanced T1-weighted fat-suppressed spin-echo images in a patient with metastatic ovarian carcinoma (*a*) and metastatic leiomyosarcoma (*b*). The enhancing "omental cake" (arrowheads, *a*, *b*) is characteristic of metastatic ovarian carcinoma but also may be seen with other malignant diseases. Enhancing peritoneal tumor deposits (arrow, *a*) are rendered very conspicuous with suppression of background fat. MRI is superior to CT imaging in detecting small peritoneum-based disease.

of contour, these masses enhance after intravenous gadolinium administration (fig. 7.23). Distinction from hypertrophied omentum due to varices in the setting of cirrhosis and portal hypertension can be made by the observation of irregular-enhancing soft tissue on gadolinium-enhanced fat-suppressed SGE images in the setting of tumor and presence of curvilinear enhancing vessels in omental hypertrophy. The concomitant use of fat suppression emphasizes the presence of ill-defined soft tissue in tumor, and the lack of soft tissue in varices, because the bulky omentum is predominantly fatty in

the latter condition, and is rendered very low in signal on fat-suppressed images, except for the thin curvilinear vessels (fig. 7.24).

Hematogenous Spread. Many malignancies including breast and lung carcinoma and melanoma may metastasize hematogenously to invade structures within the peritoneal cavity. Tumor emboli traverse the mesenteric arteries to the antimesenteric border of the bowel. Hematogenous metastasis to bowel are manifest as intramural nodules (see Chapter 6, *Gastrointestinal Tract*,

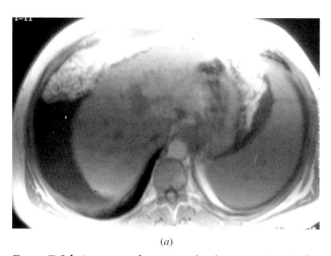

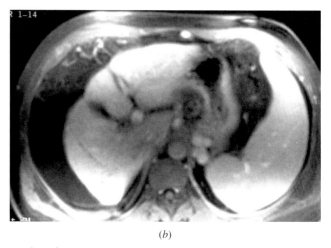

(a)   (b)

F I G . 7.24 Omentum hypertrophy due to varices in the setting of cirrhosis. SGE (*a*) and 90-s postgadolinium fat-suppressed SGE (*b*) images in a patient with cirrhosis. The omentum is enlarged on the basis of hypertrophy in the setting of portal hypertension. This is shown on postgadolinium fat-suppressed images by demonstration of suppression of the omentum and enhancement of thin curvilinear vessels. Note also that the liver is cirrhotic, and other features of portal hypertension such as splenomegaly and ascites are present.

on small bowel) [32]. These lesions appear as small enhancing nodules on gadolinium-enhanced T1-weighted fat-suppressed SGE.

Lymphatic Dissemination. Although permeation of the lymphatic system is the most common route for initial dissemination of carcinomas, sarcomas may also spread via this route. The presence of mesenteric disease is more typical of non-Hodgkin lymphoma than other malignancies. The morphologic features of involved lymph nodes is variable. Pathologic lymph nodes may form large confluent masses that encircle the splanchnic vessels, the "sandwich sign." Alternatively, a profusion of small, normal-sized, 1-cm lymph nodes may predominate [44–46]. Whereas the former pattern suggests the diagnosis of lymphoma, the latter is nonspecific. MRI has the advantage over other cross-sectional modalities in that the signal intensity of the mesenteric lymph nodes on T2-weighted images and the degree of contrast en-

hancement reflect their biological activity: tissue that is low in signal intensity on T2-weighted images with minimal contrast enhancement may suggest fibrosis rather than recurrent or persistent tumor. Evaluation of degree of contrast enhancement is aided by using T1-weighted fat-suppressed techniques. Various MRI techniques are effective at demonstrating mesenteric lymph nodes. The most consistent demonstration of lymph nodes is with 2- to 5-min gadolinium-enhanced fat-suppressed SGE. Precontrast T1-weighted fat-suppressed images show most clearly the distinction between mesenteric lymph nodes, which appear intermediate signal intensity, and pancreas, which appears high signal intensity (fig. 7.25). Imaging in multiple planes including sagittal and/or coronal help distinguish rounded lymph nodes from tubular bowel loops (see fig. 7.25).

Pseudomyxoma peritonei. Pseudomyxoma peritonei is a distinctive form of metastatic disease in which

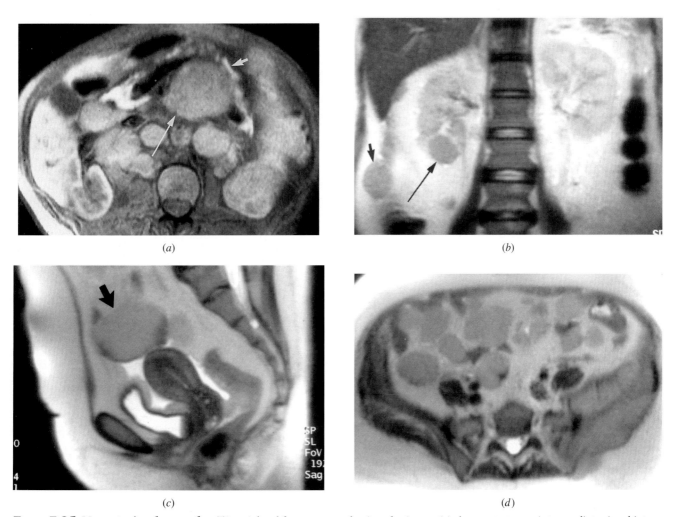

(a)

(b)

(c)

(d)

F I G . 7.25 Mesenteric adenopathy. T1-weighted fat-suppressed spin-echo image (*a*) demonstrates an intermediate-signal intensity lymph node (long arrow, *a*) that is clearly distinguished from high-signal intensity pancreas (short arrow, *a*).

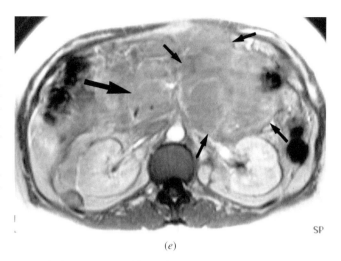

(*e*)

FIG. 7.25 (*Continued*) Coronal (*b*), sagittal (*c*) and transverse (*d*) T2-weighted SS-ETSE, and transverse 1-min postgadolinium T1-weighted SGE (*e*) images in a patient with Burkitt lymphoma demonstrate multiple masses throughout the peritoneal cavity. The largest mass within the mesentery shows heterogeneous enhancement and lies anterior to the aorta and both kidneys (arrows, *e*) and invades the anterior abdominal wall. Involvement of the head of the pancreas is also present (large arrow, *e*). Multiple additional mesenteric masses measuring up to 3.0 cm in size are also seen. Note the presence of a retroperitoneal mass (long arrow, *b*) that lies posterior to the right kidney and an abdominal wall mass (short arrow, *b*) in close proximity. The sagittal plane image demonstrates a pelvic mass (arrow, *c*) superior to the uterus.

the peritoneal cavity becomes distended with tenacious, viscous mucinous material. The primary tumor is usually a malignant neoplasm of the appendix, ovary, or pancreas [47]. The appendix is the primary site of origin of pseudomyxoma in the vast majority of cases [48]. The gelatinous deposits coat the peritoneal surfaces and characteristically indent and scallop the liver margin (fig. 7.26) [49, 50]. Septae are also common [31].

Carcinoid Tumors. Intestinal carcinoid tumor may involve the mesentery and produce a characteristic appearance [51]. The release of 5-hydroxytryptophan and

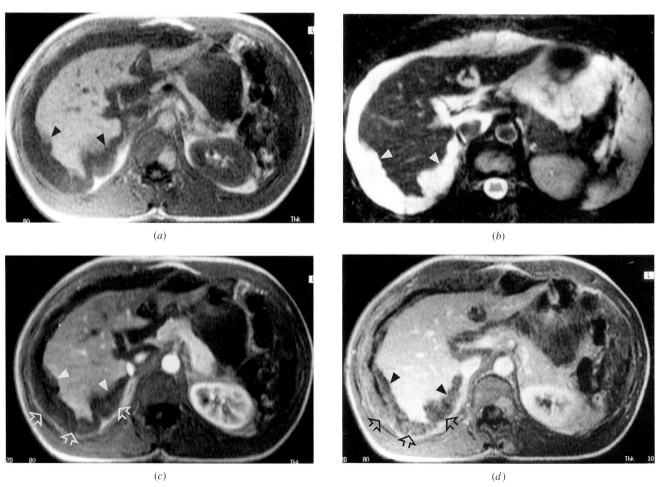

(*a*)

(*b*)

(*c*)

(*d*)

FIG. 7.26 Pseudomyxoma peritonei. SGE (*a*), T2-weighted fat-suppressed echo-train spin-echo (*b*), immediate (*c*) and interstitial-phase (*d*) postgadolinium SGE, and coronal precontrast SGE (*e*) and 5-min postgadolinium SGE (*f*) images in a patient with pseudomyxoma peritonei secondary to rupture of an appendiceal mucinous cystadenocarcinoma.

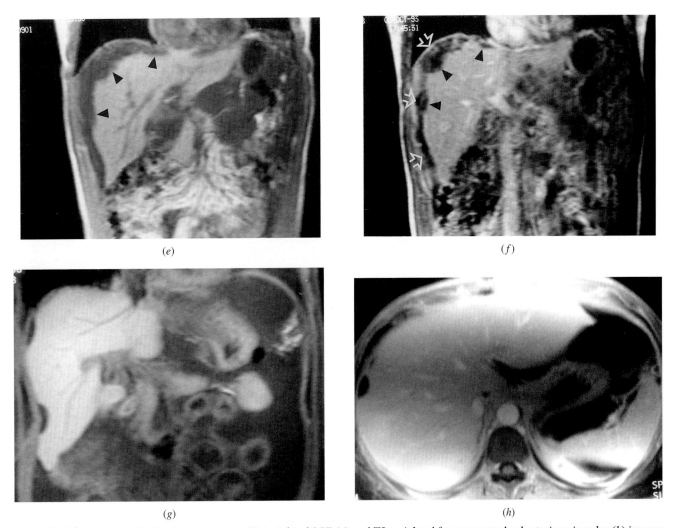

(e)   *(f)*

(g)   *(h)*

F i g . 7.26 *(Continued)* On the precontrast T1-weighted SGE (*a*) and T2-weighted fat-suppressed echo-train spin-echo (*b*) images the gelatinous material surrounding the liver has regions in which the signal intensity resembles that of simple ascites. However, the characteristic scalloping of the liver margin (arrowheads, *a–f*), coupled with the enhancement of the material (open arrows, *c, d, f*) filling the abdomen, establishes the correct diagnosis. Free fluid within the abdomen does not enhance. Coronal images (*e, f*) provide a global view of the disease extent and demonstrate subdiaphragmatic disease well.

Coronal (*g*) and transverse (*h*) interstitial-phase gadolinium-enhanced fat-suppressed SGE images in a second patient, who also has appendiceal mucinous cystadenocarcinoma. A large volume of ascites with extensive peritoneal enhancement is observed, associated with scalloping of the liver surface, features that are characteristic of pseudomyxoma peritonei.

serotonin secreted by tumor cells incites a desmoplastic reaction. The result is an irregular indurated soft tissue mass in the root of the mesentery with associated radiating soft tissue strands [52, 53]. Calcification may be present in up to 70% of tumors [54]. Non-fat-suppressed T1-weighted images are effective at showing these tumors. The tumors appear as low-signal intensity masses against the high-signal intensity mesenteric fat (fig. 7.27). T2-weighted single-shot echo-train spin-echo sequences also demonstrate low-signal intensity tissue in a background of high-signal intensity fat (see fig. 7.27). Fat-suppressed images reduce the contrast between the fibrotic tumor and fat. The desmoplastic nature of this tumor results in negligible enhancement with gadolinium (see fig. 7.27).

Intraperitoneal Fluid

Ascites

Ascites is defined as the collection of excess fluid in the peritoneal cavity. Ascites results from overproduction, impaired resorption, or leakage of fluid. It is a common manifestation of many diseases: cirrhosis, pancreatitis, obstruction (venous or lymphatic), inflammation, low-albumin states, malignancy, and trauma. The signal intensity of the fluid, a function of its protein content, coupled with its distribution, can suggest the underlying etiology. Simple transudates are low in signal intensity on T1-weighted sequences and very high in signal intensity on T2-weighted images (fig. 7.28), whereas exudates, blood, and enteric contents will have higher signal

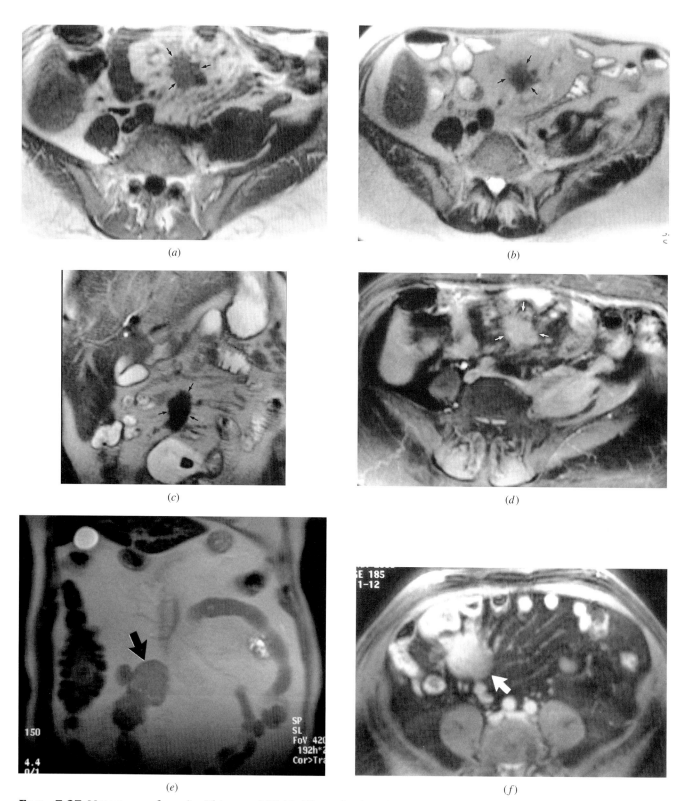

F IG . 7.27 Metastases of carcinoid tumor. SGE (*a*), T2-weighted SS-ETSE (*b*), coronal T2-weighted SS-ETSE (*c*), and 90-s post-gadolinium fat-suppressed SGE (*d*) images in a patient with a carcinoid tumor of the small bowel. Breath-hold T1-weighted SGE images are well suited for imaging the low signal intensity metastasis in the root of the small bowel mesentery (arrows, *a*); the radiating strands are highlighted by the surrounding high signal intensity of the intra-abdominal fat. The desmoplastic nature of these tumors is emphasized by its low signal intensity on T2-weighted images (arrows, *b*, *c*) and only modest enhancement after intravenous contrast (arrows, *d*).

Coronal T2-weighted SS-ETSE (*e*) and interstitial-phase gadolinium-enhanced fat-suppressed SGE (*f*) images in a second patient with mesenteric metastasis from carcinoid tumor demonstrate a spiculated mass (arrow, *e*, *f*) with thin radiating linear strands that extend into the mesentery, caused by a desmoplastic fibrous reaction in the surrounding tissue.

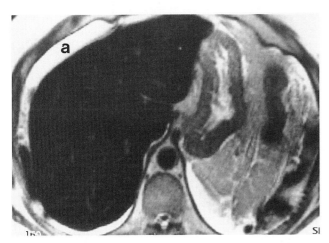

FIG. 7.28 Ascites. T2-weighted SS-ETSE image in a patient with simple transudative ascites. High-signal intensity ascites ("*a*") surrounds the abdominal viscera. The liver is low in signal intensity secondary to iron overload from multiple transfusions.

intensity on T1-weighted images and more variable signal intensity on T2-weighted images (figs. 7.29 and 7.30) [2, 55–57]. Benign processes favor the greater sac, whereas malignant fluid tends to involve the greater and lesser sacs proportionally (Fig. 7.31) [2, 3], although exceptions are common. In simple ascites, small and large bowel tend to float to the anterior abdomen in a central location (fig. 7.32). Malignant or inflammatory ascites tends to tether bowel in different locations depending on the distribution of the disease process. Breathing-independent T2-weighted imaging is effective in evaluating the distribution and presence of ascites in uncooperative patients and young children (fig. 7.33). Multiplanar imaging facilitates the evaluation of ascites distribution within various abdominal compartments (fig. 7.34).

Intraperitoneal Blood

Intraperitoneal blood most frequently occurs in the setting of trauma. MRI can readily distinguish blood from ascites. The age of hemorrhage can be determined because of the distinctive signal intensity features of hemoglobin as it undergoes progressive degradation. We have described the MR features of acute intra-abdominal hemorrhage [58]. Acute blood (<48 h), in the form of deoxyhemoglobin, is low in signal intensity on both T1- and T2-weighted images (fig. 7.35). From 48 hours to 7 days intracellular methemoglobin may be observed that is high signal on T1- and low signal on T2-weighted images. The very low signal of deoxyhemoglobin and intracellular metahemoglobin on T2-weighted images is very distinctive, and observation of very low-signal substance in the peritoneal cavity should raise the clinical concern of acute bleed. The near-signal void of these blood products can be distinguished from the signal void of air on T2-weighted images, either because of different signal on T1-weighted images or because blood tends to be observed in a dependent location, whereas air is observed in a nondependent location. Subacute blood, in the form of extracellular methemoglobin, is high in signal intensity on T1- and T2-weighted images (fig. 7.36). Fat suppression accentuates the conspicuity of this finding. Hematomas also may demonstrate heterogeneity related to hemoglobin breakdown products admixed with blood. Not infrequently, a high-signal intensity rim surrounding a low-signal intensity center is seen with subacute hematomas (fig. 7.37). A structure with a high-signal rim on noncontrast T1-weighted images is characteristic of subacute hematoma. This distinctive imaging feature represents extracellular methemoglobin encircling the retracting clot [59]. As hematomas age, a low-signal intensity rim develops around the hematoma on both

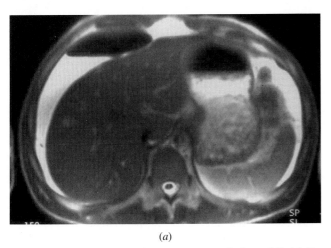

(*a*)

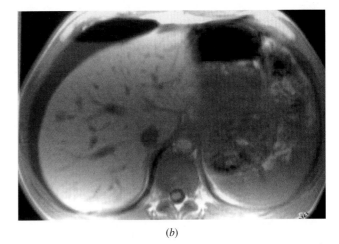

(*b*)

FIG. 7.29 Postsurgical intraperitoneal air and fluid. Transverse T2-weighted SS-ETSE (*a*) and SGE (*b*) images in a patient, with a recent history of surgery, demonstrate the presence of pneumoperitoneum and ascites. Note that air is invariably located along the nondependent surface in structures.

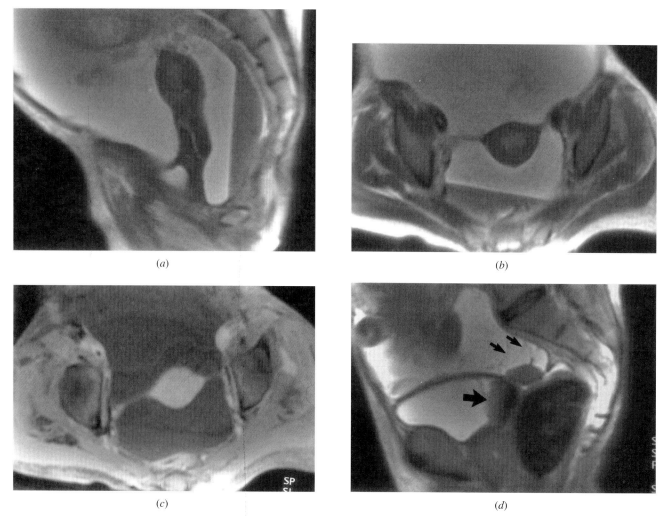

(a)

(b)

(c)

(d)

FIG. 7.30 High protein content ascites, adhesions. Sagittal (*a*) and transverse (*b*) T2-weighted SS-ETSE and transverse interstitial-phase gadolinium-enhanced fat-suppressed SGE (*c*) images. A large volume of ascites is seen within the pelvis. In the posterior cul de sac, a fluid-fluid level is seen on the T2-weighted image with the dependent fluid layer being low in signal, which is consistent with high protein content.

Sagittal T2-weighted SS-ETSE image (*d*) in a second patient demonstrates a large volume of ascites in the pelvis with multiple thin septations (arrows, *d*) and a focal collection of proteinaceous material in the vesicorectal space. Low signal in the dependent portion of the bladder (large arrow, *d*) represents gadolinium.

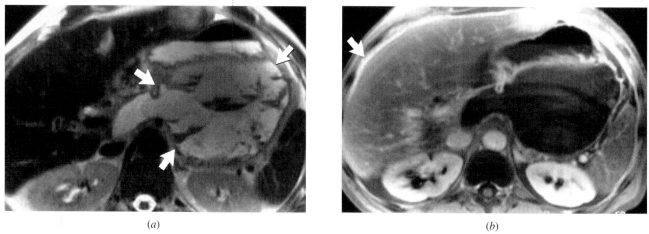

(a)

(b)

FIG. 7.31 Lesser sac involvement in malignant disease. T2-weighted SS-ETSE (*a*) and 90-s postgadolinium fat-suppressed SGE (*b*) images. There is a dominant fluid collection in the lesser sac (arrows, *a*), which contains multiple septations and multiple fluid-fluid levels from proteinaceous debris as shown on the T2-weighted image (*a*). The gadolinium-enhanced fat-suppressed image (*b*), obtained at the same anatomical level, shows the lesser sac collection but not the internal septations. A thin layer of enhancing peritoneal disease (arrow, *b*) is appreciated on the gadolinium-enhanced fat-suppressed image that is not apparent on the T2-weighted image.

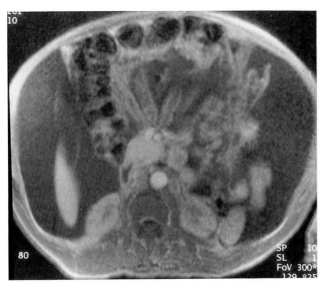

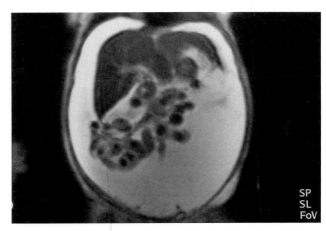

FIG. 7.32 Benign ascites. SGE image demonstrates that small and large bowel have floated anteriorly in a central location. This confirms that ascites is simple because no tethering of bowel from malignant or inflammatory adhesions has occurred.

FIG. 7.33 Ascites in a neonate. Coronal SS-ETSE image clearly shows the liver and centrally lying bowel. The central position of the bowel reflects the simple nature of the ascites.

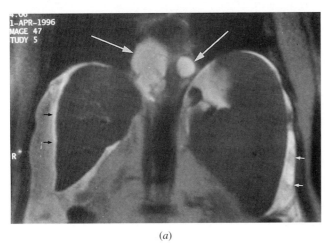

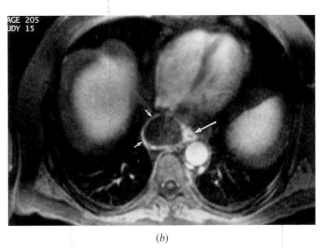

(a)   *(b)*

FIG. 7.34 Mediastinal extension of ascites. Coronal T2-weighted SS-ETSE (*a*) and transverse 45-s postgadolinium fat-suppressed SGE (*b*) images. On the coronal image, ascites is noted along the surfaces of the liver and enlarged spleen (small arrows, *a*) and mediastinal extension of the fluid is apparent (long arrows, *a*). On the gadolinium-enhanced transverse image (*b*), the encapsulated collection of ascites in the posterior mediastinum is shown (small arrow, *b*) and close approximation to the esophagus (long arrow, *b*) is apparent.

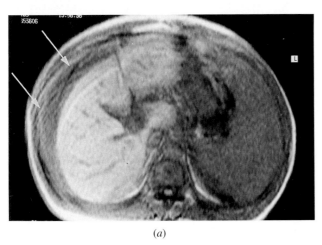

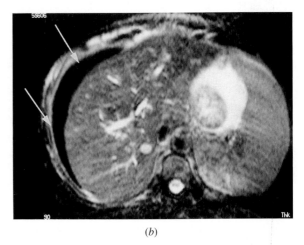

(a)   *(b)*

FIG. 7.35 Intraperitoneal acute blood. SGE (*a*), T2-weighted fat-suppressed spin-echo (*b*), and 1-min postgadolinium SGE (*c*) images in a patient status postpercutaneous liver biopsy.

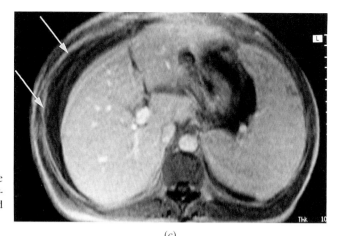

(c)

F I G . 7.35 (*Continued*) Fluid (arrows, *a–c*) surrounding the liver exhibits the signal characteristics of acute blood (deoxyhemoglobin): isointense or low signal intensity on T1-weighted images and very low signal intensity on T2-weighted images.

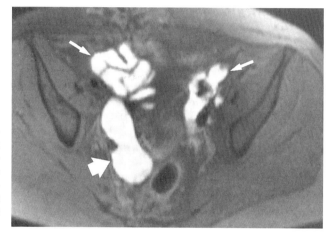

F I G . 7.36 Intraperitoneal blood. T1-weighted fat-suppressed spin-echo image in a woman 1 week after hysterectomy. There is a high-signal intensity collection in the right pelvis consistent with subacute blood (large arrow). T1-weighted fat suppression is particularly sensitive for the detection of blood, but extracellular methemoglobin must be distinguished from the high signal intensity of proteinaceous intraluminal bowel contents (small arrows).

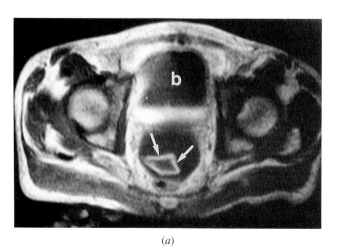

(a)

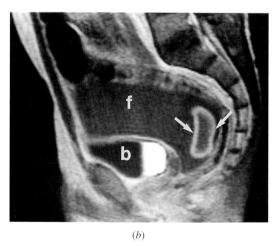

(b)

F I G . 7.37 Pelvic hematoma. Transverse (*a*) and sagittal (*b*) interstitial-phase gadolinium-enhanced T1-weighted SGE images in a patient after splenic injury. Subacute hematomas usually have a low-signal intensity core with a high-signal intensity surrounding rim (arrows, *a, b*) on T1-weighted images. These imaging characteristics reflect the retracting clot surrounded by extracellular methemoglobin. b, Bladder; f, free pelvic fluid.

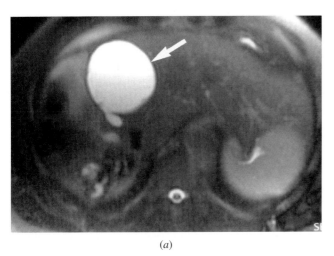
(a)

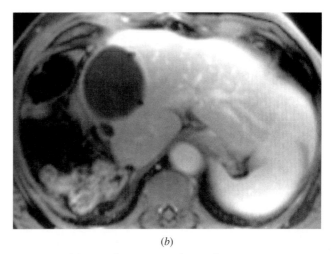
(b)

F I G . 7.38 Biloma. T2-weighted fat-suppressed SS-ETSE (*a*) and 90-s postgadolinium fat-suppressed SGE (*b*) images in a patient after right hepatectomy demonstrate a cystic mass along the resected surface of the left lobe (arrow, *a*) consistent with biloma.

T1- and T2-weighted sequences. This rim corresponds to hemosiderin and/or fibrosis.

Intraperitoneal Bile

Free intraperitoneal bile is usually the result of surgery [60]. When present in small amounts, it is clinically occult. However, in the setting of duct injury, bile leakage may result in a biloma or bile peritonitis (fig. 7.38) [60]. Free bile preferentially collects in the right upper quadrant, where it incites an inflammatory reaction. A biloma results if the bile is walled off by a pseudocapsule and adhesions. The signal intensity of a biloma is variable and mimics that of the gallbladder. Bilomas may be low, intermediate, or high in signal intensity on T1-weighted images. They are high in signal intensity on

T2-weighted images. Enhancement of peritoneum on gadolinium-enhanced T1-weighted images reflects the inflammation associated with bile leak (fig. 7.39).

Intraperitoneal Urine

Bladder rupture leads to extravasation of urine. The location of the free urine is a function of whether the dome or the bladder base is injured. If the base is compromised, urine collects extraperitoneally, whereas injury to the dome results in intraperitoneal urine, also known as urine ascites. On unenhanced images, the signal intensity of urine ascites is nonspecific. Contrast administration establishes the diagnosis as high-signal intensity gadolinium chelate in urine leaks into the peritoneal cavity.

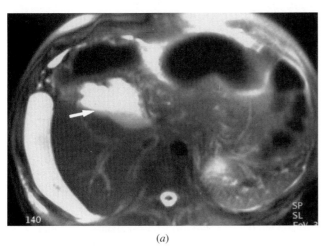
(a)

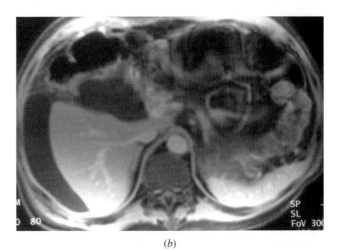
(b)

F I G . 7.39 Infected biloma. T2-weighted fat-suppressed SS-ETSE (*a*) and 90-s postgadolinium fat-suppressed SGE (*b*) images. There is a fluid collection in the region of the gallbladder fossa that appears somewhat loculated and complex, as evidenced by a fluid-debris level (arrow, *a*) on the T2-weighted image. Note that debris has an irregular linear interface with fluid, unlike high-protein-content ascites, which has a sharp linear fluid-fluid level. A moderate amount of perihepatic ascites and increased peritoneal enhancement are present. The patient had a recent history of cholecystectomy, and these findings were consistent with infected biloma with peritonitis.

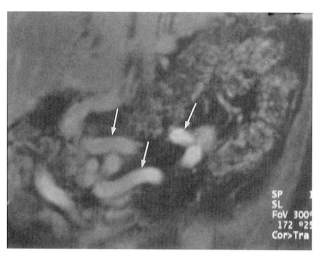

FIG. 7.40 Enlarged collateral of the superior mesenteric vein. Coronal 90-s postgadolinium fat-suppressed SGE image demonstrates an enlarged tortuous collateral vessel of the superior mesenteric vein (arrows).

Vascular Disease

In general, abnormalities in the splanchnic circulation are well shown on 2–5 min postgadolinium fat-suppressed SGE images (Fig. 7.40).

Microvarices within the peritoneal lining and omental hypertrophy are commonly observed in patients with cirrhosis and portal venous hypertension. Microvarices of the peritoneum can be difficult to distinguish from either inflammatory or neoplastic peritoneal disease. Distinctive features of microvarices on gadolinium-enhanced T1-weighted fat-suppressed SGE include the

observation of curvilinear small tubular structures and extension of some of these curvilinear structures into peritoneal fat (fig. 7.41). In contrast to microvarices, neither distinct curvilinear tubular structures nor their extension into peritoneal fat are visualized in inflammatory or malignant peritoneal disease.

Inflammation

Mesenteric Panniculitis (Isolated Lipodystrophy of the Mesentery, Retractile Mesenteritis, Sclerosing Mesenteritis)

Mesenteric panniculitis is a rare disorder characterized grossly by a diffuse, localized, or multinodular fibrofatty thickening of the mesentery of the small and/or large bowel. The disorder is notable for a spectrum of pathologic changes within the mesentery including inflammatory infiltrates, fat necrosis and fibrosis [61–63]. Although the etiology of mesenteric panniculitis is unclear, infection, trauma, ischemia, autoimmune disorders, and a history of previous abdominal surgery have been suggested as causative factors [62, 64, 65]. The diagnosis of mesenteric panniculitis is supported by the absence of pancreatitis, the most common cause of intra-abdominal fat necrosis, and inflammatory bowel disease. The changes in the mesentery may be focal or diffuse. When diffuse, the mesenteric fat is traversed by low-signal intensity strands on T1-weighted images [65] (fig. 7.42). In the focal form, heterogeneous nodular masses of fat necrosis are noted. These lesions exhibit varying amounts of fat, fluid, calcification, and soft tissue [65, 66].

A variety of malignant, inflammatory or infectious etiologies may result in inflammation of the mesentery,

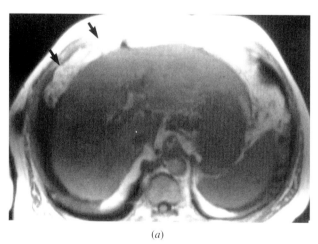

(a)

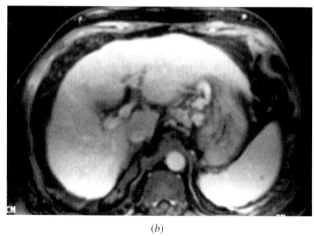

(b)

FIG. 7.41 Omental hypertrophy and peritoneal varices. SGE (*a*) and interstitial-phase gadolinium-enhanced fat-suppressed SGE (*b*) images in a cirrhotic patient demonstrate marked hypertrophy of the omentum. On the SGE image the hypertrophied omentum is high signal (arrows, *a*). On the gadolinium-enhanced fat-suppressed image (*b*), small tubular structures consistent with microvarices are identified.

Interstitial-phase gadolinium-enhanced fat-suppressed SGE (*c*) image in a second patient shows similar features as described above. Fatty tissue anterior and along the lateral liver capsule represents hypertrophied omentum containing vessels. The liver is cirrhotic, and the spleen is enlarged and contains multiple Gamna-Gandy bodies.

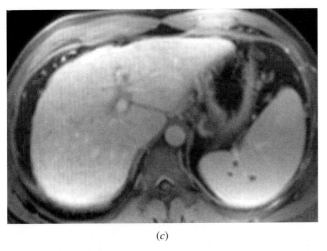

(c)

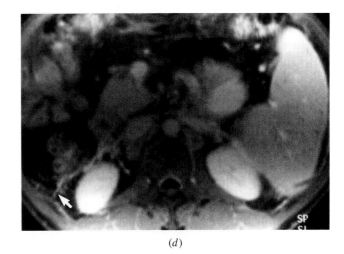

(d)

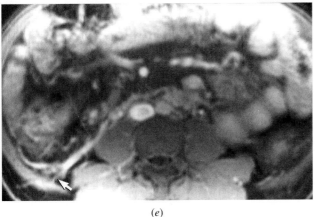

(e)

FIG. 7.41 (*Continued*) Interstitial-phase gadolinium-enhanced fat-suppressed SGE (*d, e*) images in a third cirrhotic patient demontrate the presence of peritoneal varices that appear as enhancing peritoneum in the pericolic gutters, simulating peritoneal metastases. Note that occasional vessels perforate the peritoneum and extend into the retroperitoneum (arrow, *d, e*), establishing the diagnosis of microvarices.

which may produce an imaging appearance indistinguishable from that of mesenteric panniculitis (see fig. 7.42). The differential diagnosis includes lymphoma, desmoid tumor, carcinomatosis, and carcinoid tumor. [64]

Pancreatitis

Acute pancreatitis is defined as an acute inflammatory condition of the pancreas that typically presents with abdominal pain and is associated with elevated levels of pancreatic enzymes (especially lipase and amylase) in blood and urine.

Patients with pancreatitis usually present with extrapancreatic fluid collections, preferentially in the lesser sac [2]. The enzyme-laden fluid also may dissect into the abdominal cavity and retroperitoneum. Not infrequently, fluid tracks along tissue planes to localize subcapsularly in the liver and/or spleen. Precontrast T1-weighted fat-suppressed SGE imaging is particularly effective at demonstrating the presence of blood in hemorrhagic pancreatitic ascites. The peritoneum typically enhances on gadolinium-enhanced T1-weighted fat-suppressed images because of the caustic nature of the activated pancreatic enzyme-containing fluid.

Peritonitis

Peritonitis may be caused by a variety of infectious or noninfectious causes, many of which are related to bowel perforation. Peritonitis appears as diffuse increased enhancement of the peritoneum and mesentery and is most clearly defined on interstitial-phase gadolinium-enhanced fat-suppressed SGE images (figs. 7.43 and 7.44).

Pseudocysts may develop in the setting of peritonitis as walled-off collections of fluid. In uncomplicated cases they are low in signal intensity on T1-weighted images and very high in signal intensity on T2-weighted images. Complex fluid is characterized by either increased signal on T1-, decreased or heterogeneous signal on T2-weighted images, or a combination of both. Gadolinium-enhanced T1-weighted images reveal enhancement of the pseudocapsule, which is more conspicuous in combination with fat suppression.

A localized collection of inflammatory debris may develop around tubes or catheters (e.g., CSF-peritoneal shunt or indwelling peritoneal catheters) within the peritoneal cavity, with development of a pseudocapsule. This entity is termed a cocoon (fig. 7.45).

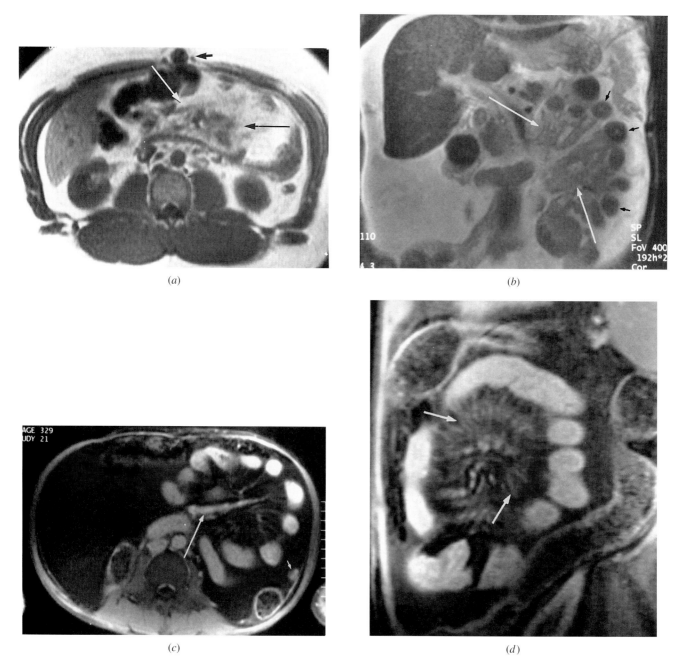

FIG. 7.42 Mesenteric lipodystrophy and tuberculous peritonitis. SGE image (*a*) demonstrates low-signal intensity strand-ing in the fat of the mesentery (long arrows, *a*), consistent with mesenteric lipodystrophy. A small ventral hernia is also present (short arrow, *a*).

Coronal T2-weighted SS-ETSE (*b*) and transverse (*c*) and sagittal (*d*) interstitial-phase fat-suppressed SGE images in a second patient, who has tuberculous peritonitis. A large volume of ascites is present. Multiple loops of thickened small bowel are appreciated (short arrows, *b*). The mesentery is infiltrated and intermediate in signal intensity (long arrows, *b*) on the T2-weighted image (*b*). The mesenteric vessels are closely bundled (long arrow, *c*), reflecting adherence of the vessels to each other secondary to the inflammatory process. Terminal branches of the mesenteric vessels (arrows, *d*) fan out to the thickened loops of small bowel creating a spoke-wheel type pattern on the sagittal image. Increased enhancement and mildly increased thickness of the peritoneum with peritoneum-based nodules (small arrow, *c*) are also appreciated. This appearance is that of retractile mesenteritis, which can be caused by a number of etiologies including tuberculosis.

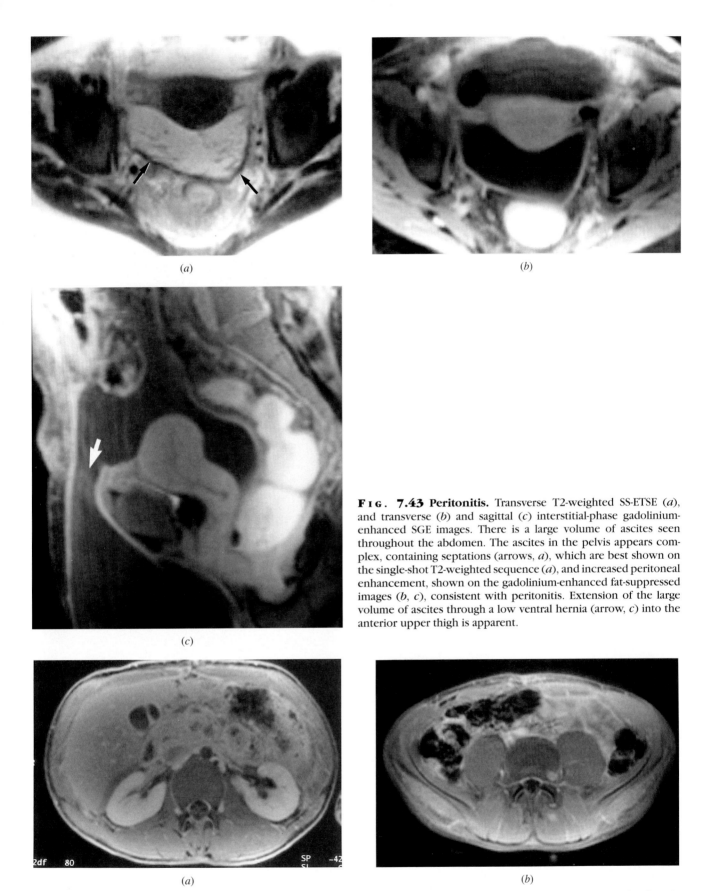

(a)

(b)

(c)

FIG. 7.43 Peritonitis. Transverse T2-weighted SS-ETSE (*a*), and transverse (*b*) and sagittal (*c*) interstitial-phase gadolinium-enhanced SGE images. There is a large volume of ascites seen throughout the abdomen. The ascites in the pelvis appears complex, containing septations (arrows, *a*), which are best shown on the single-shot T2-weighted sequence (*a*), and increased peritoneal enhancement, shown on the gadolinium-enhanced fat-suppressed images (*b*, *c*), consistent with peritonitis. Extension of the large volume of ascites through a low ventral hernia (arrow, *c*) into the anterior upper thigh is apparent.

(a)

(b)

FIG. 7.44 Chemical peritonitis. Interstitial-phase gadolinium-enhanced SGE images from the midabdomen (*a*) and pelvis (*b*) in a patient with chemical peritonitis, secondary to intraperitoneal administration of chemotherapeutic agents. Diffuse increased enhancement is present of peritoneal, mesenteric, and serosal surfaces, which has resulted in adherence of bowel loops to each other and linear enhancing strands in the mesentery. Bowel loops and mesenteric planes are ill-defined because of the generalized inflammatory process.

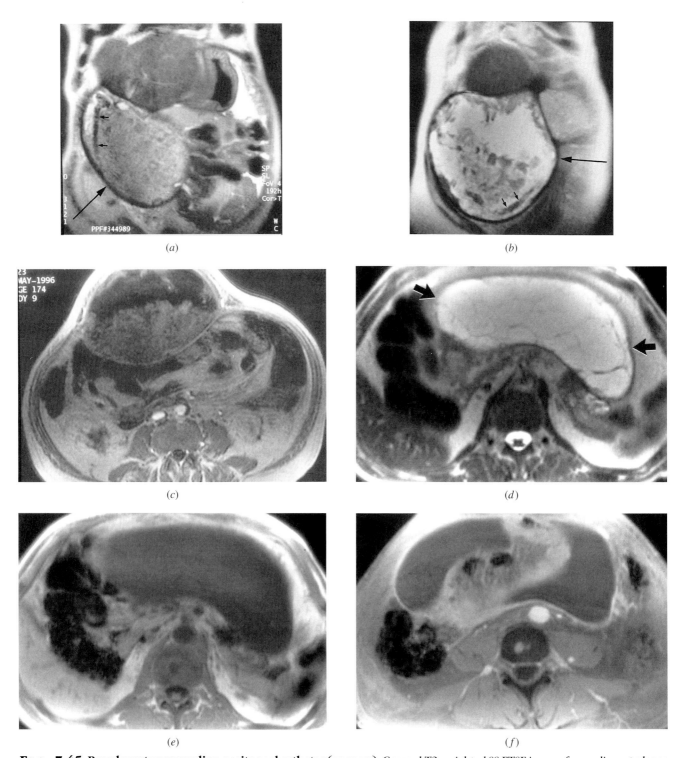

(a)   (b)

(c)   (d)

(e)   (f)

F I G . 7.45 Pseudocyst surrounding peritoneal catheter (cocoon). Coronal T2-weighted SS-ETSE images from adjacent planes (*a, b; b* is more anterior) and 90-s postgadolinium SGE (*c*) images. A 14-cm encapsulated debris-containing pseudocyst is present in the midabdomen, immediately beneath the liver. A low-signal intensity pseudocapsule surrounds the lesion (long arrows, *a, b*). The peritoneal catheter is identified within the cocoon (small arrows, *a, b*). A substantial volume of particulate debris is present (*a–c*), which is shown to layer on the transverse gadolinium-enhanced SGE image (*c*). Outside CT imaging study had been interpreted as demonstrating a hepatocellular carcinoma (HCC).

T2-weighted SS-ETSE (*d*), SGE (*e*), and 90-s postgadolinium fat-suppressed SGE (*f*) images in a second patient with a peritoneal dialysis catheter demontrate a large multiseptated encapsulated fluid collection (arrows, *d*). This fluid collection has an enhancing rim on postgadolinium images (*f*) and extends from the level of the pancreas inferiorly into the upper pelvis.

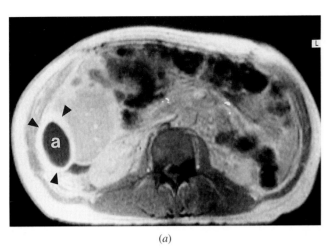

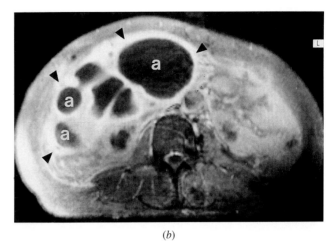

(a)   (b)

F I G . 7.46 Intra-abdominal abscess. Interstitial-phase gadolinium-enhanced T1-weighted SGE (*a*) and interstitial-phase gadolinium-enhanced T1-weighted fat-suppressed spin-echo (*b*) images in a patient with clinical suspicion of an abscess. Multiple loculated abscess collections are present along the liver capsule and in the right midabdomen ("*a*,"*a*, *b*). The thick enhancing rims (arrowheads, *a*, *b*) are characteristic of the inflammatory capsules associated with abscesses.

Abscess

Intra-abdominal abscesses are most often the sequelae of gastrointestinal or biliary surgery, diverticulitis, and Crohn disease [67]. In the appropriate clinical setting, a focal fluid collection that demonstrates rim enhance-ment on gadolinium-enhanced images suggests the correct diagnosis. The addition of fat suppression and image acquisition at 2–10 min after injection (interstitial phase) can highlight the enhancement of the abscess wall and surrounding tissues (Figs. 7.46–7.48). Layering

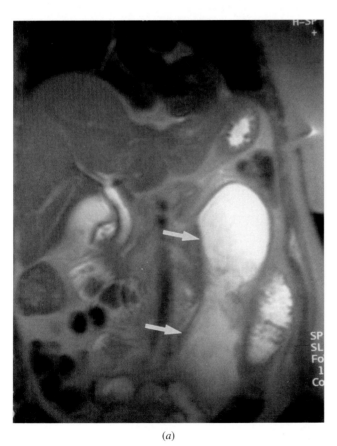

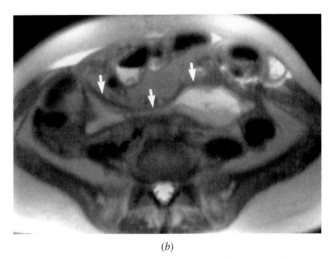

(a)   (b)

F I G . 7.47 Abdominal abscess. Coronal (*a*) and transverse (*b*) T2-weighted SS-ETSE, and transverse interstitial-phase gadolinium-enhanced fat-suppressed SGE (*c*, *d*) images. Within the left hemiabdomen, there is an extremely large fluid collection (arrows, *a*) extending from the lesser sac inferiorly into the pelvis along the left anterior pararenal space.

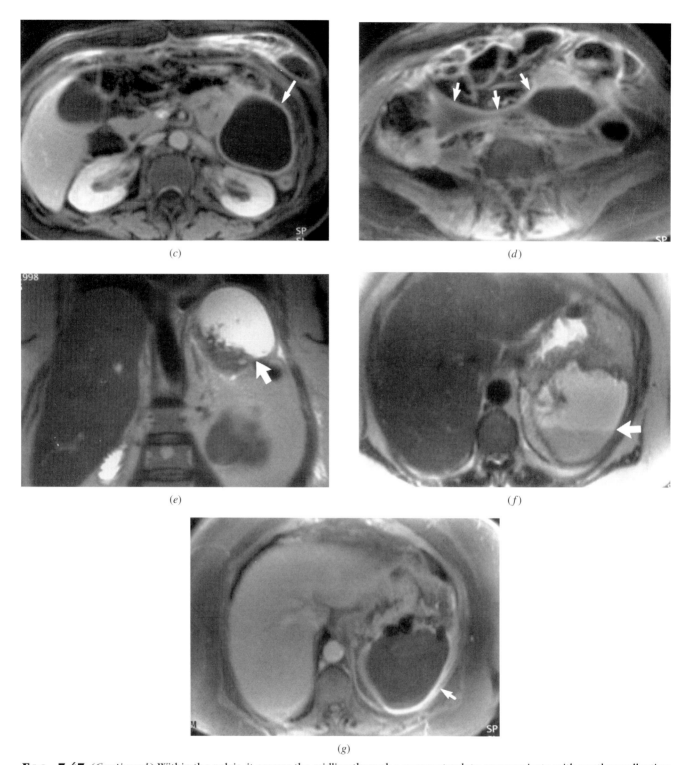

(c)

(d)

(e)

(f)

(g)

FIG. 7.47 (*Continued*) Within the pelvis, it crosses the midline through a narrow track to communicate with another collection located in the right lower quadrant. All these fluid collections possess thick enhancing walls (*c*, *d*) and have layering debris on T2-weighted images (*a*, *b*), consistent with abscesses.

Coronal (*e*) and transverse (*f*) T2-weighted SS-ETSE, and gadolinium-enhanced fat-suppressed SGE (*g*) images in a second patient, who has an abscess after splenectomy, demonstrate a large complex fluid collection adjacent to the tail of the pancreas. There is low-signal debris layering in the dependent portion of the fluid collection on the T2-weighted images (arrow, *e*, *f*) and prominent rim enhancement on the gadolinium-enhanced fat-suppressed image (arrow, *g*).

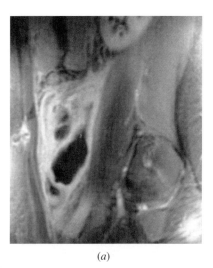

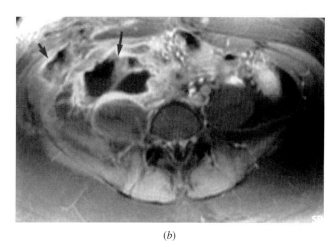

(a)   (b)

F i g . 7.48 Appendiceal abscess. Sagittal (a) and transverse (b) interstitial-phase gadolinium-enhanced fat-suppressed SGE images in a patient who underwent appendicectomy. A large multilocular fluid-containing abscess (arrows, b) is seen in the right lower quadrant of the abdomen associated with substantial enhancement of the surrounding tissues.

of lower-signal intensity debris in the dependent portion of the cystic lesion on T2-weighted images is a common finding in abscesses reflecting the layering of high protein content dependently in abscesses (fig. 7.49). This is a very specific finding for abscess. When air is identified within a fluid collection, active infection and/or fistula to the bowel (fig. 7.50) is present. The combination of breathing-independent T2-weighted echo-train spin-echo, gadolinium-enhanced capillary-phase SGE, interstitial-phase fat-suppressed SGE, and multiplanar imaging renders MRI a very accurate technique for de-

tecting intraperitoneal abscesses. MRI may be the technique of choice in patients who have dense intraluminal barium contrast, renal failure, or allergy to iodine. Noone et al. reported an accuracy of 96% in detecting intraperitoneal abscesses by MR [68]. Multiplanar imaging is also effective at showing the oval-shaped abscess collections, to distinguish them from tubule-shaped bowel [69]. The sagittal plane is essential in evaluating the pelvis for abscesses, because the relationship to pelvic organs is optimal and layering of low-signal material on T2-weighted images is clearly observed in this projection.

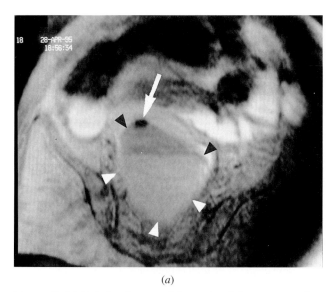

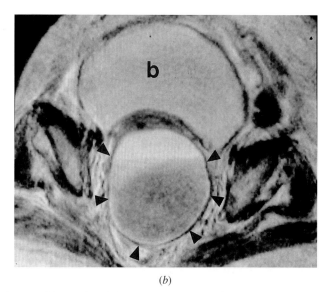

(a)   (b)

F i g . 7.49 Pelvic abscess. T1-weighted fat-suppressed spin-echo (a), T2-weighted fat-suppressed spin-echo (b), and sagittal gadolinium-enhanced T1-weighted fat-suppressed SGE (c) images in a patient with fever and an elevated white blood cell count. A complex fluid collection (arrowheads, a, b) is demonstrated in the pelvis. The variable signal intensity on the T1-weighted images reflects a high protein content (a, c). On the T2-weighted image (b), low-signal intensity debris layers in the dependent portion of the abscess. A focus of signal–void air is present (arrow, a), which is not uncommonly observed in abscesses. The wall of the abscess (arrows, c) enhances substantially after gadolinium administration. (bladder = b,b,c).

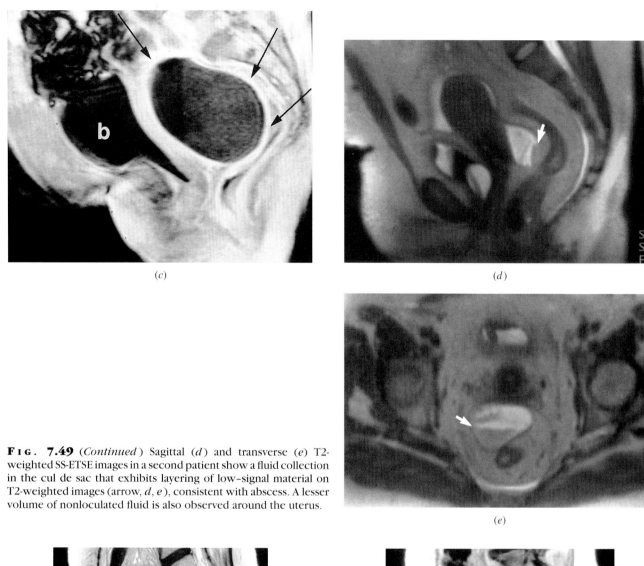

(c)

(d)

FIG. 7.49 (*Continued*) Sagittal (*d*) and transverse (*e*) T2-weighted SS-ETSE images in a second patient show a fluid collection in the cul de sac that exhibits layering of low–signal material on T2-weighted images (arrow, *d, e*), consistent with abscess. A lesser volume of nonloculated fluid is also observed around the uterus.

(e)

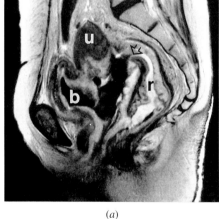

(a)

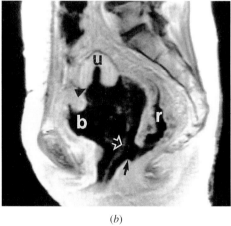

(b)

FIG. 7.50 **Pelvic abscess and fistulas.** Sagittal T2-weighted echo-train spin-echo (*a*), sagittal gadolinium-enhanced T1-weighted SGE (*b*), and transverse (*c*) and sagittal (*d*) interstitial-phase gadolinium-enhanced T1-weighted fat-suppressed spin-echo images in a patient with cervix cancer who had undergone high-dose radiation therapy. Tumor necrosis, and fistula and abscess formation are not uncommon complications of radiotherapy. A large pelvic cavity is present with communication between bladder, uterus, and rectum, which is clearly defined on the sagittal plane images (*a, b, d*). The rectal wall is substantially thickened, and submucosal edema is well shown, appearing high-signal intensity on the T2-weighted image (*a*). The signal-void regions in the abscess cavity represent air associated with the superior and low inferior rectal fistulas (open arrow, *a* and solid arrow, *d*, respectively) and superimposed infection.

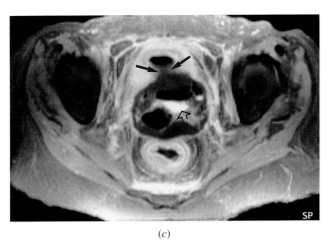
(c)

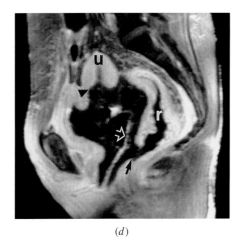
(d)

F I G . 7.50 (*Continued*) There is wide communication of the abscess cavity with the bladder. After intravenous gadolinium administration, high-signal intensity contrast (open arrow, *c*) exits the bladder through the large fistula (black arrows, *c*) and pools in the abscess. Portions of the uterine corpus and cervix have undergone necrosis; the uterine fundus remains. The posterior walls of the cervix and vagina (open arrow, *b*, *d*) are best shown on the sagittal gadolinium-enhanced T1-weighted fat-suppressed spin-echo image. r, Rectum; u, uterine fundus; b, bladder.

FUTURE DIRECTIONS

Faster scanning times coupled with open systems and MRI-compatible equipment may make routine MRI-guided percutaneous biopsies and drainages feasible, especially in patients with a contraindication for iodinated intravenous contrast [70].

CONCLUSIONS

MRI has become increasingly effective in evaluating diseases involving the peritoneum. This reflects MRI's multiplanar capabilities, robust scanning techniques, and sensitivity to intravenous contrast enhancement. The implementation of gadolinium-enhanced fat-suppressed SGE sequences and breathing-independent T2-weighted sequences has substantially improved the diagnostic usefulnes of MRI. Currently, MRI is useful for evaluating and characterizing diaphragmatic hernias, cysts, pseudocysts, endometriosis, peritoneal carcinomatosis, and intra-abdominal fluid collections.

REFERENCES

1. Williams PL, Bannister LH, Berry MM, Collins P, Dyson M, Dussek JE, Ferguson MWJ: *Gray's Anatomy* (38th ed.). New York: Churchill Livingstone, p. 1734–1746, 1995.
2. Cohen JM, Weinreb JC, Maravilla KP: Fluid collections in the intraperitoneal and extraperitoneal spaces: Comparison of MR and CT. *Radiology* 155: 705–708, 1985.
3. Gore RM, Callen PW, Filly RA: Lesser sac fluid in predicting the etiology of ascites: CT findings. *Am J Roentgenol* 139: 71–74, 1982.
4. Meyers MA: The spread and localization of acute intraperitoneal effusions. *Radiology* 95: 547–554, 1970.
5. Meyers MA: Distribution of intra-abdominal malignancy seeding dependency on dynamic of flow of ascites fluid. *Am J Roentgenol* 119: 198–206, 1973.
6. Meyers MA: *Dynamic radiology of the abdomen: Normal and pathologic anatomy* (2nd ed.). New York: Springer, 1982.
7. Ruess L, Frazier AA, Sivit CJ: CT of the mesentery, omentum and peritoneum in children. *Radiographics* 15: 89–104, 1995.
8. Gonzalez CF, Sotelo AC, de Melo DE: Primary peritoneal, omental and mesenteric tumors in childhood. *Semin Diagn Pathol* 3: 122–137, 1986.
9. Stoupis C, Ros PR, William JL: Hemorrhagic lymphangioma mimicking hemoperitoneum: MR imaging diagnosis. *J Magn Reson Imaging* 3: 541–542, 1993.
10. Lee GHM, Cohen AJ: CT imaging of abdominal hernias. *Am J Roentgenol* 161: 1209–1213, 1993.
11. Berger PE: Hernias of the abdominal wall and peritoneal cavity. In Franken EA Jr, Smith WL (eds.), *Gastrointestinal Imaging in Pediatrics*. Philadelphia: Harper & Row, p. 446–456, 1982.
12. Vanek VW, Phillips AK: Retroperitoneal, mesenteric and omental cysts. *Arch Surg* 119: 838–842, 1984.
13. Haney PF, Whitley NO: CT of benign cystic abdominal masses in children. *Am J Roentgenol* 142: 1279–1281, 1984.
14. Besson R, Hladky JP, Dhellemmes P, Debeugny P: Peritoneal pseudocyst—ventriculo-peritoneal shunt complications. *Eur J Pediatr Surg* 5(4): 195–197, 1995.
15. Kurachi H, Murakami T, Nakamura H, et al.: Imaging of peritoneal pseudocysts: Value of MR imaging compared with sonography and CT. *Am J Roentgenol* 160: 589–591, 1993.
16. Lewis VL, Shaffer HA Jr, Williamson BRJ: Pseudotumoral lipomatosis of the abdomen. *J Comput Assist Tomogr* 6: 79–82, 1982.
17. Siskind BN, Weiner FR, Frank M, Weiner SN, Bernstein RG, Luftschein S: Steroid-induced mesenteric lipomatosis. *Comput Radiol* 8(3): 175–177, 1984.
18. Gougoutas CA, Siegelman ES, Hunt J, Outwater EK: Pelvic endometriosis: various manifestations and MR imaging findings. *Am J Roentgenol* 175: 353–358, 2000.
19. Olive DL, Schwartz LB: Endometriosis. *N Eng J Med* 328: 1759–1769, 1993.

20. Arrive L, Hricak H, Martin MC: Pelvic endometriosis: MR imaging. *Radiology* 171: 687–692, 1989.

21. Sugimura K, Okizuka H, Imaoka I, Yashushi K, et al.: Pelvic endometriosis: Detection and diagnosis with chemical shift MR imaging. *Radiology* 188: 435–438, 1993.

22. Ascher SM, Agrawal R, Bis KG, Brown E, et al.: Endometriosis: Appearance and detection with conventional, fat-suppressed, and contrast-enhanced fat-suppressed spin-echo techniques. *J Magn Reson Imaging* 5: 251–257, 1995.

23. Reitamo JJ, Hayry P, Nykyri E, Saxen E: The desmoid tumor. I. Incidence, sex, age, and anatomical distribution in the Finnish population. *Am J Clin Pathol* 77(6): 665–673, 1982.

24. Hayry P, Reitamo JJ, Totterman S, Hopfner-Hallikainen D, Sivula A: The desmoid tumor. II. Analysis of factors possibly contributing to the etiology and growth behavior. *Am J Clin Pathol* 77(6): 674–680, 1982.

25. Smith AJ, Lewis JJ, Merchant NB, Leung DHY, Woodruff JM, Brennan MF: Surgical management of intra-abdominal desmoid tumors. *Br J Surg* 87(5): 608–613, 2000.

26. Daya D, McCaughey WT: Pathology of the peritoneum: A review of selected topics. *Sem Diag Pathol* 8(4): 277–289, 1991.

27. Smith TR: Malignant peritoneal mesothelioma: Marked variability of CT findings. *Abdom Imaging* 19: 27–29, 1994.

28. Whitley NO, Bohlman ME, Baker LP: CT patterns of mesenteric disease. *J Comput Assist Tomogr* 6: 490–496, 1982.

29. Whitley NO, Brenner DE, Antman KH, Grant D, et al.: CT of peritoneal mesothelioma: Analysis of eight cases. *Am J Roentgenol* 138: 531–535, 1982.

30. Furukawa T, Ueda J, Takahashi S, Higashino K, Shimura K, Tsujimura T, Araki Y: Peritoneal serous papillary carcinoma: radiological appearance. *Abdom Imaging* 24: 78–81, 1999.

31. Hamrick-Turner JE, Chiechi MV, Abbitt PL, Ros PR: Neoplastic and inflammatory processes of the peritoneum, omentum, and mesentery: Diagnosis with CT. *Radiographics* 12: 1051–1068, 1992.

32. Meyers MA, McSweeney J: Secondary neoplasms of bowel. *Radiology* 105: 1–11, 1972.

33. Daniel O: The differential diagnosis of malignant disease of the peritoneum. *Br J Surg* 39: 147–156, 1951.

34. Meyers MA, Oliphant M, Berne AS, Feldberg MAM: The peritoneal ligaments and mesenteries: Pathways of intra-abdominal spread of disease. *Radiology* 163: 593–604, 1987.

35. Oliphant M, Berne AS: Computed tomography of the subperitoneal space: Demonstration of direct spread of intra-abdominal disease. *J Comput Assist Tomogr* 6: 1127–1137, 1982.

36. Cotran RS, Kumar V, Robbins SL: *Pathologic Basis of Disease* (5th ed.). Philadelphia: W.B. Saunders, p. 250, 1994.

37. Semelka RC, Lawrence PH, Shoenut JP, Heywood M, et al.: Primary malignant ovarian disease: Prospective comparison of contrast enhanced CT and pre- and post-intravenous Gd-DTPA enhanced fat suppress and breath hold MRI with histological correlation. *J Magn Reson Imaging* 3: 99–106, 1993.

38. Cooper CR, Jeffrey RB, Silverman PM, Federle MP, et al.: Computed tomography of omental pathology. *J Comput Assist Tomogr* 10: 62–66, 1986.

39. Low RN, Semelka RC, Worawattanakul S, Altaze GD, Sigeti JS: Extrahepatic abdominal imaging in patients with malignancy: Comparison of MR imaging and helical CT, with subsequent surgical correlation. *Radiology* 210: 625–632, 1999.

40. Low RN, Carter WD, Saleh J, Sigeti JS: Ovarian cancer: Comparison of findings with perfluorocarbon-enhanced MR imaging, In-111-CYT-103 immunoscintigraphy, and CT. *Radiology* 195: 391–400, 1995.

41. Chou CK, Liu GC, Chen LT, Jaw TS: MRI manifestations of peritoneal carcinomatosis. *Gastrointest Radiol* 17: 336–338, 1992.

42. Chou CK, Liu GC, Chen LT, et al.: MRI demonstration of peritoneal implants. *Abdom Imaging* 19: 95–101, 1994.

43. Novetsky GJ, Berlin L, Epstein AJ, Lobo N, et al.: Pseudomyxoma peritonei. *J Comput Assist Tomogr* 6: 398–399, 1982.

44. Levitt RG, Sagel SS, Stanley RJ: Detection of neoplastic involvement of the mesentery and omentum by computed tomography. *Am J Roentgenol* 131: 835–838, 1978.

45. Mueller PR, Ferrucci JT Jr, Harbin WP, Kirkpatrick, et al.: Appearance of lymphomatous involvement of the mesentery by ultrasonography and body computed tomography: The "sandwich sign." *Radiology* 134: 467–473, 1980.

46. Picus D, Glazer HS, Levitt RG, Husband JE: Computed tomography of abdominal carcinoid tumors. *Am J Roentgenol* 143: 581–584, 1984.

47. Rosai J: *Ackerman's Surgical Pathology* (8th ed.). St Louis, MO: Mosby, p. 2149, 1996.

48. Young RH, Gilks CB, Scully RE: Mucinous tumors of the appendix associated with mucinous tumors of the ovary and pseudomyxoma peritonei. A clinico-pathological analysis of 22 cases supporting an origin in the appendix. *Am J Surg Pathol* 15: 415–429, 1991.

49. Dachman AH, Lichtenstein JE, Friedman AC: Mucocele of the appendix and pseudomyxoma peritonei. *Am J Roentgenol* 144: 923–929, 1985.

50. Goffinet DR, Castellino RA, Kim H, et al.: Staging laparotomies in unselected previously untreated patients with non-Hodgkin's lymphoma. *Cancer* 32: 672–681, 1973.

51. Pantongrag-Brown L, Buetow PC, Carr NJ, et al.: Calcification and fibrosis in mesenteric carcinoid tumors: CT findings and pathologic correlation. *Am J Roentgenol* 164: 387–391, 1995.

52. Cockey BM, Fishman EK, Jones B, Siegelman SS: Computed tomography of abdominal carcinoid tumor. *J Comput Assist Tomogr* 10: 953–962, 1985.

53. Terrier F, Revel D, Pajannen H, Richardson M, et al.: MR imaging of body fluid collections. *J Comput Assist Tomogr* 10: 953–962, 1986.

54. Pelage JP, Soyer P, Boudiaf M, Brocheriou-Spelle M, Dufresne AC, Coumbaras J, Rymer R: Carcinoid tumors of the abdomen: CT features. *Abdom Imaging* 24: 240–245, 1999.

55. Walls SD, Hricak H, Baily GD, Kerlan RK Jr, et al.: MR of pathologic abdominal fluid collections. *J Comput Assist Tomogr* 10: 746–750, 1986.

56. Dooms GC, Fisher MR, Hricak H, Higgins CB: MR of intramuscular hemorrhage. *J Comput Assist Tomogr* 9: 908–913, 1985.

57. Unger EC, Glazer HS, Lee JKT, Ling D: MRI of extracranial hematomas: Preliminary observations. *Am J Roentgenol* 146: 403–407, 1986.

58. Balci NC, Semelka RC, Noone TC, Asher SM: Acute and subacute liver-related hemorrhage: MRI findings. *Magn Reson Imaging* 17(2): 207–211, 1999.

59. Hahn PF, Saini S, Stark DD: Papanicolaou N, et al. Intra-abdominal hematoma: The concentric-ring sign in MR imaging. *Am J Roentgenol* 148: 115–119, 1987.

60. Zeman RK, Burrell MI: Hepatobiliary trauma. In Zeman RK, Burrell MI (eds.), *Gallbladder and Bile Duct Imaging: A Clinical Radiologic Approach.* New York: Churchill Livingstone, p. 677–704, 1987.

61. Ogden WW II, Bradburn DM, Rives JD: Mesenteric panniculitis. Review of 27 cases. *Ann Surg* 161: 864–875, 1965.

62. Bellin MF, Du LETH, Sagraty G, et al.: MRI and colour-Doppler in sclerosing mesenteritis. *Eur Radiol* 2: 373–376, 1992.

63. Patel N, Saleeb SF, Teplick SK: General case of the day. *RadioGraphics* 19: 1083–1085, 1999.

64. Sabate JM, Torrubia S, Maideu J, Franquet T, Monill JM, Perez C: Sclerosing mesenteritis: Imaging findings in 17 patients. *Am J Roentgenol* 172: 625–629, 1999.

65. Katz ME, Heiken JP, Glazer HS, Lee JKT: Intra-abdominal panniculitis: Clinical, radiographic, and CT features. *Am J Roentgenol* 145: 293–296, 1985.

66. Haynes JW, Brewer WH, Walsh JW: Focal fat necrosis presenting as a palpable abdominal mass: CT evaluation. *J Comput Assist Tomogr* 9: 568–569, 1985.

67. Wang SM, Wilson SE: Subphrenic abscess: The new epidemiology. *Arch Surg* 112: 934–936, 1977.

68. Noone TC, Semelka RC, Worawattanakul S, Marcos HB: Intraperitoneal abscesses: Diagnostic accuracy of and appearances at MR imaging. *Radiology* 208: 525–528, 1998.

69. Semelka RC, John G, Kelekis NL, Burdeny DA, Worawattanakul S, Ascher SM: Bowel-related abscesses: MR Demonstration Preliminary Results. *Magn Reson Imaging.* 16 : 855–861, 1998.

70. Anzai Y, Desalles AF, Black KL, Sinha S, et al.: Interventional MR imaging. *Radiographics* 13: 8971, 1993.

ADRENAL GLANDS

LARISSA L. NAGASE, M.D., RICHARD C. SEMELKA, M.D.,
AND DIANE ARMAO, M.D.

NORMAL ANATOMY

The adrenal glands are paired organs that lie in the retroperitoneum superomedial to the kidneys. The right adrenal gland is located medial to the right lobe of the liver, lateral to the right crus of the diaphragm, and posterior to the inferior vena cava (IVC). The left adrenal gland is situated posterior to the splenic vein and medial to the left crus of the diaphragm. The adrenal glands are a composite of two endocrine organs, cortex and medulla, the former steroid producing and the latter catecholamine producing.

MRI TECHNIQUE

Techniques that have been employed to examine the adrenal glands include T2-weighted spin-echo, T2-weighted echo-train spin-echo, T2-weighted echoplanar, T1- and T2-weighted fat-suppressed spin-echo, serial postgadolinium-enhanced gradient-echo, postgadolinium T1-weighted fat-suppressed spin-echo, and out-of-phase gradient-echo imaging [1–21]. The intention of most of these techniques has been to distinguish benign from malignant disease. The approach that appears most reliable is the combined use of in-phase and out-of-phase gradient-echo techniques [9–20]. Benign adenomas have been shown to lose signal intensity on out-of-phase images because of the presence of intracytoplasmic lipid [9–20]. Metastatic lesions do not contain intracytoplasmic lipid and therefore do not lose signal intensity on out-of-phase images [9–20]. It is important to use out-of-phase technique without concomitant use of frequency-selective fat suppression because fat suppression will cause minimization of signal dropout [22]. The best approach is to use a spoiled gradient-echo (SGE) technique for both in-phase and out-of-phase imaging. The only variation between sequences should be the echo time (TE), with an echo time of 4.2–4.5 ms for in-phase imaging and echo time of 2.2–2.7 ms for out-of-phase imaging at 1.5 T. Use of a longer echo time (e.g., 6–7 ms) for out-of-phase imaging is less ideal because it introduces T2* signal loss. Overlap, however, exists between benign and malignant masses using combined in-phase and out-of-phase techniques [11–15, 17–20]. This is because not all benign adrenal adenomas contain intracytoplasmic lipid [15–20] and benign masses of other etiologies (e.g., granulomatous disease) do not contain lipid.

Serial postgadolinium gradient-echo imaging may provide supplemental information to distinguish benign from malignant adrenal masses [6, 7]. Metastases tend to enhance more heterogeneously and retain gadolinium contrast for a more prolonged period than benign adenomas. We have recently reported on the appearance of benign and malignant adrenal masses on images acquired in the capillary phase of enhancement [23]. We observed that 70% of benign adenomas exhibited a relatively intense homogeneous capillary blush, whereas none of the malignant tumors did so. Overlap exists however, in the enhancement features of metastases and adenomas [11, 18, 23]. Adenomas and metastases may both enhance heterogeneously on immediate postgadolinium images [23], and desmoplastic metastases enhance minimally [8]. The intensity of enhancement of normal adrenal tissue and adrenal adenomas may vary [8, 18, 24].

Regarding T2-weighted imaging, metastases frequently possess a longer T2 and are brighter on T2-weighted images than adenomas. Substantial overlap exists between benign and malignant masses with this technique [4, 5, 11]. Signal intensity on T2-weighted images depends on the fluid content, predominantly in the interstitial space, of the mass. Desmoplastic neoplasms have low fluid content and therefore low signal intensity, whereas some benign lesions have high fluid content and are high in signal intensity [11]. Visual perception of signal intensity on T2-weighted images is also problematic. Most adrenal masses appear at least moderately high in signal intensity on fat-suppressed T2-weighted images because the rendering of fat low signal intensity results in rescaling of the signal intensities of abdominal organs. For similar reasons of signal intensity scaling, most adrenal masses appear moderately low in signal intensity on T2-weighted echo-train spin-echo sequences because of the high signal intensity of background fat.

Because no single technique is more than 90% accurate, a useful approach is to combine in-phase and out-of-phase images with other techniques to increase the confidence of lesion characterization. The combination with capillary-phase gadolinium-enhanced imaging may provide the most consistent results for distinguishing adenoma from metastases [23].

The demonstration of normal adrenal glands and small adrenal masses is well performed with T1-weighted fat-suppressed imaging (fig. 8.1) [8, 12]. The demonstration of renal corticomedullary difference on either noncontrast T1-weighted fat-suppressed images or immediate postgadolinium SGE images is helpful in distinguishing adrenal from renal tumors [13, 25]. The multiplanar imaging capability of MRI is also useful for assessing large tumors in the region of the upper pole of the kidney to determine intra- or extrarenal origin by imaging in the coronal or sagittal planes [25, 26]. Sagittal-plane imaging is preferred to coronal imaging [25]. The relationship between mass, kidney, and liver or spleen is shown in profile in the sagittal plane (fig. 8.2) and en face in the coronal plane. Origin of tumor is better evaluated when the orientation between these structures is viewed in profile, because partial volume effects may be observed when the organ margins are viewed en face [25]. T2-weighted images provide information on fluid content of adrenal lesions and are essential in examining for pheochromocytomas, because their fluid content is consistently higher than other adrenal masses.

MASS LESIONS

Diseases of the adrenal glands may affect the cortex or medulla. Diseases of the adrenal cortex can be divided essentially into three categories: 1) disorders associated with hyperfunction and steroid excess, 2) disorders that reduce the output of adrenal steroid, and 3) lesions that have no functional effect. Hyperfunctioning diseases may result from adrenal hyperplasia as well as from benign or malignant tumors. Many mass lesions possess a distinctive MR imaging appearance, which can be described evaluating the combination of T1, T2 and early and late postgadolinium images (Table 8.1).

Cortical Lesions

Benign

Hyperplasia. The majority (70%) of patients with Cushing syndrome have adrenal cortical hyperplasia secondary to an ACTH-producing pituitary microadenoma (Cushing disease). Adrenal hyperplasia is also identified in the context of systematic illness, acromegaly, hyperthyroidism, hypertension, diabetes, depression, and malignant disease. Hyperplasia of the adrenal cortex results secondarily to overstimulation of the cortex by ACTH. Primary hyperplasia is relatively uncommon.

Adrenal hyperplasia usually results in bilateral adrenal enlargement, diffuse or nodular, with maintenance of adrenoform shape (fig. 8.3). Unilateral adrenal enlargement may however also occur [27]. The adrenal glands may also appear normal in size [12]. Hyperplastic glands usually contain microscopic nodules, but macroscopic nodules (12 cm) may be observed [12]. Hyperplastic adrenal glands have signal intensity appearances similar to those of normal adrenals on all MR imaging sequences [12].

Adenomas. Adenomas are usually small neoplasms, less than 5 cm, characteristically solitary and well encapsulated. Adrenal adenomas are the most common adrenal masses and can be divided into two categories, nonhyperfunctioning and hyperfunctioning. Nonhyperfunctioning adenomas are more frequent than functioning adenomas. Many adrenal adenomas are found incidentally at autopsy, in 2–8% of cases, or discovered by imaging studies performed for other reasons.

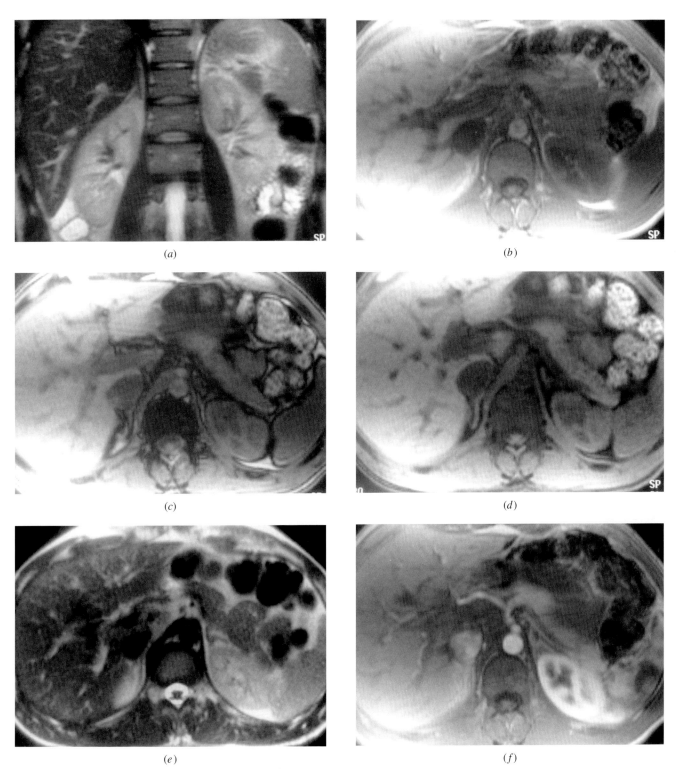

(a)

(b)

(c)

(d)

(e)

(f)

FIG. 8.1 Normal adrenals. Coronal T2-weighted single-shot echo-train spin-echo (SS-ETSE) (*a*), T1-weighted SGE (*b*), T1-weighted out-of-phase SGE (*c*), T1-weighted fat-suppressed SGE (*d*), single-shot echo-train spin-echo (SS-ETSE) (*e*), immediate postgadolinium T1 SGE (*f*), and 90-s post gadolinium T1 fat-suppressed SGE (*g*) images in one patient.

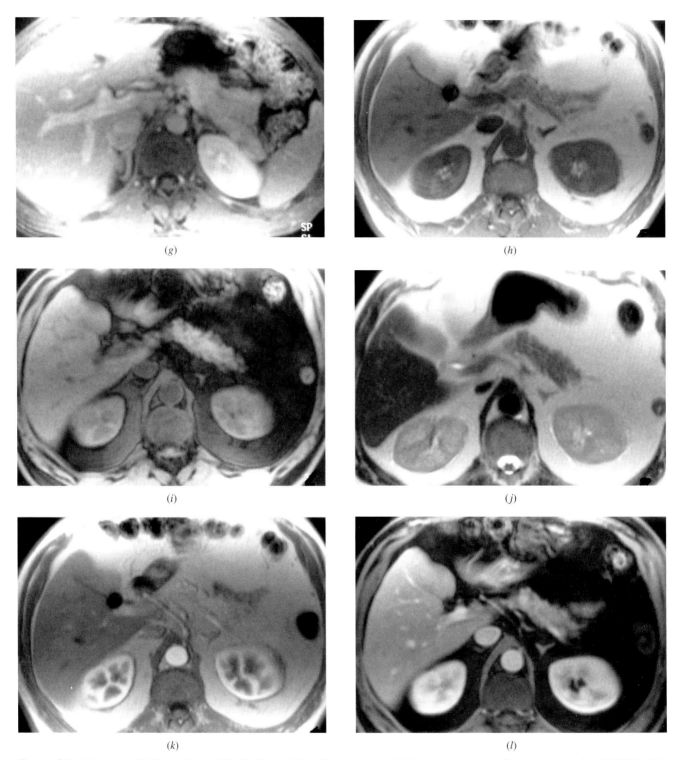

FIG. 8.1 (*Continued*) T1-weighted SGE (*h*), T1-weighted fat-suppressed SGE (*i*), single-shot echo-train spin-echo (SS-ETSE) (*j*), immediate postgadolinium T1 SGE (*k*), and 90-s postgadolinium T1 fat-suppressed SGE (*l*) images in a second patient. Relative to normal liver, normal adrenal glands are typically mildly hypointense on T1 in-phase (*b*, *h*), isointense with a signal-void rim on T1 out-of-phase (*c*), well defined and isointense on T1-weighted fat-suppressed images (*d*, *i*), isointense on T2 (*a*, *e*, *j*), enhance homogeneously on immediate postgadolinium images (*f*, *k*), and wash-out isointense with liver on delayed images (*g*, *l*).

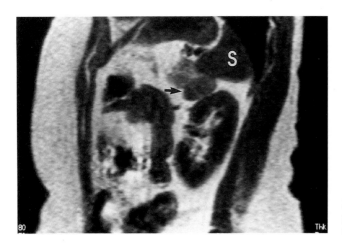

F I G . 8.2 Adrenal mass. Adrenal mass is shown in the sagittal plane. Sagittal-plane SGE image demonstrates an adrenal adenoma (arrow) that is clearly separated from kidney and spleen (s).

Increased incidence has been reported in patients who are elderly, obese, or hypertensive or who have primary malignancies of bladder, kidney, and endometrium. Hyperfunctioning adenomas are usually larger than 2 cm in diameter and commonly are cortisol secreting. The majority of adenomas are homogeneously iso- or hypointense in comparison to the normal adrenal gland on T2-weighted images (fig. 8.4), whereas adrenal metastases tend to be hyperintense [1–5]. Contrast enhancement on immediate postgadolinium images is variable and ranges from minimal (figs. 8.4–8.6) to moderately intense (figs. 8.7–8.12) [8, 11, 18]. Uniform enhancement of the entire lesion on immediate postgadolinium capillary-phase images is common for adenomas, reported in one series in 70% of cases [23], and rare for other entities. On serial postgadolinium images, rapid washout of contrast

may be a feature more typical of benign than malignant masses (fig. 8.7) [6, 7]; however, variation exists (figs. 8.10, 8.11) [11, 18]. These lesions enhance homogeneously and have regular margins on T1-weighted gadolinium-enhanced fat-suppressed images [8]. Small linear or rounded foci of low or high signal intensity may be present on various MR sequences representing small areas of cystic change, hemorrhage, or variations of vascularity (fig. 8.13). These characteristics are also present in adrenal-cortical carcinoma; however, in malignant tumors larger heterogeneous regions are generally observed [28]. Adenomas commonly possess a thin rim of enhancement, best appreciated on interstitial-phase gadolinium-enhanced images [29]. However, a thin rim of adrenal tissue may also be appreciated with small metastases, simulating this appearance.

T a b l e 8.1 Pattern Recognition: Adrenal Lesions

	T1 In phase	T1 Out of phase	T2	Early Gd	Late Gd	Other Features
Adenoma	↓–↑	↓	ϕ–↑	Homogeneous intense	Fade	80% drop in signal on out of phase; 70% have a homogeneous intense capillary blush
Metastases	↓–↑	ϕ	ϕ–↑	Heterogeneous, variable	Heterogeneous, variable	Heterogeneity increases with increase in lesion size.
Pheochromocytoma	↓–ϕ	ϕ	↑–↑↑	Variable, usually minimal	Variable	Heterogeneous and hyperintense on T2-WI; minimal enhancement with gadolinium
Adrenal Cortical Carcinoma	↓–↑	↓ (portions)	↑	↑ Heterogeneous	Fade	Hemorrhagic and necrotic areas; portions of the tumor may drop on out-of-phase images
Lymphoma	ϕ	ϕ	ϕ	Minimal	Minimal	Mild heterogeneity on all sequences.

↓ ↓, Moderately to markedly decreased; ↓, mildly decreased; ϕ, isointense; ↑, mildly increased; ↑ ↑, moderately to markedly increased.

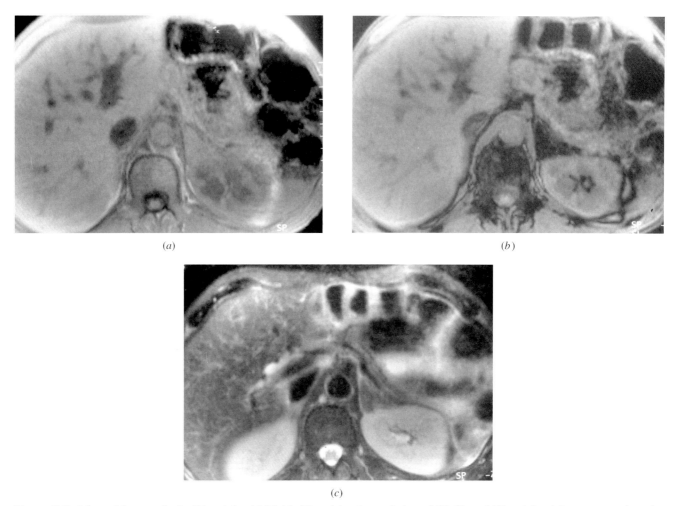

(a)

(b)

(c)

FIG. 8.3 Adrenal hyperplasia. T1-weighted SGE (*a*), T1-weighted out-of-phase SGE (*b*), and T2-weighted fat-suppressed single-shot echo-train spin-echo (SS-ETSE) (*c*) images. The left adrenal is diffusely enlarged, and the adrenaliform shape is maintained. It is isointense to the liver on T1 (*a*), drops significantly in signal intensity on out-of-phase SGE (*b*), and is slightly hypointense on T2 fat-suppressed image (*c*). The presence of water and fat in the same voxel results in the findings on out-of-phase images.

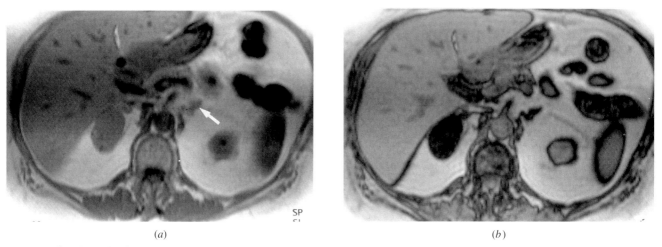

(a)

(b)

FIG. 8.4 Adrenal adenoma—mild capillary blush. T1-weighted SGE (*a*), T1-weighted out-of-phase SGE (*b*), and immediate postgadolinium SGE (*c*) images.

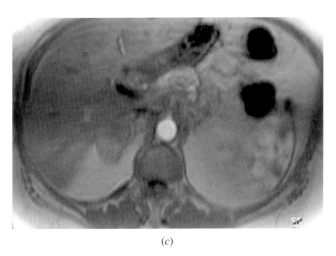

(c)

F I G . 8.4 (*Continued*) Right adrenal adenoma demonstrates signal drop on out-of-phase image and mild capillary blush on immediate postgadolinium image. Note normal left adrenal (arrow, *a*).

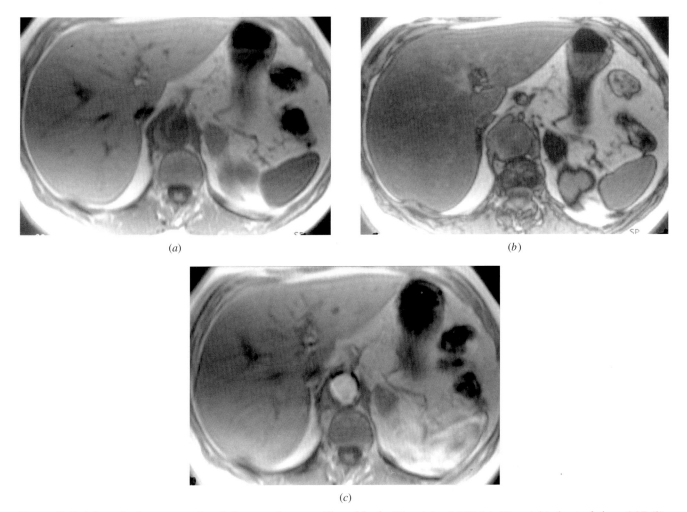

(a)　　　　　　　　　(b)

(c)

F I G . 8.5 Adrenal adenoma—signal drop and no capillary blush. T1-weighted SGE (*a*), T1-weighted out-of-phase SGE (*b*), and immediate postgadolinium SGE (*c*) images. Left adrenal adenoma demonstrates signal drop on the out-of-phase image (*b*). There is no substantial capillary blush on the immediate postgadolinium image (*c*).

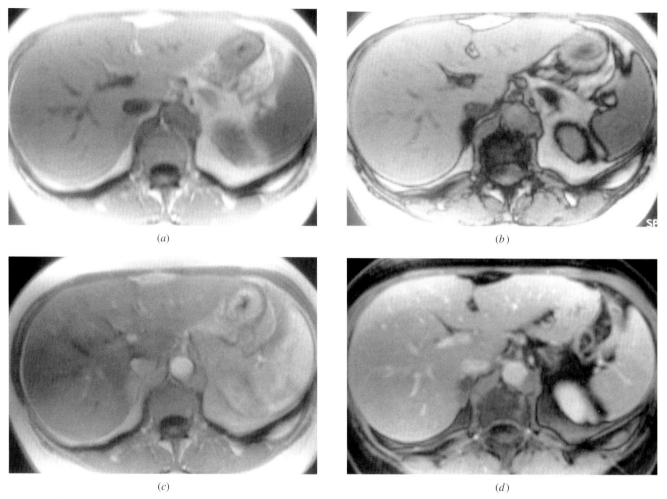

(a)   (b)

(c)   (d)

F I G . 8.6 Bilateral adrenal adenoma. T1-weighted SGE (*a*), T1-weighted out-of-phase SGE (*b*), immediate postgadolinium SGE (*c*), and 90-s postgadolinium fat-suppressed SGE (*d*) images in a patient with bilateral adrenal adenomas. Note that in this patient both adrenals show signal intensity drop on out-of-phase images, but there is no substantial capillary blush after gadolinium administration (*c*). Late enhancement is mildly heterogeneous (*d*).

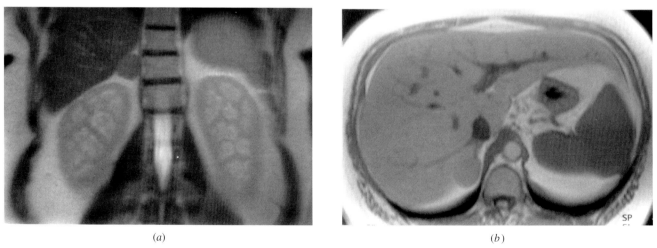

(a)   (b)

F I G . 8.7 Adrenal adenoma. Coronal T2-weighted SS-ETSE (*a*), T1-weighted SGE (*b*), T1-weighted out-of-phase SGE (*c*), immediate postgadolinium SGE (*d*), and 90-s postgadolinium fat-suppressed SGE (*e*) images. A 3 × 2-cm right adrenal mass shows signal intensity drop on the out-of-phase image (*c*) compared with the in-phase image (*b*).

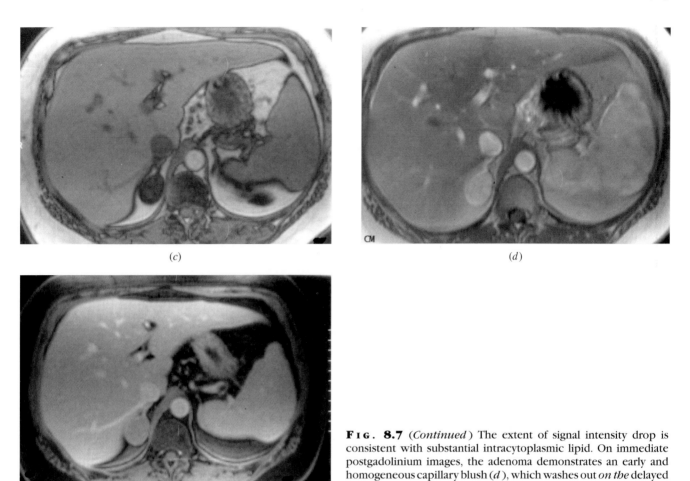

(c)

(d)

(e)

F I G .   8.7 (*Continued*) The extent of signal intensity drop is consistent with substantial intracytoplasmic lipid. On immediate postgadolinium images, the adenoma demonstrates an early and homogeneous capillary blush (*d*), which washes out *on the* delayed image (*e*).

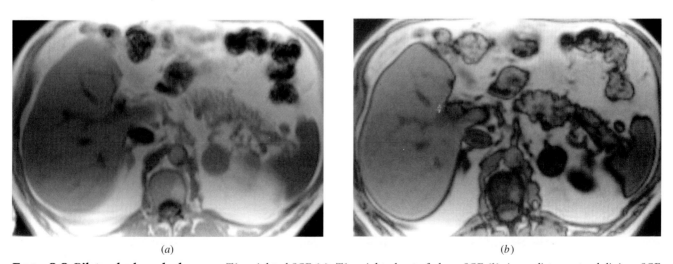

(a)

(b)

F I G .   8.8 Bilateral adrenal adenoma. T1-weighted SGE (*a*), T1-weighted out-of-phase SGE (*b*), immediate postgadolinium SGE (*c*), and 90-s postgadolinium fat-suppressed SGE (*d*) images. Bilateral adrenal adenomas, larger on the left side.

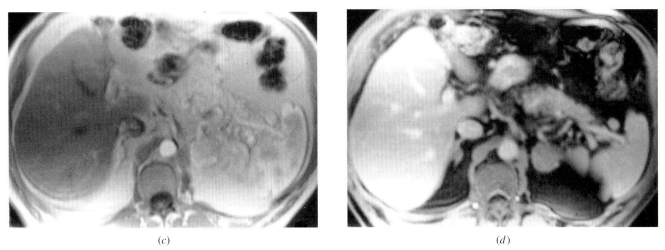

(c)   *(d)*

F I G . 8.8 *(Continued)* Both lesions have signal intensity drop on the out-of-phase image (*b*). There is an intense capillary blush on immediate postgadolinium image (*c*) and a rapid washout on delayed image (*d*).

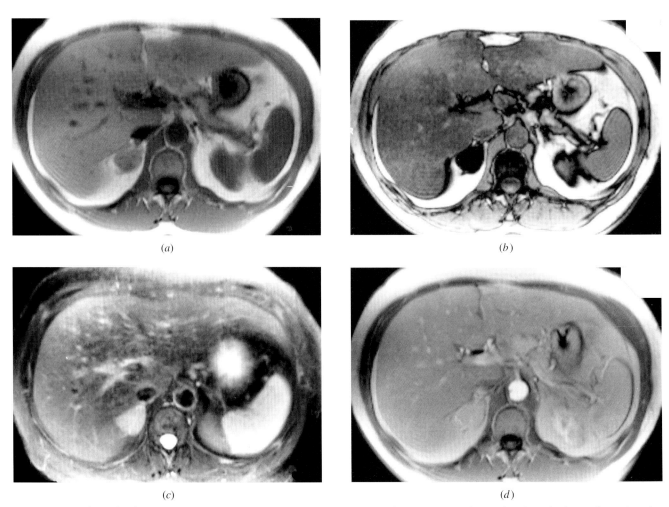

(a)   *(b)*

(c)   *(d)*

F I G . 8.9 Adrenal adenoma. T1-weighted SGE (*a*), T1-weighted out-of-phase SGE (*b*), T2-weighted single-shot echo-train spin-echo (SS-ETSE) (*c*), and 45-s postgadolinium SGE (*d*) images. Right adrenal adenoma has substantial signal drop from the in-phase (*a*) to the out-of-phase image (*b*) and moderately high signal intensity on fat-suppressed T2 image (*c*). Note the intense homogeneous capillary blush after gadolinium administration (*d*).

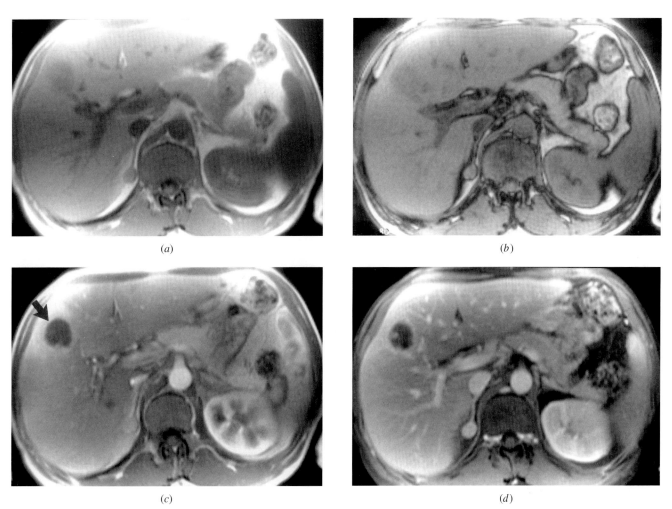

(a)   (b)

(c)   (d)

F I G . 8.10 Adrenal adenoma—no signal loss and capillary blush. T1-weighted SGE (*a*), T1-weighted out-of-phase SGE (*b*), immediate postgadolinium SGE (*c*), and 90-s postgadolinium fat-suppressed SGE (*d*) images in a patient with a nonfunctioning adenoma. The adrenal adenoma is slightly hypointense to the liver on T1 (*a*) and has no signal drop on the out-of-phase image (*b*). After gadolinium administration there is a capillary blush of the adrenal adenoma (*c*) and minimal washout of contrast material on the late image (*d*). A 3.5-cm abscess with a thin capsule is present in the liver (arrow, *c*). Note the intense perilesional enhancement on the immediate postgadolinium image.

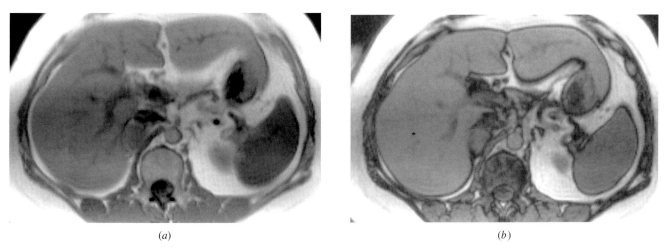

(a)   (b)

F I G . 8.11 Adrenal adenoma. T1-weighted SGE (*a*), T1-weighted out-of-phase SGE (*b*), T2-weighted fat suppressed single-shot echo-train spin-echo (SS-ETSE) (*c*), immediate postgadolinium SGE (*d*) and 90-s postgadolinium fatsuppressed SGE (*e*) images.

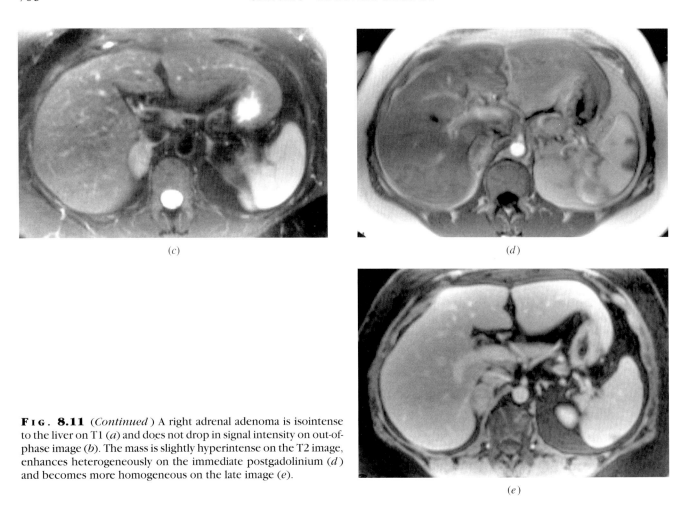

(c)

(d)

Fig. 8.11 *(Continued)* A right adrenal adenoma is isointense to the liver on T1 *(a)* and does not drop in signal intensity on out-of-phase image *(b)*. The mass is slightly hyperintense on the T2 image, enhances heterogeneously on the immediate postgadolinium *(d)* and becomes more homogeneous on the late image *(e)*.

(e)

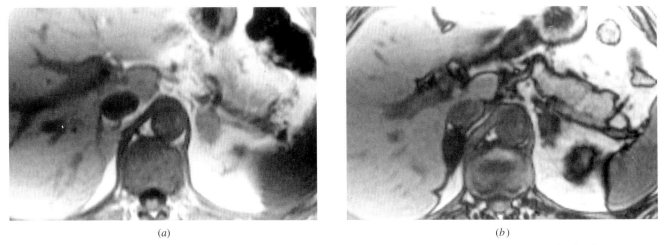

(a)

(b)

Fig. 8.12 Bilateral adrenal adenomas. T1-weighted SGE *(a)*, T1-weighted out-of-phase SGE *(b)*, T2-weighted echo train spin-echo *(c)*, immediate postgadolinium SGE *(d)*, and 90-s postgadolinium fat-suppressed SGE *(e)* images in a patient with bilateral adrenal adenomas. Bilateral adrenal adenomas drop in signal intensity from in-phase *(a)* to out-of- phase *(b)* images, and they are mildly hyperintense relative to liver on the T2 image *(c)*.

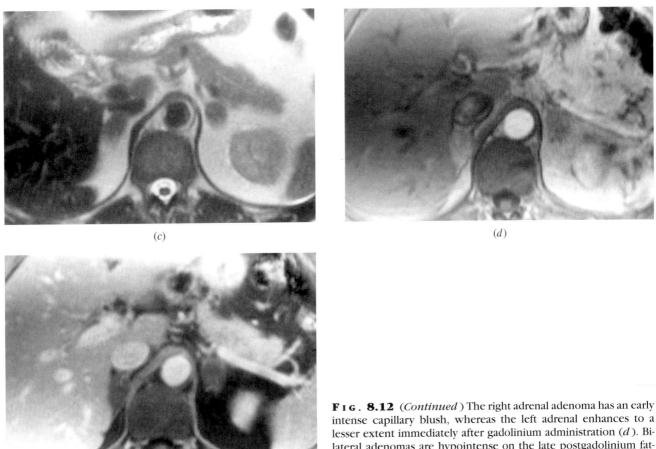

(c)

(d)

(e)

F I G . 8.12 (*Continued*) The right adrenal adenoma has an early intense capillary blush, whereas the left adrenal enhances to a lesser extent immediately after gadolinium administration (*d*). Bilateral adenomas are hypointense on the late postgadolinium fat-suppressed image (*e*).

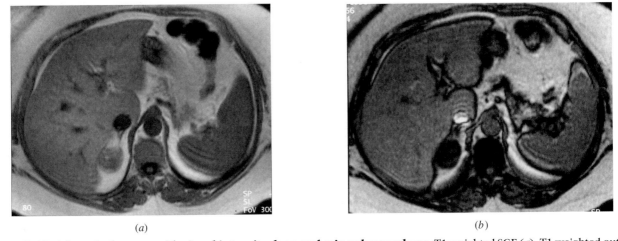

(a)

(b)

F I G . 8.13 Adrenal adenoma with signal intensity drop and minor hemorrhage. T1-weighted SGE (*a*), T1-weighted out-of-phase SGE (*b*), T2-weighted fat-suppressed spin-echo (*c*), and immediate postgadolinium SGE (*d*) images. Substantial signal intensity drop is present on the right adrenal adenoma comparing in-phase (*a*) to out-of-phase (*b*) SGE images. Small high-signal intensity foci are present on T1 (*a*) and T2-weighted (*c*) images, which is consistent with hemorrhage. The adenoma enhances intensely on the immediate postgadolinium SGE image (*d*) and contains foci of diminished enhancement that correspond to punctate regions of hemorrhage.

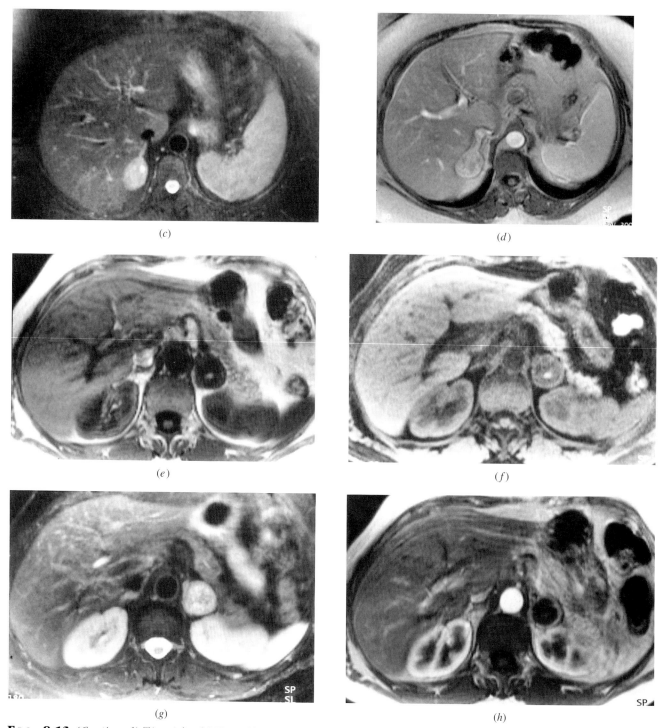

(c)

(d)

(e)

(f)

(g)

(h)

F I G . 8.13 (*Continued*) T1-weighted SGE (*e*), T1-weighted fat-suppressed SGE (*f*), T2-weighted fat-suppressed single-shot echo-train spin-echo (SS-ETSE) (*g*), immediate postgadolinium SGE (*h*), and 2-min postgadolinium fat-suppressed SGE (*i*) images in a second patient. A 3-cm left adrenal adenoma is present that contains foci of high signal intensity on the T1-weighted image (*e*), which do not suppress with fat suppression (*f*). The mass is heterogeneous on the T2-weighted image (*g*) and contains multiple high-signal intensity foci.

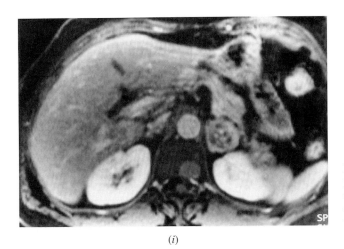

(i)

FIG. 8.13 (*Continued*) A prominent rim of enhancement is present on the immediate postgadolinium image with minimal internal enhancement (*b*). On the interstitial phase gadolinium-enhanced fat-suppressed image (*i*), central punctate high-signal intensity foci are apparent.

The most accurate method for demonstrating that a mass is an adenoma is to show loss of signal intensity on out-of-phase images (figs. 8.4–8.9, 8.12, and 8.14) [9–20]. Loss of signal intensity should parallel loss of signal in marrow of the adjacent vertebral body. Caution should be exercised in using liver as the comparative organ to determine signal intensity loss because the liver may also contain fat [17, 22]. The use of spleen may be problematic also, because the spleen may contain iron, and T2* effect will influence signal intensity changes, particularly if a longer echo time (e.g., 6–7 ms) is used for out-of-phase imaging. Renal cortex is less affected by fat or iron deposition and may be a more accurate tissue to use as a visual comparison for signal-intensity loss. An echo-time-adjusted signal intensity drop greater than 20% is diagnostic for adenomas (fig. 8.14), whereas a 10–20% signal intensity drop is suggestive of adenomas (fig. 8.15), but follow-up may be needed. Benign

lesions that do not contain intracytoplasmic lipid, do not lose signal on out-of-phase images (fig. 8.16) [11, 20]. If histological fat content is minimal, negligible signal loss may be observed on out-of-phase images, which has been reported in one series, in which this was found in two of seven resected adenomas [20]. T1-weighted fat-suppressed technique has also been useful to differentiate adenomas from malignant masses [30].

Large adenomas may undergo degenerative changes and contain foci of hemorrhage that appear as punctate high-signal intensity foci on T1-weighted and/or T2-weighted images (see fig. 8.13) [28].

Functioning adenomas with excess cortisol secretion are responsible for approximately 20% of Cushing syndrome cases. Most of these adenomas measure larger than 2 cm and are well shown on CT and MR images [31]. Hyperfunctioning and nonhyperfunctioning adenomas are presently not distinguishable on MR images because

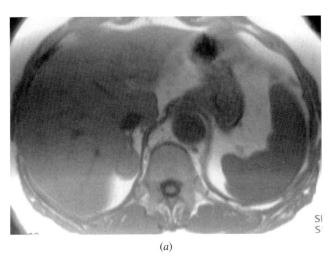

(a)

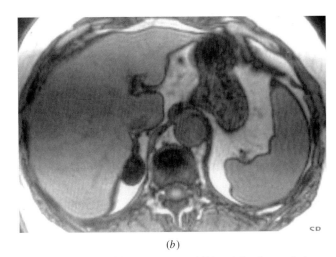

(b)

FIG. 8.14 **Adrenal adenoma with signal drop on out-of-phase image.** T1-weighted SGE (*a*) and T1-weighted out-of-phase SGE (*b*) images. Substantial signal intensity drop is present on the right adrenal adenoma comparing in-phase (*a*) to out-of-phase (*b*) SGE images, consistent with high lipid content.

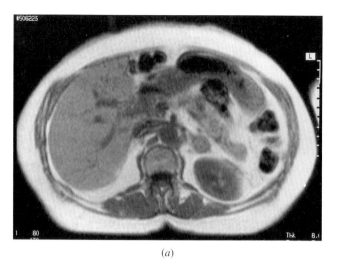

(a)

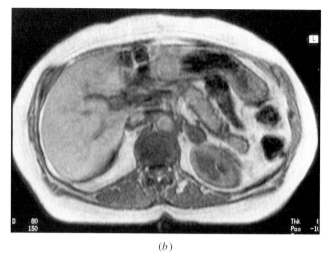

(b)

F I G . 8.15 Adrenal adenoma—mild signal drop. T1-weighted SGE (*a*) and T1-weighted out-of-phase SGE (*b*) images. Mild-signal intensity loss (approximately 15%) is noted from in-phase (*a*) to out-of-phase (*b*) images, which is in the low range for signal intensity drop to diagnose an adrenal mass as an adenoma. The extent of signal intensity drop is consistent with minimal intracytoplasmic lipid.

they have similar morphologic and signal intensity features, including the tendency of both to lose signal intensity on out-of-phase images, because they both often contain intracytoplasmic lipid [20]. Functioning adenomas may did contain negligible fat and therefore not lose signal on out-of-phase image (fig. 8.17).

Aldosterone-secreting adrenal adenomas are rare tumors, which are responsible for 75% of cases of primary aldosteronism (Conn syndrome), with adrenal hyperplasia accounting for 25% [32]. The clinical presentation includes systemic hypertension with hypokalemia, decreased plasma renin activity, and increased plasma aldosterone. These tumors are typically small, measur-

ing less than 3 cm in diameter, and the left adrenal is involved slightly more often than the right.

The distinction between adenoma and hyperplasia is important because patients with adenomas will respond to surgical management, whereas patients with hyperplasia are best treated medically [33].

Findings on tomographic images may result in diagnostic errors in patients who have a unilateral adenoma but in whom both adrenals have a nodular appearance. Doppman et al. [34] reported on 24 patients with primary aldosteronism, of whom CT images suggested the presence of hyperplasia in 6 patients, who had a unilateral aldosteronoma at surgery. T1-weighted fat-suppressed

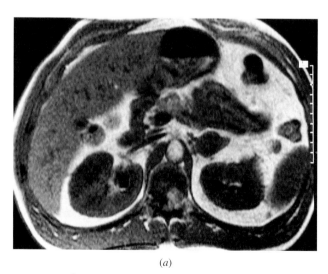

(a)

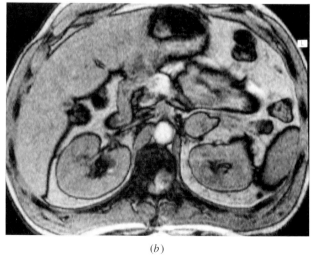

(b)

F I G . 8.16 Adrenal adenoma—no signal drop. T1-weighted SGE (*a*) and T1-weighted out-of-phase SGE (*b*) images. No signal intensity drop is noted from in-phase (*a*) to out-of-phase (*b*) images. The lack of signal intensity drop reflects the lack of appreciable intracytoplasmic lipid.

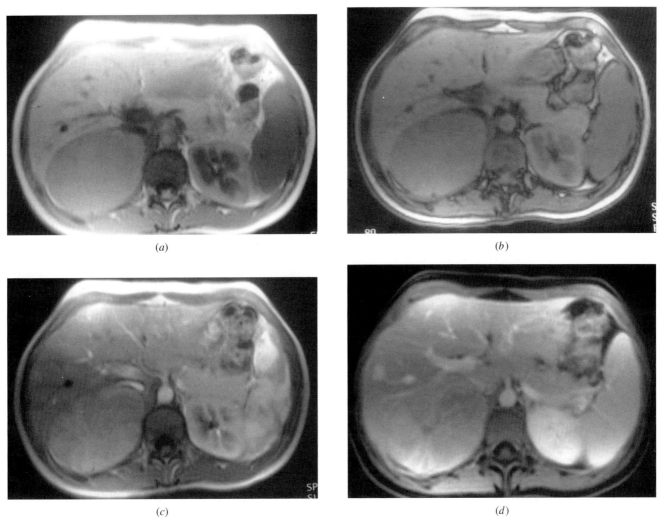

F I G . 8.17 Large functioning adrenal adenoma. T1-weighted SGE (*a*), T1-weighted out-of-phase SGE (*b*), immediate post-gadolinium SGE (*c*), and 90-s postgadolinium fat-suppressed SGE (*d*) images. A right adrenal mass appears hypointense to the liver on T1 SGE (*a*) and does not drop signal on T1 out-of-phase image (*b*). There is a heterogeneous capillary blush after contrast administration (*c*), which diminishes moderately and remains slightly hypointense on late images (*d*).

images show clear delineation of the adrenal glands and permit detection of small masses (fig. 8.18) [12]. Aldosteronomas occasionally contain intracytoplasmic lipid and may therefore lose signal intensity on out-of-phase images (see fig. 8.18) [20].

Other Benign Tumors

Myelolipoma. Myelolipomas are rare benign tumors composed of mature adult adipose tissue and hematopoietic cells [35]. These tumors are usually small and unilateral and typically have a high fat content that gives them a pathognomonic appearance on MR images [35–41]. Occasionally, myelolipomas may be large, and in these cases direct sagittal or coronal imaging may be helpful to demonstrate the extrarenal origin of these tumors [39]. The amount of fat in these lesions may vary. On the basis of T1-weighted images alone

the distinction from a hemorrhagic cyst may be difficult. The diagnosis is virtually certain if the signal of the tumor is hyperintense on T1-weighted images and decreases on fat-suppressed images (fig. 8.19) [12, 40, 41]. Because myelolipomas may be almost entirely fatcontaining, these tumors may not lose signal intensity on out-of-phase images. Signal loss using the out-of-phase technique occurs when fat and water are of similar proportions in the same voxel. Myelolipomas may exhibit a black ring phase-cancellation artifact if the tumor borders on a water-based organ, but most often, the tumor is surrounded by fat and therefore does not exhibit a black ring phase-cancellation artifact. The distinction from adenoma is based on fat content. Adenomas generally do not contain sufficient fat to result in visually apparent signal loss on fat-suppressed images. Myelolipomas generally contain such a preponderance of adipose tissue

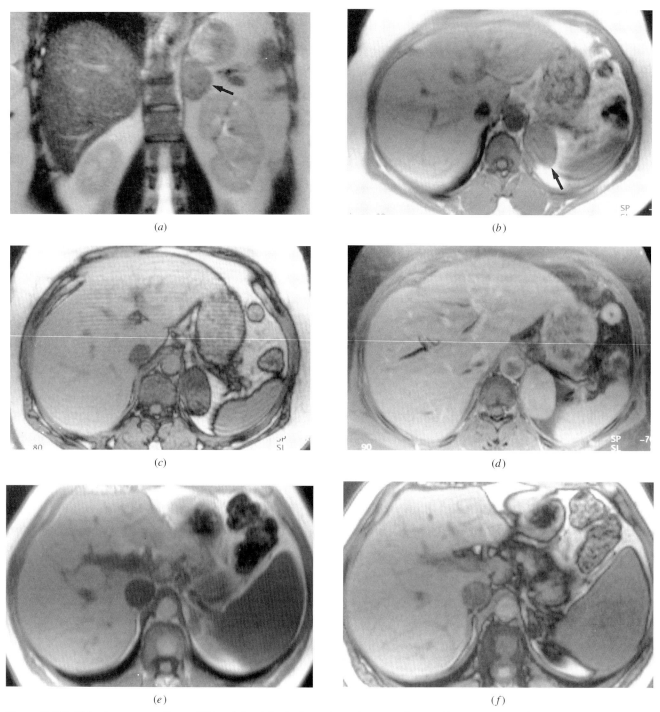

(a)   (b)

(c)   (d)

(e)   (f)

F ɪ ɢ . 8.18 Aldosteronoma. Coronal T2-weighted single-shot echo-train spin-echo (SS-ETSE) (*a*), T1-weighted SGE (*b*), T1-weighted out-of-phase SGE (*c*), and 90-s postgadolinium fat-suppressed SGE (*d*) images. A 3.5-cm left adrenal aldosteronoma is present (arrow, *a*, *b*). The mass is moderately low in signal intensity on the T2-weighted image (*a*). The mass drops in signal from in-phase (*b*) to out-of-phase (*c*) images, reflecting the presence of intracytoplasmic lipid. On the postgadolinium image (*d*) the mass enhances in a relatively homogeneous fashion.

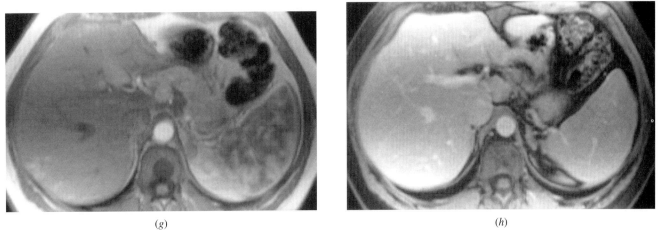

(g)   (h)

FIG. 8.18 (*Continued*) T1-weighted SGE (*e*), T1-weighted out-of-phase SGE (*f*), immediate postgadolinium T1-weighted SGE (*g*), and 90-s postgadolinium fat-suppressed SGE (*h*) images in a second patient with a small left adrenal aldosteronoma showing the same characteristics as described above.

These cases illustrate that aldosteronomas have imaging findings similar to those of other benign adrenal adenomas.

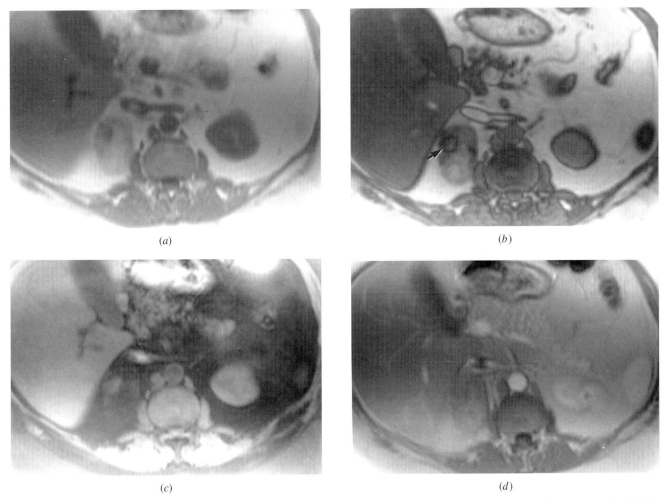

(a)   (b)

(c)   (d)

FIG. 8.19 **Adrenal myelolipoma.** T1-weighted SGE (*a*), T1-weighted out-of-phase (*b*), T1-weighted fat-suppressed SGE (*c*), immediate postgadolinium SGE (*d*), and 90-s postgadolinium SGE (*e*) images. The right adrenal myelolipoma is hyperintense on the in-phase (*a*) image and drops in signal on the out-of-phase image (*b*), except for an eccentric focal area that does not drop in signal and possesses a phase cancellation artifact (arrow, *b*).

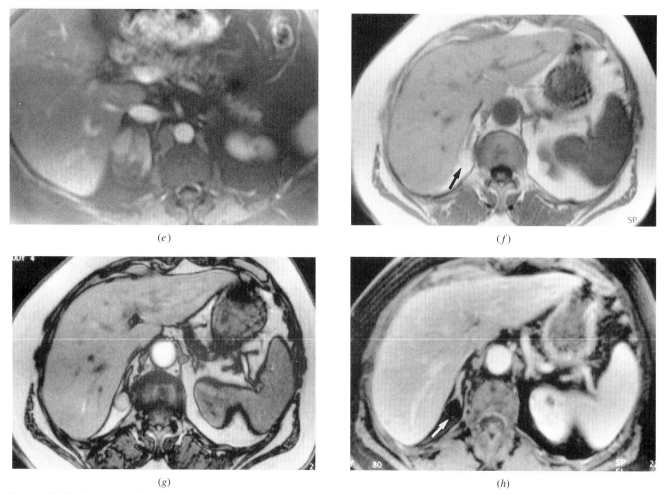

(e)   (f)

(g)   (h)

F I G. 8.19 (*Continued*) Myelolipomas may contain focal accumulation of hematopoietic cells within mature adipose tissue, which this focal region represents. The mass is hypointense on T1 fat-suppressed image (*c*), with no suppression of the same focal region. Negligible enhancement on immediate (*d*) and late (*e*) images is appreciated. The predominantly fatty portion of the tumor is low signal on the fat-suppressed image.

T1-weighted SGE (*f*), T1-weighted out-of-phase SGE (*g*), and 90-s postgadolinium fat-suppressed SGE (*h*) images in a second patient. A 1.8-cm myelolipoma (arrow, *f*) is present of the right adrenal. The tumor is high in signal intensity on the in-phase SGE image because it is composed almost entirely of fat. No drop in signal is present on the out-of-phase image (*g*), reflecting the near complete absence of water protons in the mass. On the fat-suppressed image the mass is near signal void (arrow, *h*), confirming that it is essentially all fat in composition.

that signal loss does not occur on out-of-phase images but signal loss is comparable to fat on fat-suppressed images.

Adrenal Cyst and Pseudocyst. Adrenal cysts are an uncommon, heterogeneous group of lesions, with most cases reported as an incidental finding. They have traditionally been divided into four categories: endothelial, hemorrhagic (pseudocyst), epithelial, and parasitic. Endothelial cysts and hemorrhagic pseudocysts are the most common types. Hemorrhagic pseudocysts are usually unilocular cystic masses encased in a fibrous capsule and containing amorphous abnormal material, blood, and fibrin. Microscopic examination reveals numerous irregular, thin-walled vascular channels. In contrast, endothelial cysts are usually multilocular and filled with

clear, milky fluid. Histologic examination shows a thin fibrous wall lined by a continuous layer of endothelial cells.

The majority of adrenal cysts and pseudocysts are low in signal intensity on T1-weighted images and high in signal intensity on T2-weighted images [12]. Adrenal cysts are sharply marginated and signal void on gadolinium-enhanced MR images. Because most pseudocysts result from adrenal hemorrhage, variable signal intensity on T1- and T2-weighted images may be observed (fig. 8.20) [42]. Pseudocysts that contain substantial concentration of extracellular methemoglobin from subacute hemorrhage may remain slightly hyperintense on gadolinium-enhanced images. Imaging early and late after gadolinium is useful to ensure that lesions do not enhance over time and therefore are cysts [11].

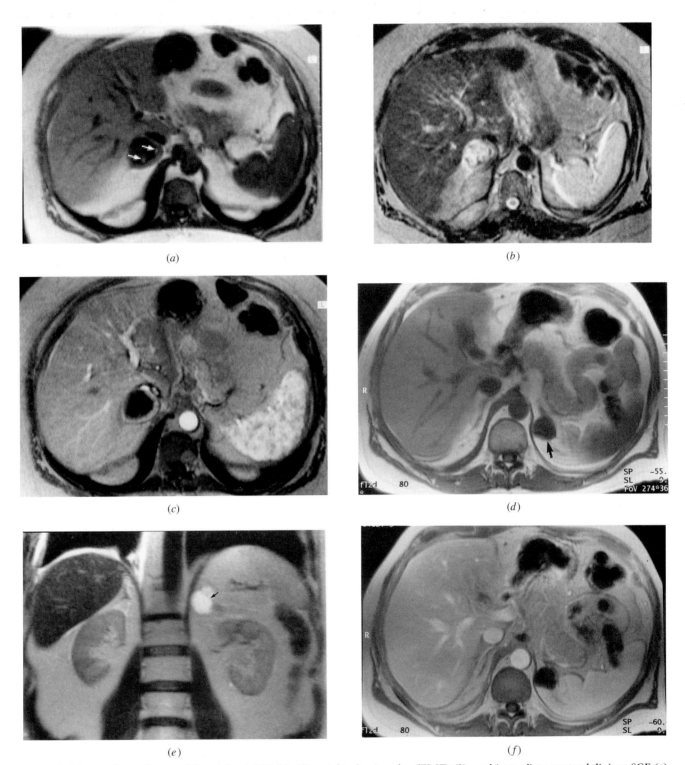

F I G . 8.20 Cyst/pseudocyst. T1-weighted SGE (*a*), T2-weighted spin-echo (T2-SE) (*b*), and immediate postgadolinium SGE (*c*) images. Small high-signal intensity foci are noted on the T1 image (arrows, *a*) within the low-signal intensity pseudocyst, a finding consistent with hemorrhage. The mass is heterogeneous and high in signal intensity on the T2-weighted image (*b*). The heterogeneity reflects the presence of blood products. The lesion is signal void on early (*c*) and late (not shown) postgadolinium images, which are diagnostic features for a cyst.

T1-weighted SGE (*d*), coronal T2-weighted single-shot echo-train spin-echo (SS-ETSE) (*e*), 45-s postgadolinium SGE (*f*), and 90-s postgadolinium fat-suppressed SGE (*g*) images in a second patient. An adrenal pseudocyst is identified arising from the left adrenal (arrow, *d*). The pseudocyst is low in signal intensity on the T1-weighted image (*d*), and high in signal intensity on the T2-weighted image (*e*) and does not enhance on early (*f*) or late (*g*) postgadolinium images.

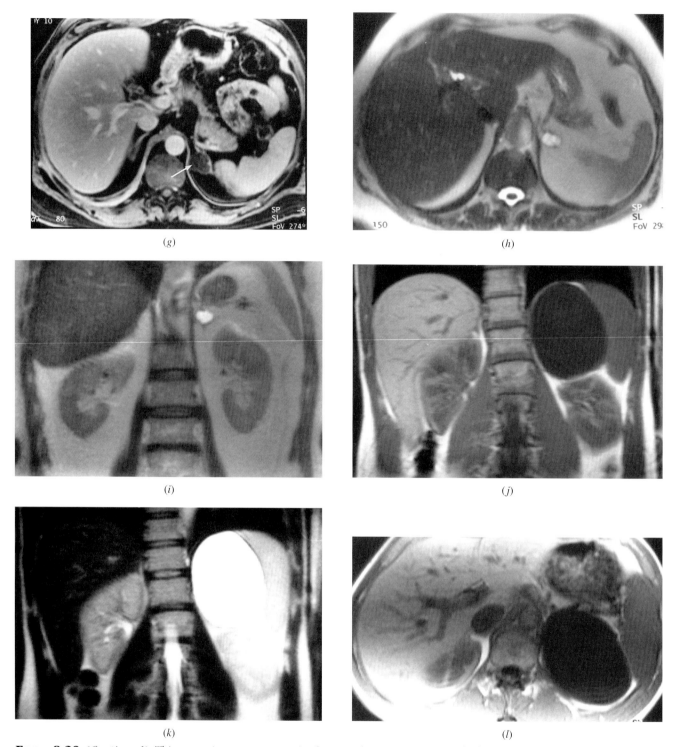

(g)

(h)

(i)

(j)

(k)

(l)

F I G .   8.20 (*Continued*) Thin septations are present in the pseudocyst (arrow, *e*), which are well shown on the breathing-independent T2-weighted image (*e*) and show faint enhancement on the interstitial-phase gadolinium-enhanced fat-suppressed image (arrow, *g*).

T2-weighted single-shot echo-train spin-echo (SS-ETSE) (*h*) and coronal T2-weighted single-shot echo-train spin-echo (SS-ETSE) (*i*) images in a third patient. A pseudocyst in the left adrenal contains septations that are well shown on the snap shot T2-weighted images (*h*, *i*) as hypointense linear structures.

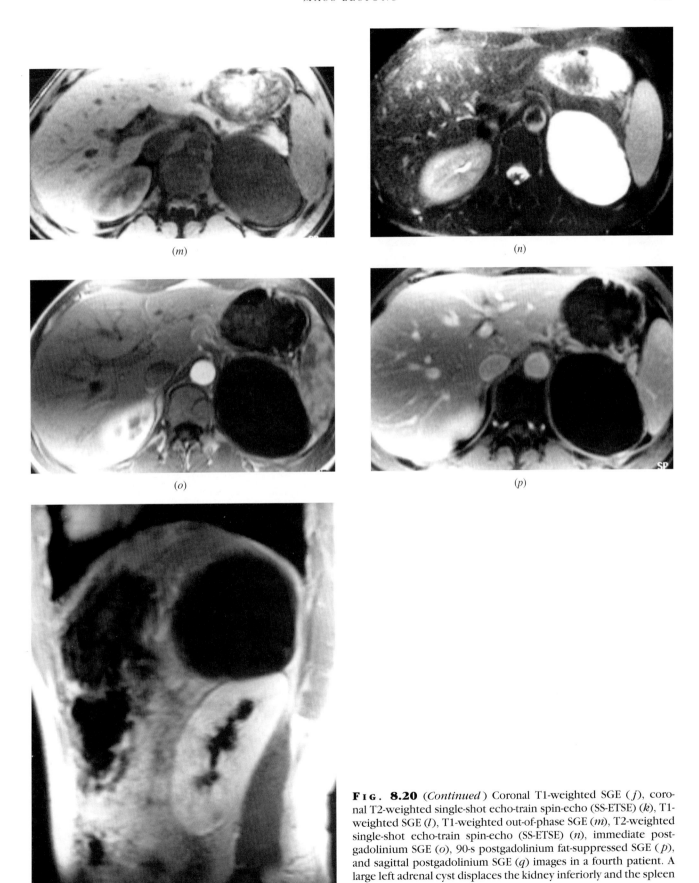

(m)

(n)

(o)

(p)

(q)

F I G. 8.20 *(Continued)* Coronal T1-weighted SGE (*j*), coronal T2-weighted single-shot echo-train spin-echo (SS-ETSE) (*k*), T1-weighted SGE (*l*), T1-weighted out-of-phase SGE (*m*), T2-weighted single-shot echo-train spin-echo (SS-ETSE) (*n*), immediate post-gadolinium SGE (*o*), 90-s postgadolinium fat-suppressed SGE (*p*), and sagittal postgadolinium SGE (*q*) images in a fourth patient. A large left adrenal cyst displaces the kidney inferiorly and the spleen anterior and laterally (*j*, *k*, *q*).

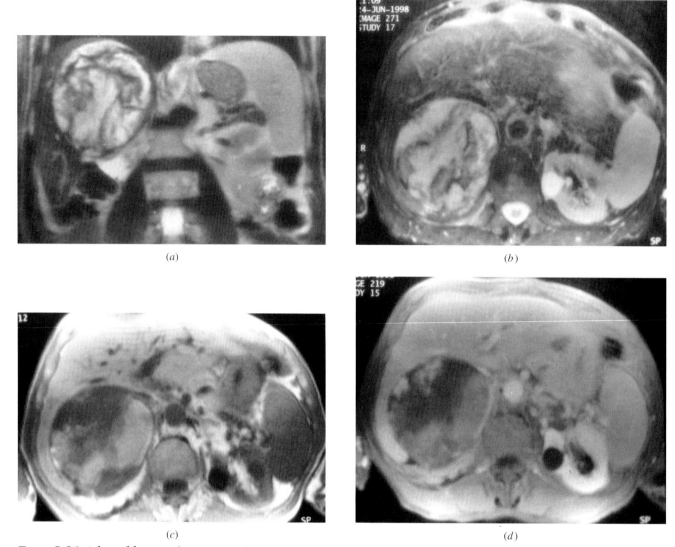

(a)   *(b)*

(c)   *(d)*

F I G . 8.21 Adrenal hemangioma. Coronal T2-weighted SS-ETSE (*a*), fat suppressed T2-weighted ETSE (*b*), T1-weighted SGE (*c*), and 90 s post gadolinium fat suppressed SGE (*d*) images. A large, 10 cm, mass is present in the right adrenal which is heterogeneous and high signal intensity on T2- (*a, b*) and T1-weighted (*c*) images, consistent with hemorrhage and central necrosis. Peripheral enhancing nodules are apparent on the gadolinium-enhanced image (*d*).

Hypovascular neoplasms may be nearly signal void on early postcontrast images but enhance on later postgadolinium images. Pseudocysts may be large in size, and sagittal-plane imaging may be useful to demonstrate the location of the mass.

> ***Hemangioma.*** Adrenal hemangioma is an uncommon, benign vascular tumor composed of mesenchymal cells. The lesions tend to be large (>10 cm) and undergo central necrosis and hemorrhage [43]. Peripheral nodules are characteristic of these masses [43]. Tumors are high in signal intensity centrally on T1- and T2-weighted images because of necrosis and hemorrhage [43]. The peripheral nodules enhance intensely with gadolinium, and the centripetal enhancement, which is characteristic of hepatic hemangiomas, is less frequently observed in adrenal

hemangiomas because of the substantial central necrosis (fig. 8.21) [44]. These tumors may resemble adrenal cortical carcinomas because of the central necrosis and hemorrhage [25].

Malignant

> ***Metastases.*** Metastases are the most frequent malignant lesions that involve the adrenal glands. The most common primary tumors originate from lung, breast, gastrointestinal tract, kidney, skin (melanoma), and thyroid gland [45].

Metastatic deposits vary in size from microscopic involvement to large tumor masses. Metastases are most frequently bilateral, but they may be unilateral. On T2-weighted images, metastases have been described as having moderately high signal intensity (fig. 8.22) [1–5].

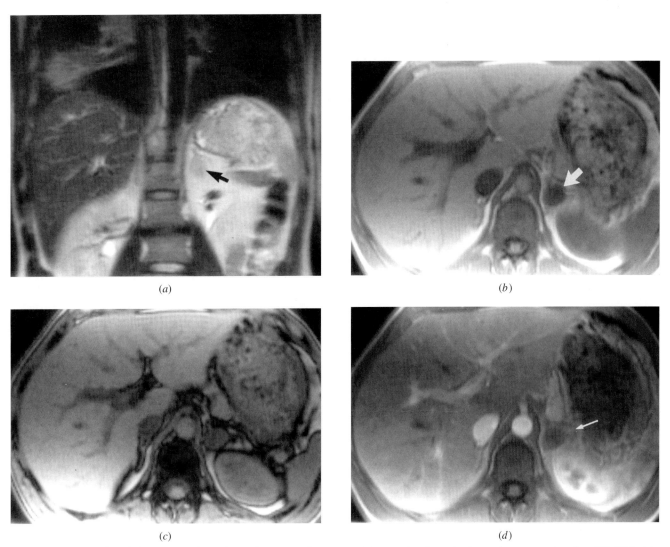

(a)

(b)

(c)

(d)

F I G . 8.22 Small left hypovascular adrenal metastasis. Coronal T2-weighted single-shot echo-train spin-echo (SS-ETSE) (*a*), T1-weighted SGE (*b*), T1-weighted out-of-phase SGE (*c*), and immediate postgadolinium SGE (*d*) images. A 1.5-cm metastasis is heterogeneous and moderately high in signal intensity on the T2-weighted image (arrow, *a*). The tumor is hypointense on T1 (*b*) and does not show signal drop on the out-of-phase image (*c*). On immediate postgadolinium image, the tumor demonstrates negligible enhancement with a thin rim (arrow, *d*).

High signal intensity on T2-weighted image should not be relied on. Many metastases, particularly those possessing significant desmoplasia, may be low signal intensity (fig. 8.23) [4, 5], whereas a number of benign lesions may be high signal [26]. Comparison of the signal intensity of the adrenal mass to either the primary tumor or other metastatic deposits may be helpful in determining if the lesion is a metastasis, because foci of tumor located in different sites frequently possess similar signal intensity [3]. Metastases frequently have irregular margins and enhance in a heterogeneous fashion, features that are well shown on gadolinium-enhanced T1-weighted fat-suppressed images [8]. Mild, heterogeneous enhancement on early postgadolinium images is commonly observed, with either progressive enhancement or minimal heterogeneous washout on more delayed interstitial-phase images. This pattern is distinct

from that manifested by adenomas which often exhibit a capillary blush. Direct extension of primary tumors may occasionally be seen. This is most frequently observed in pancreatic or renal cancer. The adrenal tumor may also invade adjacent structures or organs (fig. 8.24). Necrosis and hemorrhage are not uncommon in large metastatic deposits (figs. 8.25 and 8.26). Hemorrhage is also a feature more typical of malignant than benign masses and is better shown on MR than CT images.

The most reliable MRI feature to suggest that an adrenal mass may represent a metastasis is the demonstration that the lesion does not lose signal on out-of-phase images (see figs. 8.22–8.24) [9–10, 20]. This approach is most reliable in the investigation of patients with a known primary malignancy.

Because the accuracy of out-of-phase gradient echo images to characterize adrenal masses as benign or

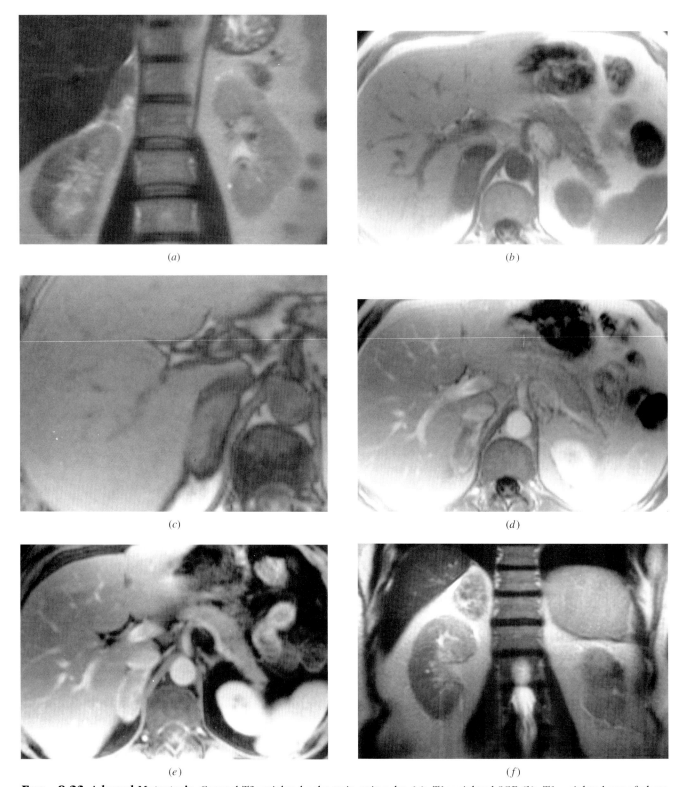

F I G . 8.23 Adrenal Metastasis. Coronal T2-weighted echo-train spin-echo (*a*), T1-weighted SGE (*b*), T1-weighted out-of-phase SGE (*c*), immediate postgadolinium SGE (*d*), and 90-s postgadolinium fat-suppressed SGE (*e*) images in a patient with primary non-small cell lung cancer. A 5.4 × 2.3-cm oval right adrenal metastasis is slightly hypointense to the liver on the in-phase image (*b*), with no drop in signal on the out-of-phase image. (*c*) After contrast administration, there is peripheral, irregular enhancement of the lesion (*d*, *e*).

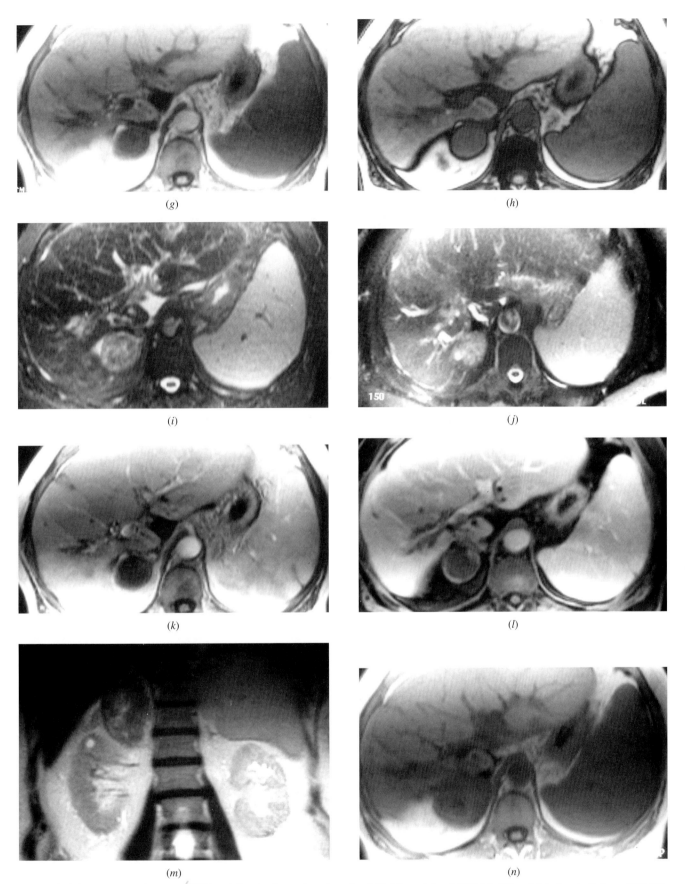

F I G . 8.23 (*Continued*) Coronal T2-weighted echo-train spin-echo (*f*), T1-weighted SGE (*g*), T1-weighted out-of-phase SGE (*h*), T2-weighted echo-train spin-echo (*i*), STIR (*j*), immediate postgadolinium SGE (*k*), and 90-s postgadolinium fat-suppressed SGE (*l*) images in a second patient, who had primary colon cancer.

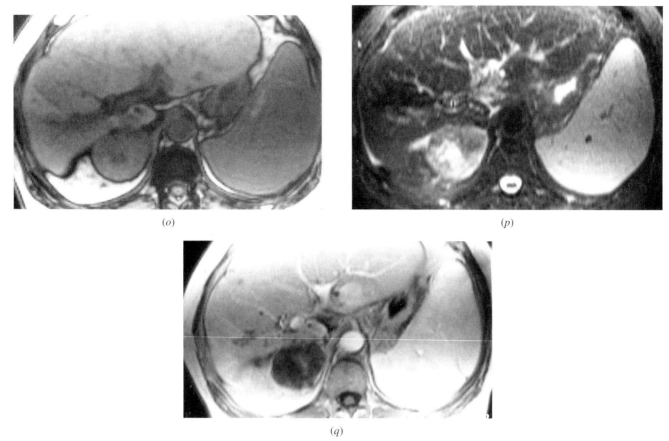

(o)   *(p)*

(q)

FIG. 8.23 (*Continued*) Coronal T2-weighted echo-train spin-echo (*m*), T1-weighted SGE (*n*), T1-weighted out-of-phase SGE (*o*), STIR (*p*), and immediate postgadolinium SGE (*q*) images in the same patient 3 months later. There is no signal loss comparing in-phase (*g*, *n*) and out-of-phase (*h*, *o*) images. On the T2-weighted images, the adrenal lesion appears heterogeneously hypointense with hyperintense foci (*f*, *i*, *j*, *m*, *p*). Interval growth has occurred after a 3-month interval (*m–q*).

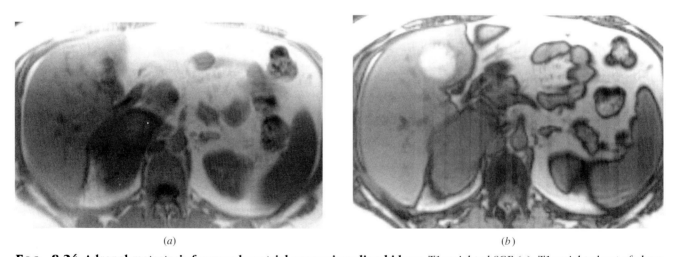

(a)   *(b)*

FIG. 8.24 Adrenal metastasis from endometrial cancer invading kidney. T1-weighted SGE (*a*), T1-weighted out-of-phase (*b*, *c*), and immediate postgadolinium SGE (*d*, *e*) images. A right adrenal metastasis is present which invades the upper pole of the right kidney. The tumor is heterogeneous and predominantly hypointense on T1 (*a*) with no signal drop on out-of-phase (*b*, *c*) images.

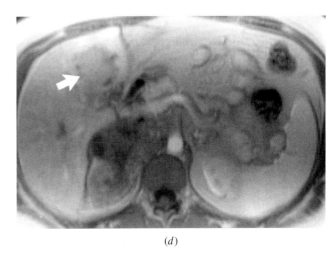

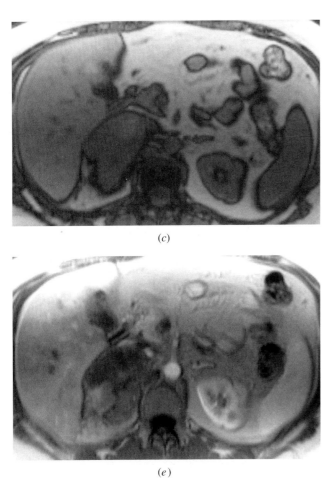

(c)

(d)

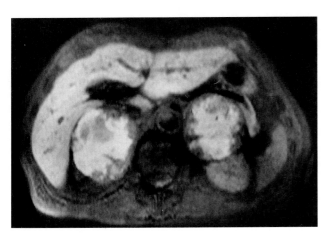

(e)

FIG. 8.24 (*Continued*) It demonstrates a diminished and heterogeneous enhancement on immediate postgadolinium images (*d, e*). Also, note hepatic metastases with irregular margins (arrow, *d*).

malignant is approximately 80%, additional information provided by T2-weighted images and postgadolinium images are useful (figs. 8.24, 8.26, and 8.27). CT-guided biopsies are at present not obviated in all cases by MRI examination. To obviate CT-guided biopsy, accuracy of MRI must approach 95% [46]. Our impression is that accuracy of MR including in-phase, out-of-phase, T2, and serial gadolinium-enhanced images, currently may be between 85 and 90%. However, not all indeterminate adrenal masses need to be biopsied. In patients with

no known primary malignancy, it is acceptable management to serially examine adrenal masses to assess change in size. Reassessment at 3 to 6 months and 1 year is performed at many centers [46–48]. It may be sufficient to acquire only in-phase and out-of-phase SGE images on follow-up examination to reduce cost.

Adrenal Cortical Carcinoma. Adrenal cortical carcinoma is a very uncommon aggressive tumor. Tumors may contain intracytoplasmic lipid or fatty regions.

FIG. 8.25 Hemorrhagic adrenal metastases. T1-weighted fat-suppressed spin-echo image demonstrates high-signal intensity subacute hemorrhage in bilateral adrenal metastases. Metastasis may undergo hemorrhage, simulating primary adrenal cortical carcinoma.

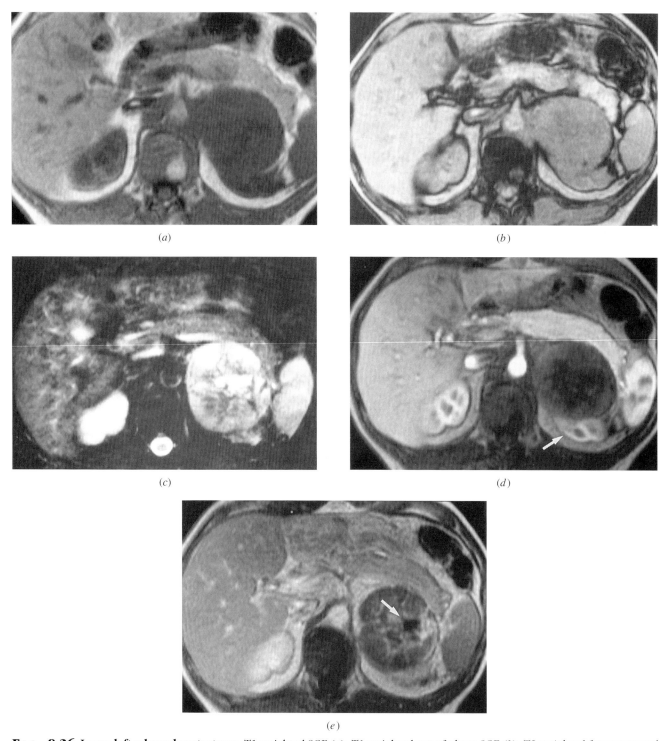

(a)   (b)

(c)   (d)

(e)

FIG. 8.26 Large left adrenal metastases. T1-weighted SGE (*a*), T1-weighted out-of-phase SGE (*b*), T2-weighted fat-suppressed spin-echo (*c*), immediate postgadolinium (*d*), and 3-min postgadolinium SGE (*e*) images. A large 8-cm left adrenal metastasis is identified that retains signal intensity from in-phase (*a*) to out-of-phase (*b*) images. The mass is heterogeneous and moderately high in signal intensity on T2-weighted images, with a central high-signal intensity region (*c*). On immediate postgadolinium image (*d*), the mass enhances minimally. On more delayed images, a central low-signal intensity signal-void region compatible with necrosis is identified (arrows, *e*) that corresponds to the region of high signal intensity on T2-weighted images. The central necrosis and heterogeneity demonstrated on T2-weighted and postgadolinium images further confirm the findings on out-of-phase images corresponding to a malignant mass. Distinction between adrenal metastasis and left kidney is best defined on the immediate postgadolinium SGE image by the demonstration of corticomedullary differentiation of the kidney (arrow, *d*).

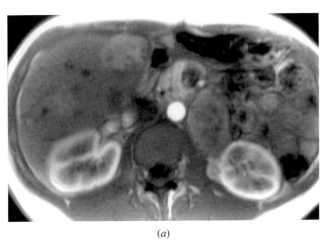
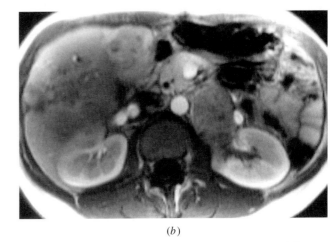

(a) (b)

FIG. 8.27 Adrenal metastasis from pancreatic gastrinoma. Immediate (a) and 45-s (b) postgadolinium SGE images. There is a 5-cm metastasis in the left adrenal with irregular patchy enhancement on the immediate postgadolinium image (a) that persists on the later image (b). Liver metastases are also appreciated.

The tumor is more common in women, and the age at presentation ranges from 20 to 70 years, although tumor occurrence in patients 20–40 years of age is not unusual [24]. Approximately 50% of the tumors are hyperfunctioning, and hypercortisolism and virilization are common presentations. In contrast to adrenal adenomas, adrenal cortical carcinomas are characteristically large encapsulated tumors, weighing over 100 g and sometimes reaching 1000 g or more before discovery. Areas of necrosis and hemorrhage are frequent [49].

Metastases are frequently found at presentation, with regional and para-aortic lymph nodes, lungs, and liver (fig. 8.28) representing common sites. Tumor thrombus into the IVC is not uncommon at presentation

(fig. 8.28). Tumors are frequently necrotic (figs. 8.28–8.30) and hemorrhagic.

In one series, MR images demonstrated central necrosis and hemorrhage in seven of eight adrenal cortical carcinomas [25]. These tumors appear heterogeneous and hyperintense on T1- and T2-weighted images, reflecting central necrosis and hemorrhage. Necrosis is well shown on gadolinium-enhanced images as signal-void regions, and hemorrhage is well shown on precontrast T1-weighted conventional or fat-suppressed images as high-signal intensity regions (fig. 8.29). Peripheral mural-based nodules may also be observed in these tumors (fig. 8.30) [25]. Although the appearance of a large mass with central hemorrhage and

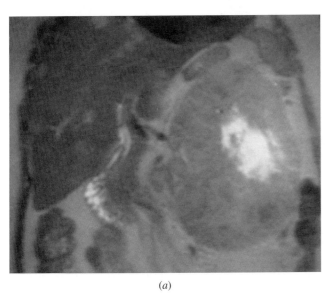
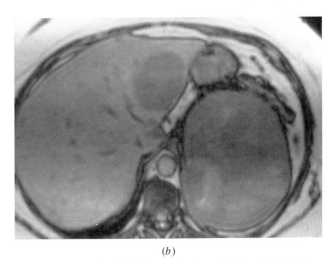

(a) (b)

FIG. 8.28 Adrenal cortical carcinoma. Coronal T2-weighted echo-train spin-echo (a), T1-weighted out-of-phase SGE (b), immediate postgadolinium SGE (c), and 90-s postgadolinium fat-suppressed SGE images (d, e). The large left adrenal cortical carcinoma is heterogeneous on T2 (a).

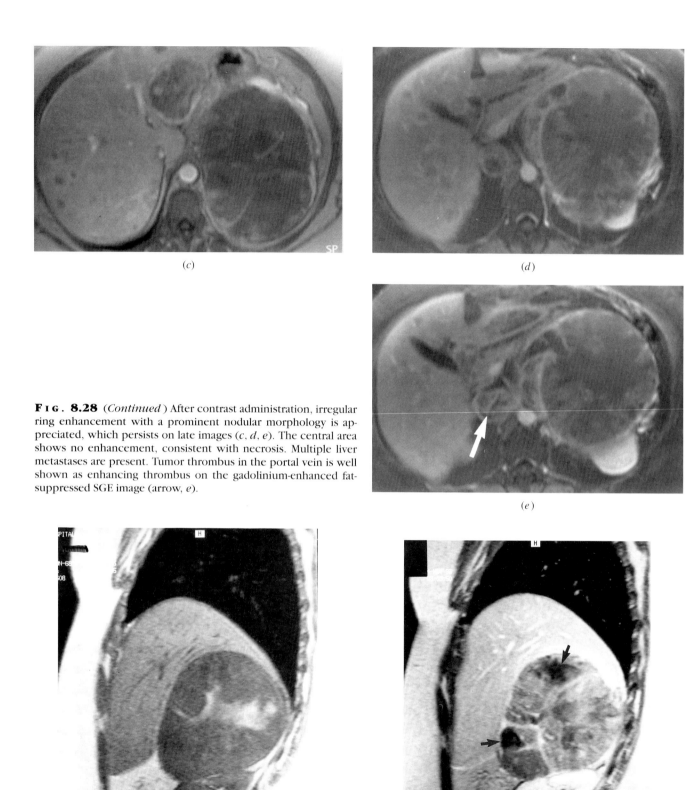

(c)

(d)

F I G . 8.28 (*Continued*) After contrast administration, irregular ring enhancement with a prominent nodular morphology is appreciated, which persists on late images (*c, d, e*). The central area shows no enhancement, consistent with necrosis. Multiple liver metastases are present. Tumor thrombus in the portal vein is well shown as enhancing thrombus on the gadolinium-enhanced fat-suppressed SGE image (arrow, *e*).

(e)

(a)

(b)

F I G . 8.29 Adrenal cortical carcinoma. Sagittal T1-weighted SGE (*a*) and 90-s postgadolinium SGE (*b*) images in a 25-year-old woman. A 7-cm mass is identified in the right upper abdomen that indents the liver and displaces the right kidney inferiorly. The relationship of the mass to the kidney and liver is clearly defined in profile in the sagittal projection, and the mass is shown to be separate from these organs. High signal intensity is present on precontrast images, a finding consistent with central hemorrhage. The mass enhances heterogeneously after contrast administration and contains signal-void regions of necrosis (arrows, *b*). (Reproduced with permission from Schlund JF, Kenney PJ, Brown ED, Ascher SM, Brown JJ, Semelka RC: Adrenocortical carcinoma: MR imaging appearance with current technique. *J Magn Reson Imaging* 5: 171–174, 1995.)

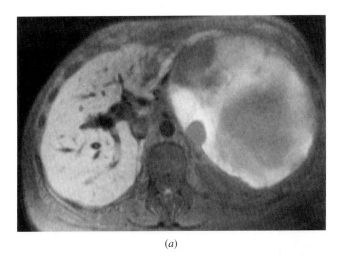

(a)

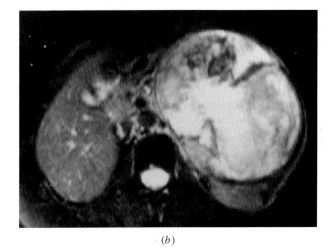

(b)

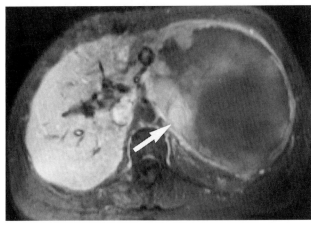

(c)

FIG. 8.30 Adrenal cortical carcinoma. T1-weighted fat-suppressed spin-echo (a), T2-weighted fat-suppressed spin-echo (b), and gadolinium-enhanced fat-suppressed spin-echo (c) images in a 41-year-old woman. On the precontrast T1-weighted image, central high signal intensity is present in the tumor, which is consistent with blood (a). On the T2-weighted image, the tumor is heterogeneous and high in signal intensity because of the presence of central necrosis and blood products of varying age (b). Peripheral nodules enhance after contrast administration (arrow, c), and the central portion of the tumor remains largely signal void. (Reproduced with permission from Schlund JF, Kenney PJ, Brown ED, Ascher SM, Brown JJ, Semelka RC: Adrenocortical carcinoma: MR imaging appearance with current technique. *J Magn Reson Imaging* 5: 171–174, 1995.)

necrosis is characteristic for adrenal cortical carcinoma, a similar appearance may be observed in other tumors including adrenal hemangioma [43] and neuroblastoma [50].

Smaller tumors also tend to have greater enhancement of the tumor periphery than of the center, possibly reflecting their propensity to undergo central

necrosis (fig. 8.31) [25]. Fat-suppressed images help delineate large tumors from adjacent pancreas and kidney. Sagittal-plane images are also useful to demonstrate that tumors do not originate from the kidney (fig. 8.29). On T2-weighted images, tumors have a high signal intensity, which partly reflects the frequent occurrence of central necrosis [3, 25, 51]. Because these tumors are functional,

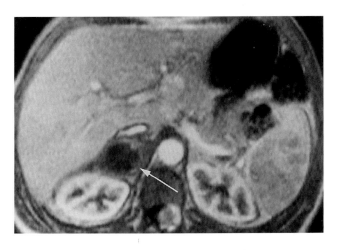

FIG. 8.31 Small adrenal cortical carcinoma. Immediate postgadolinium SGE image demonstrates a 2.5-cm right adrenal cortical carcinoma (arrow). Note that the tumor has an enhancing rim and is hypovascular centrally. (Reproduced with permission from Semelka RC, Shoenut JP: The adrenal glands. In Semelka RC, Shoenut JP (eds.), *MRI of the Abdomen with CT Correlation.* New York: Raven Press, p. 77–90, 1993.)

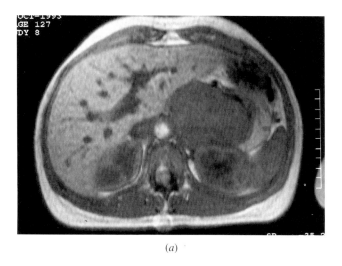

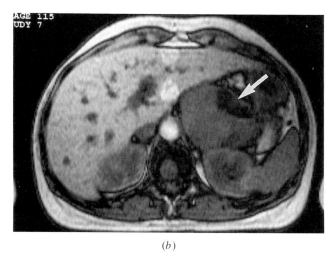

(a)

(b)

FIG. 8.32 Adrenal cortical carcinoma with signal loss on out-of-phase imaging. T1-weighted SGE (*a*), T1-weighted out-of-phase SGE (*b*), and T2-weighted fat-suppressed spin-echo (*c*) images in a 37-year-old woman. On the out-of-phase image, a moderate-sized region of the tumor loses signal (arrow, *b*) compared to the in-phase image, a finding consistent with fatty tissue. On the fat-suppressed T2-weighted image, (*c*) the tumor is hyperintense and contains a region of low signal (curved arrow, *c*) representing fat and corresponding to the region of signal drop on the out-of-phase image (*b*). (Reproduced with permission from Schlund JF, Kenney PJ, Brown ED, Ascher SM, Brown JJ, Semelka RC: Adrenocortical carcinoma: MR imaging appearance with current technique. *J Magn Reson Imaging* 5: 171–174, 1995.)

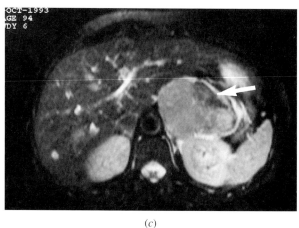

(c)

they may contain regions of intracytoplasmic lipid that result in irregular foci of signal intensity loss on out-of-phase images (fig. 8.32) [25, 52, 53]. The lack of uniform loss of signal intensity helps to distinguish these tumors from adenomas.

Medullary Masses

The adrenal medulla is composed of neuroendocrine cells derived from the neural crest. As such, it is part of the widely dispersed system of histologically and embryologically similar cells termed the paraganglion system. The most significant disorders arising in the adrenal medulla are neoplasms derived from cell types indigenous to the paraganglion system. These tumors include pheochromocytoma, neuroblastoma, and ganglioneuroma.

Pheochromocytoma

Pheochromocytoma can be defined as a paraganglioma of the adrenal medulla and is a catecholamine-producing tumor. On microscopic examination, a characteristic pattern shows tumor cells arranged in well-defined nests

("Zellballen") surrounded by fibrovascular stroma. There is no morphologic marker of malignancy for this tumor other than the presence of metastasis. Pheochromocytomas arise from the adrenal medulla in 90% of cases. The remaining 10% occur in paraganglia along the course of the sympathetic chain, most frequently in a paraaortic or paracaval location including the organs of Zuckerkandl (located at the aortic bifurcation). Mediastinal and bladder wall tumors account for 2% of pheochromocytomas. Most of the tumors are unilateral and frequently greater than 3 cm in diameter at presentation [54]. Pheochromocytomas are bilateral in 10% of cases and malignant in about 10% of cases, with metastatic spread occurring most commonly to lymph nodes, bone, and liver. Extra-adrenal origin tumors are malignant in a greater percentage of cases (40%). Patients present with sustained or paroxysmal hypertension, and the great majority of symptomatic patients have elevated levels of urinary catecholamines and their metabolites, principally vanillylmandelic acid (VMA), and metanephron. Patients with multiple endocrine neoplasia (MEN) type IIA or IIB, neurofibromatosis, von Hippel-Lindau disease, and multiple cutaneous neuromas have increased incidence

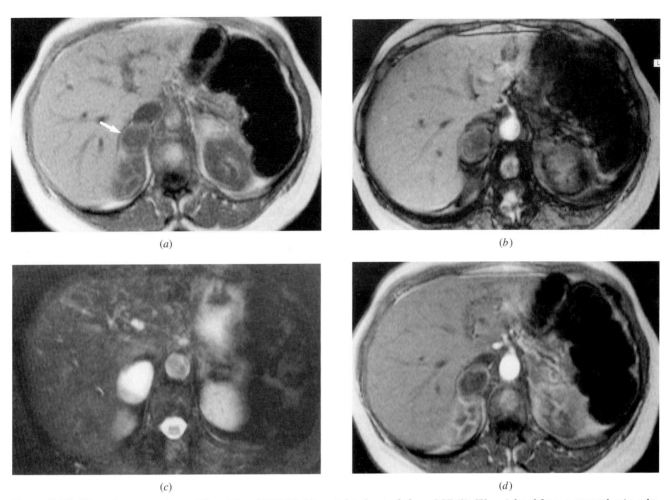

F I G . 8.33 Pheochromocytoma. T1-weighted SGE (*a*), T1-weighted out-of-phase SGE (*b*), T2-weighted fat-suppressed spin-echo (*c*), immediate postgadolinium SGE (*d*), (and 2-min postgadolinium SGE (*e*) images). A 2.5-cm pheochromocytoma arises from the right adrenal gland (arrow, *a*), which has a moderate-signal intensity peripheral rim with a low-signal intensity center on in-phase (*a*) and out-of-phase (*b*) SGE images. No appreciable drop in signal intensity is present on the out-of-phase image. On the T2-weighted image (*c*), the mass is extremely high in signal intensity, with the peripheral rim appearing slightly low in signal intensity (*c*). On the immediate postgadolinium image the tumor rim enhances intensely with minimal central enhancement (*d*).

of pheochromocytomas. Seventy-five percent of patients with MEN II have bilateral tumors, which are rarely extra-adrenal [55]. Cystic pheochromocytomas occur, and distinction from cysts may be difficult [56].

Pheochromocytomas characteristically are hypointense on T1-weighted images and hyperintense on T2-weighted images (fig. 8.33) [1] because of their high interstitial fluid space that in part may reflect necrotic, hemorrhagic, or cystic regions (fig. 8.34) that are observed on gross or microscopic pathologic analysis. Although pheochromocytomas may appear very bright (e.g., "light bulbs") on T2-weighted images, the majority are heterogeneous and moderately high signal and in rare instances, they may have moderate signal intensity [12]. A confounding variable is the signal intensity of background fat, which depends on the type of sequence employed. On echo-train spin-echo images, masses

tend to appear lower in signal intensity, whereas on fat-suppressed images masses appear higher in signal intensity. This reflects a signal intensity rescaling effect, reflecting the signal intensity of the background fat; when fat is dark the adrenal mass signal intensity is rescaled and appears brighter. MRI may be the technique of choice to examine for pheochromocytomas because these lesions are most often relatively high in signal intensity on T2-weighted images independent of tumor size and location [12, 57]. Therefore, small extra-adrenal lesions are conspicuous on T2-weighted images and are usually distinguishable from other structures such as lymph nodes and bowel, which are lower in signal intensity. Cystic pheochromocytomas are as high in signal intensity as cerebrospinal fluid (CSF) on T2-weighted images [58]. Pheochromocytomas usually enhance minimally on immediate postgadolinium images and

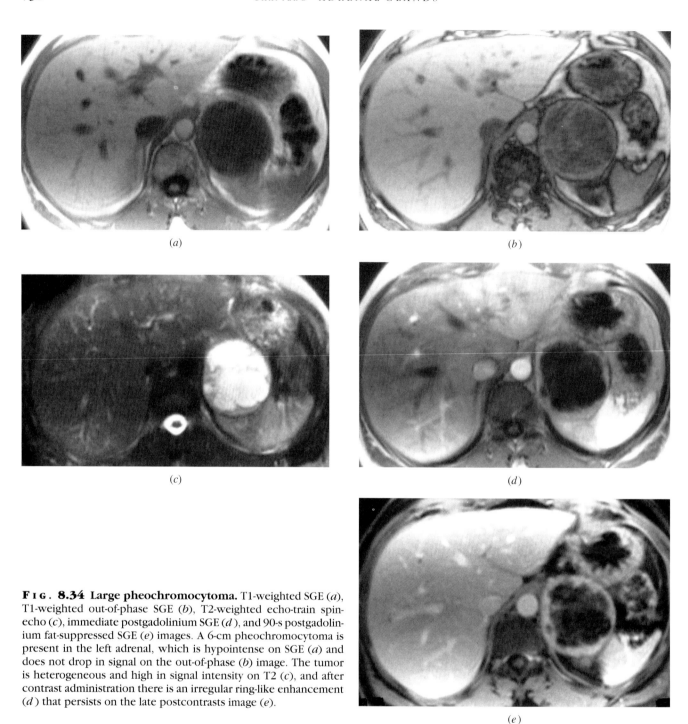

FIG. 8.34 Large pheochromocytoma. T1-weighted SGE (*a*), T1-weighted out-of-phase SGE (*b*), T2-weighted echo-train spin-echo (*c*), immediate postgadolinium SGE (*d*), and 90-s postgadolinium fat-suppressed SGE (*e*) images. A 6-cm pheochromocytoma is present in the left adrenal, which is hypointense on SGE (*a*) and does not drop in signal on the out-of-phase (*b*) image. The tumor is heterogeneous and high in signal intensity on T2 (*c*), and after contrast administration there is an irregular ring-like enhancement (*d*) that persists on the late postcontrasts image (*e*).

demonstrate progressive enhancement on later interstitial-phase images (see fig. 8.33), although relatively intense early enhancement may be observed. If early intense enhancement occurs, it reflects the capillary-rich framework within the tumor, which may also contribute to the high signal intensity on T2-weighted images (fig. 8.35). In general, pheochromocytomas do not lose signal intensity on out-of-phase images.

Neuroblastoma, Ganglioglioma, and Ganglioneuroblastoma

This group of neoplasms is distinguished by a broad range in differentiation from primitive neuroblastoma at one end of the spectrum to well-differentiated, mature ganglioneuroma at the opposite end. Tumors with intermediary cytological maturation are termed ganglioneuroblastomas.

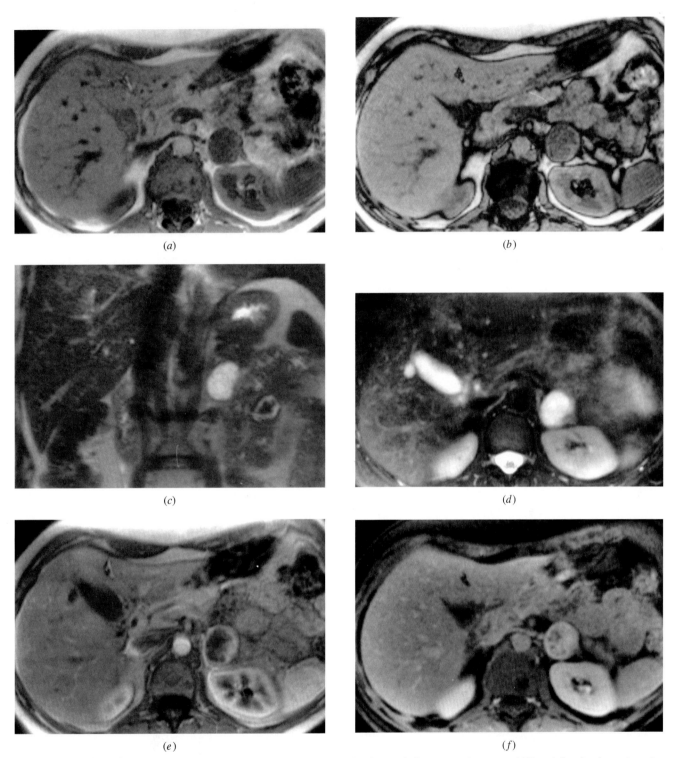

(a)

(b)

(c)

(d)

(e)

(f)

F I G . 8.35 Pheochromocytoma. T1-weighted SGE (a), T1-weighted out-of-phase SGE (b), coronal T2-weighted echo-train spin-echo (c), T2-weighted echo-train spin-echo (d), immediate postgadolinium SGE (e), and 90-s postgadolinium fat-suppressed SGE (f) images. A pheochromocytoma is present in the left adrenal, which is mildly low signal intensity on T1 (a) and does not drop in signal on the out-of-phase image (b). It appears high signal intensity on T2 (c, d), and after gadolinium administration there is irregular ringlike enhancement (e) with progressive and heterogeneous enhancement on the late image (f). The late enhancement reflects progressive passage of gadolinium into the interstitial space of the tumor.

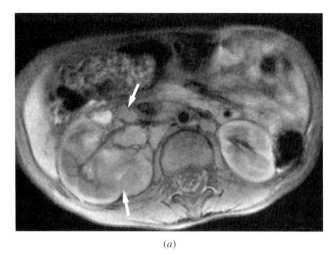
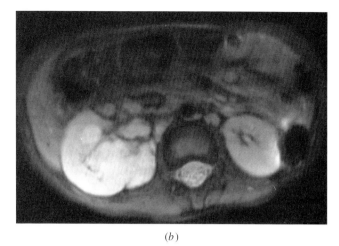

(a)   (b)

F I G . 8.36 Neuroblastoma. T1-weighted SGE (*a*) and T2-weighted fat-suppressed echo-train spin-echo (*b*) images. A right adrenal neuroblastoma is present that invades the right kidney (arrow, *a*).

Neuroblastoma is one of the most common solid tumors of children younger than 5 years of age [59]. Tumors originate from neural crest cells. Neuroblastomas most commonly arise from the adrenal medulla or cells in adjacent retroperitoneal tissue (figs. 8.36 and 8.37). In older patients, extra-adrenal sites increase in frequency [60]. As neuroblastomas occur most commonly in infants, extra-adrenal presentation, although less common than adrenal location, is still relatively frequently observed in these patients (fig. 8.38).

The most common sites of metastatic disease include the skeletal system, liver (fig. 8.39), and lymph nodes. Tumors are generally high in signal intensity on T2-weighted images and enhance with gadolinium. Extension into the neural canal is a feature of these tumors. Encasement of the aorta and IVC is a common feature of advanced disease (fig. 8.40). MRI is particularly effective at evaluating both the primary tumor and metastases in these patients, who are predominantly pediatric, because of high intrinsic soft tissue contrast resolution, which is beneficial in patients with minimal body fat. Direct multiplanar imaging renders MRI superior to CT imaging for the demonstration of extension into the neural canal, invasion of adjacent organs such as liver [59], and location relative to the diaphragm (see fig. 8.38). T2-weighted fat-suppressed

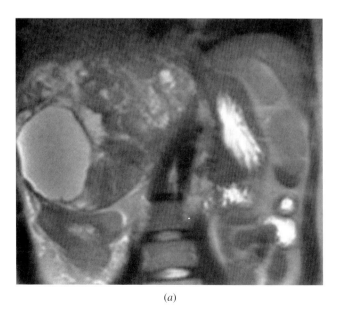
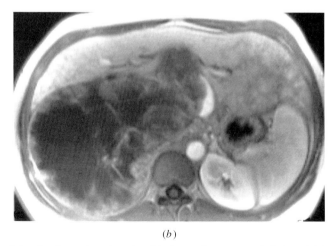

(a)   (b)

F I G . 8.37 Neuroblastoma in an adult patient. Coronal T2-weighted echo-train spin-echo (*a*), immediate postgadolinium SGE (*b*), 90-s postgadolinium fat-suppressed SGE (*c*), MRA source-coronal postcontrast fat-suppressed SGE (*d*), and MIP reconstruction-3D steady state free process postgadolinium (*e*) images. A large neuroblastoma arising from the right adrenal is present that displaces the right kidney inferiorly and compresses the liver anteriorly.

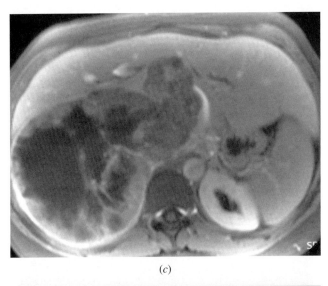

(c)

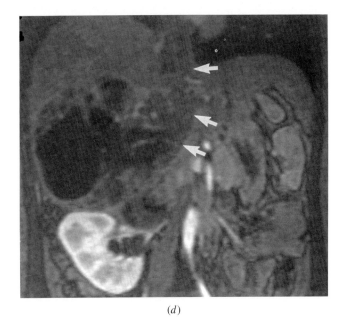

(d)

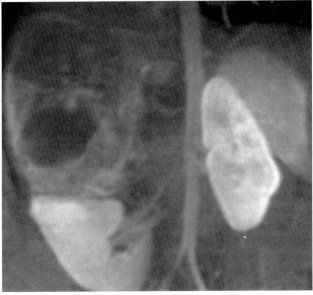

(e)

FIG. 8.37 (*Continued*) The mass is heterogeneous with hyperintense areas on T2 (*a*). After gadolinium administration there is irregular peripheral and internal septa enhancement with central nonenhancing regions that correspond to necrotic areas (*b, c*). Hemorrhage, necrosis, and cystic areas may increase as the tumor increases in size. MRA images demonstrates tumor thrombus in the IVC extending to the right atrium (arrows, *d*).

spin-echo and pre- and postcontrast T1-weighted fat-suppressed spin-echo images in transverse and sagittal planes demonstrate these tumors well (see fig. 8.40). Fat-suppressed spin-echo imaging is generally recommended rather than fat-suppressed SGE techniques in pediatric patients, because patients are often too young to cooperate with breath holding and spin-echo imaging has a higher signal-to-noise ratio, which improves image quality in small patients. Neuroblastoma may have an appearance on MRI indistinguishable from adrenal cortical carcinoma in adult patients, with one reported case [52] appearing as a large tumor with central necrosis and hemorrhage and tumor thrombus in the IVC (see fig. 8.37).

Unlike neuroblastomas, ganglioneuromas typically occur in older patients. Although each of these histologic types may encase vessels [59], ganglioneuroblastoma and ganglioneuroma uncommonly do so, and tend to be smaller and have better-defined margins (fig. 8.41). On MR images, tumors are intermediate in signal intensity on T1-weighted images and slightly heterogeneous and moderately high in signal intensity on T2-weighted images [40]. Enhancement with gadolinium is slightly heterogeneous and moderately intense.

Lymphoma

Lymphoma occasionally involves the adrenal glands secondarily in patients with disseminated malignant

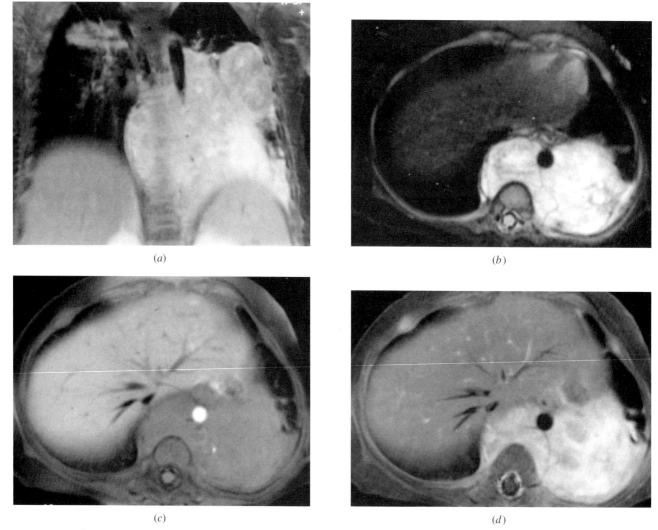

F I G . 8.38 Thoracic neuroblastoma. Coronal T2-weighted echo-train spin-echo of the chest (*a*), T2-weighted fat suppressed echo-train spin-echo (*b*), T1-weighted SGE (*c*), and 90-s fat-suppressed gadolinium-enhanced spin-echo (*d*) images. A large heterogeneously hyperintense mass arises from the left side hemithorax (*a*) and extends into the retrocrural space encasing the descending aorta (*b*, *c*, *d*). After contrast administration, the mass shows diffuse, mildly heterogeneous enhancement on interstitial-phase images (*d*). The posterior mediastinum is the second most common location of neuroblastoma, after adrenal glands.

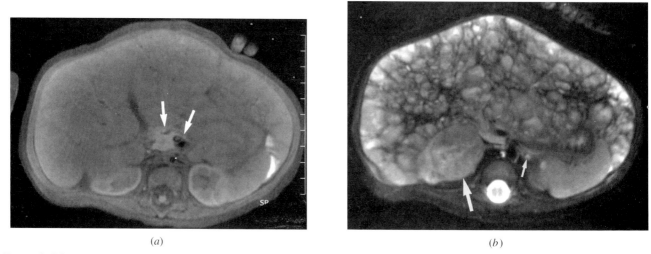

F I G . 8.39 Hepatic metastases from neuroblastoma. T1-weighted fat-suppressed spin-echo (*a*) and T2-weighted fat-suppressed echo-train spin-echo (*b*) images. The liver is massively enlarged, compressing the pancreas (arrows, *a*). Multiple liver metastases are present that appear minimally hypointense on T1 and markedly hyperintense on T2. The primary tumor in the right adrenal (large arrow, *b*) and contralateral involvement of the left adrenal (small arrow, *b*) have similar signal intensity. Neuroblastoma has a tendency to local infiltration, lymph node metastases, and hematogenous spread to liver, lungs, and bones.

lymphoma. The involvement can be uni- or bilateral. Non-Hodgkin lymphoma is the most frequent cell type [61, 62]. Retroperitoneal lymphadenopathy is frequently an associated finding [62]. Signal intensity is intermediate on T1-weighted images and usually intermediate to minimally hyperintense on T2- weighted images. Gadolinium enhancement is variable but is usually minimal on immediate postcontrast images, with increasing enhancement on delayed images (fig. 8.42), which is an enhancement pattern typically observed for lymphoma. Generally, lymphoma enhances throughout its stroma, which reflects the relatively rare occurrence of hemorrhage or necrosis even in large tumors. As with other tumors, if necrosis is present, high signal intensity is observed in this region on T2-weighted images [63], associated with lack of enhancement on postgadolinium images.

MISCELLANEOUS

Inflammatory Disease

The adrenal glands may be involved in granulomatous disease, most commonly tuberculosis, followed by histoplasmosis and blastomycosis [64–66]. Diffuse

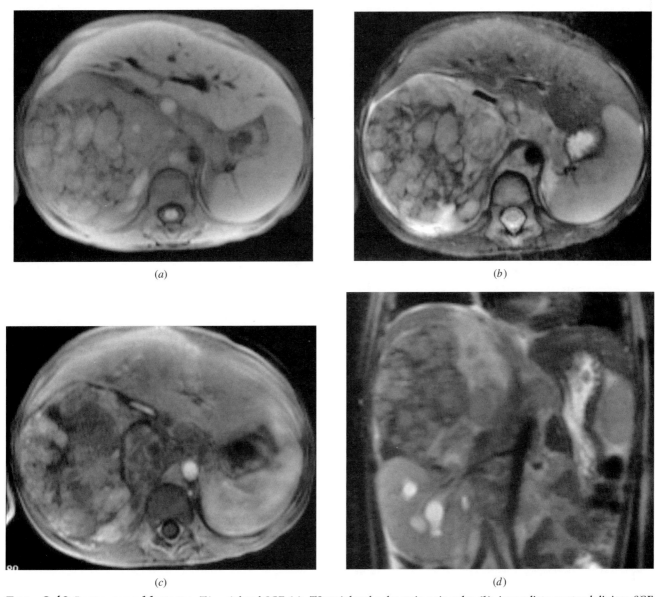

(a)

(b)

(c)

(d)

F I G . 8.40 Large neuroblastoma. T1-weighted SGE (*a*), T2-weighted echo-train spin-echo (*b*), immediate postgadolinium SGE (*c*), coronal T2-weighted echo-train spin-echo (*d*), sagittal 10-min postgadolinium SGE at the level of the left kidney (*e*) and at the level of the IVC (*f*), and immediate postgadolinium SGE at the level of the renal hilum (*g*). Neuroblastoma arising from the right adrenal displaces the right kidney inferiorly (*d*, *e*) and surrounds the IVC (arrow, *f*) and right renal hilum (arrow, *g*).

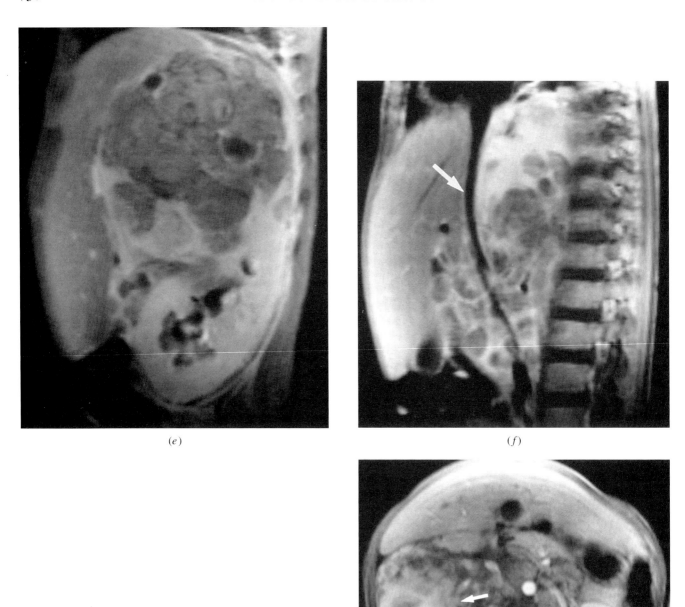

(e)

(f)

(g)

FIG. 8.40 (*Continued*) The tumor has a multinodular appearance with heterogeneous signal intensity on both T1- (*a*) and T2-(*b*) weighted images and peripheral and irregular enhancement on postgadolinium images (*c, e, f, g*).

enlargement of both adrenal glands is the most common appearance. In rare instances, massive enlargement may be seen. Slight heterogeneity of signal intensity is generally observed on T1- and T2-weighted images. Minimal heterogeneous enhancement on early postgadolinium images, which progresses over time, is also common (fig. 8.43). Signal intensity does not drop on out-of-phase images.

Adrenal Hemorrhage

Adrenal hemorrhage occurs secondary to bleeding diathesis, severe stress, blood loss with resultant hypotension (surgery, childbirth, or sepsis), or trauma [55, 67]. The MRI appearance of adrenal hemorrhage in patients with primary antiphospholipid syndrome has also been described [68]. Acute awareness of adrenal

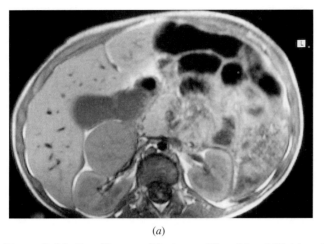

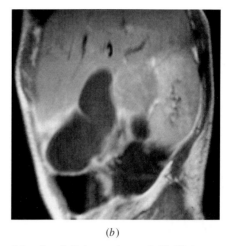

(a) *(b)*

F I G . 8.41 Ganglioneuroblastoma. T1-weighted SE (*a*) and sagittal T1-weighted gadolinium-enhanced SE (*b*) images. A well-defined 3-cm extrarenal mass is identified arising anterior to the upper pole of the right kidney. On the sagittal image (*b*), the mass is shown to abut the liver and kidney, with no evidence of invasion.

hemorrhage on tomographic images is important in that clinical findings may be nonspecific and fatal acute adrenal insufficiency may result [69]. MRI is very sensitive for the detection of adrenal hemorrhage and is superior to CT imaging. Subacute hemorrhage is high in signal intensity on T1-weighted images [68, 70–72], and the high signal intensity is more conspicuous on fat-suppressed T1-weighted images (figs. 8.44 and 8.45). Decrease in lesion size over time helps to confirm that the adrenal enlargement is due to hemorrhage (fig. 8.44).

Addison Disease

Addison disease results from adrenal insufficiency. The tomographic appearance of the adrenal glands may assist in the diagnosis of the underlying cause [65, 69,

72–74]. Autoimmune disease or pituitary insufficiency is suggested by the presence of atrophic glands [59, 60]. Adrenal hemorrhage may be readily diagnosed by the demonstration of high signal intensity substance on T1-weighted images in bilaterally enlarged glands [70–72]. Enlarged glands without hemorrhage suggest granulomatous disease [65]. Metastases may uncommonly result in adrenal insufficiency, and the adrenal glands are massive in this setting.

FUTURE DIRECTIONS

The direction of future advance for MRI of the adrenals may include echoplanar imaging [75] and new contrast agents [76, 77].

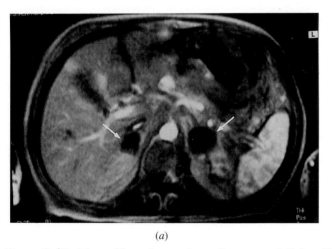

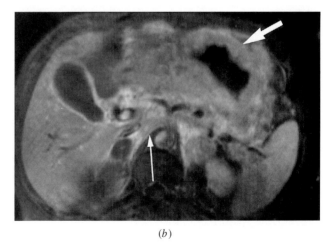

(a) *(b)*

F I G . 8.42 Adrenal lymphoma. Immediate postgadolinium SGE (*a*) and 4-min fat-suppressed gadolinium-enhanced spin-echo (*b*) images. Minimal enhancement is present of bilateral lymphomatous involvement of the adrenals on the immediate postgadolinium images (arrows, *a*). On the more delayed interstitial-phase images, mild diffuse heterogeneous enhancement is apparent (*b*). On the basis of immediate postgadolinium images alone, the adrenal masses could be confused with cysts because of the hypovascularity of the tumors. Diffuse gastric wall involvement (large arrow, *b*) and retroperitoneal adenopathy (thin arrow, *b*) are noted.

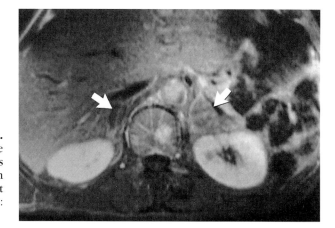

FIG. 8.43 Tuberculosis involvement of the adrenals. Gadolinium-enhanced T1-weighted fat-suppressed spin-echo image demonstrates bilateral adrenal enlargement with heterogeneous mild enhancement (arrows). (Reproduced with permission from Semelka RC, Shoenut JP: The adrenal glands. In Semelka RC, Shoenut JP (eds.), *MRI of the Abdomen with CT Correlation.* New York: Raven Press, p. 77–90, 1993.)

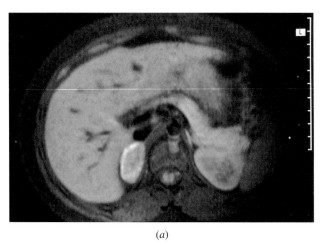

(a)

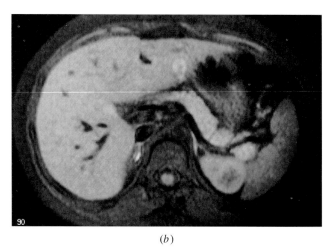

(b)

FIG. 8.44 Adrenal hemorrhage. T1-weighted fat-suppressed spin-echo (*a*) and T1-weighted fat-suppressed spin-echo image obtained 7 weeks later (*b*). The T1-weighted fat-suppressed image acquired 1 week after abdominal trauma (*a*) demonstrates a right adrenal mass with a hyperintense peripheral rim. This appearance is classic for a subacute hematoma. Seven weeks later, the mass has diminished in size and remains high in signal intensity because of persistence of extracellular methemoglobin (*b*).

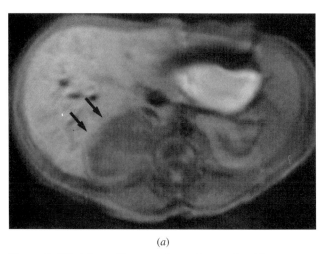

(a)

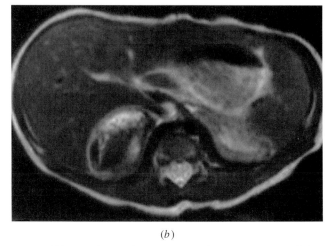

(b)

FIG. 8.45 Adrenal hemorrhage. T1-weighted fat suppressed SGE (*a*) and T2-weighted echo-train spin-echo (*b*) images in a 4-day-old patient. The mass arising from right adrenal is hypointense with a thin hyperintense rim on T1 (*a*), and heterogeneous on T2 (*b*) with hyper- and hypointense areas representing products of hemorrhage. The peripheral high-signal rim on the noncontrast T1-weighted fat-suppressed image (arrows, *a*) represents extracellular methemoglobin and is virtually pathognomonic for a subacute hematoma.

CONCLUSIONS

MRI is an effective means for evaluating adrenal pathology. The combined use of in-phase and out-of-phase SGE images is the most accurate method for distinguishing benign from malignant disease. The acquisition of other additional sequences is recommended to increase the accuracy of lesion characterization as benign or malignant, from 80% using combined in-phase and out-of-phase imaging to between 85 and 90% when T2 and gadolinium enhanced images are also used. MRI is particularly effective at detecting pheochromocytomas, which are moderately high signal on T2-weighted images. Evaluation of the primary tumor and liver metastases is well performed by MRI for adrenal cortical carcinomas and neuroblastoma.

REFERENCES

1. Reining JW, Doppman JL, Dwyer AJ, Johnson AR, Knop RH: Adrenal masses differentiated by MR. *Radiology* 158: 81–84, 1986.
2. Reinig JW, Doppman JL, Dwyer AJ, Frank J: MRI of indeterminate adrenal masses. *Am J Roentgenol* 147: 493–496, 1986.
3. Chang A, Glazer HS, Lee JKT, Ling D, Heiken JP: Adrenal gland: MR imaging. *Radiology* 163: 123–128, 1987.
4. Baker ME, Blinder R, Spritzer C, Leight GS, Herfkens RJ, Dunnick NR: MR evaluation of adrenal masses at 1.5 T. *Am J Roentgenol* 153: 307–312, 1989.
5. Kier R, McCarthy S: MR characterization of adrenal masses: Field strength and pulse sequence considerations. *Radiology* 171: 671–674, 1989.
6. Krestin GP, Steinbrich W, Friedmann G: Adrenal masses: Evaluation with fast gradient-echo MR imaging Gd-DTPA- enhanced dynamic studies. *Radiology* 171: 675–680, 1989.
7. Krestin GP, Friedmann G, Fischbach R, Neufang KFR, Allolio B: Evaluation of adrenal masses in oncologic patients: Dynamic contrast-enhanced MR vs. CT. *J Comput Assist Tomogr* 15(1): 104–110, 1991.
8. Semelka RC, Shoenut JP, Lawrence PH, Greenberg HM, Maycher B, Madden TP, Kroeker MA: Evaluation of adrenal masses with gadolinium enhancement and fat suppressed MR imaging. *J Magn Reson Imaging* 3: 337–343, 1993.
9. Mitchell DG, Grovello M, Matteucci T, Peterson RO, Miettinen MM: Benign adenocortical masses: Diagnosis with chemical shift MR imaging. *Radiology* 185: 345–351, 1992.
10. Tsushima Y, Ishizaka H, Matsumoto M: Adrenal masses: Differentiation with chemical shift, fast low-angle shot MR imaging. *Radiology* 186: 705–709, 1993.
11. Reinig JW, Stutley JE, Leonhardt CM, Spicer KM, Margolis M, Caldwell CB: Differentiation of adrenal masses with MR imaging: Comparison of techniques. *Radiology* 192: 41–46, 1994.
12. Lee MJ, Mayo-Smith WM, Hahn PF, Goldberg MA, Boland GW, Saini S, Papanicolaou N: State-of-the-art MR imaging of the adrenal gland. *Radiographics* 14: 1015–1029, 1994.
13. Bilbey JH, McLoughlin RF, Kurkjian PS, Wilkins GEL, Chan NHL, Schmidt N, Singer J: MR imaging of adrenal masses: Value of chemical-shift imaging for distinguishing adenomas from other tumors. *Am J Roentgenol* 164: 637– 642, 1995.
14. Korobkin M, Dunnick NR: Characterization of adrenal masses. (commentary) *Am J Roentgenol* 164: 643–644, 1995.
15. Outwater EK, Siegelman ES, Huang AB, Birnbaum BA: Adrenal masses: Correlation between CT attenuation value and chemical shift ratio at MR imaging with in-phase and opposed-phase sequences. *Radiology* 200: 749–752, 1996.
16. Mayo-Smith WW, Lee MJ, McNicholas MMJ, Hahn PF, Boland GW, Saini S: Characterization of adrenal masses (<5 cm) by use of chemical shift MR imaging: Observer performance versus quantitative measures. *Am J Roentgenol* 165: 91-95, 1995.
17. Outwater EK, Siegelman ES, Radecki PD, Piccoli CW, Mitchell DG: Distinction between benign and malignant adrenal masses: Value of T1-weighted chemical-shift MR imaging. *Am J Roentgenol* 165: 579–583, 1995.
18. Korobkin M, Lombardi TJ, Aisen AM, Francis IR, Quint LE, Dunnick NR: Characterization of adrenal masses with chemical shift and gadolinium-enhanced MR imaging. *Radiology* 197: 411–418, 1995.
19. McNicholas MMJ, Lee MJ, Mayo-Smith WW, Hahn PF, Boland GW, Mueller PR: An imaging algorithm for the differential diagnosis of adrenal adenomas and metastases. *Am J Roentgenol* 165: 1453–1459, 1995.
20. Korobkin M, Giordano TJ, Brodeur FJ, et al.: Adrenal adenomas: Relationship between histologic lipid and CT and MR findings. *Radiology* 200: 743–747, 1996.
21. Schwartz LH, Panicek DM, Koutcher JA, Heelan RT, Bains MS, Burt M: Echoplanar MR imaging for characterization of adrenal masses in patient with malignant neoplasms: Preliminary evaluation of calculated T2 relaxation values. *Am J Roentgenol* 164: 911–915, 1995.
22. Outwater EK, Mitchell DG: Differentiation of adrenal masses with chemical shift MR imaging (letter to the editor). *Radiology* 193: 877, 1994.
23. Chung JJ, Semelka RC, Martin DR: Adrenal adenomas: Characteristic postgadolinium capillary blush on dynamic MR imaging. *J Magn Reson Imaging* 13: 242–248, 2001.
24. Small WC, Bernardino ME: Gd-DTPA adrenal gland enhancement at 1.5 T. *Magn Reson Imaging* 9: 309–312, 1991.
25. Schlund JF, Kenney PJ, Brown ED, Ascher SM, Brown JJ, Semelka RC: Adrenocortical carcinoma: MR imaging appearance with current techniques. *J Magn Reson Imaging* 5: 171–174, 1995.
26. Falke THM, te Strake L, Shaff MI, et al.: MR imaging of the adrenals: Correlation with computed tomography. *J Comput Assist Tomogr* 10(2): 242–253, 1986.
27. McLoughlin RF, Bilbey JH: Tumors of the adrenal gland: Findings on CT and MR imaging. *Am J Roentgenol* 163: 1413–1418, 1994.
28. Newhouse JH, Heffess CS, Wagner BJ, Imray TJ, Adair CF, Davidson AJ: Large degenerated adrenal adenomas: radiologic-pathologic correlation. *Radiology* 210: 385–391, 1999.
29. Ichikawa T, Ohtomo K, Uchiyama G, Koizumi K, Monzawa S, Oba H, et al.: Adrenal adenomas: Characteristic hyperintense rim sign on fat-saturated spin-echo MR images. *Radiology* 193: 247–250, 1994.
30. Sohaib SA, Peppercorn PD, Allan C, Monson JP, Grossman AB, Besser GM, Reznek RH: Primary hyperaldosteronism (Conn syndrome): MR imaging findings. *Radiology* 214: 527–531, 2000.
31. Dunnick NR, Doppman JL, Gill JR, Strott CA, Keiser HR, Brennan MF: Localization of functional adrenal tumors by computed tomography and venous sampling. *Radiology* 142: 429–433, 1982.
32. Ikeda DM, Francis IR, Glazer GM, Amendola MA, Gross MD, Aisen AM: The detection of adrenal tumors and hyperplasia in patients with primary aldosteronism: Comparison of scintigraphy, CT, and MR imaging. *Am J Roentgenol* 153: 301–306, 1989.
33. Grant CS, Carpenter P, Van Heerden JA, Hamberger B: Primary aldosteronism. Clinical management. *Arch Surg* 119: 585–590, 1984.

34. Doppman JL, Gill JR Jr, Miller DL, et al.: Distinction between hyperaldosteronism due to bilateral hyperplasia and unilateral aldosteronoma: Reliability of CT. *Radiology* 184: 677–682, 1992.

35. Dieckmann KP, Hamm B, Pickartz H, Jonas D, Bauer HW: Adrenal myelolipoma: clinical, radiologic, and histologic features. *Urology* 29: 1–8, 1987.

36. Palmer WE, Gerard-McFarland EL, Chew FS: Adrenal myelolipoma. *Am J Roentgenol* 156: 724, 1991.

37. Musante F, Derchi LE, Bazzochi M, et al.: MR imaging of adrenal myelolipomas. *J Comput Assist Tomogr* 15: 111–114, 1991.

38. Liessi G, Cesari S, Dell'Antoni C, Spaliviero B, Avventi P: US, CT, MR and percutaneous biopsy of adrenal myelolopomas. *Eur Radiol* 5: 152–155, 1995.

39. Casey LR, Cohen AJ, Wile AG, Dietrich RB: Giant adrenal myelolipomas: CT and MRI findings. *Abdom Imaging* 19: 165–167, 1994.

40. McLoughlin RF, Bilbey JH: Tumors of the adrenal gland: Findings on CT and MR imaging. *Am J Roentgenol* 163: 1413–1418, 1994.

41. Cyran KM, Kenney PJ, Memel DS, Yacoub I: Adrenal myelolipoma. *Am J Roentgenol* 166: 395–400, 1996.

42. Aisen AM, Ohl DA, Chenevert TL, Perkins P, Mikesell W: MR of an adrenal pseudocyst. *Magn Reson Imaging* 10: 997–1000, 1992.

43. Hamrick-Turner JE, Cranston PE, Shipkey FH: Cavernous hemangiomas of the adrenal gland: MR findings. *Magn Reson Imaging* 12(8): 1263–1267, 1994.

44. Otal P, Escourrou G, Joffre F: Imaging features of uncommon adrenal masses with histopathologic correlation. *Radiographics* 19: 569–581, 1999.

45. DeAtkine AB, Dunnick NR: The adrenal glands. *Semin Oncol* 18: 131–139, 1991.

46. Silverman SG, Mueller PR, Pinkney LP, Koenker RM, Seltzer SE: Predictive value of image-guided adrenal biopsy: Analysis of results of 101 biopsies. *Radiology* 187: 715–718, 1993.

47. Belldegrun A, Hussain S, Seltzer SE, Loughlin KR, Gittes RF, Richie JP: Incidentally discovered mass of the adrenal gland. *Surg Gynecol Obstet* 163: 203–208, 1986.

48. Mitnick JS, Bosniak MA, Megibow AJ, Naidich DP: Nonfunctioning adrenal adenomas discovered incidentally on computed tomography. *Radiology* 148: 495–499, 1983.

49. Rosai J. Ackerman's surgical pathology. 8th edition. p 1020 New York, NY 1996.

50. Custodio CM, Semelka RC, Balci NC, Mitchell KM, Freeman JA: Adrenal neuroblastoma in an adult with tumor thrombus in the inferior vena cava. *J Magn Reson Imaging*. 9: 621–623, 1999.

51. Smith SM, Patel SK, Turner DA, et al.: Magnetic resonance imaging of adrenal cortical carcinoma. *Urol Radiol* 11: 1–6, 1989.

52. Ferrozzi F, Bova D: CT and MR demonstration of fat within an adrenal cortical carcinoma. *Abdom Imaging* 20: 272– 274, 1995.

53. Sato N, Watanabe Y, Saga T, Mitsudo K, Dohke M, Minami K: Adrenocortical adenoma containing a fat component CT and MR image evaluation. *Abdom Imaging* 20: 489–490, 1995.

54. Tisnado J, Amendola MA, Konerding KF, Shirazi KK, Beachley MC: Computed tomography versus angiography in the localization of pheochromocytoma. *J Comput Assist Tomogr* 4: 853–859, 1980.

55. Thomas JL, Bernardino ME: Pheochromocytoma in multiple endocrine adenomatosis. Efficacy of computed tomography. *JAMA* 245: 1467–1469, 1981.

56. Bush WH, Elder JS, Crane RE, Wales LR: Cystic pheochromocytoma. *Urology* 25: 332–334, 1985.

57. Crecelius SA, Bellah R: Pheochromocytoma of the bladder in an adolescent: Sonographic and MR imaging findings. *Am J Roentgenol* 165: 101–103, 1995.

58. Belden CJ, Powers C, Ros PR: MR demonstration of a cystic pheochromocytoma. *J Magn Reson Imaging* 5: 778–780, 1995.

59. Westra SJ, Zaninovic AC, Hall TR, Kangarloo H, Boechat MI: Imaging of the adrenal gland in children. *Radiographics* 14: 1323–1340, 1994.

60. Feinstein RS, Gatewood OMB, Fishman EK, Goldman SM, Siegelman SS: Computed tomography of adult neuroblastoma. *J Comput Assist Tomogr* 8: 720–726, 1984.

61. Paling MR, Williamson BRJ: Adrenal involvement in non-Hodgkin lymphoma. *Am J Roentgenol* 141: 303–305, 1983.

62. Glazer HS, Lee JKT, Balfe DM, Mauro MS, Griffeth R, Sagel SS: Non-Hodgkin lymphoma: Computed tomographic demonstration of unusual extranodal involvement. *Radiology* 149: 211–217, 1983.

63. Lee FT Jr, Thornbury JR, Grist TM, Kelcz F: MR imaging of adrenal lymphoma. *Abdom Imaging* 18: 95–96, 1993.

64. Hauser H, Gurret JP: Miliary tuberculosis associated with adrenal enlargement CT appearance. *J Comput Assist* Tomogr 10: 254–256, 1986.

65. Sawczuk IS, Reitelman C, Libby C, Grant D, Vita J, White RD: CT findings in Addison's disease caused by tuberculosis. *Urol Radiol* 8: 44–45, 1986.

66. Wilson DA, Muchmore HG, Tisdal RG, Fahmy A, Pitha JV: Histoplasmosis of the adrenal glands studied by CT. *Radiology* 150: 779–783, 1984.

67. Xarli VP, Steele AA, Davis PJ, Buescher ES, Rios CN, Garcia-Bunuel R: Adrenal hemorrhage in the adult. *Medicine* 57: 211–221, 1987.

68. Provenzale JM, Ortel TL, Nelson RC: Adrenal hemorrhage in patients with primary antiphospholipid syndrome: Imaging findings. *Am J Roentgenol* 165: 361–364, 1995.

69. Wolverson MK, Kannegiesser H: CT of bilateral adrenal hemorrhage with acute adrenal insufficiency in the adult. *Am J Roentgenol* 142: 311–314, 1984.

70. Koch KJ, Cory DA: Simultaneous renal vein thrombosis and bilateral adrenal hemorrhage: MR demonstration. *J Comput Assist Tomogr* 10: 681–683, 1986.

71. Brill PW, Jagannath A, Winchester P, Markisz JA, Zirinsky K: Adrenal hemorrhage and renal vein thrombosis in the newborn: MR imaging. *Radiology* 170: 95–96, 1989.

72. Wilms G, Tits J, Vanstraelen D, Marchal G, Baert AL: Addison's disease due to bilateral post-traumatic adrenal hemorrhage: CT and MR findings. *Eur Radiol* 1: 172–174, 1991.

73. Doppman JL, Gill JR Jr, Nienhuis AW, Earll JM, Long JA Jr: CT findings in Addison's disease. *J Comput Assist* Tomogr 6: 757–761, 1982.

74. McMurry JF Jr, Long D, McClure R, Kotchen TA: Addison's disease with adrenal enlargement on computed tomographic scanning. *Am J Med* 77: 365–368, 1984.

75. Schwartz LH, Panicek DM, Koutcher JA, Brown KT, Getrajdman GI, Heelan RT, et al.: Adrenal masses in patients with malignancy: Prospective comparsion of echo-planar, fast spin-echo, and chemical shift MR imaging. *Radiology* 197: 421–425, 1995.

76. Mitchell DG, Outwater EK, Matteucci T, Rubin DL, Chezmar JL, Saini S: Adrenal gland enhancement at MR imaging with Mn-DPDP. *Radiology* 194: 783–787, 1995.

77. Weissleder T, Wang YM, Papisov M, et al.: Polymeric contrast agents for MR imaging of adrenal glands. *J Magn Reson Imaging* 3: 93–97, 1993.

KIDNEYS

RICHARD C. SEMELKA, M.D., LARISSA BRAGA, M.D., DIANE ARMAO, M.D., AND HECTOR COOPER, M.D.

What is man, when you come to think upon him, but
a minutely set, ingenious machine for turning, with
infinitive artfulness, the red wine of Shiraz into urine?
    Isak Dinesen, *Seven Gothic Tales* (1934)
        "The Dreamers."

NORMAL ANATOMY

The kidneys are paired organs that lie in the retroperitoneum. They are situated within the perirenal space, which contains abundant fat. Kidney and adipose tissue together are enclosed within renal fascia (Gerota fascia). The kidney is surrounded by a fibroelastic capsule, usually not visible on tomographic images. The renal capsule is connected to the renal fascia through fibrous trabeculae that traverse perirenal fat. At the lateral renal borders, the anterior and posterior fascial layers fuse to form the lateral conal fascia. Superiorly, the fascia fuse, whereas inferiorly they are open, forming a potential communication with the anterior and posterior perirenal spaces.

The medial surface of the kidney shows the hilum containing vessels, nerves, and the renal pelvis of the ureter. The hilum leads into a larger space, or renal sinus, containing the calyces, vessels, and fat. The renal parenchyma contains an external cortex and internal medulla. The cortex contains glomeruli and convoluted tubules. The medulla contains conical structures or pyramids. The cortex arches over the bases of the pyramids and extends between them towards the renal sinus as a renal column of Bertin. The apices of the renal pyramids converge to the renal sinus, where they project into calyces as papillae.

MRI TECHNIQUE

The basic magnetic resonance imaging (MRI) examination of the kidneys involves single-shot T2-weighted sequences with precontrast and postgadolinium chelate T1-weighted images acquired as nonsuppressed and fat-suppressed sequences. The immediate postgadolinium images should be acquired as an immediate postgadolinium capillary-phase SGE sequence. A diagnostically useful protocol is as follows: 1) coronal T2-weighted single-shot echo-train spin-echo, 2) precontrast T1-weighted breath-hold spoiled gradient-echo (SGE), 3) precontrast breath-hold T1-weighted fat-suppressed SGE, 4) dynamic capillary-phase gadolinium-enhanced T1-weighted SGE, and 5) gadolinium-enhanced interstitial-phase

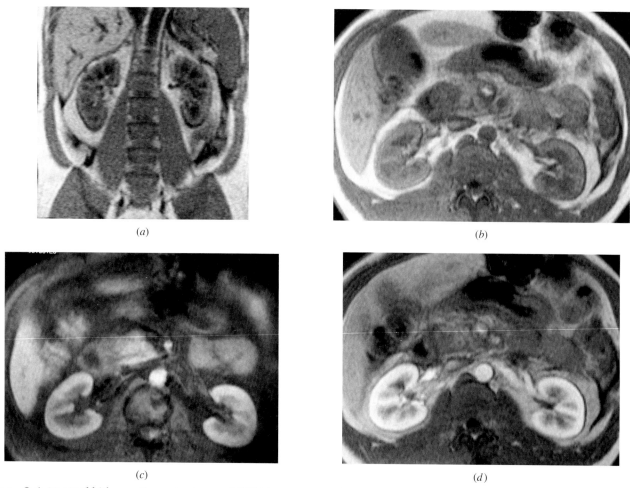

(a)

(b)

(c)

(d)

FIG. 9.1 Normal kidneys. Precontrast coronal SGE (*a*), precontrast SGE (*b*), T1-weighted fat-suppressed spin-echo (*c*), immediate postgadolinium SGE (*d*), gadolinium-enhanced T1-weighted fat-suppressed spin-echo (*e*), 8-min postgadolinium transverse (*f*), and 8.5-min coronal (*g*) gadolinium-enhanced SGE images. Corticomedullary differentiation is shown on precontrast T1-weighted images (*a–c*), and on immediate postgadolinium SGE (*d*) images. Corticomedullary differentiation is most clearly defined on the precontrast T1-weighted fat-suppressed image (*c*) and the immediate postgadolinium SGE image (*d*).

T1-weighted fat-suppressed SGE (fig. 9.1) techniques [1]. Precontrast and postcontrast image acquisition in the sagittal or coronal plane frequently is helpful to 1) evaluate the superior and inferior borders of renal lesions, 2) characterize lesions as cystic or solid, or 3) demonstrate renal/perirenal location and extension.

MR angiography (MRA) has achieved diagnostically sufficient image quality to reproducibly demonstrate main renal arterial disease (fig. 9.2) [2,3]. Reproducible demonstration of intraparenchymal small vessel disease has not yet been realized.

The echo-train spin-echo (ETSE) technique may be tailored to generate an MR urogram effect, which in early reports has been shown to be effective at elucidating causes of a dilated renal collecting system [4]. Temporal changes in signal intensity (SI) of renal cortex and medulla after contrast injection provides information on renal function [5–7]. The ability to generate diverse imaging information on tissue morphology, renal vessels, collecting system, and function renders MRI a comprehensive diagnostic modality for investigating renal disease [8].

Gadolinium chelates are freely filtered by renal glomeruli and undergo excretion by renal tubules with no tubular reabsorption or excretion [9]. Because of this elimination pathway, gadolinium chelates are ideal for studying morphology and function of the kidneys. Gadolinium possesses the additional property of changing signal intensity based on concentration. When dilute, gadolinium enhances T1 relaxation and renders urine high in signal intensity. When concentrated, gadolinium induces magnetic susceptibility and signal intensity loss, causing urine to be low in signal intensity [5–7]. The concentrating ability of the kidneys can be evaluated by gadolinium-enhanced MRI, a property that cannot be assessed by dynamic iodine-enhanced CT imaging.

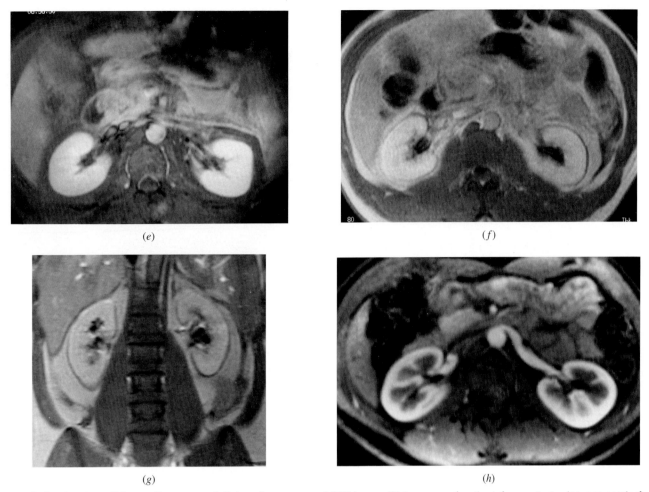

(e)

(f)

(g)

(h)

FIG. 9.1 (*Continued*) Immediate postgadolinium fat-suppressed SGE image (*h*) in a second patient demonstrates intense cortical enhancement and good demonstration of high-signal intensity gadolinium-containing left renal vein. Sharp definition of the outer renal cortex is shown because of the suppression of fat.

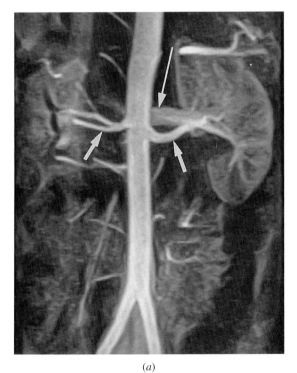

(a)

FIG. 9.2 MRA of normal kidneys. Coronal MIP of bolus gadolinium-enhanced 3D gradient echo demonstrates normal renal arteries in sharp detail (short arrows). The left renal vein is also opacified (long arrow).

743

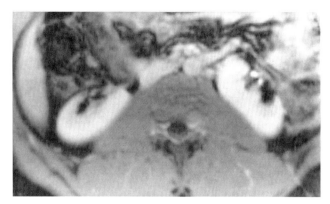

FIG. 9.3 Malrotation. Postgadolinium T1-weighted fat-suppressed SGE image. The most common form of malrotation is anterior orientation of the pelvis.

NORMAL VARIANTS AND CONGENITAL ANOMALIES

Initially in utero the kidneys are located in the pelvis, but through growth of the caudal region of the embryo they "ascend" to the abdomen. About 10% of the population are born with potentially significant malformations of the urinary tract [10].

The organogenesis of the kidney is complex, and a diverse array of anomalies affect the urinary tract. The majority relate to abnormalities of renal position (fig. 9.3), form, mass, and number.

Prominent columns of Bertin are frequently observed in kidneys, and it may be difficult to distinguish these from renal masses on other imaging modalities. Columns will follow the signal intensity of renal cortex on all pre- and postgadolinium images. An important observation is that on immediate postgadolinium images the column enhances to the same extent as renal cortex

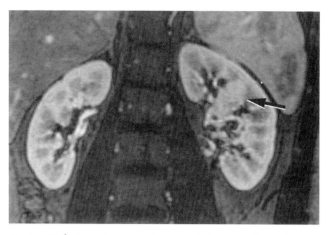

FIG. 9.4 Prominent column of Bertin. Coronal postgadolinium gradient-echo image. Bertin column (arrow) follows a continuous contour and remains isointense with the renal cortex.

and follows a smooth continuous contour with cortex. On more delayed images the enhancement of the column remains isointense with cortex (fig. 9.4).

Persistent fetal lobulation is another common normal variant. Coronal images demonstrate the undulating contour of the kidney. Immediate postgadolinium images show uniform cortical thickening, which excludes the presence of a mass (fig. 9.5).

Ectopic kidney refers to the malposition of one or both kidneys. Pelvic kidney accounts for most cases of ectopic kidney. In this case, the kidneys are often malformed (fig. 9.6). The presence of intense uptake of gadolinium chelates by renal cortex and identification of renal corticomedullary organization allow confident diagnosis of this entity.

Horseshoe kidney occurs in about 1 in every 600 persons and is the most common form of renal

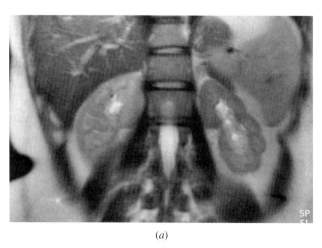

(a)

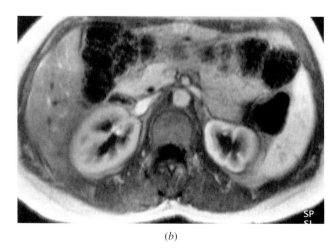

(b)

FIG. 9.5 Fetal lobulation. Coronal single-shot echo-train spin-echo (SS-ETSE) (a), and transverse immediate postgadolinium SGE (b) images. The coronal SS-ETSE image (a) demonstrates an undulating contour of the entire left kidney. The immediate postgadolinium SGE image demonstrates uniform cortical thickness, excluding the presence of a mass.

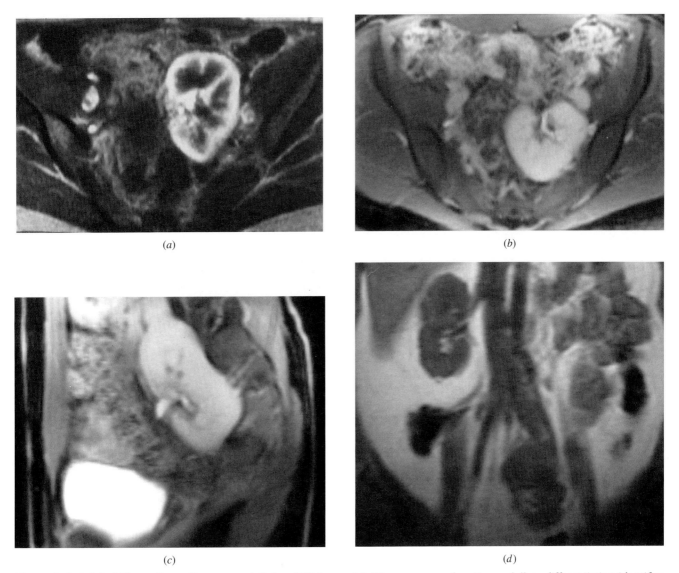

(a)

(b)

(c)

(d)

FIG. 9.6 Pelvic kidney. Immediate postgadolinium SGE image (*a*). The presence of corticomedullary differentiation identifies the pelvic mass as a kidney.

Axial (*b*) and sagittal (*c*) gadolinium-enhanced T1-weighted fat-suppressed SGE in a second patient and coronal SS-ETSE image (*d*) in a third patient demonstrate other examples of a pelvic kidney.

fusion. It is defined as the midline fusion of two distinct renal masses, each with its own ureter and pelvis. This entity is demonstrated on tomographic images by the fusion of the lower poles of both kidneys across the midline, immediately anterior to vertebral bodies (fig. 9.7).

Crossed fused ectopia is an uncommon entity. In crossed ectopia the ectopic kidney is situated opposite the side of insertion of its ureter in the trigone. Fusion with the other kidney is present in 90% of cases. Crossed fused ectopy can be diagnosed on MR images by the identification of corticomedullary organization in the mass. Direct coronal imaging is helpful in demonstrating the fused renal moieties (fig. 9.8). Extrarenal anomalies (genital, skeletal, and anorectal) occur in up to 25% of patients [11].

Duplication of the collecting system is a relatively common anomaly, which may sometimes be difficult to detect on transverse tomographic images (fig. 9.9).

Hypoplastic kidney. Renal hypoplasia is defined as failure of the kidney to develop to a normal size. The hypoplastic kidney is a congenitally small (<50% of normal) but otherwise normally developed kidney. The small size of the kidney is usually a manifestation of a marked reduction in the number of renal lobes. The normal adult kidney has a minimum of 10 lobes, each composed of a medullary pyramid surrounded by a cap of cortex. Hypoplastic kidney possesses only one to five lobes. Hypoplastic kidneys have an intact collecting system and normal cortical enhancement. The renal artery,

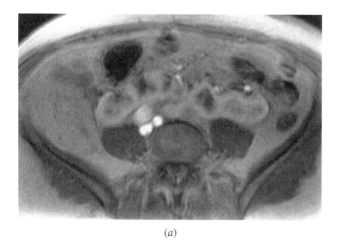

(a)

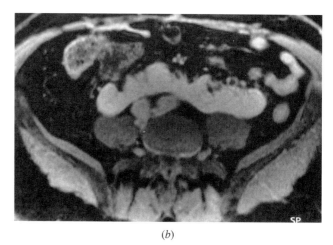

(b)

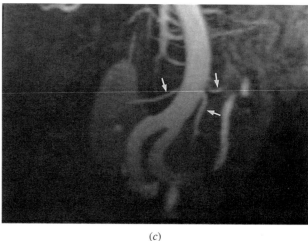

(c)

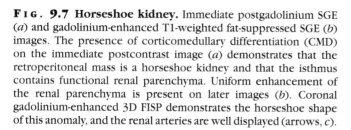

F I G . 9.7 Horseshoe kidney. Immediate postgadolinium SGE (*a*) and gadolinium-enhanced T1-weighted fat-suppressed SGE (*b*) images. The presence of corticomedullary differentiation (CMD) on the immediate postcontrast image (*a*) demonstrates that the retroperitoneal mass is a horseshoe kidney and that the isthmus contains functional renal parenchyma. Uniform enhancement of the renal parenchyma is present on later images (*b*). Coronal gadolinium-enhanced 3D FISP demonstrates the horseshoe shape of this anomaly, and the renal arteries are well displayed (arrows, *c*).

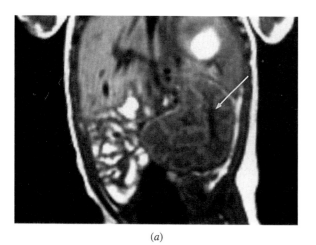

(a)

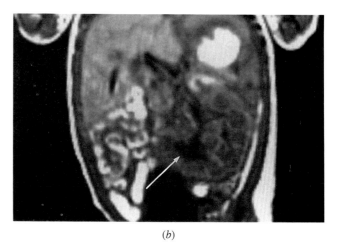

(b)

F I G . 9.8 Crossed-fused ectopy. Coronal T1-weighted spin-echo images (*a*, *b*) demonstrate fusion of a small inferomedial kidney to the normal-sized and -positioned left kidney. Clear depiction is rendered by the definition of CMD. The collecting system of the normally positioned left kidney is normal in size (arrow, *a*), whereas the crossed-fused right kidney has a mildly dilated collecting system (arrow, *b*).

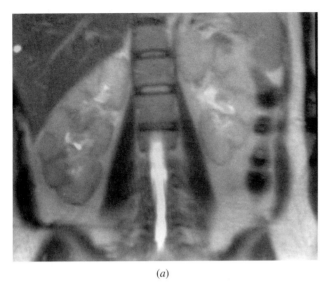

(a)

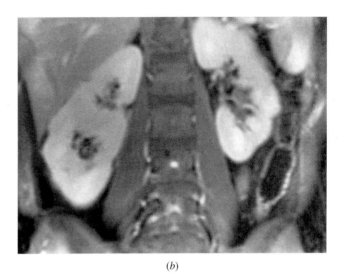

(b)

F I G . 9.9 Duplex collecting system. Coronal SS-ETSE (*a*) and postgadolinium T1-weighted fat-suppressed SGE (*b*) images demonstrate a patient with a duplicated collecting system in the right kidney. Note the thick column of Bertin separating the two pelves.

however, is diminutive, suggesting that in utero vascular compromise may be the underlying cause. Renal injury sustained in childhood such as surgery, radiation, or reflux may result in a small, smooth kidney similar in appearance to a true hypoplastic kidney (fig. 9.10).

Hyperplastic (hypertrophic) kidney. Renal hyperplasia that results in renal enlargement occurs in the setting of longstanding compromise or absence of the contralateral kidney. Hyperplasia is most pronounced if the original stimulus for renal enlargement occurs in

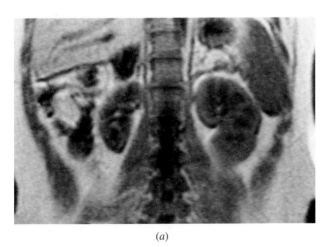

(a)

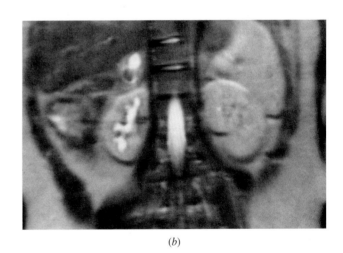

(b)

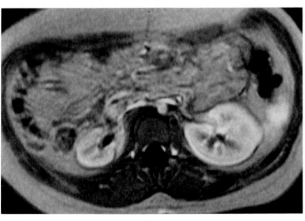

(c)

F I G . 9.10 Hypoplastic Kidney. Small kidney secondary to ureter reimplantation in infancy. Coronal SGE (*a*), coronal single-shot echo-train spin-echo (*b*), and immediate postgadolinium SGE (*c*) images. The right kidney is small and smooth in contour and has uniform cortical thickness (*a–c*). Corticomedullary differentiation is preserved on precontrast T1-weighted images. Mild caliectasis with dilatation of the intrarenal collecting system is demonstrated on the T2-weighted image (*b*), reflecting the underlying disease of the collecting system. On the immediate postgadolinium SGE image (*c*), the renal cortex is thin but uniform in thickness, and enhancement is symmetric with the normal left kidney.

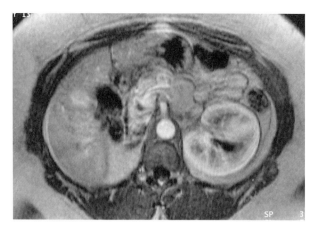

Fig. 9.11 Renal hypertrophy. Immediate postgadolinium SGE image demonstrates generalized enlargement of the left kidney with uniform thickness of renal cortex. This adult patient had undergone a right nephrectomy.

childhood. Generalized, globular renal enlargement with increased thickness of renal cortex is observed on immediate postgadolinium SGE images (fig. 9.11).

DISEASE OF THE RENAL PARENCHYMA

Mass Lesions

A number of renal masses as have distinctive MR imaging appearance that can be described on T1, T2, and early and late postgadolinium images (Table 9.1).

Benign Masses

Cysts. Benign cystic disease of the kidney are a heterogeneous group comprising both hereditary and acquired disorders. These lesions are an important clinical entity [12] for reasons which include:

1) They are common and sometimes present diagnostic challenges for clinicians, radiologists and pathologists.
2) Forms such as adult polycystic disease are important causes of renal failure.
3) Cysts can occasionally be confused with malignant tumors.

■ SIMPLE CYSTS

Simple renal cysts are the most common renal lesion in the adult. Simple cysts occur as single, sometimes multiple, fluid-filled, oval-shaped structures in the cortex [13]. Simple cysts do not enhance with gadolinium and are sharply demarcated from adjacent renal parenchyma [1,14]. Simple cysts are very low in signal intensity on T1-weighted images and very high in signal intensity on T2-weighted images. Cysts are considered simple when they contain clear to amber-colored serous fluid, similar in composition to urine, are signal void on T1-weighted images, and have no definable wall when they extend beyond the renal cortex [1]. Simple cysts may be observed as nearly signal-void lesions on postgadolinium images even when they measure 3–4 mm in diameter

Table 9.1   Pattern Recognition of Common Renal Lesions on T1, T2, and Early and Late Postgadolinium Images

Lesion	T1	T2	Early	Late	Other
Simple cyst	↓↓	↑↑	○	○	No definable wall
Complex cyst	↓–↑	↓–↑	○	○	Mural enhancement may be present
Angiomyolipoma	↑	∅	○–↑	○–↑	On out-of-phase T1-weighted images AML shows a black ring phase cancellation artifact; lesions diminish in signal on T1-weighted fat-suppressed images.
Renal cell	↓–↑	∅–↑	↑	↓	The majority are hypervascular. The majority washout on delayed images relative to renal parenchyma.
Lymphoma	∅–↑	∅–↑	Minimal	Minimal	Lymphoma rarely has central necrosis. Most often, the tumor has a large extrarenal retroperitoneal component.

↓↓ moderately to greatly decreased signal intensity
↓ mildly decreased signal intensity
∅ isointense
↑ mildly increased
↑↑ greatly increased
○ absent

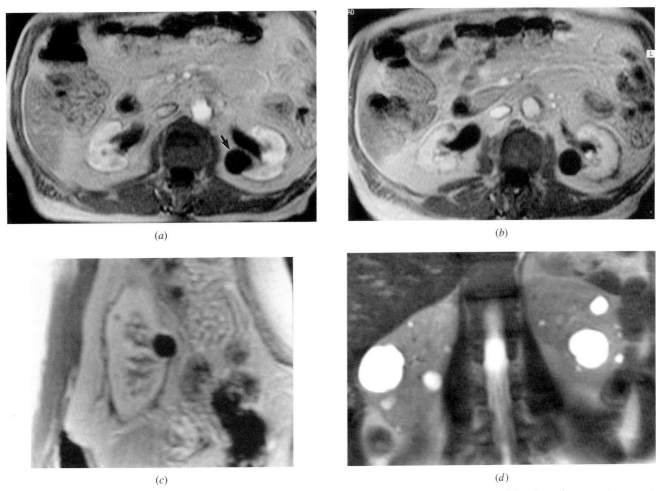

(a)

(b)

(c)

(d)

F I G . 9.12 Renal cyst. Immediate (*a*) and 5-min (*b*) postgadolinium SGE images. A cyst is present arising from the posterior aspect of the left kidney. The cyst demonstrates signal void, sharply marginated, and has no definable wall on the immediate postgadolinium image (arrow, *a*). No change in the appearance of the cyst occurs on the delayed postcontrast image (*b*).

Sagittal 5-min postgadolinium SGE image (*c*) of the left kidney in a second patient demonstrates a sharp superior and inferior margin of the renal cyst confirming that it is a simple cyst.

SS-ETSE image (*d*) in a third patient shows multiple bilateral simple renal cysts.

(fig. 9.12). Sagittal or coronal images permit direct visualization of the superior and inferior margins of cysts.

COMPLEX CYSTS

Cysts are considered complex when they contain hemorrhage, septations, calcifications, or thickened wall. Region of interest measurements on pre- and postgadolinium T1-weighted images are useful to ensure lack of contrast enhancement in cysts that are high in signal intensity on pre- and postcontrast images.

A recent series compared the MR imaging appearance of complex cysts and cystic renal neoplasms [15]. In that series, the combination of mural irregularity and intense mural enhancement in renal cystic lesions was a strong predictor of malignancy (P = 0.0002). In compar-

ison, benign cysts that possessed a thickened enhancing wall, had more uniform mural thickening. Rarely, benign cysts may contain nodules (fig. 9.13), which renders them suspicious for renal cancer.

HEMORRHAGIC CYST

Hemorrhagic cysts are commonly encountered on MRI examinations. Many of these cysts are not identified as hemorrhagic on CT examinations, which reflects the higher sensitivity of MRI for the detection of blood. The majority of hemorrhagic cysts are high in signal intensity on T1- and T2-weighted images because imaging studies are often acquired in the subacute phase of hemorrhage, which lasts from 1 to 26 weeks after bleeding (fig. 9.14). The observation that most hemorrhagic cysts are high

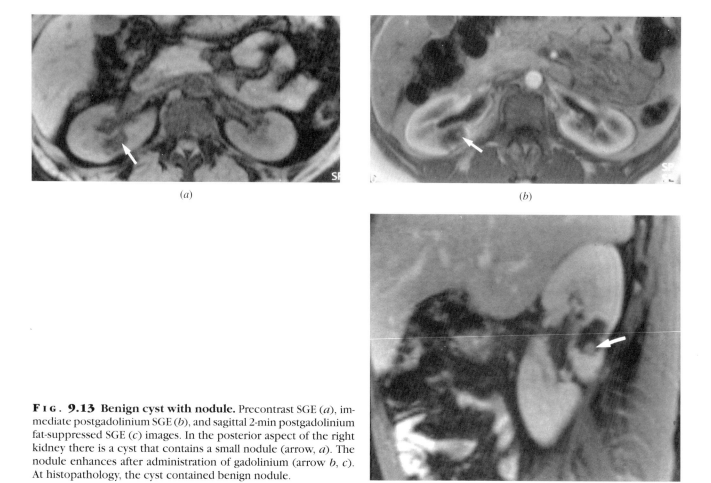

(a)

(b)

(c)

F I G . 9.13 Benign cyst with nodule. Precontrast SGE (*a*), immediate postgadolinium SGE (*b*), and sagittal 2-min postgadolinium fat-suppressed SGE (*c*) images. In the posterior aspect of the right kidney there is a cyst that contains a small nodule (arrow, *a*). The nodule enhances after administration of gadolinium (arrow *b*, *c*). At histopathology, the cyst contained benign nodule.

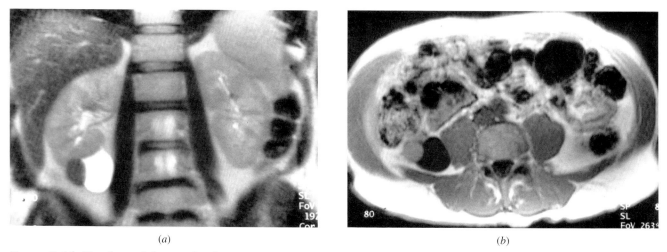

(a)

(b)

F I G . 9.14 Simple and hemorrhagic cysts. Coronal SS-ETSE (*a*), axial precontrast T1-weighted SGE (*b*), precontrast T1 weighted fat-suppressed SGE (*c*), and 90-s gadolinium-enhanced T1 weighted fat-suppressed SGE (*d*) images. Exophytic simple and hemorrhagic renal cysts are side-by-side arising from the lower pole of the right kidney. The hemorrhagic cyst shows increased T1 signal (*b*, *c*) and decreased T2 signal (*a*), signal behavior opposite that of the simple cyst.

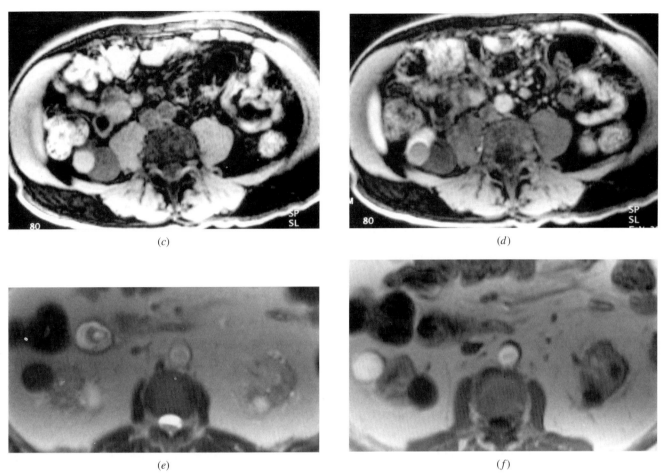

(c)

(d)

(e)

(f)

F I G . 9.14 (*Continued*) SS-ETSE (*e*) and immediate postgadolinium SGE (*f*) images in a second patient show bilateral simple renal cysts and, at the same tomographic level arising from the lateral aspect of the right kidney, another cyst with increased signal on T1-weighted images (*f*), and low signal on T2 (*e*), consistent with increased protein content or hemorrhage.

signal intensity on T1- and T2-weighted images reflects the long time period in which blood is present as extracellular methemoglobin. Hemorrhagic cysts may be readily diagnosed as benign if they are homogeneously high in signal intensity on both T1- and T2-weighted images or if they show a fluid-fluid level (fig. 9.15) and have a smooth, thin wall. Many cysts that are high in signal intensity on precontrast T1-weighted images are rendered low in signal intensity after gadolinium administration because of rescaling of abdominal tissue signal intensities with the presence of gadolinium (fig. 9.16). Occasionally, organizing hemorrhage contains fibrous strands that make distinction from solid neoplasms difficult.

Acute or early subacute hemorrhage that contains intracellular deoxyhemoglobin or intracellular methemoglobin may pose a diagnostic problem. On T2-weighted images, these cysts may be low in signal intensity and have an appearance resembling solid neoplasms (fig. 9.17). Proteinaceous cysts have a similar appearance. Because of the occasional occurrence of rel-

atively acute blood or protein in cysts, caution must be exercised in using T2-weighted information to determine whether lesions are cystic or solid. In cysts containing acute hemorrhage, the demonstration of lack of lesion enhancement, and sharp margination with no internal change, on serial postgadolinium images acquired up to 5 min after contrast injection are important imaging findings to show that they are cysts (see fig. 9.17). Clinical history and follow-up MRI at 3–6 months also may be required.

SEPTATED CYSTS

Septations in cysts may occur as a result of various events, including fibrin strands after hemorrhage or inflammation, or close juxtaposition of two or more cysts. Demonstration that septations are uniform and thin (2 mm) without enhancing nodular components helps to ascertain that septated cysts are not malignant (fig. 9.18).

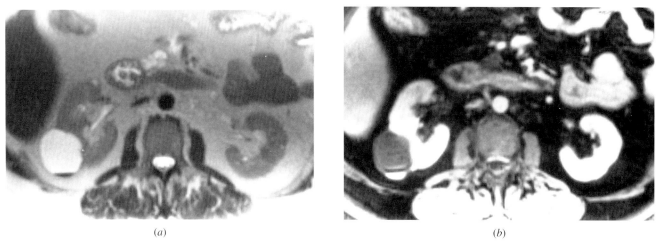

(a)   (b)

F I G . 9.15 Hemorrhagic cyst. SS-ETSE (*a*) and postgadolinium T1-weighted fat-suppressed SGE (*b*) images. A cyst in the right kidney demonstrates layering material that is low signal on T2 (*a*) and increased signal on T1 (*b*), consistent with hemorrhage.

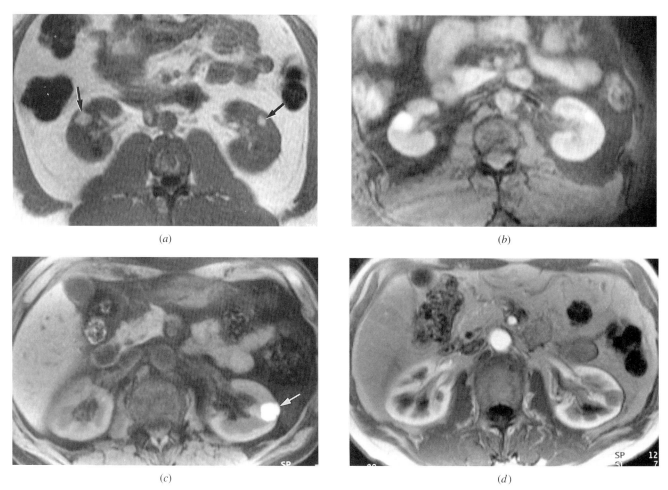

(a)   (b)

(c)   (d)

F I G . 9.16 Hemorrhagic renal cysts. Precontrast SGE (*a*) and T1-weighted fat-suppressed images. Bilateral renal cysts are apparent on the T1-weighted SGE image (*a*), which are high in signal intensity (arrows, *a*), a finding consistent with subacute blood or fat. The T1-weighted image with fat suppression (*b*) demonstrates that these lesions remain high in signal intensity and therefore are not fat containing. Fat suppression accentuates the high signal intensity of these cysts.

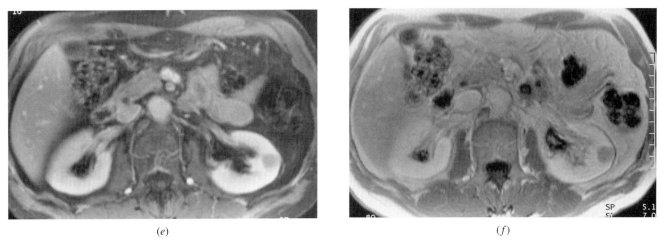

(e)   *(f)*

F I G . 9.16 (*Continued*) Fat-suppressed SGE (*c*), immediate postgadolinium SGE (*d*) 90-s postgadolinium fat-suppressed SGE (*e*), and 5-min postgadolinium SGE (*f*) images in a second patient. A well-defined, uniformly high-signal intensity hemorrhagic cyst is present in the left kidney on the fat-suppressed image (arrow, *c*). The cyst does not change in size or shape and does not demonstrate internal enhancement on serial postgadolinium images. Because of the intrinsic high signal intensity of the hemorrhage, the cyst is low in signal but not signal void on the postcontrast images.

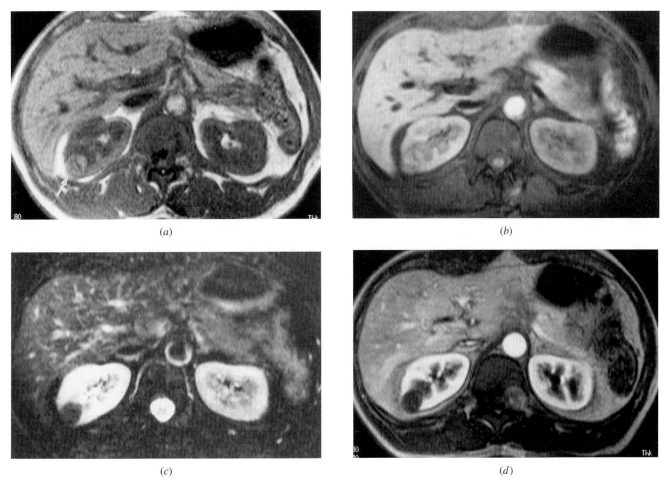

(a)   *(b)*

(c)   *(d)*

F I G . 9.17 Hemorrhagic cyst containing relatively acute blood (intracellular methemoglobin). Precontrast SGE (*a*), precontrast T1-weighted fat-suppressed spin-echo (*b*), T2-weighted fat-suppressed spin-echo (*c*), immediate postgadolinium SGE (*d*), gadolinium-enhanced T1-weighted fat-suppressed spin-echo (*e*), 8-min transverse (*f*), and 8.5-min sagittal (*g*) postgadolinium SGE images.

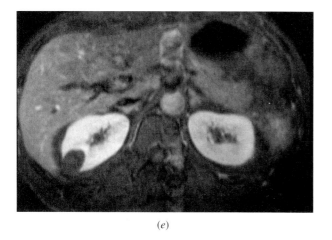

(e)

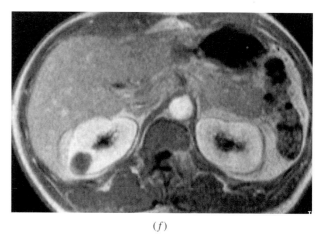

(f)

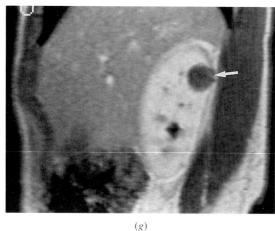

(g)

F I G . 9.17 (*Continued*) A lesion is present in the right kidney (arrow, *a*), which is mixed high signal intensity on precontrast T1-weighted images (*a*, *b*), low in signal intensity on T2-weighted image (*c*), and low in signal intensity on early (*d*) and delayed (*e–g*) images. The low signal intensity on the T2-weighted image (*c*) may mimic a solid lesion. Although the lesion is low in signal intensity and not signal void on postcontrast images, it is sharply marginated, has no definable wall or nodularity, and does not change in size and shape between early (*d*) and late (*e–g*) postcontrast images. The postcontrast sagittal plane image demonstrates that the superior and inferior margins of the cyst (arrow, *g*) are sharply defined.

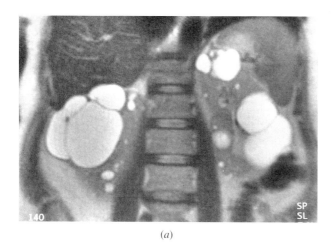

(a)

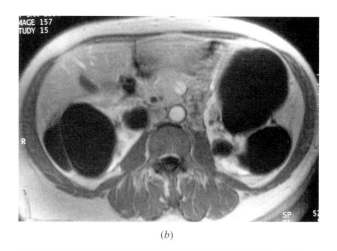

(b)

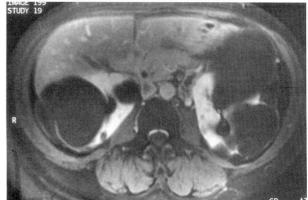

(c)

F I G . 9.18 Septated renal cysts. Coronal SS-ETSE (*a*), immediate postgadolinium SGE (*b*), and 90-s postgadolinium fat-suppressed SGE (*c*) images. Multiple closely grouped cysts are presented in both kidneys, which create an appearance of multicystic masses (*a*). Renal parenchyma enhances normally (*b*), and the cysts do not change in size and shape on serial postgadolinium images (*b*, *c*) with no internal enhancement demonstrated.

CALCIFIED CYSTS

Calcium is generally signal void on MR images. Although calcium is difficult to appreciate on MR images, the lack of signal allows clear visualization of surrounding tissue and internal morphology [14]. Therefore, the presence of tumor tissue is readily determined. An advantage of MRI over CT imaging and ultrasound in the evaluation of calcified cysts is that calcium does not interfere with the evaluation of adjacent soft tissue. MRI is therefore indicated for the evaluation of calcified cysts.

CYSTS WITH THICKENED WALLS

Some cysts possess thickened walls that by MR imaging are usually regular in thickness and contour but may be irregular. Cyst contents are occasionally moderate to high in signal intensity on T1-weighted images because of the presence of protein or subacute blood (fig. 9.19).

The thickened cyst wall may enhance moderately with gadolinium (fig. 9.20). Histopathologic examination of this category of complex cysts shows prominent reactive macrophage infiltration of either the cyst wall or adjacent renal parenchyma [15]. These cysts occasionally have a prominent perinephric component of inflammatory tissue, greater than that typically seen for cystic renal cancers. However, it is often not possible to distinguish these cysts from cystic renal cancers. Surgery, therefore, cannot be avoided for many of these lesions. If surgery is not performed, close imaging follow-up is recommended.

PERINEPHRIC PSEUDOCYSTS (PARAPELVIC CYSTS)

Perinephric pseudocysts are formed from extravasation of urine into perinephric fat in the region of the renal sinus (fig. 9.21). These lesions may result from blunt trauma to the kidney or surgical procedures in which the

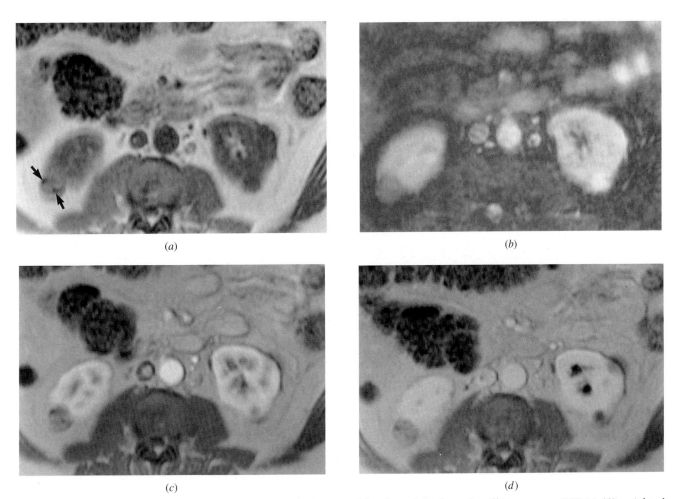

(a)

(b)

(c)

(d)

F I G . 9.19 Cyst complicated by the presence of calcification, blood, and thickened wall. Precontrast SGE (*a*), T2-weighted fat-suppressed spin-echo (*b*), immediate (*c*) and 8-min transverse (*d*), and 8.5-min sagittal (*e*) postgadolinium SGE images.

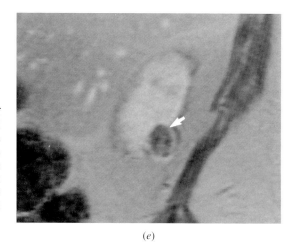

(*e*)

FIG. 9.19 (*Continued*) A lesion arises from the posterior aspect of the right kidney, which is mixed in signal intensity and contains signal void calcifications (arrows, *a*) on the precontrast SGE image. The lesion is mildly low in signal intensity on the T2-weighted image (*b*), which mimics the appearance of a solid tumor. The complicated cyst remains moderate in signal intensity on postcontrast images, but it is sharply defined from adjacent cortex and does not change in size or shape between early (*c*) and late (*d*, *e*) postcontrast images. The superior margin of the cyst is well defined on the sagittal image (arrow, *e*).

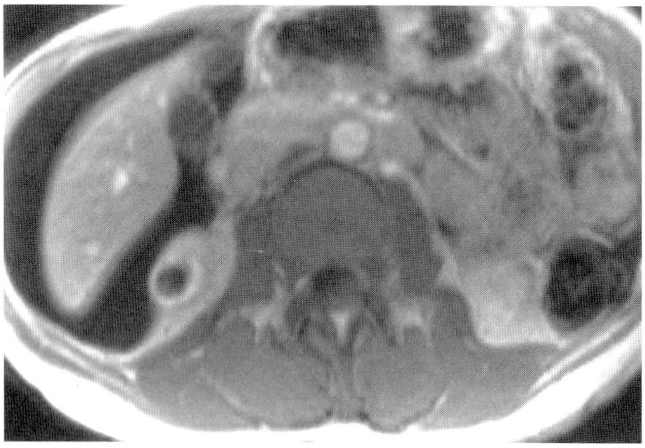

(*a*)

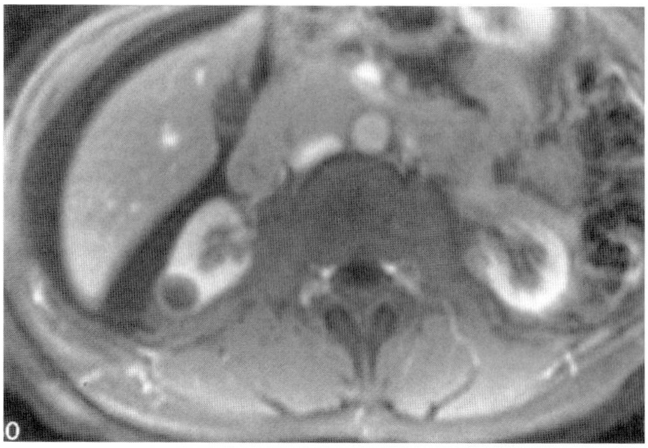

(*b*)

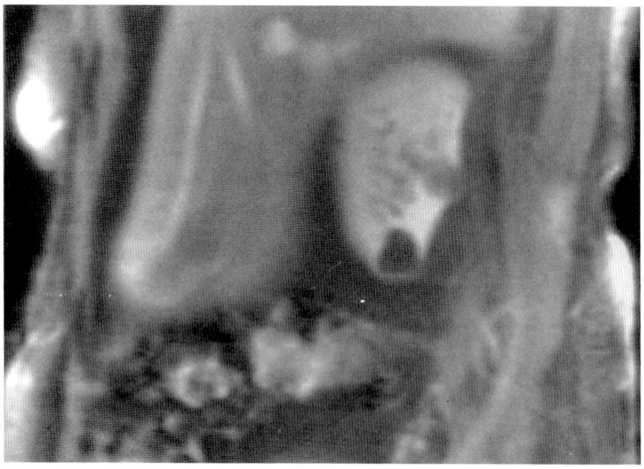

(*c*)

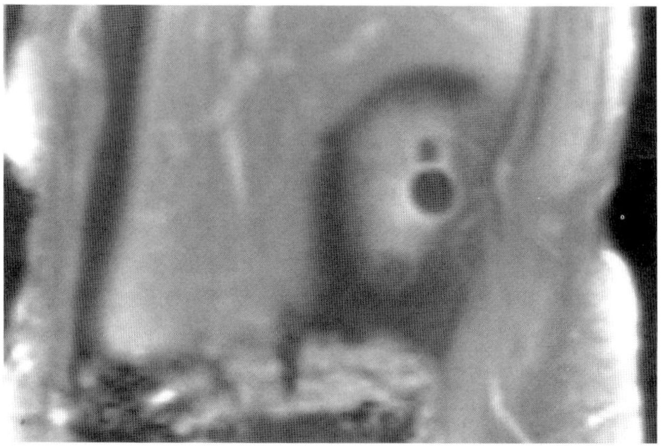

(*d*)

FIG. 9.20 Cyst with thickened wall and reactive cellular infiltrate. Postgadolinium 45 s T1-weighted SGE (*a*), axial (*b*) and sagittal (*c*, *d*) 3- to 4-min interstitial-phase gadolinium-enhanced T1-weighted fat-suppressed SGE images. Note 3 cysts in the right kidney which have thick enhancing walls that show no mural irregularity.

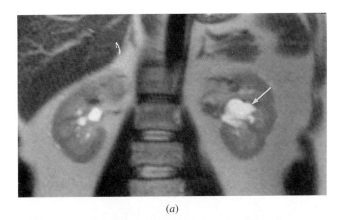

(a)

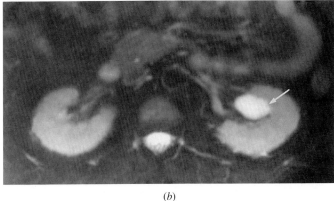

(b)

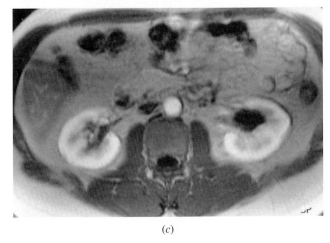

(c)

FIG. 9.21 Parapelvic cyst. Coronal SS-ETSE (*a*), T2-weighted fat-suppressed spin-echo (*b*), and immediate postgadolinium SGE (*c*) images. An oval-shaped parapelvic cyst is present in the left renal sinus (arrow, *a*, *b*). The parapelvic cyst is separate from the collecting system, is high in signal intensity on T2-weighted images (*a*, *b*), signal void and well defined on the postgadolinium image (*c*).

renal pelvis or calyces are damaged or the renal capsule is torn, but often the underlying cause is unknown and they are observed as incidental finding more common in elderly patients. Some degree of accompanying urinary obstruction is not uncommon, and occasionally these cysts may present with urinary obstruction [16]. They may be solitary or, more commonly, multiple and bilateral. At times these lesions may be difficult to distinguish from a dilated renal collecting system. Images acquired 10–20 min after gadolinium demonstrate that cystic structures in the area of the renal sinus represent parapelvic cysts and not dilated collecting system. Gadolinium is sufficiently dilute on late postcontrast images to render urine high in signal intensity, which allows differentiation between high-signal intensity dilute gadolinium-containing urine in the collecting system and low-signal intensity fluid in parapelvic cysts. A MR urogram may also demonstrate that these oval-shaped cystic lesions do not communicate with the renal collecting system.

On MRI, they appear as perinephric cystic lesions most commonly located in the renal sinus.

Autosomal Dominant Polycystic Kidney Disease. Autosomal dominant polycystic kidney disease is characterized by the development of variably sized re-

nal cysts in both kidneys, which progress over time [17]. The disease usually becomes manifest in adult patients, which explains the alternate designation of adult polycystic kidney disease. Patients usually present late in the course of the condition with abdominal masses or hypertension or after trauma (17). Renal failure is a late event. The disease is almost always bilateral, although unilateral disease has been described. Cysts are frequently present in other organs including liver, spleen, and pancreas. Patients are at risk of subarachnoid hemorrhage from ruptured berry aneurysms in the circle of Willis.

The typical MRI appearance is that of bilaterally enlarged kidneys with multiple renal cysts of varying sizes involving all portions of the renal parenchyma, distorting the normal renal shape and architecture. Early in the course of the disease the cysts are small (fig. 9.22). Over time, kidneys enlarge massively (fig. 9.23). Cysts characteristically have varying signal intensities on all sequences because of the presence of blood products of differing ages [18] (fig. 9.23). The liver is the organ in which extrarenal cysts are most commonly observed. Liver cysts range in number from solitary to numerous. Even with extensive liver involvement, cysts tend not to distort the hepatic architecture and usually are <2 cm in diameter.

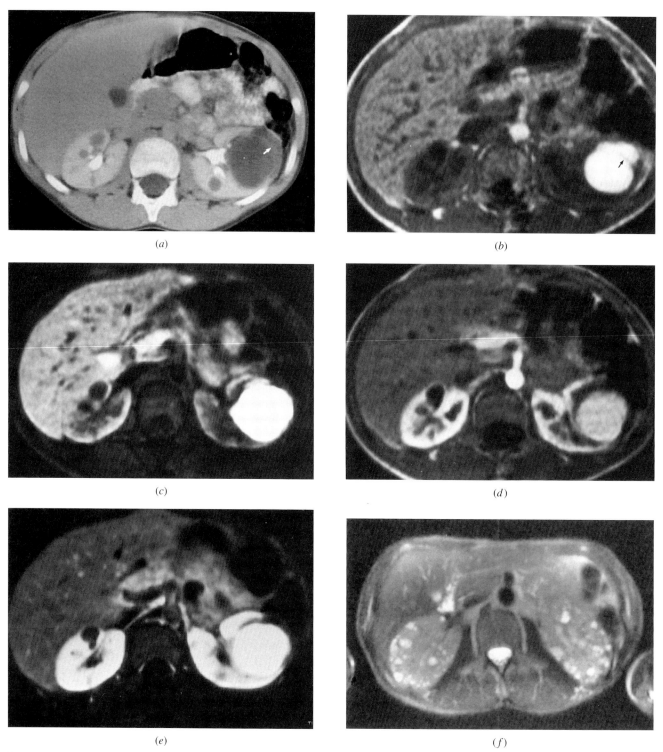

(a)

(b)

(c)

(d)

(e)

(f)

F I G . 9.22 Autosomal dominant polycystic kidney disease in the early stage of development. Contrast-enhanced CT (*a*), SGE (*b*), T1-weighted fat-suppressed spin-echo (*c*), immediate postgadolinium SGE (*d*), and gadolinium-enhanced T1-weighted fat-suppressed spin-echo (*e*) images. Multiple small bilateral renal cysts and a large left renal cyst are present. The majority of cysts are <1 cm in diameter, and the renal parenchyma is of normal thickness and not substantially distorted. These findings are consistent with early changes of autosomal dominant polycystic kidney disease. A large left renal cyst contains an internal septation on the CT image (arrow, *a*). Precontrast SGE image (*b*) shows that the cyst is high in signal intensity and contains a low-signal-intensity reticular strand (arrow, *b*). This cyst does not suppress with fat suppression (*c*) and does not enhance with gadolinium (*d*), which is consistent with subacute blood in a hemorrhagic cyst. A signal-void rim is appreciated on the postcontrast T1-FS image (*e*), which probably represents hemosiderin deposition.

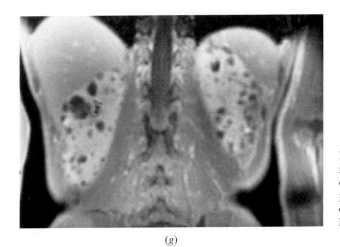

(g)

FIG. 9.22 (*Continued*) Fat-suppressed SS-ETSE (*f*) and coronal 90-s postgadolinium SGE (*g*) images in a second patient demonstrate multiple <2-cm cysts scattered throughout the renal parenchyma consistent with early stage autosomal dominant polycystic kidney disease. Note that kidneys are not substantially enlarged at this point.

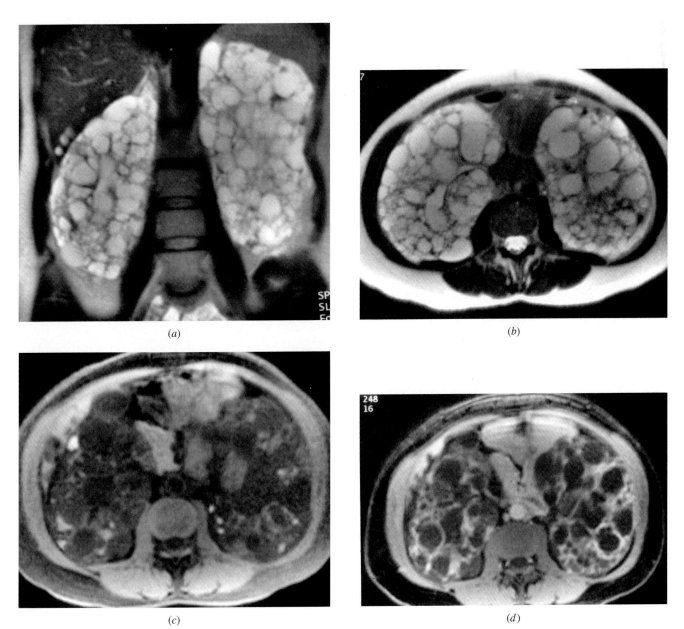

(a)

(b)

(c)

(d)

FIG. 9.23 Autosomal dominant polycystic kidney disease. Coronal (*a*) and transverse (*b*) SS-ETSE and precontrast (*c*), and postgadolinium (*d*) T1-weighted fat-suppressed SGE images. The kidneys are greatly enlarged with numerous cysts.

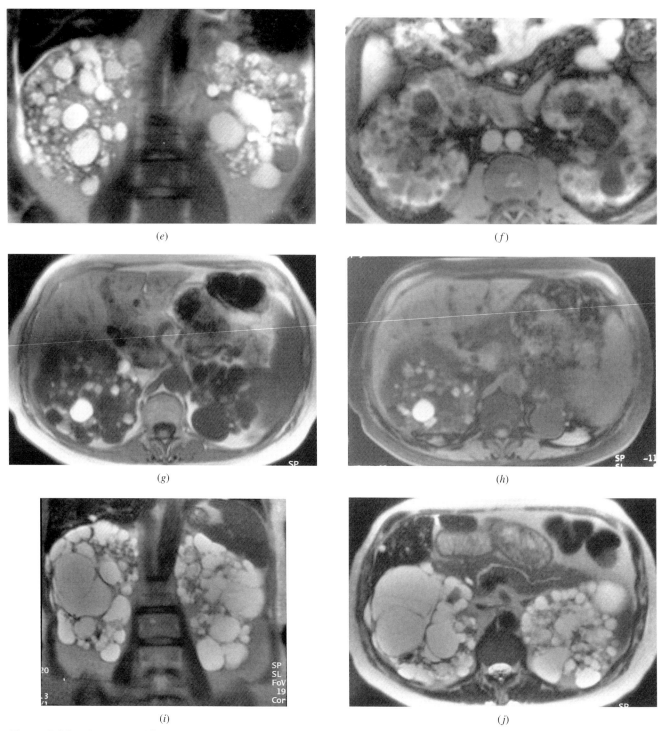

(e)

(f)

(g)

(h)

(i)

(j)

FIG. 9.23 (*Continued*) The majority of the cysts demonstrate increased T2 signal and decreased T1 signal consistent with simple cysts, but a sizable fraction have varying signal consistent with blood products of differing age. Postgadolinium images demonstrate no dominant enhancing areas worrisome for neoplasm.

Coronal SS-ETSE (*e*) and axial postcontrast fat-suppressed SGE (*f*) images in a second patient show the same findings described above. Evaluation for neoplasm in cystic kidneys such as these is difficult because of the varying signal of cysts.

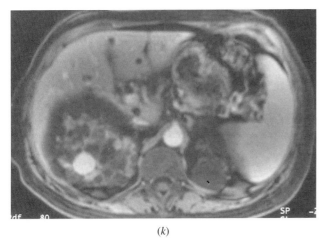

(k)

F I G . 9.23 (*Continued*) SGE (*g*), fat-suppressed SGE (*h*), coronal SS-ETSE (*i*), transverse SS-ETSE (*j*), and 90-s postgadolinium fat-suppressed SGE (*k*) images in a third patient. The kidneys are massively enlarged and contain multiple cysts of varying sizes scattered throughout the renal parenchyma, distorting renal architecture. Several cysts are high in signal intensity on T1-weighted images (*g*), and the high signal intensity is accentuated on the fat-suppressed T1-weighted image (*h*). The hemorrhagic cysts vary in signal intensity on T2-weighted images (*h, i*), consistent with blood products of varying age. Minimal enhancing parenchyma is apparent after gadolinium (*k*).

Autosomal Recessive Polycystic Kidney Disease. Autosomal recessive polycystic kidney disease (ARPKD) is a heritable but phenotypically heterogeneous disorder characterized by nonobstructive renal collecting duct ectasia, hepatic biliary duct ectasia and malformation, and fibrosis of kidneys and liver. Liver pathology is referred to as congenital hepatic fibrosis and is always present in ARPKD [16].

Kidneys are bilaterally enlarged with varying number of usually <1-cm cysts scattered through both kidneys (fig. 9.24). Patients often expire in infancy because of the effects of renal failure. In patients with less severe renal disease, progressive liver disease tends to result in patient death at less than 10 years of age. On MR images, multiple parenchymal cysts <1 cm in diameter are apparent on postgadolinium images.

Multicystic Dysplastic Kidney. Multicystic dysplastic kidney results from a congenital failure of fusion of the metanephrosis and ureteric bud resulting in a nonfunctional cystic renal mass. The ureter is typically atretic. Multicystic dysplastic kidney typically is large in infancy and, if left untreated, atrophies with time. The cyst wall often calcifies during the atrophic process. Multicystic dysplastic kidney may be diagnosed in childhood as a large multicystic mass that lacks organization of a collecting system and shows no evidence of normal renal parenchyma (fig. 9.25). Lesions also may be diagnosed in utero using breathing-independent T2-weighted single-shot echo-train spin-echo (fig. 9.26) images. Occasionally, a large multicystic dysplastic kidney may be observed in adolescent or adult patients.

Medullary Cystic Disease (Nephronophthisis— Uremic Medullary Cystic Disease Complex). Patients with medullary cystic disease typically present in adolescence with salt-wasting nephropathy and renal failure. On imaging studies, the renal medulla is extensively replaced by 1- to 2-cm cysts [20] (fig. 9.27). As renal failure progresses, smooth cortical atrophy develops.

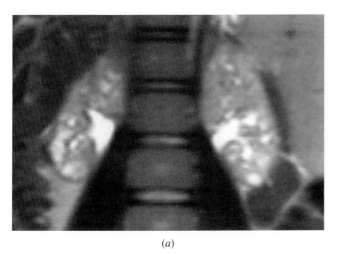

(a)

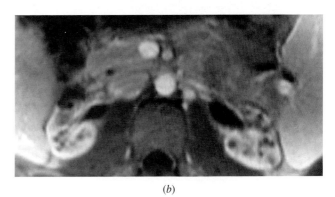

(b)

F I G . 9.24 Autosomal recessive polycystic kidney disease. Coronal SS-ETSE (*a*), immediate postgadolinium SGE (*b*), and interstitial phase postgadolinium fat-suppressed SGE (*c*) images in a patient with autosomal recessive polycystic kidney disease.

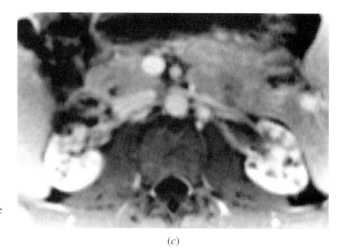

(c)

F i g . 9.24 (*Continued*) The kidneys are small, with multiple tiny cysts, scattered throughout the renal parenchyma.

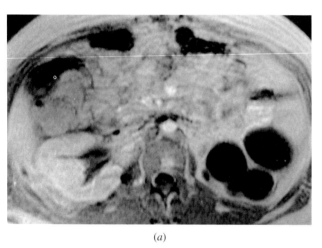

(a)

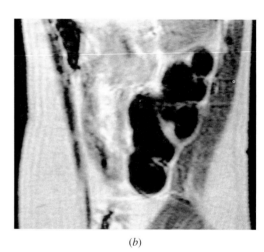

(b)

F i g . 9.25 **Multicystic dysplastic kidney.** Transverse 2-min (*a*) and sagittal 2.5-min (*b*) postgadolinium SGE images. A multicystic dysplastic kidney is present in the left renal fossa that has an cluster of grapes appearance with no evidence of organization into a renal collecting system and no renal parenchyma evident.

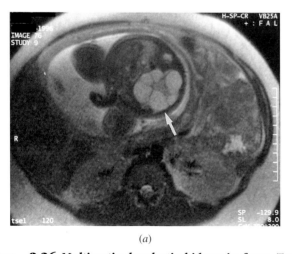

(a)

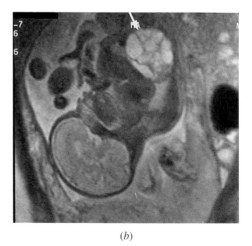

(b)

F i g . 9.26 **Multicystic dysplastic kidney in fetus.** Transverse (*a*) and sagittal (*b*) SS-ETSE images of a fetus demonstrate a multicystic mass in the left renal fossa (arrow, *a, b*) with no evidence of organization into a renal collecting system.

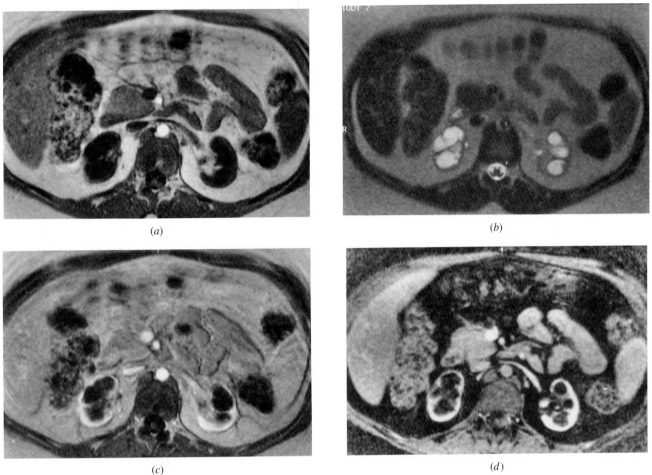

F I G . 9.27 Medullary cystic disease. SGE (*a*) SS-ETSE (*b*), immediate postgadolinium SGE (*c*), and 90-s postgadolinium T1-weighted fat-suppressed SGE (*d*) images. Multiple cysts measuring <2 cm in diameter occupy the majority of the renal medulla. These simulate the appearance of corticomedullary differentiation on precontrast images (*a*) in this patient with chronic renal failure. The cysts are homogeneously high in signal intensity on the T2-weighted image (*b*). After gadolinium administration, cysts in the renal medulla do not enhance and appear nearly signal void (*c, d*).

Medullary Sponge Kidney. Medullary sponge kidney (MSK) is characterized by multiple cystic dilatations of the papillary collecting ducts. Calculi are frequently present in the cystic cavities. The disease is usually bilateral but may be unilateral or segmental. Patients present with calculi, obstruction, infection, or hematuria. Tubular ectasia is considered a precursor of MSK. On intravenous urography, tubular ectasia appears as contrast-filled tubular structures that radiate from the calyx into the papilla. A similar appearance may be appreciated on interstitial-phase gadolinium-enhanced MR images, with prominent radiating, enhancing tubular structures demonstrated in the renal papillae (fig. 9.28).

Acquired Cystic Disease of Dialysis. Approximately 50% of patients on long-term hemodialysis develop multiple renal cysts [21–23]. The etiology is uncertain but may relate to ischemia or fibrosis. Kidneys are usually atrophic at the time of development of cystic disease. Cysts tend to be predominantly superficial in location in the renal cortex and tend not to expand the kidney substantially in size, in contrast to autosomal dominant cystic kidney disease, in which cysts are scattered throughout the parenchyma and renal size is usually massive. Cysts generally are smaller in size than in autosomal dominant polycystic kidney disease, measuring <2 cm in diameter. Uncommonly, cysts may also be >2 cm and/or scattered throughout renal parenchyma. Hemorrhage is frequently present in renal cysts in patients with chronic renal failure.

On MR images multiple small cysts are present in both kidneys, mainly in a superficial renal cortical location (figs. 9.29 and 9.30). Cysts are frequently high in signal intensity on precontrast T1-weighted images because of the presence of subacute blood (fig. 9.31).

MRI is well suited for detection of renal cancer and discrimination between nonenhancing cysts and

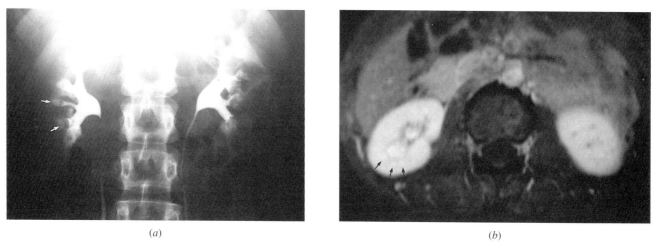

(a)   (b)

F I G . 9.28 Medullary sponge kidney. Five-minute intravenous urogram (*a*) and interstitial-phase gadolinium-enhanced T1-weighted fat-suppressed spin-echo (*b*) images. Tubular ectasia is apparent on the intravenous urogram (arrows, *a*). On the interstitial-phase gadolinium-enhanced image (*b*), prominent papillary enhancement is present (arrows, *b*).

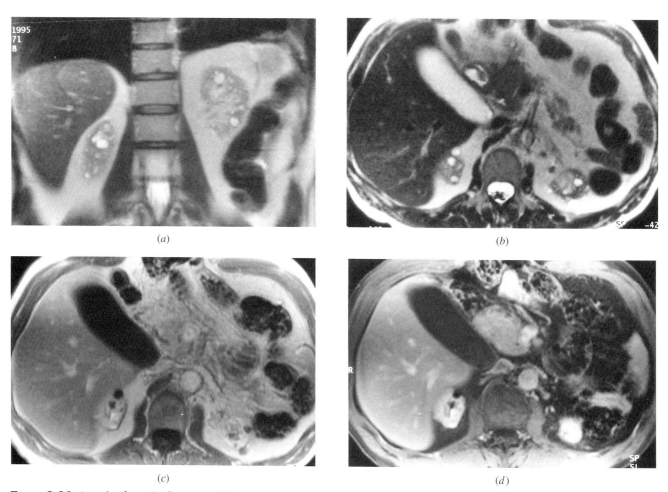

(a)   (b)

(c)   (d)

F I G . 9.29 Acquired cystic disease of dialysis. Coronal SS-ETSE (*a*), transverse SS-ETSE (*b*), immediate postgadolinium SGE (*c*), and gadolinium-enhanced T1-weighted fat-suppressed SGE (*d*) images. Multiple cysts <2 cm in diameter are present in both kidneys located predominantly in a superficial cortical location. The capillary phase of enhancement (*c*) demonstrates minimal parenchymal enhancement and no corticomedullary differentiation. On the gadolinium-enhanced T1-weighted fat-suppressed spin-echo image (*d*), multiple renal cysts are well shown in a background of moderately enhanced atrophic parenchymal tissue.

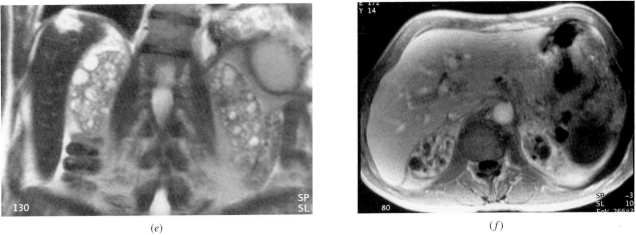

FIG. 9.29 (*Continued*) Coronal SS-ETSE (*e*) and interstitial-phase gadolinium-enhanced fat-suppressed SGE (*f*) images in a second patient on chronic hemodialysis with Alport syndrome. Multiple small cysts are scattered throughout the kidneys.

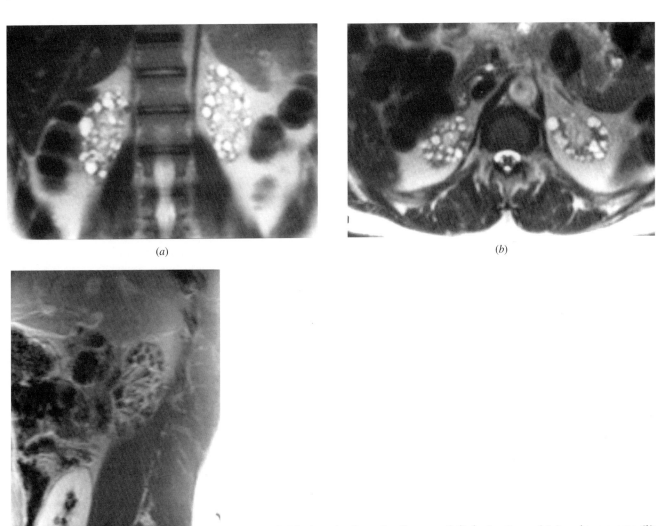

FIG. 9.30 Acquired cystic disease of dialysis. Coronal (*a*) and transverse (*b*) SS-ETSE, and sagittal postgadolinium T1-weighted SGE (*c*) images. Extensive multiple bilateral renal cysts with high signal on T2 (*a, b*) and low signal on postgadolinium T1-weighted images (*c*) are present in atrophic native kidneys. Note also transplanted kidney in the right pelvis (*c*).

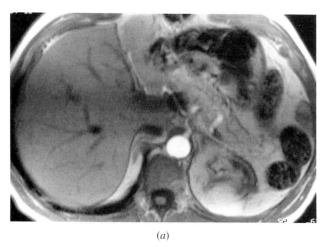

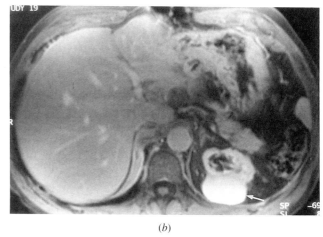

(a)   (b)

F I G . 9.31 Hemorrhagic large renal cyst in cystic disease of dialysis. Immediate postgadolinium SGE (*a*) and interstitial-phase gadolinium-enhanced fat-suppressed SGE (*b*) images demonstrate a homogeneously high-signal intensity superficial 4-cm cyst arising from the posterior left renal cortex (arrow, *b*).

enhancing cancers. Cysts demonstrate no evidence of enhancement and do not change in morphology on serial postcontrast images, whereas cancers and renal parenchyma will demonstrate evidence of enhancement.

Multilocular Cystic Nephroma (Cystic Nephroma).

Multilocular cystic nephroma is an uncommon benign lesion, which is usually unilateral, solitary, and sharply demarcated from surrounding uninvolved renal tissue. Cystic nephromas are composed of multiple non-communicating cysts separated by a fibrous stroma. This lesion has been described as occurring most frequently in boys aged 2 months to 4 years as well as adults, predominantly women, aged 40 years and older [24]. In a recent MRI study, adult-type multilocular cystic nephromas were observed in men and women in their 20s and 30s in an approximately equivalent gender distribution [25]. The diagnosis of multilocular cystic nephroma on MR images requires the demonstration of a multi-cystic renal mass that bulges into the renal pelvis and has relatively thick (2–4 mm), relatively uniform, fibrous septations (fig. 9.32) [25,26]. Septations are well defined and moderately low in signal intensity on T2-weighted images and enhance on postgadolinium images [25]. Transverse plane images should be supplemented with sagittal or coronal images to demonstrate indentation into the renal pelvis. Usually cysts are low in signal intensity on T1-weighted images, but not uncommonly they are high in signal intensity, presumably reflecting the presence of proteinaceous material or blood (fig. 9.33) [25, 26].

Angiomyolipoma.

Angiomyolipomas are benign tumors composed of variable amounts of three elements: 1) thick-walled blood vessels, 2) smooth muscle, and 3) mature fat. The fat component is usually substantial,

permitting characterization on CT images and on combined T1-weighted regular (in phase) and fat-suppressed images or combined T1-weighted in-phase and out-of-phase SGE images [27]. Although benign, these tumors may increase in size over time, with larger tumors having a greater propensity to bleed [28–31]. Angiomyolipomas have a greater tendency to increase in size when they are multiple than when they are solitary [29, 31]. Lesions may be detected and characterized, even when they are 1 cm in diameter, because of the high signal intensity of fat on T1-weighted images that attenuates on fat-suppressed images (fig. 9.34). Out-of-phase images are a useful addition to an imaging protocol performed to characterize renal masses as angiomyolipomas (figs. 9.35 and 9.36). A fat-water signal-void phase cancellation occurs at the boundary between the angiomyolipoma and the adjacent renal parenchyma [18]. When angiomyolipomas are very small (<1 cm) the phase cancellation may occupy the entire lesion and render it signal void [32]. In a small number of cases, when muscle or vascular components predominate, distinction from renal cell cancer may be difficult. When the diagnosis, based on imaging findings, is certain and tumors are <4 cm in size and asymptomatic, imaging follow-up is adequate management [30, 33]. Case reports have described renal cell cancers which contain a small volume of fat [34]. Uniform distribution of a high concentration of fat in renal cell cancer has not been described, unlike angiomyolipoma, in which fat content is usually relatively uniform and prominent. A heterogeneous-appearing mass with foci of fat should be considered an indeterminant lesion.

Tuberous Sclerosis (Bourneville Disease).

Tuberous sclerosis is a neurocutaneous syndrome, part of the general category of phakomatoses with autosomal dominant inheritance, although approximately 50% arise

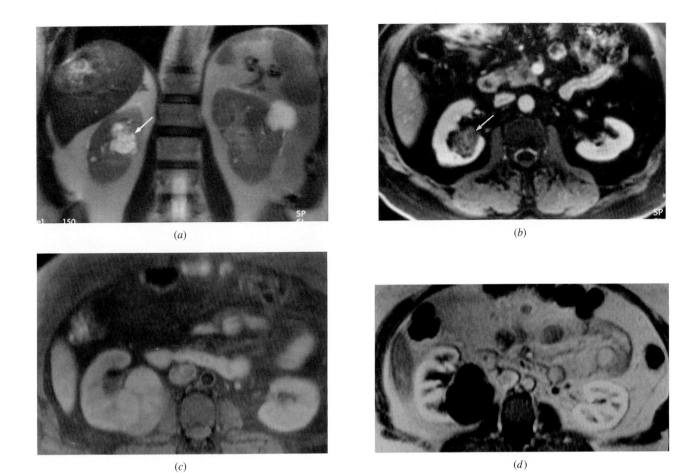

(a)

(b)

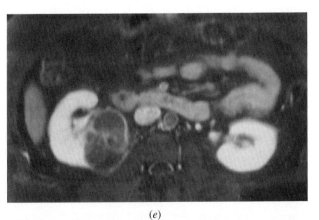

(c)

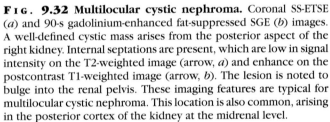

(d)

F I G . 9.32 Multilocular cystic nephroma. Coronal SS-ETSE (*a*) and 90-s gadolinium-enhanced fat-suppressed SGE (*b*) images. A well-defined cystic mass arises from the posterior aspect of the right kidney. Internal septations are present, which are low in signal intensity on the T2-weighted image (arrow, *a*) and enhance on the postcontrast T1-weighted image (arrow, *b*). The lesion is noted to bulge into the renal pelvis. These imaging features are typical for multilocular cystic nephroma. This location is also common, arising in the posterior cortex of the kidney at the midrenal level.

T1-weighted fat-suppressed spin-echo (*c*), immediate post-gadolinium SGE (*d*), and gadolinium-enhanced T1-weighted fat-suppressed spin-echo images (*e*) in a second patient with multilocular cystic nephroma demonstrate a similar-appearing cystic mass that bulges into the renal pelvis and contains enhancing internal septations. Note that the cyst contents are intermediate in signal intensity on the precontrast T1-weighted image (*c*).

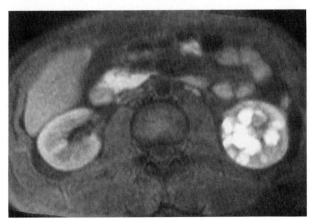

(e)

F I G . 9.33 Multilocular cystic nephroma. Precontrast T1-weighted fat-suppressed spin-echo image demonstrates a multilocular cystic nephroma in the lower pole of the left kidney. Many of the cysts are high in signal intensity compatible with either subacute blood or protein. Cysts are not uncommonly high in signal intensity on T1-weighted images in multilocular cystic nephroma.

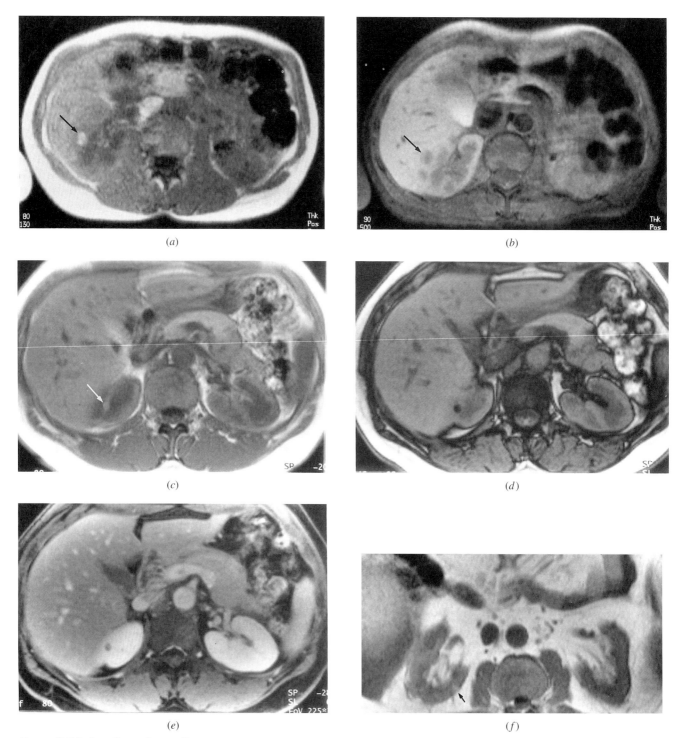

(a)

(b)

(c)

(d)

(e)

(f)

F I G . 9.34 Small angiomyolipoma. SGE (*a*) and T1-weighted fat-suppressed spin-echo (*b*) images. A small high-signal-intensity lesion arises from the upper pole of the right kidney on the SGE image (arrow, *a*). Fat suppression decreases the signal intensity of this lesion (arrow, *b*), confirming that it represents and angiomyolipoma.

SGE (*c*), out-of-phase SGE (*d*), and interstitial-phase gadolinium-enhanced fat-suppressed SGE (*e*) images in a second patient demonstrate a high signal intensity tumor on the in-phase image (arrow, *c*) that becomes signal void on the out-of-phase image (*d*) due to phase-cancellation artifact. The lesion is very low in signal on the post-gadolinium fat-suppressed SGE image (*e*).

SGE (*f*), fat-suppressed SGE (*g*) and out-of-phase SGE (*h*) images in a third patient. A 6 mm angiomyolipoma is present in the right kidney that is high in signal intensity on the in-phase image (arrow, *f*), suppresses to low signal intensity on the fat-suppressed image (arrow, *g*), and is signal void on the out-of-phase image (arrow, *h*).

SGE (*i*), fat-suppressed SGE (*j*) and out-of-phase SGE (*k*) images in a forth patient demonstrate tiny lesions that arise in a subcapsular location in the mid right kidney. These lesions are high signal on T1, signal void on the out-of-phase image (phase cancellation), and low signal on fat-suppressed images (fat suppression effect).

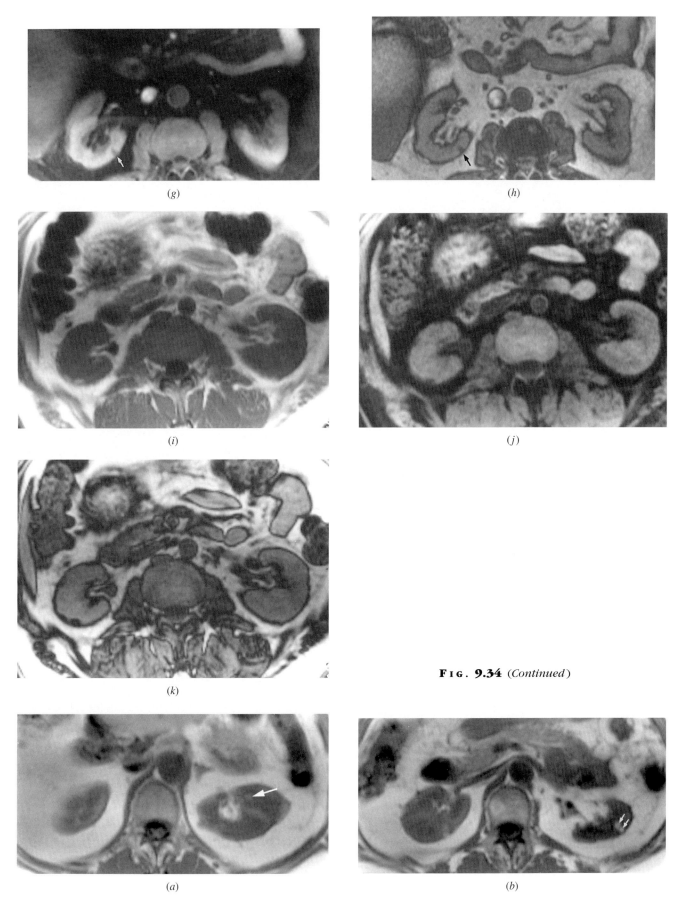

(g)

(h)

(i)

(j)

(k)

FIG. 9.34 (*Continued*)

(a)

(b)

FIG. 9.35 Angiomyolipoma and hemorrhagic cyst. Precontrast T1-weighted SGE (*a, b*) and T1-weighted out-of-phase SGE (*c, d*) images.

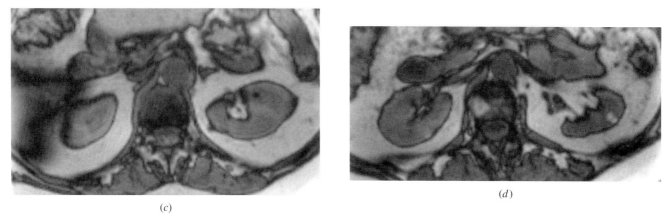

(c)

(d)

F I G . 9.35 (*Continued*) The angiomyolipoma (arrow, *a*) is high signal on in-phase and signal void on out-of-phase (*c*). The hemorrhagic cysts (arrows, *b*) are high signal on in-phase (*b*) and out-of-phase (*d*) images.

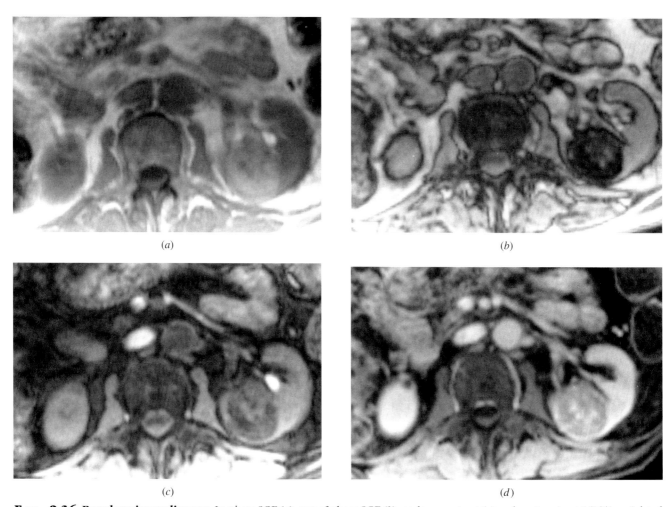

(a)

(b)

(c)

(d)

F I G . 9.36 Renal angiomyolipoma. *In-phase* SGE (*a*), out-of-phase SGE (*b*), and precontrast (*c*) and postcontrast (*d*) T1-weighted fat-suppressed SGE images. A 4-cm lesion with predominantly high signal on T1-weighted images (*a*) is present in the left kidney, which demonstrates regions of phase cancellation on out-of-phase images (*b*) and decreased signal on fat-suppressed images (*c*) diagnostic for the presence of substantial fat, confirming that the lesion represents an angiomyolipoma.

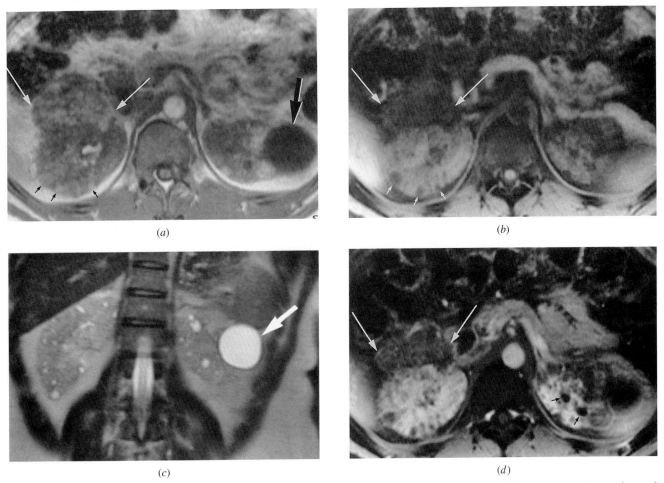

FIG. 9.37 Tuberous sclerosis. SGE (*a*), fat-suppressed SGE (*b*), SS-ETSE (*c*), and interstitial-phase gadolinium-enhanced transverse (*d*) and sagittal (*e*) fat-suppressed SGE images. Numerous varying-size angiomyolipomas are present throughout both kidneys (small arrows, *a*) including a large exophytic angiomyolipoma with multiple high-signal intensity punctuate foci of fat (long arrows, *a*). Multiple cysts are also present (large arrow, *a*). On the precontrast fat-suppressed image, the numerous small angiomyolipomas (small arrows, *b*) and the large angiomyolipoma (long arrows, *b*) decrease in signal intensity. The numerous angiomyolipomas and cysts (arrow, *c*) are high in signal intensity on the SS-ETSE image (*c*). After gadolinium administration the kidneys are shown to be extensively replaced by angiomyolipomas and cysts (small arrows, *d*). The large exophytic angiomyolipoma (long arrows, *d*, *e*) is well shown on transverse (*d*) and sagittal (*e*) postgadolinium fat-suppressed SGE-images.

from spontaneous mutation. This disorder is characterized by mental retardation, epilepsy, and cutaneous lesions [35].

Patients with tuberous sclerosis have an increased incidence of renal cysts and angiomyolipomas [28, 36]. Cystic disease varies considerably in extent and is usually multiple. Renal architecture is not uncommonly distorted. Cysts disease may be so extensive that the kidneys may resemble those of patients with autosomal dominant polycystic kidney disease. The incidence of angiomyolipomas is 70–95% [35], and they frequently are multiple and bilateral (fig. 9.37). Angiomyolipomas in patients with tuberous sclerosis have a tendency to increase in size over time, and be at increased risk of hemorrhage [28, 29, 35]. It is uncertain whether there is an increased incidence of renal cell carcinoma [35].

von Hippel-Lindau Disease. von Hippel-Lindau disease is a neurocutaneous syndrome, part of the general category of phakomatoses with autosomal dominant inheritance. Patients with von Hippel-Lindau disease have an increased incidence of renal cysts, adenomas, and carcinoma [37]. Carcinomas tend to be multicentric and bilateral (fig. 9.38) [37]. T1-weighted fat-suppressed imaging with gadolinium enhancement is the most sensitive technique for detecting multiple tumors, many of which are 1 cm in diameter.

Adenoma. Renal adenomas are benign tumors of renal cell origin and typically are small solid neoplasms [38]. The relationship of adenomas to renal cell carcinomas is uncertain [31]. Adenomas cannot be distinguished from papillary renal cell cancers on imaging

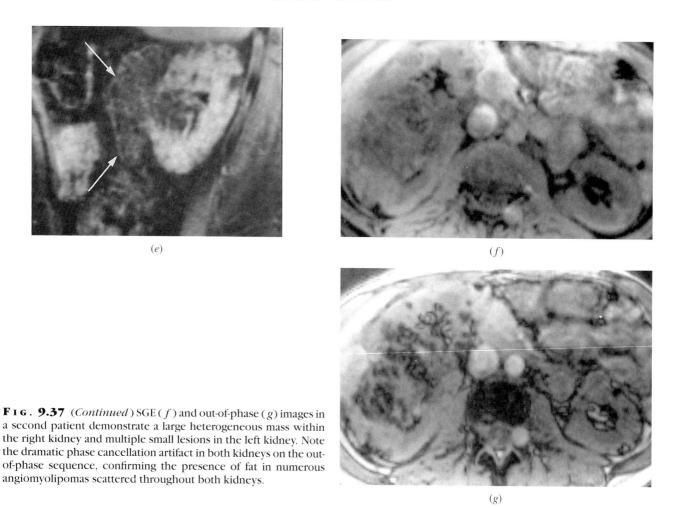

(e)

(f)

FIG. 9.37 (*Continued*) SGE (*f*) and out-of-phase (*g*) images in a second patient demonstrate a large heterogeneous mass within the right kidney and multiple small lesions in the left kidney. Note the dramatic phase cancellation artifact in both kidneys on the out-of-phase sequence, confirming the presence of fat in numerous angiomyolipomas scattered throughout both kidneys.

(g)

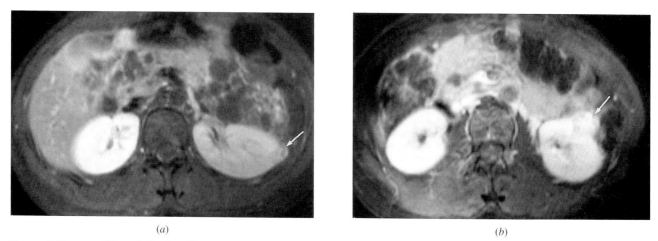

(a)

(b)

FIG. 9.38 von Hippel-Lindau disease. Gadolinium-enhanced T1-weighted fat-suppressed spin-echo images (*a, b*). Two small renal cancers are present in the mid (arrow, *a*) and lower (arrow, *b*) pole of the left kidney. Multiple pancreatic cysts are also appreciated (*a*).

studies [39, 40]. Depending on the clinical picture, patients with small solid tumors may benefit from serial reassessment to detect tumor growth. Tumor growth raises the concern of malignancy [26, 33–38]. It may be reasonable to follow a mass at 3 months, 6 months, 1 year, and yearly thereafter. Particularly in elderly patients, close observation likely results in the least patient morbidity [45, 46]. On MR images, adenomas are typically small (<4 cm), round masses that are slightly hypointense on T1-weighted images and slightly hyperintense on T2-weighted images and enhance in a diffuse intense fashion on capillary-phase images [18].

Oncocytomas are benign epithelial tumors that are generally solid and well encapsulated. A central stellate fibrous scar is often present [47]. Their incidence has been reported as 2–15% [48]. MRI reveals spherical masses that are relatively homogeneous with substantial central enhancement on capillary-phase images

(fig. 9.39) [48]. The characteristic early enhancement pattern is described as "spoke wheel" [18] but may not be commonly observed. In comparison, renal cancers tend to exhibit greater peripheral enhancement. Neither pattern of enhancement nor presence of central scar may be specific enough to permit reliable distinction from renal cell carcinoma [40, 49].

Myelofibrosis with Extramedullary Hematopoiesis. Myelofibrosis is a disorder classified as a chronic myeloproliferative disease, characterized by proliferation of bone marrow connective tissue and development of extramedullary hematopoiesis [50].

Extramedullary hematopoiesis (EMH) is defined as the formation and development of blood cells within an ectopic site outside the bone marrow. EMH is not always associated with myelofibrosis, and either of these processes may occur in the absence of a hematologic disorder. The liver and spleen are affected most commonly

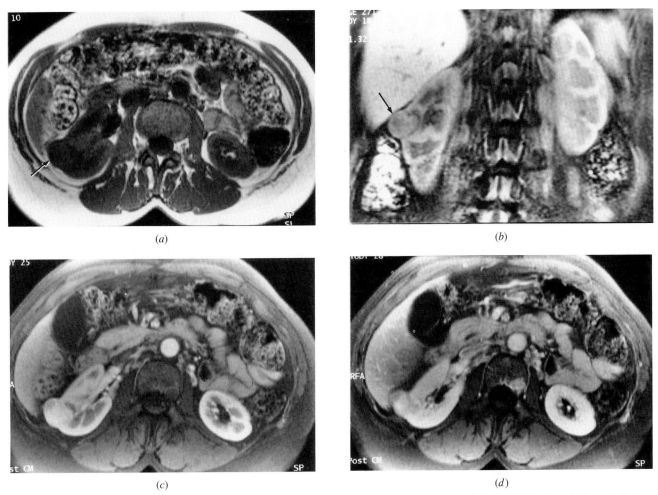

(a)

(b)

(c)

(d)

F i g . 9.39 **Renal oncocytoma.** SGE (*a*), coronal fat-suppressed SGE (*b*), immediate postgadolinium SGE (*c*), and 90-s gadolinium-enhanced fat-suppressed SGE (*d*) images. A well defined 2-cm mass is present in the right kidney (arrow, *a, b*). The majority of the tumor enhances in a moderately intense fashion on the immediate postgadolinium image (*c*) and shows mild peripheral washout by 90 s (*d*). The appearance is indistinguishable from that of a small renal cancer.

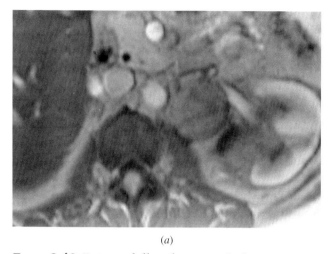
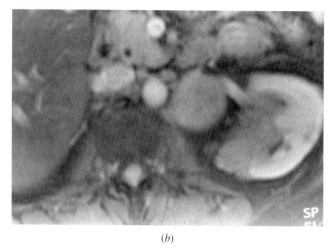

(a)   (b)

FIG. 9.40 Extramedullary hematopoiesis. Immediate postgadolinium SGE images (*a*) and 90 s postgadolinium T1-weighted fat-suppressed SGE (*b*) images in a patient with myelofibrosis. The left kidney demonstrates an infiltrating soft tissue mass involving the hilum and extending into the renal parenchyma. A large lymph node is also observed in the left para-aortic region.

resulting in hepatosplenomegaly [51]. Reports of renal involvement are rare in the literature [50].

The disease runs a chronic course and typically presents with symptoms related to anemia and splenomegaly that may be observed years before the diagnosis. When extramedullary hematopoiesis involves the kidneys it may lead to renal failure due to either ureteral obstruction or extensive parenchymal involvement [50]. The recognition of EMH as the cause of renal failure is important in these circumstances, as this entity may respond to radiotherapy [52].

In general, the differential diagnosis of a mass encasing the renal pelvis includes transitional cell carcinoma, lymphoma, lipomatosis, and renal cell carcinoma [52]. In the proper clinical setting, renal extramedullary hematopoiesis should be considered in the differential diagnosis. On MR images, EH tends to show mild early and late post contrast enhancement (fig. 9.40).

Malignant Masses

Renal Cell Carcinoma. More than 28,000 new cases of renal neoplasm were diagnosed in 1997, and 11,300 deaths occurred in the United States. Renal cell carcinoma is the predominant histology (80–85%) [53]. The peak age of incidence is 50–60 years of age with a male to female ratio of 2 to 1 [54]. Tumors are usually solitary. In approximately 5% of patients tumors are multiple. Patients usually present late in the course of the disease when tumors are large and in an advanced stage because of a lack of symptoms with small tumors. Renal cell cancer is associated with a myriad of presenting features including paraneoplastic phenomena.

Staging of renal cell cancer can be performed by either Robson's or TNM classification. Robson's classification is frequently used and is described in this text

(See below). Both MRI and current-generation CT scanners are able to detect renal cancers that measure 1 cm in diameter. In a study comparing dynamic contrast-enhanced CT imaging and MRI, these techniques detected 54 and 58 of 61 renal tumors that were present in 53 patients, respectively [55]. CT imaging and MRI correctly staged 24 and 29, respectively, of 31 renal cancers that were resected [55].

Although conventional MRI sequences may be useful in evaluating large renal tumors to assess the presence of tumor thrombus or extension of tumor to adjacent organs [56], consistent demonstration of small tumors, distinction between cysts and tumors, and reliable evaluation of tumor thrombus and metastases requires the use of intravenous gadolinium. MRI using gadolinium-enhanced breath-hold SGE and fat-suppressed sequences is superior to CT imaging in differentiating cysts from solid tumors because of the higher sensitivity of MRI for gadolinium than CT imaging for iodine contrast [1, 14, 55].

The typical appearance of a renal cell cancer is an irregular mass with ill-defined margins. Tumors are generally slightly hypointense on T1-weighted images and slightly hyperintense on T2-weighted images relative to renal cortex [56]. The minimal signal difference from renal cortex renders tumors poorly visualized on noncontrast images. After gadolinium administration, heterogeneous enhancement is apparent on immediate postgadolinium images, and enhancement diminishes on more delayed postcontrast images. Tumors are frequently hypervascular and demonstrate intense enhancement on immediate postgadolinium capillary-phase images, usually in a heterogeneous fashion with more intense peripheral enhancement [1, 14, 55–58]. Homogeneous enhancement does occur and is typical of small, low-grade cancers [55]. Homogeneously enhancing small tumors may be difficult to distinguish from renal cortex on immediate postgadolinium images. As a result, it is important that a renal MRI protocol include not only immediate postgadolinium capillary-phase images but also more delayed interstitial-phase images (fig. 9.41). Diminished enhancement on interstitial-phase images is observed for the great majority of tumors. Hypervascular cancers tend to wash out of contrast, whereas renal cortex remains high in signal intensity because of retention of contrast in renal tubules (see fig. 9.41). Large, >5-cm, hypervascular cancers most commonly demonstrate central necrosis.

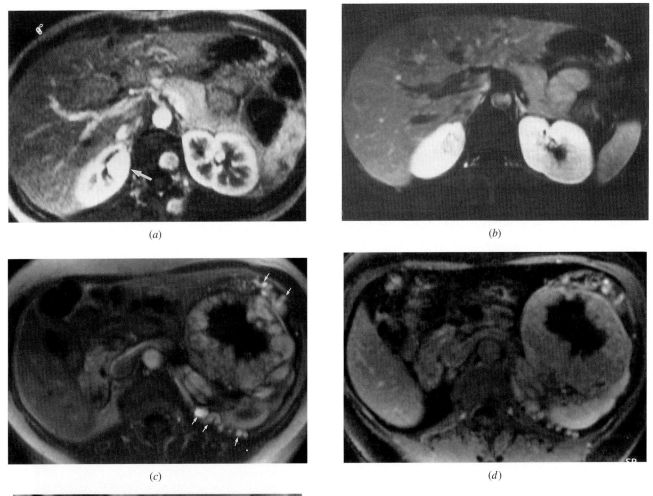

(a)

(b)

(c)

(d)

(e)

F I G . 9.41 Hypervascular renal cell cancer. Immediate postgadolinium SGE (*a*) and gadolinium-enhanced T1-weighted fat-suppressed spin-echo (*b*) images demonstrate a small uniform-enhancing Stage I renal cell cancer. A 2-cm renal cancer arises from the upper pole of the right kidney. The cancer enhances in a uniform intense fashion (arrow, *a*) on the immediate postgadolinium image, comparable in signal intensity to renal cortex. On the later interstitial-phase image the tumor is heterogeneous and lower in signal intensity than cortex.

Immediate postgadolinium SGE (*c*), 90-s postgadolinium fat-suppressed SGE (*d*) and sagittal 5-min postgadolinium SGE (*e*) images in a second patient demonstrate a 7-cm hypervascular renal cell cancer arising from the left kidney. On the immediate postgadolinium image (*c*), viable tumor enhances intensely with lack of enhancement of the central portion of the tumor. Intense enhancement of multiple enlarged feeding vessels is present (arrows, *c*). On the 90-s postgadolinium image (*d*) the tumor has diminished in signal lower than renal cortex. The sagittal image (*e*) displays the location of the tumor in the midportion of the kidney.

Approximately 20% of renal carcinomas may be hypovascular. This MRI finding may be related to a subset of renal cell carcinoma termed papillary renal cell carcinoma (approximately 15% of all cases). These tumors tend to be large, solid, well-demarcated lesions that are slow growing and show hypovascularity or avascularity on angiography [59]. Hypovascular renal cancers enhance minimally on capillary-phase images and remain low in signal intensity relative to cortex on interstitial-phase images. These tumors may be sharply marginated and may resemble cysts on contrast-enhanced CT images. Diagnosis of a hypovascular renal cancer requires identification of small, short, curvilinear enhanced structures that are present on postgadolinium images but not apparent on precontrast images. Interstitial-phase images acquired with fat suppression are the most reliable at demonstrating these enhancing structures (fig. 9.42). A recent study [60] demonstrated that negligible enhancement of a renal lesion, particularly a small lesion (<1 cm), after administration of gadolinium, may not exclude malignancy in occasional small (<1 cm) hemorrhagic tumors. Careful attention should be paid to the heterogeneity of

signal intensity of these lesions on all MR sequences, as this may be an indicator of their solid composition.

Hemorrhage occurs occasionally in tumors in patients with normal renal function. This is different from tumors in patients with chronic renal failure, in which hemorrhage is relatively common (see below). Hemorrhage appears high in signal intensity on noncontrast T1-weighted images (fig. 9.43).

Tumor size is not a reliable criterion for diagnosing renal cancer nor for distinguishing cancer from adenoma [40–46]. Renal cell cancers occasionally show no change in size in intervals of greater than 1 year [42, 45]. Any solid renal tumor that is nonfatty should be considered a possible renal cell carcinoma and should, at a minimum, be followed by serial imaging.

Robson's staging classifications for Renal Cell Carcinoma

Stage 1 renal carcinomas are confined within the renal capsule (figs. 9.44 and 9.45).

Stage 2 carcinomas extend beyond the renal capsule but are confined by Gerota fascia (figs. 9.46 and 9.47). Carcinomas that are completely intraparenchymal

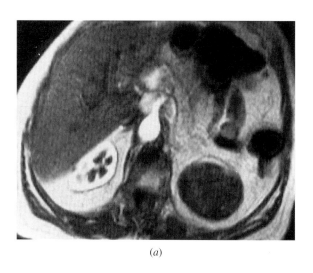

(a)

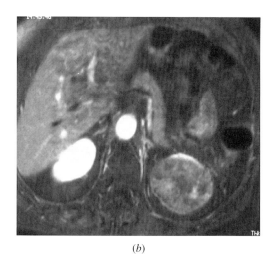

(b)

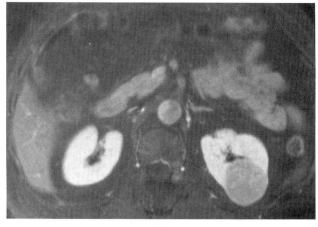

(c)

F I G . 9.42 Hypovascular Stage 2 renal cell cancer. Immediate postgadolinium SGE (*a*) and gadolinium-enhanced T1-weighted fat-suppressed spin-echo (*b*) images. The tumor shows diminished enhancement immediately after contrast (*a*). The interstitial-phase fat-suppressed image demonstrates small irregular enhancing structures within the mass (*b*), which distinguishes this lesion from a complicated cyst.

Interstitial-phase gadolinium-enhanced T1-weighted fat-suppressed spin-echo image (*c*) in a second patient shows small irregular enhancing structures in a hypovascular renal cancer arising from the left kidney. The great majority of hypovascular renal cell cancers are of papillary subtype.

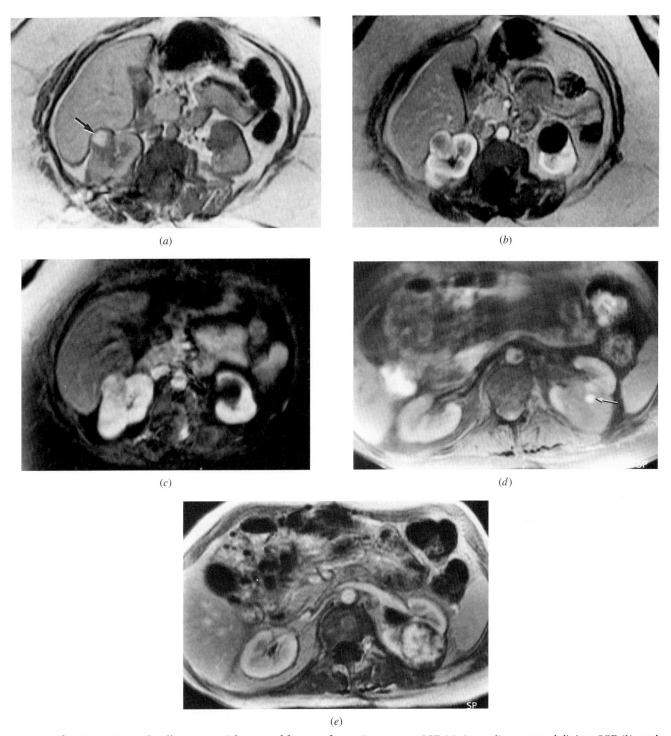

(a)   *(b)*

(c)   *(d)*

(e)

F I G . 9.43 Stage 2 renal cell cancer with central hemorrhage. Precontrast SGE (*a*), immediate postgadolinium SGE (*b*), and gadolinium-enhanced T1-weighted fat-suppressed spin-echo (*c*) images. Hemorrhage is present in a 2.5-cm Stage 2 renal cancer arising from the right kidney, which appears as high-signal intensity substance on the precontrast T1-weighted image (arrow, *a*). The tumor shows intense rim enhancement on the immediate postgadolinium image (*b*). Heterogeneous enhancement of the tumor is apparent on the interstitial-phase fat-suppressed image (*c*).

   Precontrast fat-suppressed SGE (*d*) and immediate postgadolinium SGE (*e*) images in a second patient demonstrate a 5-cm tumor arising in the left kidney. Foci of central high signal intensity on the precontrast image (arrow, *d*) are consistent with hemorrhage. The tumor exhibits an unusual central radiating enhancement pattern on the immediate postgadolinium SGE image (*e*). This pattern of enhancement may be more typical of oncocytoma but was present in this renal cell cancer.

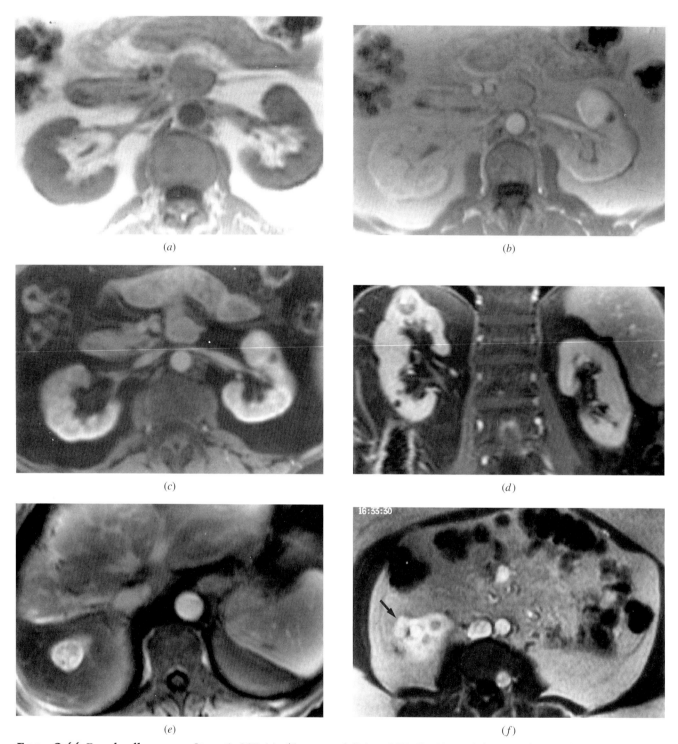

F I G . 9.44 Renal cell cancer—Stage 1. SGE (*a*), 45-s postgadolinium SGE (*b*), 90-s gadolinium-enhanced fat-suppressed SGE (*c*) images. There is a lesion in the anterior aspect of the mid pole of the left kidney that is heterogeneous in signal intensity on T1-weighted images and enhances markedly post-gadolinium administration, consistent with a renal cell carcinoma. Adjacent to this lesion, a tiny simple cyst is noted.

Coronal (*d*) and transverse (*e*) 2- to 3-min postgadolinium fat-suppressed SGE images in a second patient. A 2-cm renal cell cancer arises from the upper pole of the right kidney that exhibits heterogeneous enhancement on interstitial phase images.

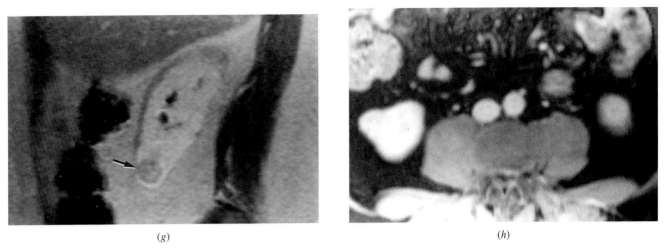

(g) (h)

F I G . 9.44 (*Continued*) Immediate postgadolinium SGE (*f*) and 7-min postgadolinium sagittal SGE (*g*) images in a third patient. A small renal cancer arises from the lower pole of the right kidney. The tumor demonstrates marked enhancement immediately after contrast administration (arrow, *f*) and diminished enhancement on the delayed postcontrast SGE image (arrow, *g*).

Ninety-second postgadolinium fat-suppressed SGE image (*h*) in a fourth patient. There is a small lesion in the upper pole of the right kidney that shows marked enhancement after administration of gadolinium.

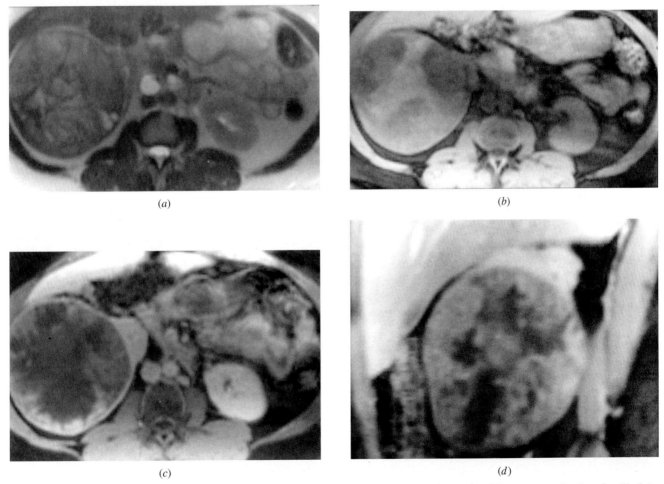

(a) (b)

(c) (d)

F I G . 9.45 Large renal cell cancer—Stage 1. Transverse SS-ETSE (*a*), precontrast T1-weighted fat-suppressed spin-echo (*b*), 2- to 3-min postgadolinium transverse (*c*) and sagittal (*d*) fat-suppressed SGE images. A large, well-encapsulated mass is seen involving the mid to lower portion of the right kidney with marked heterogeneity in signal on T1- and T2-weighted images, and on postgadolinium images. Despite the relatively large tumor size this represented a stage 1 renal cancer. Small areas of central low signal on postgadolinium images represent foci of necrosis.

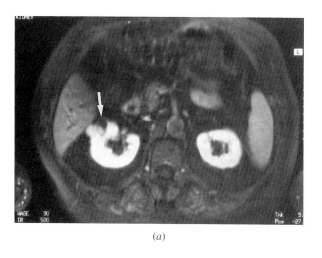

(a)

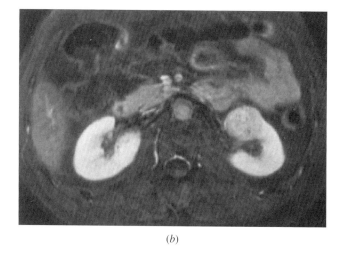

(b)

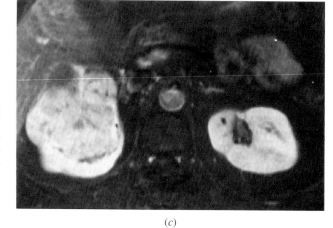

(c)

F I G . 9.46 Renal cell cancer—Stage 2. Gadolinium-enhanced T1-weighted fat-suppressed spin-echo images in 3 patients (*a–c*). Stage 2 cancer can vary in size from small (*a*) to large (*c*). Tumors are heterogeneous and lower in signal intensity than adjacent cortex on interstitial-phase images. Larger cancers have a propensity to undergo regions of necrosis that appear nearly signal void on postcontrast images (*c*). A simple renal cyst (arrows, *a*) adjacent to the renal cancer is present in the first of these patients.

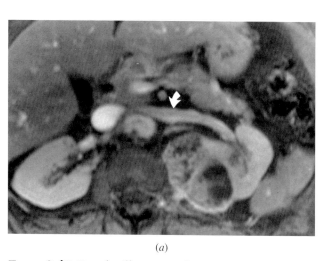

(a)

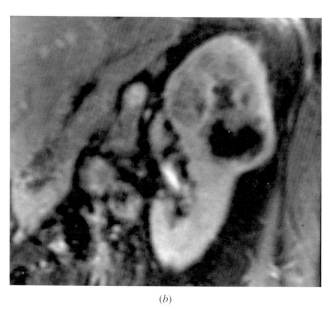

(b)

F I G . 9.47 Renal cell cancer—Stage 2. Transverse (*a*) and sagittal (*b*) 2-to 3-min postgadolinium T1-weighted fat-suppressed SGE images. A large renal cancer arises from the upper pole of the left kidney. This mass demonstrates marked heterogeneity of signal on the postgadolinium images, with central areas of necrosis. The renal vein is clearly shown as free of thrombus on the gadolinium-enhanced fat-suppressed image (arrow, *a*). There is no evidence of perinephretic fat infiltration.

are Stage 1 carcinomas. On the basis of imaging features, distinction between Stage 1 and Stage 2 carcinomas cannot be reliably made for tumors that extend beyond the cortical margins. Large exophytic tumors may be Stage 1, and tumors with a small extrarenal component may be Stage 2. Surgical management is identical for disease Stages 1 and 2, so differentiation by imaging is not essential. Renal cell carcinomas Stages 1 and 2 are associated with a high survival rate because the tumor is amenable to complete resection.

Stage 3a renal carcinoma is defined by tumor extension into the renal vein. Tumor thrombus frequently extends into the inferior vena cava (IVC) and grows superiorly with the direction of blood flow toward (fig. 9.48) and, in advanced cases, into the right atrium. Symptoms directly attributable to tumor thrombus are rare, even in the presence of total IVC occlusion, because venous collateralization occurs through the azygos and lumbar

systems. Hence, the presence of IVC thrombus is often detected incidentally by radiologic imaging [61].

MRI is superior to CT imaging in determining the presence and superior extent of thrombus. In one series of 431 patients, the sensitivity of MR imaging (90%) for detecting IVC thrombus was greater than that of either CT (79%) or conventional sonography (68%) [61].

Modern-generation CT imaging is not substantially inferior to MRI in detecting the presence of thrombus. However, the major advantages of MRI are demonstration of the superior extent of thrombus and determination whether thrombus is tumor or blood thrombus.

Direct coronal or sagittal plane images are important for the demonstration of the superior extent of thrombus. This information is useful in that it assists in surgical planning for thrombus extraction. Thrombus extension above the hepatic veins requires a thoracoabdominal approach rather than an abdominal approach, whereas the

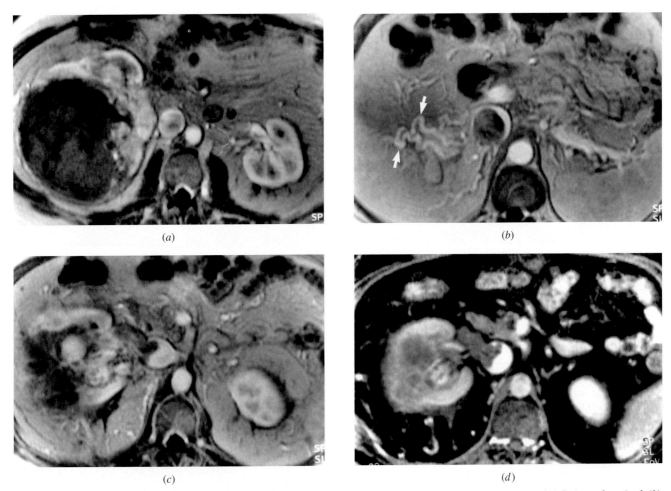

(a)

(b)

(c)

(d)

F I G. 9.48 Renal cell cancer—Stage 3-A. Immediate (*a*) and 45-s (*b, c*) and transverse (*d, e*), coronal (*f, g*), and sagittal (*h*) gadolinium-enhanced T1-weighted fat-suppressed SGE images. A heterogeneous enhancing large renal cancer is present, which originates from the lower two-thirds of the right kidney. An enhancing tumor thrombus is seen within the right renal vein that extends into the inferior vena cava. Direct coronal (*f, g*) and sagittal (*h*) images permit evaluation of the superior extent of thrombus (arrow, *f*).

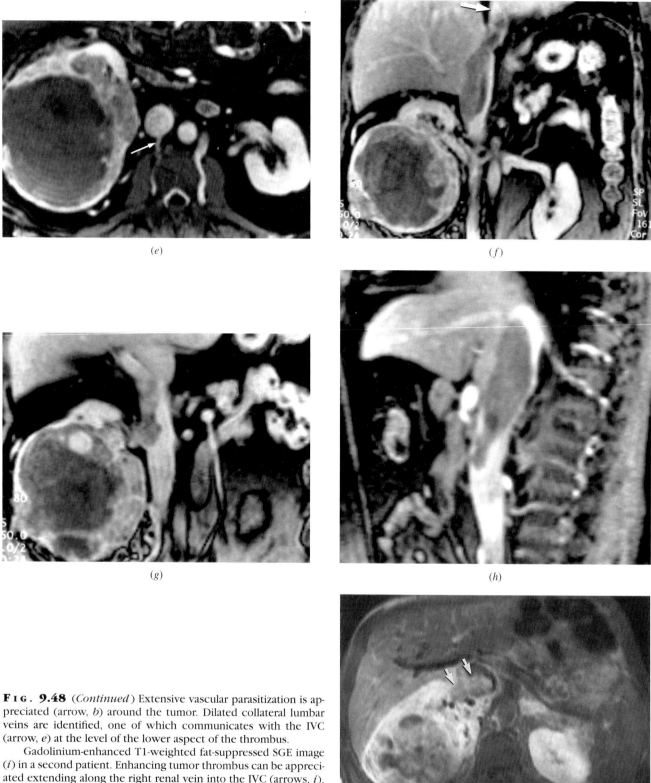

(e)

(f)

(g)

(h)

(i)

F I G . 9.48 (*Continued*) Extensive vascular parasitization is appreciated (arrow, *b*) around the tumor. Dilated collateral lumbar veins are identified, one of which communicates with the IVC (arrow, *e*) at the level of the lower aspect of the thrombus.

Gadolinium-enhanced T1-weighted fat-suppressed SGE image (*i*) in a second patient. Enhancing tumor thrombus can be appreciated extending along the right renal vein into the IVC (arrows, *i*). Enhancement of tumor thrombus is well shown on fat-suppressed postgadolinium images acquired in the interstitial phase.

latter approach is used if thrombus extends below the hepatic veins.

Gadolinium administration is generally useful for the evaluation of thrombus composition because tumor thrombus virtually always enhances with gadolinium. Although differentiation of tumor thrombus from bland thrombus may not change surgical treatment, it is an important distinction because the neovascular bed of the tumor thrombus may adhere to the venous wall, whereas a simple tumor clot will not [61], and patient prognosis and likelihood of lung metastases are affected. In comparison, in one CT imaging series, tumor thrombus was correctly detected in 18 of 19 patients on CT images of the patients, but only three of these thrombi demonstrated appreciable enhancement [62]. A gradient-echo technique that refocuses the signal of flowing blood (e.g., gradient recalled acquisition in steady state) has been proposed as another method for evaluating tumor thrombus [63]. On these images, tumor thrombus is intermediate in signal intensity (i.e., soft tissue signal intensity) whereas blood thrombus is low in signal intensity because of the presence of blood breakdown products. Because contrast enhancement should be rou-

tinely employed in evaluating kidneys and flow-sensitive gradient-echo is rapid to perform, it may be reasonable to use both methods to evaluate thrombus to increase confidence of characterization.

Stage 3b renal carcinoma is defined by the presence of malignant nodes (fig. 9.49). MRI is occasionally able to detect necrosis in lymph nodes, which appears as irregular low-signal intensity centers that may not be apparent on CT images. In the presence of a necrotic primary tumor, necrosis of lymph nodes may be specific for nodal involvement. The presence of enlarged lymph nodes does not necessarily indicate Stage 3b or 3c disease because adenopathy also may be benign. Studer et al. [64] reported that 58% of 163 patients with renal cell carcinoma had enlarged hyperplastic lymph nodes.

Stage 3c is tumor extension into the renal vein and nodal involvement (fig. 9.50).

Stage 4 disease is extension to local (**4a**) or distant (**4b**) sites. Even when renal cancers are large and have a long interface with adjacent organs (e.g., liver), direct tumor invasion is relatively uncommon (fig. 9.51). Direct multiplanar imaging facilitates recognition of smooth interfaces, implying no invasion, and

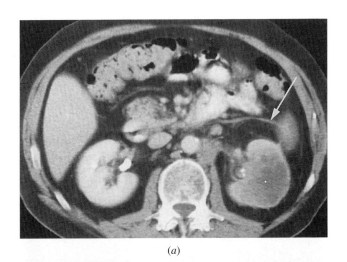

(a)

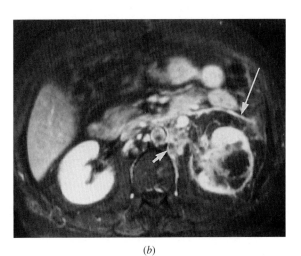

(b)

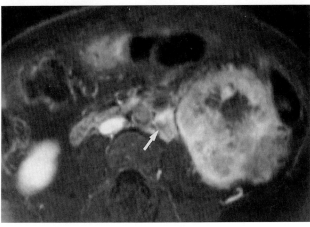

(c)

FIG. 9.49 Renal cell cancer—Stage 3-B. Contrast-enhanced CT (*a*) and interstial-phase gadolinium-enhanced T1-weighted fat-suppressed spin-echo (*b*) images. A necrotic 6-cm tumor is present in the left kidney. Enlarged para-aortic nodes are identified on the CT scan. On the postcontrast T1-weighted fat-suppressed image the nodes enhance in a heterogeneous fashion with central low signal intensity (short arrow, *b*), with an appearance similar to that of the primary tumor. Note the thickening of Gerota fascia (long arrows, *a, b*) shown on the CT and MR images.

Gadolinium-enhanced T1-weighted fat-suppressed image (*c*) of a Stage 3-B cancer in a second patient demonstrates a heterogeneous necrotic primary renal cancer of the left kidney with central necrosis and para-aorta lymph nodes with a similar heterogeneous appearance (arrow, *c*).

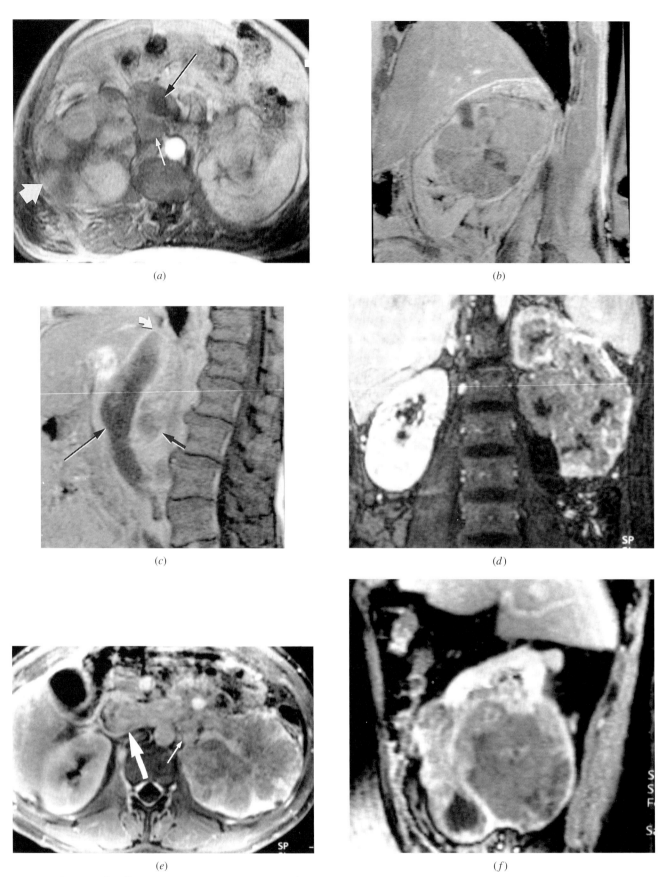

FIG. 9.50 Renal cell cancer—Stage 3-C. Transverse 45 s (*a*) and sagittal 90-second (*b, c*) postgadolinium SGE images. A 7-cm heterogeneously enhancing renal cancer is present in the right kidney (arrow, *a*). Thrombus is present in the IVC (long arrow, *a, c*). Retrocaval (short arrows *a, c*) and paracaval nodes are identified. The thrombus (long arrow, *c*) is noted to terminate approximately 1 cm below the level of the diaphragm on the sagittal projection (curved arrow, *c*).

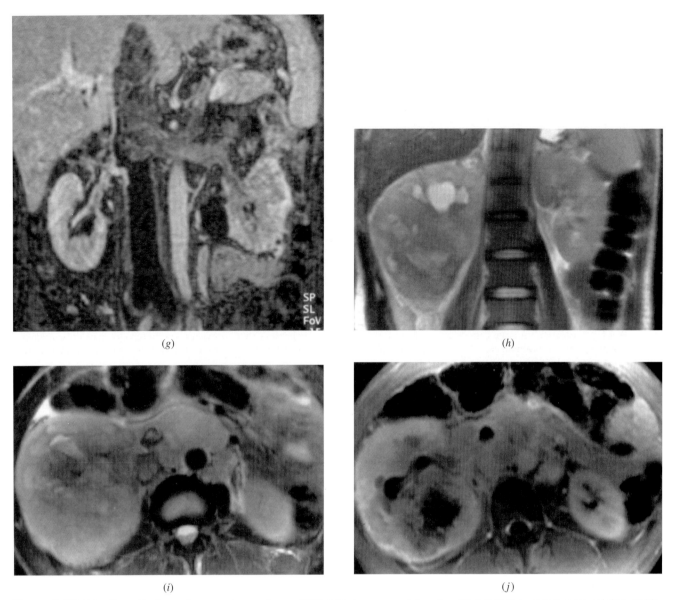

(g)　　　　　　　　　　　　　　　(h)

(i)　　　　　　　　　　　　　　　(j)

FIG. 9.50 (*Continued*) Coronal source image for an MRA (*d*), transverse (*e*) and sagittal (*f*) 2- to 3-min postgadolinium T1-weighted fat-suppressed SGE and coronal 3D MIP reconstructed MRA (*g*) images in a second patient. A large heterogeneous infiltrative mass is seen involving the lower two-thirds of the left kidney, which invades the left renal vein and extends into the IVC (large arrow, *e*). Regional lymph node metastases are present (small arrow, *e*).

Coronal (*b*) and transverse (*i*) SS-ETSE and 90-s postgadolinium fat-suppressed (*j*) SGE images in a third patient shows a large heterogeneous mass in the right kidney associated with IVC thrombosis and extensive enlarged retroperitoneal lymph nodes.

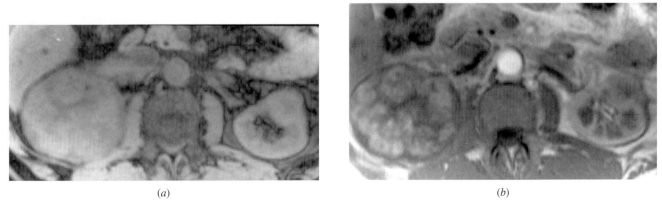

(a)　　　　　　　　　　　　　　　(b)

FIG. 9.51 Renal cell cancer—Stage 4-A. Precontrast T1-weighted fat-suppressed SGE (*a*), immediate postgadolinium SGE (*b*), 2-min postgadolinium fat-suppressed SGE (*c*), and coronal source image for MRA (*d*) images.

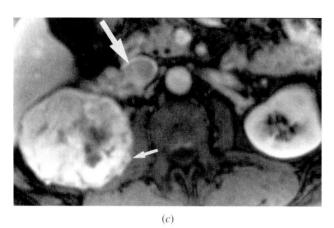

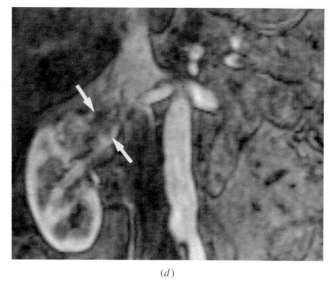

(c)   *(d)*

F I G . 9.51 *(Continued)* A large cancer arising from the right kidney is present that shows intense heterogeneous enhancement on immediate postgadolinium images (*b*), foci of central necrosis (*c*), tumor thrombus (long arrow, *c*; arrows, *d*), and invasion of the right psoas muscle (short arrow, *c*).

irregularly marginated interfaces, consistent with invasion. The sagittal plane is particularly effective at evaluating the interface with the liver. Renal cancer metastasizes to lung, adrenal glands, mediastinum, axial skeleton (fig. 9.52), and liver. The lung is the most common site of metastases. Lung metastases measuring 3 mm in diameter are detected on CT images. Reliable detection of metastases measuring 3 mm in diameter may be made using a gadolinium-enhanced modified MRA sequence termed VIBE. Advantages of this sequence include minimal phase-encoding artifact posterior to the heart, good

opacification of pulmonary vessels, and consistent image quality [65].

In rare instances, renal cell carcinoma is visualized on MRI as largely or completely cystic (fig. 9.53). This radiologic appearance may be best correlated pathologically with a distinct subtype of renal cell carcinoma termed multilocular cystic renal cell carcinoma. This rare form of renal cell carcinoma has a characteristic gross appearance. In contrast to many renal cell carcinomas, which are primarily solid masses with focal cystic degeneration, multilocular cystic renal cell carcinoma is

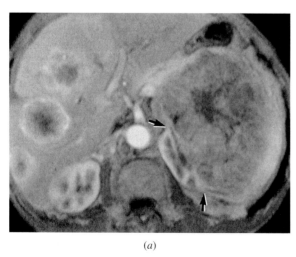

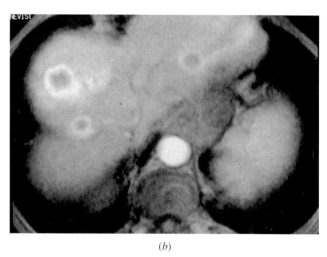

(a)   *(b)*

F I G . 9.52 Renal cell cancer—Stage 4-B. Immediate postgadolinium SGE images (*a, b*) demonstrate a 12-cm renal cancer arising from the left kidney (arrows, *a*). Multiple hypervascular ring-enhancing liver metastases are noted. Renal cancer metastases to the liver are frequently hypervascular.

Transverse (*c, d*) and sagittal (*e*) 2- to 3-min postgadolinium T1-weighted fat-suppressed SGE images in a second patient. There is a large heterogeneous mass in the lateral aspect of the right kidney that invades the renal vein and extends into the IVC (arrows, *c*). Extensive retroperitoneal adenopathy is also present (arrow, *d*).

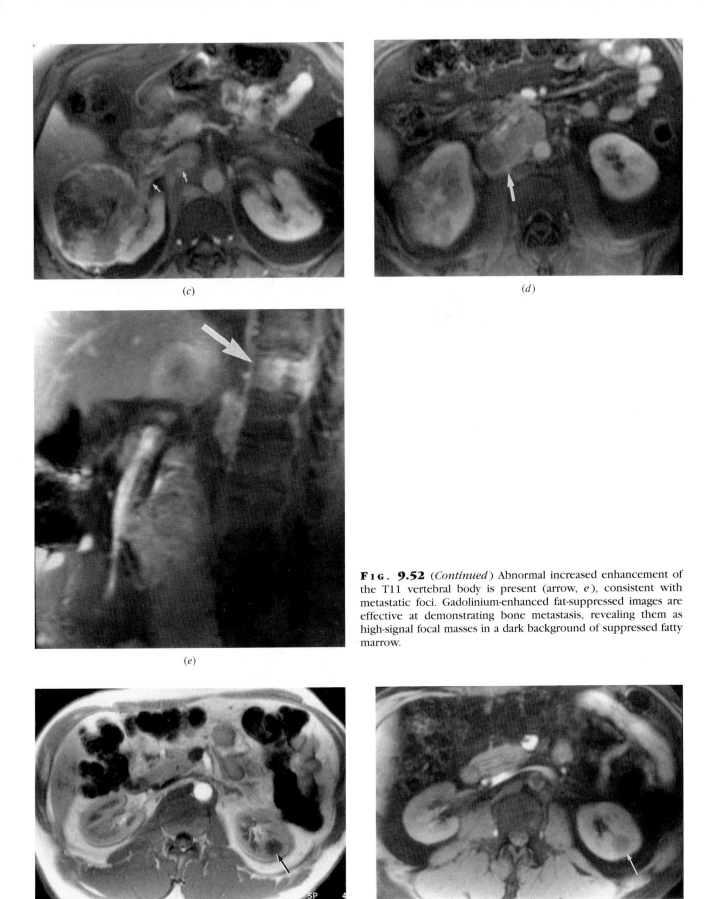

(c)

(d)

(e)

FIG. 9.52 (*Continued*) Abnormal increased enhancement of the T11 vertebral body is present (arrow, *e*), consistent with metastatic foci. Gadolinium-enhanced fat-suppressed images are effective at demonstrating bone metastasis, revealing them as high-signal focal masses in a dark background of suppressed fatty marrow.

(a)

(b)

FIG. 9.53 Purely cystic renal cell cancer. SGE (*a*), fat-suppressed SGE (*b*), coronal SS-ETSE (*c*), T2-weighted echo-train spin-echo (*d*), immediate postgadolinium SGE (*e*), and interstitial-phase gadolinium-enhanced fat-suppressed SGE (*f*) images.

787

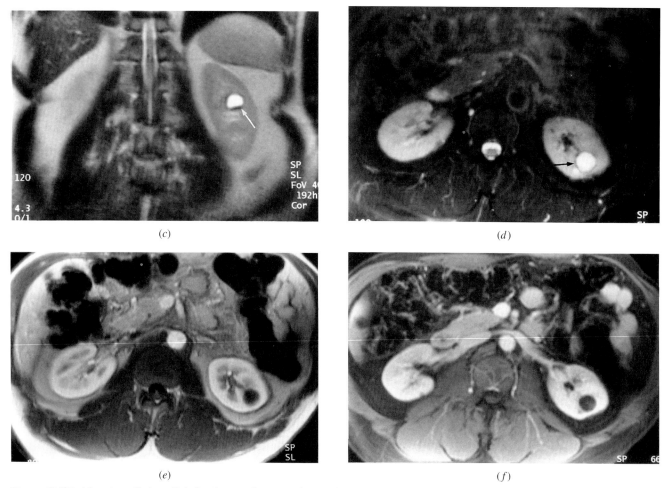

(c)

(d)

(e)

(f)

F I G . 9.53 (*Continued*) A well-defined cystic lesion with mural calcification was demonstrated on CT images (not shown). The lesion is well circumscribed and low in signal intensity on T1-weighted images (arrow, *a, b*) and high in signal intensity on T2-weighted images and does not enhance after gadolinium administration (*e, f*). A low-signal intensity mural rim on the T2-weighted images (arrow, *c, d*) corresponds to calcification as shown on the CT image. At surgery the lesion was considered to represent a cyst, but at histologic examination a thin sheet of tumor cells was present in part of the cyst wall.

predominantly cystic with only a modicum of a solid component. Cyst walls are often densely fibrotic with focal calcifications. Microscopically, tumor cells generally show low-grade cytologic features. Multilocular cystic renal cell carcinoma appears to be an extremely low-grade form of renal cell carcinoma that, if treated early, may be curable. [66]. This renal cell carcinoma may have a septated cystic appearance resembling multilocular cystic nephroma on MRI (fig. 9.56). Septations tend to be thicker and more irregular than those observed in multilocular cystic nephroma and hemorrhage is common (fig. 9.53).

Cystic changes are relatively common in renal cancer. Rarely lesions may appear virtually identical to a cyst, with a thin layer of tumor cells within the wall (fig. 9.54). We have observed a propensity for cystic change in tumors in the setting of multifocal or bilateral renal cancers (fig. 9.55).

Other features that may be observed with renal cancer include substantial hemorrhage in the perinephric

space (fig. 9.56), secondary to the extensive vascularity, friable vessels, and large size these tumors can attain. Although renal cancers usually grow as focal cortical based neoplasms, poorly differentiated tumors may demonstrate extensive, ill-defined renal parenchymal infiltration (fig. 9.57) resembling transitional cell cancer, lymphoma, or metastases from poorly differentiated tumors.

Recent studies have reported that occasionally some clear cell carcinomas and, less commonly, granular cell carcinomas, may show a relative focal or diffuse loss of signal intensity on opposed-phase MR images [67, 68]. These lesions have microscopic fat that is not detected on CT or on conventional T1-weighted images. One series demonstrated that mean opposed-phase/in-phase signal intensity ratio of clear cell carcinomas was significantly different from that of other renal cancers (P < 0.0002) [67]. This study demonstrated that clear cell carcinoma, when compared with other renal cancers, may show a relative focal or diffuse loss of signal intensity. In renal masses, this signal intensity loss, consistent with

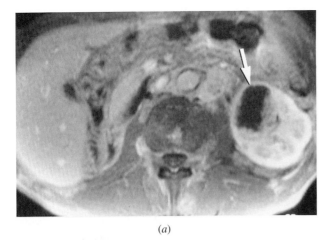

(a)

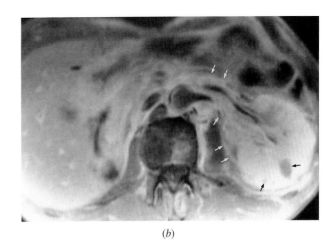

(b)

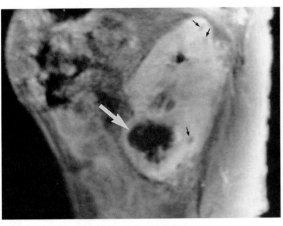

(c)

F I G . 9.54 Multifocal renal cell cancer with cystic tumor and Sheetlike tumor infiltration. Immediate postgadolinium SGE (*a*), interstitial-phase fat-suppressed SGE (*b*), and sagittal interstitial-phase SGE (*c*) images in a patient with prior right nephrectomy for renal cancer. A predominantly cystic renal cancer is present in the lower pole of the left kidney (large arrow, *a, c*). Extensive tumor infiltration in a sheetlike pattern is identified along the renal capsule and into the renal hilum (small white arrows, *b*). Numerous small cysts are also present (small black arrows, *b, c*), which are seeded with tumor.

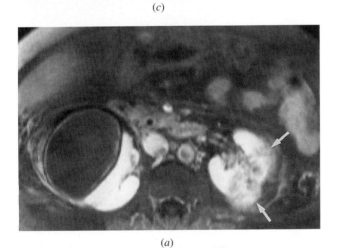

(a)

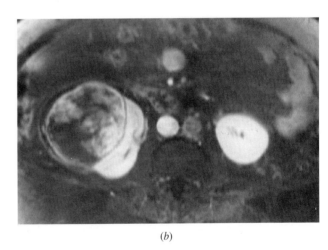

(b)

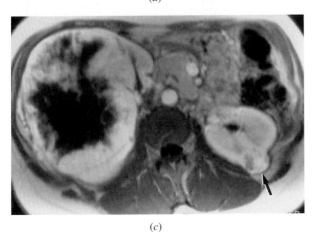

(c)

F I G . 9.55 Bilateral renal cell cancer. Interstitial-phase gadolinium-enhanced T1-weighted fat-suppressed spin-echo images from midrenal (*a*) and lower renal (*b*) levels. A large cystic/solid renal cancer arises from the right kidney. Two smaller renal cancers (arrows, *a*) are identified at the level of the renal hilum in the left kidney.

Immediate postgadolinium SGE image (*c*) in a second patient demonstrates bilateral hypervascular renal cell cancers. The large right renal cancer demonstrates a necrotic center, whereas the 2-cm left renal cancer (arrow, *c*) demonstrates intense heterogeneous enhancement.

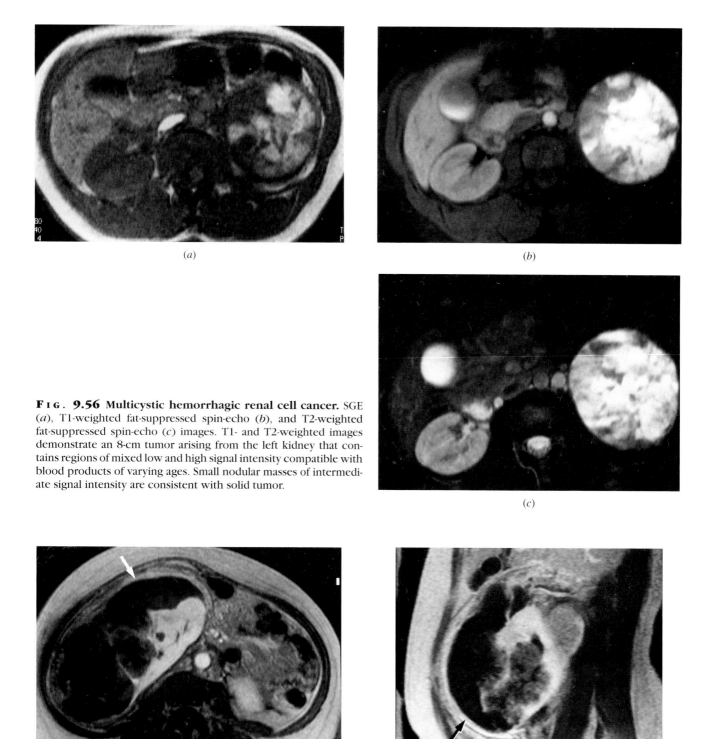

F I G . 9.56 Multicystic hemorrhagic renal cell cancer. SGE (*a*), T1-weighted fat-suppressed spin-echo (*b*), and T2-weighted fat-suppressed spin-echo (*c*) images. T1- and T2-weighted images demonstrate an 8-cm tumor arising from the left kidney that contains regions of mixed low and high signal intensity compatible with blood products of varying ages. Small nodular masses of intermediate signal intensity are consistent with solid tumor.

(*a*)   (*b*)   (*c*)

(*a*)   (*b*)

F I G . 9.57 Renal cell cancer with perirenal hemorrhage. Transverse 90 s (*a*) and sagittal 120-second (*b*) postgadolinium SGE images. An 8-cm irregular cystic/solid renal cancer arises from the lower the lower two-thirds of the right kidney. A large perirenal collection of blood surrounds the kidney (arrows *a*, *b*). The blood appears low in signal intensity on postcontrast images because of rescaling of abdominal tissue signal intensities.

Precontrast T1-weighted fat-suppressed SGE (*c*) and sagittal 3-min postgadolinium T1-weighted fat-suppressed SGE (*d*) images in a second patient. A large mass arises in the upper pole of the right kidney. The tumor is heterogeneous on the 3-min postgadolinium fat-suppressed SGE image (arrow, *d*).

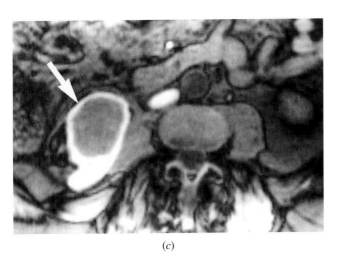

(c)

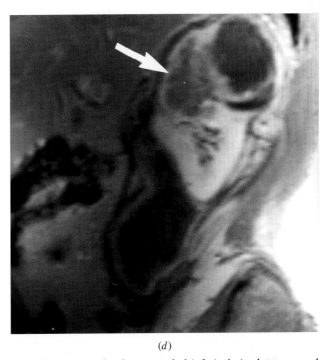

(d)

FIG. 9.57 (*Continued*) The tumor has resulted in a large perinephric hematoma that has extended inferiorly in the pararenal space (arrow, *c*). The peripheral rim of high signal on the noncontrast T1-weighted image is diagnostic for hemorrhage.

lipid, does not necessarily indicate angiomyolipoma. It should be noted that fat content in these reported cancers was minimal and/or focal, which contrasts with the majority of angiomyolipomas, in which the fat content is substantial and diffuse. The differential diagnosis is angiomyolipoma with minimal fat content [68].

Recurrent renal cancer. Renal cancer recurrence occurs most commonly in the resection bed of the resected cancer. Distinction from resection bed fibrosis is usually feasible, as fibrosis tends to appear as lin-

ear, small volume tissue that exhibits minimal contrast enhancement, whereas tumor recurrence appears more nodular or masslike with relatively substantial irregular contrast enhancement. Involvement of adjacent organs by the recurrent tumor may be shown. Recurrence may also be manifest as tumor involvement of distant sites (fig. 9.58).

Renal Cancer in Chronic Renal Failure. Patients with chronic renal failure have a substantial risk of developing renal cell carcinoma, which has a reported

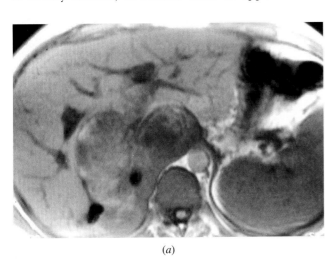

(a)

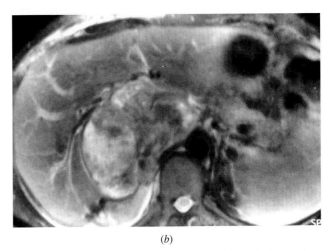

(b)

FIG. 9.58 Recurrent Renal-cell Cancer. Precontrast T1-weighted SGE (*a*), T2-weighted fat-suppressed SGE (*b*), immediate postgadolinium SGE (*c*), and 2-min postgadolinium T1-weighted fat-suppressed SGE (*d*) images. There is a large heterogeneous mass in the right nephrectomy space consistent with tumor recurrence. The large tumor mass compresses the right lobe of the liver and portal vein with invasion of the IVC.

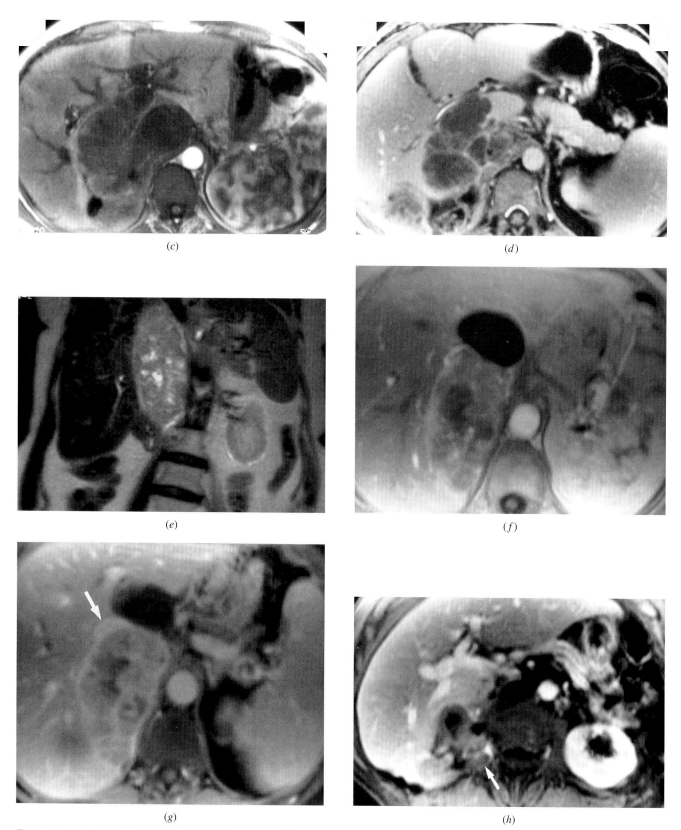

(c)

(d)

(e)

(f)

(g)

(h)

F I G . 9.58 (*Continued*) Coronal SS-ETSE (*e*), immediate postgadolinium SGE (*f*), and 2-min postgadolinium fat-suppressed SGE (*g*) images in a second patient. There is a large mass in the right upper quadrant that compresses the IVC anteriorly (arrow, *g*). This mass is heterogeneously increased signal on T2 weighted sequences and demonstrates mild heterogenous enhancement after gadolinium administration.

Postgadolinium T1 weighted fat-suppressed SGE (*h*) image in a third patient. An irregular heterogeneous mass is evident in the superior aspect of the right renal fossa. This lesion invades the right psoas muscle (arrow, *h*) and the right hepatic lobe. The tumor also abuts the posterior branch of the right portal vein and the main portal vein.

incidence of approximately 7% [23]. Tumors in patients with chronic renal failure are much more commonly hypovascular than tumors in patients with normal renal function. The frequent occurrence of hypovascular cancers and the suboptimal enhancement of renal parenchyma in patients with chronic renal failure on iodine contrast-enhanced CT images renders chronic renal failure patients difficult to evaluate with CT. In comparison, MRI is able to demonstrate diminished heterogeneous enhancement of tumors and moderate enhancement of background renal parenchyma, thereby improving detection of cancer in this patient group (fig. 9.59). Cancers in patients with diminished renal function have a great propensity to undergo hemorrhage [69] (fig. 9.60), which may be so extensive that the cancer can resemble a hemorrhagic cyst (fig. 9.61). Therefore,

caution must be exercised in describing hemorrhagic renal lesions as cysts in patients with chronic renal failure. Renal cancer also may arise in patients with other underlying renal diseases such as polycystic kidney disease (fig. 9.62).

Renal Cancer-Role of MRI. MRI is slightly superior to dynamic contrast-enhanced CT imaging for the detection, characterization, and staging of renal cancer [1, 14, 55]. There is, however, little difference between dual-phase spiral or multidetector CT imaging and MRI in the routine investigation of renal masses. There are definite indications for the use of MRI, which include 1) allergy to iodine contrast, 2) indeterminate, particularly calcified renal masses, and 3) renal failure [69–72]. The greater enhancement of renal parenchyma in

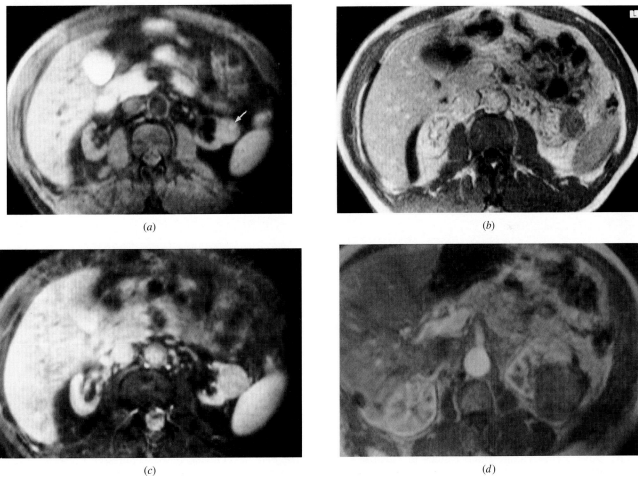

(a)　　　　　　　　　　(b)

(c)　　　　　　　　　　(d)

F I G . 9.59 Hypovascular renal cell cancer in chronic renal failure. T1-weighted fat-suppressed spin-echo (*a*), 90-s postgadolinium SGE (*b*), and interstitial-phase gadolinium-enhanced T1-weighted fat-suppressed spin-echo (*c*) images. The kidneys are chronically failed and appear atrophic with no corticomedullary differentiation on the precontrast image. A 2.5-cm renal cancer arises from the lateral aspect of the left kidney and contains a punctate high-signal intensity focus on the noncontrast T1-weighted image consistent with hemorrhage (arrow, *a*). The tumor enhances minimally on the 90-s postgadolinium SGE image (*b*). Small irregular enhancing structures are apparent on the gadolinium-enhanced T1-weighted fat-suppressed image (*c*), which represent enhancing stroma in a hypovascular renal cancer.

　　Immediate postgadolinium SGE image (*d*) in a second patient in chronic renal failure with a hypovascular 5.5-cm renal cancer in the left kidney.

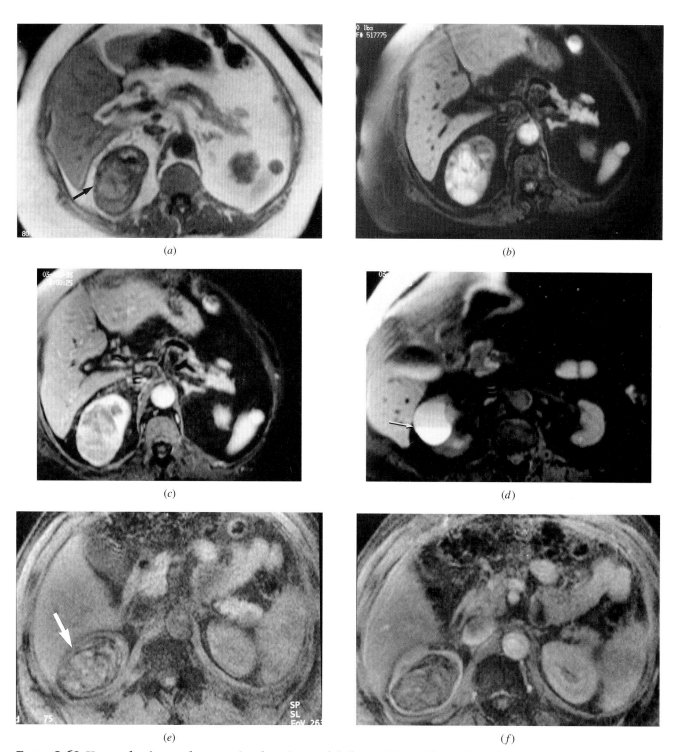

(a)

(b)

(c)

(d)

(e)

(f)

F I G . 9.60 Hemorrhagic renal cancer in chronic renal failure. SGE (*a*), T1-weighted fat-suppressed spin-echo (*b*), and interstitial-phase gadolinium-enhanced T1-weighted fat-suppressed spin-echo (*c*) images. A 5-cm renal cancer is present in the right kidney (arrow, *a*) that is heterogeneously high in signal intensity on precontrast T1-weighted images (*a, b*), consistent with hemorrhage, and shows heterogeneous high-signal intensity stroma on the postgadolinium image (*c*). T1-weighted fat-suppressed spin-echo image (*d*) at a level immediately inferior to the renal cancer shows a hemorrhagic renal cyst with a fluid level (arrow, *d*).

Fat-suppressed SGE (*e*) and 90-s postgadolinium SGE (*f*) images in a second patient demonstrate a 5-cm tumor that is heterogeneously high in signal intensity on the precontrast fat-suppressed image (arrow, *e*) and is heterogeneously diminished in signal intensity on the postgadolinium image (*f*).

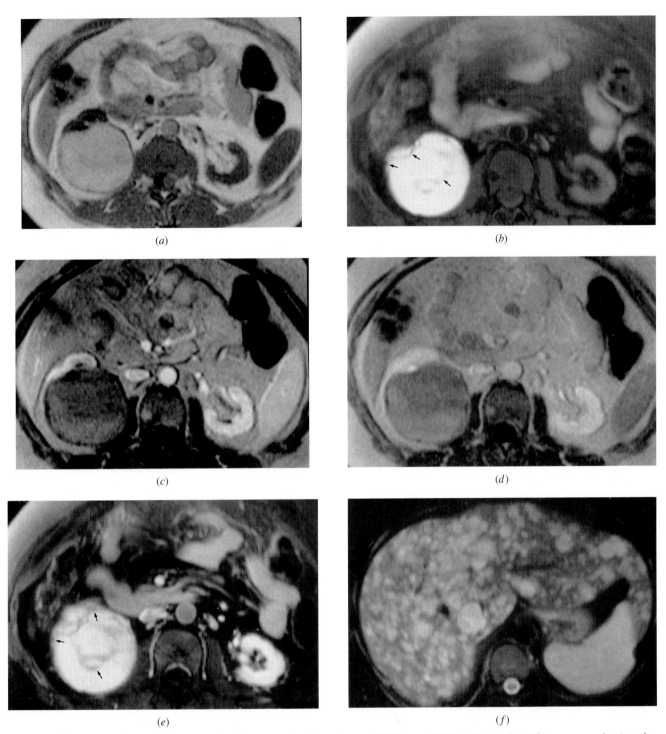

(a)   *(b)*

(c)   *(d)*

(e)   *(f)*

F I G . 9.61 Hemorrhagic cystic renal cell cancer in chronic renal failure. SGE (*a*), T1-weighted fat-suppressed spin-echo (*b*), immediate postgadolinium SGE (*c*), 1 minute postgadolinium SGE (*d*), and interstitial-phase gadolinium-enhanced T1-weighted fat-suppressed spin-echo (*e*) images. A largely cystic hemorrhagic renal mass is noted arising from the lower pole of the right kidney. Small murally based nodular densities and reticular markings are apparent on precontrast and postcontrast images, which are best shown on the fat-suppressed images (arrows, *b*, *e*).

Multiple surgical biopsies did not reveal renal cancer. T2-weighted fat-suppressed spin-echo (*f*), immediate postgadolinium SGE (*g*, *h*), and interstitial-phase gadolinium-enhanced T1-weighted fat-suppressed spin-echo (*i*) images obtained 2-1/2 years later.

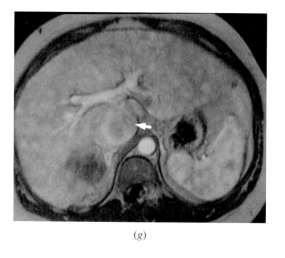

(g)

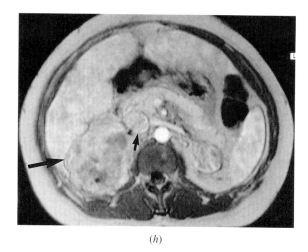

(h)

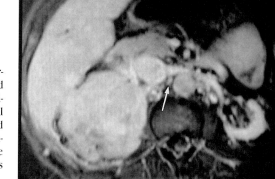

(i)

FIG. 9.61 (*Continued*) Numerous liver metastases are apparent, which are small, and high in signal intensity on T2-weighted images (*f*) and enhance in a uniform intense fashion on immediate postgadolinium SGE images (*g*, *h*). An 8-cm hypervascular renal cancer has developed from the cystic cancer (large arrows, *h*), and tumor thrombus expands the IVC (small arrow, *g*, *h*). Gadolinium-enhanced T1-weighted fat-suppressed spin-echo image shows the heterogeneous cancer, tumor thrombus, and small lymph nodes (arrow, *i*).

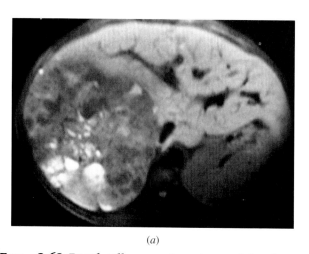

(a)

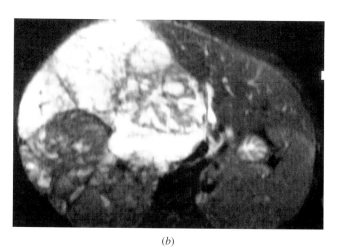

(b)

FIG. 9.62 Renal cell cancer in autosomal dominant polycystic kidney disease. T1-weighted fat-suppressed spin-echo (*a*), T2-weighted fat-suppressed spin-echo (*b*), interstitial-phase gadolinium-enhanced T1-weighted fat-suppressed spin-echo (*c*), and sagittal interstitial-phase gadolinium-enhanced SGE (*d*) images. A large multilocular renal mass is present involving the entire right kidney. Cystic spaces vary in signal on T1-weighted (*a*) and T2-weighted (*b*) images, consistent with blood products of differing age. Enhancement of septations and more solid tissue is present on postgadolinium images (*c*, *d*). The superior-inferior extent of the massive tumor is shown on the sagittal-plane image (arrows, *d*). Tumor infiltration of the entire kidney was present at histopathology. The left kidney had been removed with the same histologic findings.

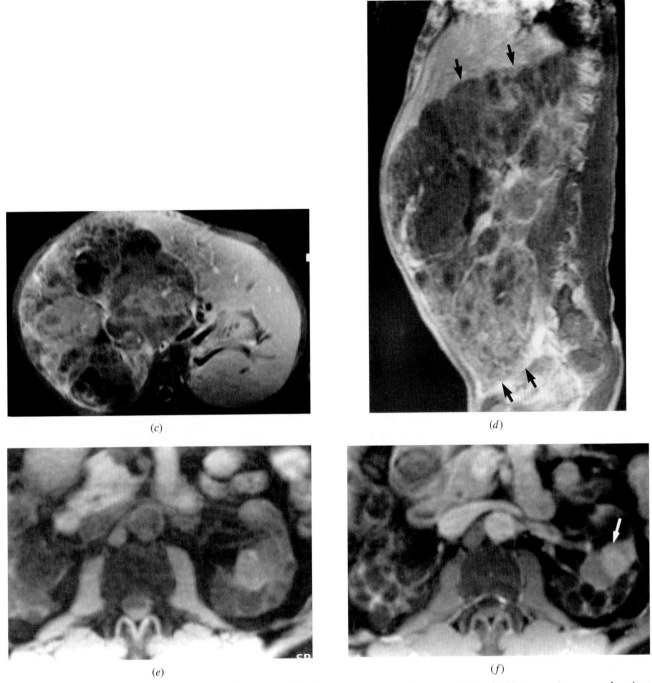

(c)

(d)

(e)

(f)

FIG. 9.62 (*Continued*) Precontrast (*e*) and 90-s postgadolinium (*f*) T1-weighted fat-suppressed SGE images in a second patient demonstrate a mass in the left kidney. The tumor is not identified on the T1-weighted image and enhances moderately on postgadolinium images (arrow, *f*). This mass represented renal cell cancer. In patients with autosomal dominant polycystic kidney disease it is essential to carefully compare pre- and postgadolinium images to identify areas that show enhancement.

patients with renal failure, the smaller volume of contrast, and lesser renal toxicity, justify the routine use of contrast-enhanced MRI in these patients [69–72]. If necessary, gadolinium also may be hemodialyzed [73]. There may be no indication to perform noncontrast CT imaging alone in the investigation of renal masses. MRI may also be superior for the evaluation of tumor thrombus and liver metastases. Early detection of renal cancer is critical

to improving patient survival [41, 74, 75]. Because of the ability of MRI to detect renal tumors smaller than 1 cm in diameter, the role of MRI in detecting and characterizing renal masses may become increasingly important in patients with bilateral renal tumors or in patients scheduled for renal-sparing surgery because both CT imaging and ultrasound miss at least 50 percent of tumors smaller than 1 cm [76]. This may have a greater impact in the future, as renal-sparing surgery becomes a more prevalent practice [77, 80].

Wilms Tumor (Nephroblastoma). Wilms tumor is the most common primary renal tumor in childhood. The tumor is diagnosed most frequently in children between the ages of 2 and 5 years. Gross pathologic characteristics of the tumor include a large homogeneous, well-circumscribed mass that tends to be solitary. Bilaterality or multicentricity occurs in 10% of cases. Areas of hemorrhage, cyst formation, and necrosis are sometimes encountered. Microscopically, the classic triphasic composition of cell types is usually identified; namely, blastemal ("small, round blue cells"), epithelial, and stromal. Wilms tumors calcify in only 5% of cases, in contrast to neuroblastomas, which calcify in 50% of cases. Unilateral Wilms tumor is associated with a 41% incidence of nephrogenic rests, whereas multifocal Wilms has a 99% incidence of nephrogenic rests [81]. The risk of Wilms tumor is increased in association with at least three recognizable groups of congenital syndromes. The first group, or WAGR syndrome, is characterized by aniridia, genital anomalies, and mental retardation with a high risk of developing wilms tumor. The second group has the Denys-Drash syndrome, consisting of gonadal dysgenesis (male pseudohermaphroditism) and nephropathy leading to renal failure. The third group consists of children with Beckwith-Wiedemann syndrome characterized by enlargement of body organs, hemihypertrophy, renal medullary cysts, and abnormal cells in the adrenal cortex. Current staging of Wilms tumors involves a five-stage system in which Stage 1 is a tumor confined to the kidney that has been completely excised; Stage 2 is a tumor that has extended locally beyond the kidney and has been completely excised;

Stage 3 is the presence of residual tumor after surgery that was confined to the abdomen without hematogeneous spread; Stage 4 is hematogeneous metastases; and Stage 5 is bilateral renal involvement [82]. Metastases occur to the lungs, liver, and lymph nodes. Wilms tumor, in rare instances, may be highly cystic. Tumors arise from the kidney with an appearance at times indistinguishable from that of renal cell cancer. Age therefore constitutes a criterion for predicting the diagnosis, because the most common renal malignancy in the pediatric patient is Wilms tumor. A transition occurs in the midteens, after which renal cell cancer is the most common renal tumor. Features suggestive of Wilms tumor are large renal tumors that cross the midline. Central necrosis and tumor thrombus are less common in large Wilms tumors compared to renal cell cancer, but this does not provide consistent differentiating information. Wilms tumors commonly contain central hemorrhage.

Wilms tumors are slightly hypointense on T1-weighted images and slightly hyperintense on T2-weighted images [81]. Large cancers are frequently heterogeneous with regions of high signal intensity on T1-weighted images because of the presence of hemorrhage (fig. 9.63). Tumors enhance heterogeneously on postgadolinium images but tend to be less intensely enhanced and less heterogeneous than renal-cell cancer on early postcontrast images. Nephrogenic rests are typically <2 cm and enhance minimally on postgadolinium images [81]. As with renal cancer, tumor thrombus in Wilms tumor is well shown using gadolinium-enhanced MR images (fig. 9.64) and is better defined than on CT images [83].

Lymphoma. Lymphomatous involvement of the kidneys generally occurs in the context of widespread

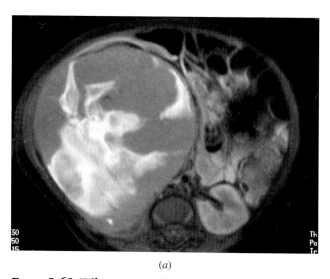

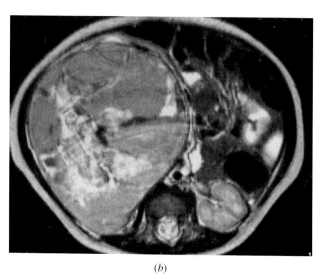

(a)   (b)

FIG. 9.63 Wilms tumor. T1-weighted fat-suppressed spin-echo (*a*), T2-weighted echo-train spin-echo (*b*), and interstitial-phase gadolinium-enhanced T1-weighted fat-suppressed spin-echo (*c*) images.

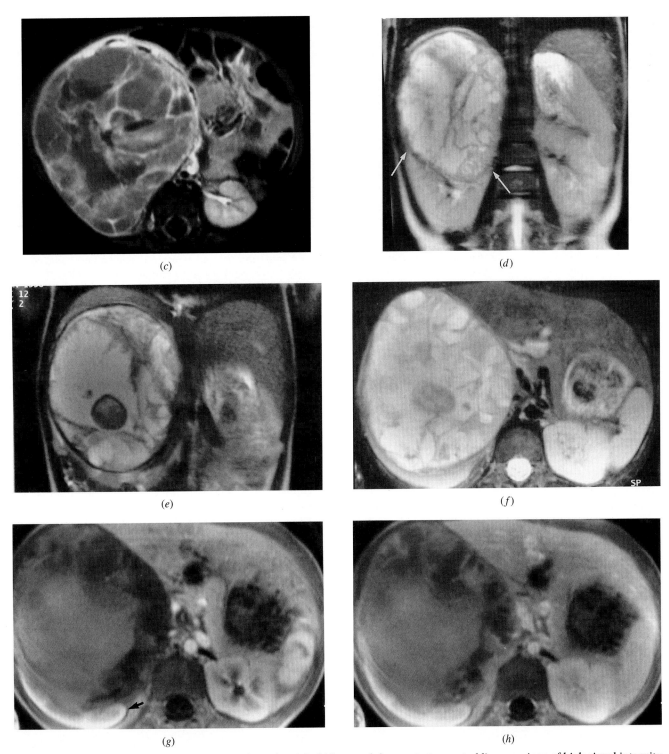

(c)

(d)

(e)

(f)

(g)

(h)

FIG. 9.63 (*Continued*) A large mass arises from the right kidney and demonstrates central linear regions of high signal intensity on T1- and T2-weighted images, consistent with blood. No substantial central necrosis is identified on the postcontrast images despite the large size of the tumor.

Coronal SS-ETSE (*d*, *e*), T2-weighted fat-suppressed spin-echo (*f*) and immediate (*g*), and 90-s (*h*) postgadolinium SGE images in a second patient. A large heterogeneous Wilms tumor arises from the upper pole of the right kidney (arrows, *d*). A rim of posterior normal renal cortex is apparent (arrow, *g*).

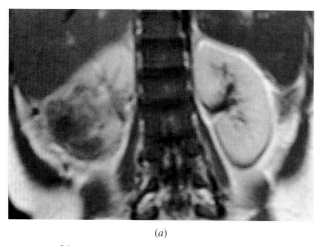

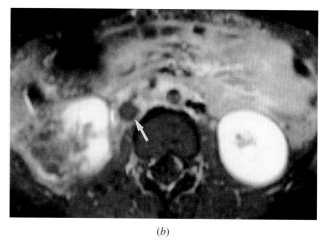

(a)   (b)

FIG. 9.64 Wilms tumor. Coronal gadolinium-enhanced T1-weighted spin-echo (a) and transverse gadolinium-enhanced T1-weighted fat-suppressed spin-echo (b) images. A heterogeneously enhancing tumor is present arising from the lower half of the right kidney (a, b). Thrombus is noted in the IVC (arrow, b), which represents blood thrombus at this tomographic section inferior to the renal vein.

disease. However, isolated focal involvement of the kidney does occur [84–86]. Non-Hodgkin lymphoma more commonly involves the kidneys than Hodgkin lymphoma and is most commonly the B cell type [84]. Three basic patterns of involvement occur, which are 1) direct invasion from adjacent disease, most commonly large retroperitoneal masses (fig. 9.65); 2) focal masses that may be solitary or multiple (figs. 9.66 and 9.67); and 3) diffuse infiltration (fig. 9.68) [84–86]. Lymphoma commonly extends along the subcapsular surface of the kidney, particularly in the setting of invasion from adjacent disease. Renal parenchyma lacks lymphoid tissue, so primary renal lymphoma usually arises from lymphatic tissue in the renal sinus. Direct invasion of the kidney by a large retroperitoneal nodal mass, is the most common form of renal disease and is often observed at initial presentation.

Lymphoma is generally slightly hypointense relative to renal cortex on T1-weighted images and heterogeneous and slightly hypointense to isointense on T2-weighted images. Gadolinium enhancement of most lymphomas is mildly heterogeneous and minimal on early postcontrast images and remains minimal on late postcontrast images [86].

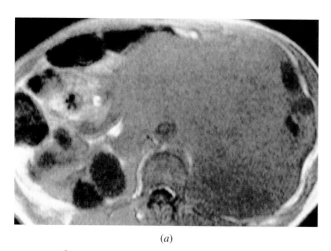

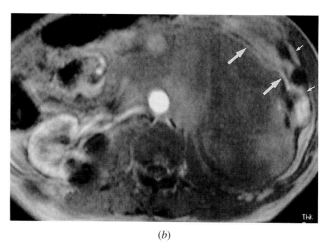

(a)   (b)

FIG. 9.65 Renal lymphoma, large retroperitoneal mass invading kidney. SGE (a), immediate postgadolinium SGE (b), and gadolinium-enhanced T1-weighted fat-suppressed spin-echo (c) images. A large retroperitoneal mass is present that is homogeneous and soft tissue signal intensity on the SGE image (a), and enhances minimally on capillary-phase (b) and interstitial-phase (c) images. On postcontrast images lymphoma is moderately heterogeneous with no evidence of necrosis. A thin rim of spared renal cortex is evident (small arrows, b), and the kidney is displaced anterolaterally. Tumor invades through the renal pelvis into the renal medulla. The renal artery is patent (arrows, b, c) but encased by lymphoma. Patency is shown by the presence of high-signal intensity gadolinium in the artery on the immediate postgadolinium SGE image (b) and by flow void on the spin-echo image (c).

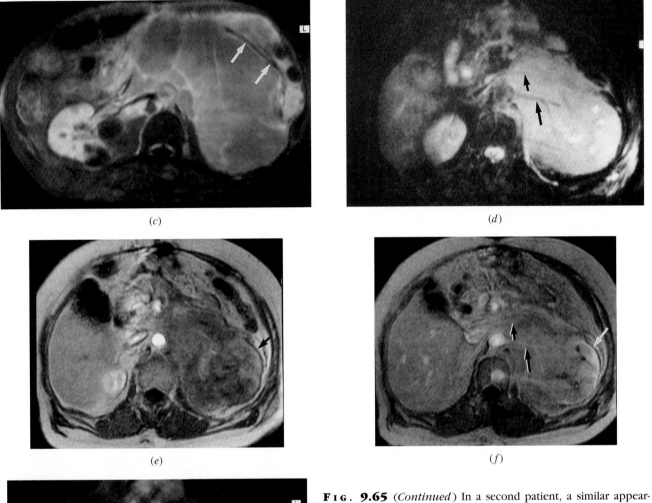

(c)

(d)

(e)

(f)

(g)

FIG. 9.65 (*Continued*) In a second patient, a similar appearance of lymphoma is shown on T2-weighted fat-suppressed spin-echo (*d*), immediate (*e*) and 90-s (*f*) postgadolinium SGE, and gadolinium-enhanced T1-weighted fat-suppressed spin-echo (*g*) images. Lymphoma is mildly hyperintense on the T2-weighted image (*d*) and heterogeneous and mildly enhanced on capillary-phase (*e*) and interstitial-phase (*f, g*) gadolinium-enhanced images. The renal artery (arrow *d, f, g*) and renal vein (small arrow *d, f, g*) are encased by tumor but patent. Patency is demonstrated by the presence of high signal intensity on the SGE image (*f*) and signal void on the spin-echo images (*d, g*). The involved kidney demonstrates diminished cortical enhancement (arrow, *e*) relative to the normal contralateral right kidney on the capillary-phase image (*e*). Lymphoma has extensively invaded the medulla, but relative sparing of cortex is observed (white arrow, *f, g*).

Lymphoma tends to infiltrate the renal medulla. Retroperitoneal lymphoma that invades the kidney usually extends through the renal sinus into the renal medulla (see fig. 9.65). Diffuse infiltration of the kidney predominantly affects the medulla, with relative sparing of the renal cortex (see fig. 9.68) [83]. Focal masses arise in the renal medulla or cortex (see fig. 9.66) [86, 87]. Cortex-based masses tend to enhance more intensely than other forms of renal involvement [86, 87], which

may reflect the greater blood supply of the cortex. As most forms of lymphoma involve the medulla, these tumors can be distinguished from renal carcinoma because renal carcinomas originate in the renal cortex. Other distinguishing features include: 1) the degree of vascularity (lymphoma shows mild diffuse heterogeneous enhancement, whereas renal cancer shows intense early heterogeneous enhancement), 2) the presence of necrosis (necrosis is uncommon in lymphoma, even in large

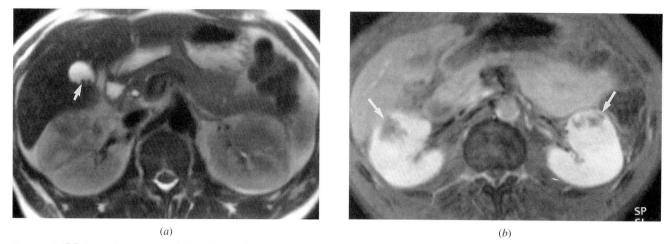

(a)

(b)

F I G . 9.66 Lymphoma—multifocal renal involvement. T2-weighted breathing-independent SS-ETSE (*a*) and gadolinium-enhanced T1-weighted fat-suppressed spin-echo (*b*) images. Lymphoma masses are midly hypo- to isointense on T2-weighted images (*a*) and heterogeneous with low signal intensity centers (arrows, *b*) on interstitial-phase gadolinium-enhanced T1-weighted images (*b*). Incidental note is made of gallstones, which are well shown on the breathing-independent T2-weighted image (arrow, *a*).

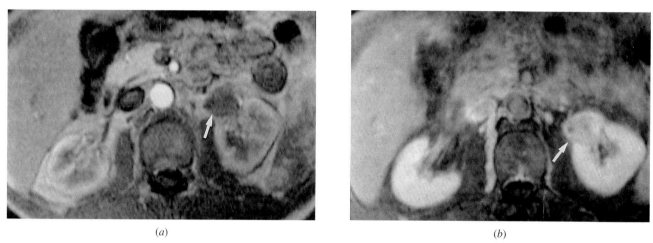

(a)

(b)

F I G . 9.67 Lymphoma, solitary mass. Immediate postgadolinium SGE (*a*) and gadolinium-enhanced T1-weighted fat-suppressed spin-echo (*b*) images. A solitary lymphoma mass is present in the left kidney (arrow *a*, *b*) that is minimally enhanced on the capillary-phase image (*a*) and heterogeneous and moderately enhanced on the interstitial phase image (*b*). (Reproduced with permission from Semelka RC, Kelekis NL, Burdeny DA, Mitchell DG, Brown JJ, Siegelman ES: Renal lymphoma: Demonstration by MR imaging. *Am J Roentgenol* 166: 823–827, 1996.)

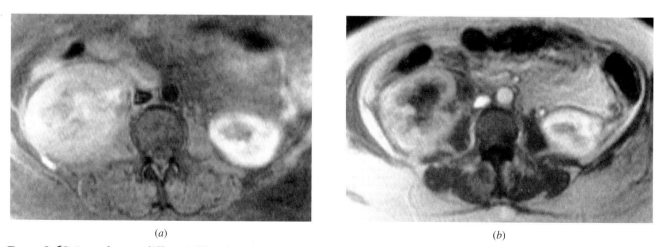

(a)

(b)

F I G . 9.68 Lymphoma, diffuse infiltration. T1-weighted fat-suppressed spin-echo (*a*), immediate postgadolinium SGE (*b*), and gadolinium-enhanced T1-weighted fat-suppressed spin-echo (*c*) images. The right kidney is enlarged in a generalized fashion (*a–c*). CMD is not well shown on the precontrast T1-weighted image (*a*).

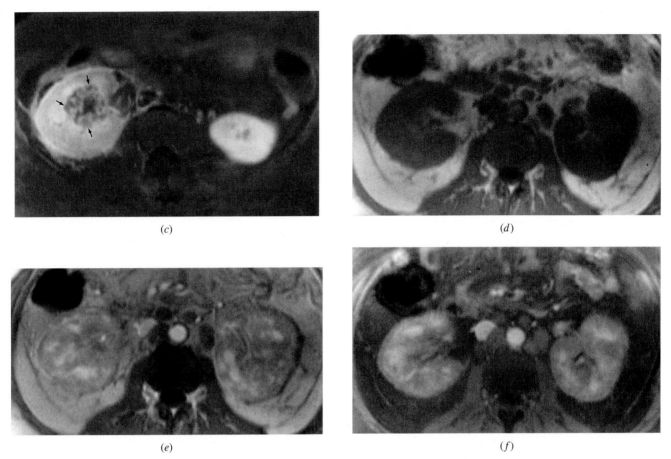

F I G. 9.68 (*Continued*) On the immediate postgadolinium image (*b*), diminished enhancement of the renal cortex is present. However, the cortex has a normal thickness and uniformity. On the later interstitial phase image increased enhancement is present in the outer medulla, and multiple low signal intensity foci (arrows, *c*) are present in the inner medulla, which likely represent focal aggregates of lymphoma. (Reproduced with permission from Semelka RC, Kelekis NL, Burdeny DA, Mitchell DG, Brown JJ, Siegelman ES: Renal lymphoma: Demonstration by MR imaging. *Am J Roentgenol* 166: 823–827, 1996.)

Precontrast (*d*), 45-s postcontrast (*e*), and interstitial-phase fat-suppressed (*f*) T1-weighted SGE images in a second patient. The kidneys show decreased CMD on noncontrast T1-weighted images. There is also decreased, cortical enhancement on the 45-s postcontrast image, with heterogeneous medullary enhancement. The extent of renal enhancement shows negligible changes on the later postcontrast image.

masses, whereas central necrosis is very common in large renal carcinomas), 3) the presence of tumor thrombus (lymphoma rarely results in tumor thrombus, whereas tumor thrombus is common in large renal carcinomas), 4) the location of the center of the tumor (in lymphoma the center is most often outside the contour of the kidney, whereas in renal cancer it is in the renal cortex), 5) the presence of renal artery encasement with diminished capillary-phase enhancement of the entire kidney (Large retroperitoneal mass and diffusely infiltrative patterns of lymphoma commonly encase the renal artery and result in generalized diminished renal enhancement [86], which is a rare finding in renal carcinoma), and 6) the presence of direct extension and involvement of the psoas muscle (common in lymphoma and rare in renal carcinoma). Solitary focal renal cortical involvement of lymphoma, however, may resemble renal carcinoma. Focal masses usually arise

in the setting of recurrent disease, so the history of lymphoma is known, and diagnosis can be established on the basis of clinical history.

Granulocytic Sarcoma (Chloroma). Granulocytic sarcoma or chloroma (from the Greek *chloros*, meaning green) is an uncommon malignant neoplasm that develops in 3–10% of patients with acute myeloblastic leukemia and less commonly in patients with acute lymphocytic leukemia. The incidence of granulocytic sarcomas has increased in recent times because of more prolonged leukemic remission.

Abdominal granulocytic sarcomas show moderately low signal intensity on T1-weighted, mildly high signal intensity on T2-weighted, and minimal enhancement on postgadolinium images (fig. 9.69). The MR appearance is consistent with hypovascular solid tissue.

Renal carcinomas usually have a different appearance in that they are cortex based and generally enhance in an early heterogenous intense fashion. Hypovascular renal cancers may be difficult to distinguish from granulocytic sarcoma on the basis of imaging appearance, although granulocytic sarcomas usually do not have as regular a spherical shape, fine pattern of small internal vessels, or clear origin from renal cortex as generally observed in hypovascular renal cell cancers. The appearance of granulocytic sarcoma is distinct from renal abscesses and hemorrhage, which are in the differential diagnosis of renal masses in leukemia patients [88].

Metastases. Metastases to the kidney are a late manifestation of advanced disease. The most common primary tumors to metastasize to the kidneys are lung (19.8–23.3% of cases), breast (12.3% of cases), and gastric carcinomas, as reported in large autopsy series [89], but metastases may occur in the setting of many malignant diseases (fig. 9.70). Metastases usually appear as multiple bilateral renal masses, but solitary masses may occur (fig. 9.71). Poorly differentiated adenocarcinomas

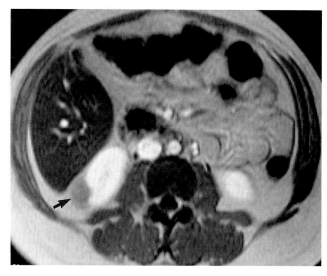

F I G . 9.69 Granulocytic sarcoma. Transverse 90-s postgadolinium SGE image in a patient with acute myelogenous leukemia. A homogeneous minimally enhanced 2-cm granulocytic sarcoma (arrow) arises from the upper pole of the right kidney. The liver is low in signal intensity secondary to transfusional hemosiderosis.

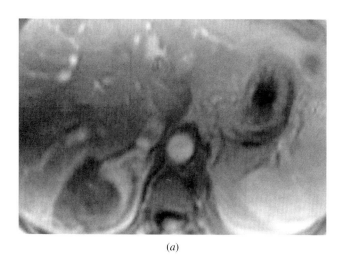

(a)

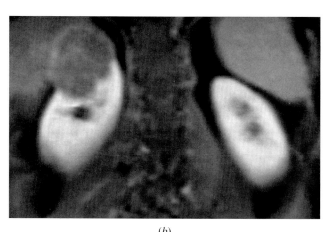

(b)

F I G . 9.70 Renal metastases from ovarian cancer. Transverse 45-s postgadolinium SGE (*a*), and coronal (*b*) and transverse (*c*) 2- to 3-min postgadolinium T1-weighted fat-suppressed SGE images. A tumor is present in the upper pole of the right kidney that demonstrates mild and heterogeneous enhancement.

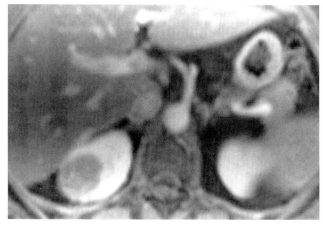

(c)

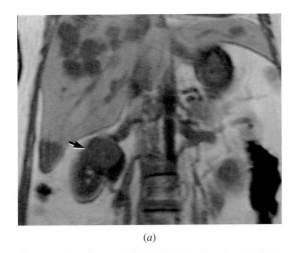

(a)

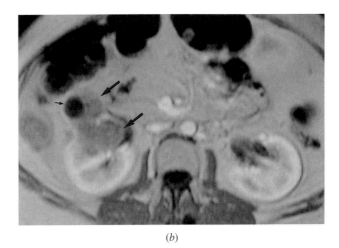

(b)

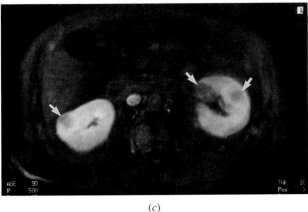

(c)

FIG. 9.71 Renal metastases. Coronal SGE (a) and immediate postgadolinium transverse SGE (b) images. On the precontrast image (a), a homogeneous intermediate-signal intensity mass is noted in the right kidney (arrow, a). In addition, multiple leiomyosarcoma liver metastases are present. On the immediate postcontrast image the renal metastasis (arrow, b) is noted to involve cortex and medulla (arrow, b) and extends into the perirenal space. The mass contains a small cystic component (small arrow, b).

Gadolinium-enhanced T1-weighted fat-suppressed image (c) in a second patient, who has renal metastases from lung cancer, and demonstrates multiple low-signal intensity metastatic lesions in both kidneys (arrows, c).

may diffusely infiltrate the kidneys with a similar appearance to that of lymphoma (fig. 9.72).

Diffuse Renal Parenchymal Disease

Diffuse renal parenchymal diseases are common medical conditions. A variety of disease processes may result in parenchymal disease, and they may be classified into the following broad categories: glomerular disease; acute and chronic tubulointerstitial disease; diabetic nephropathy and nephrosclerosis and other forms of microvascular disease; ischemic nephropathy caused by disease of the main renal arteries; obstructive nephropathy; and infectious renal disease [90].

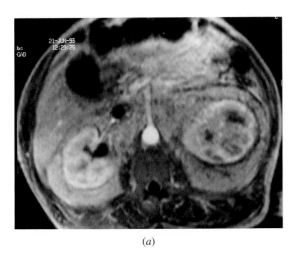

(a)

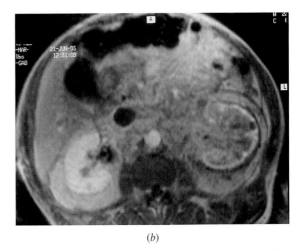

(b)

FIG. 9.72 Renal metastases, undifferentiated adenocarcinoma. Immediate (a) and 90-s (b) postgadolinium SGE and interstitial-phase gadolinium-enhanced T1-weighted fat-suppressed spin-echo (c) images.

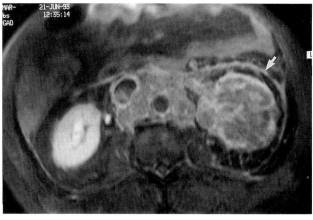

(*c*)

F I G . 9.72 (*Continued*) Massive retroperitoneal adenopathy with extension through the renal hilum and invasion of the renal medulla is present (*a–c*). Extensive infiltration of the medulla with relative sparing of the cortex is well shown on interstitial-phase images (*b, c*). This appearance of renal involvement resembles lymphoma. Thickening of Gerota fascia (arrow, *c*) and retroperitoneal adenopathy are best shown on the gadolinium-enhanced fat-suppressed image, reflecting good conspicuity of enhanced malignant tissue in a background of suppressed fat.

MRI has played a limited role in the evaluation of diffuse renal parenchymal disease. The intrinsic high soft tissue contrast resolution of breath-hold SGE and fat-suppressed images and the clear definition of the renal cortex on immediate postgadolinium images does provide useful information for the evaluation of morphologic changes associated with these entities [90]. The renal cortex is most distinctly shown on immediate postgadolinium SGE images, and alterations of thickness, regularity, and temporal enhancement of the cortex provide information that correlates with underlying pathophysiology [90]. A study of 121 patients with renal disease [90] described MRI findings for diffuse parenchymal diseases. The presence of corticomedullary differentiation demonstrated a strong inverse relationship with serum creatinine (sCr) ($r = -0.568$, $P < 0.001$). The mean cortex thickness for normal kidney and kidneys with glomerular disease was 8.4 and 7.8 mm, respectively, which were significantly thicker ($P < 0.01$) than renal cortex in patients with microvascular disease (5.2 mm), tubulointerstitial disease secondary to antineoplastic chemotherapy (5.6 mm), ischemic nephropathy (5.5 mm), and obstructive nephropathy (4.3 mm). Irregularity of the renal cortex was common in microvascular disease (60.9%), infectious renal disease (62.5%), obstructive nephropathy (55.6%), and nonchemotherapy tubulointerstitial disease (53.8%) compared with chemotherapy-induced tubulointerstitial disease (5.9%), glomerular disease (3.8%), and normal kidneys (0%). Diffuse high signal intensity of the entire medulla on delayed postcontrast images was observed in 20.7% of patients with diffuse renal disease and in none of the patients with normal kidneys. Combining this information with other imaging findings, such as dilation of the renal collecting system in obstructive nephropathy or atherosclerotic disease of the aorta in ischemic nephropathy and microvascular disease, allows prediction of the probable underlying type of diffuse renal parenchymal disease. Dynamic changes of temporal enhancement of the cortex and medulla in normal kidneys, obstructive nephropathy, and postextracorporeal shock wave lithotripsy for renal calculous disease have been described [5, 18, 70]. Temporal changes in other causes of diffuse renal parenchymal disease remain to be established.

Diminished Renal Function

Loss of corticomedullary differentiation (CMD) on T1-weighted images in patients with elevated sCr has been described [91]. This is a nonspecific finding observed in virtually all renal diseases that result in diminished renal function [91]. Demonstration of CMD is best made on precontrast T1-weighted fat-suppressed images [91]. Fat-suppressed SGE imaging may be superior to fat-suppressed spin-echo imaging because breath-holding results in greater image sharpness. In one study that described the relationship of CMD to the level of sCr using precontrast T1-weighted fat-suppressed spin-echo and immediate postgadolinium SGE imaging, all patients with sCr of >3.0 mg/dL showed loss of CMD on precontrast images (fig. 9.73) [91]. In patients with sCr of 1.5–2.9 mg/dL, the loss of CMD occurred in approximately half of the patients. The loss of CMD on immediate postgadolinium SGE images was not observed until sCr exceeded 8.5 mg/dL. Changes in fluid content between cortex and medulla likely account for the changes on precontrast images. This reflects some combination of increased fluid in cortex and decreased fluid in the medulla. CMD on immediate postgadolinium images reflects autoregulatory blood flow distribution in the kidney that may be lost in advanced renal disease. This may reflect irreversible renal parenchymal damage [91].

Not all patients with elevated sCr show loss of CMD. Loss of CMD on precontrast images presumably develops over some period of time. Patients with acute renal failure who are imaged within 1 week of onset may show preservation of CMD. A recent study, which evaluated

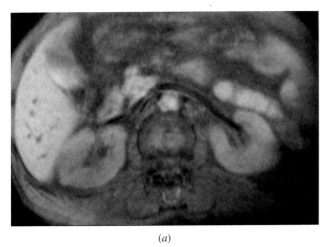
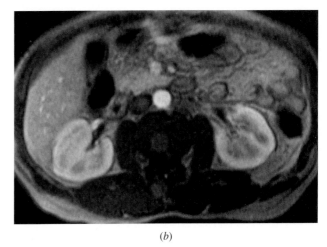

(a)   (b)

F I G . 9.73 Elevated serum creatinine (3 mg/dL) with loss of CMD. T1-weighted fat-suppressed spin-echo (a) and immediate postgadolinium SGE (b) images. Loss of corticomedullary differentiation (CMD) on the precontrast image (a) is noted with preservation of CMD on the immediate postgadolinium SGE (b) image. Loss of CMD on precontrast T1-weighted images is a nonspecific finding of diminished renal function.

the appearance of CMD in patients with acute renal failure (defined as onset within 2 weeks of the MRI exam) showed that 21 patients with acute renal failure had preservation of CMD on noncontrast T1-weighted images [92]. The conclusion of this study is that caution should be exercised in interpreting renal function based on CMD in patients with acute renal failure, as CMD may be preserved in the setting of severely compromised kidneys [92]. Careful consideration must be given to the evaluation of renal function based on CMD in patients with acute renal failure, because CMD may be preserved initially in the setting of severely compromised kidneys.

Glomerular Disease

The clinical manifestations of glomerular disease are varied and range from asymptomatic urinary abnormalities to acute nephritis, nephrotic syndrome, and chronic renal failure. In patients with nephrotic syndrome, the majority have membranous nephropathy and MRI findings are generally minimal (fig. 9.74) [90]. Diffuse increased enhancement resulting in high signal intensity of the medulla may be observed on delayed postgadolinium images. In chronic disease, cortical thinning is smooth and regular in contour and medullary atrophy may be substantial (fig. 9.75). Nephrotic syndrome may also be associated with renal vein thrombosis. Renal vein thrombus may be well shown using a number of MRI techniques [55, 63, 90, 93]. SGE images acquired 45–120 s after gadolinium serve as an effective technique for demonstrating renal vein thrombus (fig. 9.76). Detection of thrombus is important because it is treatable with thrombolytic agents and successful treatment may result in improvement of the condition.

Tubulointerstitial Disease

A variety of underlying etiologies may result in tubulointerstitial disease, of which drug-related causes are among the most common. Tubulointerstitial disease secondary to analgesic drug overuse results in irregular cortical thinning (fig. 9.77) [90]. The irregularity presumably reflects the intermittent nature of the insult because drug intake is sporadic. Tubulointerstitial disease from antineoplastic chemotherapy results in more uniform cortical thinning (fig. 9.78) [90]. This presumably reflects the fact that the cortical insult is more constant because of the regular rate of chemotherapy drug administration.

Acute Tubular Necrosis

Acute tubular necrosis results from metabolic or toxic etiologies in the majority of cases. Within 1 week of onset of this condition CMD may be preserved despite substantial elevation of sCr (fig. 9.79). This likely reflects the fact that the loss of CMD may take more than 1 week to develop.

Tubular Blockage

A number of etiological agents may result in tubular blockage. Renal failure may result from blockage of a substantial portion of the renal tubules by various substances. The classic example of diffuse tubular blockage is by Bence Jones proteinuria in multiple myeloma (fig. 9.80).

Another example of renal tubular injury is with high levels of urinary pigments (myoglobinuria), especially in the setting of renal hypoperfusion and ischemia [94]. Many disorders in which myoglobinuria develops result from severe and excessive stress or overuse of striated muscles (see fig. 9.80) [95].

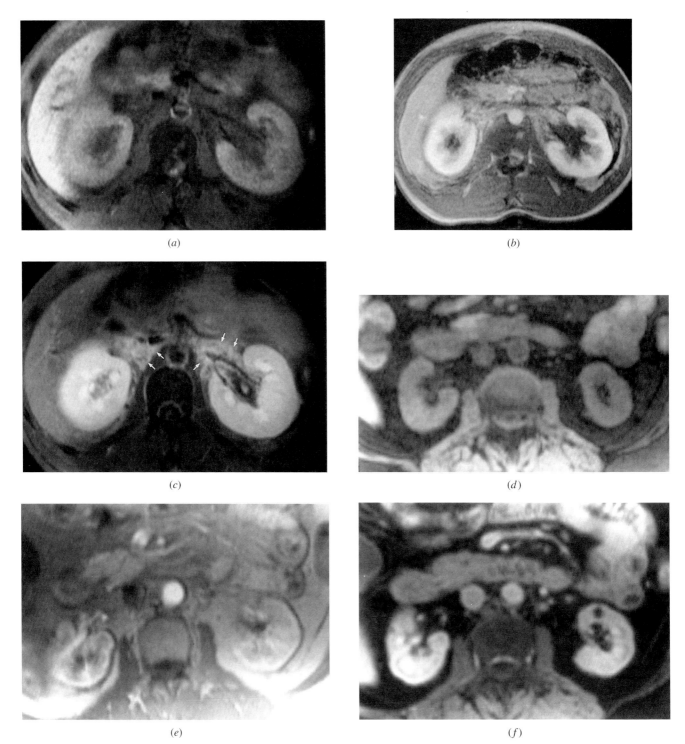

(a)

(b)

(c)

(d)

(e)

(f)

FIG. 9.74 Recent-onset membranous nephropathy. T1-weighted fat-suppressed spin-echo (*a*), immediate postgadolinium SGE (*b*), and gadolinium-enhanced T1-weighted fat-suppressed spin-echo (*c*) images. CMD is diminished on the precontrast image (*a*). Renal cortex is uniform and of normal thickness on the immediate postgadolinium image (*b*). Diffuse increased enhancement of the medulla is noted on the interstitial-phase image (*c*). Enhancing platelike retroperitoneal tissue is present that extends into the left renal hilum (arrows, *c*). This represents acute benign retroperitoneal fibrosis.

T1-weighted fat-suppressed SGE (*d*), immediate postgadolinium SGE (*e*), and 90 s postgadolinium T1-weighted fat-suppressed SGE (*f*) images in a second patient with chronic renal failure. Decreased corticomedullary differentiation is present on the precontrast fat-suppressed image (*d*), and increased medullary enhancement is appreciated on the interstitial-phase image (*f*). Note also a small simple cyst in the left kidney.

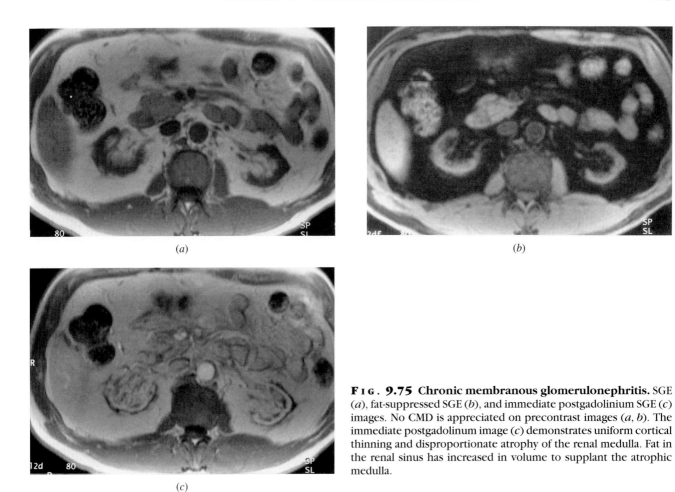

(a)

(b)

(c)

FIG. 9.75 Chronic membranous glomerulonephritis. SGE (a), fat-suppressed SGE (b), and immediate postgadolinium SGE (c) images. No CMD is appreciated on precontrast images (a, b). The immediate postgadolinum image (c) demonstrates uniform cortical thinning and disproportionate atrophy of the renal medulla. Fat in the renal sinus has increased in volume to supplant the atrophic medulla.

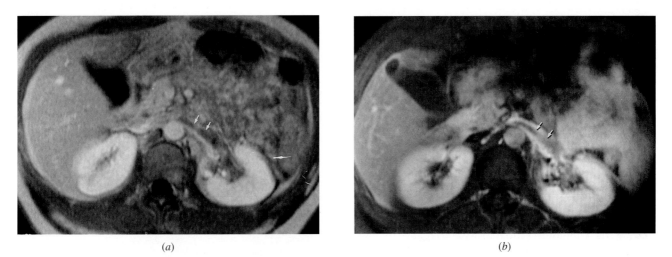

(a)

(b)

FIG. 9.76 Renal vein thrombosis with nephrotic syndrome. Ninety-second gadolinium-enhanced SGE (a) and gadolinium-enhanced T1-weighted fat-suppressed spin-echo (b) images. Low signal bland thrombus is identified in the left renal vein (arrows a, b). Flow in the vein surrounding the thrombus is identified as high signal intensity on these images. Greater conspicuity of gadolinium in the patent periphery of the vein is apparent on the fat-suppressed image because of suppression of the competing signal intensity of fat (b).

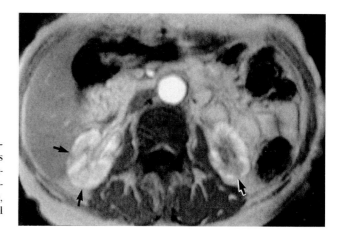

FIG. 9.77 Tubulointerstitial disease secondary to analgesic abuse. Immediate postgadolinium SGE image demonstrates irregular cortical thinning ranging in thickness from 1 to 4 mm. Regions of extreme cortical thinning are apparent (arrows). (Reproduced with permission from Kettritz U, Semelka RC, Brown ED, Sharp TJ, Lawing WL, Colindres RE: MR findings in diffuse renal parenchymal disease. *J Magn Reson Imaging.* 6: 36–144, 1996.)

Other Parenchymal Diseases

Iron Deposition

Iron deposition occurs in the renal cortex in the setting of intravascular hemolysis with hemoglobin accumulation in renal glomeruli. Sickle cell disease is the most common entity to result in this condition [96, 97]. The usual appearance is low signal intensity of the renal cortex caused by the T2*-shortening effects of iron. This is best appreciated on gradient-echo or T2-weighted images (fig. 9.81). On immediate postgadolinium images the T1-shortening effects of gadolinium usually exceed the T2-shortening effects of the iron in the renal cortex, resulting in high-signal intensity enhanced renal cortex. On interstitial-phase images, passage of contrast into

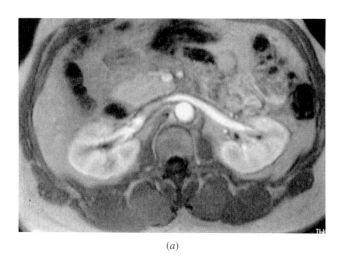

(a)

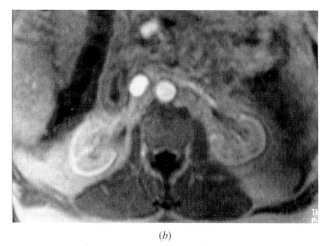

(b)

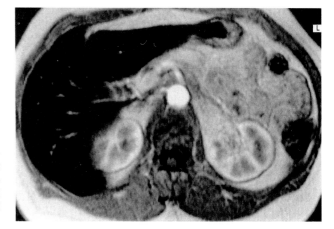

(c)

FIG. 9.78 Tubulointerstitial disease secondary to chemotherapy. Immediate postgadolinium images in 3 patients (a-c) who have a remote history of antineoplastic chemotherapy. Regular cortical thinning is present in all patients. Note the low signal intensity of the liver in the third patient (c) due to transfusional siderosis.

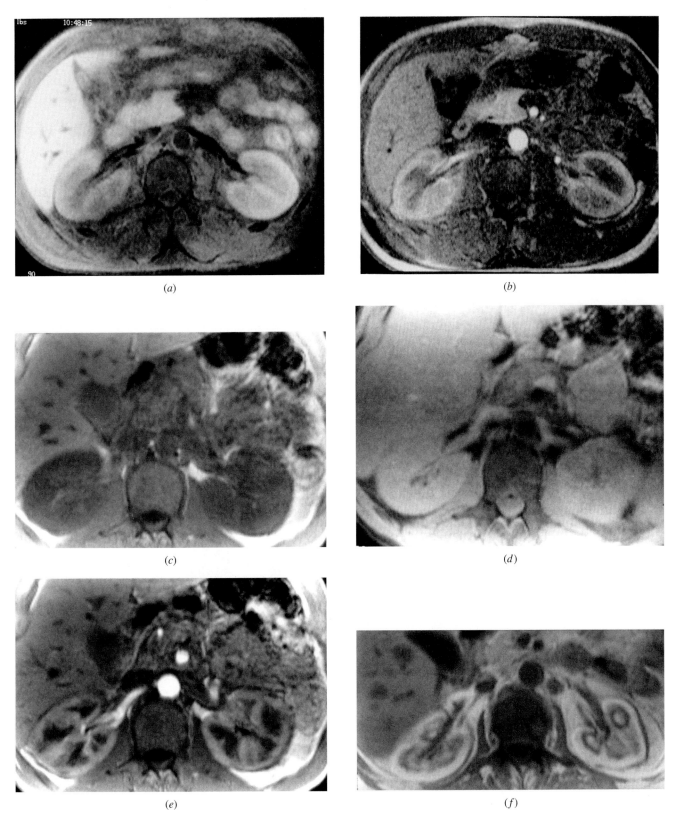

(a)

(b)

(c)

(d)

(e)

(f)

F I G . 9.79 Acute tubular necrosis. T1-weighted fat-suppressed spin-echo (*a*) and immediate postgadolinium SGE (*b*) images. Corticomedullary differentiation is demonstrated on both precontrast (*a*) and immediate postcontrast (*b*) images in a patient with acute tubular necrosis and serum creatinine of 6.3 mg/dL. Acute tubular necrosis developed within 1 week before to MRI examination, and the acute nature of the injury presumably accounts for the presence of CMD on the precontrast image.

Precontrast T1-weighted SGE (*c*), T1-weighted fat-suppressed SGE (*d*), and immediate post-gadolinium SGE (*e*) images in a second patient, with acute tubular necrosis of 1-week duration, demonstrates globular-shaped kidneys with decreased CMD on precontrast images.

Precontrast T1-weighted SGE image (*f*) in a third patient shows high signal intensity in the medullar of kidneys on noncontrast T1-weighted images, suggesting infiltration with blood or protein.

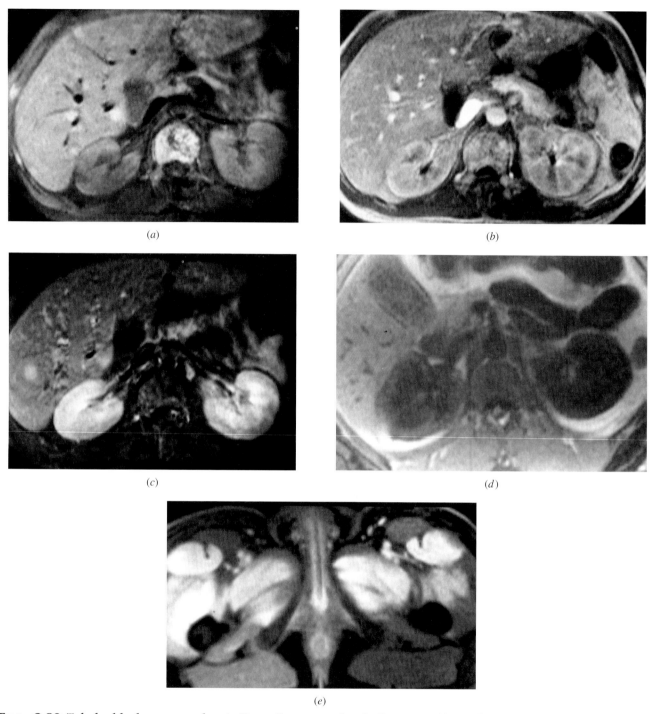

(a)

(b)

(c)

(d)

(e)

FIG. 9.80 Tubular blockage. secondary to Bence Jones proteinuria. Precontrast T1-weighted fat-suppressed spin-echo (*a*), immediate postgadolinium SGE (*b*), and gadolinium-enhanced T1-weighted fat-suppressed spin-echo (*c*) images. This patient with multiple myeloma has high-signal intensity lesions in the bone marrow and liver and absent corticomedullary differentiation on pre-contrast T1-weighted fat-suppressed spin-echo images (*a*). On immediate postgadolinium images (*b*) corticomedullary differentiation is present, but cortical enhancement is not intense. On interstitial-phase T1-weighted fat-suppressed spin-echo images (*c*) diffuse high signal intensity is present in the renal medulla, suggesting the presence of tubular leakage of gadolinium.

   Secondary to rhabdomyolysis. Precontrast T1-weighted SGE (*d*) and precontrast T1 weighted fat-suppressed SGE (*e*) images. The kidneys are enlarged with diminished corticomedullary differentiation on the precontrast image. Extensive high signal is present in the muscles of the upper thighs (*e*), which on this noncontrast image reflects diffuse hemorrhagic changes.

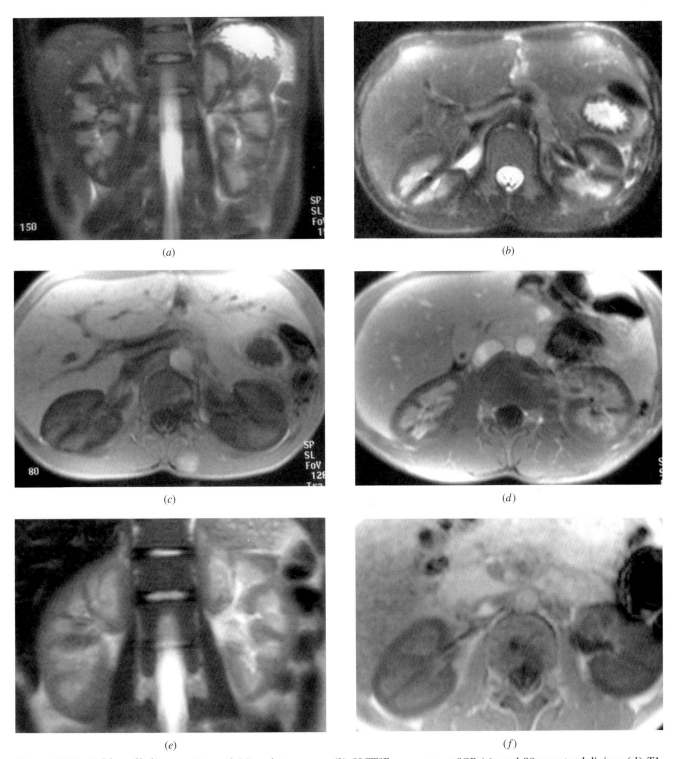

F I G . 9.81 Sickle cell disease. Coronal (*a*) and transverse (*b*) SS-ETSE, precontrast SGE (*c*), and 90-s postgadolinium (*d*) T1-weighted fat-suppressed SGE (*d*) images. The kidneys are globular-shaped, and the renal cortices are low signal on T1-and T2-weighted images, consistent with iron deposition.

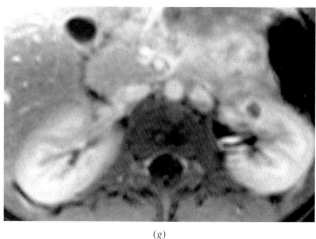

(g)

FIG. 9.81 (*Continued*) Coronal SS-ETSE (*e*), precontrast T1-weighted SGE (*f*) and postgadolinium T1 weighted fat-suppressed spin-echo (*g*) images in a second patient reveal similar findings.

the tubules and enhancement of the medulla result in signal reversal, with the cortex becoming lower in signal intensity than the medulla. Less commonly, dilute-concentration iron in the glomeruli may result in a high-signal intensity renal cortex on precontrast T1-weighted images (fig. 9.82). The spleen in sickle cell disease is also affected with iron deposition, and splenic infarcts are observed.

Paroxysmal nocturnal hemoglobinuria results in iron deposition in the renal cortex [98]. Iron deposition in the liver and spleen are variable and related to blood transfusions or portal hypertension [98].

Parenchymal Changes From Obstruction

Acute and chronic obstructions are well shown on MR images. In acute obstruction kidney size is enlarged, and contrast persists in the renal parenchyma for a prolonged period of time, resulting in a prolonged nephrogram phase (fig. 9.83). The concentration of gadolinium in the collecting system is usually dilute, resulting in high signal. This is caused by the combination of the excretion of dilute urine, which occurs in the setting of acute severe obstruction, and the dilutional effect of gadolinium within a large volume of urine in a dilated collecting system. Corticomedullary differentiation is diminished on immediate postgadolinium images [5]. In chronic obstruction, the kidney, which is initially enlarged, over time gradually decreases in size and develops diminished renal perfusion (fig. 9.84) [5]. Renal cortical thinning occurs and, in pure renal obstruction, is usually uniform. Irregular cortical thinning, however, is not unusual. The regularity of cortical thinning presumably reflects the tissue pressure experienced in different portions of the kidney. Uniform cortical thinning may reflect a relatively uniform increased pressure throughout the kidney. Irregular thinning may be related to variations in calyceal dilatation and pressure. The presence of associated reflux in some conditions also contributes to irregular cortical thinning (fig. 9.85). The collecting

system generally remains dilated when the kidney atrophies, which permits distinction from chronic ischemia in which the collecting system is not dilated.

Reflux Nephropathy and Chronic Pyelonephritis

Reflux nephropathy represents renal parenchymal changes secondary to urine reflux into the renal collecting system. Changes of reflux nephropathy are more common in the upper or lower pole regions of the kidneys because of the presence of compound papillae or fused tips of the medullary pyramids. Owing to the fusion of multiple papillae, the papillary tip is flattered or concave. Normally, large terminal collecting ducts open into the calyces in the area of the papillary tip. In compound papillae, collecting duct orifices are wide, gaping, and permanently opened and are unable to be compressed in the presence of vesicoureteral reflux. This situation can lead to backflow of urine via the gaping collecting duct openings into the renal tubular system. In simple (unfused) papillae, collecting ducts open in slitlike fashion onto sharply convex papillary tips. This condition favors closure of the ducts when pelvic pressure rises—a protective measure that prevents intrarenal reflux.

Renal scarring is a frequent sequela of reflux nephropathy and occurs superficial to dilated calyces (fig. 9.86). The renal cortex is thin and usually very irregular [90]. The hallmark of chronic pyelonephritis is a coarse, discrete corticomedullary scar overlying a dilated, blunted, or deformed calyx. Most scars are in the upper and lower poles, consistent with the presence of compound papillae and resulting reflux at these sites [99].

Renal Arterial Disease

Disease of the renal arterial system may be thrombotic/arterial wall or embolic in nature. Thrombosis/arterial wall disease may be further subdivided into large vessel, medium vessel, and small vessel disease.

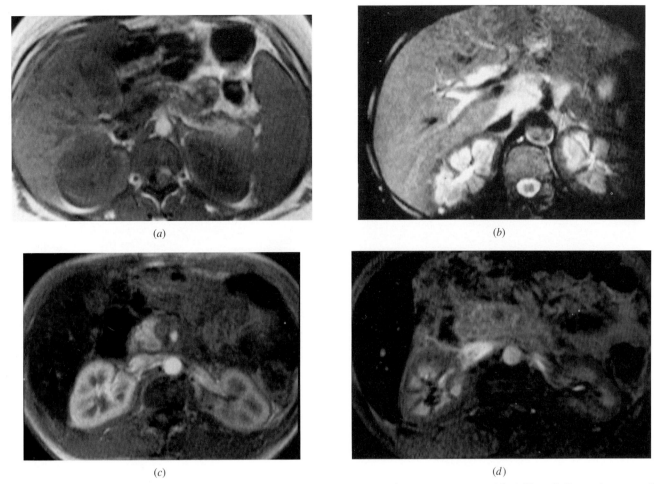

F I G . 9.82 Sickle cell disease. SGE (*a*) image demonstrates preservation of CMD in a patient with sickle cell disease because of the presence of dilute iron in the renal cortex that results in a T1-shortening paramagnetic effect.

T2-weighted fat-suppressed spin-echo image (*b*) in a second patient demonstrates low signal intensity of renal cortex secondary to accumulation of free hemoglobin. High-signal intensity celiac and porta hepatic nodes are also present.

Immediate (*c*) and 2-min (*d*) postgadolinium SGE images in a third patient. On the immediate postgadolinium image (*c*), the renal cortex is high in signal intensity, which reflects that the T1-shortening effect of gadolinium exceeds the T2-shortening effects of iron. At 2 min after injection (*d*), the T2 shortening of iron in the cortex exceeds the T1 shortening of gadolinium, causing diminished signal intensity of the cortex. The relative washout of gadolinium from the cortex coupled with the transit of gadolinium into the medulla results in this signal reversal of cortex and medulla. Signal intensity changes in renal parenchyma on postgadolinium images in patients with sickle cell disease reflect the changing balance on T2-shortening effects of iron and T1-shortening effects of gadolinium.

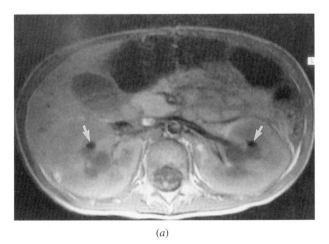

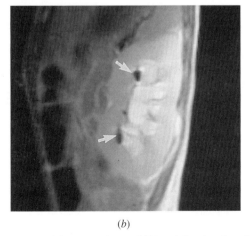

F I G . 9.83 Acute obstruction. T1-weighted spin-echo (*a*) and sagittal-plane gadolinium-enhanced T1-weighted spin-echo (*b*) images. The kidneys are enlarged in a globular fashion. CMD is preserved, reflecting the acuteness of the obstruction (*a*). Gadolinium excreted into the collecting system is dilute and high in signal intensity (*b*). Signal-void foci located in the nondependent portions of the renal collecting system demonstrate blooming artifact (arrows *a*, *b*) that represents air introduced by Foley catheterization.

815

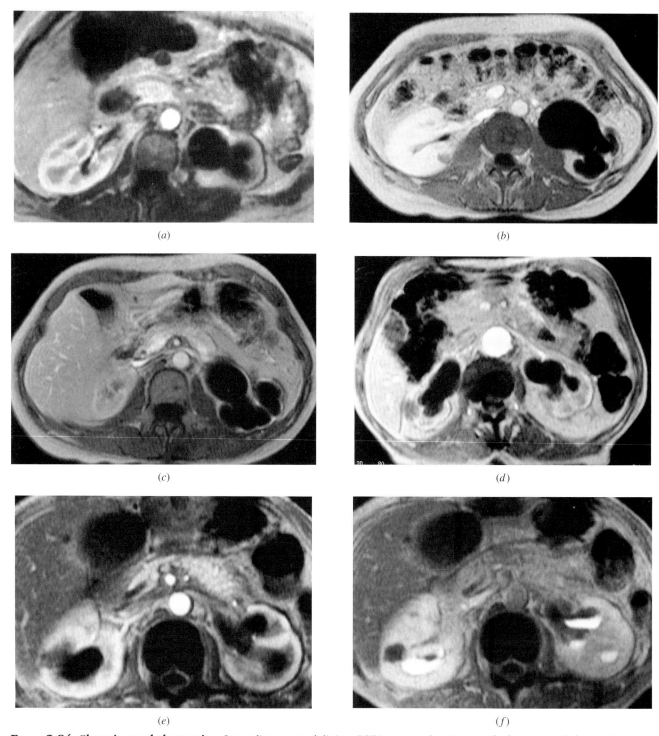

(a)

(b)

(c)

(d)

(e)

(f)

F I G . 9.84 Chronic renal obstruction. Immediate postgadolinium SGE images in 5 patients with chronic renal obstruction (*a-e*). In all cases of unilateral obstruction (*a-c*) the degree of cortical enhancement is less than that of the contralateral normal kidney. Substantial pelvicalyceal dilatation is present in all cases. CMD is diminished, and the cortex is thinned and relatively smooth. These factors reflect the duration and severity of obstruction. Excreted urine is dilute in the setting of chronic obstruction because kidneys lose concentrating ability. Excretion of dilute gadolinium is shown on a 4-min postgadolinium SGE image (*f*) obtained in the same patient illustrated in (*e*).

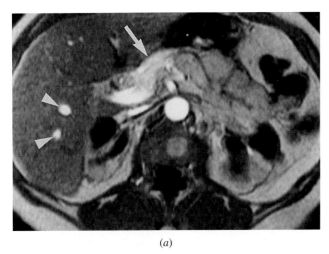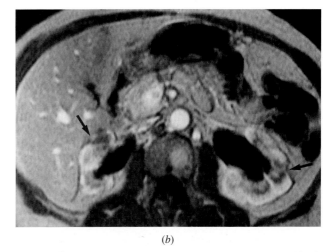

(a)   *(b)*

F I G . 9.85 Complicated chronic renal obstruction. Immediate (*a*) and 45-s (*b*) postgadolinium SGE images. Dilatation of both renal collecting systems has resulted from multiple urological procedures, including creation of an ileal conduit for obstruction of the distal ureters. Minimal cortical enhancement is shown on the immediate postgadolinium image. Image acquisition has been timed in the capillary phase of enhancement as evidenced by high signal intensity of the body of the pancreas (arrow, *a*) and contrast in portal veins (arrowheads, *a*). Cortical enhancement has developed in a delayed fashion and is apparent at 45 s. The combination of obstruction associated with reflux has resulted in variation in calyceal dilatation and tissue pressure experienced by the different regions of the kidneys. The result is severe irregularity of the renal cortex (arow, *b*). (Reproduced with permission from Kettritz U, Semelka RC, Brown ED, Sharp TJ, Lawing WL, Colindres RE: MR findings in diffuse renal parenchymal disease. *J Magn Reson Imaging* 1: 136–144, 1996.)

Ischemic nephropathy results from atherosclerotic disease of the main renal artery. Concomitant changes of atherosclerotic disease of the abdominal aorta are virtually always present. MRI studies can be tailored to demonstrate both the anatomic change of renal artery disease and the functional consequences of renal artery perfusion and contrast excretion. Anatomic changes of renal artery disease are shown on MR angiographic sequences. The most reproducible technique for demonstrating changes of main artery disease is gadolinium-

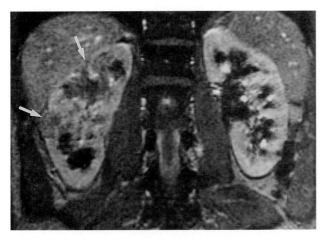

F I G . 9.86 Reflux nephropathy. Coronal 2.5-min postgadolinium gradient-echo image. Reflux nephropathy of the right kidney is shown by irregular thinning of the renal cortex overlying renal calyces. Damage in this patient is most severe in the upper and midrenal regions (arrows).

enhanced 3D gradient-echo MRA [2, 3]. It is critical that, in addition to the 3D reconstructed images, the source images be examined to determine normal arteries (fig. 9.87), the number of arteries, and the presence of stenosis (fig. 9.88). Reconstruction of images in both the coronal and transverse planes is useful. A recent article described that gadolinium-enhanced MR angiography was an accurate method for the diagnosis of renal artery stenosis, with sensitivities and specificities ranging from 97% to 98% and 90% to 100%, respectively. Sensitivity and specificity were calculated for detection of only grade 2 stenosis and for detection of stenotic or occlusive disease (e.g., stenosis >50%, including occlusions) [100]. Another study assessed the ability of dynamic gadolinium administration to demonstrate renal artery stenosis and renal stent patency using conventional angiography as the gold standard. Severity of renal artery stenosis was classified correctly with an accuracy of 98%, yielding 98% specificity and 100% sensitivity. The renal stents were visualized with 100% accurate patency documentation [101]. The renal arteries are more clearly demonstrated if fat suppression is added to the MRA sequence to remove the competing high signal intensity of fat and render small enhanced vessels more conspicuous. Imaging with 3D sequence acquisition achieves section thickness of 2 mm, which markedly improves detection of stenosis. Kidneys with chronic ischemic nephropathy typically are small and smooth and show minimal early enhancement on immediate postgadolinium images with delayed development and persistence of corticomedullary

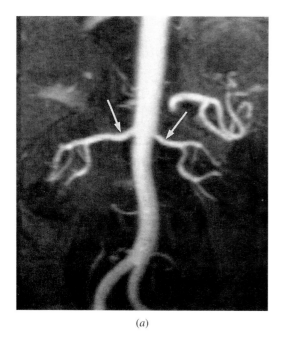

(a)

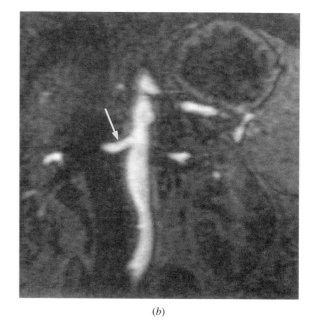

(b)

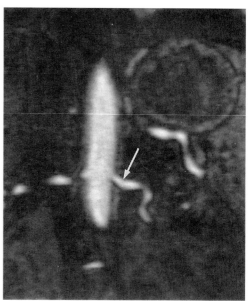

(c)

FIG. 9.87 MR angiogram with coronal 3D GE. Coronal maximum-intensity projection (MIP) reconstructed image (*a*) and individual 2-mm-thin 3D GE source images of right (*b*) and left (*c*) renal artery origin. The MIP reconstructed image displays a normal aorta and renal arteries (arrows, *a*). Areas of stenosis, however, can be masked in reconstructed images. The individual source images of the right (arrow, *b*) and left (arrow, *c*) renal artery are normal.

differentiation (fig. 9.89) [90,101]. The renal cortex is uniformly thin and frequently smooth, which reflects the global and chronic nature of the ischemic injury (fig. 9.90).

Aortic dissection also may result in changes of diminished renal arterial blood flow to the kidney fed by the false lumen [102]. This may occur either by occlusion/thrombosis of the renal artery by the intimal flap or false channel or by decreased arterial flow through the renal artery fed by the false lumen. Capillary-phase gadolinium-enhanced imaging is effective at demonstrating differences in enhancement between the kidneys, where one is fed by the true lumen and the other (usually the left) is fed by the false lumen (fig. 9.91) [103].

Renal artery pseudoaneurysms are not rare. They may undergo rupture or may come to clinical attention because of pressure effects on other structures. MRA is an effective technique to evaluate size, location, and appearance of pseudoaneurysms (fig. 9.92).

Renal artery injury sustained by trauma or surgery may result in changes of ischemic nephropathy (fig. 9.93). This may result in an acute or chronic ischemic process depending on the time of occurrence. The degree of renal artery compromise effects the extent of renal parenchymal changes. Associated perirenal hemorrhage is usually present.

Fibromuscular dysplasia is a disease that affects the main renal arteries. The disease is characterized by fibrous or fibromuscular thickening affecting any layer of the blood vessel wall. Stenoses of fibromuscular dysplasia often can be differentiated from atherosclerotic stenosis based on the segmental nature of the former, with alternating portions of luminal expansions and narrowings. Gadolinium-enhanced 3D MRA may be the most accurate MRI method for demonstrating this entity. Controlled comparisons with conventional angiography, however, are lacking. Care should be exercised not to misinterpret stepladder image reconstruction artifact for fibromuscular displasia. At the present time, MRA may not be a consistent enough technique to demonstrate

subtle changes of fibromuscular displasia to supplant angiographic approaches.

Medium vessel disease is often observed in combination with large- or small vessel disease. Atherosclerotic disease, for example, results in disease of all three types of vessels (fig. 9.94). Various immunologic vasculitides such as Wegener granulomatosis or polyarteritis nodosa involve medium and small vessels.

Small vessel disease is a very common cause of renal vascular disease. Nephrosclerosis caused by hypertension and/or diabetic angiopathy are the most frequently observed disease entities, but a variety of vasculitises

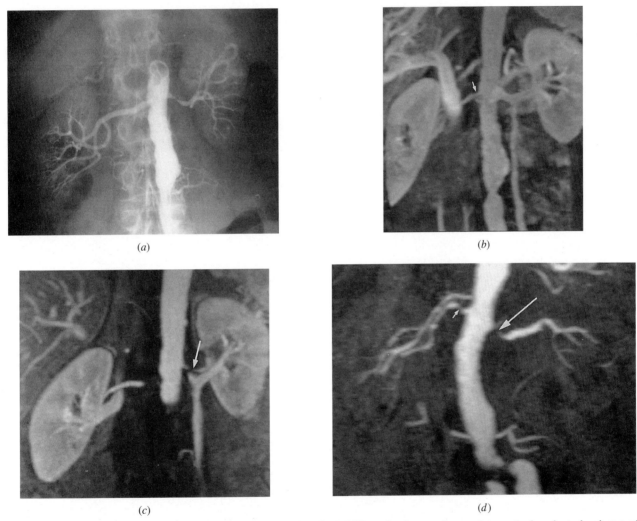

(a)

(b)

(c)

(d)

F I G . 9.88 Renal artery stenosis. Angiogram (*a*) and tailored 3D MIP projections, using an interactively selected volume of interest of a gadolinium-enhanced 3D GE sequence (*b, c*). Mild stenosis of the right and severe stenosis of the left renal arteries are shown on the angiogram. MIP tailored for the right renal artery demonstrates minimal stenosis (arrow, *b*). MIP tailored for the left renal artery demonstrates severe stenosis (arrow, *c*).

Coronal 3D MIP gadolinium-enhanced 3D GE (*d*) in a second patient demonstrates 2 right renal arteries with moderate stenosis of the lower artery (short arrow, *d*) and moderately severe stenosis of a solitary left renal artery (long arrow, *d*). Breath-hold gadolinium-enhanced MR angiography is efficient at depicting the main as well as accessory renal arteries, which is important for preoperative planning (e.g., surgical repair of atherosclerotic aneurysms of the abdominal aorta).

MIP reconstructed MRA projection (*e*) and coronal 3D thin section source (*f*) images. On the MIP reconstructed image a short segment of right renal artery is not visualized. On the basis of this image it is not clear whether this represents stenosis or occlusion.

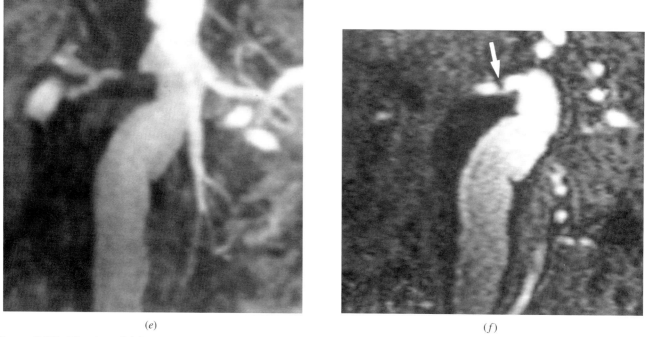

(e)   (f)

FIG. 9.88 (*Continued*) The source image (*f*) demonstrates that there is a short segment of high-grade stenosis (arrow, *f*).

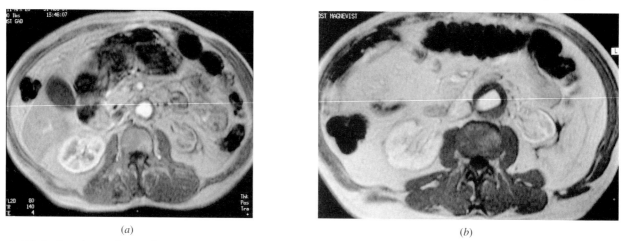

(a)   (b)

FIG. 9.89 Ischemic nephropathy. Immediate postgadolinium SGE (*a*) and 2-min postgadolinium SGE (*b*) images in 2 patients. In these patients atherosclerotic disease of the aorta is present, and the involved left kidney is small, smooth and has uniform cortical thinning. The diseased kidneys enhance in a diminished fashion compared to the normal right kidneys on immediate postgadolinium images (*a*). CMD develops later and persists in a more prolonged fashion on interstitial-phase images (*b*). The renal collecting systems are normal in caliber, which is an important observation to exclude obstructive nephropathy.

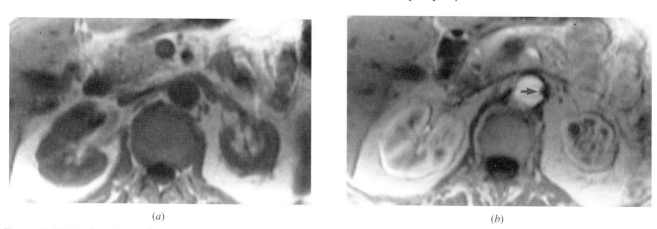

(a)   (b)

FIG. 9.90 Ischemic nephropathy. Precontrast T1-weighted SGE (*a*), immediate postgadolinium (*b*), and 90-s postgadolinium fat-suppressed SGE (*c*) images.

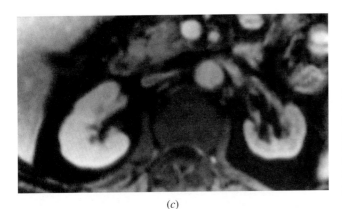

(c)

F I G . 9.90 (*Continued*) The left kidney is uniformly small, with uniform thinning of the renal cortex observed on postcontrast images (*b, c*). Cortical enhancement of the ischemic kidney is diminished on the immediate postgadolinium image but shows prolonged and increasing intensity at 90 s (*c*) when CMD in the contralateral kidney has faded. Note a small, low-signal focus along the left aspect of the aortic wall, which represents atheromatosis plaque at origin of the left renal artery (arrow, *b*).

also results in this pattern of renal vascular disease. Antiphospholipase deficiency has more currently received recognition as a cause of severe small vessel disease. Changes of small vessel disease are best shown on immediate postgadolinium SGE images as irregular areas of focal cortical thinning or focal perfusion defects [90].

As diabetes and hypertension tend to be chronic and progressive in nature, cortical irregularity is due to irreversible scarring. On serial postgadolinium MR images areas of cortical thinning appear as fixed irregularities that are unchanged from capillary-phase to interstitial-phase images (fig. 9.95). Vasculitis may be secondary to

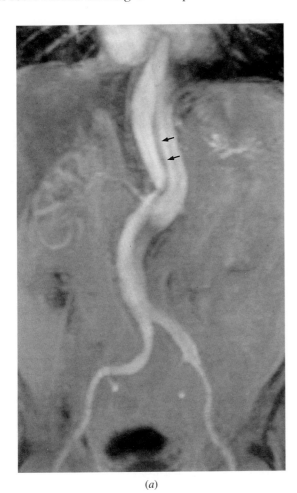

(a)

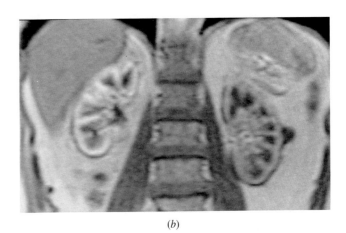

(b)

F I G . 9.91 Aortic dissection with differential renal perfusion. Coronal MIP reconstructed projection of coronal immediate postgadolinium 2D SGE images (*a*) and coronal 2D immediate postgadolinium source SGE image (*b*). Aortic dissection (small arrows, *a*) is shown on the MIP reconstructed gadolinium-enhanced SGE image (*a*). On a individual coronal source SGE image (*b*), lesser enhancement of the left renal cortex is present, reflecting diminished perfusion of the kidney due to its blood supply arising from the false lumen, which has slower flow.

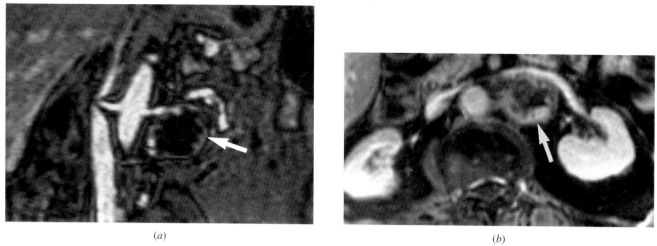

(a)   (b)

FIG. 9.92 Thrombosed left renal artery pseudoaneurysm. Coronal 3D source (*a*) and 3-min gadolinium-enhanced fat-suppressed SGE (*b*) images. A pseudoaneurysm is identified projecting posteroinferiorly from the left renal artery (arrow, *a, b*). The pseudoaneurysm does not fill with contrast on early or late postcontrast images, consistent with thrombosis.

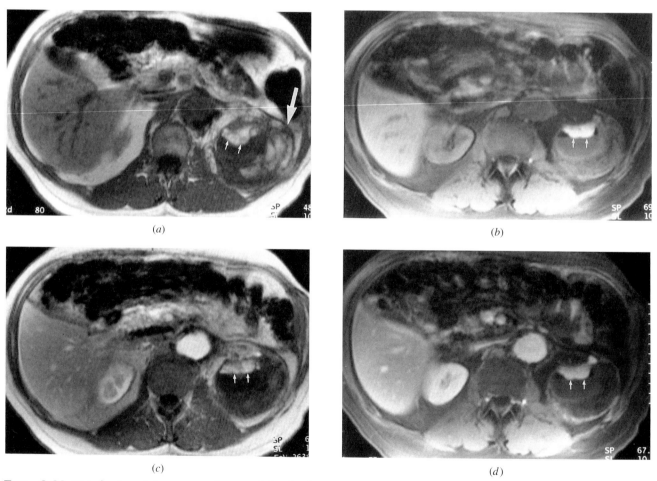

(a)   (b)

(c)   (d)

FIG. 9.93 Renal artery injury secondary to abdominal aortic aneurysm surgical repair. SGE (*a*), fat-suppressed SGE (*b*), immediate postgadolinium SGE (*c*), and 90-s postgadolinium fat-suppressed SGE (*d*) images. Abdominal aortic surgery was performed 1 year earlier, in which the left renal artery was injured. The left kidney is atrophic and high in signal intensity on T1-weighted images (small arrows, *a, b*), reflecting intraparenchymal hemorrhage. Associated subcapsular fluid collection and high-signal intensity perirenal fluid (large arrow, *a*) are present. The kidney remains unchanged in signal intensity on postcontrast images (small arrows, *c, d*).

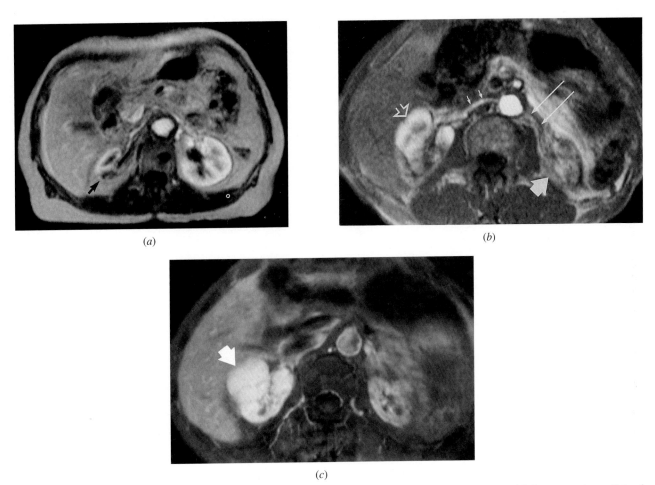

(a)

(b)

(c)

F I G . **9.94 Mixed large, medium-, and small vessel disease.** Immediate postgadolinium SGE image (*a*) demonstrates unilateral renovascular disease. The right kidney is noted to be globally small in size with a thin renal cortex. Cortical thinning is greater in the posterior aspect of the kidney (arrow, *a*) associated with greater decrease in enchancement.

Immediate postgadolinium SGE (*b*) and gadolinium-enhanced T1-weighted fat-suppressed SGE (*c*) images in a second patient demonstrate bilateral renovascular disease. Global severe diminished enhancement of the left kidney and asymmetric renovascular disease of the right kidney are apparent. The posterior portion of the right kidney has severe disease as shown by severe cortical thinning and diminished enhancement (*b*). The main right renal artery is normal in caliber for most of its length, reflecting the presence of predominant medium- and small vessel disease. The main left renal artery is small in caliber (long arrows, *b*) and, combined with global diminished enhancement of the left kidney (large arrow, *b*), reflects the severity of the main renal artery disease. Hypertrophy of the anterior cortex of the right kidney has developed (hollow arrow, *b*) in compensation for the renovascular disease of the posterior aspect of the kidney. Uniform cortical thickness with presence of corticomedullary differentiation of the anterior portion of the right kidney on the immediate postgadolinium image shows that the enlargement is due to hypertrophy and not tumor. Later interstitial-phase gadolinium-enhanced T1-weighted fat-suppressed spin-echo image (*c*) in this patient demonstrates relatively uniform enhancement of this region of renal hypertrophy (large arrow, *c*), which mimics the appearance of a tumor. Atherosclerotic disease of the aorta is apparent in both patients.

a number of etiologies, the most common of which are drug effects or collagen vascular diseases. Onset of vascular changes is typically more acute than with diabetes or hypertension. Early in the course of vasculitis, MR images may demonstrate multiple transient perfusional defects that are observed on immediate postgadolinium images and that resolve on more delayed images (fig. 9.96), which reflect ischemic changes. Acute cortical necrosis may result from rapid-onset diffuse small vessel disease (fig. 9.97).

Aortic atheroemboli are the most frequent cause of renal emboli [11]. The next common cause of renal emboli is embolism of mural thrombi in patients with atrial arrhythmias or prior myocardial infarction emboli because the kidneys receive approximately 20% of the cardiac output. Renal infarction from embolic events tends to occur between calyces and demonstrates well-defined wedge-shaped defects in the renal outline. A thin enhancing peripheral rim is present because of enhancement of small vessels in the renal capsule. (fig. 9.98) [102].

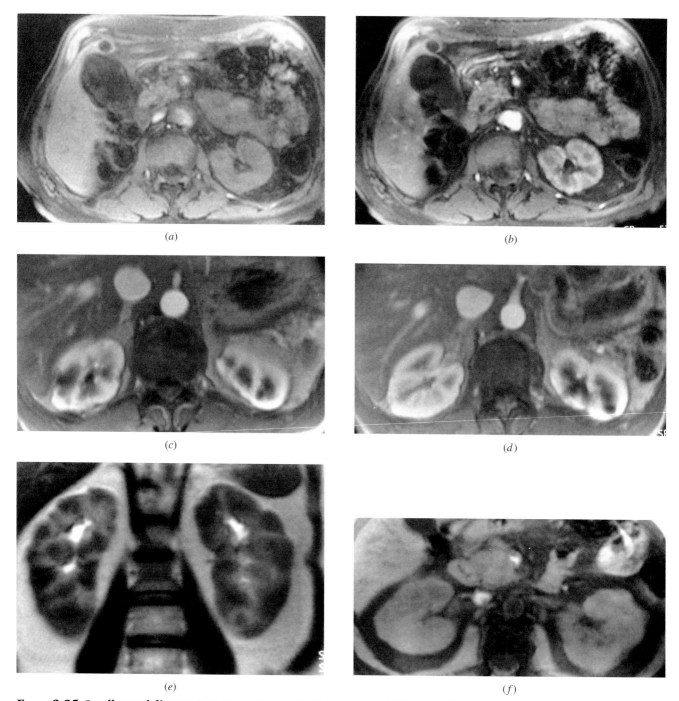

(a)

(b)

(c)

(d)

(e)

(f)

F I G . 9.95 Small vessel disease. Precontrast T1-weighted fat-suppressed SGE (*a*) and immediate postgadolinium T1-weighted fat-suppressed SGE (*b*) images. Loss of corticomedullary differentiation in the left kidney is apparent on the precontrast image, consistent with diminished renal function (*a*). On the immediate postgadolinium image (*b*), multiple small cortical defects are present because of small vessel disease.

Transverse immediate postgadolinium SGE images (*c, d*) in a second patient demonsrate bilateral small irregular renal cortical defects. These changes represent small vessel disease in this diabetic patient.

Coronal SS-ETSE (*e*), precontrast T1-weighted fat-suppressed SGE (*f*), immediate postgadolinium SGE (*g*), and 90-s postgadolinium fat-suppressed SGE (*h*) images in a third patient with small vessel disease. This patient is in renal failure, as evidenced by loss of CMD on precontrast images.

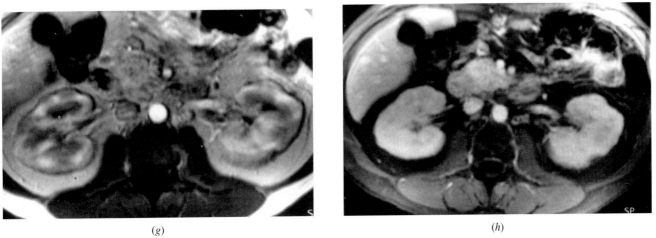

(g)

(h)

FIG. 9.95 (*Continue*) Focal patchy areas of diminished enhancement are appreciated on immediate postgadolinium images (*g*), many of which show enhancement by 90 s (*h*). This pattern of enhancement reflects ischemic changes.

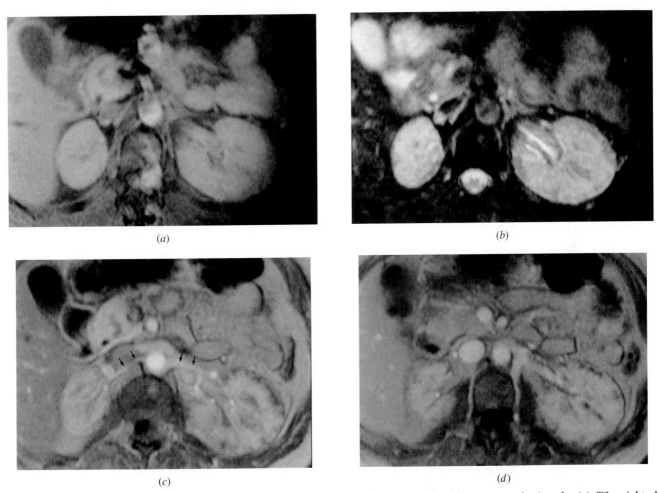

(a)

(b)

(c)

(d)

FIG. 9.96 Small vessel disease due to thrombotic microangiopathy. T1-weighted fat-suppressed spin-echo (*a*), T2-weighted fat-suppressed spin-echo (*b*), and immediate (*c*) and 90-s (*d*) postgadolinium SGE images. No corticomedullary differentiation is apparent on the precontrast T1-weighted fat-suppressed spin-echo image (*a*). On the T2-weighted image (*b*), numerous 5-mm cortical defects are present. Multiple cortical defects are clearly shown on the immediate postgadolinium image (*c*). In addition, the main renal arteries are noted to be normal (arrows, *c*). On the more delayed image (*d*) some defects have resolved. However, many defects persist consistent with necrosis. Histology revealed thrombotic microangiopathy with acute tubular necrosis and cortical necrosis.

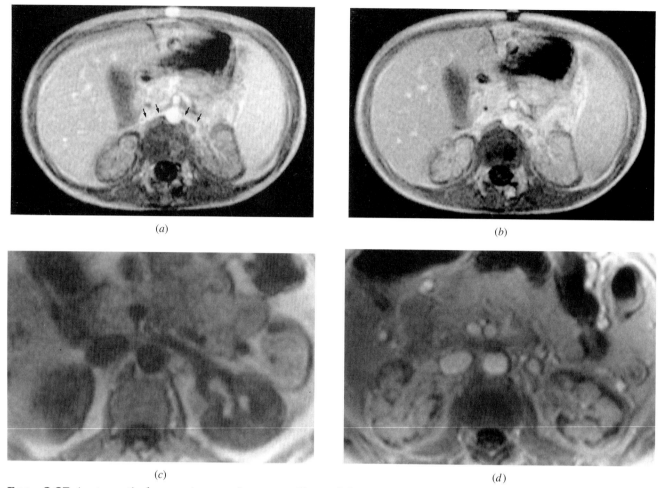

(a)   (b)

(c)   (d)

F I G . 9.97 Acute cortical necrosis secondary to small vessel disease from mixed connective tissue disease. Immediate (*a*) and 45-s (*b*) postgadolinium SGE images demonstrate low-signal intensity renal cortex due to lack of contrast enhancement. This appearance reflects acute cortical necrosis. Normal-appearing main renal arteries are present (arrows, *a*). (Reproduced with permission from Kettritz U, Semelka RC, Brown ED, Sharp TJ, Lawing WL, Colindres RE: MR findings in diffuse renal parenchymal disease. *J Magn Reson Imaging* 1: 136–144, 1996.)

Precontrast (*c*) and immediate postgadolinium (*d*) T1-weighted SGE images in a second patient with acute cortical necrosis. Extensive irregular linear regions that exhibit lack of enhancement are appreciated on the postcontrast image (*d*).

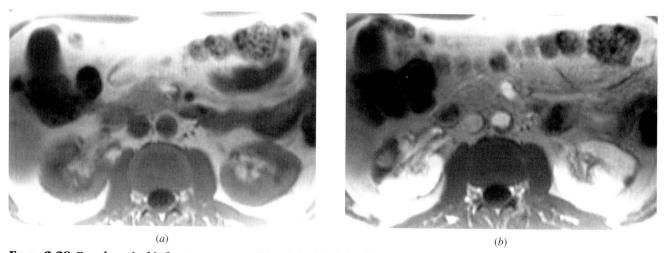

(a)   (b)

F I G . 9.98 Renal cortical infarcts. Precontrast T1-weighted SGE (*a*), 45-s postgadolinium SGE (*b*), and 90-s (*c, d*) postgadolinium fat-suppressed SGE images. There are multiple, peripheral, wedge-shaped areas of decreased enhancement within the kidneys.

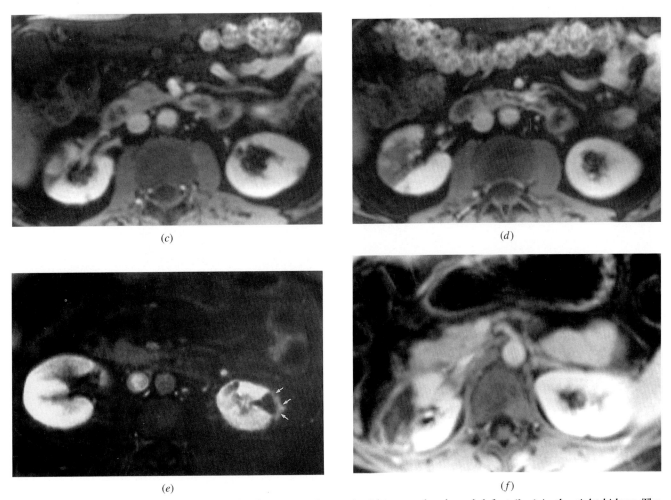

(c)

(d)

(e)

(f)

F I G . 9.98 (*Continued*) A focus of central enhancement is noted within a wedge-shaped defect (*b, c*) in the right kidney. The wedge-shaped defects are consistent with areas of infarct, with central sparing in one of the infarcts.

Interstitial-phase gadolinium-enhanced T1-weighted fat-suppressed spin-echo image (*e*) in a second patient demonstrates a nearly signal-void wedge-shaped defect in the inferior pole of the left kidney. Linear enhancement peripheral to the wedge-shaped defect (arrows) is due to enhancement of capsular based vessels. This is a classic feature of renal emboli. (Reproduced with permission from Semelka RC, Shoenut JP, Greenberg HM. The Kidney. In: Semelka RC, Shoenut JP (eds.), *MRI of the abdomen with CT correlation.* New York: Raven Press, 1993, p. 91–118.)

Transverse 90-s postgadolinium T1 weighted fat-suppressed spin-echo image (*f*) in a third patient. There is a wedge-shaped defect in the mid aspect of the right kidney consistent with a renal infarction. Note thin capsular enhancement along the outer margin of the defect.

Renal Vein Thrombosis

Renal vein thrombosis may occur as bland or tumor thrombus (see Renal Carcinoma section). Bland thrombus may occur as an acute or chronic process. Acute renal vein thrombosis may be observed in the setting of various hypercoagulable states. In the acute setting the kidney enlarges because of tissue swelling secondary to the obstruction of egress of blood flow. A progressive and persistent nephrogram is also observed (fig. 9.99). In the setting of chronic thrombosis, the kidney is often normal in size. Association membranous glomerulonepritis (see Glomerular Disease section) may be observed.

Renal Scarring

Renal scarring results from irreversible damage to renal parenchyma with regional loss of cortex. Scarring arises from a great variety of renal insults, which include vascular and collecting system disease. Scarring defects are well shown on postgadolinium images, with immediate postgadolinium images clearly defining the extent of cortical loss (figs. 9.100 and 9.101).

End-Stage Kidney

End-stage kidney appears as an atrophic diminutive kidney reflecting severe hypovascularity secondary to the loss of renal arterial supply. A variety of diffuse renal

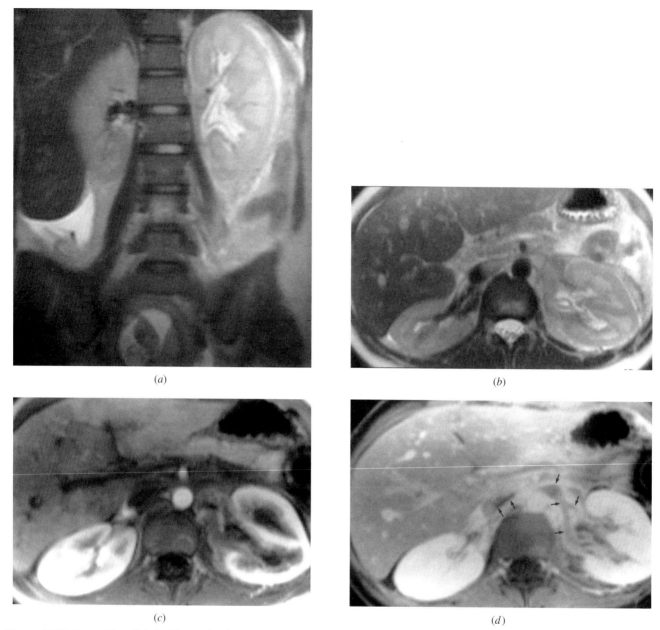

(a)

(b)

(c)

(d)

F I G . 9.99 Acute Renal Vein Thrombosis. Coronal (a) and transverse (b) SS-ETSE, immediate postgadolinium SGE (c), and 90-s postgadolinium T1-weighed fat-suppressed SGE (d) images. This pregnant patient presented with severe left flank pain. The left kidney is enlarged, and fluid surrounds the collecting system, consistent with edema. Intraluminal clot is appreciated within the left renal vein extending into the IVC (arrows, d).

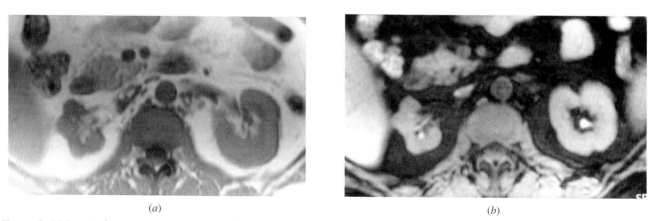

(a)

(b)

F I G . 9.100 Renal Scarring. Precontrast SGE (a), fat-suppressed SGE (b), immediate postgadolinium SGE (c) and 90-s postgadolinium fat-suppressed SGE (d) images.

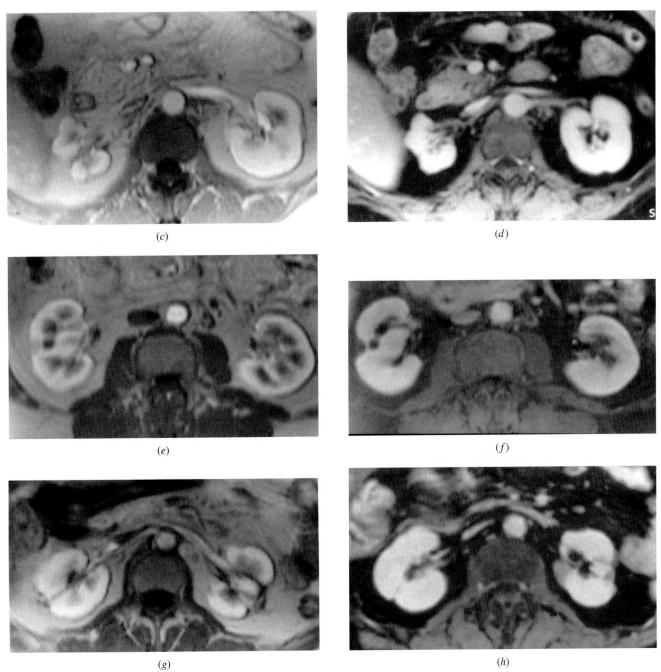

(c)

(d)

(e)

(f)

(g)

(h)

FIG. 9.100 *(Continued)* The right kidney is small and irregular in contour, consistent with chronic vascular injury, and the left kidney demonstrates compensatory hypertrophy.

Immediate postgadolinium SGE (*e*) and T1-weighted fat-suppressed SGE (*f*) images in a second patient demonstrate a cortical defect in the right kidney consistent with a scar. A cyst is noted deep to the infarct.

Immediate postgadolinium SGE (*g*) and 90-s postgadolinium fat-suppressed SGE (*h*) images in a third patient reveal bilateral renal cortical scars more extensive in the left kidney.

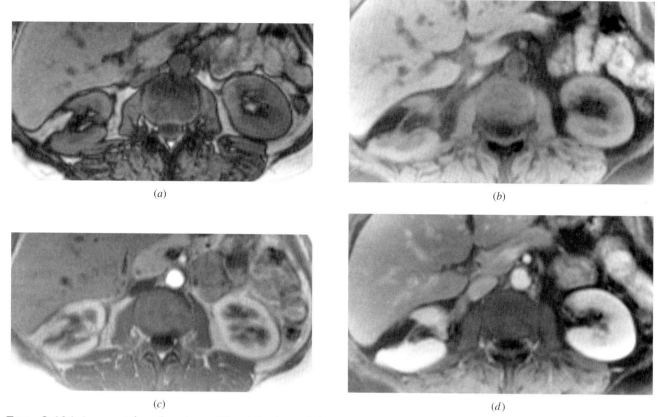

(a)

(b)

(c)

(d)

F I G . 9.101 Segmental nephrectomy. T1-weighted out-of-phase (a), T1-weighted fat-suppressed SGE (b), immediate postgadolinium SGE (c), and 90-s postgadolinium T1-weighted fatsuppressed SGE (d) images. There is a surgical defect in the midpole of the right kidney that has been filled by perirenal fat.

parenchymal diseases will result in end-stage kidneys, with hypertensive nephropathy likely the most common cause. Kidneys may be markedly atrophied on MR images and demonstrate the enhancement pattern of scar tissue, negligible capillary-phase enhancement with slight enhancement on later postcontrast images (fig. 9.102).

Infection

Acute Infection

Acute pyelonephritis is defined as acute suppurative inflammation of the kidney caused by bacterial infection and usually results in enlargement of the infected kidney [104]. The infection is most commonly caused by

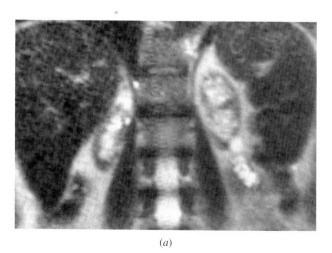

(a)

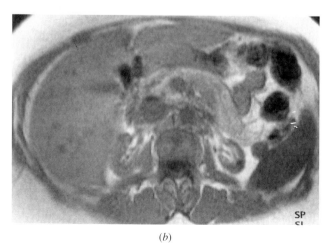

(b)

F I G . 9.102 End-stage kidney secondary to sustained hypertension. Coronal SS-ETSE (a), SGE (b), immediate postgadolinium SGE (c), and 2-min postgadolinium fat-suppressed SGE (d) images.

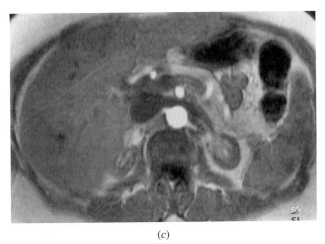

(c)

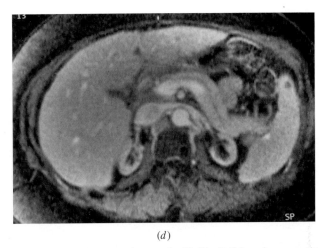

(d)

FIG. 9.102 (*Continued*) Bilateral diminutive atrophic kidneys are apparent on precontrast images (*a, b*). Negligible enhancement is appreciated on the immediate postgadolinium SGE image (*c*). On more delayed images (*d*), renal parenchymal enhancement has increased. This enhancement pattern is observed in fibrotic tissue.

Gram-negative bacilli as an ascending infection from the lower urinary tract. Perinephric fluid may be observed, which is best shown on postgadolinium images (fig. 9.103). Proteinaceous material in the renal tubules may occasionally be visualized as high-signal intensity sub-stance in the renal medulla on noncontrast T1-weighted fat-suppressed images (see fig. 9.103). MR findings of acute pyelonephritis include a striated nephrogram that radiates from the renal medulla to the cortex, globular renal enlargement, and perinephric fluid (fig. 9.104).

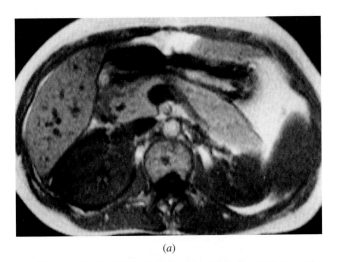

(a)

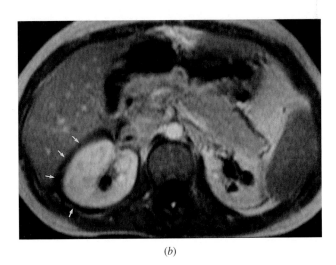

(b)

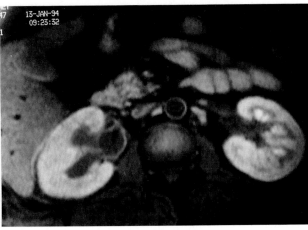

(c)

FIG. 9.103 Acute pyelonephritis. SGE (*a*) and 2-min post-gadolinium SGE (*b*) images. The right kidney is swollen, and perinephric fluid (arrows, *b*) is present. No focal parenchymal abnormalities are identified.

Precontrast T1-weighted fat-suppressed spin-echo image (*c*) in a second patient demonstrates striated, cone-shaped regions of high signal intensity in the medulla of the left kidney, consistent with proteinaceous material in acute pyelonephritis. Hydronephrosis of the right kidney is identified.

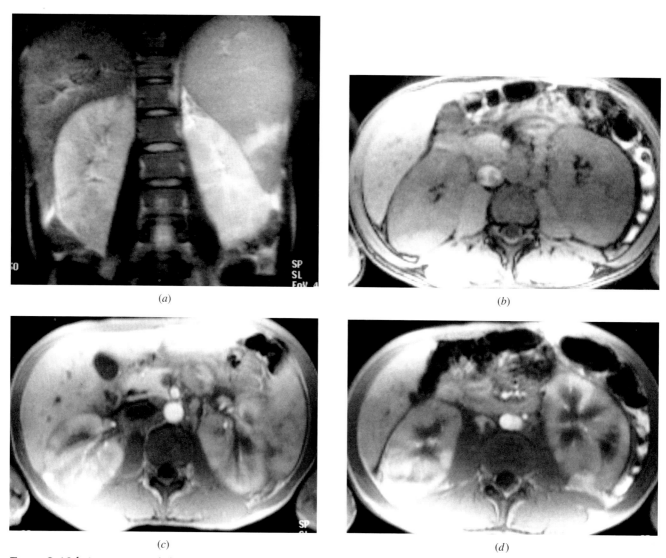

F I G . 9.104 Severe acute bilateral pyelonephritis. Coronal SS-ETSE (*a*), precontrast SGE (*b*), and immediate postgadolinium SGE (*c, d*) images. The kidneys are enlarged and demonstrate heterogeneous signal intensity on T1- and T2-weighted images, and heterogeneous enhancement after administration of gadolinium. Note that the heterogeneous enhancement has a striated nephrogram appearance, which is a feature that may be observed in acute pyelonephritis.

Abscess

Renal abscess usually occurs as a complication of an ascending urinary tract infection, but hematogenous infections also occur [105]. Hematogenous infection may be seen in tuberculosis secondary to disseminated infection or in the setting of intravenous drug use. On MR images, renal abscesses appear as irregular mass lesions with a signal void center (figs. 9.105 and 9.106) [106]. Perinephric stranding is frequently prominent [106]. Perinephric linear densities are more prominent in renal abscesses than in necrotic renal cancers because these reflect inflammatory tissue. It may not, however, always be possible to distinguish abscesses from cancer based on imaging findings, and follow-up studies may be needed to ensure resolution after treatment [107]. Patients with multifocal or diffuse renal abscesses frequently have

elevated serum creatinine (see figs. 9.105 and 9.106). Ultrasound and noncontrast CT imaging perform poorly at detecting renal abscesses; therefore, in patients with renal dysfunction, MRI is the procedure of choice [106].

Xanthogranulomatous Pyelonephritis

Xanthogranulomatous pyelonephritis (XGPN) is an unusual form of chronic pyelonephritis that represents the inflammatory sequela of recurrent suppurative renal infections that develop in the setting of chronic urinary obstruction [108]. The disorder is characterized pathologically by collections of foamy macrophages, "xanthoma cells," acute and chronic inflammatory cells, and multinucleated giant cells. Sixty percent of cases are associated with proteus infection, which usually involves the

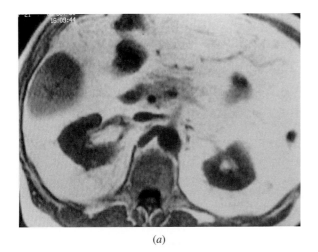

(a)

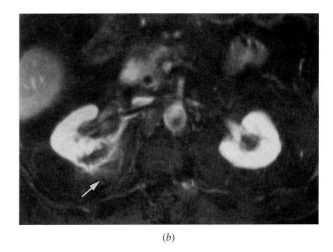

(b)

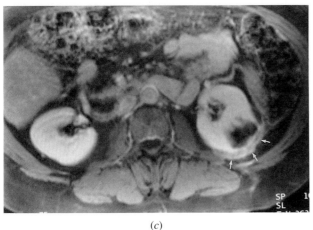

(c)

F I G . 9.105 Solitary renal abscess. SGE (a) and gadolinium-enhanced T1-weighted fat-suppressed spin-echo (b) images in a patient with a solitary abscess in the posterior aspect of the right kidney. Perirenal stranding is noted on the precontrast image, but the abscess is not well seen. On the gadolinium-enhanced fat-suppressed spin-echo image a signal-void intraparenchymal renal abscess is noted. The inner aspect of the abscess wall is irregular. Prominent perirenal stranding (arrow, b) is an important imaging feature of renal abscess.

Three-minute postgadolinium fat-suppressed SGE image (c) in a second patient who is a diabetic. A left renal abscess is present that appears as a low-signal intensity cystic lesion with an irregular wall. Prominent thickening and increased enhancement of adjacent fascia (small arrows, c) is present.

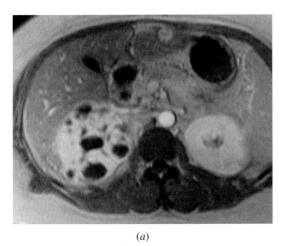

(a)

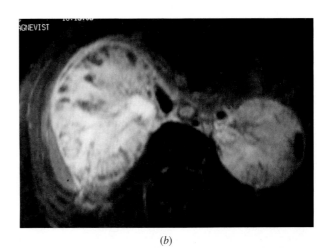

(b)

F I G . 9.106 Multiple renal abscess. Ninety-second postgadolinium SGE image (a) demonstrates multiple signal-void abscesses in the right kidney.

Bilateral renal abscesses with substantial renal enlargement are demonstrated on a gadolinium-enhanced T1-weighted fat-suppressed spin-echo image (b) in a second patient with HIV infection and elevated serum creatinine. Ultrasound and noncontrast CT imaging demonstrated renal enlargement with no definition of abscesses. In the same patient, a repeat MRI study was performed after a 15-day course of antibilitics. The gadolinium-enhanced T1-weighted fat-suppressed spin-echo image (c) demonstrates decrease in renal size with decrease in size and number of abscesses.

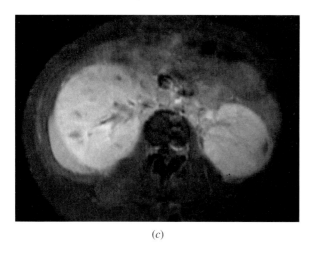

(c)

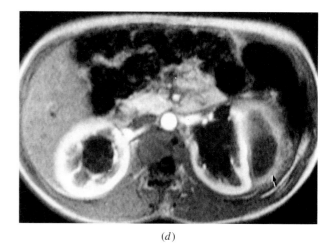

(d)

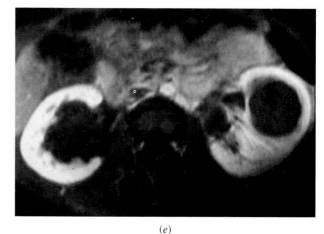

(e)

FIG. 9.106 (*Continued*) Immediate postgadolinium SGE (*d*) and gadolinium-enhanced T1-weighted fat-suppressed spin-echo (*e*) images in a third patient demonstrate a renal abscess with a prominent extrarenal component (arrow, *d*). Multiple parapelvic cysts are present in both kidneys.

kidney globally, although focal XGPN has been described [108].

On MR images, the kidney usually is enlarged. After gadolinium administration, minimal enhancement is present on capillary-phase images with progressively intense enhancement on interstitial-phase images (fig. 9.107). This enhancement pattern reflects poor renal perfusion (minimal early enhancement) with substantial capillary leakage due to inflammatory change (increased delayed enhancement). Perinephric inflammatory changes are prominent, with extension to the psoas muscle commonly present. The renal collecting system

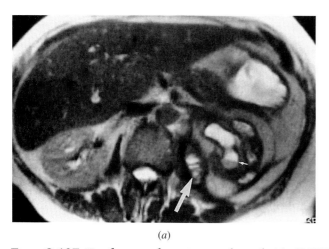

(a)

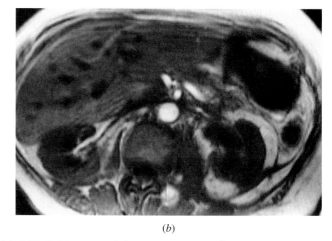

(b)

FIG. 9.107 Xanthogranulomatous pyelonephritis. SS-ETSE (*a*), SGE (*b*) 90-s postgadolinium SGE (*c*), and 4-min postgadolinium fat-suppressed SGE (*d*) images. The left renal collecting system is noted to be dilated (*a–d*). A large extrarenal component of the infection is noted in the psoas muscle (arrow, *a, d*).

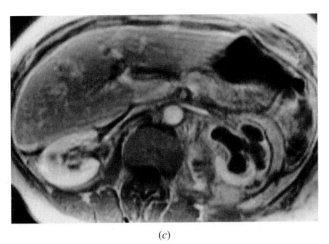

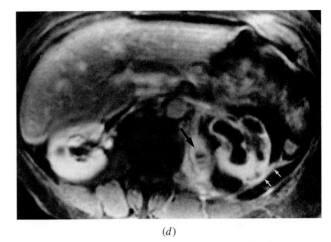

(c) *(d)*

F I G . 9.107 (*Continued*) Layering of low-signal intensity material (small arrow, *a*) is noted in calyces on the T2-weighted image (*a*). No excretion of gadolinium by the involved kidney is apparent on the 4-min postgadolinium image. Inflammatory changes in Gerota fascia and lateral conal fascia (small arrows, *d*) and psoas abscess are most clearly defined on the gadolinium-enhanced fat-suppressed image (*d*). The combination of dilatation of the collecting system, lack of contrast excretion, and prominent extrarenal inflammatory changes are features observed for xanthogranulomatous pyelonephritis.

almost invariably is dilated, and signal void calculi may be identified. No evidence of gadolinium excretion in the collecting system is appreciated.

Malakoplakia:

Malakoplakia (*malakos* = soft and *plakos* = plaques) is a rare chronic granulomatous inflammatory process often affecting immunocompromised hosts. The disease is most frequently observed in the urinary tract of middle-aged women as a complication of recurrent urinary tract infections (coliforms, 90%; *E. coli*, 75%) [109].

The lower urinary tract is more commonly affected, with renal parenchymal involvement being unusual (16% of cases) [109]. The typical mucosal lesion of malakoplakia is a yellow-brown soft plaque with central umbilication. Parenchymal lesions are characterized by nodules of variable size that may be discrete, coalesce to become diffuse, or undergo suppuration with abscess formation. Renal parenchymal malakoplakia can be multifocal or unifocal. In multifocal malakoplakia the kidneys are enlarged with solid infiltration and, when the disease is unifocal, a nonspecific mass identified [110].

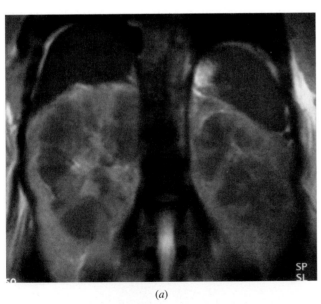

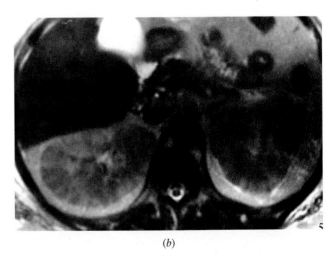

(a) *(b)*

F I G . 9.108 Malakoplakia. Coronal (*a*) and axial (*b*) SS-ETSE, precontrast SGE (*c*) and 1-min postgadolinium SGE (*d*) images. The kidneys are enlarged with an extensive multinodular appearance. High-signal septations are appreciated on the T2-weighted sequences (*a*, *b*), which enhance after gadolinium administration (*d*).

T2-weighted fat-suppressed echo-train spin-echo (*e*), T1-weighted SGE (*f*), and transverse (*g*) and sagittal (*h*) T1-weighted postgadolinium fat-suppressed SGE images in a second patient.

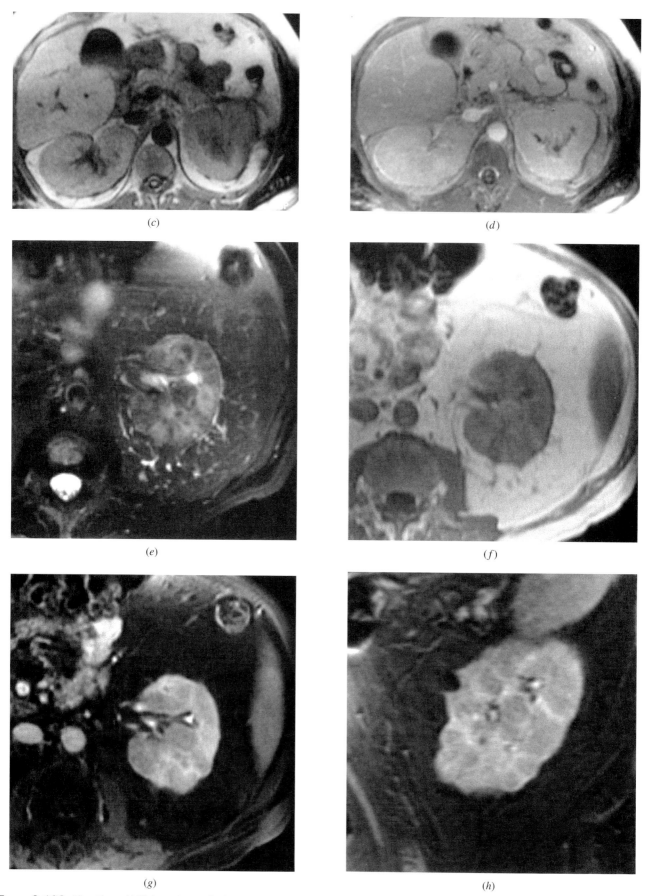

(c)

(d)

(e)

(f)

(g)

(h)

F I G . 9.108 (*Continued*) This patient, who had undergone liver transplantation, has a similar appearance of extensive multinodular infiltrate in the kidneys with intervening linear stroma that is high signal on T2 (*e*) and enhances with gadolinium (*g*, *h*). (Courtsey of Eric Outwater, MD, University of Arizona.)

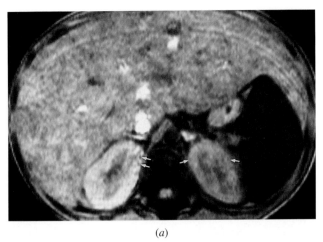

(a)

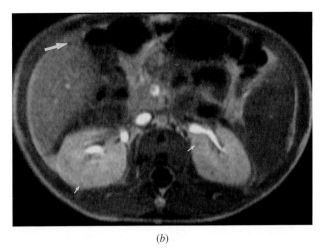

(b)

F I G . 9.109 Renal candidiasis. Immediate (a) and 90-s (b) postgadolinium SGE images, in 2 patients with renal candidiasis. Multiple low-signal intensity lesions, <5 mm in size, are present in the kidneys of both patients (small arrows, a, b). Extensive hepatic involvement is apparent in the first patient (a), whereas fewer liver lesions are apparent in the second patient (arrow, b).

The clinical presentation and radiologic appearance are often suggestive of a neoplasm. The diagnosis is established on the basis of histopathology. The characteristic histologic feature of the lesion is the presence of Michaelis-Gutmann bodies [111].

Multifocal malakoplakia appears as multiple ill-defined regions of lower signal intensity with intervening linear stroma in a mildly enlarged kidney on T2-weighted and postgadolinium SGE images (fig. 9.108). There is currently insufficient experience with MRI, to determine the specificity of this finding.

Candidiasis
Renal candidiasis occurs in the context of hepatosplenic candidiasis. These lesions are typically small (5 mm) and well defined. Lesions are best shown on gadolinium-

enhanced T1-weighted interstitial-phase fat-suppressed images (fig. 9.109) [112].

Fungus balls also may develop in the collecting system. Diabetes predisposes to this condition.

Pyonephrosis
Pyonephrosis is a complication of acute pyelonephritis and occurs in the setting of total or almost complete urinary tract obstruction, when the suppurative exudate is unable to drain, thus filling the renal pelvis and calyces. MRI features consistent with pyonephrosis include debris layering in the obstructed renal pelvis, most clearly defined on T2-weighted single-shot echo-train spin-echo as dependently layering low-signal intensity fluid, and enhancement of the wall of the renal pelvis on gadolinium-enhanced images (fig. 9.110).

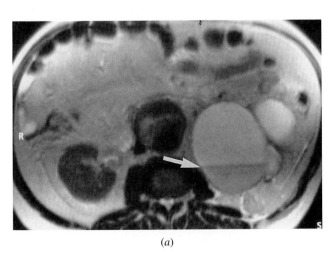

(a)

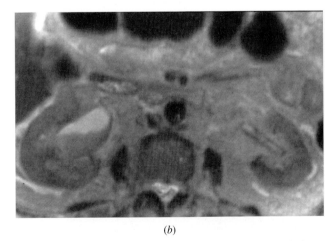

(b)

F I G . 9.110 Pyonephrosis. Transverse SS-ETSE image (a) demonstrates severe dilatation of the collecting system of the left kidney. Layering of low-signal intensity debris (arrow, a) in the dependent portion of the renal pelvis is a common appearance in infection.

Transverse SS-ETSE image (b) in a second patient. There is hydronephrosis of the right kidney with layering of low-signal material consistent with infection within the dilated collecting system. Note also perinephric fluid stranding.

Hemorrhage

Renal/perirenal hemorrhage occurs in the context of bleeding disorders, trauma, and neoplasms. Large perinephric hematomas may occur in patients who have undergone renal lithotripsy or renal biopsy. MRI is more sensitive than CT imaging to the presence of hemor-

rhage in fluid collections. Parenchymal or subcapsular hemorrhage appears as high- or mixed high-signal intensity fluid on both T1- and T2-weighted images (fig. 9.111) [18]. Perirenal hemorrhage frequently has an unusual multilayered appearance because of extravasation of blood along the fibrous trabeculae which traverse perirenal fat.

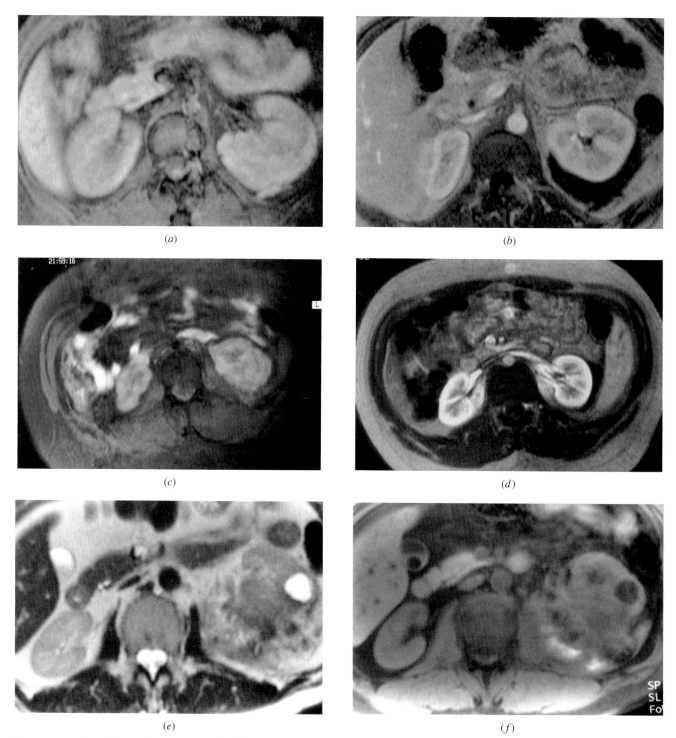

(a)

(b)

(c)

(d)

(e)

(f)

F I G . 9.111 Perirenal hematoma after biopsy. T1-weighted fat-suppressed spin-echo (a) and immediate postgadolinium SGE (b) images in 1 patient and the same sequences (c, d), respectively in a second patient.

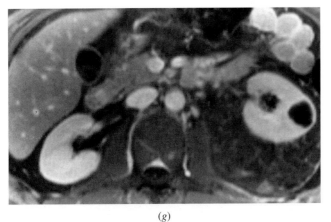

(g)

On the precontrast fat-suppressed spin-echo images (*a, c*) high-signal intensity fluid is present in the perirenal space of the left kidney, consistent with subacute blood. On the immediate postgadolinium SGE images (*b, d*) the fluid appears low in signal intensity because of rescaling of the tissue signal intensities after gadolinium administration.

Transverse SS-ETSE (*e*), precontrast fat-suppressed SGE (*f*), and postgadolinium T1-weighted fat-suppressed SGE (*g*) images in a third patient. There is heterogeneous signal intensity fluid in the left perinephric space on T1- (*f*) and T2- (*e*) weighted images, displacing the kidney anterior and laterally, consistent with a perirenal hematoma, after renal biopsy. Note also a thick-walled cyst within the left kidney, which is of uniform thickness but has prominent mural enhancement (*g*).

DISEASE OF THE RENAL COLLECTING SYSTEM: RENAL PELVIS AND URETER

Mass Lesions

Primary Tumors
Primary neoplasms of the ureter or renal pelvis are uncommon and collectively are only one-tenth as common as primary neoplasm of the bladder.

Transitional Cell Carcinoma (Urothelial Carcinoma).
The majority of primary tumors of the urothelium are malignant. Transitional cell carcinoma (TCC) is the most common malignancy of the urothelium, accounting for more than 90% of tumors [113]. Squamous cell cancer accounts for 8%, and adenocarcinoma for less than 1% [113]. TCC represents 8% of all renal tumors, rarely occurring in patients younger than 30 years of age. TCC of the upper tract is epidemiologically similar to that of the bladder. Males are more commonly affected,

in a 3 to 1 ratio with females. Risk factors include analgesics, tobacco, caffeine, chronic infection, and urolithiasis. Staging of transitional cell cancer is as follows: Stage 1, limited to urothelial mucosa and lamina propria; Stage 2, invasion of, but not beyond, pelvic/ureteral muscularis; Stage 3, invasion beyond muscularis into adventitial fat or renal parenchyma; and Stage 4, distant metastasis. Tumors usually appear as eccentric filling defects in the renal pelvis (fig. 9.112) [113, 114]. On occasion, they may cause concentric wall thickening (113, 114). Tumors usually spread superficially (fig. 9.113), but in rare instances they may be large focal masses. TCC has a propensity to invade renal parenchyma, but invasion may be difficult to detect. Invasion of or along the IVC may occur and is well depicted on MR images (fig. 9.114) [114, 115]. Although these tumors are hypovascular, they may be moderately high in signal intensity on gadolinium-enhanced interstitial-phase T1-weighted fat-suppressed images, presumably because of diminished clearance of contrast from the interstitial space [115]. Tumors tend to invade locally, with spread to adjacent lymph nodes. There is a great propensity for the tumor to be

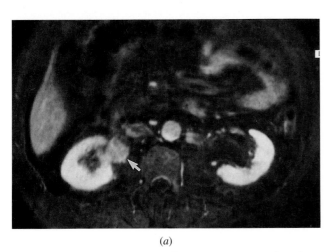

(a)

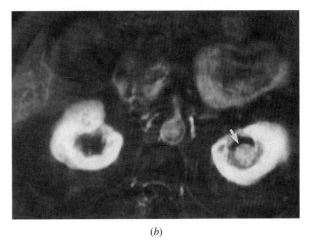

(b)

F I G . 9.112 Transitional cell cancer—Stage 2, focal mass type. Gadolinium-enhanced T1-weighted fat-suppressed spin-echo images in 3 patients with transitional cell cancer.

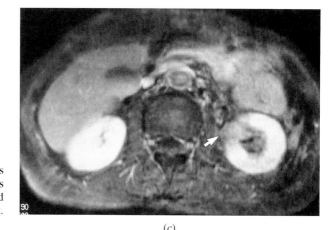

(c)

F I G . 9.112 (*Continued*) Tumors are focal rounded masses (arrow, *a–c*) that show heterogeneous mottled enhancement less than neighboring renal cortex. Note that masses have well-defined margins that correspond to lack of infiltration into surrounding fat.

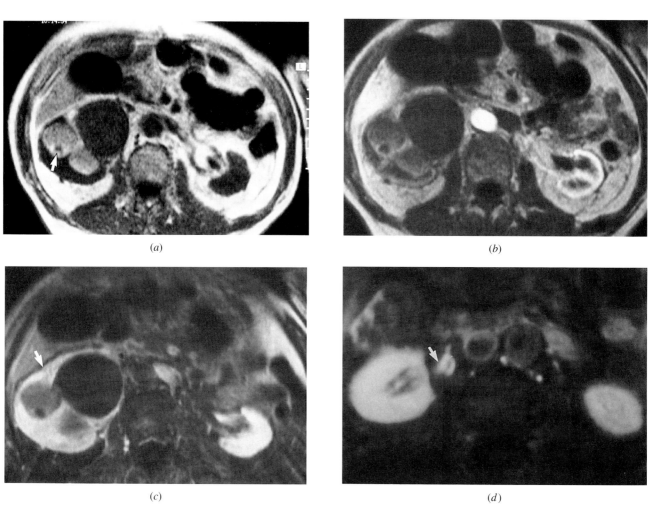

(a)

(b)

(c)

(d)

F I G . 9.113 Transitional cell cancer—Stage 3, superficially spreading pattern. SGE (*a*), immediate postgadolinium SGE (*b*), and gadolinium-enhanced T1-weighted fat-suppressed spin-echo (*c*) images. Severe dilatation of the right renal collecting system is present (*a–c*). Blood is identified as high-signal intensity substance in dilated calyces on the precontrast image (*a*), and a small low-signal intensity blood clot is also apparent (arrow, *a*). The renal pelvis is filled with a large signal-void blood clot. Diminished cortical enhancement is present on the immediate postgadolinium image (*b*). Thickening of the proximal aspect of the renal pelvis urothelium is noted with invasion of the renal cortex (arrow, *c*), which is best appreciated on the gadolinium-enhanced T1-weighted fat-suppressed spin-echo images (*c*).

Gadolinium-enhanced T1-weighted fat-suppressed spin-echo image (*d*) in a second patient shows increased thickness and intense enhancement of the proximal ureter. Ill-defined external margin of the tumor (arrow, *d*) on the lateral aspect of the ureter wall is consistent with tumor extension into the periureteral fat.

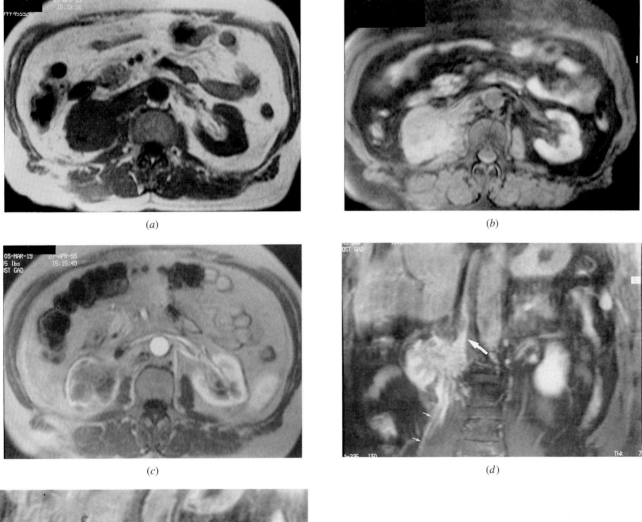

(a)

(b)

(c)

(d)

(e)

F IG . 9.114 Transitional—cell carcinoma—Stage 4. SGE (*a*), T1-weighted fat-suppressed spin-echo (*b*), immediate post-gadolinium SGE (*c*), and coronal gadolinium-enhanced images. T1-weighted fat-suppressed spin-echo images from posterior (*d*) and anterior (*e*) locations. Low-signal intensity tumor is seen involving kidney and extending posterior to the IVC on the precontrast images (*a*, *b*). On the immediate postgadolinium image (*c*), the tumor is noted to involve predominantly the medulla with relative sparing of the renal cortex. The extent of tumor is best displayed on the coronal images, in which tumor is shown to extend along the psoas muscle and ureter inferiorly (small arrows, *d*, *e*) and along the vertebral bodies and IVC superiorly (arrows, *d*, *e*).

multifocal; 30–50% of cases are multifocal, and 15–25% are bilateral. Evaluation of the entire urothelium with retrograde pyelography is essential to establish the full extent of disease. The role of MR urography is not established at present. Liver metastases from TCC tend to be hypovascular (fig. 9.115). In rare instances, TCC may have poorly differentiated histology and act as a locally aggressive malignancy (fig. 9.116).

Squamous Cell Carcinoma. A predisposing cause for squamous cell malignancy is usually present. Calculi are present in 50–60% of cases, and chronic infection, leukoplakia, and chronic drug overuse (e.g., phenacetin) are also associated with this malignancy [113]. Squamous cell carcinoma cannot be distinguished from transitional cell cancer on the basis of imaging findings. Early tumors tend to spread superficially [113]. As tumors enlarge

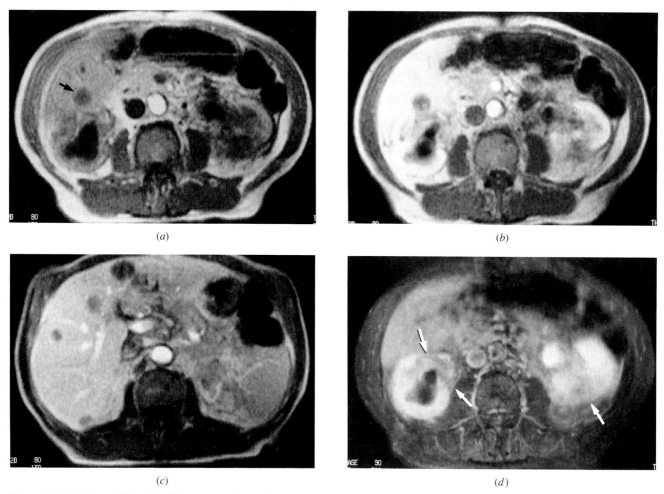

(a)

(b)

(c)

(d)

F I G . 9.115 Transitional cell cancer—Stage 4. SGE (*a*), immediate (*b*) and 90-s (*c*) postgadolinium SGE, and gadolinium-enhanced T1-weighted fat-suppressed spin-echo (*d*) images. Bilateral infiltrative tumors are present arising from the collection system of both kidneys (*a, b, d*). The transitional cell tumors are low in signal intensity on precontrast T1-weighted images (*a*), enhance minimally on immediate postgadolinium images (*b*), and show heterogeneous enhancement less than renal parenchyma on later images (arrow, *d*). Liver metastases are also present (*c*). Liver metastases from transitional cell cancer are generally hypovascular and are low in signal intensity on precontrast T1-weighted images (arrow, *a*), show faint rim enhancement on immediate postgadolinium images (*b*), and often remain well defined and hypointense on later postcontrast images (*c*). Liver metastases frequently are poorly seen on T2-weighted images (not shown) because of their hypovascularity.

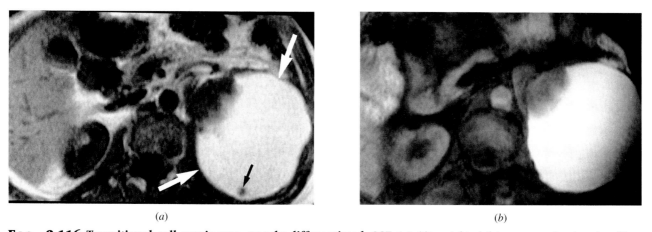

(a)

(b)

F I G . 9.116 Transitional cell carcinoma, poorly differentiated. SGE (*a*), T1-weighted fat-suppressed spin-echo (*b*), and gadolinium-enhanced T1-weighted fat-suppressed spin-echo (*c, d*) images. An irregular tumor arises from the midportion of the kidney and is associated with a large hemorrhagic fluid collection (large arrows, *a*).

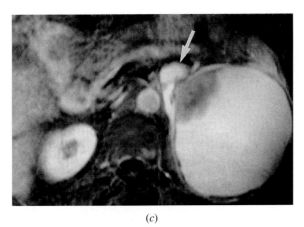
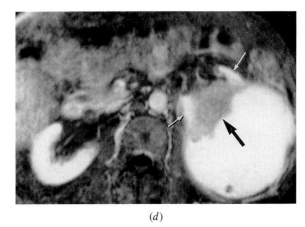

(c) *(d)*

F I G . 9.116 (*Continued*) A small tumor nodule is present in the cystic hemorrhagic component (small arrow, *a*). On the gadolinium-enhanced image, renal parenchyma is well defined as uniformly enhancing tissue (arrow, *c*). The tumor mass extends from the renal pelvis through the renal parenchyma into the cystic space. Anterior and posterior cortices (arrows, *d*) are splayed by the irregular tumor mass (black arrow, *d*).

they may develop irregular margins (fig. 9.117), which is somewhat uncommon for transitional cell carcinoma.

Secondary Tumors

Lymphoma. Lymphoma is the most common secondary tumor to invade the urothelium. Direct coronal imaging with MRI allows visualization of the extent of disease [90].

Metastases from Other Primary Tumors.

Metastases to the ureter are rare. Breast, gastrointestinal tract, prostate, cervix, and kidney are the malignancies that most frequently metastasize to the ureters [113]. Small enhancing nodules of tumor may be appreciated on gadolinium-enhanced fat-suppressed images.

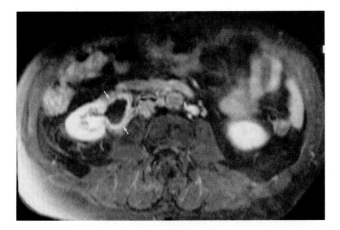

F I G . 9.117 Squamous cell cancer. Gadolinium-enhanced T1-weighted fat-suppressed spin-echo image demonstrates dilatation of the right renal pelvis with irregularly thickened and intensely enhancing urothelium, which represents squamous cell cancer (arrows). Surrounding peripelvic fat contains ill-defined enhancing tissue consistent with tumor extension.

Filling Defects in the Collecting System

Calculi are the most common filling defects in the renal collecting system. Calcium oxalate stones are the most common form of renal calculi in North America, accounting for approximately 65% of cases (fig. 9.118) [116]. Regardless of calcium composition, renal calculi are signal void on MR images (fig. 9.119). To maximize conspicuity of signal-void calculi, they are best displayed on sequences in which urine is high in signal intensity. T2-weighted single-shot echo-train spin-echo sequences generate MR urographic images that can be reconstructed to resemble conventional intravenous urography [4, 118]. MR urography may be effective at demonstrating ureteric calculi because of the high contrast between high-signal intensity urine in dilated ureter and obstructing low-signal intensity calculus (fig. 9.120). Because T2-weighted single-shot echo-train spin-echo images have <1-s temporal resolution, MRI may be a very time-efficient and cost-effective method of evaluating obstructing calculi. After gadolinium administration, detection of calculi is feasible when gadolinium is sufficiently dilute to render urine high in signal intensity. This is best accomplished by ensuring that the patient is well hydrated and by delay of image acquisition 10–30 min after injection [5]. Signal-void calculi may be detected as small as 1–2 mm in diameter in a background of high-signal intensity urine. Obstruction by calculi causes alteration in renal parenchymal enhancement and in the transit of contrast material within the kidney, which is well shown on MR images (see section on Renal Function). Because renal calculi are radiopaque in the great majority of cases on noncontrast spiral CT, and are therefore well shown even when minute and nonobstructing, CT is the procedure of choice for evaluating renal calculi.

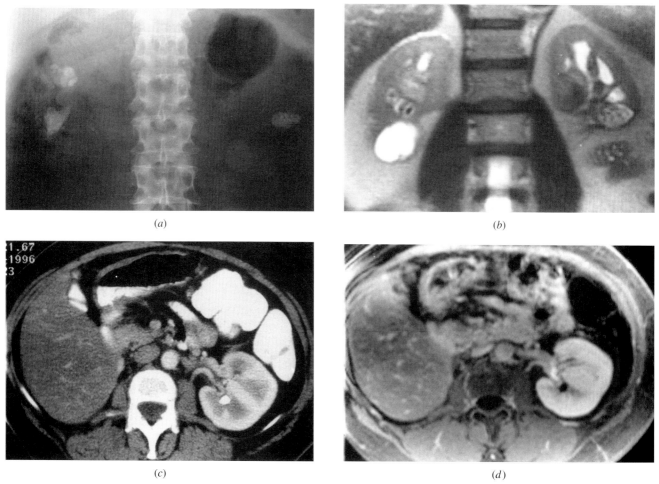

(a)

(b)

(c)

(d)

FIG. 9.118 Renal calculi. Abdominal radiographic (*a*) and coronal SS-ETSE (*b*) images. Radiopaque renal calculi seen on the abdominal radiograph appear as signal-void defects in high-signal fluid-filled renal collecting systems on the single-shot T2-weighted sequence.

Contrast-enhanced CT (*c*) and 90-s postgadolinium T1-weighted fat-suppressed (*d*) images in a second patient. The radiopaque calculus is clearly shown on CT (*c*), and is apparent as a signal-void focus on the MR image (*d*). The calculus is difficult to appreciate on the MR image.

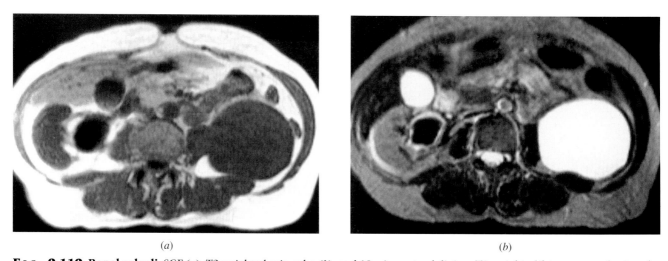

(a)

(b)

FIG. 9.119 Renal calculi. SGE (*a*), T2-weighted spin-echo (*b*), and 10-min postgadolinium T1-weighted fat-suppressed spin-echo (*c*) images. The renal calculus in the right renal pelvis is signal void on all sequences (*a*–*c*). Conspicuity of the calculus is greatest on the T2-weighted image and the dilute gadolinium (high signal intensity)-enhanced image. Urine is high in signal intensity on these sequences and contrasts well with the signal-void calculus.

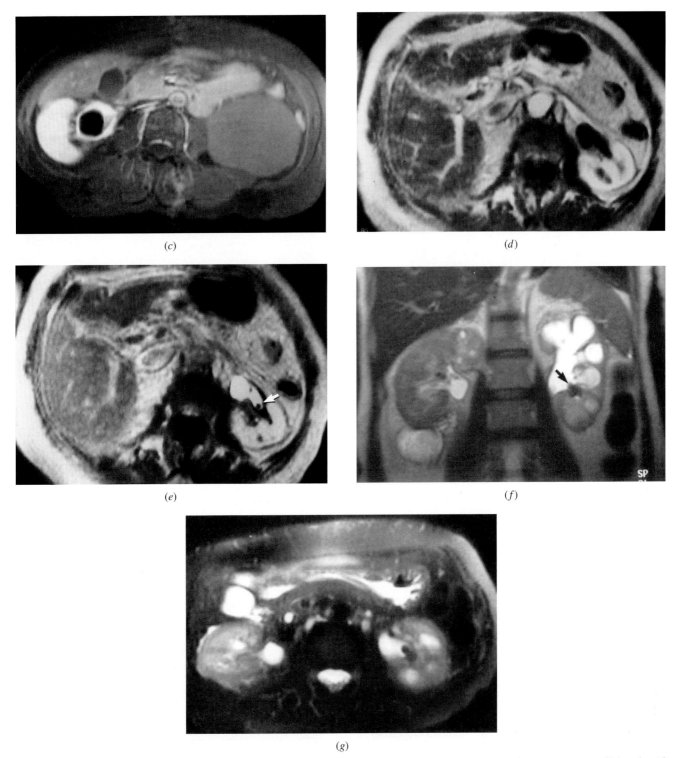

(c)

(d)

(e)

(f)

(g)

F I G . 9.119 (*Continued*) Immediate (*d*) and 10-min (*e*) postgadolinium images in a second patient demonstrate a small signal-void calculus, which is not apparent in gadolinium-free signal-void urine (*d*) but is well shown on late postgadolinium image (arrow, *e*) because of the high signal intensity of dilute gadolinium-containing urine.

Coronal (*f*) and transverse fat-suppressed (*g*) SS-ETSE in a third patient. A signal-void calculus (arrow, *f*) is present in the lower pole infundibulum of the left kidney. Hydronephrosis is also present.

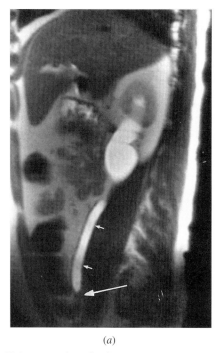

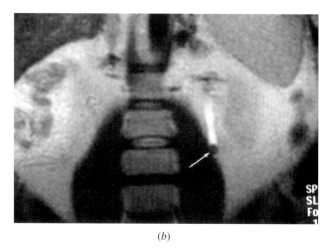

(a)   (b)

F I G . 9.120 Ureteric calculi. Sagittal (*a*) SS-ETSE image. The proximal two-thirds of the ureter are dilated and urine filled, resulting in high signal intensity on the SS-ETSE image (small arrows, *a*). A low-signal intensity calculus is demonstrated obstructing the ureter (long arrow, *a*), which forms a convex meniscus sign within the urine-filled ureter.

Coronal SS-ETSE (*b*) image in a second patient demonstrates mild to moderate left-sided hydronephrosis with an obstructing stone in the proximal left ureter.

Other filling defects such as blood clots or fungus balls are also demonstrable as low-signal intensity mass lesions in high-signal intensity urine on T2-weighted sequences and as nonenhancing mass lesions situated in the high-signal intensity contrast-filled collecting system on delayed postgadolinium SGE images. Foci of air in the collecting system may be distinguished from solid lesions by the presence of susceptibility artifact surrounding the defect and by the observation that air foci locate

in nondependent positions and solid lesions tend to layer in dependent positions (fig. 9.121).

Dilation of the Collecting System

Dilation of the renal collecting system may arise as a normal variant (fig. 9.122), congenital anomaly, obstruction, reflux related or after obstruction. MR urography adequately reveals the severity and the level of obstruction

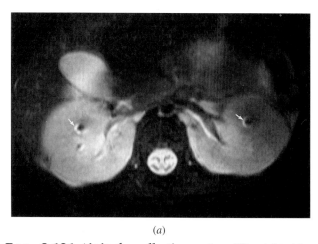

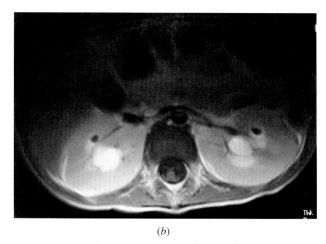

(a)   (b)

F I G . 9.121 Air in the collecting system. T2-weighted fat-suppressed spin-echo (*a*) and gadolinium-enhanced T1-SE (*b*) images. Multiple foci are present in the nondependent portions of the renal collecting system, demonstrating signal void on both T2-weighted (*a*) and gadolinium-enhanced T1-weighted (*b*) images. These foci possess bright external rings on the T2-weighted images from air-fluid magnetic susceptibility artifact (arrows, *a*).

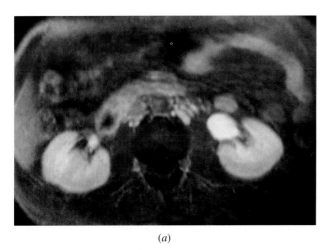

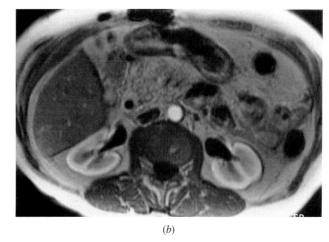

(a)   (b)

F I G . 9.122 Extrarenal pelvis. Gadolinium-enhanced T1-weighted fat-suppressed spin-echo image (*a*). Dilute, high signal intensity gadolinium is present in a prominent extrarenal pelvis of the left kidney. The calyces are normal and small in size, reflecting the absence of obstruction. This establishes the diagnosis of extrarenal pelvis.

Immediate postgadolinium SGE image (*b*) in a second patient demonstrates bilateral extrarenal pelves. Calyces are normal in size, and cortical enhancement is symmetric and normal.

of the collecting system (fig. 9.123). The combination of MR urography, tissue imaging sequences to evaluate renal cortex, and dynamic serial postcontrast imaging to assess renal function provides comprehensive information on the morphologic and functional status of kidneys with dilated collecting systems (fig. 9.124). As with intravenous urography and CT imaging, gadolinium-enhanced SGE images can demonstrate delayed excretion of contrast (fig. 9.125).

Calyceal Diverticulum

Calyceal diverticula may be shown on MR images with a combination of MR urography and delayed gadolinium-

enhanced images. The MR urogram demonstrates the fluid-filled structure (fig. 9.126), but the communication with the collecting system is confirmed by demonstration of high-signal intensity fluid in the diverticulum on delayed postgadolinium images due to the presence of dilute gadolinium. Calyceal diverticula frequently contain calculi, which may be well shown using sequences that result in high-signal intensity urine. Diverticula may uncommonly extend to the cortical surface.

JUXTARENAL PROCESSES

Tumor, hemorrhage, abscesses, and urine leaks all may occur in a juxtarenal location. Urine extravasation most

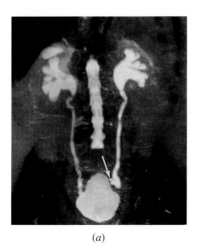

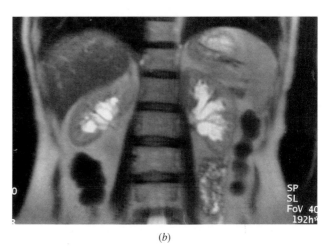

(a)   (b)

F I G . 9.123 MR urogram. Coronal MIP reconstructed MR urogram from 20 multisection coronal echo-train spin-echo sections (*a*) demonstrates bilateral severe dilatation of the renal collecting systems secondary to bladder outlet obstruction from prostate cancer. Superior deviation of the left ureter (arrow) results from superior extension of cancer.

Coronal SS-ETSE image (*b*) in a second patient demonstrates moderate calicectasis bilaterally from chronic ureteropelvic junction obstruction.

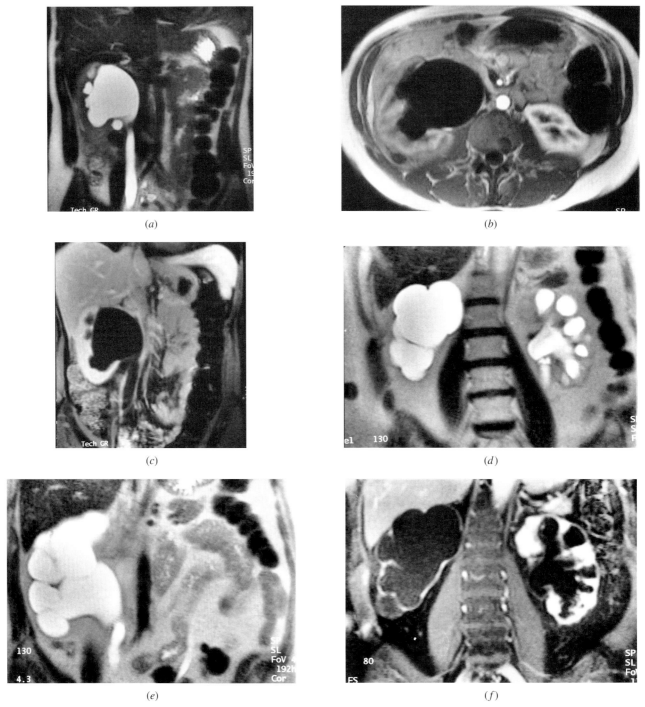

(a)

(b)

(c)

(d)

(e)

(f)

F I G . 9.124 Comprehensive evaluation of renal obstruction. Coronal SS-ETSE (*a*), immediate postgadolinium SGE (*b*), and coronal 3-min postgadolinium fat-suppressed SGE (*c*) images in a patient with distal ureteral obstruction secondary to gynecological malignancy. The coronal SS-ETSE image (*a*) demonstrates the severe dilatation of the renal collecting system and ureter. The immediate postgadolinium SGE image (*b*) demonstrates diminished cortical enhancement of the obstructed right kidney compared to the left. The thickness of the renal cortex is well preserved. The coronal gadolinium-enhanced SGE image (*c*) demonstrates signal-void urine in the ureter and renal pelvis and enhanced renal cortex.

Coronal SS-ETSE (*d, e*) and coronal 2-min postgadolinium fat-suppressed SGE image (*f*) in a second patient with bilateral distal ureteral obstruction. Massive hydronephrosis is present in the right renal collecting system, and severe dilatation is present in left (*d, e*). After gadolinium administration (*f*), essentially no renal parenchyma is identified in the right kidney, whereas moderately severe thinning is present in the left kidney.

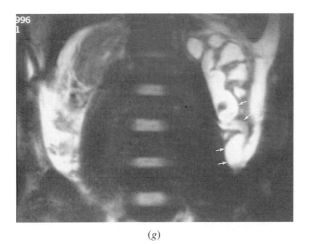

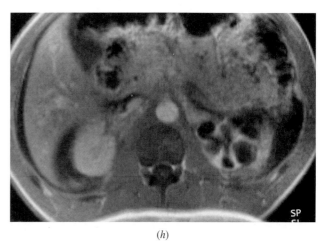

(g)   (h)

F I G . 9.124 (*Continued*) Coronal SS-ETSE (*g*) and 90-s postgadolinium SGE (*h*) images in a third patient with longstanding ureterovesical obstruction secondary to childhood ureteric reimplantation. Coronal SS-ETSE (*g*) shows severe hydronephrosis and tortuosity of the ureter (small arrows, *g*) of the left kidney. The transverse gadolinium-enhanced image demonstrates extreme thinning of the renal parenchyma in the left kidney, which is effectively nonfunctioning. A normal-appearing right kidney is seen. Intraperitoneal high signal intensity on the T2-weighted image (*g*) and low signal intensity on the postgadolinium T1-weighted image (*h*) represent ascites.

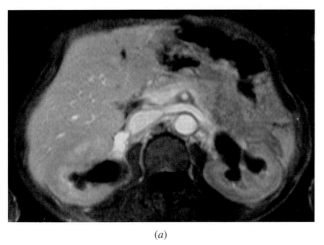

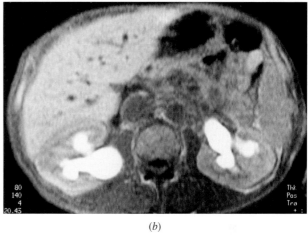

(a)   (b)

F I G . 9.125 Delayed excretion in high-grade obstruction. Transverse 2-min postgadolinium fat-suppressed SGE image (*a*) demonstrates severe dilatation of the renal collecting system secondary to bladder cancer. SGE image (*b*) obtained 24 h later demonstrates delayed excretion of gadolinium.

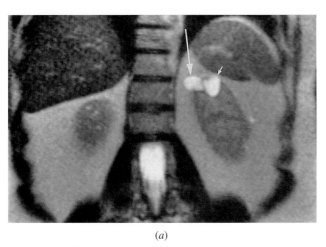

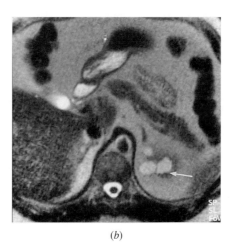

(a)   (b)

F I G . 9.126 Calyceal diverticulum. Coronal (*a*) and transverse (*b*) SS-ETSE images. The coronal image demonstrates a calyceal diverticulum (small arrow, *a*) adjacent to a renal cyst (long arrow, *a*). The calyceal diverticulum extends to the surface of the kidney and contains low-signal intensity milk of calcium, which is commonly observed in these lesions. Minute low-signal intensity calculi are apparent in the dependent portion of the diverticulum (arrow, *b*) on the transverse image (*b*). Atrophy of the overlying renal cortex is apparent.

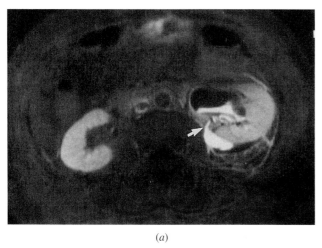

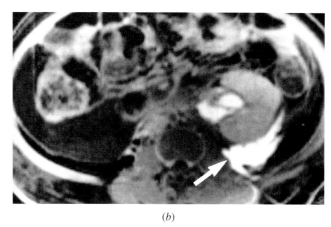

(a)   (b)

FIG. 9.127 Pyelosinus rupture. Gadolinium-enhanced T1-weighted fat-suppressed spin-echo image demonstrates leakage of dilute high-signal intensity gadolinium (arrow) from a dilated, obstructed left renal collecting system.

Transverse 3-min postgadolinium T1-weighted fat-suppressed SGE image (b) in a second patient with a history of trauma. High-signal fluid extravasates into the perinephric space (arrow, b) at the same time as high-signal fluid appears in the collecting system.

commonly occurs either as a result of trauma or secondary to calyceal rupture due to elevated intracollecting system pressure. Although acute obstruction on the basis of renal calculi is the most common cause of calyceal rupture, this also may be seen in other causes of obstruction (fig. 9.127).

TRAUMA

Renal trauma is a common occurrence in abdominal injury. Tomographic imaging is the most accurate method for assessing the severity of injury, which is generally classified as mild (contusion), moderate (laceration into the collection system), or severe (disruption of renal pedicle or complete crush). Precontrast T1-weighted images, especially fat suppressed, are sensitive to the presence of blood. Dynamic gadolinium-enhanced images demonstrate patent renal vessels as high in signal intensity and are useful for assessing their integrity. Degree of renal injury is well shown on postgadolinium images by the demonstration of lacerations, hemorrhage, or areas of diminished enhancement (fig. 9.128).

Early perinephric leak of contrast material is consistent with vascular injury, whereas >2-min postcontrast leak is indicative of collecting system injury [118].

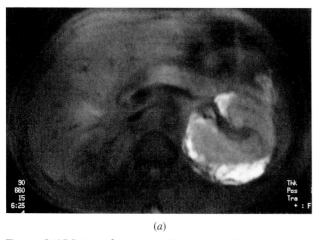

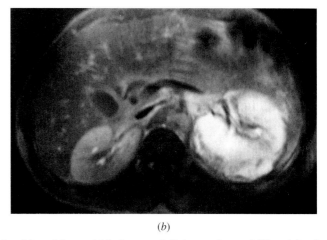

(a)   (b)

FIG. 9.128 Renal trauma. T1-weighted fat-suppressed spin-echo (a) and interstitial-phase gadolinium-enhanced T1-weighted fat-suppressed spin-echo (b) images. High-signal intensity perirenal hematoma is present surrounding an enlarged left kidney on the precontrast image. The interstitial-phase gadolinium-enhanced image demonstrates greater enhancement of the left kidney compared with the normal right kidney. This excludes renal artery compromise but implies increased intrarenal tissue pressure, capillary leakage, and/or renal vein compromise.

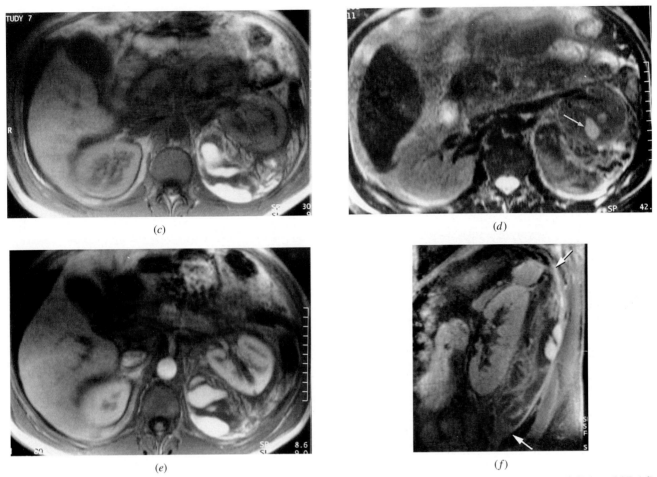

(c)   *(d)*

(e)   *(f)*

F i g . 9.128 (*Continued*) SGE (*c*), SS-ETSE (*d*), immediate postgadolinium SGE (*e*), and sagittal 90-s postgadolinium SGE (*f*) images in a second patient who sustained abdominal trauma. High-signal intensity hemorrhage is noted in the perirenal and posterior pararenal space in the left kidney with a multilayered appearance (*c*). Mixed high signal intensity is apparent on the T2-weighted image (*d*), which is consistent with blood products of varying age. In addition a tubule-shaped focus of high signal intensity is present in the renal parenchyma, a finding consistent with an intraparenchymal laceration (arrow, *d*). The kidney enhances normally immediately after contrast administration, excluding a major renal arterial injury. The sagittal image (*f*) demonstrates the full renal length and the volume of posterior pararenal blood (arrows, *f*).

RENAL FUNCTION

Gadolinium-enhanced dynamic serial imaging of the kidneys demonstrates distinct phases of contrast enhancement based on the location of the bulk of the contrast agent. The phases of enhancement can be separated into 1) capillary, 2) early tubular, 3) ductal, and 4) excretory [5]. Evaluation of the concentrating ability of the kidneys may be made by the observation of signal intensity changes in renal tissue based on the presence of gadolinium of varying concentrations (fig. 9.129). When dilute, gadolinium renders tissues high in signal intensity, and when concentrated, gadolinium renders tissues signal void. The assessment of these phases of enhancement has been shown to distinguish normal kidneys and those with dilated nonobstructed collecting

systems from acute and chronic obstruction. Patients must be mildly dehydrated to provide the physiologic condition for renal concentration. This can be achieved by a 5-h fast. Dilated, nonobstructed kidneys have a temporal pattern of signal intensity changes similar to that of normal kidneys because renal transit is not abnormal (fig. 9.130). Acutely obstructed kidneys are enlarged and have increased renal transit time. This corresponds to an appearance of a prolonged increasing-signal intensity nephrogram and delayed appearance of contrast in the renal ducts and collecting system (fig. 9.131). Chronic obstruction has diminished cortical enhancement and increased transit time (fig. 9.132).

Functional changes of cortical and medullary enhancement also may be observed in the context of renal ischemia [119].

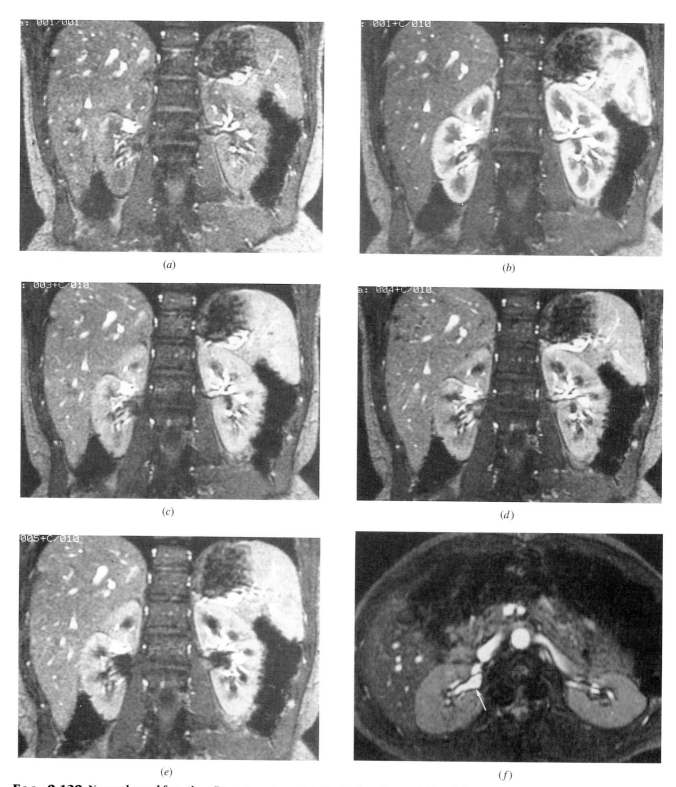

(a)

(b)

(c)

(d)

(e)

(f)

F I G . 9.129 Normal renal function. Precontrast image (*a*). Minimal corticomedullary differentiation is present. Cortical enhance-ment (capillary)-phase image (*b*). Cortex signal intensity is increased by 17%. Corticomedullary differentiation is distinct because of differential blood flow and increased delivery of gadolinium to the renal cortex. Early tubular-phase (*c*) image. Signal intensity of medulla is transiently increased, whereas there is little change in cortical signal intensity. Ductal-phase image (*d*). Signal intensity of medulla is decreased (6% from vascular phase) because of the concentration of gadolinium in distal convoluted tubules and collecting ducts. There is minimal decrease in cortical signal intensity (2%). Decreased signal intensity is apparent in the inner medulla and therefore mainly represents concentrated gadolinium in collecting ducts. Excretory-phase image (*e*). Urine containing concentrated gadolinium appears in renal collecting systems as signal-void fluid. Excretory-phase image (*f*) obtained 15 min after injection. No corticomedullary differentiation is present. Urine contains dilute (high signal intensity) gadolinium (arrows, *f*) because of rapid clear-ance of gadolinium from the body. (Reprinted with permission from Semelka RC, Hricak H, Tomei E, Floth A, Stoller M: Obstructive nephropathy: Evaluation with dynamic Gd-DTPA enhanced MR imaging. *Radiology* 175: 797–803, 1990.)

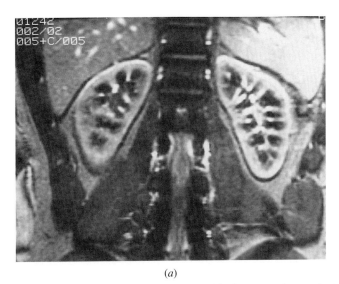 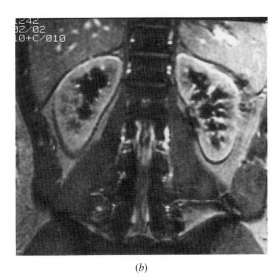

(a)   (b)

FIG. 9.130 Dilated nonobstructed kidney. Gradient-echo images of subject with a dilated nonobstructed right kidney. Ductal-phase image (a). Low signal intensity of the medulla appears simultaneously in the dilated nonobstructed right kidney and in the normal left kidney. In the excretory-phase image (b), excretion of concentrated urine is bilaterally symmetric. Susceptibility-induced image distortion of the renal collecting systems is caused by the high concentration of gadolinium. (Reprinted with permission from Semelka RC, Hricak H, Tomei E, Floth A, Stoller M: Obstructive nephropathy: Evaluation with dynamic Gd-DTPA enhanced MR imaging. *Radiology* 175: 797–803, 1990.)

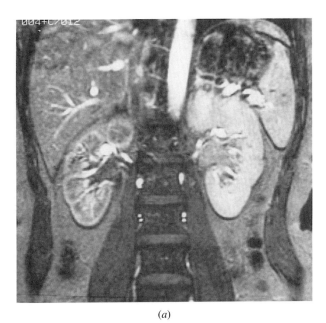 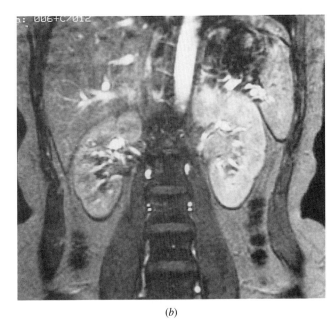

(a)   (b)

FIG. 9.131 Acute obstruction. Gradient-echo images of subject with an acutely obstructed left kidney and normal right kidney. Cortical enhancement (capillary)-phase image (a). The acutely obstructed left kidney is larger and swollen compared with the right kidney. Obstruction to venous drainage results in an abnormal pattern of contrast enhancement of the obstructed kidney. The parenchymal signal intensity is greater, and corticomedullary differentiation is diminished. Ductal-phase image (b). Tubular concentration is apparent in the normal right kidney but not in the obstructed left kidney. Cortical enhancement is persistent on the obstructed side, analogous to the persistent nephrogram on intravenous urogram (IVU) examination. Excretory-phase image (c). The delayed image obtained at 3.5 min shows dilute (high signal intensity) urine in dilated calyces (arrows, c) of the left kidney. Concentrated (low signal intensity) urine is excreted from the right kidney. Excretory-phase image (d) obtained 15 min after injection. Dilute urine is excreted by the normal right kidney.

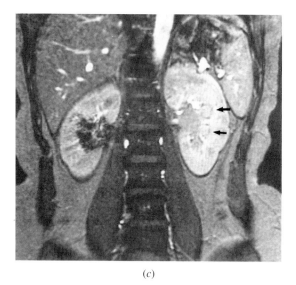

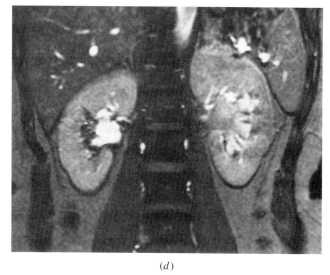

(c)   (d)

FIG. 9.131 (*Continued*) Further excretion into the dilated left renal collecting system can be appreciated. (Reprinted with permission from Semelka RC, Hricak H, Tomei E, Floth A, Stoller M: Obstructive nephropathy: Evaluation with dynamic Gd-DTPA enhanced MR imaging. *Radiology* 175: 797–803, 1990.)

RENAL TRANSPLANTS

In the United States, 11,000 renal transplants are performed annually [120]. MRI has been used to evaluate potential donors, potential recipients, and recipients after transplantation.

In the evaluation of donors, pretransplantation assessment of the renal vascular anatomy of the potential renal donor is important. The incidence of variant arterial anatomy of the kidney is 40%, including early renal artery division or branches, multiple renal arteries (aberrant and accessory renal arteries), and multiple renal veins [120]. Angiography has been the primary modality for the evaluation of renal vascular anatomy. However, in recent studies, excellent sensitivity and accuracy in the depiction of accessory renal arteries has been demonstrated by gadolinium-enhanced 3D MRA. In these studies, conventional angiography was used as

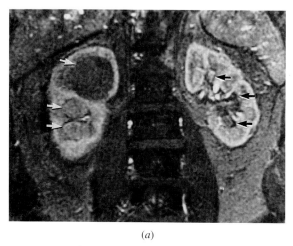

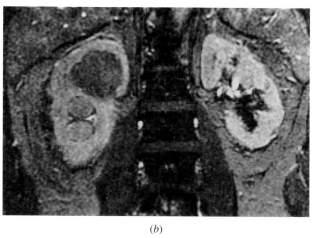

(a)   (b)

FIG. 9.132 Chronic obstruction. Gradient-echo images of a subject with a chronically obstructed right kidney and a dilated nonobstructed left kidney. Cortical enhancement (capillary)-phase image (*a*). Normal cortical enhancement is appreciated in the left kidney, which demonstrates corticomedullary distinction. Cortical enhancement is lower in the chronically obstructed right kidney with no definition of CMD. Low-signal intensity gadolinium-free urine is present in both collecting systems (arrows, *a*). On the excretory-phase image (*b*), concentrated urine is excreted by the dilated nonobstructed left kidney. There is no apparent excretion by the chronically obstructed right kidney, no development of corticomedullary differentiation, and no significant changes in parenchymal signal intensity from the cortical enhancement phase. (Reprinted with permission from Semelka RC, Hricak H, Tomei E, Floth A, Stoller M: Obstructive nephropathy: Evaluation with dynamic Gd-DTPA enhanced MR imaging, *Radiology* 175: 797–803, 1990.)

the standard of reference [120, 121]. A current article shows that combined gadolinium-enhanced 3D MRA, MR urography, and MR nephrography can accurately depict the arterial supply, collecting system, and renal parenchyma of the donor kidney [121]. In our experience however, depiction of small anomalous renal arteries, particularly when they arise in unusual locations (e.g., distal abdominal aorta, common iliac artery) may elude detection with current MRA technique and yet be clearly defined on angiography.

In the evaluation of potential recipients, MRI may be used to evaluate the native kidneys for disease processes (e.g., development of renal cancer) and the appearance of the common iliac arteries, which are used as the site for anastomosis of the renal transplant artery, for mural disease or luminal narrowing, particularly if there is a history of prior transplants that have failed.

In the evaluation of recipients after transplantation, normal-functioning transplants have good CMD on pre-contrast T1-weighted fat-suppressed images and immediate postgadolinium images (figs. 9.133 and 9.134).

Some immediate complications may be associated with surgical difficulties; these include renal artery thro-mbosis or stenosis, renal vein thrombosis, urinary leak, or lymphocele. Others complications include rejection, cyclosporine toxicity, acute tubular necrosis, infection (figs. 9.135 and 9.136), and transplantation-related malignancies such as post-transplantation lymphoproliferative disorder and lymphoma [120].

Regarding immediate complications, allograft renal artery stenosis occurs in 2–10% of cases and may occur as early as 2 days or as late as several years [120]. Gadolinium-enhanced 3D MRA technique is an accurate reproducible technique for evaluating renal artery complications [2, 3, 120]. Normal transplant arteries and veins are clearly identified (fig. 9.137). Stenosis or thrombosis of artery or vein is similarly demonstrated in a reproducible fashion with this technique (fig. 9.138).

In renal transplant patients, lymphoceles are defined histopathologically as collections of lymphatic fluid (i.e., nonsanguinous and not purulent) in the perinephric space (fig. 9.139) [120]. The fluid is derived from the renal lymph vessels that are not reanastomosed with recipient lymphatics. Clinical differential diagnosis includes urine leak, hematoma and, rarely, posttransplant lymphoproliferative disorder [122]. The incidence of

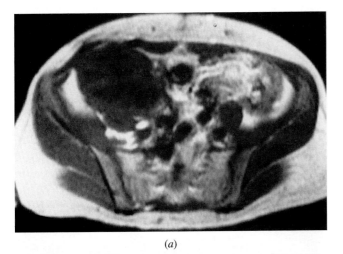

(a)

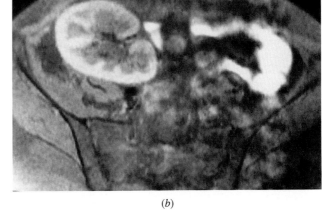

(b)

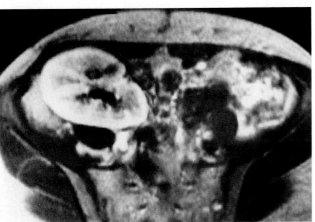

(c)

F I G . 9.133 Normal transplant kidney. SGE (a), T1-weighted fat-suppressed spin-echo (b), and immediate postgadolinium SGE (c) images of a functioning renal transplant. Normal corticomedullary differentiation is apparent on the SGE image (a), which is clearly defined on the T1-weighted fat-suppressed image (b). Corticomedullary differentiation on the immediate postgadolinium image (c) is consistent with a normal pattern of renal blood flow. (Reprinted with permission from Semelka RC, Shoenut JP, Greenberg HM. The Kidney. In: Semelka RC, Shoenut JP, (eds.), *MRI of the Abdomen with CT Correlation.* New York: Raven Press, 1993, p. 91–118.)

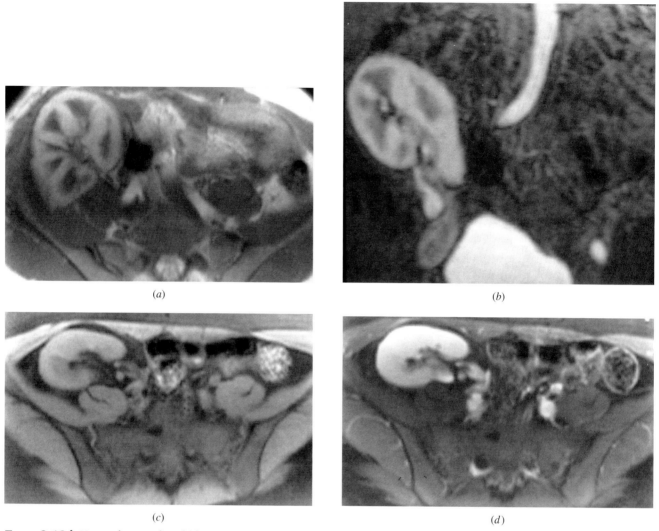

(a)   *(b)*

(c)   *(d)*

FIG. 9.134 Normal transplant kidney. Transverse immediate postgadolinium SGE (*a*) and coronal 3D MRA source (*b*) image. The kidney transplant in the right lower quadrant demonstrates normal capillary phase enhancement. No complications were identified.

Precontrast (*c*) and postgadolinium (*d*) T1-weighted fat-suppressed SGE images in a second patient. CMD is present on the noncontrast image. No complications are evident.

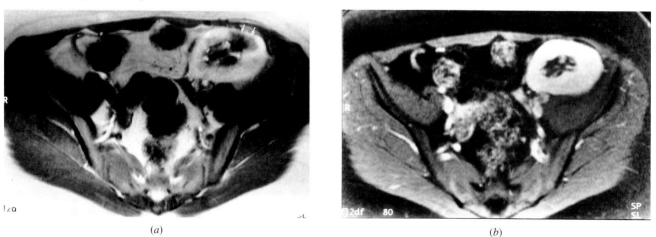

(a)   *(b)*

FIG. 9.135 Acute focal pyelonephritis in a renal transplant. Immediate postgadolinium SGE (*a*) and 90-s postgadolinium T1-weighted fat-suppressed SGE (*b*) images demonstrate a focal region anteriorly in the transplant kidney that shows a striated nephrogram appearance on the capillary-phase image (arrows, *a*), which resolves on the interstitial-phase image (*b*). This appearance is consistent with acute focal pyelonephritis without abscess formation.

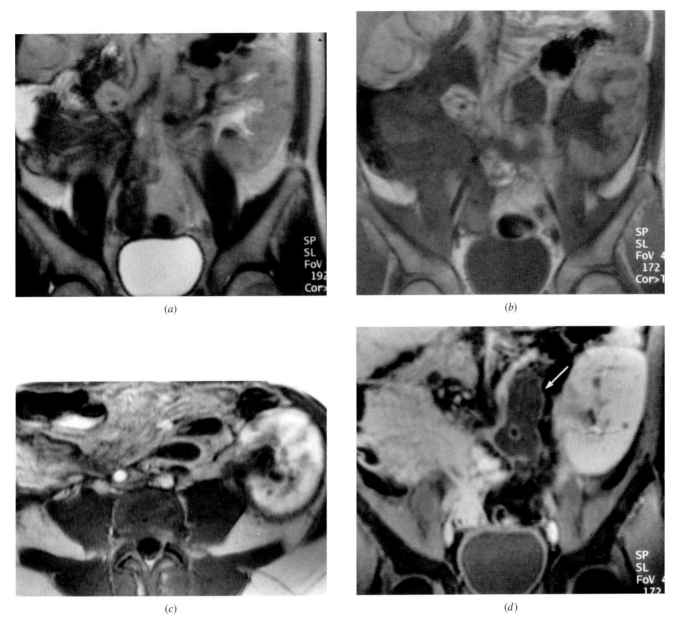

FIG. 9.136 **Renal transplant with abscesses.** Coronal SS-ETSE (*a*), immediate postgadolinium SGE (*b*), and transverse (*c*) and coronal (*d*) 90-s postgadolinium T1-weighted fat-suppressed SGE images. There are multiple low-signal intensity lesions present in the renal transplant. These demonstrate decreased T2 signal and no definite enhancement. These represent small abscesses based on their appearance combined with clinical history. There is also a well-circumscribed 3-cm fluid collection present in the central midabdomen, which represents a loculated fluid collection or seroma (arrow, *d*).

lymphoceles after renal transplantation is between 1–18% of cases. This is considered the most common cause of peritransplant fluid collection. Lymphoceles that occur in the first month are often related to surgery. Late occurrence is often related to rejection. Lymphoceles are low signal on T1 and high signal on T2. Urinoma is a complication occurring early, in the first 5 weeks, after transplantation, and is caused by the leakage of urine from the pyeloureteral anastomotic site, which creates a cystlike fluid-filled structure. There are in general two surgical techniques used for ureter anastomosis in renal

transplantation, implantation of the donor ureter into the recipient bladder and anastomosis of the donor pelvis to the recipient ureter (pyeloureteral anastomosis). Urine leaks are more common in the latter procedure [123]. The incidence of this varies between 3 and 10%. The signal characteristic of the urinoma is nonspecific and is low on T1- and high on T2-weighted images. Lymphocele and seroma have similar signal intensities.

Regarding rejection, loss of renal CMD on T1-weighted images is an observation found in renal allografts undergoing rejection (fig. 9.140) [124–126]. In

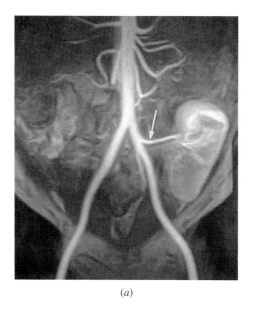

(a)

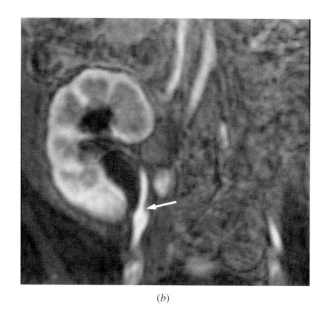

(b)

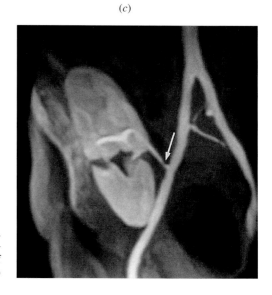

(c)

F I G . 9.137 Normal renal artery of a renal transplant. Coronal 3D source image (*a*). The artery is patent, and its anastomosis with the left common iliac artery is well visualized on the source image (arrow, *a*).

Coronal 3D source image (*b*) and MIP reconstruction (*c*) image in a second patient demonstrate a normal-caliber renal artery (arrow, *b*). It is important to examine source images in addition to the reconstructed images.

F I G . 9.138 Renal artery stenosis in a transplant kidney. Coronal MRA MIP reconstruction demonstrates stenosis of the renal artery (arrow) approximately 2 cm distal to the anastomosis with the internal iliac artery. (Courtesy of Susan M. Ascher MD, Dept of Radiology, Georgetown University Medical Center)

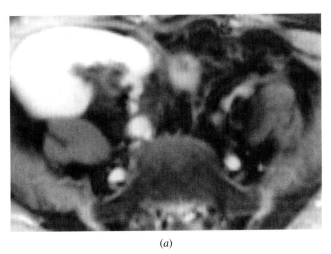 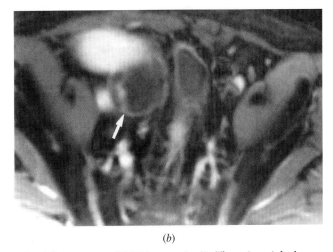

(a)   (b)

F I G . 9.139 Lymphocele. Transverse 90-s postgadolinium T1-weighted fat-suppressed SGE images (*a, b*). There is a right lower quadrant kidney transplant, and projecting inferiorly from the renal hilum there is a well-delineated collection with a thin enhancing capsule (arrow, *b*) that represents a lymphocele.

a study comparing the accuracy of MRI, quantitative scintigraphy, and sonography for the detection of renal transplant rejection, the sensitivities for these modalities were 97%, 80%, and 70%, respectively [125]. Loss of CMD, however, is nonspecific and observed also in cyclosporine toxicity and other infiltrative or diffuse renal parenchymal diseases [90, 127]. Chronic rejection results in loss of CMD on T1-weighted fat-suppressed images (fig. 9.141). The degree of loss of CMD on dynamic contrast-enhanced images may correlate with the severity of rejection. Longstanding severe rejection may result in morphologic alterations of the kidney (fig. 9.142).

MR UROGRAPHY

MR Urography (MRU) has been performed as a complementary tool to evaluate for urinary tract abnormalities. The common principle of these techniques is based on the acquisition of a heavily T2-weighted pulse sequence, which results in solid organs and moving fluids having a low signal intensity, whereas stationary fluids including bile, urine, cerebrospinal fluid, and bowel fluid have a high signal intensity. In selected cases, postprocessing is performed with a maximum-intensity projection (MIP), which permits 3D rotation, producing views of

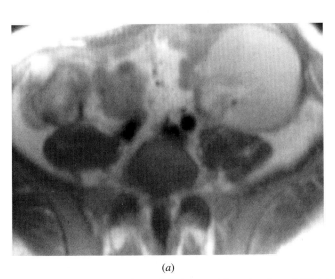 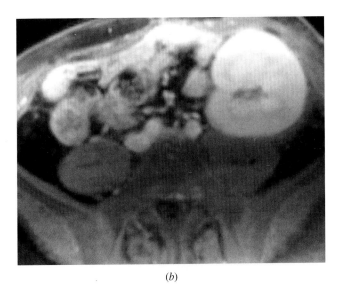

(a)   (b)

F I G . 9.140 Transplanted kidney with rejection. SGE (*a*) and 90-s gadolinium-enhanced T1-weighted fat-suppressed SGE (*b*) images. The renal transplant in the left pelvic fossa demonstrates decreased CMD on the precontrast image (*a*) and appears globular or swollen. These findings are consistent with chronic rejection.

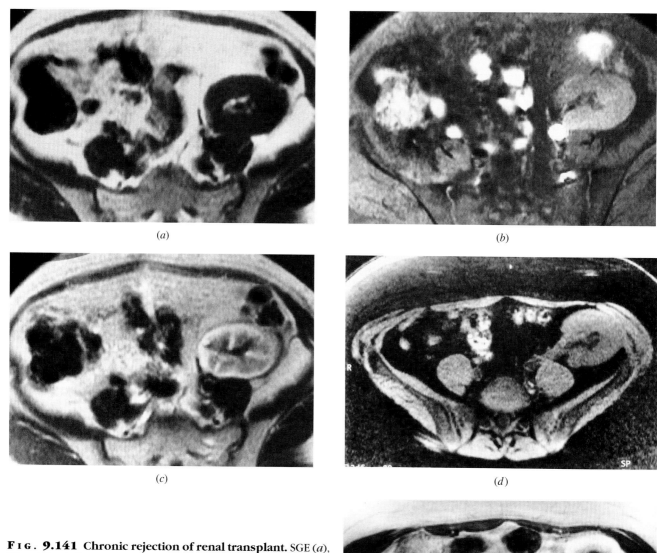

(a)

(b)

(c)

(d)

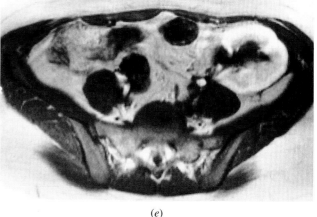

(e)

F I G . 9.141 Chronic rejection of renal transplant. SGE (*a*), T1-weighted fat-suppressed spin-echo (*b*), and immediate post-gadolinium SGE (*c*) images in a renal transplant undergoing chronic rejection. Loss of CMD is apparent on precontrast T1-weighted images (*a*, *b*). The presence of CMD on the capillary-phase image shows persistence of a normal pattern of renal blood flow, which is consistent with preservation of some renal function.

Fat-suppressed SGE (*d*) and immediate postgadolinium SGE (*e*) images in a second patient with chronic rejection. Loss of visualization of the CMD is apparent on the precontrast T1-weighted fat-suppressed image (*d*). CMD is present on the immediate postgadolinium SGE image, which is consistent with preservation of some renal function.

suspected areas of disease without superimposition of structures.

A recent article reported that the accuracy of MRU is excellent in the detection of ureterohydronephrosis and superior to conventional intravenous urography (IVU) in cases of renal failure. MRU was equivalent to IVU for the diagnosis of ureterohydronephosis in patients with normal renal function, with an accuracy of 100%. No difference was observed in the extent of dilatation between IVU and MRU [128].

MRU has proved to be efficient in detecting the level of obstruction and permitting an analysis of the type of obstruction. The main disadvantage is the inability of the technique to demonstrate small calculi in a consistent fashion, especially small, nonobstructing calculi.

MRU has also been described acquiring images late after gadolinium administration using a 3D gradient-echo technique. High-signal gadolinium is shown in the collecting system on these T1-weighted images. Advantages of this technique include lesser problems with

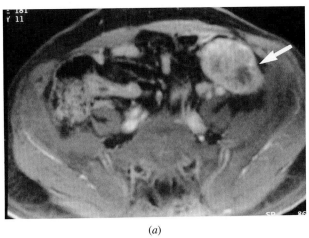

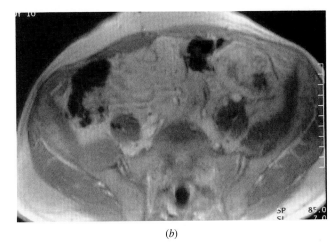

(a)   (b)

F I G . 9.142 Severe chronic rejection. Transverse 45-s postgadolinium fat-suppressed SGE (*a*) and 90-s postgadolinium SGE (*b*) images. The transplanted kidney has an irregular contour (arrow, *a*). Irregularly margined central areas of diminished enhancement are present on 45- and 90-s images. By 90 s, enhancement of renal medulla should equilibrate with the cortex, therefore this central diminished enhancement does not reflect normal medulla.

image reconstruction because adjacent competing high-signal fluid is not present, which may be observed on T2-weighted images, and it provides information on renal function.

FUTURE DIRECTIONS

Anatomic display of kidneys is accurate using current imaging techniques and phased-array multicoil imaging. Although gadolinium-enhanced 3D MRA is the most reproducible technique, advances in noncontrast MRA continue to develop [129–131]. It remains to be determined whether noncontrast MRA may be sufficiently accurate to assess renal transplant donors. Renal function and functional and morphologic disturbance caused by various renal diseases are currently under investigation [132–138]. Fast imaging techniques such as turboFLASH and echoplanar imaging [134, 135, 139], new contrast agents [133], or a combination of both [134, 35] are being employed to examine renal function. Flow quantification may provide useful information on renal perfusion [136, 137]. Pharmacological stresses also may develop into a clinical routine for evaluating renal vascular disease [138]. Futher advances in MRA is needed to improve visualization of small vessels and intrarenal vessels.

CONCLUSIONS

MRI performs well at detecting and characterizing renal masses and staging renal cancer. Because CT imaging is also an effective modality and greater clinical experience has been established with this modality, the current role

of MRI is to study patients who are not ideal candidates for CT imaging or to solve problems. Indications for MRI include 1) evaluation of tumor thrombus, 2) characterization of complicated renal lesions, particularly calcified cysts, 3) allergy to iodinated contrast, 4) elevated sCr (to avoid worsening renal failure and because of adequate contrast enhancement of diseased renal parenchyma), and 5) evaluation of chronically impaired kidneys for renal cancer. In diffuse renal parenchymal disease MRI is able to provide useful information that can help to determine underlying etiology. Current high-quality MRA using gadolinium-enhanced 3D gradient echo and 3D fat-suppressed SGE allows adequate evaluation of many patients with renal artery disease. MR urography evaluates dilatation of the renal collection system in a rapid, noninvasive fashion. The combination of tissue-imaging sequences, MRA, and MR urography, makes MRI a modality that can comprehensively evaluate the full spectrum of renal diseases.

REFERENCES

1. Semelka RC, Shoenut JP, Kroeker MA, MacMahon RG, Greenberg HM: Renal lesions: Controlled comparison between CT and 1.5 T MR imaging with nonenhanced- and gadolinium-enhanced fat-suppressed spin-echo and breath-hold FLASH techniques. *Radiology* 182: 425–430, 1992.
2. Prince MR, Narasimham DL, Stanley JC, Chenevert TL, Williams DM, Marx MV, Cho KJ: Breath-hold gadolinium-enhanced MR angiography of the abdominal aorta and its major branches. *Radiology* 197: 785–792, 1995.
3. Snidow JJ, Johnson MS, Harris VJ, Margosian PM, Aisen AM, Lalka SG, Cikrit DF, Trerotola SO: Three-dimensional gadolinium-enhanced MR angiography for aortoiliac inflow assessment plus renal artery screening in a single breath-hold. *Radiology* 198: 725–732, 1996.

4. Rothpearl A, Frager D, Subramanian A, Bashist B, Baer J, Kay C, Cooke K, Raia C: MR urography: Technique and application. *Radiology* 194: 125–130, 1995.

5. Semelka RC, Hricak H, Tomei E, Floth A, Stoller M: Obstructive nephropathy: Evaluation with dynamic Gd-DTPA-enhanced MR imaging. *Radiology* 175: 797–803, 1990.

6. Choyke PL, Frank JA, Girton ME, et al.: Dynamic Gd-DTPA-enhanced MR imaging of the kidney: Experimental results. *Radiology* 170: 713–720, 1989.

7. Kikinis R, von Schulthess GK, Jager P, et al.: Normal and hydronephrotic kidney: Evaluation of renal function with contrast-enhanced MR imaging. *Radiology* 165: 837–842, 1987.

8. Ros PR, Gauger J, Stoupis C, Burton SS, Mao J, Wilcox C, Rosenber EB, Briggs RW: Diagnosis of renal artery stenosis: Feasibility of combining MR angiography, MR renography, and gadopentetate-based measurements of glomerular filtration rate. *Am J Roentgenol* 165: 1447–1457, 1995.

9. Barnhart JL, Kuhnert N, Douglas BA, et al.: Biodistribution of Gd-CL and Gd-DTPA and their influence on proton magnetic relaxation in rat tissues. *Magn Reson Imaging* 5: 221–231, 1987.

10. Jennete JL, Olson JL, Schwartz MM, Silva FG: *Heptinstall's Pathology of the Kidney* (5th ed.). Volume 2. Philadelphia: Lippincott-Raven, 1998, p. 1149.

11. Bostwick DG, Eble JN: *Urologic surgical pathology* (1st ed.). London, Mosby, 1997, p. 14.

12. Cotran RS, Kumar V, Robbins SL: *Pathology basis of disease* (5th ed.). Philadelphia: Saunders, 1994.

13. Dalton D, Neiman H, Grayhack JT: The natural history of simple renal cysts: A preliminary study. *J Urol* 135: 905–908, 1986.

14. Semelka RC, Hricak H, Stevens SK, Fingold R, Tomei E, Carroll PR: Combined gadolinium-enhanced and fat saturation MR imaging of renal masses. *Radiology* 178: 803–809, 1991.

15. Balci NC, Semelka RC, Patt RH, Dubois D, Freeman JA, Gomez-Caminero A, Woosley JT: Complex renal cysts: Findings on MR imaging. *Am J Roentgenol* 172: 1485–1500, 1999.

16. Jennete JC; Olson JL; Schwartz MM; Silva FG: *Heptinstall's Pathology of the Kidney* (5th ed.). Vol. 2. Philadelphia: Lippincott-Raven, 1998, p. 1196.

17. Gabow PA: Autosomal dominant polycystic kidney disease. *N Engl J Med* 329: 332–342, 1993.

18. Huch Boni RA, Debatin JF, Krestin GP: Contrast-enhanced MR imaging of the kidneys and adrenal glands. Contrast agents for body MR Imaging. *MRI Clin N A* 1064–1089, 1996.

19. Lonergan GJ, Rice RR, Suarez ES: Autosomal recessive polycystic kidney disease: Radiology-pathologic correlation. *Radiographics* 20: 837–855, 2000.

20. Wise SW, Hartman DS, Hardesty LA, Mosher TJ. Renal medullary cystic disease: Assessment by MRI. *Abdom Imag* 23 (6): 649–651, 1998.

21. Cho C, Friedland GW, Swenson RS: Acquired renal cystic disease and renal neoplasms in hemodialysis patients. *Urol Radiol* 6: 153–157, 1984.

22. Ishikawa I: Uremic acquired cystic disease of kidney. *Urology* 26: 101–107, 1985.

23. Levine E, Grantham JJ, Slucher SL, Greathouse JL, Krohn BP: CT of acquired cystic kidney disease and renal tumors in long term dialysis patients. *Am J Roentgenol* 142: 125–131, 1984.

24. Agrons GA, Wagner BJ, Davidson AJ, Suarez ES: Multilocular cystic renal tumor in children: Radiologic-pathologic correlation. *Radiographics* 15: 653–669, 1995.

25. Kettritz U, Semelka RC, Siegelman ES, Shoenut JP, Mithell DG: Multilocular cystic nephroma: MR imaging appearance with current techniques, including gadolinium enhancement. *J Magn Reson Imaging* 1: 145–148, 1996.

26. Dikengil A, Benson M, Sanders L, Newhouse JH: MRI of multilocular cystic nephroma. *Urol Radiol* 10: 95–99, 1988.

27. Bellin MF, Richard F, Attias S, et al.: Renal angiomyolipoma: Comparison of MRI and CT results for diagnosis. *Eur Radiol* 2: 465–472, 1992.

28. Van Ball JG, Smits NJ, Keeman JN, et al.: The evolution of renal angiomylipomas in patients with tuberous sclerosis. *J Urol* 152: 35–38, 1994.

29. Lemaitre L, Robert Y, Dubrulle F, Claudon M, Duhamel A, Danjou P, Mazeman E: Renal angiomyolipoma: Growth followed up with CT and/or US. *Radiology* 197: 598–602, 1995.

30. Steiner MS, Goldman SM, Fishman EK, Marshall FF: The natural history of renal angiomyolipoma. *J Urol* 150: 1782–1786, 1993.

31. Wills, JS: Management of small renal neoplasms and angiomyolipoma: A growing problem. *Radiology* 197: 583–586, 1995.

32. Burdeny DA, Semelka RC, Kelekis NL, Reinhold C, Ascher SM: Small (<1.5 cm) angiomyolipomas of the kidney: Characterization by combined use of in-phase and fat attenuated MR techniques. *Magn Reson Imaging* 15 (2): 141–145, 1997.

33. Osterling JE, Fishman EK, Goldman SM, Marshall FF: The management of renal angiomyolipoma. *J Urol* 135: 1121–1124, 1986.

34. Strotzer M, Lehner KB, Becker K: Detection of fat in a renal cell carcinoma mimicking angiomyolipoma. *Radiology* 188: 427–428, 1993.

35. Reichard EA, Roubidoux MA, Dunnick NR: Renal neoplasms in patients with renal cystic diseases. *Abdom Imaging* 23: 237–248, 1998.

36. Mitnick JS, Bosniak MA, Mitton S, Raghavendra BN, Subramanyan BR, Genieser NB: Cystic renal disease in tuberous sclerosis. *Radiology* 147: 85–87, 1983.

37. Choyke PL, Glenn GM, Wlather MM, Patronas NJ, Linehan WM, Zbar B: von Hippel-Lindau disease: Genetic, clinical, and imaging features. *Radiology* 194: 629–642, 1995.

38. Quinn MJ, Hartman DS, Friedman AC, et al.: Renal oncocytoma: New observations. *Radiology* 153: 49–53, 1984.

39. Press GA, McClennan BL, Melson GL, Weyman PJ, Mauro MA, Lee JKT: Papillary renal cell carcinoma: CT and sonographic evaluation. *Am J Roentgenol* 143: 1005–1010, 1984.

40. Davidson AJ, Hayews WS, Hartman DS, McCarthy WF, Davis CJ: Renal oncocytoma and carcinoma: Failure of differentiation with CT. *Radiology* 186: 693–696, 1993.

41. Bosniak MA: The small (≤3.0 cm) renal parenchymal tumor: Detection, diagnosis, and controversies. *Radiology* 179: 307–317, 1991.

42. Birnbaum BA, Bosniak MA, Megibow AJ, Lubat E, Gordon RB: Observations on the growth of renal neoplasms. *Radiology* 176: 695–701, 1990.

43. Levine E, Huntrakoon M, Wetzel LH: Small renal neoplasms: Clinical, pathologic, and imaging features. *Am J Roentgenol* 153: 69–73, 1989.

44. Curry NS: Small renal masses (lesions smaller than 3 cm): Imaging evaluation and managment. *Am J Roentgenol* 164: 355–362, 1995.

45. Bosniak MA, Birnbaum BA, Krinsky GA, Waisman J: Small renal parenchymal neoplasms: Further observations on growth. *Radiology* 197: 589–597, 1995.

46. Bosniak MA, Rofsky NM: Problems in the detection and characterization of small renal masses. *Radiology* 198: 638–641, 1996.

47. Jennete JC, Olson JL, Schwartz MM, Silva FG: *Heptinstall's Pathology of the Kidney* (5th ed.). Vol. 2. Philadelphia: Lippincott-Raven, 1998, p. 1548.

48. Newhouse JH, Wagner BJ: Renal oncocytomas. *Abdom Imaging* 23: 249–255, 1998.

49. Ball DS, Friedman AC, Hartman DS, Radecki PD, Caroline DF: Scar sign of renal oncocytoma: Magnetic resonance imaging appearance and lack of specificity. *Urol Radiol* 8: 46–48, 1986.

50. Schnuelle P, Waldhen R, Lehmann KJ, Woenckhaus J, Back W, et al.: Idiopathic myelofibrosis with extramedullary hematopoiesis in the kidneys. *Clin Nephrol* 52 (4): 256–262, 1999.

51. Tefferi A: Myelofibrosis with myeloid metaplasia—Review articles. *N Engl J Med* 342 (17): 1255–65, 2000.

52. Gryspeerdt S, Oyen R, Baert AL, Boogaerts M: Extramedullary hematopoiesis encasing the pelvicalyceal system: CT findings. *Ann Hematol* 71: 53–56, 1995.

53. Marshall FF, Stewart AK, Menck HR: The national cancer data base—Report on kidney cancers. *Cancer* 80 (11): 2167–2174, 1997.

54. Boring CC, Squires TS, Tony T: Cancer statistics, 1991. *CA Cancer J Clin* 41: 19, 1991.

55. Semelka RC, Shoenut JP, Magro CM, Kroeker MA, MacMahon R, Greenberg HM: Renal cancer staging: Comparison of contrast-enhanced CT and gadolinium-enhanced fat-suppressed spin-echo and gradient-echo MR imaging. *J Magn Reson Imaging* 3: 597–602, 1993.

56. Hricak H, Thoeni RF, Carroll PR, Demas BE, Marotti M, Tanagho EA: Detection and staging of renal neoplasms: A reassessment of MR imaging. *Radiology* 166: 643–649, 1988.

57. Eilenberg SS, Lee JKT, Brown JJ, Mirowitz SA, Tartar VM: Renal masses: Evaluation with gradient-echo Gd-DTPA-enhanced dynamic MR imaging. *Radiology* 176: 333–338, 1990.

58. Rominger MB, Kenney PJ, Morgan DE, Bernreuter WK, Listinsky JJ: Gadolinium-enhanced MR imaging of renal masses. *Radiographics* 12: 1097–1116, 1992.

59. Bard RH, Lord B, Fromowitz F: Papillary adenocarcinoma of kidney. *Urology* 19: 16–20, 1982.

60. Tello R, Davison BD, Malley M, Fenlon H, Thomson KR, Witte DJ, Harewood L: MR imaging of renal masses interpreted on CT to be suspicious. *Am J Roentgenol* 174: 1017–1022, 2000.

61. Oto A, Herts BR, Remer EM, Novick AC: Inferior vena cava tumor thrombus in renal cell carcinoma: Staging by MR imaging and impact on surgical treatment. *Am J Roentgenol* 171: 1619–1624, 1998.

62. Zeman RK, Cronan JJ, Rosenfield AT, Lynch JH, Jaffe MH, Clark LR: Renal cell carcinoma: Dynamic thin-section CT assessment of vascular invasion and tumor vascularity. *Radiology* 167: 393–396, 1988.

63. Roubidoux MA, Dunnick NR, Sostman HD, Leder RA: Renal carcinoma: Detection of venous extension with gradient echo MR imaging. *Radiology* 182: 269–272, 1992.

64. Studer UE, Scherz S, Scheidegger J, et al.: Enlargement of regional lymph nodes in renal cell carcinoma is often not due to metastases. *J Urol* 144: 243–245, 1990.

65. Bader TR, Semelka RC, Pedro MS, Armao DM, Molina PL: MR imaging of pulmonary parenchymal disease with a breath-hold 3D gradient-echo technique. J Magn Reson Imaging (in press).

66. Murad T, Komako W, Oyesu R, Bauer K: Multilocular cystic renal cell carcinoma. *Am J Clin Pathol* 95 (5): 633–637, 1991.

67. Outwater EK, Bhatia M, Siegelman ES, Burke MA, Mitchell DG: Lipid in renal clear cell carcinoma: Detection on opposed-phase gradient-echo MR images. *Radiology* 205: 103–107, 1997.

68. Yoshimitsu K, Honda H, Kuroiwa T, Irie H, Tajima T, Jimi M, Kuroiwa K, et al.: Fat detection in granular-cell renal cell carcinoma using chemical-shift gradient-echo MR imaging: another renal tumor that contains fat. *Abdom Imaging* 25: 100–102, 2000.

69. John G, Semelka RC, Burdeny DA, Kelekis NL, Kettritz U, Freeman JA: Renal cell cancer: Incidence of hemorrhage on MR images in patients with renal insufficiency. *J Magn Reson Imag* 7: 157–160, 1997.

70. Terens WL, Gluck R, Golimbu M, Rofsky NM: Use of gadolinium-DTPA-enhanced MRI to characterize renal masses in patient with renal insufficiency. *Urology* 40: 152–154, 1992.

71. Rofsky NM, Weinreb JC, Bosniak MA, Libes RB, Birnbaum BA: Renal lesion characterization with gadolinium-enhanced MR imaging: Efficacy and safety in patients with renal insufficiency. *Radiology* 180: 85–89, 1991.

72. Haustein J, Niendorf HP, Krestin G, et al.: Renal tolerance of gadolinium-DTPA/dimeglumine in patients with chronic renal failure. *Invest Radiol* 27: 153–156, 1992.

73. Choyke PL, Girton ME, Vaughn EM, Frank JA, Austin HA: Clearance of gadolinium chelates by hemodialysis: An in vitro study. *J Magn Reson Imaging* 4: 470–472, 1995.

74. Thompson IM, Peek M: Improvement in survival of patients with renal cell carcinoma: The role of the serendipitous detected tumor. *J Urol* 140: 487–490, 1988.

75. Smith SJ, Bosniak MA, Megibow AJ, Hulnick DH, Horii SC, Raghavendra BN: Renal cell carcinoma: Earlier detection and increased detection. *Radiology* 170: 699–703, 1989.

76. Jamis-Dow CA, Choyke PL, Jennings SB, Linehan WM, Thakore KN, Walther MM: Small (≤3 cm) renal masses: Detection with CT versus US and pathologic correlation. *Radiology* 198: 785–788, 1996.

77. Butler BP, Novick AC, Miller DP, et al.: Management of small unilateral renal cell carcinomas: Radical versus nephron-sparing surgery. *Urology* 45: 34–41, 1995.

78. Novick AC: Partial nephrectomy for renal cell carcinoma. *Urology* 46: 149–152, 1995.

79. Nissenkorn I, Bernheim J: Multicentricity in renal cell carcinoma. *J Urol* 153: 620–622, 1995.

80. Pronet J, Tessler A, Brown J, Golimbu M, Bosniak M, Morales P: Partial nephrectomy for renal cell carcinoma: Indications, results and implications. *J Urol* 145: 472–476, 1991.

81. Gylys-Morin V, Hoffer FA, Kozakewich H, Shamberger RC: Wilms tumor and nephroblastomatosis: Imaging characteristics at gadolinium-enhanced MR imaging. *Radiology* 188: 517–521, 1993.

82. Cohen MD: Staging of Wilms' tumour. *Clin Radiol* 14: 77–81, 1993.

83. Weese DL, Applebaum H, Taber P: Mapping intravascular extension of Wilms' tumor with magnetic resonance imaging. *J Pediatr Surg* 1: 64–67, 1991.

84. Richards MA, Mootoosamy I, Reznek RH, Webb JA, Lister TA: Renal involvement in patients with non-Hodgkin's lymphoma: Clinical and pathological features in 23 cases. *Hematol Oncol* 8: 105–110, 1990.

85. Heiken JP, McClennan BL, Gold RP: Renal lymphoma. *Semin Ultrasound CT MR* 7: 58–66, 1986.

86. Semelka RC, Kelekis NL, Burdeny DA, Mitchell DG, Brown JJ, Siegelman ES: Renal lymphoma: Demonstration by MR imaging. *Am J Roentgenol* 166: 823–827, 1996.

87. Hauser M, Krestin GP, Hagspiel KD: Bilateral solid multifocal intrarenal and perirenal lesions: Differentiation with ultrasonography, computed tomography and magnetic resonance imaging. *Clin Radiol* 50: 288–294, 1995.

88. Marcos HB, Semelka RC, Woosley JT: Abdominal granulocytic sarcomas: Demostration by MRI. *Magn Reson Imaging* 15 (7): 873–876, 1997.

89. Bailey JE, Roubidoux MA, Dunnick NR: Secondary renal neoplasms. *Imaging* 23: 266–274, 1998.

90. Kettritz U, Semelka RC, Brown ED, Sharp TJ, Lawing WL, Colindres RE: MR findings in diffuse renal parenchymal disease. *J Magn Reson Imaging* 6: 136–144, 1996.

91. Semelka RC, Corrigan K, Ascher SM, Brown JJ, Colindres RE: Renal corticomedullary differentiation: Observation in patient with differing serum creatinine levels. *Radiology* 190: 149–152, 1994.

92. Chung JJ, Semelka RC, Martin DR: Acute renal failure: common occurrence of preservation of corticomedullary differentiation on MR images. Magn Reson Imaging 19: 789–793, 2001.

93. Tempany CMC, Morton RA, Marshall FF: MRI of the renal veins: Assessment of nonneoplastic venous thrombosis. *J Comput Assist Tomogr* 16 (6): 929–934, 1992.

94. Wyngaarden JB, Smith LH, Bennett JC: *Cecil Textbook of Medicine* (19th ed.). Philadelphia: WB Saunders, 1992, p. 2263.

95. Engel AG, Franzini C: *Myology* (2nd ed.). New York: McGraw-Hill, 1994, p. 1681.

96. Lande IM, Glazer GM, Sarnaik S, Aisen A, Rucknagel D, Martel W: Sickle-cell nephropathy: MR imaging. *Radiology* 158: 379–383, 1986.

97. Siegelman ES, Outwater E, Hanau CA, Ballas SK, Steiner RM, Rao VM, Mitchell DG: Abdominal iron distribution in sickle cell disease: MR finding in transfusion and nontransfusion dependent patients. *J Comput Assist Tomogr* 18 (1): 63–67, 1994.

98. Roubidouz MA: MR of the kidneys, liver, and spleen in paroxysmal nocturnal hemoglobinuria. *Abdom Imaging* 19: 168–173, 1994.

99. Cotran RS, Kumar V, Robbins SL. *Pathology basis of disease* (5th ed.). Philadelphia: Saunders, 1994.

100. Bakker J, Beek FJA, Beutler JJ, Hene' RJ, Kort GAP, Lange EE, et al.: Renal artery stenosis and accessory renal arteries: Accuracy of detection and visualization with gadolinium-enhanced breath-hold MR angiography. *Radiology* 207: 497–504, 1998.

101. Tello R, Thomson KR, Witte D, Becker GJ, Tress BM: Standard dose Gd-DTPA dynamic MR of renal arteries. *J Magn Reson Imaging* 8: 421–426, 1998.

102. Saunders HS, Dyer RB, Shifrin RY, Scharling ES, Bechtold RE, Zagoria RJ: The CT nephrogram: Implications for evaluation of urinary tract disease. *Radiographics* 15: 1069–1085, 1995.

103. Kelekis NL, Semelka RC, Molina P, Warshauer DM: Immediate postgadolinium spoiled gradient-echo MRI for evaluating the abdominal aorta in the setting of abdominal MR examination. *J Magn Reson Imaging* 7: 652–656, 1997.

104. Goldman SM, Fishman EK: Upper urinary tract infection: The current role of CT, ultrasound, and MRI. *Semin Ultrasound CT MR* 4: 335–360, 1991.

105. Fowler JE Jr, Perkins T: Presentation, diagnosis and treatment of renal abscesses: 1972–1988. *J Urol* 151: 847–851, 1994.

106. Brown ED, Semelka RC: Renal abscesses: Appearance on gadolinium-enhanced magnetic resonance images. *Abdom Imaging* 21: 172–176, 1996.

107. Bova JG, Potter JL, Arevalos E, Hopens T, Goldstein HM, Radwin HM: Renal and perirenal infection: The role of computerized tomography. *J Urol* 133: 375–378, 1985.

108. Mulopulos GP, Patel SK, Pessis D: MR imaging of xanthogranulomatous pyelonephritis. *J Comput Assist Tomogr* 10: 154–156, 1986.

109. Ling BN, Delaney VB, Campbell WG: Acute renal failure due to bilateral renal parenchymal malakoplakia. *Am J Kidney Di* 13 (5): 430–433, 1989.

110. Pamilo M, Kalatunga A: Renal parenchymal malakoplakia. A report of two cases. The radiological and ultrasound images. *Br J Radiol* 57: 751–755, 1984.

111. Esparza AR, McKay DB, Cronan JJ, Chazan JA: Renal parenchymal malakoplakia. Histologic spectrum and its relationship to megalocytic intersticial nephritis an xantnogranulomatous pyelonephritis. *Am J Surg Pathol* 13 (3): 225–236, 1989.

112. Semelka RC, Shoenut JP, Greenberg HM, Bow EJ: Detection of acute and treated lesions of hepatosplenic candidiasis: Comparison of dynamic contrast-enhanced CT and MR imaging. *J Magn Reson Imaging* 2: 414–420, 1992.

113. Winalski CS, Lipman JC, Tumeh SS: Ureteral neoplasms. *Radiographics* 10: 271–283, 1990.

114. Weeks SM, Brown ED, Brown JJ, Adamis MK, Eisenberg LB, Semelka RC: Transitional cell carcinoma of the upper urinary tract staging by MRI. *Abdom Imaging* 20: 365–367, 1995.

115. Leo ME, Petrou SP, Barrett DM: Transitional cell carcinoma of the kidney with vena caval involvement: Report of 3 cases and a review of the literature. *J Urol* 148: 398–400, 1992.

116. Coe FL, Parks JH, Asplin JR: The pathogenesis and treatment of kidney stones. *N Engl J Med* 327: 1141–1152, 1992.

117. Regan F, Bohlman ME, Khazan R, Rodriguez R, Schultze-Haakh H: MR urography using HASTE imaging in the assessment of ureteric obstruction. *Am J Roentgenol* 167: 1115–1120, 1996.

118. Hani BM, Noone TC, Semelka RC: MRI evaluation of acute renal trauma. *J Magn Reson Imaging* 8: 989–990, 1998.

119. Laissy J-P, Faraggi M, Lebtahi R, et al.: Functional evaluation of normal and ischemic kidney by means of gadolinium-DOTA enhanced TurboFLASH MR imaging: A preliminary comparison with 99mTc-MAG3 dynamic scintigraphy. *Magn Reson Imaging* 12: 413–419, 1994.

120. Neimatallah MA, Dong Q, Schoenberg SO, Cho KJ, Prince MR: Magnetic Resonance Imaging in renal transplantation. *J Magn Reson Imaging* 10: 357–368, 1999.

121. Low RN, Martinz AG, Steinberg SM, Alzate GD, et al.: Potencial renal transplant donors: Evaluation with gadolinium-enhanced MR angiography and MR urography. *Radiology* 207: 165–172, 1998.

122. Jennete JC; Olson JL; Schwartz MM; Silva FG: *Heptinstall's Pathology of the Kidney* (5th ed.). Vol. 2. Philadelphia: Lippincott-Raven, 1998, p. 1497.

123. Jennete JC, Olson JL, Schwartz MM, Silva FG: *Heptinstall's Pathology of the Kidney* (5th ed.). Vol. 2. Philadelphia: Lippincott-Raven, 1998, p. 1412.

124. McCreath GT, McMillan N, Patterson J, et al.: Magnetic resonance imaging of renal transplants: Initial experience. *Br J Radiol* 61: 113–118, 1988.

125. Hricak H, Terrier F, Marotti M, et al.: Post-transplant renal rejection: Comparison of quantitative scintigraphy, ultrasonography and magnetic resonance imaging. *Radiology* 162: 685–688, 1987.

126. Hanna S, Helenon O, Legendre C, et al.: MR imaging of renal transplant rejection. *Acta Radiol* 32: 42–46, 1991.

127. Liou JTS, Lee JKT, Heiken JP, Totty WG, Molina PL, Flye WM: Renal transplants: Can acute rejection and acute tubular necrosis be differentiated with MR imaging? *Radiology* 179: 61–65, 1991.

128. Roy C, Saussine C, Guth S, Horviller S, Tuchmann C, Vasilescu C, Le Bras Y, Jacqmin D: MR Urography in the evaluation of urinary tract obstruction. *Abdom Imaging* 23: 27–34, 1998.

129. Edelman RR, Siewert B, Adamis M, Gaa J, Laub G, Wielopolski P: Signal targeting with alternating radiofrequency (STAR) sequences. *Magn Reson Med* 31: 233–238, 1994.

130. Li D, Haacke EM, Muyler JP III, Berr S, Brookeman JR, Hutton MC: Three-dimensional time-of-flight MR angiography using selective inversion recovery RAGE with fat saturation and ECG-triggering: Application to renal arteries. *Magn Reson Med* 31: 414–422, 1994.

131. Yucel EK, Kaufman JA, Prince M, Bazari H, Fang LST, Waltman AC: Time-of-flight renal MR angiography: Utility in patients with renal insufficiency. *Magn Reson Imaging* 11: 925–930, 1993.

132. Kim SH, Byun H, Park JH, Han JK, Lee JS: Renal parenchymal abnormalities associated with renal vein thrombosis: Correlation between MR imaging and pathologic findings in rabbits. *Am J Roentgenol* 162: 1361–1365, 1994.

133. Vexler VS, Bethezene Y, Clement O, Muhler A, Rosenau W, Moseley ME, Brasch RC: Detection of zonal renal ischemia with contrast-enhanced MR imaging with a macromolecular blood pool contrast agent. *J Magn Reson Imaging* 2: 311–319, 1992.

134. Trillaud H, Grenier N, Degreze P, Louail C, Chambon C, Francoi J: First-pass evaluation of renal perfusion with TurboFLASH MR imaging and superparamagnetic iron oxide particles. *J Magn Reson Imaging* 3: 83–91, 1993.

135. Wolf GL, Hoop B, Cannillo JA, Rogowska JA, Halpern EF: Measurement of renal transit of gadopentetate dimeglumine with echo-planar MR imaging. *J Magn Reson Imaging* 4: 365–372, 1994.

136. Wolf RL, King BF, Torres VE, Wilson DM, Ehman RL: Measurement of normal renal arterial blood flow: Cine phase-contrast MR imaging vs. clearance of *p*-aminohippurate. *Am J Roentgenol* 161: 995–1002, 1993.

137. Debatin JF, Ting RH, Wegmuller H, et al.: Renal artery blood flow: Quantification with phase-contrast MR imaging with and without breath holding. *Radiology* 190: 371–378, 1994.

138. Trillaud H, Roques F, Degreze P, Combe C, Grenier N: Gd-DOTA tubular transit asymmetry induced by angiotensin-converting enzyme inhibitor in experimental renovascular hypertension. *J Magn Reson Imaging* 1: 149–155, 1996.

139. Muller MR, Prasad PV, Bimmler D, Kaiser A, Edelman RR: Functional imaging of the kidney by means of measurement of the apparent diffusion coefficient. *Radiology* 193: 711–715, 1994.

CHAPTER 10

RETROPERITONEUM

DIEGO R. MARTIN, M.D., P.H.D., RICHARD C. SEMELKA, M.D., MONICA S. PEDRO, M.D., AND NIKOLAOS L. KELEKIS, M.D.

NORMAL ANATOMY

The retroperitoneum is limited anteriorly by the parietal peritoneum and posteriorly by the transversalis fascia, extending from the level of the diaphragm to the level of the pelvic inlet. It is divided into the perirenal, anterior pararenal, and posterior pararenal spaces. Additional potential dissection planes exist between the retroperitoneal spaces: the retromesenteric plane, formed by retromesenteric fusion planes anteriorly and the anterior renal (Gerota) fascia posteriorly, and the retrorenal plane formed by retromesenteric fusion planes and the posterior renal (Zuckerkandl) fascia. These potential spaces may form the pathway by which rapidly accumulating fluid collections in the retroperitoneal space may extend to the pelvis [1].

The kidneys, adrenals, and pancreas are retroperitoneal structures and are discussed separately in individual chapters.

Other structures contained within the retroperitoneum include lymph nodes and lymphatic vessels, fat, and nerves. Major vessels include the aorta and inferior vena cava, and major skeletal muscles include the psoas. Neoplastic, infectious, inflammatory, idiopathic, and hemorrhagic processes can arise from, or involve, these particular retroperitoneal structures and are discussed in this chapter.

MRI TECHNIQUE

The retroperitoneum can be reliably assessed by MRI. An imaging protocol should be designed to 1) maximize the signal intensity differences between suspected pathology and background tissues, 2) directly image the full extent of disease processes, and 3) define their boundaries with adjacent organs. The combination of breath-hold and breathing-independent sequences acquired in at least two different planes can achieve these goals without substantially prolonging the examination time. In the investigation of abnormal retroperitoneal tissue, the imaging protocol should include precontrast spoiled gradient-echo (SGE), fat-suppressed T2-weighted, and postgadolinium fat-suppressed SGE images. In the investigation of retroperitoneal hemorrhage, precontrast fat-suppressed SGE images should be obtained because this technique has the greatest sensitivity for subacute hemorrhage. Postcontrast fat-suppressed SGE images, using intravenously administered gadolinium chelate, are important for delineation and characterization of retroperitoneal lymph nodes, other masses, inflammation or infection, and fibrosis. Vascular structures are also well defined on postcontrast fat-suppressed SGE images. Image acquisition in two orthogonal planes permits direct evaluation of the extent of retroperitoneal disease.

Oral contrast also may be used in selected cases to provide better delineation of bowel and to facilitate distinction of bowel from retroperitoneal tissue. Orally administered water provides adequate bowel opacification as a positive contrast medium for short-duration T2-weighted, echo-train spin-echo [e.g., half-Fourier single-shot turbo spin-echo (HASTE)] sequences and as a negative contrast medium for breath-hold T1-weighted (e.g., SGE) sequences. The selection of sequences may vary according to the clinical history, the other organs that are examined, and the capabilities of the equipment.

MR angiographic techniques, particularly breath-hold three-dimensional (3D) gradient-echo sequences, play an important role in imaging the aorta and its branches. The combined use of 3D gradient-echo MR angiography (MRA) and tissue-imaging sequences provides information on vessel lumen, vessel wall, and surrounding organs.

RETROPERITONEAL VESSELS

MR Angiography (MRA)

The aorta and its branches are well evaluated by MRA using currently available techniques. Generally, techniques can be classified as black blood (flowing blood appears as signal void) or bright blood (flowing blood appears as high signal intensity). Conventional T1- and T2-weighted spin-echo images will generally display the aortic lumen as a signal void (dark-blood technique) because the excited blood leaves the slice in the time interval between excitation pulse and echo sampling. Despite the use of presaturation pulses and a long echo time, slow blood flow, as can be seen during diastole in the infrarenal aorta, may appear bright on T1-weighted spin-echo images, which has the potential of appearing similar to thrombus. Cardiac gating can be used to reduce pulsatile motion artifacts and can reduce diastolic slow flow effects by acquiring SE images from inferior to superior, thus obtaining infrarenal aorta images during systole.

Bright-blood techniques include sequences that refocus blood signal intensity with gradient pulses or gadolinium-enhanced gradient-echo sequences. Sequences that refocus blood signal include cine gradient-echo, time-of-flight MR angiography, and phase-contrast MR angiography. Time-of-flight MRA techniques [3–9] rely on the inflow of unsaturated spins into the examined slice (2D) or volume (3D). Although these techniques have been used for head and neck applications, they do not achieve reproducible image quality in the abdomen because of respiratory and peristaltic motion and because of the large volume of examined tissues and vessels. As the majority of these techniques are non-breath hold they have limited reproducibility in patients who are uncooperative, a circumstance that may be observed in patients with substantial disease. Furthermore, slow or turbulent flow in aortic aneurysms and poststenotic turbulent flow (e.g., in aortic occlusive disease or renal artery stenosis) cause dephasing that leads to signal loss and impaired vessel visualization [6, 9–11]. Phase-contrast techniques may be used when flow velocity and direction information is required (fig. 10.1). They require cardiac triggering and can be relatively long acquisition sequences, predominantly used for assessment of critical aortic stenosis or for assessment of cardiac valvular disease.

The disadvantages of the time-of-flight techniques include signal loss in low-flow and turbulent-flow states and saturation of in-plane flow. To overcome these disadvantages of time-of-flight techniques, gadolinium enhancement has been employed in conjunction with 2D or 3D fast gradient-echo acquisitions, yielding good, reproducible results [10–16]. The 3D gadolinium-enhanced

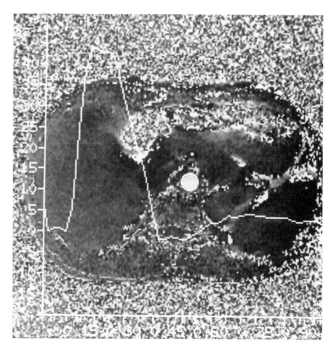

F I G . 10.1 Phase map of the normal aorta. The abdominal aorta (encircled) appears high in signal intensity on this phase map in the systolic phase of antegrade blood flow. A blood velocity tracing obtained throughout the cardiac cycle is superimposed on the phase image, demonstrating the normal velocity profile of blood in the abdominal aorta. (Reproduced with permission from Semelka RC, Shoenut JP, Kroeker MA: The retroperitoneum and the abdominal wall. In: Semelka RC, Shoenut JP (eds.), *MRI of the Abdomen with CT Correlation.* New York: Raven Press, p. 13–41, 1993.)

gradient-echo MRA technique does not rely on time-of-flight effects but rather on the T1 shortening provided by gadolinium. Advantages compared with 2D techniques include a high signal-to-noise ratio permitting nearly isotropic resolution (typically 2-mm effective slice thickness), acquisition of the central phase-encoding steps at the same time point for all the slices, and avoidance of slice misregistration [11]. Recent advances in MRI, including the use of phased-array coils that increase the signal-to-noise ratio and faster-rising gradient times, have led to the implementation of fast 3D gradient-echo acquisitions in a breath hold [17]. Typically, 0.1–0.2 mmol/kg body weight of gadolinium is administered into an arm vein using a dual-chamber power injector at a rate of 2–3 cc/s, followed by 15 cc of saline to clear lines and veins. A tight bolus technique is useful when examining renal arteries because the venous return from the kidneys is rapid and overlap from renal veins is more difficult to control with infusion techniques. A slower infusion technique may be used when smaller and/or distal vessels are imaged, as in combined examinations of aortoiliac and lower extremity vessels. Timing of the injection depends on the vessels studied, the patient cardiac output, and the total acquisition time of the 3D gradient sequence, with the objective being to maximize intravascular gadolinium concentration during acquisition of the central phase-encoding steps [13]. It is these central encoding steps that are responsible for generating image contrast. To simplify timing, 3D gradient-echo sequences have been designed to reorder phase-encoding steps, obtaining image contrast information at the beginning of the acquisition. Such techniques include helical, helicocentric, or elliptocentric 3D gradient sequences.

For aortic imaging, the time interval between initiating contrast injection and initiating the imaging sequence can be determined using a timed bolus technique. This is accomplished by placing a sagittal gradient-echo slice centered on the descending thoracic aorta and imaging one image every 2 s as a 2- or 3-cc gadolinium injection is administered. Alternatively, an automated system can be employed such that the control software measures signal intensity arising from within a region of interest, placed within the aortic lumen, and the entire 40-cc intravenous gadolinium bolus is then administered such that a prescribed 3D gradient acquisition is triggered when the system detects a rise in intraluminal aortic signal intensity.

Automation has progressed further such that a bolus-chase technique, similar in concept to conventional fluoroscopic angiography, is now possible. This is performed by prescribing up to three consecutive fields of view having three separate centering points, which can extend from the aortic arch to the vessels of both lower extremities and feet (fig. 10.2). Each field of view can overlap slightly with the neighboring field by 2 cm,

with each field typically measuring between 34 and 40 cm in length. Imaging of the superior field is acquired with initiation determined using a timed-bolus or automated preparation technique. Subsequent middle and lower fields are imaged as previously prescribed, with the table moving the patient to the appropriate new center point automatically. In this way, the bolus of arterial gadolinium contrast can be chased into the lower extremities. Venous filling can then be chased in reverse sequence from the feet to the IVC. Although the time interval between initiating contrast injection and initiating imaging of the superior first station can be determined by prior bolus timing or by automated bolus detection, the subsequent imaging at the second and third inferior stations are timed empirically. To include the aorta, bilateral iliac, and bilateral lower extremity vessels, coronal 3D volumes are used. The ankles may be elevated to keep the calf arteries within a level horizontal plane. More recent faster image acquisition sequencing, such as true free induction in steady-state precession (e.g, true FISP or FIESTA) sequences, in combination with gadolinium, can be used for obtaining high spatial resolution, high contrast, and high temporal resolution, allowing more eloquent bolus-chase imaging. For example, a single bolus of contrast can now be imaged as the contrast first passes through the respective right heart, pulmonary arteries and veins, left heart, and then into the aorta (fig. 10.3). Generally, as temporal resolution improves, optimal image timing becomes easier, arterial-venous delineation is superior, and the required dose of contrast decreases. Previously, an aortic run-off study would require a combination of two or three stations, each treated as an individual exam requiring a total of two or three doses of gadolinium, typically at 0.1 mmol/kg each.

Another development necessary for multiple consecutive field-of-view imaging for aortic run-off exams has been specialized peripheral vascular phased-array coils that can cover from the chest to the feet (see fig. 10.2). Without such coil designs, a solitary phased-array torso coil would require repositioning, or more simply, the built-in body coil could be used. However, signal-to-noise ratio is significantly improved using surface coils.

The data acquired can be postprocessed either by multiplanar reconstructions or by 3D reconstruction using a maximum-intensity projection (MIP) algorithm. The small size of the individual slices permits reconstructions and 3D MIP projections at any level without image degradation. MIP images provide a quick overview and are useful in tracking vessels that have a tortuous course in and out of the section plane. They are also useful for identifying smaller vessels (e.g., accessory renal arteries) (fig. 10.4). The diagnosis, however, is usually based on the individual source sections, and evaluation

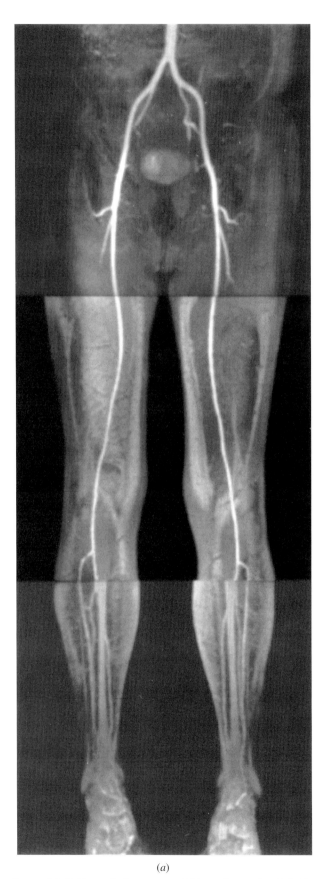

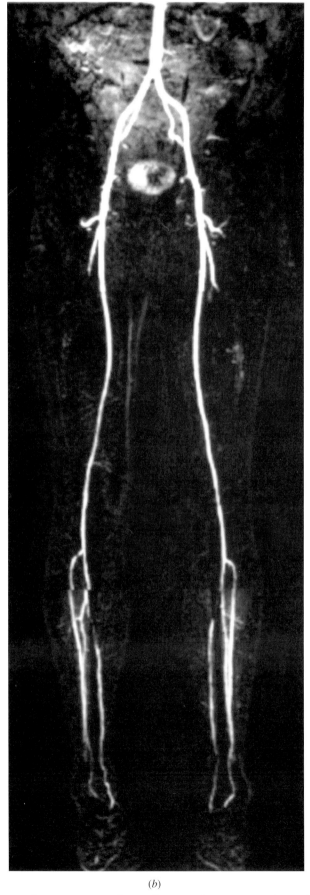

(a)   (b)

F I G . 10.2 Extended-coverage MR angiography (MRA). Aortic run-off 3-station 3D gradient-echo MRA showing normal (*a* and *b*), abnormal (*c*, right side), and conventional fluoroscopic digital subtraction angiogram (c, left side).

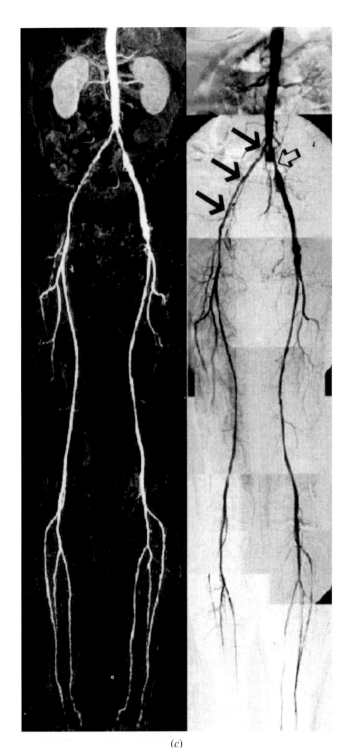

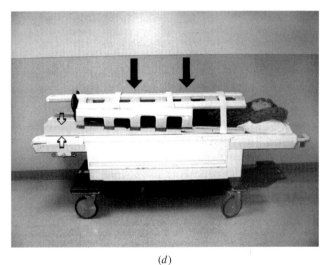

(c)   (d)

Fig. 10.2 (*Continued*) A normal patient was scanned using a peripheral vascular 3-station phased-array coil (*d*) having 2-cm overlaps between upper and middle (junction at the midsuperficial femoral artery), and again between middle and bifurcation into the peroneal and posterior tibial arteries). A bolus of 0 lower stations (junction at the distal end of the common peroneal trunk, just above 0.2 mmol/kg gadolinium was administered intravenously at a rate of 2 cc/s after a 15-s timed injection, based on bolus timing (see text). Each acquisition required 32 s, using 4-mm slice thickness constructions. The data was processed by maximum intensity projection (MIP) software analysis and is shown with no background subtraction and with soft tissue window and level (*a*), and after background subtraction using a high-contrast window and level (*b*) to eliminate soft tissues. Surgical planning often requires soft tissue visualization for spatial reference (*a*), although vascular detail may be more easily appreciated after removal of the soft tissue (*b*). Image *c* compares an MRA run-off study performed as in *a* and *b*, but with atherosclerotic irregular narrowing demonstrated over a long segment of right common and external iliac artery, and a short segment of proximal to mid-left common iliac artery. Nearly identical results are demonstrated on a conventional fluoroscopic angiogram using iodinated contrast agent, performed on the same patient, and shown on the right (arrows, right common and external iliac artery, hollow arrow: proximal left common iliac artery).

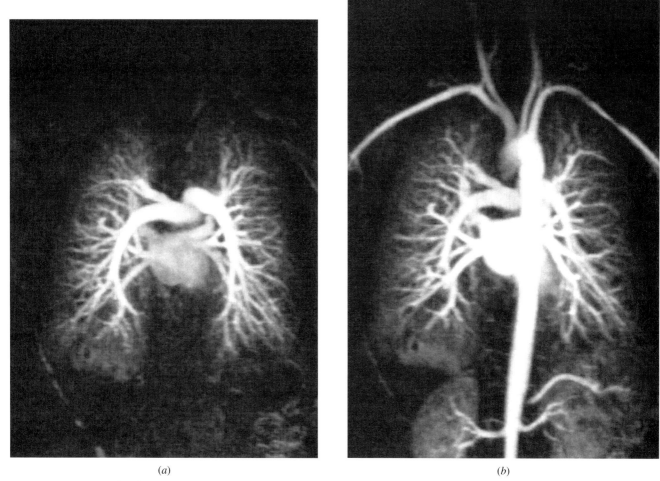

(a)   (b)

F I G . 10.3 Normal pulmonary MRA. Coronal 3D gradient-echo (*a* and *b*) images. The acquisition of image data over a short time period, after rapid injection of a small volume of gadolinium contrast, allows better temporal resolution, obtaining an image with contrast predominantly within the pulmonary arteries and just starting to fill pulmonary veins and left atrium. The image acquired immediately after the pulmonary angiogram (*b*) shows contrast within the pulmonary veins, left atrium, aorta, and major aortic arch vessels and starting to fill the renal arteries.

should not rely solely on the MIP images. The source images are superior to MIP reconstructions in the depiction of vessel wall, presence of mural thrombus, renal artery ostia, and intimal flap in aortic dissections [4]. Of critical importance for viewing and interpretation of large MRA data sets is a picture archival computing system (PACS) that has viewing workstations with software capable of image stacking and scrolling (i.e, rapid paging from one image slice to the next).

A useful adjunct, particularly in uncooperative patients, is a single-shot echo-train spin-echo technique (e.g: HASTE) combined with a set of preparatory inversion pulses (black-blood technique): A non-slice-selective 180° inversion pulse is applied, which is followed by a slice-selective 180° inversion pulse before the start of the echo-train sequence. The first pulse inverts the longitudinal magnetization of the whole body, whereas the second pulse selectively restores the lon-

gitudinal magnetization of the examined slice. The time delay of the first inversion pulse is selected so that the central phase-encoding steps are acquired when blood reaches the null point, resulting in no signal from blood [18].

For clinical examinations, it may be of value to obtain a bright-blood and a black-blood technique for studying the aorta [5, 19]. An attractive feature of MRI is its ability to image the aorta along its longitudinal length, which has a particular advantage in studying the length of a disease process such as aneurysm [5, 16, 19].

For the assessment of aortic pathology, early (up to 2 min after injection) postgadolinium images obtained for investigation of diseases of solid abdominal organs provide a fast and reproducible technique incorporated into the routine abdominal MRI protocol. Immediate postgadolinium SGE images also generate information on capillary blood flow, which may provide important

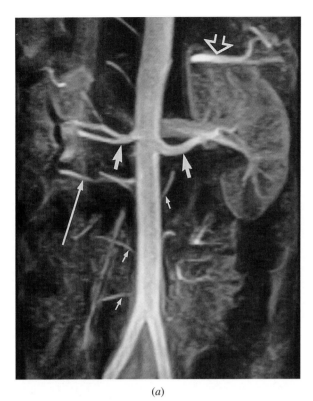

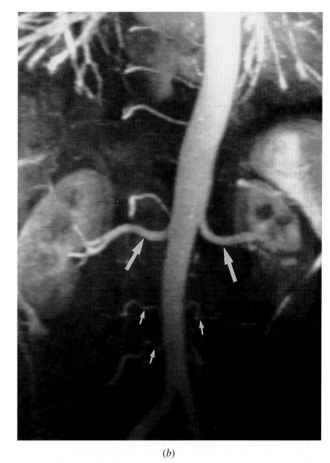

(a)   (b)

F i g . 10.4 Normal abdominal aorta and iliac vessels. Anteroposterior projection (*a*) from a 3D MIP reconstruction of a set of immediate postgadolinium coronal breath-hold 3D gradient-echo sections with effective slice thickness of 2 mm. The abdominal aorta, left and right renal arteries (arrows, *a*) and a right accessory lower pole renal artery (long arrow, *a*), common iliac arteries, and lumbar arteries (small arrows, *a*) are well visualized with good lumen enhancement and smooth contours. The celiac axis and superior mesenteric artery are not visualized because they course outside the narrow (4 cm) coronal slab. A segment of the splenic artery is identified reentering the acquired slab in its posterior course toward the hilum of the spleen (hollow arrow, *a*).

Anteroposterior projection (*b*) from a 3D MIP reconstruction of a set of immediate postgadolinium coronal breath-hold 3D gradient-echo sections with effective slice thickness of 2 mm in a second patient. The normal aorta, renal arteries (arrows, *b*), and lumbar arteries (small arrows, *b*) are well demonstrated.

insight into the impact of anatomical vessel abnormalities on organ perfusion. When angiographic sequences are not available, an anteroposterior projection of an MIP reconstruction using immediate postgadolinium coronal SGE sections (6–8 mm thick) results in angiograph-like images.

Aorta

Aortic Aneurysm

Abdominal aortic aneurysm (AAA) is a common disease entity in North America. The incidence is 21.1 per 100,000, and men are five times more likely than women to be affected by AAA. The median age at diagnosis is 69 years for men and 78 years for women [20]. Important diagnostic information for patient management includes diameter of the aneurysm, its longitudinal length, and

its relationship to renal, common iliac, and femoral arteries. Spontaneous rupture is a frequent complication of aneurysms 6 cm or more in diameter, but it is relatively uncommon for AAAs smaller than 5 cm [21, 22]. MR images with black-blood and bright-blood techniques are successful at demonstrating aneurysms [5, 16, 19, 23–27]. Gadolinium-enhanced 3D gradient-echo MR angiography (e.g., 3D FISP) demonstrates the full extent of the aneurysm and its relationship to the renal arteries, celiac axis, and superior mesenteric artery (SMA) (fig. 10.5). In patients with atherosclerotic disease, renal artery stenosis may coexist and is well depicted on gadolinium-enhanced 3D FISP images. Stenosis of the SMA also can be assessed reliably, and this is of importance in patients with suprarenal aortic aneurysms because postoperative bowel ischemia may complicate the aneurysm repair [27]. Assessment of the aortic wall,

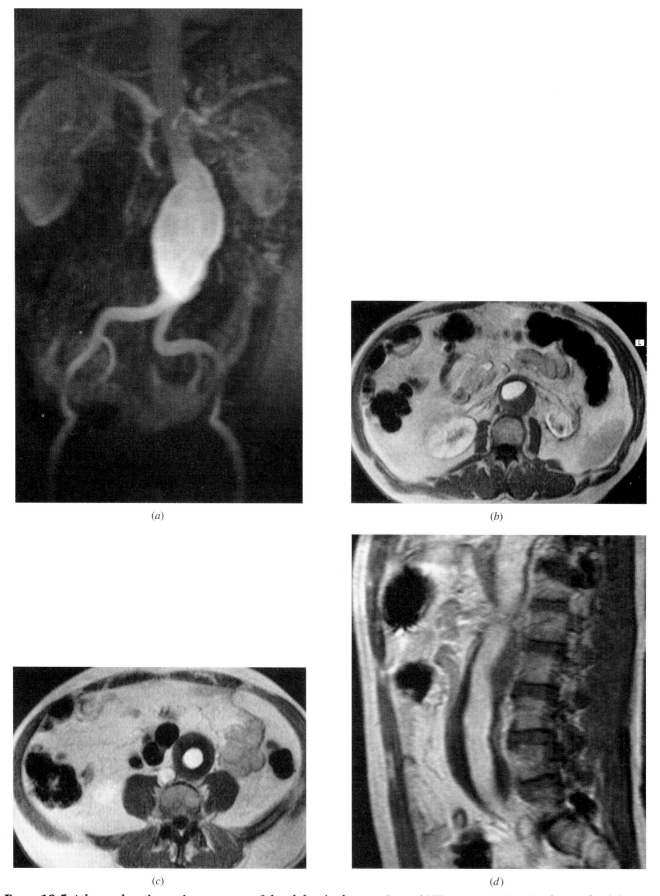

(a)

(b)

(c)

(d)

FIG. 10.5 Atherosclerotic aortic aneurysm of the abdominal aorta. Coronal MIP reconstruction (*a*) of a set of gadolinium-enhanced 2-mm thin-section coronal 3D gradient-echo sections in a patient with an infrarenal aortic aneurysm. The MIP images demonstrate a large fusiform infrarenal aortic aneurysm. The aneurysm is shown not to extend into the common iliac arteries.

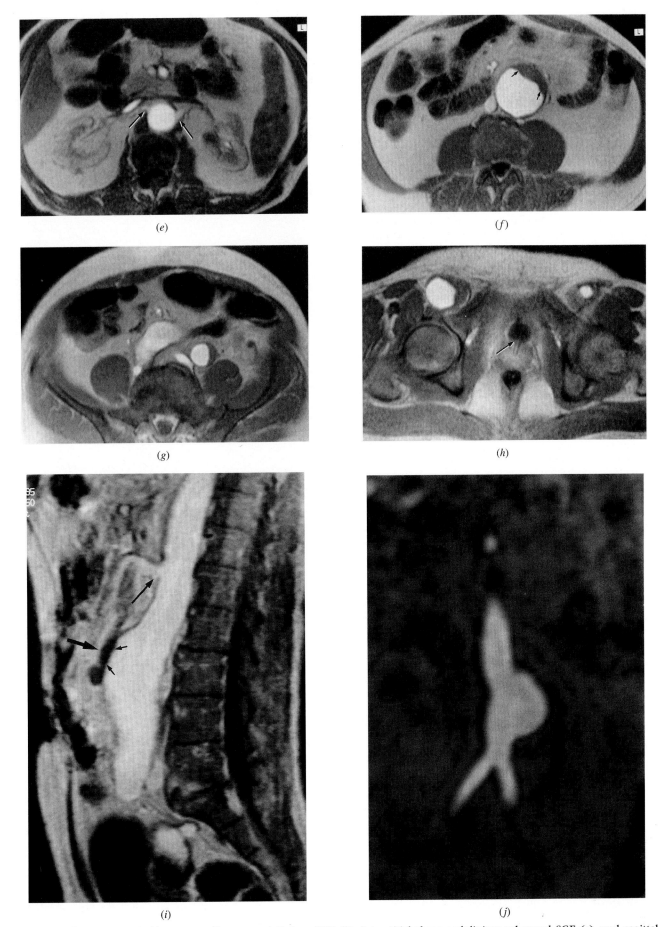

(e)

(f)

(g)

(h)

(i)

(j)

F I G . 10.5 (*Continued*) Transverse 45-s postgadolinium SGE (*b*), interstitial-phase gadolinium-enhanced SGE (*c*), and sagittal interstitial-phase SGE (*d*) images in a second patient.

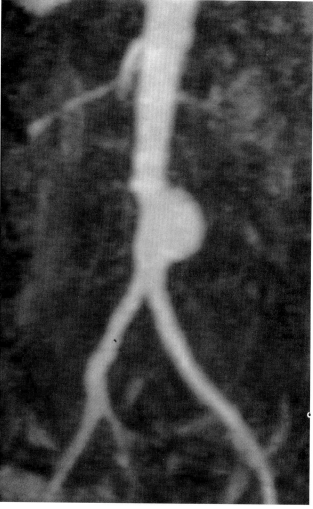

(k)

F I G . 10.5 (*Continued*) An abdominal aortic aneurysm containing high-signal intensity gadolinium in the lumen and low-signal intensity wall thrombus is evident on the 45-s postgadolinium SGE image (*b*). The left kidney is small and demonstrates delayed enhancement of a uniform thin cortex, findings consistent with left renal artery stenosis. Note that the signal intensity of the cortex and medulla of the right kidney has equilibrated at this tubular phase of enhancement. Good delineation of the patent lumen and mural thrombus is provided by gadolinium enhancement on early postgadolinium SGE images (*b*, *c*), whereas imaging in the sagittal plane demonstrates the longitudinal extent of disease.

Immediate postgadolinium (*e*) and transverse (*f*, *g*, *h*) and sagittal (*i*) interstitial-phase gadolinium-enhanced SGE images in a third patient. The abdominal aorta is normal in diameter at the level of the origins (arrows, *e*) of the renal arteries. At lower tomographic levels (*f–h*), enlargement of the aortic lumen with sharp demarcation of the high-signal intensity patent lumen and low-signal intensity wall thrombus (small arrows, *f*) is noted. Involvement of the infrarenal aorta (*f*), common iliac arteries (*g*), and common femoral arteries (*h*) is demonstrated. A Foley catheter is also noted in place (arrow, *h*). The sagittal interstitial-phase image provides direct visualization of the site of maximal anteroposterior diameter (arrow, *i*) with depiction of low-signal intensity thrombus (small arrows, *i*) in the anterior aortic wall. The origin of the superior mesenteric artery (thin arrow, *i*) is also demonstrated.

Coronal 2-mm gadolinium-enhanced 3D gradient-echo source image (*j*) and MIP reconstruction of the 2-mm 3D gradient echo sections (*k*) in a fourth patient. The source image (*j*) most clearly define the vascular abnormalities, whereas the MIP reconstructed image provides the overall topographic display (*k*). In this patient, a saccular infrarenal aortic aneurysm is clearly shown.

mural thrombus, and abdominal viscera is accomplished on the postgadolinium SGE (fig. 10.6) or fat-suppressed SGE images after the 3D acquisition (see fig. 10.5).

Inflammatory aortitis, also termed inflammatory aortic aneurysm, is an uncommon entity in which an inflammatory reaction develops around an aortic aneurysm [28]. Etiologic factors proposed by some investigators include an immune response to ceroid produced in atheromatous plaque [25], whereas other investigators have found evidence of vasculitis involving the aortic wall in patients with inflammatory aortic aneurysms and have postulated that the combination of retroperitoneal fibrosis, vasculitis, and aortic aneurysm may represent a distinct pathological entity [28]. Gadolinium-enhanced fat-suppressed SGE images demonstrate infiltrative enhancing tissue surrounding an aortic aneurysm (fig. 10.7).

Aortic Dissection

Aortic dissection usually originates in the thoracic aorta. MRI with MRA has been shown to be accurate in the detection of aortic dissection [27, 29, 30]. The noninvasive nature of the technique and the lack of nephrotoxicity are important features of MRI. Because patients may frequently have compromised renal function, the lack of nephrotoxicity is an advantage over angiography and CT imaging. Strengths of MRI include the ability to demonstrate the intimal flap [29] and entry site [11], to examine the whole length of the aorta, and occasionally to demonstrate so-called "aortic cobwebs," which are fibroelastic bands formed during the dissection process that project from the false lumen wall [31]. The detection of these bands facilitates the distinction of the false from the true lumen because they are located in the false lumen. On spin-echo images, flow in the true lumen is usually signal void, whereas flow in the false lumen can be signal void or high in signal intensity depending upon the velocity of blood flow (fig. 10.8). Slow flow in the false lumen of a dissection may be difficult to differentiate from thrombosis on spin-echo images.

The role of conventional spin-echo imaging is limited because gadolinium-enhanced SGE (2D or 3D),

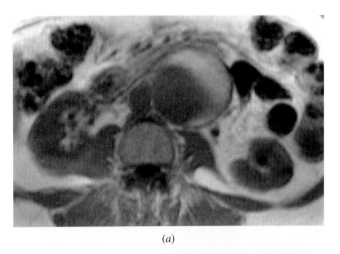

(a)

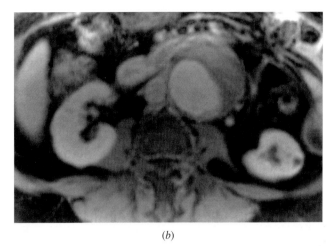

(b)

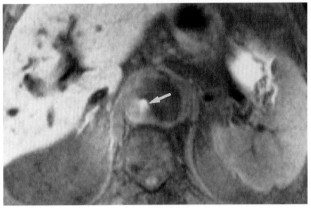

(c)

FIG. 10.6 High-signal intensity mural thrombus. Precontrast SGE (*a*) and gadolinium-enhanced fat-suppressed SGE (*b*) images. An abdominal aortic aneurysm containing high-signal intensity thrombus (arrow, *a*) is observed on the precontrast SGE image. On the postcontrast image, the lumen is opacified and the thrombus becomes relatively low signal.

T1-weighted fat-suppressed spin-echo image (*c*) in a second patient with aortic aneurysm demonstrates an aortic aneurysm with atherosclerotic plaque in its right posterior aortic wall with a high-signal intensity focus (arrow, *c*) representing clot of more recent origin.

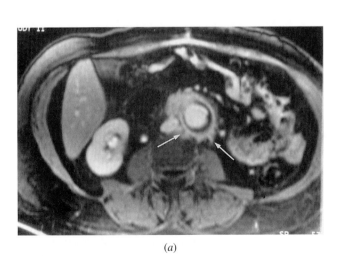

(a)

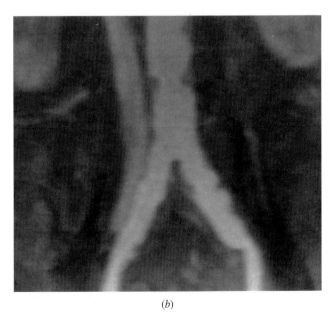

(b)

FIG. 10.7 Inflammatory aortitis. Interstitial-phase gadolinium-enhanced fat-suppressed SGE image (*a*). An aortic aneurysm is present with diffusely thickened wall and enhancing ill-defined tissue that projects (arrows) into the retroperitoneal fat surrounding the aneurysm. Enhancement of the lumen and nearly signal-void mural thrombus are also shown.

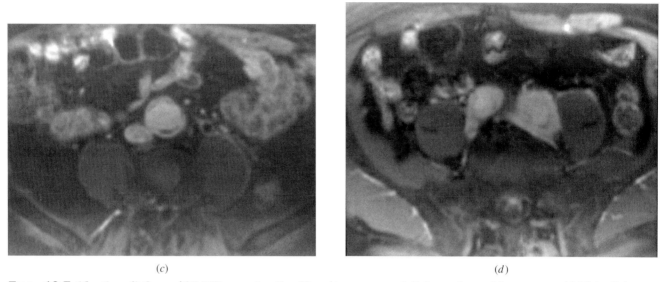

(c)   (d)

FIG. 10.7 (*Continued*) Coronal 3D MIP reconstruction (*b*) and transverse gadolinium-enhanced fat-suppressed SGE (*c, d*) images in a second patient demonstrate dilatation of the infrarenal aorta and common iliac arteries. Note the homogeneous enhancing tissue surrounding these vessels, consistent with perianeurysmal inflammation.

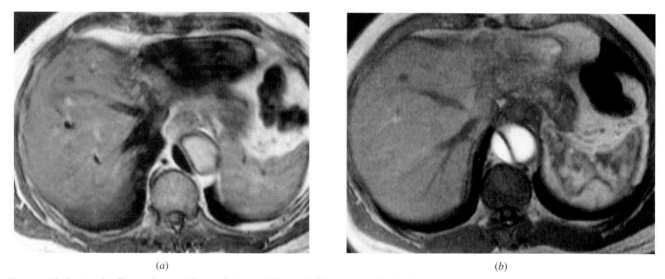

(a)   (b)

FIG. 10.8 Aortic dissection with perfusion differential between the kidneys. T1-weighted spin-echo (*a*) and immediate (*b, c*) and 90-s (*d*) postgadolinium SGE images. The T1-weighted spin-echo image (*a*) shows enlargement of the abdominal aorta, which contains an intimal flap and has a true and a false lumen. High signal intensity is noted in the false lumen because of slow flow. Note that the true lumen has a biconvex configuration because of the higher blood pressure. The immediate postgadolinium SGE image (*b*) acquired at the same tomographic level shows enhancement of both lumens with sharp demarcation of the intimal flap. The false lumen enhances substantially less than the true lumen on the immediate postgadolinium SGE image (*c*) at a lower tomographic level because of diminished contrast delivery secondary to slow flow in the false lumen. The right renal artery (arrow, *c*) is demonstrated originating from the true lumen. Intense cortical enhancement of the right kidney and minimal cortical enhancement of the left kidney is evident, reflecting the origin of the left renal artery from the false lumen. Note that on the 90-s postgadolinium SGE image (*d*) lumen and kidneys enhance to the same extent.

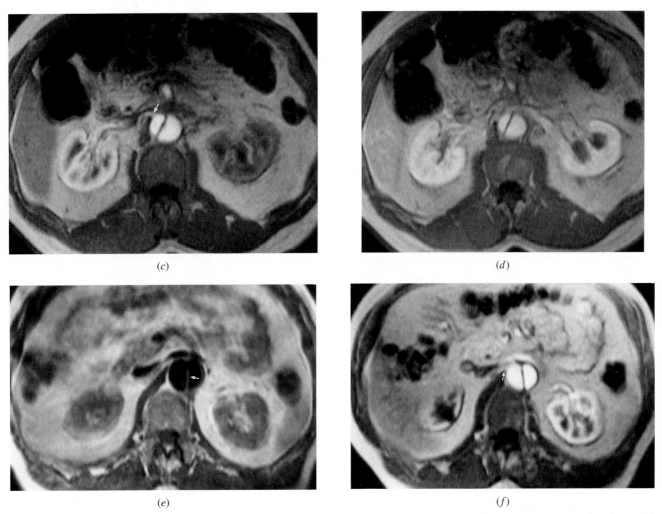

(c)

(d)

(e)

(f)

FIG. 10.8 (*Continued*) T1-weighted spin-echo (*e*) and immediate postgadolinium SGE (*f*) images in a second patient with aortic dissection. The T1-weighted spin-echo image shows an aortic aneurysm with an intimal flap (arrow, *e*). Both lumen are signal void on this image, reflecting higher blood velocity in the false lumen than observed in the first patient. The right lumen has a biconvex configuration consistent with the true lumen. High flow in both lumen is also reflected as equal enhancement on the immediate postgadolinium SGE image. The origin of the right renal artery (arrow, *f*) from the true lumen is well shown. Immediate postgadolinium SGE images in patients with aortic dissection provide hemodynamic information that is helpful in determining true and false lumens and abdominal organ arterial perfusion.

gadolinium-enhanced 3D gradient-echo (e.g., 3D FISP), and gadolinium-enhanced fat-suppressed SGE (2D or 3D) imaging are all fast, accurate, and reproducible techniques for the demonstration of dissection. Gadolinium-enhanced SGE and 3D gradient-echo techniques reliably differentiate slow flow, which is high in signal intensity on these images, from thrombus, which is low to intermediate in signal intensity (fig. 10.8). Breath-hold gadolinium-enhanced 3D gradient-echo images provide sharp detail and demonstrate the full extent of dissection, the entry site, the location of the intimal flap, and the relation of the visceral vessels to the true and false lumen (fig. 10.9). The entry site, intimal flap, and origins of the vessels are better shown on the individual sections than on the 3D MIP reconstructions. The acquisition of

two data sets provides dynamic flow information, which often demonstrates delayed enhancement of the false lumen (see fig. 10.9), which is apparent in cases with slow flow. Breath-hold immediate postgadolinium SGE images may also provide this information. Postgadolinium SGE and fat-suppressed SGE images delineate the intimal flap, demonstrate the origins of the aortic branches, and can assess extension of the dissection into the splanchnic vessels (fig. 10.10). This extension is evaluated better on transverse- than on sagittal- or coronal-plane images.

In rare instances the only finding may be wall thickening with or without high-signal intensity foci on T1-weighted images [32, 33]. The high-signal intensity foci on T1-weighted images reflect the presence of intramural hematoma. This pattern may be missed on angiography

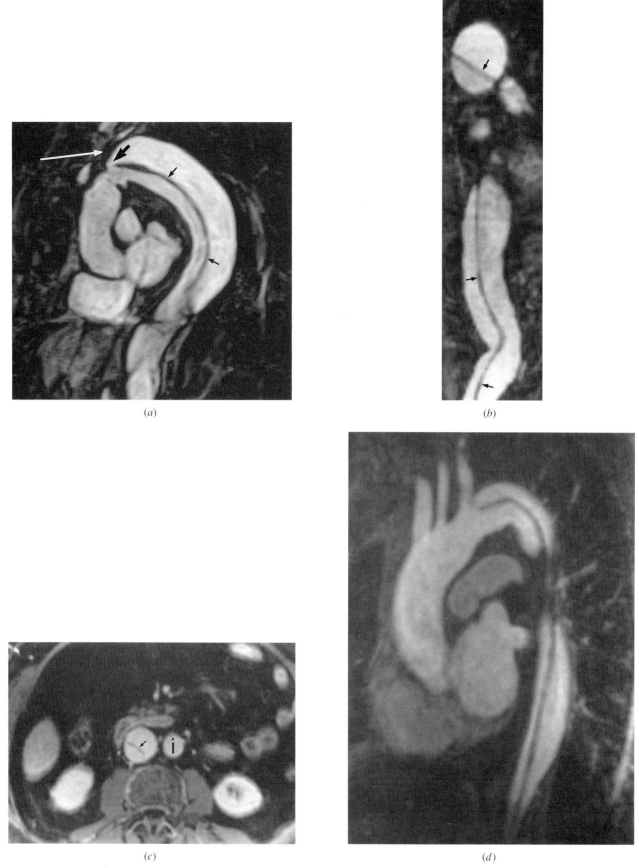

F I G . 10.9 Aortic dissection. Gadolinium-enhanced 2-mm thin-section 3D gradient-echo image (*a*) obtained in an oblique sagittal plane through the center of the lumen of the aortic arch, coronal multiplanar reconstruction (*b*) from the set of gadolinium enhanced 2-mm thin oblique sagittal 3D gradient-echo sections, and transverse interstitial-phase gadolinium-enhanced fat-suppressed SGE images (*c*) in a patient with type B aortic dissection.

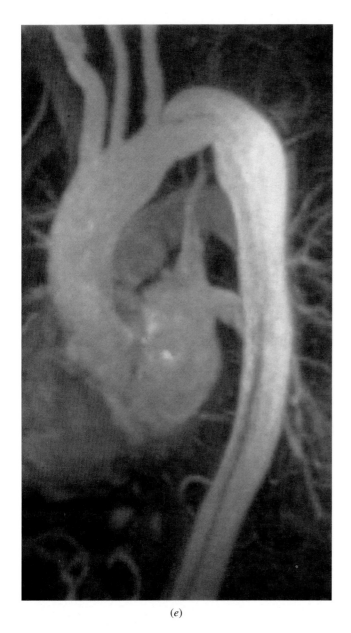

(e)

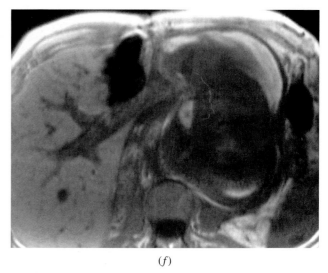

(f)

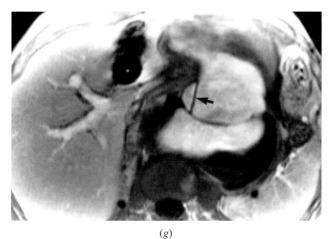

(g)

FIG. 10.9 (*Continued*) The oblique sagittal gadolinium-enhanced 3D gradient-echo image (*a*) demonstrates an aortic dissection originating in the thoracic aorta. The intimal flap (small arrows, *a–c*) is readily demonstrated as a low-signal intensity curvilinear structure. The entry site (arrow, *a*) is identified immediately distal to the origin of the left subclavian artery (long arrow, *a*). The multiplanar reconstruction (*b*) outlines the course of the dissection and demonstrates the intimal flap (small arrows, *b*) from the thoracic to the abdominal aorta. The intimal flap is well seen on the interstitial-phase gadolinium-enhanced fat suppressed SGE image (*c*) at the level of the abdominal aorta. Incidental note is made of a left-sided IVC ("*i*," *c*).

Coronal 2-mm gadolinium-enhanced 3D gradient-echo source image (*d*) and 3D MIP reconstruction of the 2-mm 3D gradient-echo sections (*e*) from a second patient show similar features of an aortic dissection.

Transverse SGE (*f*), and immediate postgadolinium SGE (*g*) images in a third patient. There is a large complex abdominal aortic saccular aneurysm associated with thrombus and dissection. The intimal flap is clearly shown (arrow, *g*) after contrast administration.

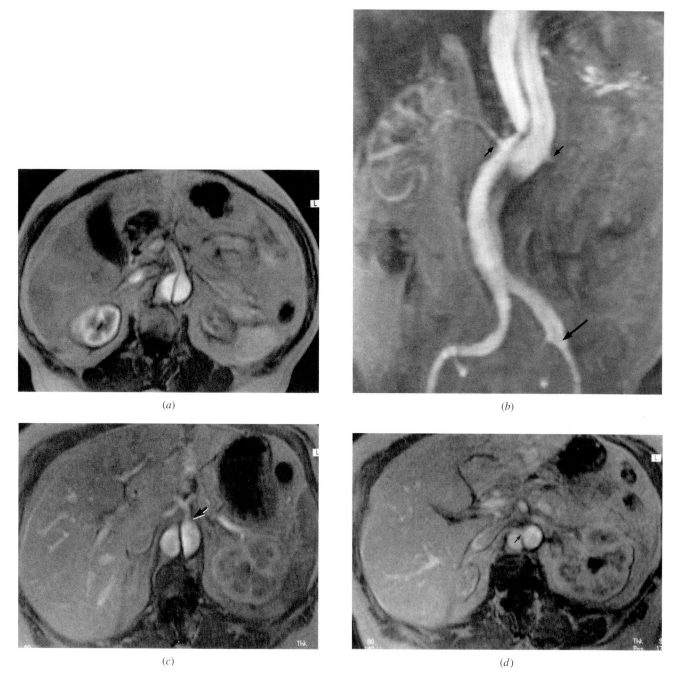

(a)

(b)

(c)

(d)

F I G . 10.10 Aortic dissection with extension into the superior mesenteric artery. Immediate postgadolinium SGE image (*a*) and coronal projection (*b*) from 3D MIP reconstruction of a set of coronal immediate postgadolinium SGE images obtained in a follow-up study. The immediate postgadolinium SGE image (*a*) at the level of the origin of the superior mesenteric artery shows high signal intensity, gadolinium-containing true (right) and false (left) lumens, and extension of the intimal flap into the superior mesenteric artery. The coronal projection from the 3D MIP reconstruction shows the abdominal aorta and iliac arteries, with the intimal flap extending into the external iliac artery (arrow, *b*). The ostia of the renal arteries are clearly depicted (small arrows, *b*), whereas the left renal artery and kidney are not visualized because of decreased enhancement from slow blood flow in the false lumen.

Immediate postgadolinium SGE images (*c, d*) at two tomographic levels in a second patient. The high-signal intensity gadolinium-containing aorta is clearly shown on both images. The intimal flap is well shown as are the origins of the celiac axis (arrow, *c*) and right renal artery (small arrow, *d*) from the true lumen.

and has been postulated to represent the early stage of dissection with hemorrhage from the vasa vasorum that leads to aortic wall weakening and subsequent intimal rupture [32, 33]. In one report, the transition from this appearance to classic dissection with intimal flap and blood flow in the false lumen was documented on follow-up studies in two patients [33].

Penetrating Aortic Ulcers and Intramural Dissecting Hematoma

Penetrating aortic ulcers result from ulcerated atherosclerotic plaques that penetrate the internal elastic lamina and may lead to hematoma formation within the media of the aortic wall, false aneurysm, and finally transmural rupture of the aorta. They are more commonly located in the descending thoracic or upper abdominal aorta (fig. 10.11) [34]. In cases of intramural dissecting hematoma the intimal flap is not often seen and is irregular and thick. The intramural hematoma rarely fills with contrast and is usually seen to extend both cephalad and caudal to the entry site, which is at the penetrating atherosclerotic ulcer. Extensive atherosclerotic changes are usually present in the aorta [34]. It is important to differentiate this entity from aortic dissection because management may be different. MRI can demonstrate intramural hematoma, atherosclerotic ulcer, and false aneurysm [34, 35] and is superior to angiography in depicting the extent of intramural thrombus. MRI may be similar or superior to CT imaging in differentiating acute hematoma from atherosclerotic plaque and chronic thrombus [35]. Intramural hematoma is high in signal intensity on both T1- and T2-weighted images and can be differentiated from chronic mural thrombus, which is low in signal intensity [35]. The combination of gadolinium-enhanced

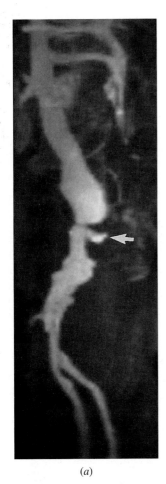

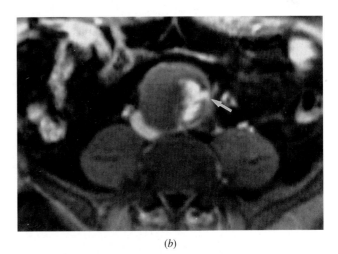

(a)   (b)

F I G . 10.11 Penetrating aortic ulcer. Lateral MIP projection of a set of gadolinium-enhanced 2-mm coronal 3D gradient-echo sections (a), and transverse interstitial-phase gadolinium-enhanced fat-suppressed SGE (b) images. An atherosclerotic aneurysm of the infrarenal abdominal aorta is present. An ulceration of the atherosclerotic plaque (arrow, a, b) is demonstrated on the lateral MIP projection. On the interstitial-phase gadolinium-enhanced fat-suppressed SGE image (b) the diameter of the aortic aneurysm and the presence of mural thrombus are well evaluated. The depth of the ulceration in relation to the outer aortic wall is appreciated. Interstitial-phase gadolinium-enhanced fat-suppressed SGE images provide information on the aortic wall and the surrounding tissues that are not available on MR angiographic images.

3D gradient-echo images to define the aortic lumen and gadolinium-enhanced fat-suppressed SGE images to demonstrate the wall thickness in deep aortic ulcers may be the most effective means for evaluating this entity (see fig. 10.11).

Aortoiliac Atherosclerotic Disease—Thrombosis

Gadolinium-enhanced SGE or fat-suppressed SGE images may demonstrate gross atherosclerotic changes of the aorta and iliac arteries. Gadolinium-enhanced 3D gradient-echo images can reliably assess atherosclerotic changes and stenosis of the aorta (fig. 10.12) and iliac arteries (figs. 10.13 and 10.14) and are able to demonstrate the lumen of the stenotic segment and the immediate

poststenotic area (see fig. 10.13) because they do not suffer from dephasing, reverse flow or in-plane saturation phenomena compared with time-of-flight techniques.

Occlusion of the abdominal aorta and its branches may occur in advanced thrombotic disease or dissection. Gadolinium-enhanced SGE images permit clear distinction between high-signal intensity patent lumen and low-signal intensity thrombosed lumen (fig. 10.15). Coronal or sagittal images are useful to confirm the level of occlusion (figs. 10.15 and 10.16).

Postoperative Aortic Graft Evaluation

Postoperative complications of abdominal aortic graft surgery include occlusion, hemorrhage with false

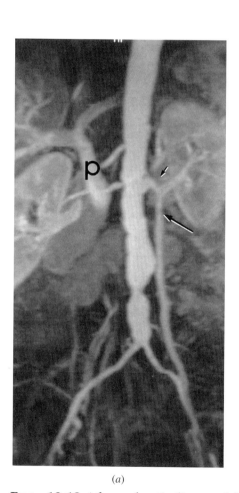

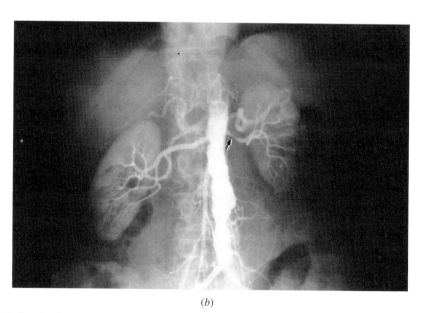

(a)   *(b)*

F I G . 10.12 Atherosclerotic disease of the abdominal aorta. Coronal 3D MIP reconstruction of gadolinium enhanced 2 mm source images (*a*) and anteroposterior conventional arteriography image (*b*). Diffuse atherosclerotic disease of the abdominal aorta with irregularity of the contour and focal stenotic and dilated segments is demonstrated on the 3D MIP image (*a*). Close correlation of the MRI findings with the intra-arterial catheter angiographic image (*b*) is present. The image acquisition timing in this case was slightly delayed, and the 3D gradient echo images were acquired during the capillary rather than the arterial phase of enhancement, as evidenced by the presence of enhanced portal vein (*p, a*) and right renal vein. Enhancement of the left renal vein partially masks a stenosis (small arrow, *a, b*) of the left renal artery. Targeted 3D MIP reconstructions of the left renal artery revealed this stenosis. Note early retrograde filling of the left ovarian vein (arrow, *a*).

Coronal 3D MIP reconstruction of gadolinium enhanced 2 mm source images (*c*) in a second patient shows irregular contour of the aorta (small arrows, *c*) due to diffuse atherosclerotic changes. Note normal renal arteries (long arrows, *c*) bilaterally. The common hepatic artery (short arrow, *c*) and splenic artery (hollow arrow, *c*) are also demonstrated.

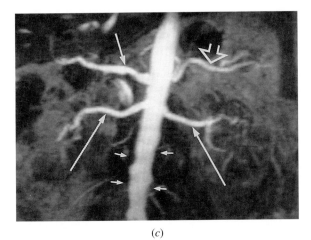

(c)

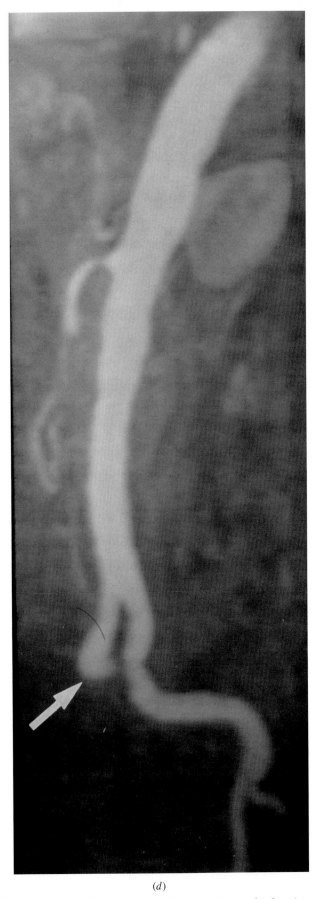

(d)

F I G. 10.12 (*Continued*) Coronal 3D MIP reconstruction of gadolinium enhanced 2 mm source images (*d*) in a third patient demonstrates slight irregularity of the abdominal aorta associated with stenoses of the celiac axis and superior mesenteric artery and occlusion of the right common iliac artery (arrow, *d*).

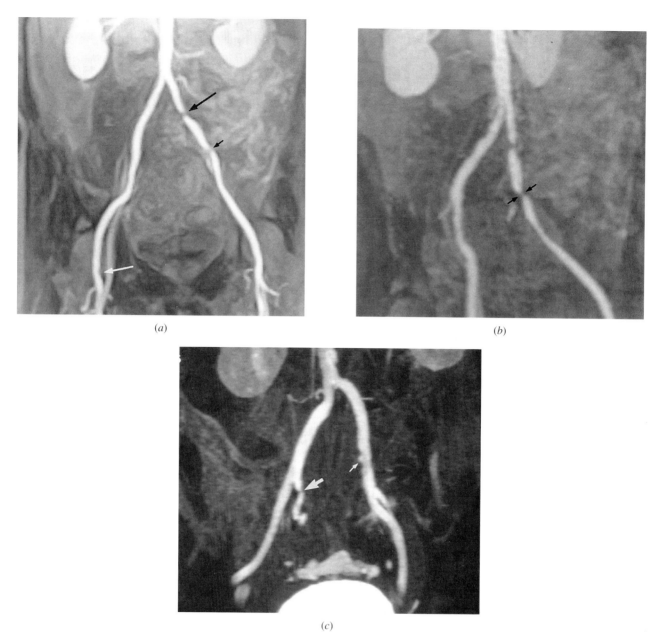

(a)

(b)

(c)

F I G . 10.13 Stenosis of the left common and external iliac arteries. Coronal (*a*) and right anterior oblique (*b*) 3D MIP reconstructions of gadolinium enhanced 2 mm source images. High-grade stenoses are demonstrated of the left common iliac (black arrow, *a*) and left external iliac (small black arrow, *a*) arteries. Irregularity of the vessel contour from diffuse atherosclerotic disease and a more prominent eccentric plaque at the right common femoral artery (white arrow, *a*) are also noted. On the oblique image (*b*) vessel lumen distal to the high-grade stenoses and the lumen of the stenotic segment (small arrows, *b*) are well visualized, reflecting negligible signal loss from dephasing. This is due to the very short echo time of the sequence combined with the T1 shortening from gadolinium enhancement. The internal iliac arteries are not adequately visualized because of their location outside the obtained 3D slab.

Coronal 3D MIP reconstruction of gadolinium enhanced 2 mm source images (*c*) in a second patient with diabetes mellitus and recent onset of impotence. A high-grade stenosis (arrow, *c*) of the right internal iliac artery is demonstrated 1 cm from its origin. The lumen immediately distal to the stenotic area is well visualized because of minimized dephasing despite turbulent flow. An ulcerated atherosclerotic plaque (small arrow, *c*) in the left common iliac artery is also present. The peripheral segments of the internal iliac arteries are not visualized because of their course outside the acquired 3D slab.

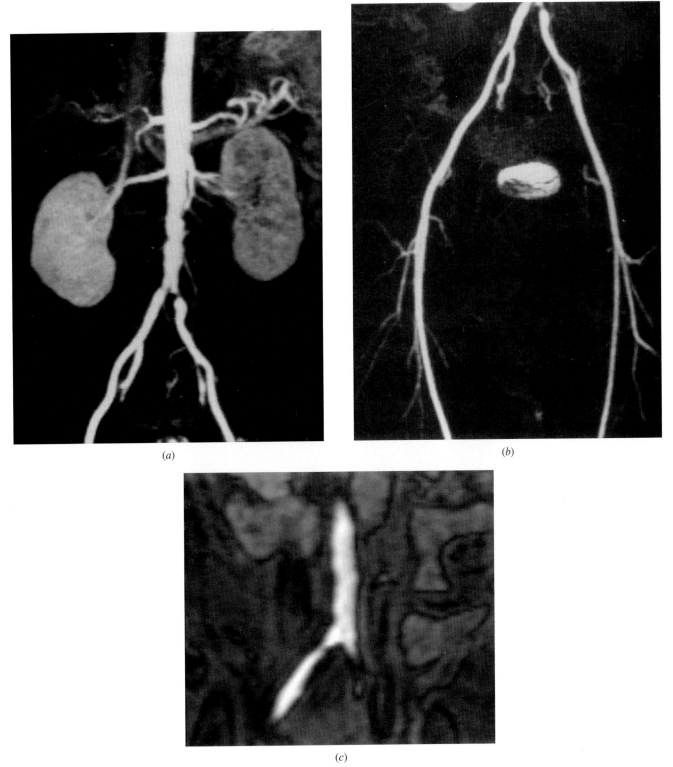

(a)

(b)

(c)

F I G . 10.14 Stenosis of the iliac arteries. Coronal 3D MIP reconstructions of gadolinium enhanced 2 mm source images from abdominal (*a*) and pelvic (*b*) acquisitions demonstrate stenosis of the left common and left internal left iliac arteries. Note irregularity of the infrarenal abdominal aorta from atherosclerotic disease.

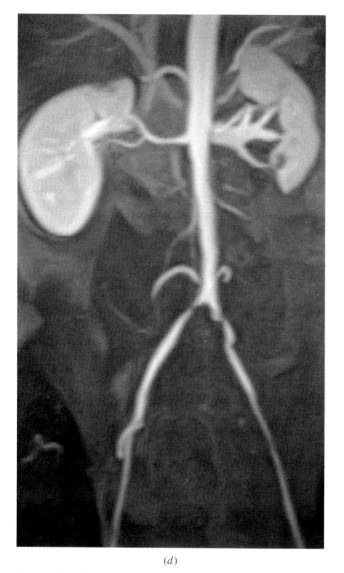

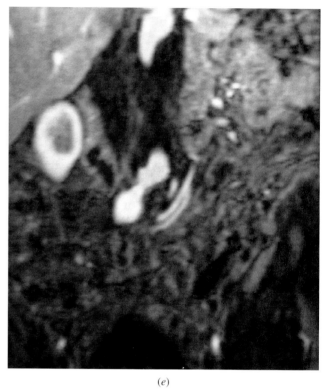

(d)   (e)

F I G . 10.14 (*Continued*) Coronal gadolinium-enhanced 2-mm 3D gradient-echo source image (*c*) and 3D MIP reconstruction of the 3D gradient-echo images (*d*) in a second patient. There are bilateral stenoses of the common iliac arteries, more severe on the left. The source image better defines the severity of stenosis.

Coronal gadolinium-enhanced 2-mm 3D gradient-echo source image (*e*) and 3D MIP reconstruction of the 3D gradient-echo images (*f*) in a third patient. Moderate stenosis at the bifurcation of the abdominal aorta is seen associated with severe stenosis at the origin of the right common iliac artery. There is a fusiform expansion of the right common iliac artery just distal to the stenosis, with another segment of severe stenosis more distal.

aneurysm formation, infection, and aortoenteric fistula formation. Complications are well shown on MR images [19]. Although some of these complications can occur acutely in the postoperative period, it is generally agreed that MR imaging should not be performed before 4–6 weeks after surgery to allow endothelial repair and reduction of risk for injury due to surgical clip dislodgement. Fluid is frequently present surrounding the graft within 3 months after surgery (fig. 10.17). Fluid surrounding the graft beyond 3 months or an

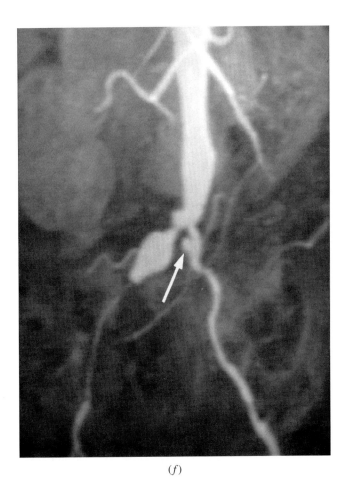

(f)

FIG. 10.14 (*Continued*) Note also a moderate stenosis of the origin of the left common iliac artery, with a small saccular aneurysm (arrow, *f*). The source image (*e*) identifies the true extent of stenosis.

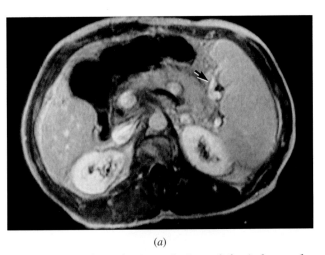

(a)

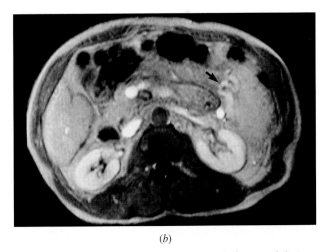

(b)

FIG. 10.15 Thrombotic occlusion of the infrarenal aorta. Transverse (*a, b*) and coronal (*c*) interstitial-phase gadolinium-enhanced SGE images. The lumen of the abdominal aorta demonstrates normal enhancement at the level of celiac axis origin (*a*). On the SGE image at a lower tomographic level (*b*), lack of enhancement of the aortic lumen reflects thrombotic occlusion. The abrupt transition (arrows, *c*) of enhancing patent to low-signal intensity thrombosed lumen is demonstrated on the coronal image. This patient was assessed for multifocal hepatocellular carcinoma, and a tumor nodule (hollow arrow, *c*) is demonstrated in the right lobe of the liver. Splenomegaly with varices (arrows, *a, b*) is also present in this patient because of portal hypertension secondary to alcoholic cirrhosis.

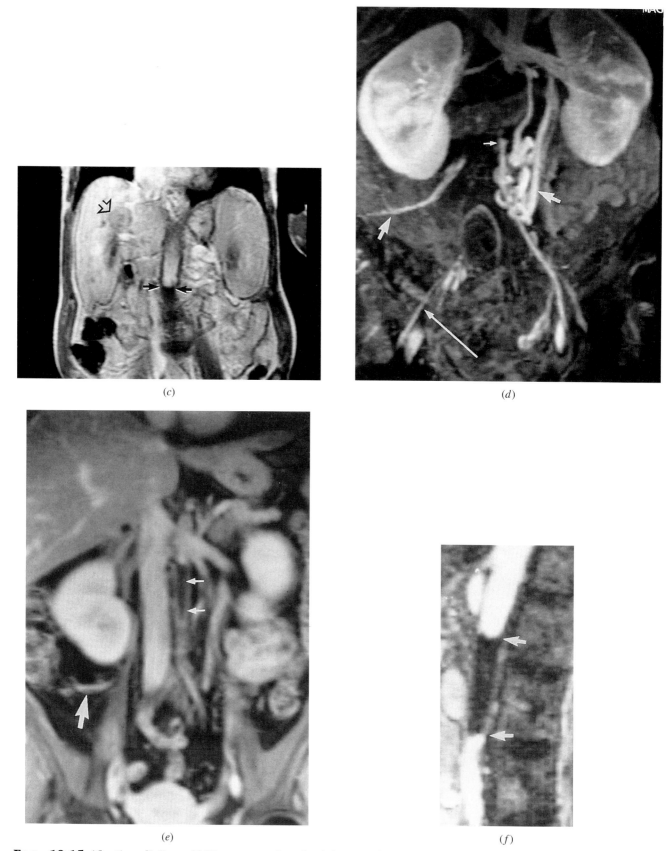

FIG. 10.15 (*Continued*) Coronal MIP reconstruction of gadolinium enhanced 2 mm source images (*d*) coronal interstitial-phase gadolinium-enhanced fat-suppressed SGE image (*e*), and sagittal multiplanar reconstruction of gadolinium enhanced 2 mm source images (*f*) in a second patient with infrarenal aortic occlusion.

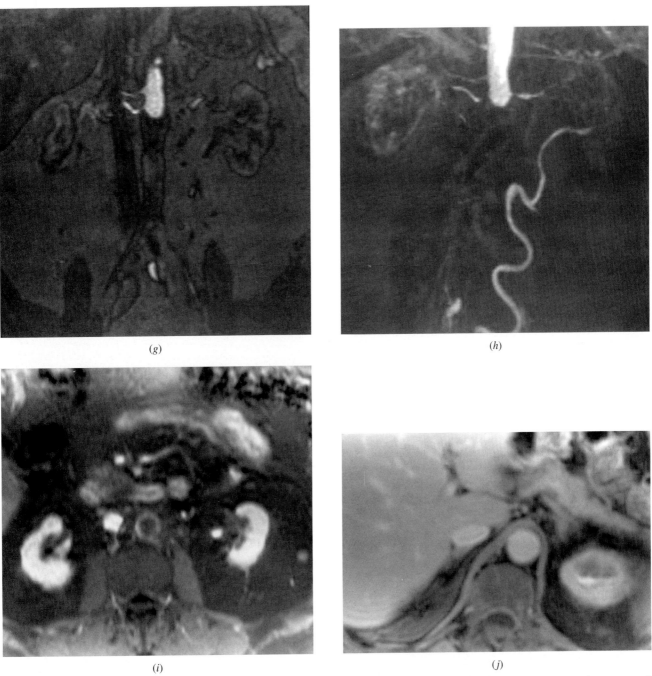

(g)

(h)

(i)

(j)

F I G. 10.15 (*Continued*) Complete occlusion of the infrarenal aorta 1 cm below the level of the renal arteries is demonstrated on the coronal MIP image (*d*). The lumen of the aorta (small arrow, *d*) is reconstituted distally, through numerous retroperitoneal collateral vessels (arrows, *d*). The left common iliac artery is patent, whereas the right common iliac artery is occluded at its origin with reconstitution at the level of the distal external iliac artery (long arrow, *d*). Thrombus (small arrows, *e*) in the infrarenal aorta and a large retroperitoneal collateral (arrow, *e*) are demonstrated on the interstitial-phase gadolinium-enhanced fat-suppressed SGE image (*e*). The sagittal 2-mm thin reconstruction (*f*) through the center of the aortic lumen clearly demonstrates the superior and inferior margins (arrows, *f*) of the near signal-void thrombus against the homogeneous high-signal intensity gadolinium-enhanced patent lumen. The acquisition of a volume of data with thin sections permits excellent resolution for multiplanar reconstructions.

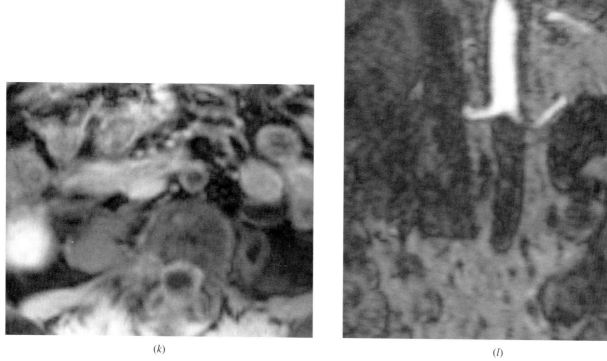

(k)   (l)

FIG. 10.15 (*Continued*) Coronal gadolinium-enhanced 2-mm 3D gradient-echo source image (*g*), 3D MIP reconstruction of the 3D gradient-echo images (*h*) and transverse interstitial-phase gadolinium-enhanced fat-suppressed SGE (*i*) images in a third patient also demonstrate complete aortic obstruction. Note the lack of enhancement of the distal abdominal aorta (*i*). The MRA images demonstrate that the renal arteries are patent, there are two right renal arteries, and bilateral moderate renal artery stenosis is present.

Transverse interstitial-phase gadolinium-enhanced fat-suppressed SGE (*j*, *k*) and coronal gadolinium-enhanced 2-mm 3D gradient-echo source (*l*) images in a fourth patient. Note the transition of opacified (*j*) to nonopacified (*k*) lumen on transverse images, which is clearly shown in the coronal plane.

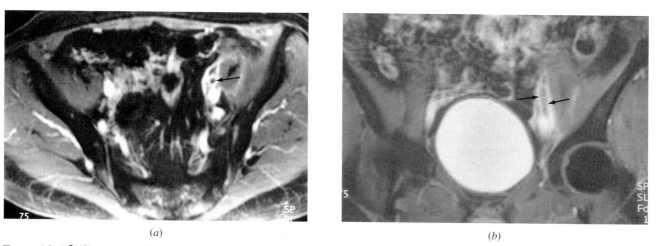

(a)   (b)

FIG. 10.16 **Iliac artery thrombosis.** Transverse (*a*) and coronal (*b*) interstitial-phase gadolinium-enhanced fat-suppressed SGE images. The left external iliac artery is identified medial to the psoas muscle on the transverse image (*a*) and contains low signal intensity thrombus (arrow, *a*). The presence of intraluminal thrombus (arrows, *b*) is confirmed on the coronal image. Postgadolinium SGE images, acquired within 2 min after gadolinium injection and performed as part of routine abdominal and pelvic MR imaging protocols, provide a reproducible technique for the assessment of the patency of large and medium-sized arteries and veins.

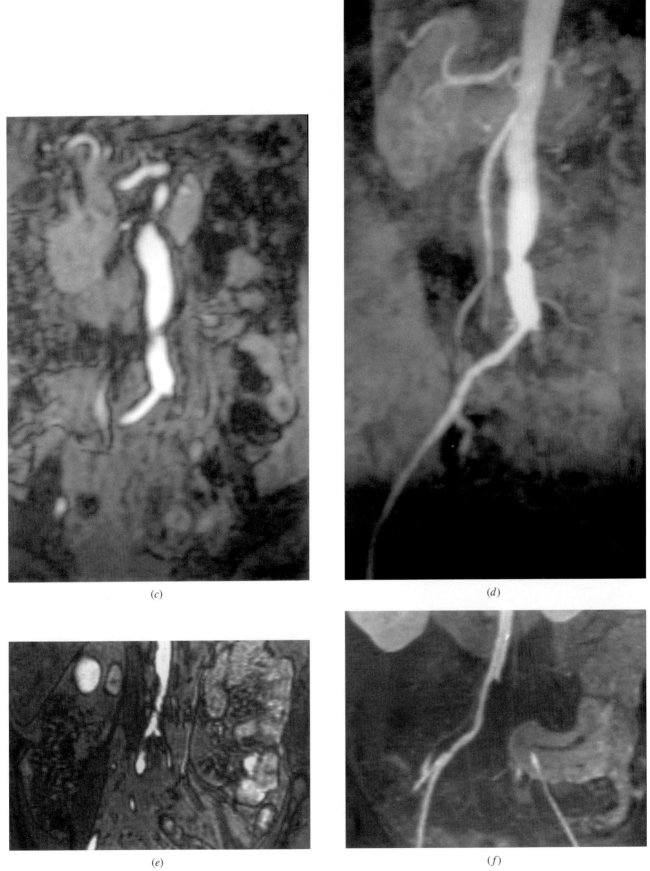

(c)

(d)

(e)

(f)

F I G . 10.16 (*Continued*) Coronal gadolinium-enhanced 2-mm 3D gradient-echo source image (*c*) and 3D MIP reconstruction of the 3D gradient-echo images (*d*) in a second patient demonstrate distal abdominal aortic stenosis and occlusion of the left common iliac artery.

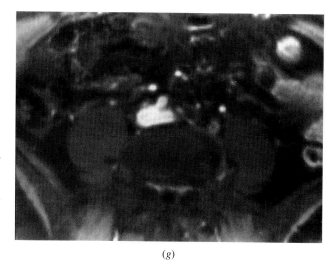

(g)

FIG. 10.16 (*Continued*) Careful attention to the source images (*c*) reveal no contiguous distal opacification of the vessel.

Coronal gadolinium-enhanced 2-mm 3D gradient-echo source (*e*), 3D MIP reconstruction of the 3D gradient-echo images (*f*), and transverse interstitial-phase gadolinium-enhanced fat-suppressed SGE (*g*) images in a fourth patient show obstruction of the left common iliac artery.

increasing volume of perigraft fluid after 3 months is suggestive of infection on T1- and T2-weighted images [19, 36, 37]. Gadolinium-enhanced fat-suppressed imaging may also be an ideal technique for evaluating inflammatory enhancement in aortic graft infections

(fig. 10.18). Gadolinium-enhanced fat-suppressed SGE images are preferable to gadolinium-enhanced T1-weighted fat-suppressed spin-echo images because patency of the graft lumen can also be assessed reliably with the SGE sequence. Patent lumen is high in signal

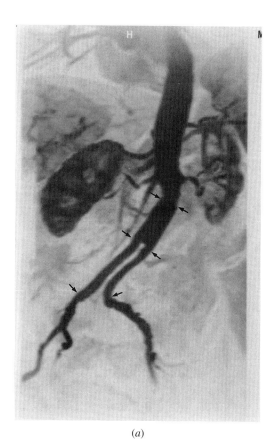

(a)

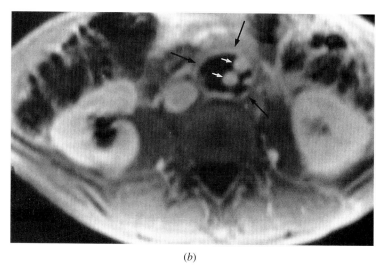

(b)

FIG. 10.17 Aortobifemoral graft after surgery. A 3D MIP reconstruction of gadolinium enhanced 2 mm source images (*a*) and transverse (*b*) and coronal (*c*) interstitial-phase gadolinium-enhanced fat-suppressed SGE images in a patient with Marfan's syndrome 1 month after surgery.

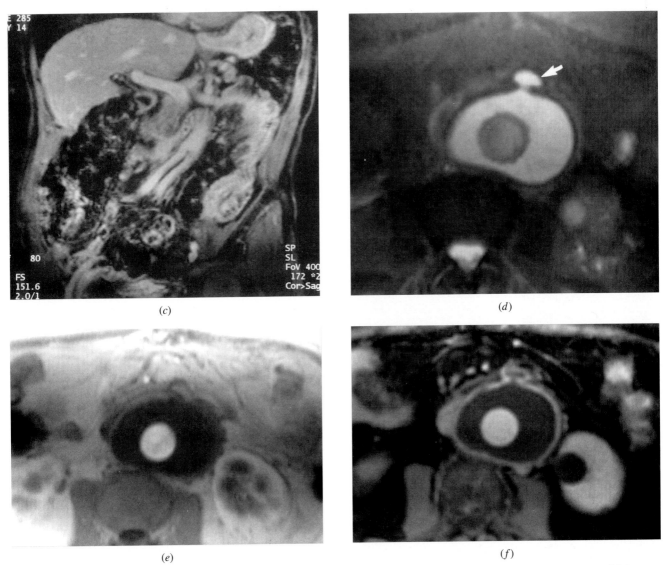

(c)

(d)

(e)

(f)

F I G . 10.17 (*Continued*) The MIP image (*a*) demonstrates an abdominal aortic aneurysm with a maximal diameter of 4.5 cm at the level of the upper pole of the left kidney. More distally within the abdominal aorta, an aortoiliac graft is identified (small arrows, *a*). Irregularity of the luminal contour is noted distal to the graft because of atherosclerotic disease. The transverse 1-min postgadolinium fat-suppressed SGE image shows the patent lumens of the limbs of the graft (small arrows, *b*) surrounded by low-signal intensity postoperative fluid contained within the wall (arrows, *b*) of the native aorta. The patency of the graft is also shown on the coronal interstitial-phase gadolinium-enhanced fat-suppressed SGE image (*c*).

T2-weighted fat-suppressed SS-ETSE (*d*), immediate postgadolinium SGE (*e*) and interstitial-phase gadolinium-enhanced fat-suppressed SGE (*f*) images in a second patient, with recent history of aortobifemoral graft surgery, demonstrate the presence of perigraft fluid. A small pocket of fluid is noted along the incision margin of the aneurysm (arrow, *d*).

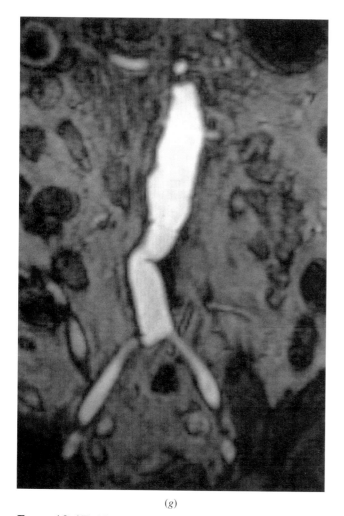

(g)

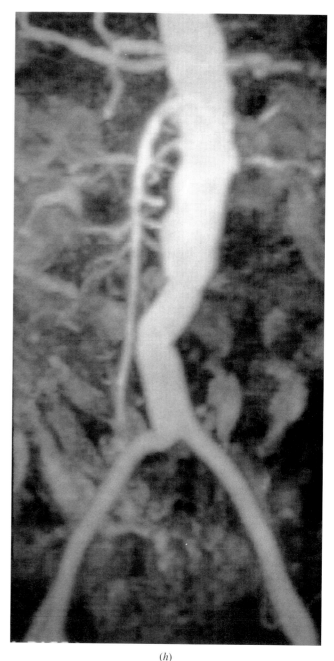

(h)

FIG. 10.17 (*Continued*) Coronal immediate postgadolinium 2-mm 3D gradient-echo source image (*g*) and MIP reconstruction of the 2-mm 3D source images (*h*) demonstrate a normal appearance for the vascular graft.

intensity, and intraluminal thrombus is low to inter-mediate in signal intensity. Inflammatory tissue shows substantial enhancement, and fluid collections/abscesses will have low central signal intensity.

Endoluminal placement of aortic grafts is a proce-dure that is gaining in popularity because of the lower risks associated with this procedure compared with open surgical graft placement. MRI may be used to ensure ad-equate position of the graft (figs. 10.19 and 10.20) and to examine for complications.

Inferior Vena Cava

As with the aorta, the IVC may be evaluated with bright-blood and black-blood techniques [38, 39]. The IVC may be evaluated for the presence of thrombus, differenti-ation of blood from tumor thrombus, and in rare in-stances, for the evaluation of primary tumors. In the vast majority of cases an abdominal protocol employ-ing precontrast SGE and postgadolinium SGE and/or fat-suppressed SGE images provides sufficient evaluation

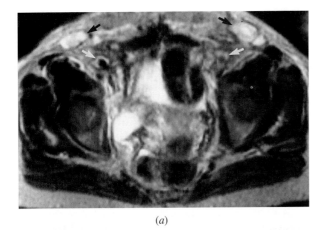

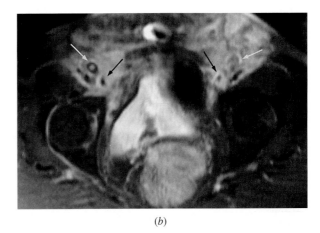

(a)

(b)

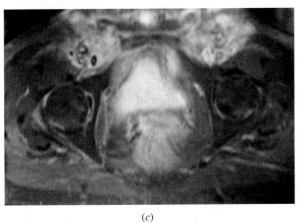

(c)

FIG. 10.18 Infected aortobifemoral graft. T2-weighted spin-echo (*a*) and gadolinium-enhanced T1-weighted fat-suppressed spin-echo (*b, c*) images. High-signal intensity fluid (white arrows, *a*) is demonstrated on the T2-weighted image (*a*) surrounding the wall of the infected graft. The subcutaneous fat in the groins and anterior abdominal wall is heterogeneously high in signal intensity reflecting the presence of inflammation, and bilateral enlarged inguinal lymph nodes (black arrows, *a*) are noted. Intense enhancement of the surrounding soft tissue and the walls of the grafts (black arrows, *b*) as well as the walls of the common femoral veins (white arrows, *b*) is demonstrated on gadolinium-enhanced T1-weighted fat-suppressed spin-echo images, reflecting severe inflammatory changes.

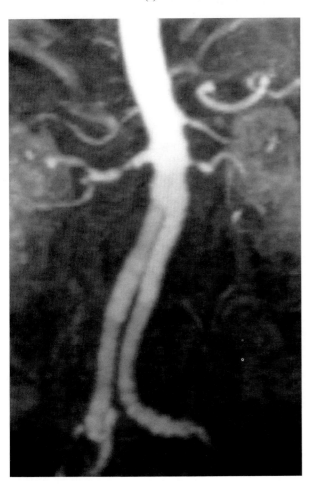

FIG. 10.19 Endovascular graft. Coronal 3D MIP reconstruction of gadolinium enhanced 2-mm source images demonstrates an abdominal aortic aneurysm and the presence of a patent endovascular stent graft.

897

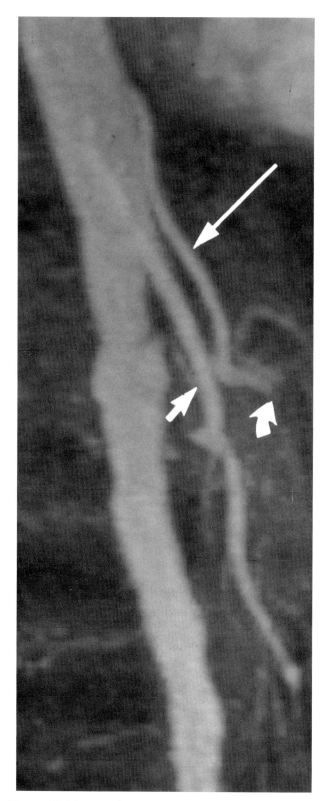

FIG. 10.20 Vascular graft to branch vessel. Sagittal 3D MIP reconstruction of gadolinium enhanced 2 mm source images in a patient with thoracic aortic grafts, one to the celiac axis (long arrow) and another to the SMA (short arrow). The SMA distal to the graft is patent. The splenic artery distal to the celiac graft is thrombosed (curved arrow).

of the IVC for patient management. At least one sequence should be performed in the sagittal or coronal plane, such as gadolinium-enhanced SGE or, preferably, fat-suppressed SGE images, because it permits direct visualization of the longitudinal extent of the IVC, which is ideal in examining for the extent of blood or tumor thrombus. Breath-hold time-of-flight techniques are less effective at demonstrating slow flow than gadolinium-enhanced SGE techniques. Gadolinium-enhanced MRA of the IVC is not usually performed because preferential venous enhancement requires suppression of the arterial signal by presaturation pulses, which are not effective at overcoming the extreme T1 shortening caused by gadolinium. Alternatively when 3D venography-like images are required to answer complicated clinical problems, immediate postgadolinium breath-hold 3D gradient-echo techniques (e.g., breath-hold coronal 3D FISP acquisition) may be performed during the simultaneous injection of gadolinium in peripheral veins of both legs. This technique provides thin (2 mm) slice resolution but is seldom needed in routine clinical practice. There is also the theoretical risk of dislodgement of deep venous thrombi leading to pulmonary emboli, particularly in nonambulatory patients.

Congenital Abnormalities

Congenital abnormalities of the inferior vena cava and related veins are common [38–42]. The most common venous anomalies are those of the left renal vein. Retroaortic left renal vein is the most common (fig. 10.21) [40–42], with other anomalies such as circumaortic left renal vein (fig. 10.22) being less common. A combination of a black-blood technique (e.g., T1-weighted spin-echo or SGE with inferior presaturation pulses) and a bright-blood technique (dynamic gadolinium-enhanced SGE or, preferably, fat-suppressed SGE imaging)

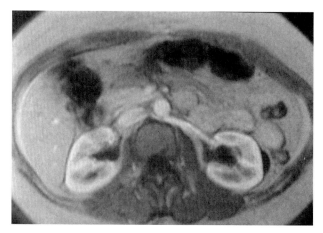

FIG. 10.21 Retroaortic left renal vein. The immediate postgadolinium SGE image demonstrates a retroaortic left renal vein entering the IVC.

is useful to determine whether rounded or tubular retroperitoneal structures are vascular in nature [43]. Left-sided vena cava (fig. 10.23), duplicated vena cava (fig. 10.24), and IVC interruption with azygous/ hemi-azygous continuation are not uncommon anomalies, which are well shown by MRI. Gadolinium enhancement is useful because in noncontrast images duplicated IVC, thrombophlebitis of the left-sided IVC, and existing retroperitoneal collateral vessels may mimic retroperitoneal lymphadenopathy [44].

Venous Thrombosis

MRI performs well in evaluating IVC thrombosis [45, 46] and distinguishing tumor from blood thrombus. Gadolinium-enhanced SGE or fat-suppressed SGE images are useful for these determinations. Tumor thrombus enhances, whereas blood (also termed bland)

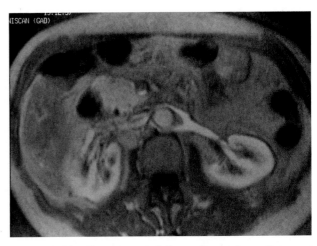

F I G . 10.22 Circumaortic left renal vein. Immediate post-gadolinium SGE image clearly defines both limbs of the circumaortic left renal vein with their entry into the IVC.

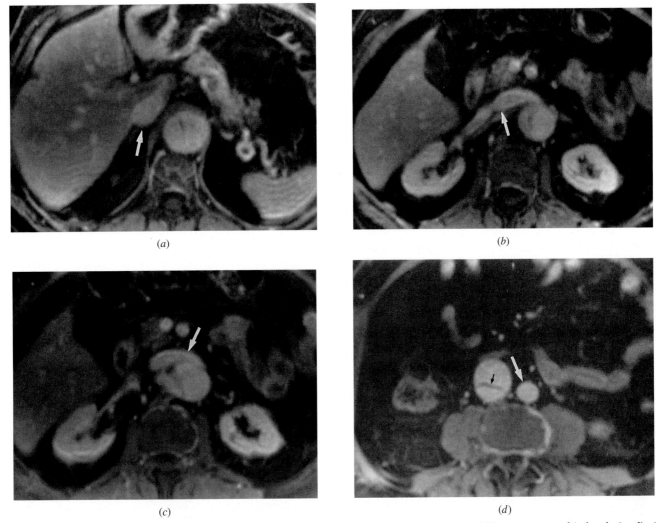

(a)

(b)

(c)

(d)

F I G . 10.23 Left-sided IVC. Transverse 90-s postgadolinium fat-suppressed SGE images at different tomographic levels (*a–d*). A right-sided suprarenal IVC is demonstrated on the most cranial image (arrow, *a*). At the level of the renal veins, the IVC (arrow, *b*) crosses over the aorta to the left and the infrarenal IVC (arrow, *c, d*) is left-sided (*c*). An aortic dissection is also present with the intimal flap (small arrow, *d*) shown in the contrast-enhanced aortic lumen.

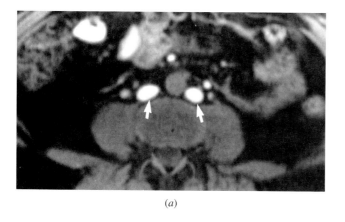

(a)

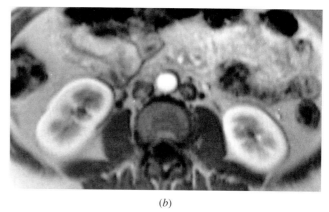

(b)

FIG. 10.24 Duplicated IVC. Noncontrast fat-suppressed SGE (a), immediate postgadolinium (b), and interstitial-phase gadolinium-enhanced SGE (c) images in a patient with duplicated IVC. The noncontrast T1-weighted image shows high-signal time-of-flight effects in venous structures on the inferior sections of the data acquisition. The bilateral IVC's (arrows, a) are clearly appreciated with the time-of-flight effects. The capillary phase image (b) shows lack of enhancement of the IVC's early postcontrast, which then become opacified on the interstitial-phase image (c). Combining morphologic and directional flow information on the precontrast images with dynamic temporal flow information on serial postgadolinium SGE images permits evaluation of congenital vascular variations and malformations.

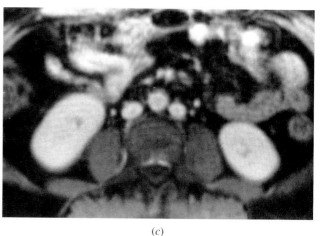

(c)

thrombus does not enhance with contrast (figs. 10.25–10.27) [47]. Signal intensity measurements of thrombus before and after gadolinium administration may be necessary because blood thrombus, which is subacute or responding to anticoagulant therapy, may be high in signal intensity on precontrast images. Lack of increase

in signal intensity on postcontrast images would confirm the blood nature of the thrombus. Flow-sensitive gradient-echo techniques with a lower flip angle (30–45°) may distinguish tumor from blood thrombus. Tumor thrombus is intermediate (soft tissue) in signal intensity on these sequences, whereas blood thrombus is

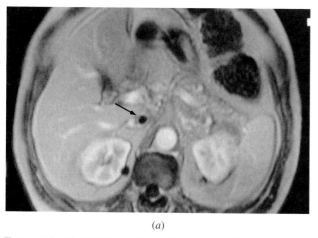

(a)

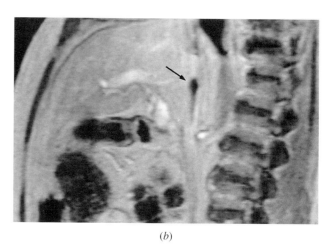

(b)

FIG. 10.25 IVC thrombosis. Transverse 45-s (a) and sagittal 90-s (b) postgadolinium SGE images. Bland thrombus (arrow, a, b) appears nearly signal void on gadolinium-enhanced SGE images.

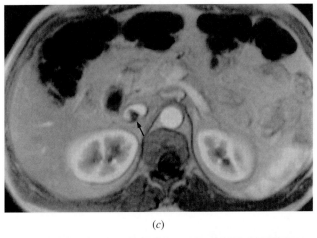

(c)

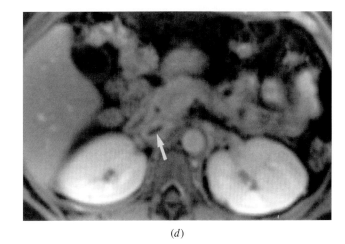

(d)

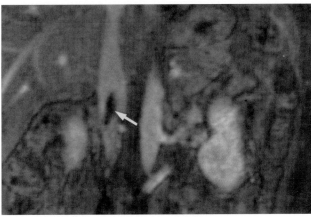

(e)

F I G . 10.25 (*Continued*) The 45-s postgadolinium SGE image (*c*) in a second patient demonstrates low- to intermediate-signal intensity thrombus (arrow, *c*) attached to the posterior wall of the IVC. The combination of intense enhancement of the IVC on gadolinium-enhanced SGE images with multiplanar imaging renders MRI an excellent, minimally invasive modality for the assessment of venous thrombosis.

Gadolinium-enhanced interstitial-phase SGE images (*d, e*) in a third patient show a nonocclusive low-signal intensity structure (arrows, *d, e*) within the lumen of the infrahepatic IVC consistent with thrombus. Imaging in two planes is useful to verify patency or thrombosis of vessels.

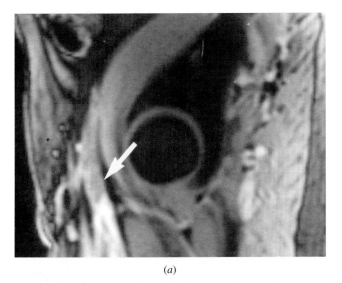

(a)

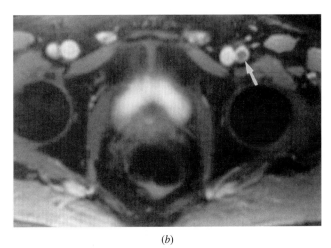

(b)

F I G . 10.26 Venous thrombosis. Sagittal (*a*) and transverse (*b*) interstitial-phase gadolinium-enhanced fat-suppressed SGE images demonstrate nonenhancing very low-signal intensity tissue (arrows, *a, b*) within the lumen of the left external iliac vein consistent with venous thrombus.

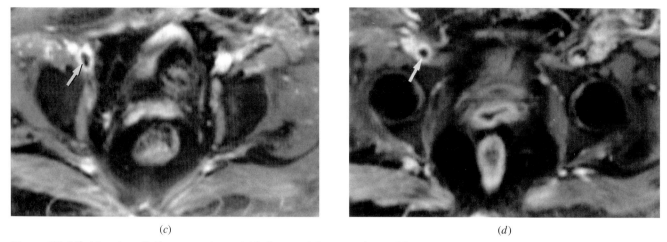

(c)   (d)

F I G . 10.26 (*Continued*) Transverse interstitial-phase gadolinium-enhanced fat-suppressed SGE images (*c, d*) in a second patient show the same finding within the right common femoral vein (arrows, *c, d*).

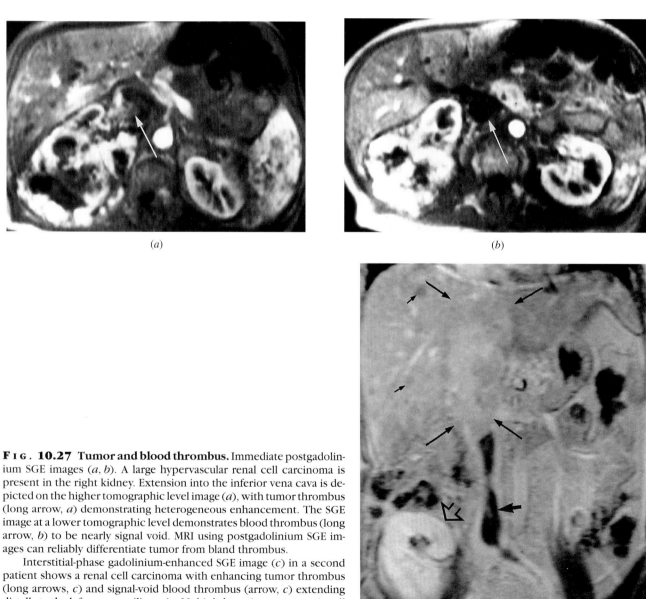

(a)   (b)

F I G . 10.27 Tumor and blood thrombus. Immediate postgadolinium SGE images (*a, b*). A large hypervascular renal cell carcinoma is present in the right kidney. Extension into the inferior vena cava is depicted on the higher tomographic level image (*a*), with tumor thrombus (long arrow, *a*) demonstrating heterogeneous enhancement. The SGE image at a lower tomographic level demonstrates blood thrombus (long arrow, *b*) to be nearly signal void. MRI using postgadolinium SGE images can reliably differentiate tumor from bland thrombus.

Interstitial-phase gadolinium-enhanced SGE image (*c*) in a second patient shows a renal cell carcinoma with enhancing tumor thrombus (long arrows, *c*) and signal-void blood thrombus (arrow, *c*) extending distally to the left common iliac vein. Multiple hepatic metastases (small arrows, *c*) and a renal transplant (hollow arrow, *c*) are also noted.

(c)

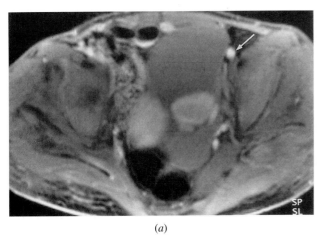
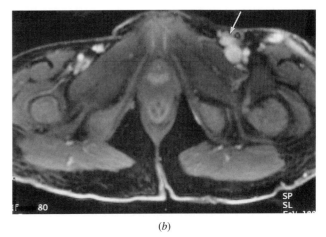

(a)   (b)

F I G . 10.28 Chronic venous thrombosis. Interstitial-phase gadolinium-enhanced fat-suppressed SGE images at superior (a) and more inferior (b) tomographic levels. At the level of the midpelvis, only the left external iliac artery (arrow, a) is identified, whereas the chronically thrombosed left external iliac vein appears as linear nonenhancing tissue immediately posterior to the artery. A collateral enhancing vessel (arrow, b) is noted, reconstituting the left common femoral vein at a lower tomographic level (b). SGE images obtained from 45 s to 2 min after gadolinium administration provide reproducible uniform intense enhancement of normal veins, rendering this technique sensitive to the presence of thrombus even in medium- and small-diameter vessels. Imaging within 40 s permits evaluation of arteries, often without the presence of contrast in veins.

generally very low in signal intensity [48]. Blood thrombus frequently exists at the tail of tumor thrombus (see fig. 10.27), and the two components can be distinguished readily on postgadolinium SGE and fat-suppressed SGE images. Thus the combination of gadolinium-enhanced and flow-sensitive techniques to assess thrombus may be useful. Evaluation of the degree of expansion of the IVC is also contributory as pronounced expansion of the lumen is characteristic of tumor thrombus but atypical of blood thrombus. MRI, because of direct multiplanar and serial dynamic postcontrast imaging capability, is superior to CT imaging in determining the presence and extent of tumor thrombus. MRI outperforms CT imaging in detecting the extension of tumor thrombus supradiaphragmatically into the right atrium. This is an important evaluation in the preoperative setting, as supradiaphragmatic thrombus requires combined thoracoabdominal surgery, whereas tumor thrombus with superior extension that ends below the hepatic veins may require only an abdominal approach.

In cases of chronic venous thrombosis the affected vessel may not be identified if the thrombus is organized and the vein highly contracted. In these cases careful evaluation may reveal the absence of a vein in its expected location in combination with the presence of collateral vessel networks (fig. 10.28). IVC filters can be recognized by the symmetric arrangement of their elements and the magnetic susceptibility artifact on SGE images (fig. 10.29).

In a fashion similar to that of IVC evaluation, MRI is effective at demonstrating renal and gonadal veins as well as retroperitoneal collaterals in cases of venous thrombosis [39]. Compression of the left renal vein between the aorta and superior mesenteric artery may result in the "nutcracker syndrome," and, when a pressure gradient is present, it may occasionally lead to the development of a varicocele, ovarian vein or pelviureteral varices, hematuria, and flank pain [49]. Thrombosed, enlarged retroperitoneal collateral veins may mimic lymphadenopathy on imaging studies [44]. In these cases, careful visual assessment of the course of the structures on transverse images may indicate the vascular nature of the masses [44]. Direct coronal or sagittal imaging is also helpful because these planes demonstrate the tubular shape of these vessels. Gadolinium-enhanced

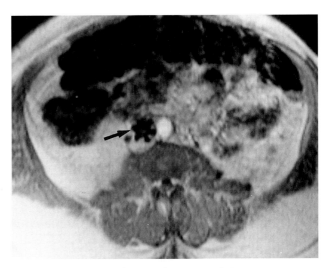

F I G . 10.29 IVC filter. A 45-s postgadolinium SGE image demonstrates a Gianturco IVC filter (arrow) in the inferior vena cava. The filter is readily recognized by the magnetic susceptibility effect and the symmetric configuration of its pedicles.

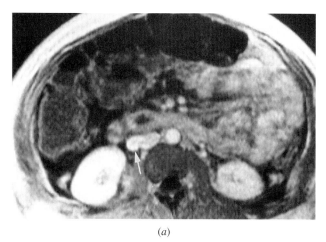
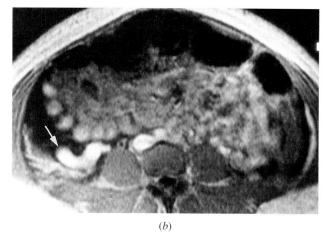

(a)   (b)

F I G . 10.30 Dilated gonadal vein. Transverse 90-s postgadolinium SGE images at superior (*a*) and more inferior (*b*) tomographic levels. A dilated right gonadal vein is demonstrated at its drainage into the IVC (arrow, *a*). At the lower tomographic level, the enhancing vessel (arrow, *b*) follows a serpiginous course. Low-signal intensity ascites with centrally displaced bowel loops is also identified.

fat-suppressed SGE images provide a definitive answer because they demonstrate lack of enhancement in thrombosed vessels compared with moderate enhancement of lymph nodes. Gonadal veins may be enlarged in cases of varicoceles in men and varices of the ovarian venous plexus in women (fig. 10.30). Early retrograde filling of a large and/or tortuous gonadal vein may be demonstrated on immediate postgadolinium SGE or arterial-phase bolus-enhanced 3D gradient-echo images (see fig. 10.12). Markedly enlarged ovarian veins are commonly encountered during pregnancy because of compression by the pregnant uterus and increased venous flow (fig. 10.31). Thrombosis of the ovarian veins may complicate puerperal infection and is readily detected on gadolinium-enhanced fat-suppressed SGE

images. Congenital abnormalities of lymphatic channels are relatively rare. Dilatation of the cisterna chyli is one example (fig. 10.32). Lymphangioma and lymphangioma/hemangioma are described below. Postsurgical changes of lymphatic obstruction or lymphoceles are not uncommon complications, which usually do not have long-term morbidity complications.

Primary Malignant Tumors

Primary malignant tumors of the IVC are rare. The most common histologic type is leiomyosarcoma, followed by angiosarcoma [50]. In a review of leiomyosarcomas of the retroperitoneum and inferior vena cava, leiomyosarcomas involving the IVC have been classified as Pattern 2 when completely intraluminal and Pattern 3 in

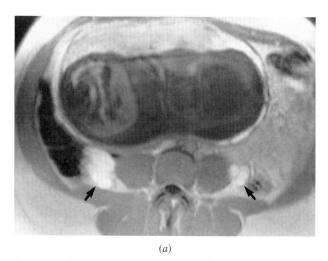
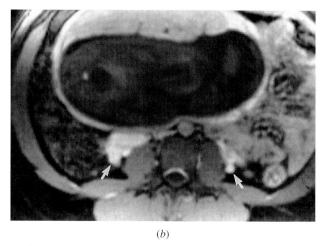

(a)   (b)

F I G . 10.31 Dilated ovarian veins during pregnancy. Interstitial-phase gadolinium-enhanced SGE (*a*) and fat-suppressed SGE (*b*) images in a pregnant woman. The inferior vena cava is compressed by the pregnant uterus, and the ovarian veins (arrows, *a, b*) are enlarged, more prominent on the right. The patient was scanned for evaluation of persistent right flank pain, and her pain was attributed to the venous engorgement.

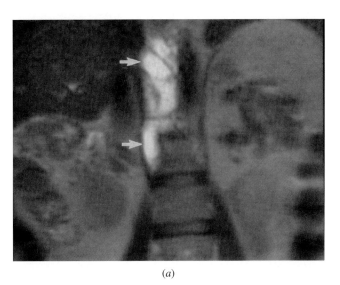

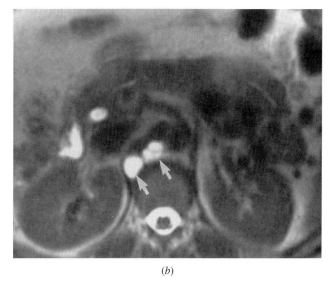

(a)   *(b)*

F I G . 10.32 Dilated cysterna chyli. Coronal (*a*) and transverse (*b*) SS-ETSE images demonstrate multiple tortuous dilated tubular structures (arrows, *a, b*) that do not conform to arteries or veins and are situated in the location of the cysterna chyli.

cases of combined extraluminal and intraluminal components, which comprise 5% and 33%, respectively, of the total cases [16]. Pattern 1 has no major IVC component and will be discussed below in the primary retroperitoneal neoplasm subsection. These tumors are frequently large at presentation (fig. 10.33) but tend to present earlier than their completely extraluminal counterparts, because of symptoms related to obstruction of the IVC. Signal intensity of these tumors is moderately low on T1-weighted images and mixed moderate to high on T2-weighted images. Areas of intermixed tumor and blood thrombus may have bright signal intensity on the T1-weighted images, a finding accentuated on fat-suppressed images (see fig. 10.33). These tumors, which are usually hypervascular, demonstrate intense heterogeneous enhancement on gadolinium-enhanced images [51]. Bright-blood MRI techniques are useful for demonstrating IVC patency and extent of tumor [51].

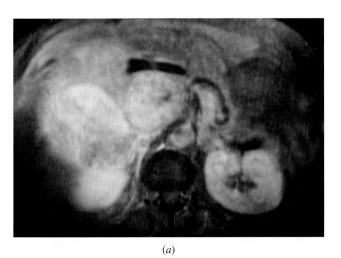

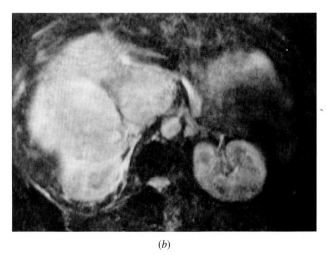

(a)   *(b)*

F I G . 10.33 Leiomyosarcoma of the IVC. T1-weighted fat-suppressed spin-echo (*a*), T2-weighted fat-suppressed spin-echo (*b*), sagittal gradient-refocused (time-of-flight) SGE (*c*), immediate (*d, e*) postgadolinium SGE, and sagittal 90-s postgadolinium SGE (*f*) images. A large tumor is present with a large IVC component and a large retroperitoneal component. The tumor is heterogeneous on both T1- (*a*) and T2-weighted (*b*) images. The hyperintense areas on the noncontrast T1-weighted fat-suppressed image (*a*) reflect the presence of subacute blood products admixed in the tumor thrombus. The superior extent of the tumor within the IVC (arrow, *c*) is immediately below the diaphragm. The IVC and the anteriorly displaced left hepatic vein (small arrow, *c*) immediately above the tumor are patent as shown by the presence of high signal intensity on the flow-sensitive SGE image (*c*). On the immediate postgadolinium SGE images (*d, e*) the mass (long arrows, *d*) enhances in a diffuse heterogeneous fashion. The sagittal 90-s postgadolinium SGE image (*f*) demonstrates the mass (arrows, *f*) invading and compressing the kidney posteriorly. An intense enhancing tumor containing central nonenhancing areas of necrosis is a common appearance for leiomyosarcomas.

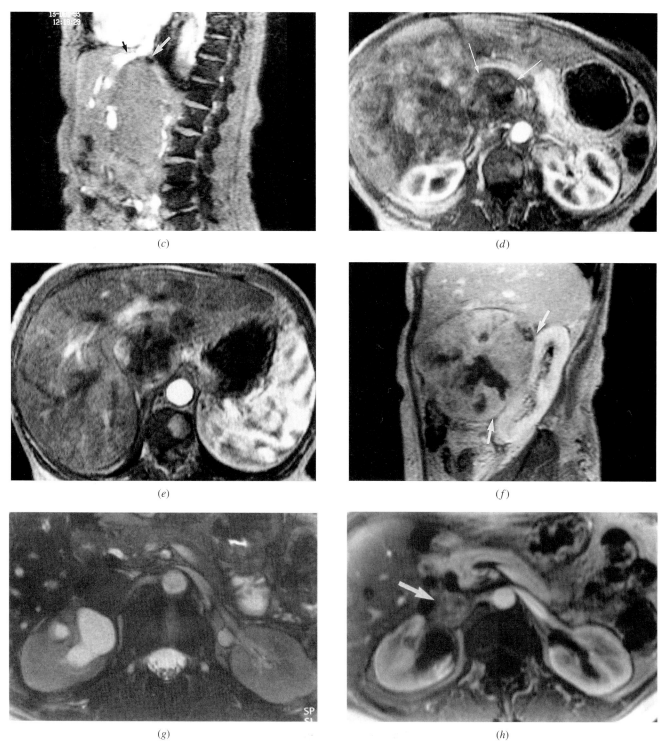

(c)

(d)

(e)

(f)

(g)

(h)

FIG. 10.33 (*Continued*) T2-weighted fat-suppressed SS-ETSE (*g*), immediate postgadolinium SGE (*h*), and interstitial-phase gadolinium-enhanced fat-suppressed SGE (*i*) images in a second patient. The IVC is enlarged by the presence of a mass that is hypointense on the T2-weighted image (*g*) and enhances heterogeneously on early (arrow, *h*) and late postgadolinium images.

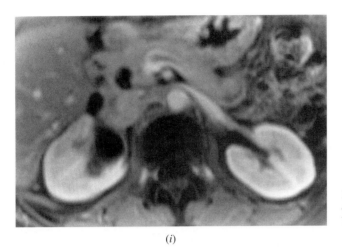

(i)

FIG. 10.33 (*Continued*) Note also the presence of hydronephrosis of the right kidney, secondary to ureteral involvement by the mass.

Gadolinium-enhanced 3D MRA may demonstrate the extent of tumor well using MIP reconstructions. On occasion, it may be difficult to distinguish neoplasm, with completely intraluminal growth, from tumor thrombus. Expansion of the IVC and enhancement on postgadolinium SGE images are features favoring neoplasm and tumor thrombus. In rare cases of hypovascular neoplasms (e.g., malignant fibrous histiocytoma) IVC expansion and demonstration of arterial feeders on immediate postgadolinium SGE images may help to distinguish the neoplasm from blood thrombus (Fig. 10.34) [51]. In rare instances, leiomyosarcomas originating in the renal veins may extend intraluminally into the IVC, and they may appear as tumors in the medial portion of the kidney with tumor thrombus in the renal vein and IVC [53].

RETROPERITONEAL MASSES

Benign Masses

Retroperitoneal Fibrosis

Retroperitoneal fibrosis is most frequently an idiopathic disease [2]. Benign retroperitoneal fibrosis also may arise secondary to certain drugs (classically methysergide), inflammatory aortic aneurysm, retroperitoneal hemorrhage, infection, surgery, or radiation therapy [54]. Idiopathic retroperitoneal fibrosis is considered part of a more extensive systemic fibrotic disorder related to mediastinal fibrosis, sclerosing cholangitis, Riedel thyroiditis, orbital and sinus pseudotumors [55, 56], and pulmonary hyalinizing granulomas [57].

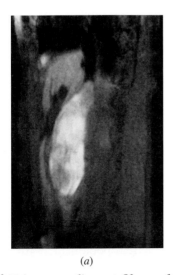

(a)

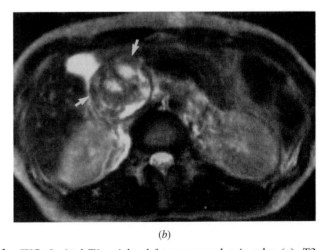

(b)

FIG. 10.34 Primary malignant fibrous histiocytoma of the IVC. Sagittal T1-weighted fat-suppressed spin-echo (*a*), T2-weighted spin-echo (*b*), sagittal gradient-refocused (time-of-flight) SGE (*c*), immediate (*d*) and 90-s (*e*) postgadolinium SGE, and transverse gadolinium-enhanced T1-weighted fat-suppressed spin-echo (*f*) images. The tumor (arrows, *b*) is heterogeneous in signal intensity on the T1- (*a*) and T2-weighted (*b*) images and contains areas of high signal intensity on the T1-weighted fat-suppressed spin-echo image (*a*), reflecting the presence of subacute methemoglobin in the thrombus. The neoplasm expands the IVC but is contained within the vessel lumen, which is consistent with its primary origin from the vessel wall.

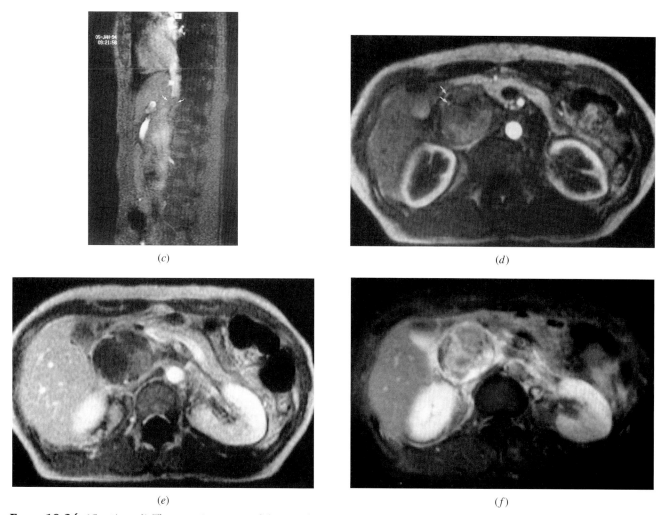

(c)

(d)

(e)

(f)

F I G . 10.34 (*Continued*) The superior extent of the neoplasm (small arrows, *c*) is clearly depicted at the level of the intrahepatic IVC, the patent portion of which is high in signal on the flow-sensitive gradient-refocused SGE image (c). Feeding arterioles (small arrows, *d*) within the tumor are demonstrated as tubular enhancing structures on the immediate postgadolinium SGE image (*d*). The neoplasm enhances minimally in a heterogeneous fashion on the immediate (*d*) and 90-s (*e*) postgadolinium SGE images, reflecting its hypovascular nature. Progressive enhancement is noted on the more delayed T1-weighted fat-suppressed spin-echo image (*f*), which is consistent with delayed enhancement of fibrotic tumor components. The superior extension of tumor thrombus in the IVC is important for surgical planning because the demonstration of supradiaphragmatic extension requires a combined abdominothoracic surgical approach. Sagittal images are superior to transverse sections for demonstrating the craniocaudal extent and defining the superior border of tumor thrombus in the IVC.

The most important differential diagnosis is between idiopathic benign and malignant retroperitoneal fibrosis, particularly as malignant neoplasms may coexist with benign retroperitoneal fibrosis [58]. Retroperitoneal fibrosis most commonly appears as oval-shaped tissue that encases the aorta. The extent of disease may vary from a focal region of fibrosis to dense infiltration of the retroperitoneum encasing the aorta, inferior vena cava (IVC), and ureters. The disease in its acute stage may present as a focal unilateral mass in the region of the common iliac vessels. Over time, fibrosis extends superiorly in the retroperitoneum along the major vessels. In rare instances, thrombosis of the iliac veins [59] and portal vein [60] may be encountered. In the majority of cases the fibrous tissue is located around the abdominal aorta below the level of the renal vessels. A feature distinguishing retroperitoneal fibrosis from retroperitoneal malignant adenopathy and lymphomas is that the fibrous tissue envelopes the aorta, IVC, and ureters but does not displace the aorta substantially anteriorly. Lymph nodes have a rounded, nodular configuration of retroperitoneal masses, whereas retroperitoneal fibrosis has a more platelike, curvilinear morphology.

Early reports suggested that MRI may be able to distinguish benign from malignant retroperitoneal fibrosis [54, 61]. Acute benign retroperitoneal fibrosis may, however, resemble malignant retroperitoneal fibrosis because both may enhance substantially with contrast and may be high in signal intensity on T2-weighted sequences (fig. 10.35) [62–64]. This enhancement pattern is due to the extensive capillary network of acute benign granulation tissue, comparable to that in the postoperative spine [65]. Morphologically, acute benign retroperitoneal fibrosis has very infiltrative margins, and may be very extensive throughout the retroperitoneum. Over, time, the margins of benign retroperitoneal fibrosis become better defined and the tissue becomes more confluent and contracted around the aorta, IVC, and ureters. Eventually, the granulation tissue alters to a more collagenous fibrotic form after approximately 1 year of

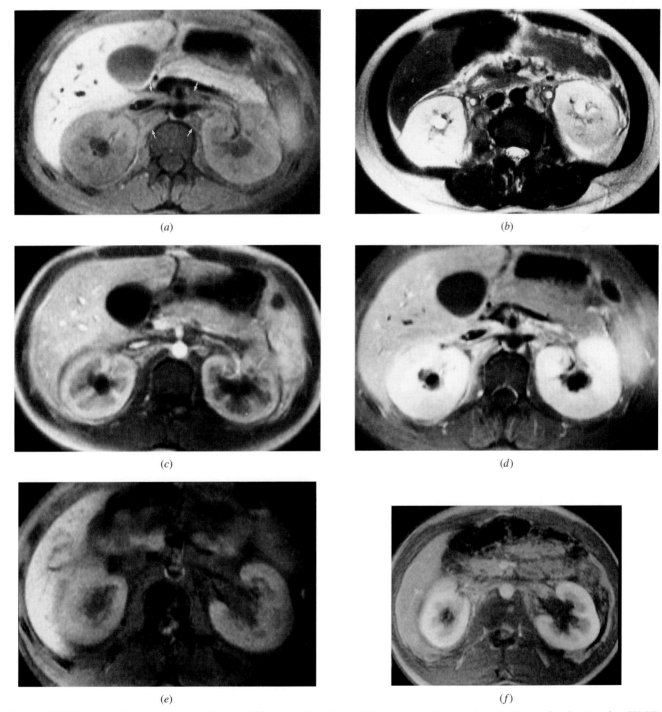

F I G . 10.35 Acute benign retroperitoneal fibrosis. T1-weighted fat-suppressed spin-echo (*a*), T2-weighted spin-echo (T2-SE) (*b*), immediate postgadolinium SGE (*c*), and delayed postgadolinium T1-weighted fat-suppressed spin-echo (*d*) images. The aorta, IVC, renal arteries, and ureters are encased by soft tissue (arrows, *a*), which is low in signal intensity on T1-weighted (*a*) and heterogeneously high in signal intensity on T2-weighted (*b*) images and has ill-defined margins.

FIG. 10.35 (*Continued*) There is bilateral hydronephrosis and ureteral dilatation (*b*) caused by ureteral obstruction at a lower level. The fibrous tissue demonstrates heterogeneous enhancement on the immediate postgadolinium SGE image (*c*), which progresses on the more delayed T1-weighted fat-suppressed spin-echo image (*d*).

Precontrast T1-weighted fat-suppressed spin-echo (*e*), immediate postgadolinium SGE (*f*), and gadolinium-enhanced T1-weighted fat-suppressed spin-echo (*g*) images in a second patient with biopsy-proven membranous glomerulonephritis and benign retroperitoneal fibrosis. Ill-defined extensive infiltrative soft tissue is present in the retroperitoneum. The fibrous tissue is low signal on the precontrast T1-weighted image (*e*), demonstrates moderate heterogeneous enhancement on the immediate postgadolinium image (*f*), and is more conspicuous on the gadolinium-enhanced T1-weighted fat-suppressed spin-echo image (*g*) because of the removal of the competing high signal intensity of the fat and progressive enhancement of the fibrous tissue. Corticomedullary differentiation is absent in both kidneys on the precontrast T1-weighted fat-suppressed spin-echo image (*e*) because of elevated serum creatinine level. Corticomedullary differentiation, however, is present on the immediate postgadolinium SGE image (*f*), reflecting some preservation of renal function. Increased medullary enhancement is shown in both kidneys on the gadolinium-enhanced T1-weighted fat-suppressed spin-echo image (*g*), reflecting tubulointerstitial damage.

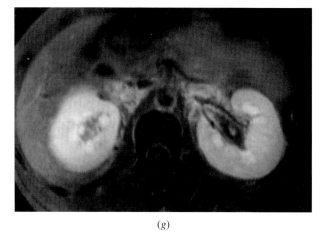

(*g*)

development. During the course of maturation, signal intensity on T2-weighted images decreases, enhancement on immediate postgadolinium SGE images decreases, and the pattern of enhancement appears as a delayed, progressive increase in signal intensity (see fig. 10.35). Granulation tissue on T2-weighted images generally shows decrease in signal intensity after approximately 1 year. Interstitial-phase gadolinium-enhanced fat-suppressed SGE images may show enhancement of fibrous tissue for approximately 1.5 years from onset. Mature chronic benign retroperitoneal fibrosis is low in signal intensity on T2-weighted images and demonstrates negligible contrast enhancement (fig. 10.36), facil-

itating differentiation from malignancy. Imaging findings that may favor benign fibrosis include a well-marginated mass with smooth borders and a decrease in size and/or progressive smoothing of the borders on follow-up examinations.

Benign Retroperitoneal Neoplasms

Benign retroperitoneal tumors are rare [50, 66]. Therefore, any retroperitoneal tumor should initially be considered malignant. Retroperitoneal neurilemoma may have a characteristic high signal intensity on T2-weighted images [67]. Retroperitoneal plexiform neurofibromas are usually bilateral [68], slightly higher in signal

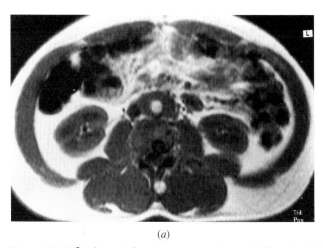

(*a*)

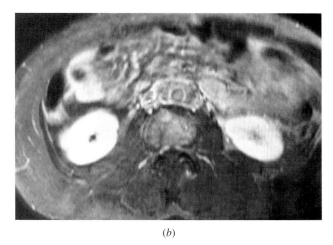

(*b*)

FIG. 10.36 Chronic benign retroperitoneal fibrosis. SGE (*a*) and interstitial-phase gadolinium-enhanced fat-suppressed spin-echo (*b*) images. Low-signal intensity oval-shaped tissue surrounds the aorta. The fibrous tissue has well-defined margins and shows minimal enhancement on the gadolinium-enhanced T1-weighted fat-suppressed spin-echo image (*b*), findings that are typical of mature fibrous tissue.

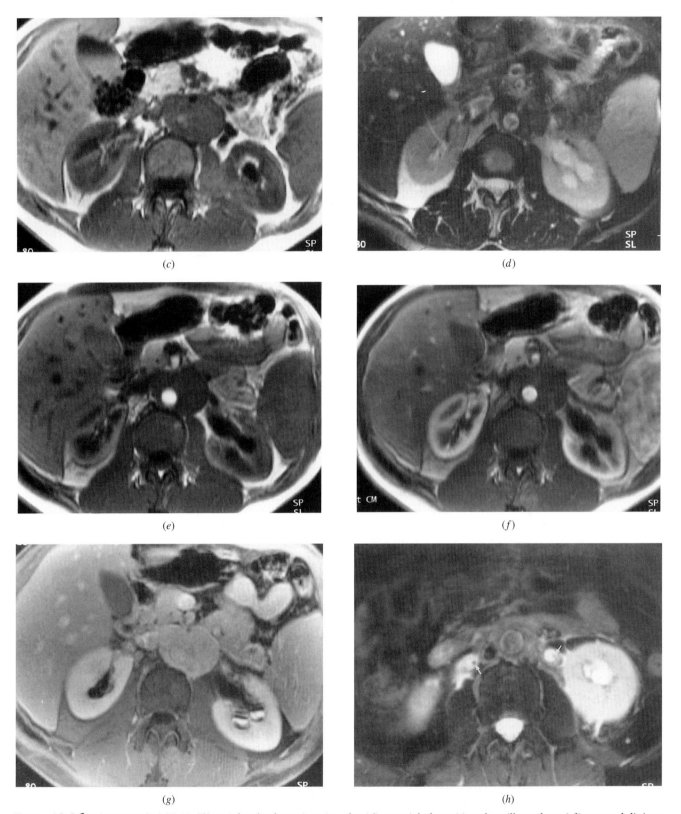

(c)

(d)

(e)

(f)

(g)

(h)

F I G . 10.36 (*Continued*) SGE (*c*), T2-weighted echo-train spin-echo (*d*), arterial-phase (*e*) and capillary-phase (*f*) postgadolinium SGE, and 90-s postgadolinium fat-suppressed SGE (*g*) images in a second patient. The fibrotic tissue is oval-shaped with well-defined margins and encases the aorta. Note that, despite its size, the tissue does not substantially displace the aorta anteriorly. The fibrotic tissue is low in signal intensity on the T1-weighted image (*c*) and heterogeneously low with focal areas of high signal intensity on the T2-weighted image (*d*), demonstrates minimal enhancement on the arterial-phase (*e*) and capillary-phase (*f*) postgadolinium SGE images, and enhances moderately on the more delayed fat-suppressed SGE (*g*) image.

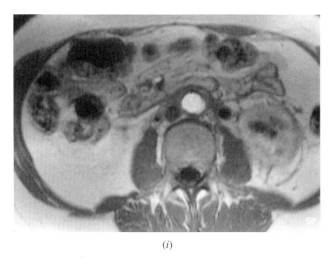

(i)

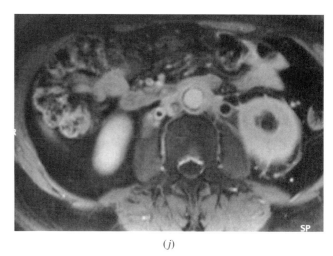

(j)

FIG. 10.36 (*Continued*) Delayed enhancement is characteristic of relatively mature fibrous tissue. Greater enhancement of the fibrotic tissue in the second patient reflects a more active stage in the transition between acute and chronic fibrosis than in the first patient. The pyelocalyceal system of the left kidney is dilated because of concomitant ureteral obstruction.

T2-weighted echo-train spin-echo (*h*), immediate postgadolinium SGE (*i*), and interstitial-phase gadolinium-enhanced fat-suppressed SGE (*j*) images in a third patient. Again noted is relatively well-marginated oval tissue encasing the aorta, IVC, and both ureters. The fibrous tissue is heterogeneously low in signal intensity on the T2-weighted image (*h*) and demonstrates minimal enhancement on the immediate postgadolinium SGE image (*i*), progressing to moderate enhancement on the interstitial-phase gadolinium-enhanced fat-suppressed SGE image (*j*), indicating mature fibrous tissue. Bilateral ureteral obstruction with hydronephrosis is present and signal-void ureteral stents (arrows, *h*) are demonstrated in both ureters on the T2-weighted image (*h*). The majority of the fibrous tissue is located anterior to the aorta and IVC, and these vessels are not displaced substantially anteriorly.

intensity than muscles on T1-weighted images, and high in signal intensity on T2-weighted images [69–71] (fig. 10.37). Other rare neoplasms include paragangliomas, hemangiomas/lymphangiomas, and lipomas [65]. Paragangliomas of Zuckerkandl's organ may be hormone secreting. Imaging follow-up after surgery is advisable because 30% of these tumors are malignant and show late manifestation of remote disease [72]. Inflammatory pseudotumor is a rare benign mass lesion that is minimally low in signal intensity on T1-weighted images and

heterogeneous and moderately high in signal intensity on T2-weighted images and demonstrates moderately intense diffuse heterogeneous enhancement on immediate postgadolinium SGE images (fig. 10.37). This appearance may mimic that of malignant tumors.

Benign Lymphadenopathy
Benign lymphadenopathy may occur secondary to inflammatory or infectious disease. Sequences suited for detection of lymph nodes include precontrast T1-weighted

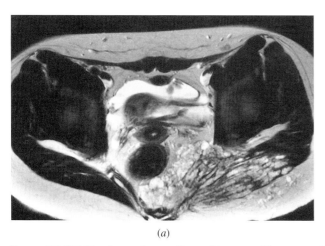

(a)

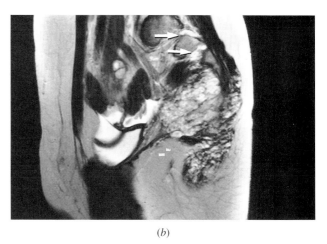

(b)

FIG. 10.37 Benign retroperitoneal tumors. Transverse (*a*) and sagittal (*b*) 512-resolution T2-weighted echo-train spin-echo images in a patient with plexiform neurofibroma of the pelvis and neurofibromatosis Type 1. The plexiform neurofibroma appears as a large heterogeneous mass that occupies the majority of the left posterior pelvis and infiltrates the left gluteus maximus and pyriformis muscles. Extension into the sacral neural foramina is present (arrows, *b*).

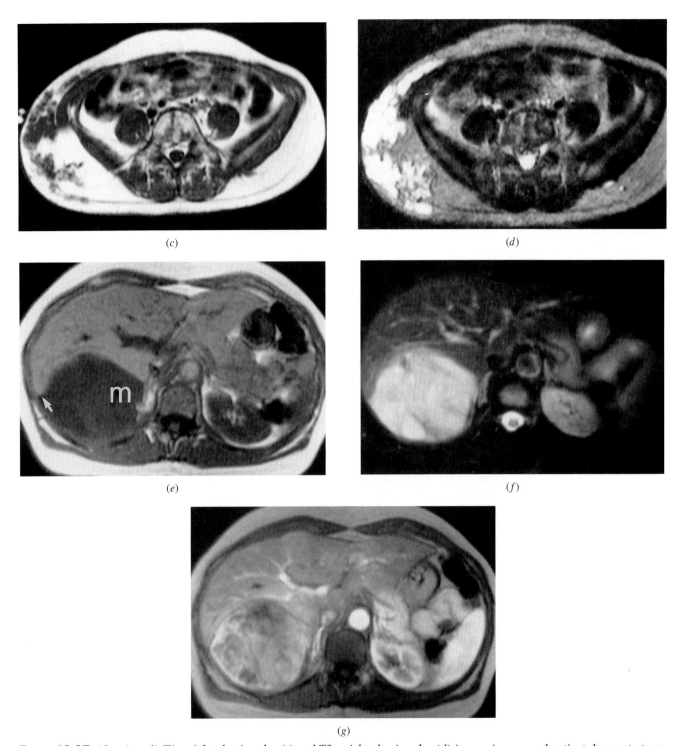

(c)

(d)

(e)

(f)

(g)

F I G . 10.37 (*Continued*) T1-weighted spin-echo (*c*) and T2-weighted spin-echo (*d*) images in a second patient demonstrate an extensive plexiform neurofibroma in the right subcutaneous tissues that is low in signal intensity on the T1-weighted image (*c*) and high in signal intensity on the T2-weighted image (*d*). The tumors are high in signal intensity on the T2-weighted images in both patients, which is characteristic for tumors of neural origin.

SGE (*e*), T2-weighted fat-suppressed echo-train spin-echo (*f*) and immediate postgadolinium SGE (*g*) images in a patient with inflammatory pseudotumor arising from the renal capsule. A large mass (mass = m, *e*) is noted posterior to the liver. The mass is well-marginated, heterogeneous, and low in signal intensity on the T1-weighted image (*e*) and moderately high in signal on the T2-weighted image (*f*) and demonstrates intense diffuse heterogeneous enhancement on the immediate postgadolinium SGE image (*g*). The posterior liver margin at the interface with the mass forms an obtuse angle consistent with an extrahepatic origin of the mass. The right kidney (not shown) was displaced but not invaded by the mass. Inflammatory pseudotumor may have an aggressive appearance that mimics the appearance of a malignant tumor.

SE or SGE, fat-suppressed T2-weighted spin-echo or echo-train spin-echo, and gadolinium-enhanced fat-suppressed SGE techniques. In each of these techniques the signal difference between lymph nodes and background tissue is substantial. The enlarged lymph nodes appear low in signal on precontrast SGE in a background of high-signal fat, and nodes are moderately high in signal on fat-suppressed T2-weighted and gadolinium-enhanced T1-weighted images, set in a background of low-signal suppressed fat. Fat-suppressed T2-weighted images are very sensitive for the detection of lymph nodes and exceed CT imaging, particularly in pediatric patients or other patients with minimal retroperitoneal fat (fig. 10.38).

Mycobacterium avium intracellulare infection is not uncommon in immunocompromised patients and may exhibit enlarged lymph nodes and evidence of liver involvement (fig. 10.39). Massive retroperitoneal adenopathy mimicking lymphoma may be an uncommon manifestation of sarcoidosis (fig. 10.40). Lymph nodes enhance with gadolinium and may have a speckled appearance on T2-weighted images [73–75]. Substantial benign adenopathy resembling malignant disease may also be found in Castleman disease (fig. 10.41), also known as giant lymph node hyperplasia. The lymph nodes have a heterogeneous appearance on MR images and may show increased vascularity of the adjacent fat [76]. Retroperitoneal adenopathy is commonly observed in Kawasaki disease, and involved lymph nodes are often hemorrhagic, demonstrating characteristic high signal intensity on T1-weighted images (fig. 10.42).

Miscellaneous

Masses of extramedullary hematopoiesis are most commonly found in patients with hereditary hemolytic anemias, particularly thalassemia major, but may be encountered in chronic leukemias, polycythemia vera, and diseases with extensive bone marrow infiltration [77].

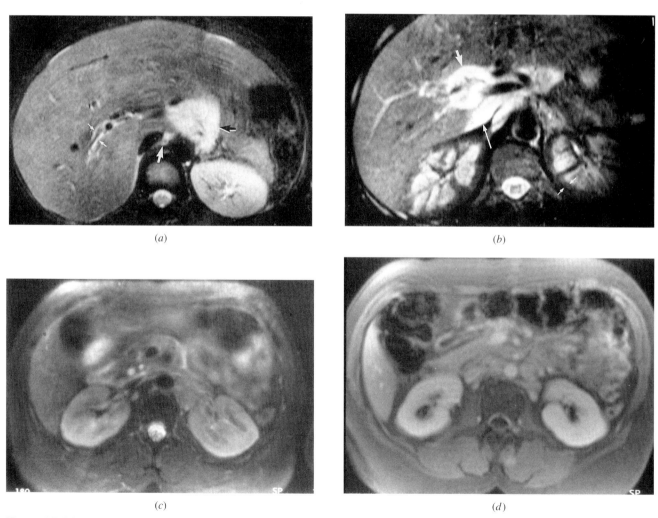

(a)   (b)

(c)   (d)

F I G . 10.38 Benign retroperitoneal adenopathy. T2-weighted fat-suppressed spin-echo image (*a*) in a patient with sclerosing cholangitis demonstrates para-aortic (black arrow) and aortocaval (white arrow) lymphadenopathy. Enlarged lymph nodes are readily distinguished in a dark background. Periportal high signal intensity is also noted (small arrows).

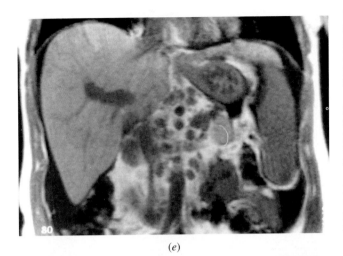

(e)

F I G . 10.38 (*Continued*) T2-weighted fat-suppressed image in a second patient (*b*) shows inflammatory portal (arrow, *b*) and portocaval (thin arrow, *b*) nodes as high-signal intensity structures. Note also that the cortex of the kidneys (small arrows, *b*) in this patient with sickle cell anemia is low in signal intensity secondary to iron deposition.

Transverse T2-weighted fat-suppressed SS-ETSE (*c*) and interstitial-phase gadolinium-enhanced fat-suppressed SGE (*d*) images in a third patient demonstrate extensive retroperitoneal lymphadenopathy. These two sequences allow good distinction between low-signal background tissue and moderate signal lymph nodes.

Coronal SGE (*e*) image in a fourth patient shows multiple enlarged retroperitoneal lymph nodes that are low signal intensity compared to the background fat. The coronal plane is effective at showing rounded retroperitoneal nodes, which are distinguishable from tubule-shaped vessels.

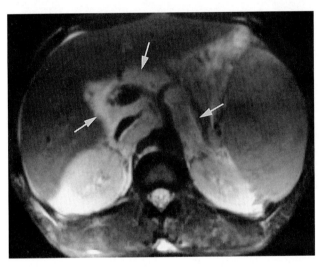

F I G . 10.39 Retroperitoneal lymphadenopathy from *Mycobacterium avium intracellulare* in a 13-year-old female patient. T2-weighted fat-suppressed echo-train spin-echo image shows extensive para-aortic, aortocaval, paracaval, portocaval, and celiac lymphadenopathy (arrows). Retroperitoneal lymph nodes are conspicuous on T2-weighted fat-suppressed images as high-signal intensity masses, and this permits detection of small lymph nodes, which appear moderate signal, in thin or pediatric patients, who have little retroperitoneal fat.

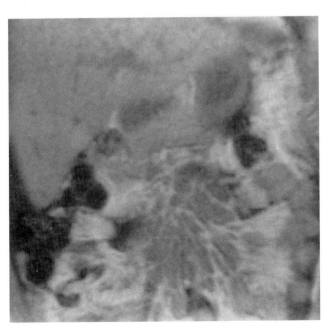

F I G . 10.40 Sarcoidosis. Coronal SGE image demonstrates diffuse mesenteric lymphadenopathy in a patient with sarcoidosis.

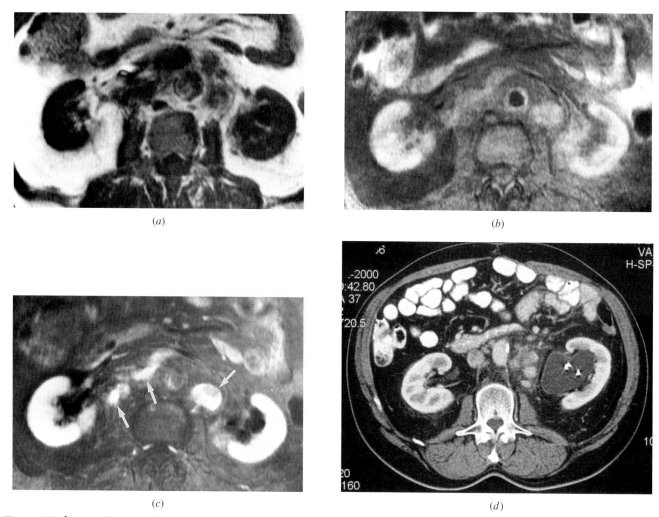

(a)

(b)

(c)

(d)

F I G . 10.41 Castleman's disease. SGE (*a*), T1-weighted fat-suppressed spin-echo (*b*), and gadolinium-enhanced T1-weighted fat-suppressed spin-echo (*c*) images. Enlarged retroperitoneal lymph nodes are present. The lymph nodes are low in signal intensity on the SGE image (*a*) and intermediate to moderate in signal intensity on the T1-weighted fat-suppressed spin-echo image (*b*), with several of them demonstrating substantial enhancement (arrows, *c*) on the gadolinium-enhanced image (*c*). Ill-defined stranding is also present in the retroperitoneum (*a*). (Reproduced with permission from Semelka RC, Shoenut JP, Kroeker MA: The retroperitoneum and the abdominal wall. In Semelka RC, Shoenut JP (eds.), *MRI of the Abdomen with CT Correlation.* New York: Raven Press, p. 13–41, 1993.)

Iodine-contrast enhanced spiral CT image (*d*) in a second patient demonstrates enlarged lymph nodes and ill-defined retroperitoneal tissue. Associated hydronephrosis is present because of entrapment of the ureters by strandy tissue. (Courtesy of Andrea Baur, M.D., Klinikum Grosshadern, University of Munich.)

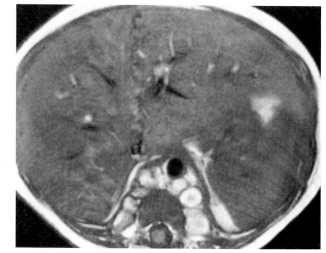

F I G . 10.42 Hemorrhagic lymph nodes in Kawasaki disease. T1-SE image shows multiple retrocrural lymph nodes that are high in signal intensity because of the presence of subacute blood. (Reproduced with permission from Semelka RC, Shoenut JP, Kroeker MA: The retroperitoneum and the abdominal wall. In Semelka RC, Shoenut JP (eds.), *MRI of the Abdomen with CT Correlation.* New York: Raven Press, p. 13–41, 1993.)

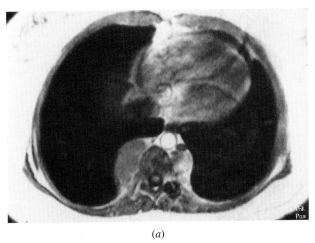 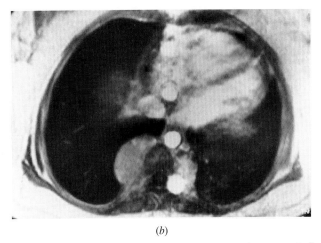

(a)   (b)

F I G . 10.43 Extramedullary hematopoiesis in thalassemia major. SGE (*a*) and immediate postgadolinium SGE (*b*) images. Soft tissue paravertebral masses in the lower thorax and abdomen are demonstrated. The hematopoietic masses are low in signal intensity on the SGE image (*a*) and demonstrate moderate enhancement on the immediate postgadolinium SGE image (*b*). (Reproduced with permission from Semelka RC, Shoenut JP, Kroeker MA: The retroperitoneum and the abdominal wall. In Semelka RC, Shoenut JP (eds.), *MRI of the Abdomen with CT Correlation.* New York: Raven Press, p. 13–41, 1993.)

Common retroperitoneal locations are the retrocrural and presacral spaces. Occasionally, they have an aggressive appearance and may result in bone destruction [77]. The masses are intermediate in signal intensity on T1-weighted images and intermediate to moderately high in signal intensity on T2-weighted images and enhance moderately after gadolinium administration (fig. 10.43).

Retroperitoneal hematomas may occur in patients with coagulation disorders or hemophilia, and after renal biopsy (fig. 10.44). Hematomas have a characteristic appearance of a focal collection of fluid with a high-signal peripheral rim on noncontrast T1-weighted images, which is pronounced with fat suppression.

Malignant Masses

Malignant Retroperitoneal Fibrosis

Malignant retroperitoneal fibrosis is most commonly associated with cervical, bowel, breast, prostate, lung, and kidney cancers [53, 78]. The tumor consists of malignant cell infiltration of the retroperitoneum with associated

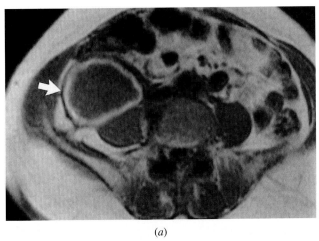 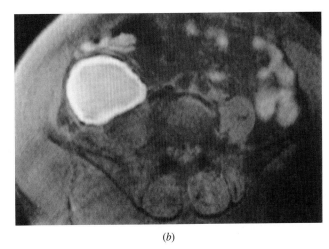

(a)   (b)

F I G . 10.44 Retroperitoneal hematoma. SGE (*a*), fat-suppressed T1-weighted spin-echo (*b*), and interstitial-phase gadolinium-enhanced SGE (*c*) images. A 7.5-cm well-defined hematoma (arrow, *a*) is noted along the anterior margin of the right psoas muscle. The periphery of the hematoma is hyperintense on the precontrast SGE image (*a*). The hyperintensity is markedly accentuated on the T1-weighted fat-suppressed spin-echo image (*b*), confirming that fat is not the cause of hyperintensity. A thin rim that is low in signal intensity on both T1- and T2-weighted (not shown) images reflects the presence of hemosiderin and suggests chronicity of the hematoma.

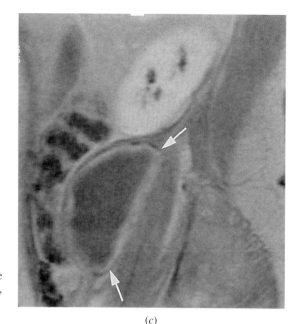

(c)

FIG. 10.44 (*Continued*) After gadolinium administration, there are no enhancing tissue components identified in the hematoma (arrows, *c*), which excludes tumor as the cause.

desmoplastic reaction that often encases the aorta, IVC, and ureters. The contour of the mass is not lobular, distinguishing malignant retroperitoneal fibrosis from adenopathy, and may be infiltrative and irregular (fig. 10.45), a finding that favors malignant rather than benign retroperitoneal fibrosis. Ureteral obstruction with bilateral hydronephrosis is common. Malignant retroperitoneal fibrosis is usually moderately high in signal intensity on T2-weighted images, exhibiting moderately intense enhancement with gadolinium [53, 60, 61]. Malignant retroperitoneal fibrosis will usually demonstrate enhancement on immediate postgadolinium images. MRI can distinguish chronic benign from

malignant retroperitoneal fibrosis, but distinction from acute benign retroperitoneal fibrosis is not always possible. Findings favoring malignancy include a more irregular contour and increase in size and irregularity on follow-up examinations. Acute benign retroperitoneal fibrosis has a more wispy infiltrative pattern compared to malignant disease, which is more solid and irregular. Clinical history is also helpful as acute benign retroperitoneal fibrosis is often observed in younger patients (20–40 yrs) with no pre-existent malignant disease, and malignant retroperitoneal fibrosis is, more commonly observed in older patients (>40 years). In indeterminate cases that have somewhat well-defined borders, high

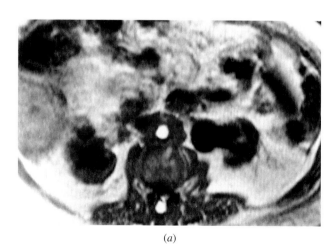

(a)

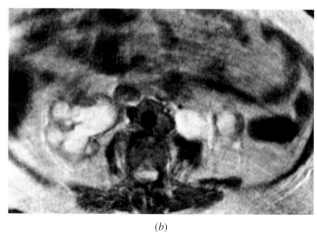

(b)

FIG. 10.45 Malignant retroperitoneal fibrosis from cervical cancer. SGE (*a*), T2-weighted echo-train spin-echo (*b*) and immediate postgadolinium SGE (*c*) images. The aorta is encased by abnormal soft tissue, which has slightly ill-defined margins. The soft tissue is low in signal intensity on the SGE image (*a*) and heterogeneous and moderate in signal intensity on the T2-weighted echo-train spin-echo image (*b*) and demonstrates diffuse heterogeneous enhancement after gadolinium administration (*c*). This appearance is compatible with active malignant rather than chronic benign retroperitoneal fibrosis. Note bilateral hydronephrosis resulting from ureteral obstruction at a lower level.

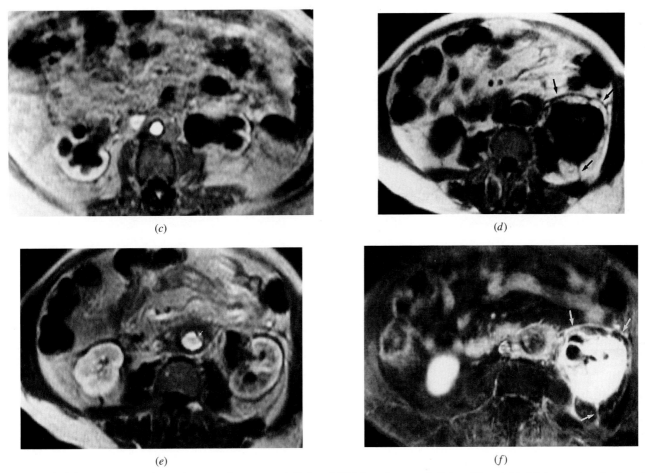

F I G . 10.45 (*Continued*) SGE (*d*), immediate postgadolinium SGE (*e*), and postgadolinium T1-weighted fat-suppressed spin-echo (*f*) images in a second patient with malignant retroperitoneal fibrosis. An oval-shaped mass encases the aorta. The mass is low in signal intensity on the SGE image (*d*), and demonstrates moderate heterogeneous enhancement on the immediate postgadolinium image (*e*) that progresses on the postgadolinium T1-weighted fat-suppressed spin-echo image (*f*). The mass has aggressive infiltrating margins (arrows, *f*). The left perirenal fascia and perirenal septae are thickened (arrows, *d*) and demonstrate enhancement (arrows, *f*) on the gadolinium-enhanced T1-weighted fat-suppressed spin-echo (*f*) image. Also noted is a dissection involving the abdominal aorta with good demonstration of the intimal flap (small arrow, *e*).

signal intensity on T2-weighted images and increased enhancement on immediate postgadolinium SGE images are findings that should be evaluated with caution. Biopsies from multiple sites should be obtained because benign retroperitoneal fibrosis may coexist with malignant neoplasms that are known to induce malignant retroperitoneal fibrosis [57].

Lymphoma

Lymphoma is the most common retroperitoneal malignancy, and both Hodgkin and non-Hodgkin lymphomas may involve the retroperitoneum [79–83]. Non-Hodgkin lymphoma more commonly involves a variety of nodal groups, (in particular, mesenteric nodes are involved in >50% of the cases), and extranodal sites [80]. Intra-abdominal Hodgkin lymphoma tends to be limited to the spleen and retroperitoneum, with spread of disease to contiguous nodes [79].

MRI performs well in the demonstration of enlarged lymph nodes (figs. 10.46–10.48) [83–85] and outperforms CT imaging in the evaluation of the upper abdominal para-aortic and portar hepatis regions, and thin patients [83]. Short tau inversion recovery (STIR) and T2-weighted fat-suppressed spin-echo, or echo-train spin-echo techniques result in excellent conspicuity of moderately high-signal intensity nodes in a suppressed background. The fat-suppressed single-shot echo-train spin-echo sequence may be used as an alternative in uncooperative or pediatric patients, and results are generally good with this technique. Persistent tissue after therapy also may be better characterized by MRI as recurrent disease or fibrosis [81, 82, 86]. After approximately 1 year, fibrotic tissue is low in signal intensity on T2-weighted images, unlike recurrent disease, which is high or mixed high in signal intensity on T2-weighted images. Chronic fibrotic tissue will enhance minimally with gadolinium

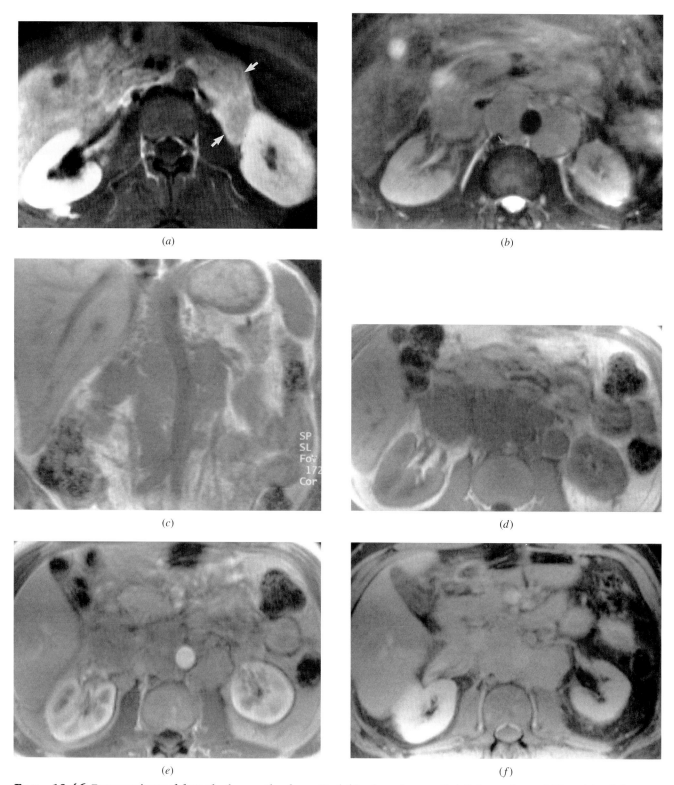

(a)

(b)

(c)

(d)

(e)

(f)

FIG. 10.46 Retroperitoneal lymphadenopathy from Hodgkin lymphoma. Gadolinium-enhanced T1-weighted fat-suppressed spin-echo image (*a*) shows a 4-cm moderately enhancing lymphomatous nodal mass (arrows) in a left periaortic location at the level of the left renal hilum. (Reproduced with permission from Semelka RC, Shoenut JP, Kroeker MA: The retroperitoneum and the abdominal wall. In Semelka RC, Shoenut JP (eds.), *MRI of the Abdomen with CT Correlation*. New York: Raven Press, p. 13–41, 1993.)

Transverse fat-suppressed T2-weighted SS-ETSE (*b*), coronal (*c*), and transverse (*d*) SGE, immediate postgadolinium SGE (*e*), and gadolinium-enhanced fat-suppressed SGE (*f*) images in a second patient with Hodgkin lymphoma. Extensive retroperitoeal adenopathy is shown.

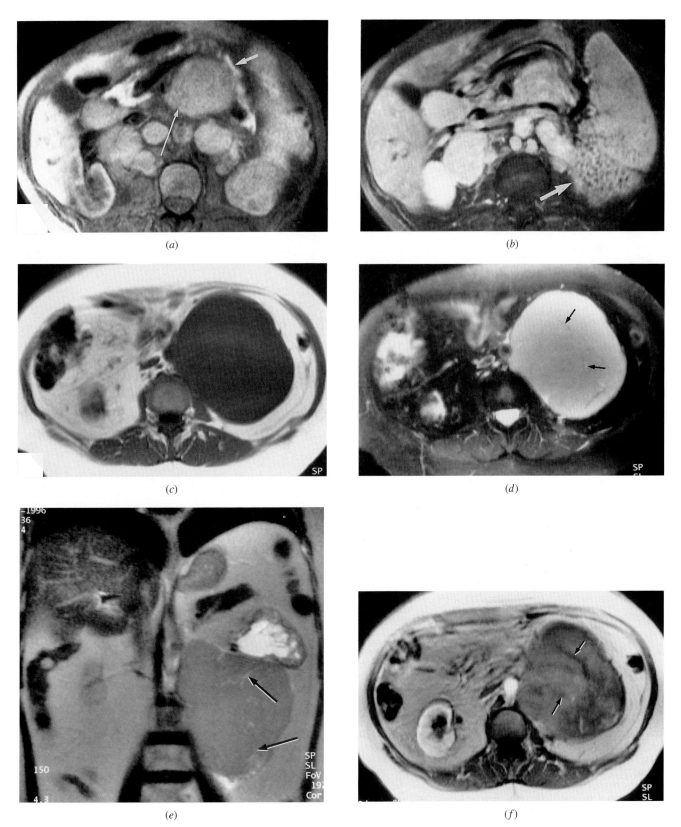

F I G . 10.47 Non-Hodgkin lymphoma. Precontrast (*a*) and gadolinium-enhanced (*b*) T1-weighted fat-suppressed spin-echo images in a patient with retroperitoneal lymphadenopathy from non-Hodgkin lymphoma. Extensive retroperitoneal and mesenteric lymphadenopathy is noted. The precontrast T1-weighted fat-suppressed spin-echo image (*a*) permits distinction of the normal high-signal intensity pancreas (short white arrow, *a*) from the retropancreatic nodal mass (long white arrow, *a*) and documents the extrapancreatic location of the mass. The nodal masses show moderate to intense enhancement on the gadolinium-enhanced image (*b*), whereas abnormal enhancement of the spleen (arrow, *b*) reflects lymphomatous infiltration. (Reproduced with permission from Semelka RC, Shoenut JP, Kroeker MA: The retroperitoneum and the abdominal wall. In Semelka RC, Shoenut JP (eds.), *MRI of the Abdomen with CT Correlation.* New York: Raven Press, p. 13–41, 1993.)

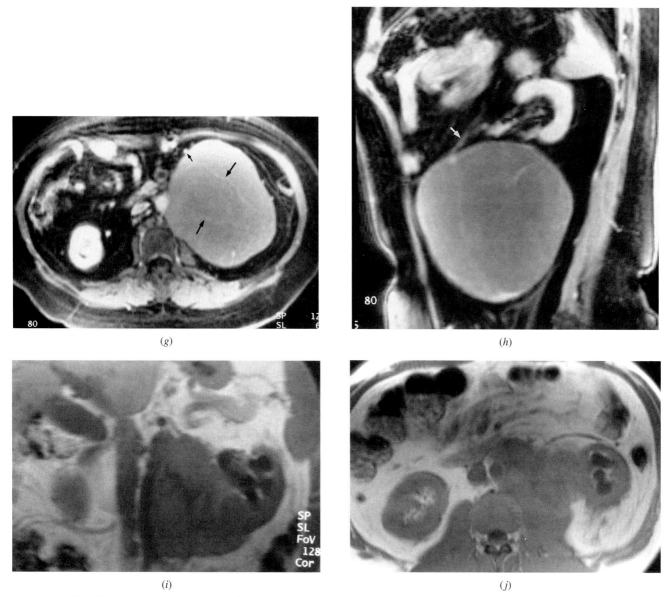

(g)

(h)

(i)

(j)

FIG. 10.47 (*Continued*) SGE (*c*), T2-weighted fat-suppressed echo-train spin-echo (*d*), coronal T2-weighted SS-ETSE (*e*), immediate postgadolinium SGE (*f*), and transverse (*g*) and sagittal (*h*) interstitial phase gadolinium-enhanced fat-suppressed SGE images in a patient with lymphoma presenting as a solitary retroperitoneal mass. A large, well-defined retroperitoneal mass is present. The mass is mildly heterogeneous and low in signal intensity on the T1-weighted image (*c*) and moderately high signal intensity on the T2-weighted image (*d*). Thin septations (arrows, *d*, *e*) are present in the mass. The coronal T2-weighted SS-ETSE image demonstrates superior displacement and hydronephrosis of the left kidney secondary to ureteral compression caused by the mass. The lymphoma mass demonstrates mild to moderate diffuse heterogeneous enhancement on the immediate postgadolinium SGE image (*f*), which becomes more homogeneous over time on the interstitial-phase fat-suppressed SGE image (*g*). Note that the internal septations (arrows, *f*, *g*) show minimal enhancement on the immediate postgadolinium SGE image (*f*) and show progressive enhancement on the more delayed fat-suppressed SGE images (*g*, *h*), consistent with fibrous tissue. The anteriorly displaced ureter is identified at the anterior margin of the mass on the interstitial-phase fat-suppressed SGE image (small arrow, *g*). Note that the sagittal image clearly demonstrates the fat plane between the kidney and the mass and depicts a segment of the anterosuperiorly displaced ureter (small arrow, *h*). A solitary mass lesion with no evidence of other sites of nodal or organ disease is a rare appearance for lymphoma.

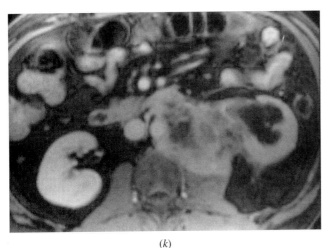

(k)

FIG. 10.47 (*Continued*) Coronal (*i*) and transverse (*j*) SGE and 90-s gadolinium-enhanced fat-suppressed SGE (*k*) images. There is a large heterogeneous mass originating in the retroperitoneum on the left that extends from the celiac axis inferiorly to the aortic bifurcation. This mass is isointense on noncontrast T1-weighted images (*i, j*) and enhances heterogeneously (*k*). The mass encases the left renal artery and vein, as well as the ureter, resulting in hydronephrosis. This pattern is the most common form of kidney involvement by lymphoma. The psoas muscle is also compressed. This lesion represented large cell lymphoma at histopathology.

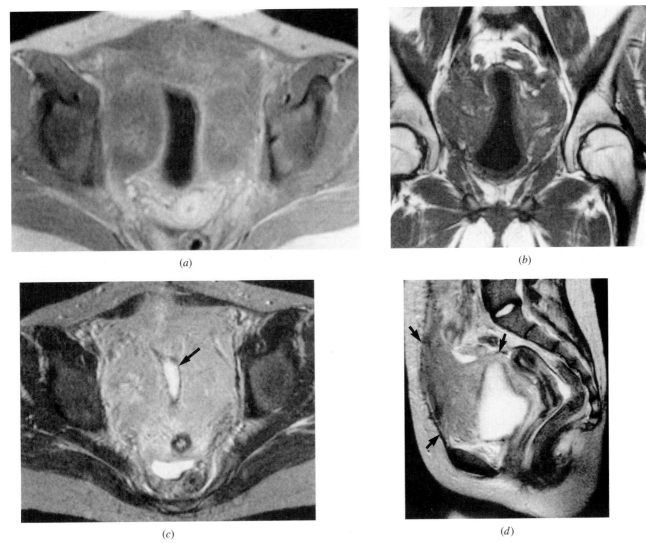

(a)   (b)

(c)   (d)

FIG. 10.48 Burkitt lymphoma of the pelvis. SGE (*a*), coronal T1-SE (*b*), T2-SE (*c*), sagittal T2-SE (*d*), and gadolinium-enhanced fat-suppressed T1-weighted spin-echo (*e*) images. Large lymphoma masses are present in the pelvis that cause compression of the urinary bladder (arrow, *c*), which has an hourglass configuration, well shown on the coronal T1-SE image (*b*).

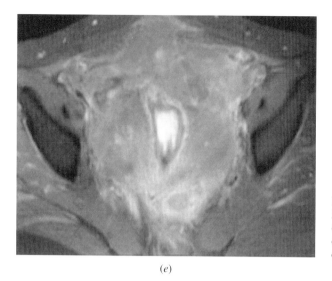

(e)

FIG. 10.48 (*Continued*) The sagittal T2-SE image depicts the large lymphomatous mass (arrows, *d*) that extends along the dome of the bladder into the uterovesicular space. The masses are heterogeneous on both T1- and T2-weighted images and show minimal enhancement after gadolinium administration (*e*).

compared with the enhancement of persistent or recurrent disease, which is moderate or marked and often heterogeneous. In rare instances, lymphoma may appear as a large solitary retroperitoneal mass (fig. 10.47) that mimics the appearance of a primary malignant retroperitoneal tumor.

Malignant Metastatic Lymphadenopathy

Carcinomas associated with retroperitoneal lymphadenopathy include kidney, colon, pancreas, lung, breast, testes, prostate, cervix, and melanoma [84, 87, 88]. Enlarged lymph nodes are usually moderate in signal intensity on T2-weighted images and higher than adjacent psoas muscle (figs. 10.49 and 10.50). T2-weighted

fat-suppressed spin-echo or echo-train spin-echo images are particularly effective at demonstrating nodes in patients who are thin. The addition of fat suppression is important, particularly when echo-train spin-echo sequences are used, because fat is high in signal intensity on these images (fig. 10.49). Adenopathy, whether benign or malignant, will enhance on postgadolinium SGE images. A feature favoring malignancy is the depiction of necrotic lymph nodes (fig. 10.51) in a patient in whom the primary tumor is also necrotic. The MRI and CT imaging criteria for describing lymph nodes as pathologically enlarged is lymph node minimum transverse diameter greater than 1.5 cm. Unfortunately, sensitivity and specificity of measurements are not high, as benign

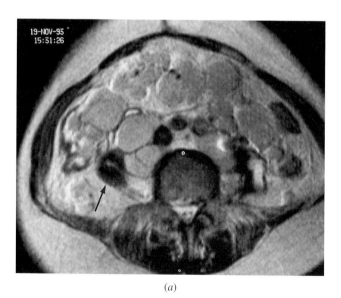

(a)

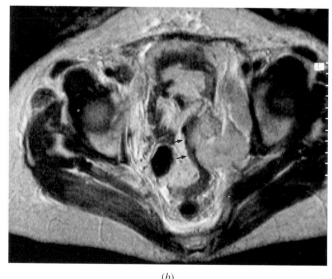

(b)

FIG. 10.49 Malignant retroperitoneal adenopathy. T2-weighted spin-echo images from cranial (*a*) and more caudal (*b*) levels. Enlarged retroperitoneal lymph nodes are demonstrated as rounded, well-defined masses of moderate signal intensity on both images. Note lateral displacement of the right psoas muscle (arrow, *a*) by enlarged paracaval lymph nodes, and medial displacement of the sigmoid colon (arrows, b) by enlarged left obturator lymph nodes.

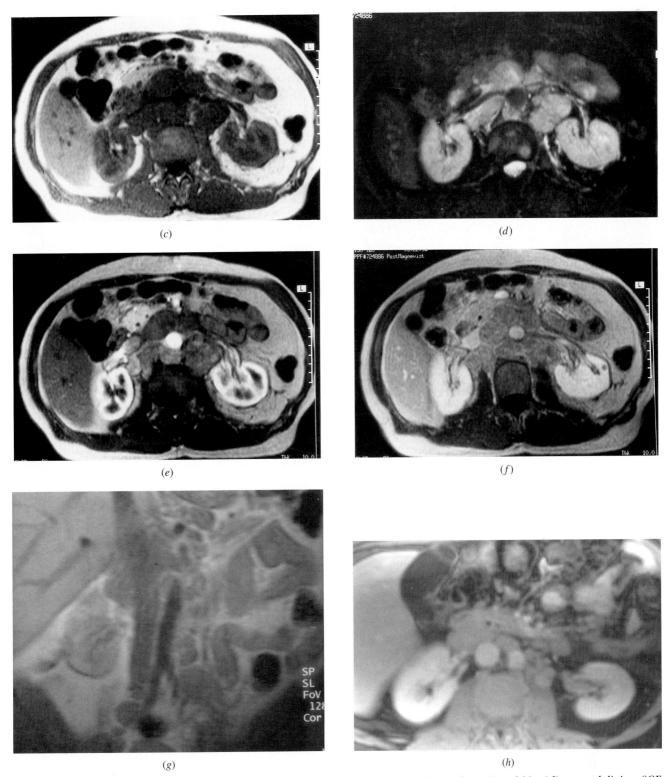

(c)

(d)

(e)

(f)

(g)

(h)

F I G. 10.49 (*Continued*) SGE (*c*), T2-weighted fat-suppressed spin-echo (*d*), and immediate (*e*) and 90-s (*f*) postgadolinium SGE images in a second patient who has prostate cancer. Multiple enlarged lymph nodes are present in the retroperitoneum displacing the aorta and the IVC anteriorly. The lymph nodes are low in signal intensity on the SGE image (*c*) and high in signal intensity on the T2-weighted fat-suppressed spin-echo image (*d*). Fat suppression removes the competing high signal intensity of fat and renders the lymph nodes particularly conspicuous on the T2-weighted image. The lymph nodes enhance minimally on the immediate postgadolinium SGE image (*e*) and show progressive enhancement on the 90-s postgadolinium SGE image (*f*).

Coronal SGE (*g*) and interstitial-phase gadolinium-enhanced fat-suppressed SGE (*h*) images in third patient who has chronic lymphocytic leukemia. Diffuse abdominal adenopathy is appreciate in portocaval, periaortic, and iliac chains.

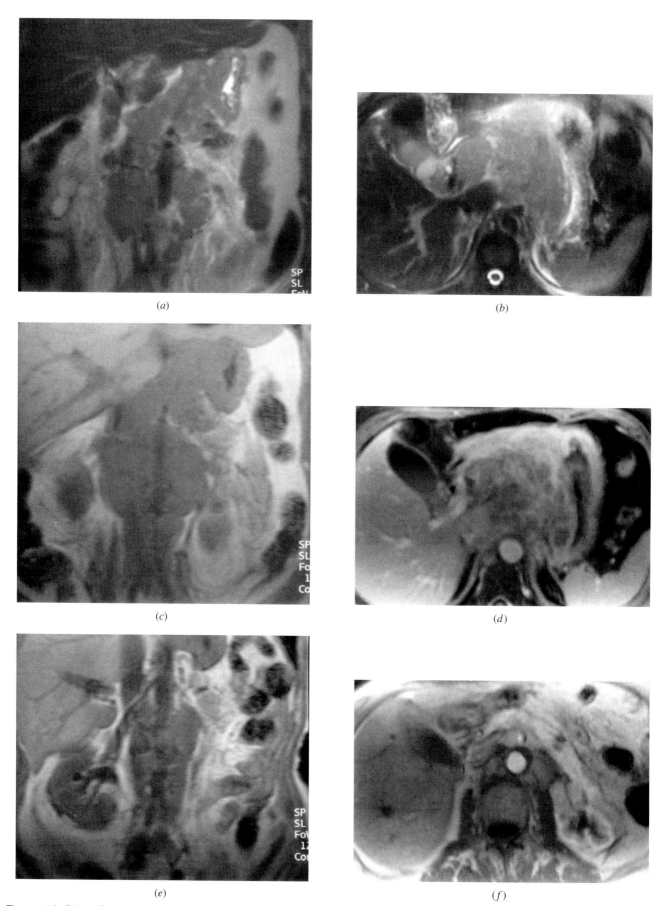

FIG. 10.50 Malignant retroperitoneal lymphadenopathy. Coronal T2-weighted SS-ETSE (*a*), transverse fat-suppressed T2-weighted SS-ETSE (*b*), coronal SGE (*c*), and interstitial-phase gadolinium-enhanced fat-suppressed SGE (*d*) images in a patient with gastric adenocarcinoma.

926

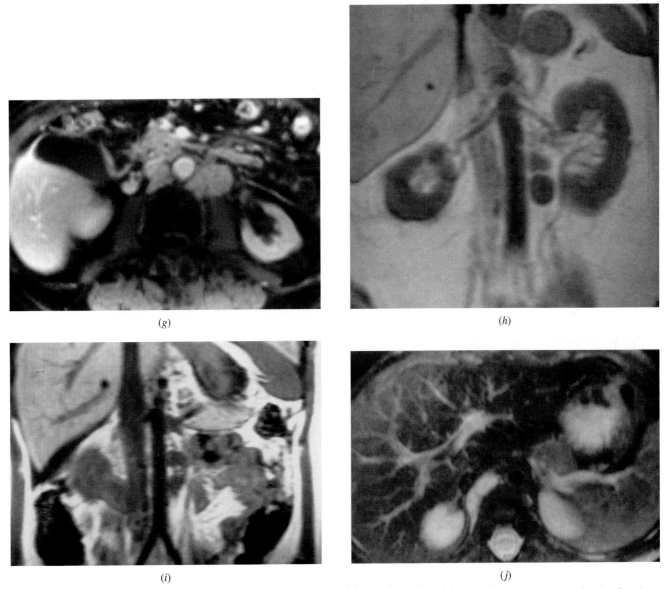

(g)

(h)

(i)

(j)

F I G . 10.50 (*Continued*) There is a large, mildly heterogeneous lobulated mass involving the lesser curvature and extending into the gastrohepatic ligament (*d*). Extensive retroperitoneal lymph nodes are also appreciated.

Coronal SGE (*e*), immediate post-gadolinium SGE (*f*), and interstitial-phase gadolinium-enhanced fat-suppressed SGE (*g*) images in a second patient with recurrent colon cancer demonstrate the presence of aortocaval and left para-aortic bulky lymphadenopathy that extend superiorly to the level of the kidneys.

Coronal SGE image (*h*) in a third patient, who has carcinoma of the uterus, shows enlarged left para-aortic lymph nodes consistent with metastatic lymphadenopathy.

Coronal SGE image (*i*) in a fourth patient, who has endometrial stromal sarcoma, also demonstrates left para-aortic retroperitoneal adenopathy.

Transverse T2-weighted fat-suppressed SS-ETSE image (*j*) in a fifth patient with neuroblastoma shows the presence of retrocrural lymph nodes that represent recurrent disease.

reactive lymph nodes may exceed 2 cm in diameter in the vicinity of malignant neoplasms and gastrointestinal and pancreatic cancers and cholangiocarcinoma usually involve lymph nodes without causing nodal enlargement. Tissue-specific contrast agents may increase the diagnostic accuracy of MRI in characterizing retroperitoneal lymphadenopathy. MR lymphography using iron oxide particles is currently under investigation. This technique has been shown to distinguish contrast-enhanced, low-signal intensity benign lymph nodes from nonenhanced, intermediate, heterogeneous signal intensity malignant nodes on T2-weighted images in animal models [89]; initial clinical trials are promising [90].

Testicular Cancer

Testicular cancer may arise in an undescended testis located in the retroperitoneum [91], in the mediastinum or the retroperitoneum without evidence of primary testicular tumor [65], or in the testicles, metastasizing along the lymphatic pathway of testicular arteries and veins into para-aortic and paracaval nodes at the level of the renal hila (fig. 10.52). It is the most common solid cancer in men between the ages of 15 and 34 years, and in 95% of the cases it is of germ cell origin, either seminomatous (40%) or nonseminomatous (embryonal cell tumors, teratocarcinomas, teratomas, choriocarcinomas, and mixed histology tumors). The remaining 5% are of stromal origin (Sertoli, Leydig, or mesenchymal cell carcinomas). MRI and CT imaging have comparable abil-

ity to detect lymphadenopathy associated with testicular cancer [92]. MRI is useful in detecting undescended testes, which may be the site of origin of testicular neoplasms. T2-weighted fat-suppressed images may show the undescended testis as a moderate- to high-signal intensity structure along the anatomic course of the spermatic vessels. In tumors arising in undescended testes, MRI may perform better than CT imaging in lesion characterization [91].

Primary Retroperitoneal Neoplasms

The majority of primary retroperitoneal tumors (70–90%) are malignant (figs. 10.53–10.56) [85, 86, 93, 94]. The most common histological type is liposarcoma, followed by leiomyosarcoma and malignant fibrous histiocytoma

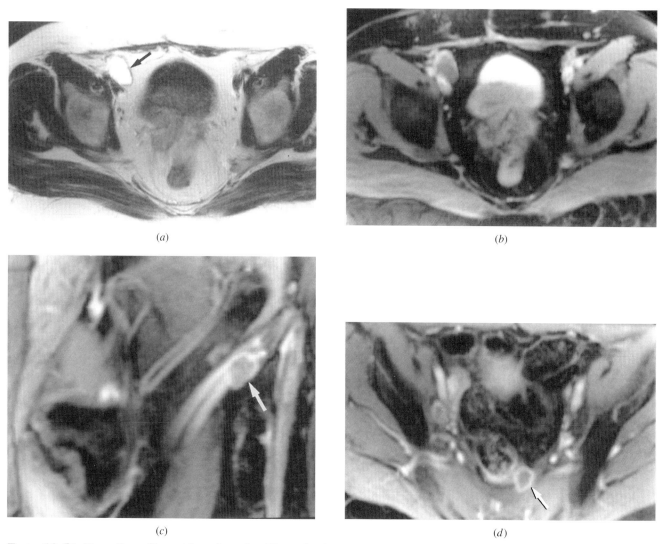

(a)

(b)

(c)

(d)

F I G . 10.51 Necrotic malignant lymph nodes. T2-weighted ETSE (*a*) and interstitial-phase gadolinium-enhanced fat-suppressed SGE (*b*) images in a patient with ovarian cancer. There is a large right external iliac lymph node (arrow, *a*) that is high signal on T2 (*a*) and is centrally near signal void with a thin peripheral rim of enhancement on the postgadolinium image (*b*).

Sagittal (*c*) and transverse (*d*) interstitial-phase gadolinium-enhanced fat-suppressed SGE images in a second patient, who has cervical cancer, demonstrate a left perirectal lymph node that is low signal and has a thin rim enhancement (arrow *c*, *d*). The combination of sagittal- and transverse-plane images permit identification of the rounded configuration of the mass in multiple planes.

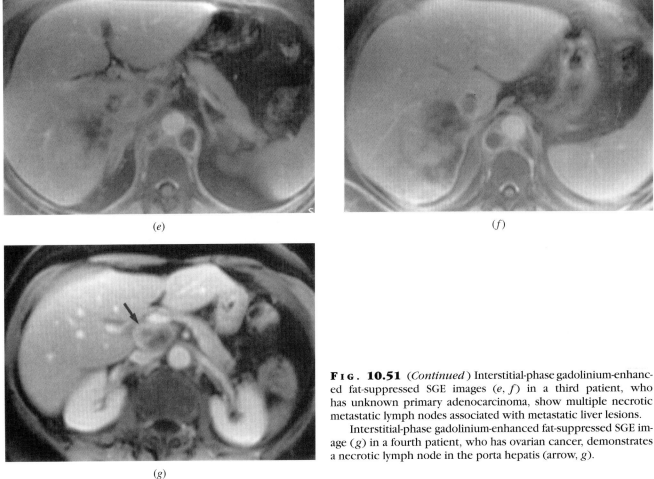

(e)

(f)

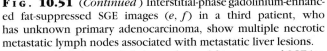

(g)

FIG. 10.51 (*Continued*) Interstitial-phase gadolinium-enhanced fat-suppressed SGE images (*e, f*) in a third patient, who has unknown primary adenocarcinoma, show multiple necrotic metastatic lymph nodes associated with metastatic liver lesions.

Interstitial-phase gadolinium-enhanced fat-suppressed SGE image (*g*) in a fourth patient, who has ovarian cancer, demonstrates a necrotic lymph node in the porta hepatis (arrow, *g*).

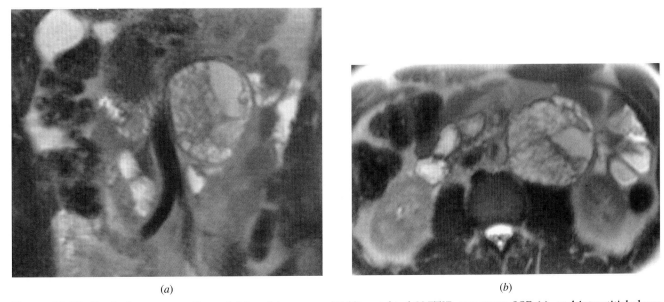

(a)

(b)

FIG. 10.52 Testicular cancer. Coronal (*a*) and transverse (*b*) T2-weighted SS-ETSE, transverse SGE (*c*), and interstitial-phase gadolinium-enhanced fat-suppressed SGE (*d*) images. There is a large left retroperitoneal mass that demonstrates heterogeneous internal signal on T1- and T2-weighted images and possesses thin septations that enhance after contrast administration. This is consistent with a large nodal mass secondary to nonseminomatous testicular cancer.

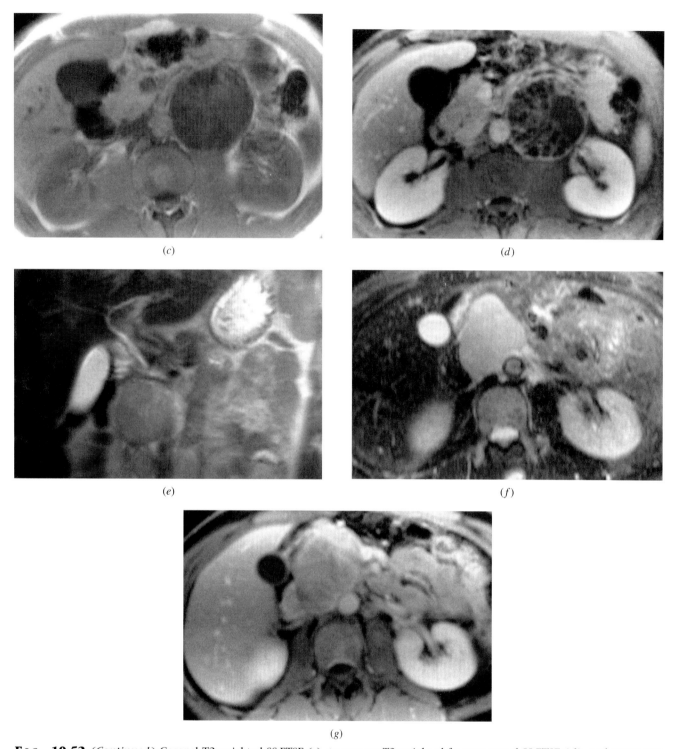

(c)

(d)

(e)

(f)

(g)

FIG. 10.52 (*Continued*) Coronal T2-weighted SS-ETSE (*e*), transverse T2-weighted fat-suppressed SS-ETSE (*f*), and transverse interstitial-phase gadolinium-enhanced SGE (*g*) images in a second patient, who has right testis rhabdomyosarcoma. There is a nodal mass in the aortocaval region that displaces the pancreas anteriorly and the inferior vena cava laterally. Left para-aortic lymph nodes are also identified.

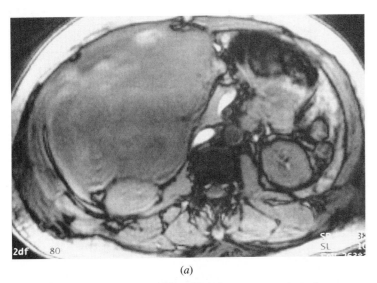

(a)

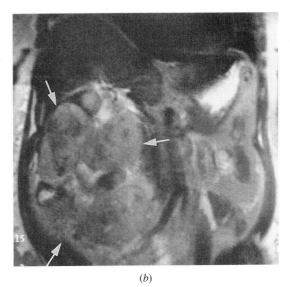

(b)

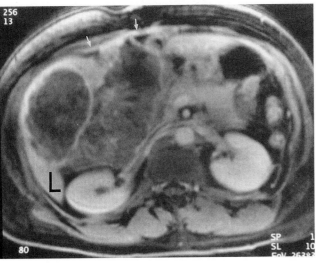

(c)

FIG. 10.53 Retroperitoneal carcinoma. Out-of-phase SGE (*a*), coronal T2-weighted SS-ETSE (*b*), and interstitial-phase gadolinium-enhanced fat-suppressed SGE (*c*) images. A large, lobulated, heterogeneous mass is located in the right abdomen. The mass is heterogenous on both T1- (*a*) and T2-weighted (arrows, *b*) images, displacing the aorta and IVC medially and the right kidney posteriorly. Areas of high signal intensity on the T2-weighted image (*b*) represent necrotic areas. The mass demonstrates peripheral and patchy heterogeneous enhancement on the interstitial-phase gadolinium-enhanced fat-suppressed SGE image (*c*). Invasion of the right lobe of the liver ("*l*," *c*) is clearly demonstrated. The mass abuts the anterior abdominal wall, and enhancement of the anterior peritoneum (small arrows, *c*) is evident secondary to recent laparotomy attempt, which was aborted because of the large size of the mass.

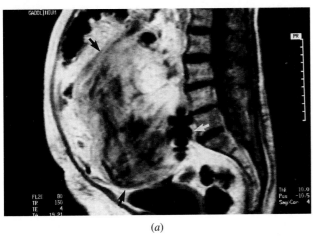

(a)

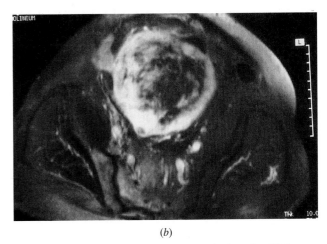

(b)

FIG. 10.54 Retroperitoneal sarcoma. Sagittal T1-SE (*a*) and postgadolinium T1-weighted fat-suppressed spin-echo (*b*) images in a patient with recurrent retroperitoneal leiomyosarcoma. A large, markedly heterogeneous mass (arrows, *a*) arises in the retroperitoneum immediately anterior to the lumbar spine and extends inferiorly to the pelvis. The mass demonstrates intense heterogeneous enhancement on interstitial-phase gadolinium-enhanced images. Magnetic susceptibility artifacts are present caused by surgical clips (white arrow, *a*).

Transverse interstitial-phase gadolinium-enhanced fat-suppressed SGE image (*c*) in a second patient, who has retroperitoneal leiomyosarcoma, demonstrates a large left-sided retroperitoneal mass that is heterogeneous in appearance and invades the lower and medial aspect of the left kidney.

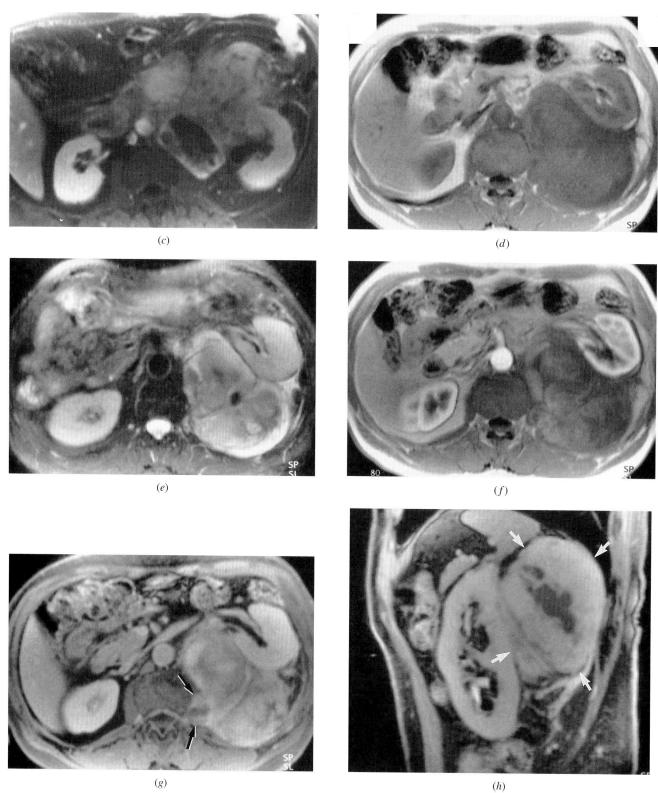

(c)

(d)

(e)

(f)

(g)

(h)

F I G . 10.54 (*Continued*) SGE (*d*), T2-weighted fat-suppressed echo-train spin-echo (*e*), immediate postgadolinium SGE (*f*), and transverse (*g*) and sagittal (*h*) interstitial-phase gadolinium-enhanced fat-suppressed SGE images in a third patient, who has pleomorphic rhabdomyosarcoma. A large, left-sided retroperitoneal rhabdomyosarcoma mass is present. The mass displaces the left kidney anterolaterally, consistent with the retroperitoneal origin of the mass. The mass is heterogeneous and low in signal intensity on the precontrast SGE image (*d*) and heterogeneous and mixed high signal intensity on the T2-weighted image (*e*). The mass demonstrates moderate and heterogeneous enhancement on the immediate postgadolinium SGE image (*f*) with progressive enhancement on the interstitial-phase fat-suppressed SGE images (*g*, *h*). Invasion of the left psoas muscle (arrows, *g*) is well shown on the interstitial-phase fat-suppressed SGE image (*g*) as an enhancing area with irregular margins within the muscle. The sagittal image demonstrates the longitudinal extent of the mass (arrows, *h*) and anterior displacement of the kidney. Central necrosis is present that appears as a central area of lack of enhancement within the mass.

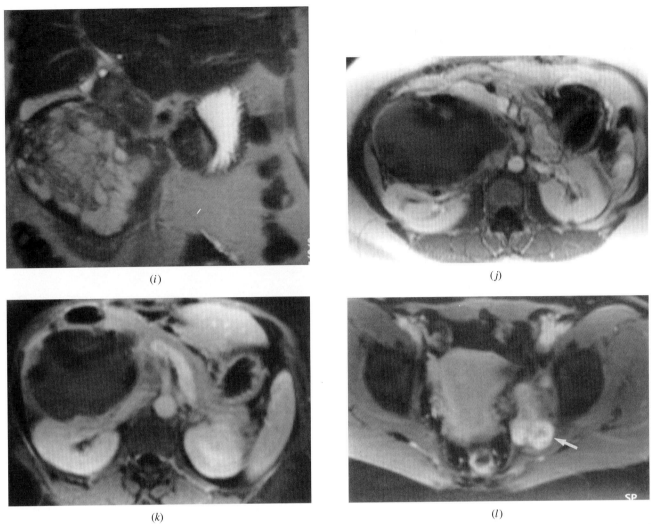

(i)

(j)

(k)

(l)

FIG. 10.54 (*Continued*) Coronal SS-ETSE (*i*), immediate postgadolinium SGE (*j*), and interstitial-phase gadolinium-enhanced fat-suppressed SGE (*k*) in a fourth patient, who has retroperitoneal sarcoma. A large and heterogeneously enhancing tumor with septations and necrosis is seen in the right abdomen, abutting the head of the pancreas, porta hepatis, the right kidney, and the inferior vena cava.

Interstitial-phase gadolinium-enhanced fat-suppressed SGE (*l*) image in a fifth patient, who has retroperitoneal sarcoma. A heterogeneous, moderately intense mass (arrow, *l*) is present in the left pelvis. Involvement of the obturator internus and pyriformis muscles is apparent.

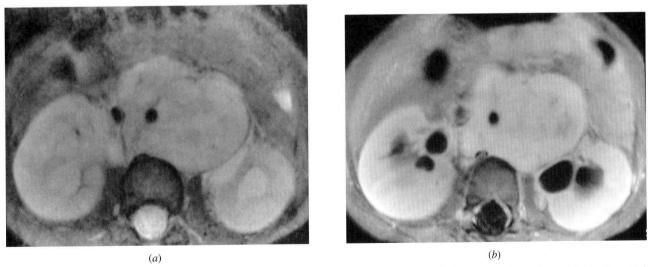

(a)

(b)

FIG. 10.55 Embryonal rhabdomyosarcoma. T2-weighted ETSE fat-suppressed (*a*), and transverse (*b*) and sagittal (*c*) interstitial-phase gadolinium-enhanced T1-weighted fat-suppressed SE images in a 21-month-old patient with embryonal rhabdomyosarcoma.

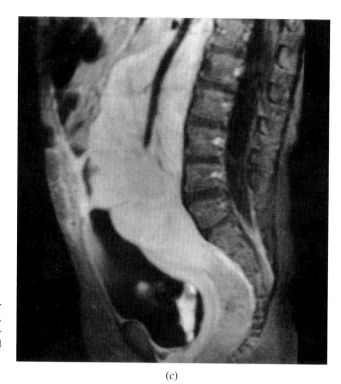

(c)

FIG. 10.55 (*Continued*) There is massive enhancing retroperitoneal adenopathy that lifts and encases the aorta, iliac vessels, and IVC. The lymph nodes are moderately hyperintense on T2-weighted images (*a*) and enhance moderately intensely with mild heterogeneity on postgadolinium images (*b*, *c*).

[65, 66, 93, 94]. A male predominance exists for liposarcomas and malignant fibrous histiocytomas, whereas leiomyosarcomas are more common in women [65, 66]. Tumors are typically large at presentation (see figs. 10.53 and 10.54), because of their silent clinical course. Presenting symptoms include abdominal mass, pain, weight loss, and nausea and vomiting [66]. In a review of leiomyosarcomas of the retroperitoneum and IVC, leiomyosarcomas with no major vascular involvement have been classified as Pattern 1 and comprise 62% of

the total cases [66]. On MR images, tumors are generally mixed low and intermediate in signal intensity on T1-weighted images and mixed medium and high in signal intensity on T2-weighted images [66, 94]. Tumors enhance in a heterogeneous fashion, and leiomyosarcomas, in particular, are hypervascular and demonstrate intense enhancement (fig. 10.54). Areas of necrosis may be present, which is common in leiomyosarcomas [65, 66], and are demonstrated as areas that are low signal intensity on T1-weighted images, high signal intensity on

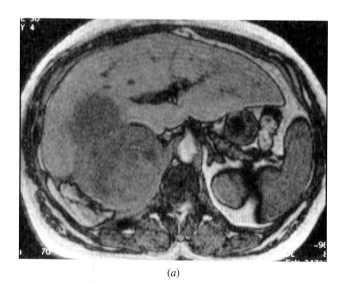

(a)

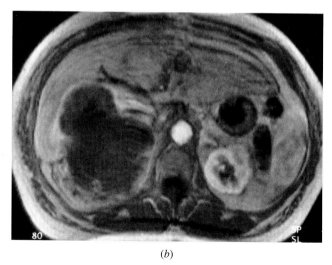

(b)

FIG. 10.56 Hemangiopericytoma. Transverse out-of-phase SGE (*a*) and immediate postgadolinium SGE (*b*) images show a large lobulated necrotic mass in the right abdomen that invades the right kidney and the liver. Histopathologic examination established the diagnosis of hemangiopericytoma.

T2-weighted images, and lack enhancement on post-gadolinium images. Hemorrhage occasionally occurs in the liquefied necrotic areas and appears mixed high signal intensity on T1-weighted images and mixed low and high signal intensity on T2-weighted images, with occasional demonstration of a dependent low-signal layer on T2-weighted images [66]. The various histologic types share common MRI appearances, and differentiation may not be feasible. In rare cases liposarcomas may be sufficiently well differentiated (lipogenic liposarcoma) to contain mature fat, which is high in signal intensity on T1- and T2-weighted echo-train spin-echo images, intermediate in signal intensity on T2-weighted spin-echo images, and suppresses on fat-suppressed images. In these cases, soft tissue strands are present within the fatty mass, and tumor nodules may enhance after gadolinium administration. These tumors are well assessed by MRI, which provides direct imaging of the craniocaudal and transverse extent of the tumor.

Neuroblastoma and ganglioneuroblastoma are tumors discussed in Chapter 8, Adrenal Glands. Extra-adrenal involvement increases with age [95]. MRI with the use of phased-array multicoil, T2-weighted fat-suppressed echo-train spin-echo, and gadolinium-enhanced T1-weighted fat-suppressed images provides excellent morphologic detail and tumor/background contrast. MRI may be superior to CT imaging because CT may not detect small tumor masses or involved lymph nodes in this mainly pediatric population due to small patient size and lack of retroperitoneal fat. The T2-weighted single-shot echo train spin-echo sequence should be part of the imaging protocol as it is very resistant to motion artifacts from movement or respiration. This is important in pediatric patients, who may move during the acquisition, and in problematic areas such as the subdiaphragmatic paraspinal retroperitoneum. Added advantages of MRI include the lack of ionizing radiation and direct imaging in the coronal and sagittal plane, which provides direct evaluation of the craniocaudal extent of tumor and facilitates detection of tumor extension into the neural foramina, a common feature of these neoplasms. Furthermore, MRI is the method of choice for imaging of the spine and delineation of tumor involving neural and perineural structures.

PSOAS MUSCLE

Diseases affecting the psoas muscle more commonly originate from adjacent structures and involve the muscle by direct extension. These include malignant and infectious processes of the spine, kidney, bowel, pancreas, and retroperitoneal lymph nodes [96, 97]. Atrophy of the iliopsoas from neuromuscular disease can occur. Spontaneous hemorrhage may also occur in the iliopsoas muscle and is most frequently observed in patients on anticoagulant therapy or in hemophiliacs. Primary tumors of the muscle are rare, but the psoas can be the site of metastatic deposits.

The psoas muscle is well evaluated by MRI. The normal muscle is low in signal intensity on T2-weighted images. As most disease processes are high in signal intensity on T2-weighted images (fig. 10.57), they are usually clearly shown [96, 97]. Imaging in the coronal or sagittal planes provides direct evaluation of the full craniocaudal extent of the muscle. Lymph nodes are well evaluated on precontrast sagittal SGE images in a background of retroperitoneal fat, but they are isointense with psoas muscle. Lymph nodes are readily distinguished from psoas muscle on T2-weighted images because muscle is low in signal intensity compared to the moderate signal intensity of lymph nodes [96, 97]. Metastatic disease to

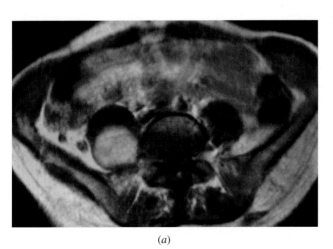

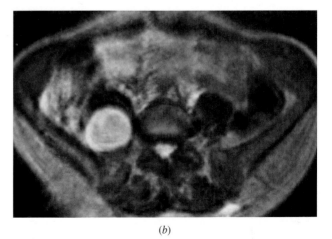

(a)   (b)

F I G. 10.57 Neurogenic psoas tumor. T1-weighted spin-echo (*a*) and T2-weighted spin-echo (*b*) images. A well-defined rounded tumor is noted in the right psoas muscle. The tumor is moderate in signal intensity on the T1-weighted image and high in signal intensity on the T2-weighted image. High signal intensity on T2-weighted images is a common feature of tumors of neural origin.

the iliopsoas muscle is moderate to high in signal intensity on T2-weighted images and shows substantial enhancement on gadolinium-enhanced fat-suppressed T1-weighted SGE images (figs. 10.58 and 10.59). Infection is well shown on MR images as high-signal intensity areas on fat-suppressed T2-weighted images and intense enhancement on gadolinium-enhanced fat-suppressed SGE images (fig. 10.60). Destruction of adjacent vertebral body is common with associated extension into the disk space. Disk space involvement is more typical of infection than of malignancy. On postgadolinium images, abscesses are shown as expansile lesions with signal-void centers, intense peripheral enhancement, and enhancement of the periabscess tissues (see fig. 10.60).

Hemorrhage is well shown on MR images because the high signal intensity of subacute blood on T1-weighted images [98–100]. The appearance of a fluid structure that possesses a high-signal peripheral rim in noncontrast T1-weighted fat suppressed images is

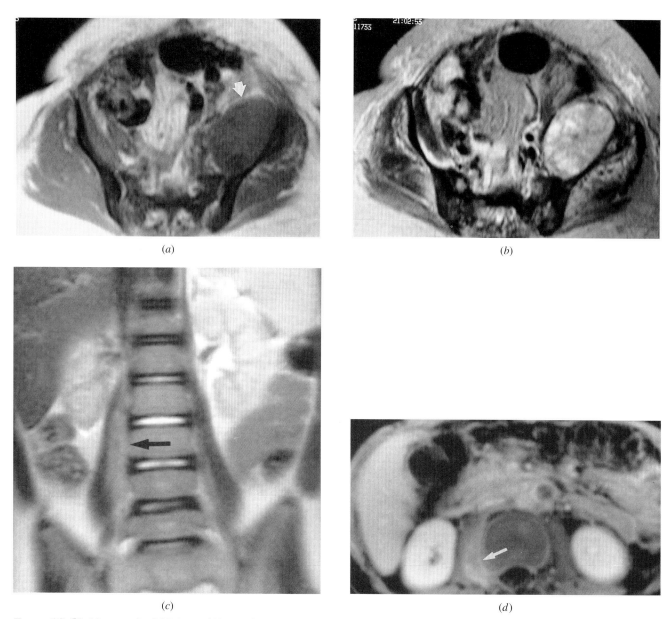

(a)

(b)

(c)

(d)

F I G . 10.58 Metastasis. SGE (*a*) and T2-weighted spin-echo (*b*) images. A large heterogeneous mass (arrow, *a*) is present in the left iliopsoas muscle, consistent with metastasis from breast cancer. The metastasis is low in signal intensity on the SGE image (*a*) and high in signal intensity on the T2-weighted spin-echo image (*b*).

Coronal T2-weighted SS-ETSE (*c*) and transverse 90-s gadolinium-enhanced fat-suppressed SGE (*d*) images in a second patient, who has a history of neuroblastoma, demonstrate an area within the medial right psoas muscle with high signal on the T2-weighted image (arrow, *c*) and peripheral enhancement after contrast administration (*d*), which represents a metastasis.

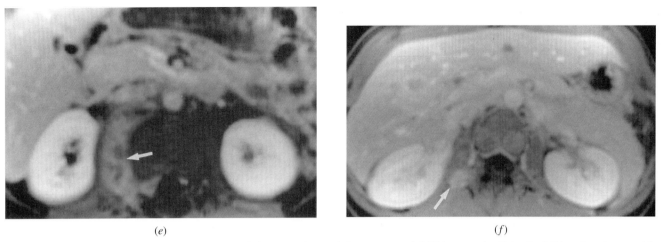

(e)   *(f)*

F ɪ ɢ . 10.58 *(Continued)* Transverse 90-s gadolinium-enhanced fat-suppressed SGE images *(e, f)* in 2 additional patients with cancer demonstrate metastatic masses (arrow, *e, f*) involving the right psoas muscle. The greater enhancement of the metastases relative to the psoas muscle increases their conspicuity.

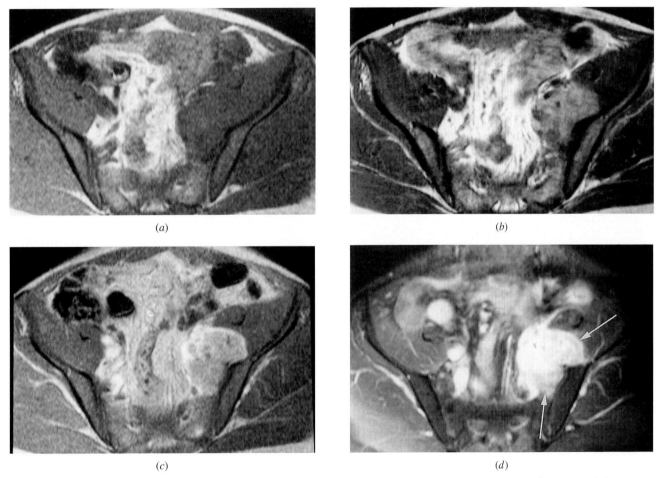

(a)   *(b)*

(c)   *(d)*

F ɪ ɢ . 10.59 Metastasis to the iliacus muscle from melanoma. SGE *(a)*, T2-weighted spin-echo *(b)*, 45-s postgadolinium *(c)*, and gadolinium-enhanced T1-weighted fat-suppressed spin-echo *(d)* images. A mass is identified in the posterior portion of the left iliacus muscle. The mass is isointense to muscle on the SGE image *(a)* and heterogeneously high in signal intensity on the T2-weighted image *(b)* and enhances in a heterogeneous fashion after gadolinium administration *(c, d)*. The degree of enhancement and delineation of its borders are best appreciated on the postgadolinium T1-weighted fat-suppressed spin-echo image (arrows, *d*).

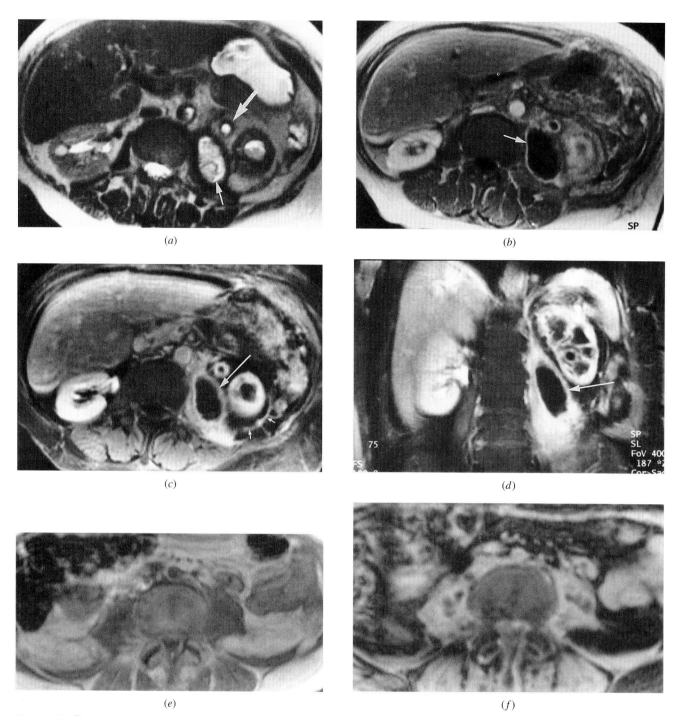

(a)

(b)

(c)

(d)

(e)

(f)

FIG. 10.60 Psoas abscess. T2-weighted SS-ETSE (*a*), 45-s postgadolinium SGE (*b*), and transverse (*c*) and coronal (*d*) interstitial-phase gadolinium-enhanced fat-suppressed SGE images. A complex fluid collection is present in an enlarged left psoas muscle. The fluid is heterogeneously high in signal intensity on the T2-weighted image (arrow, *a*) and contains low-signal intensity necrotic debris. The left ureter (large arrow, *a*) is dilated and has a thick wall. The abscess wall (arrow, *b*) and the ureteral wall demonstrate enhancement on the 45-s postgadolinium SGE image (*b*), which progresses on the interstitial-phase images (*c*, *d*) to intense enhancement of the abscess-containing psoas muscle (long arrows, *c*, *d*) and the ureteral wall. Ill-defined borders with linear enhancing strands reflect the extension of the inflammation into the pararenal and perirenal fat. Enhancement of the thickened left perirenal fascia (small arrows, *c*) is also noted. The contents of the abscess are signal void on the postgadolinium images (*b*–*d*). Imaging in the coronal plane (*d*) provides direct evaluation of the craniocaudal extent of the abscess. The right psoas muscle is uninvolved and remains low in signal intensity on the postgadolinium images. The collecting system of the left kidney is dilated and low in signal intensity on the interstitial-phase gadolinium-enhanced fat-suppressed SGE images (*c*, *d*) because of absent gadolinium excretion in a kidney with xanthogranulomatous pyelonephritis.

SGE (*e*) and interstitial-phase gadolinium-enhanced fat-suppressed SGE (*f*) images in a second patient demonstrate increased enhancement of the psoas muscles bilaterally, which contain fluid collections that have central low-signal areas with peripheral rim enhancement, consistent with abscesses.

virtually pathognomonic for subacute hematoma. The use of fat suppression permits the detection of even small amounts of blood, and imaging in different planes provides direct evaluation of the dimensions and extent of the hematoma (fig. 10.61).

THE BODY WALL

Neoplasms

Benign Tumors

Cysts and desmoid tumors are two common benign body wall tumors [101]. Desmoids may be encountered in the setting of Gardner syndrome and are relatively avascular, locally aggressive masses with a propensity for recurrence, occurring more commonly in middle-aged women [102]. They arise most commonly from the aponeurosis of the rectus abdominis muscle and may

on occasion be very large, mimicking intra-abdominal masses [102]. They are readily detected on T1-weighted images as low-signal intensity masses in a background of high-signal intensity fat (fig. 10.62). In mature desmoids, areas of abundant fibrosis result in low signal intensity on T2-weighted images [102].

The body wall also may be involved in cases of endometriosis, occurring almost exclusively along scars from previous surgery. Endometriomas are generally shown best on noncontrast T1-weighted fat-suppressed SGE images as high-signal intensity foci.

Malignant Tumors

Direct tumor spread, hematogenous metastases (figs. 10.63 and 10.64), sarcomas (figs. 10.65 and 10.66), and lymphomas can involve the body wall. Tumors are medium-signal intensity masses that are well defined in the background of high-signal intensity subcutaneous

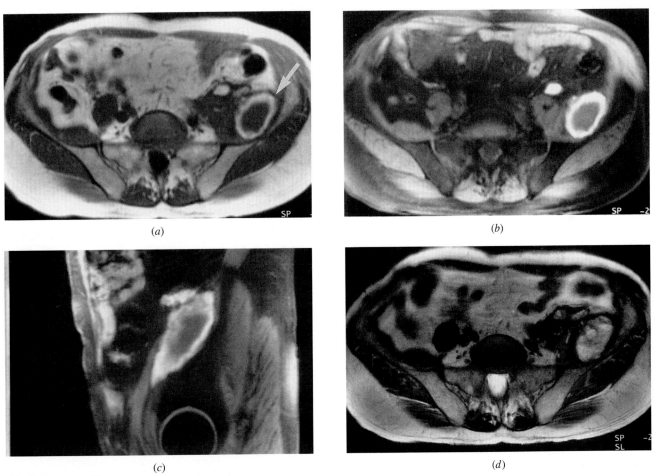

(a)

(b)

(c)

(d)

F I G. 10.61 Hematoma in the right iliacus muscle. SGE (*a*), transverse (*b*) and sagittal (*c*) fat-suppressed SGE, T2-weighted echo-train spin-echo (*d*), and T2-weighted fat-suppressed echo-train spin-echo (*e*) images. The left iliacus is enlarged and contains a complex fluid collection that is low in signal intensity centrally with a high-signal intensity peripheral rim (arrow, *a*) on the T1-weighted images (*a–c*) and heterogeneously high in signal intensity on the T2-weighted images (*d, e*). The hyperintensity of the peripheral rim is accentuated with the use of fat suppression on the T1-weighted images (*b, c*). The sagittal fat-suppressed SGE image (*c*) demonstrates the craniocaudal extent of the hematoma. The mixed signal intensity of the hematoma reflects blood products in different stages of degradation.

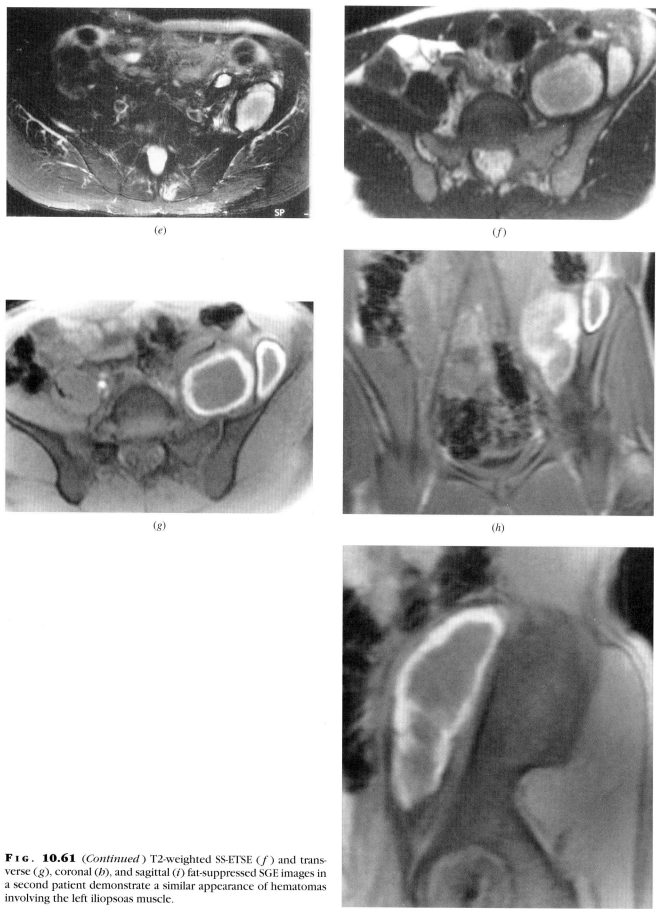

(e)

(f)

(g)

(h)

(i)

FIG. 10.61 (*Continued*) T2-weighted SS-ETSE (*f*) and transverse (*g*), coronal (*h*), and sagittal (*i*) fat-suppressed SGE images in a second patient demonstrate a similar appearance of hematomas involving the left iliopsoas muscle.

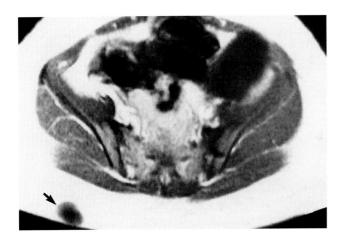

F I G . 10.62 Desmoid. SGE image in a patient with Gardner syndrome demonstrates a subcutaneous desmoid (arrow) in the right gluteal region. Fibrous tumors are low in signal intensity on T1-weighted images and are readily detected against a background of high-signal intensity fat.

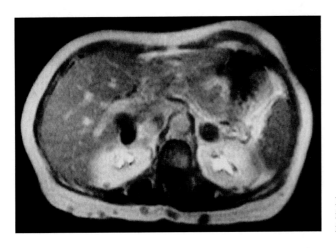

F I G . 10.63 Subcutaneous metastases. Delayed postgadolinium SGE image demonstrates multiple subcutaneous metastases from breast cancer.

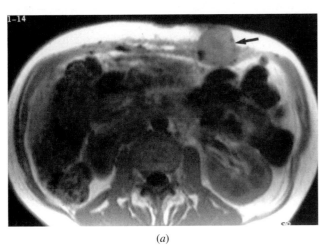

(a)

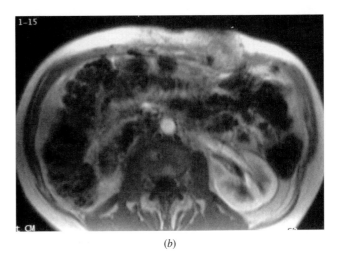

(b)

F I G . 10.64 Abdominal wall metastases from hepatocellular carcinoma (HCC). SGE (a), immediate postgadolinium SGE (b), and 90-s gadolinium-enhanced fat-suppressed SGE (c) images. An abdominal wall metastasis is present (arrow, a) that is isointense in T1 (a) and demonstrates moderate enhancement with mild heterogeneity on immediate postgadolinium image (b) and heterogeneous enhancement on delayed fat-suppressed image (c). The mass is well shown on sequences that have good contrast between tumor and background tissue, such as SGE and gadolinium-enhanced fat-suppressed SGE.

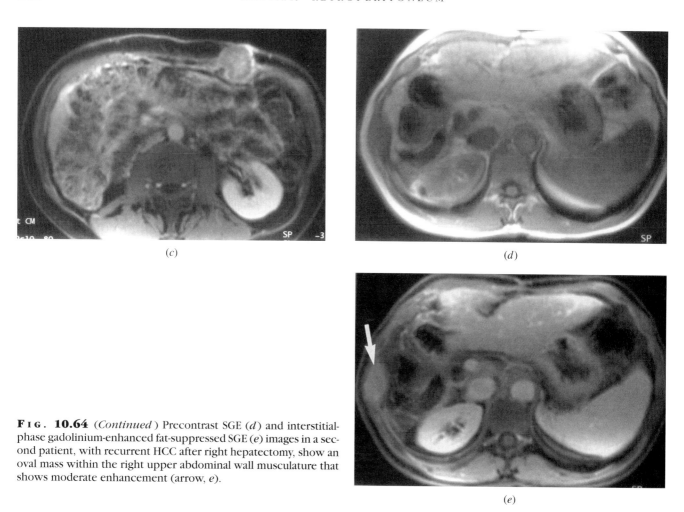

(c)

(d)

FIG. 10.64 (*Continued*) Precontrast SGE (*d*) and interstitial-phase gadolinium-enhanced fat-suppressed SGE (*e*) images in a second patient, with recurrent HCC after right hepatectomy, show an oval mass within the right upper abdominal wall musculature that shows moderate enhancement (arrow, *e*).

(e)

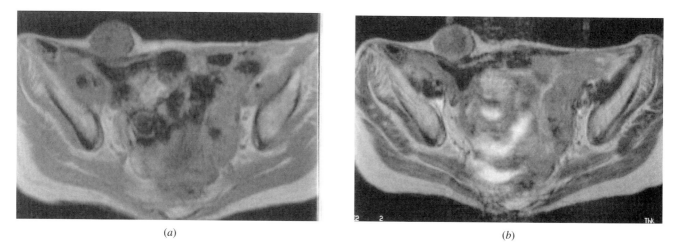

(a)

(b)

FIG. 10.65 **Malignant fibrous histiocytoma of the right anterior abdominal wall.** SGE (*a*), transverse (*b*) and sagittal (*c*) T2-weighted echo-train spin-echo, 90-s postgadolinium SGE at superior (*d*) and inferior (*e*) tomographic levels, and gadolinium-enhanced T1-weighted fat-suppressed spin-echo (*f*) images. The tumor is readily identified as a low-signal intensity well-defined mass against the high-signal intensity background of subcutaneous fat on the T1-weighted image (*a*) and is heterogeneously low to intermediate in signal intensity on the T2-weighted images (*b*, *c*). The tumor abuts and displaces the right rectus abdominis muscle, which is well shown on the sagittal T2-weighted image (*c*).

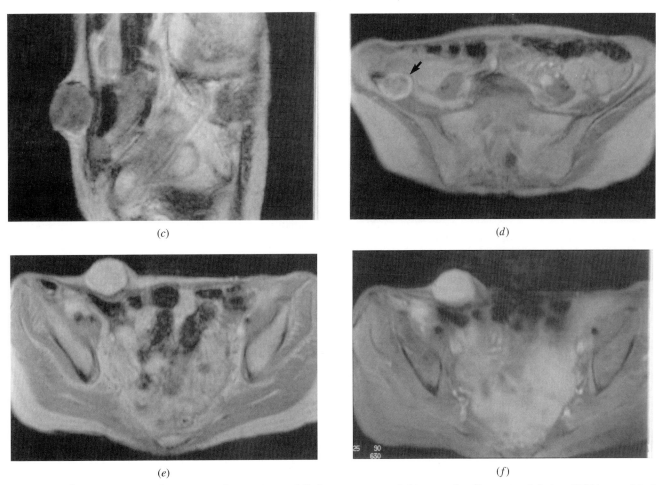

(c)   (d)

(e)   (f)

F I G . 10.65 (*Continued*) The tumor enhances in a mildly heterogeneous fashion on the 45-s postgadolinium SGE image (*e*). A metastatic tumor nodule (arrow, *d*) with predominantly peripheral heterogeneous enhancement is also present at a higher tomographic level (*d*) in the right iliacus muscle. Enhancement of the tumor is more uniform on the more delayed gadolinium-enhanced T1-weighted fat-suppressed spin-echo image (*f*), reflecting delayed enhancement of the fibrotic components of the tumor. The use of fat suppression increases the conspicuity of the abnormally enhancing tumor.

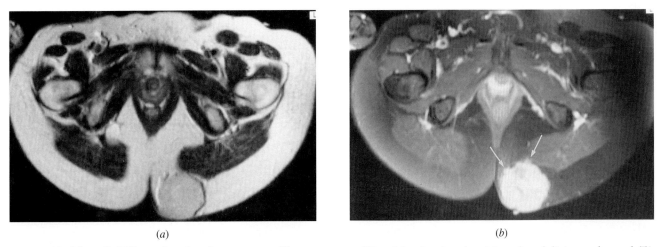

(a)   (b)

F I G . 10.66 Well-differentiated subcutaneous fibrosarcoma. T2-weighted spin-echo (*a*) and gadolinium-enhanced T1-weighted fat-suppressed spin-echo (*b*) images. The tumor is located in the subcutaneous tissue of the left buttock, is moderate in signal intensity on the T2-weighted image (*a*), and shows intense enhancement on the gadolinium-enhanced T1-weighted fat-suppressed image (*b*). The anterior margin of the mass appears irregular (arrows, *b*) and abuts the gluteus maximus muscle. Note the presence of chemical-shift artifact on the lateral edges of the mass on the T2-weighted image (*a*).

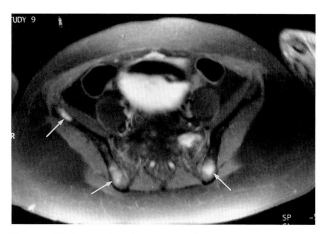

Fig. 10.67 Leukemic bone infiltrates. Gadolinium-enhanced T1-weighted fat-suppressed spin-echo image in a patient with leukemia shows focal enhancing leukemic lesions (arrows) in the bone marrow of the iliac bones bilaterally. Normal fat-containing marrow is low in signal intensity, rendering enhancing tumors conspicuous.

fat on T1-weighted SE or SGE images. On gadolinium-enhanced fat-suppressed T1-weighted images they are moderate to high in signal intensity in a background of low-signal intensity fat. Imaging in the sagittal plane permits direct visualization of the extent of the tumor and its relationship to the abdominal wall muscles.

Tumors arising in or involving the skeletal structures of the abdomen and pelvis are well shown on a combination of T1-weighted images, T2-weighted fat-suppressed images, and gadolinium-enhanced fat-suppressed SGE images (figs. 10.67 and 10.68).

Miscellaneous

Hernias, hematomas, infection, arteriovenous malformations, and varices (fig. 10.69) may involve the abdominal wall. (Hernias are discussed in Chapter 7, Peritoneal Cavity.) Malignant or vascular lesions are well shown on SGE and gadolinium-enhanced fat-suppressed SGE images. Vascular structures are shown as low-signal intensity structures on SGE images and enhance after gadolinium administration. The enhancement is rendered more conspicuous with the addition of fat suppression on postcontrast images. Involvement of the abdominal wall in cases of hemangiomas or lymphangiomas is not infrequent and may be part of a larger mass, usually of congenital origin. MRI demonstrates multiple ovoid and tubular structures infiltrating subcutaneous tissue and abdominal wall muscles (fig. 10.70). The hemangiomatous component is comprised of smaller vascular spaces that may enhance after gadolinium administration, whereas the lymphangiomatous components are generally cystic, larger in size, and high in signal intensity on T1-weighted images and demonstrate dependent low-signal intensity layers on T2-weighted images (see fig. 10.70). MRI using multiplanar imaging demonstrates the extent of the abnormality and degree of infiltration of muscles and abdominal structures. Heavily T2-weighted echo-train spin-echo images have been used to image patients with generalized lymphangiomatosis, because the fluid-filled cystic spaces are high in signal intensity on these images. Differentiation from hemangiomatous malformations or the hemangiomatous component of mixed malformations may also be possible with this technique because the vascular hemangiomatous spaces will be lower in signal intensity on these images [103].

Cellulitis can be differentiated from abscess on MR images by the demonstration of a signal-void center in an abscess. The extent of inflammatory or infectious disease is well defined on gadolinium-enhanced fat-suppressed SGE images by the extent and intensity of high-signal enhancing tissue.

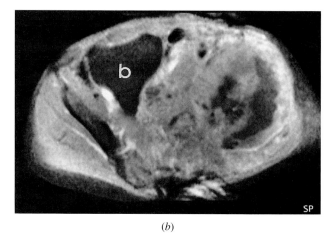

(a)　　　　　(b)

Fig. 10.68 Extensive Ewing sarcoma of the pelvis. T2-weighted fat-suppressed echo-train spin-echo (a) and gadolinium-enhanced fat-suppressed SGE (b) images. An extensive heterogeneous mass originating from the left iliac bone is demonstrated. The mass invades all the muscles of the left pelvis and displaces the bladder ("b," a, b) to the right. The tumor is heterogeneous with mixed high-signal intensity areas on the T2-weighted image (a) and demonstrates heterogeneous enhancement after gadolinium administration (b).

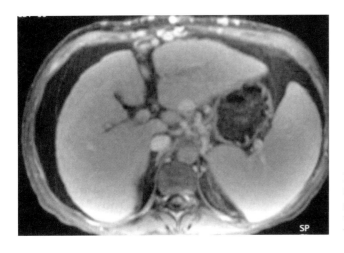

FIG. 10.69 Subcutaneous varices in a patient with cirrhosis. Interstitial-phase gadolinium-enhanced fat-suppressed SGE image demonstrates numerous enhancing serpiginous vessels within the anterior abdominal wall, consistent with varices. Multiple varices at the gastroesophageal junction are also present.

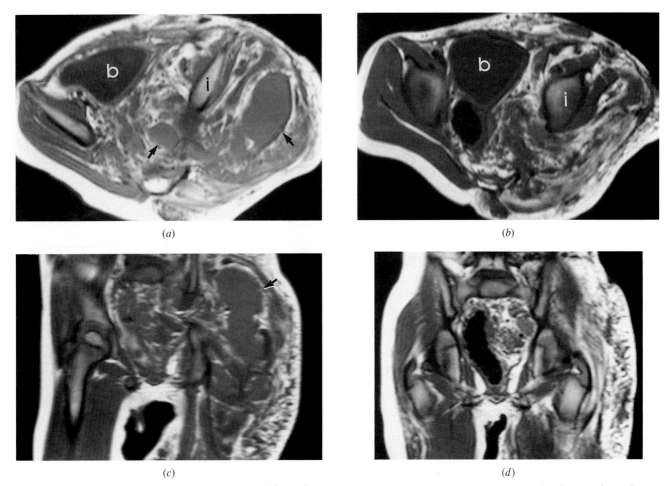

(a)

(b)

(c)

(d)

FIG. 10.70 Lymphangioma-hemangioma of the pelvis. Transverse (a, b) and coronal (c, d) T1-weighted spin-echo and transverse (e, f) and sagittal (g) T2-weighted spin-echo images. An extensive heterogeneous mass is present in the left and central pelvis. The mass infiltrates the subcutaneous tissue of the entire left hemipelvis, the gluteus maximus, intermedius, and minor muscles and extends into the true pelvis, causing extensive deformity and displacing the bladder ("b," a, b, e–g) and left iliac bone ("i," a, b, e, f) anteriorly to the right.

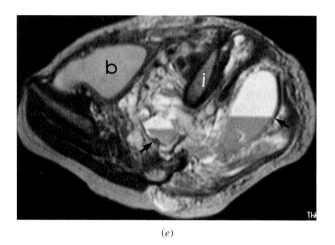

(e)

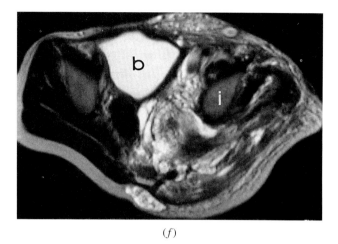

(f)

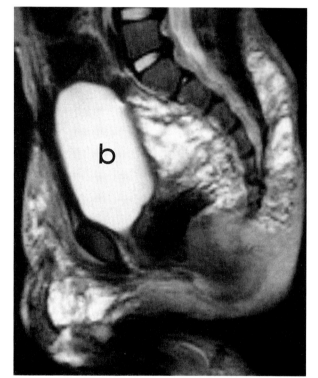

(g)

F I G . 10.70 (*Continued*) The mass consists of numerous tubular and ovoid cystic structures, representing malformed blood and lymph vessels. The cystic spaces are low in signal intensity on the T1-weighted images and high in signal intensity on the T2-weighted images, reflecting their fluid content. Larger fluid-filled cystic spaces (arrows, *a, c, e*) have fluid-fluid levels on the T2-weighted image (*e*) with the dependent lower-signal intensity level representing fluid of higher protein concentration. The presence of large fluid-filled cystic spaces is characteristic of lymphangiomatous rather than hemangiomatous malformations. The coronal images (*c, d*) demonstrate the extent of the pelvic deformity and extension of the vascular malformation to the muscles and subcutaneous tissues of the left thigh, which are enlarged compared with the contralateral side.

CONCLUSION

MRI should be considered as a primary diagnostic technique for assessment of most benign and malignant disease processes affecting the retroperitoneum and body wall. Continued advances in MRA, with improvements in dynamic gadolinium-enhanced gradient-echo and true FISP sequencing techniques, and improved automated multistation surface phased-array coil and table movement systems, have resulted in an increasing role for MRI in the diagnosis of aortoiliac disease

REFERENCES

1. Molmenti EP, Balfe DM, Kanterman RY, Bennet HF: Anatomy of the retroperitoneum: Observations of the distribution of pathologic fluid collections. *Radiology* 200: 95–103, 1996.
2. Lepor H, Walsh PC: Idiopathic retroperitoneal fibrosis. *J Urol* 122: 1–6, 1979.
3. Swan JS, Grist TM, Weber DM, Sproat IA, Wojtowycz MM: MR angiography of the pelvis with variable velocity encoding and a phased-array coil. *Radiology* 190: 363–369, 1994.
4. Arlart IP, Guhl L, Edelman RR: Magnetic resonance angiography of the abdominal aorta. *Cardiovasc Intervent Radiol* 15: 43–50, 1992.

5. Sallevelt PE, Barentsz JO, Ruijs SJ, Heijstraten FM, Buskens FG, Strijk SP: Role of MR imaging in the preoperative evaluation of atherosclerotic abdominal aortic aneurysms. *Radiographics* 14: 87–98; 1994.

6. Kim D, Edelman RR, Kent KC, Porter DH, Skillman JJ: Abdominal aorta and renal artery stenosis: Evaluation with MR angiography. *Radiology* 174: 727–731, 1990.

7. Mulligan SA, Doyle M, Matsuda T, Koslin DB, Kenney PJ, Barton RE, Pohost GM: Aortoiliac disease: Two-dimensional inflow MR angiography with lipid suppression. *J Magn Reson Imaging* 3: 829–834, 1993.

8. Ecklund K, Hartnell GG, Hughes LA, Stokes KR, Finn JP: MR angiography as the sole method in evaluating abdominal aortic aneurysms: Correlation with conventional techniques and surgery [see comments]. *Radiology* 192: 345–350, 1994.

9. Durham JR, Hackworth CA, Tober JC, Bova JG, Bennett WF, Schmalbrock P, Van Aman ME, Horowitz JD, Wright JG, Smead WL: Magnetic resonance angiography in the preoperative evaluation of abdominal aortic aneurysms. *Am J Surg* 166: 173–177, 1993.

10. Kaufman JA, Geller SC, Petersen MJ, Cambria RP, Prince MR, Waltman AC: MR imaging (including MR angiography) of abdominal aortic aneurysms: Comparison with conventional angiography. *Am J Roentgenol* 163: 203–210, 1994.

11. Prince MR, Narasimham DL, Jacoby WT, Williams DM, Cho KJ, Marx MV, Deeb GM: Three-dimensional gadolinium enhanced MR angiography of the thoracic aorta. *Am J Roentgenol* 166: 1387–1397, 1996.

12. Douek PC, Revel D, Chazel S, Falise B, Villard J, Amiel M: Fast MR angiography of the aortoiliac arteries and arteries of the lower extremity: Value of bolus-enhanced, whole-volume subtraction technique. *Am J Roentgenol* 165: 431–437, 1995.

13. Prince MR, Yucel EK, Kaufman JA, Harrison DC, Geller SC: Dynamic gadolinium-enhanced three-dimensional abdominal MR arteriography. *J Magn Reson Imaging* 3: 877–881, 1993.

14. Snidow JJ, Aisen AM, Harris VJ, Trerotola SO, Johnson MS, Sawchuk AP, Dalsing MC: Iliac artery MR angiography: Comparison of three-dimensional gadolinium-enhanced and two-dimensional time-of-flight techniques. *Radiology* 196: 371–378, 1995.

15. Sivananthan UM, Ridgway JP, Bann K, Verma SP, Cullingworth J, Ward J, Rees MR: Fast magnetic resonance angiography using turbo-FLASH sequences in advanced aortoiliac disease. *Br J Radiol* 66: 1103–1110, 1993.

16. Prince MR: Gadolinium-enhanced MR aortography. *Radiology* 191: 155–164, 1994.

17. Leung DA, McKinnon GC, Davis CP, Pfammatter T, Krestin GP, Debatin JF: Breath-hold, contrast-enhanced, three-dimensional MR angiography. *Radiology* 200: 562–571, 1996.

18. Edelman RR, Chien D, Kim D. Fast selective black blood MR. imaging. *Radiology* 181: 655–660, 1991.

19. Auffermann W, Olofsson P, Stoney R, Higgins CB: MR imaging of complications of aortic surgery. *J Comput Assist Tomogr* 11: 982–989, 1987.

20. Bickerstaff LK, Hollier LH, Van Peenen HJ, Melton LJd, Pairolero PC, Cherry KJ: Abdominal aortic aneurysms: The changing natural history. *J Vasc Surg* 1: 6–12, 1984.

21. Szilagyi DE, Elliott JP, Smith RF: Clinical fate of the patient with asymptomatic abdominal aortic aneurysm and unfit for surgical treatment. *Arch Surg* 104: 600–606, 1972.

22. Dinsmore RE, Wedeen VJ, Miller SW, Rosen BR, Fifer M, Vlahakes GJ, Edelman RR, Brady TJ: MRI of dissection of the aorta: Recognition of the intimal tear and differential flow velocities. *Am J Roentgenol* 146: 1286–1288, 1986.

23. Herfkens RJ, Higgins CB, Hricak H, Lipton MJ, Crooks LE, Sheldon PE, Kaufman L: Nuclear magnetic resonance imaging of atherosclerotic disease. *Radiology* 148: 161–166, 1983.

24. Lee JK, Ling D, Heiken JP, Glazer HS, Sicard GA, Totty WG, Levitt RG, Murphy WA: Magnetic resonance imaging of abdominal aortic aneurysms. *Am J Roentgenol* 143: 1197–1202, 1984.

25. Flak B, Li DK, Ho BY, Knickerbocker WJ, Fache S, Mayo J, Chung W: Magnetic resonance imaging of aneurysms of the abdominal aorta. *Am J Roentgenol* 144: 991–996, 1985.

26. Evancho AM, Osbakken M, Weidner W: Comparison of NMR imaging and aortography for preoperative evaluation of abdominal aortic aneurysm. *Magn Reson Med* 2: 41–55, 1985.

27. LaRoy LL, Cormier PJ, Matalon TA, Patel SK, Turner DA, Silver B: Imaging of abdominal aortic aneurysms. *Am J Roentgenol* 152: 785–792, 1989.

28. Lindell OI, Sariola HV, Lehtonen TA: The occurrence of vasculitis in perianeurysmal fibrosis. *J Urol* 138: 727–729, 1987.

29. Amparo EG, Higgins CB, Hricak H, Sollitto R: Aortic dissection: Magnetic resonance imaging. *Radiology* 155: 399–406, 1985.

30. Geisinger MA, Risius B, JA OD, Zelch MG, Moodie DS, Graor RA, George CR: Thoracic aortic dissections: Magnetic resonance imaging. *Radiology* 155: 407–412, 1985.

31. Williams DM, Joshi A, Dake MD, Deeb GM, Miller DC, Abrams GD: Aortic cobwebs: An anatomic marker identifying the false lumen in aortic dissection—imaging and pathologic correlation *Radiology* 190: 167–174, 1994.

32. Yamada T, Tada S, Harada J: Aortic dissection without intimal rupture: Diagnosis with MR imaging and CT. *Radiology* 168: 347–352, 1988.

33. Wolff KA, Herold CJ, Tempany CM, Parravano JG, Zerhouni EA: Aortic dissection: Atypical patterns seen at MR imaging. *Radiology* 181: 489–495, 1991.

34. Welch TJ, Stanson AW, Sheedy PFD, Johnson CM, McKusick MA: Radiologic evaluation of penetrating aortic atherosclerotic ulcer. *Radiographics* 10: 675–685, 1990.

35. Yucel EK, Steinberg FL, Egglin TK, Geller SC, Waltman AC, Athanasoulis CA: Penetrating aortic ulcers: Diagnosis with MR imaging. *Radiology* 177: 779–781, 1990.

36. Justich E, Amparo EG, Hricak H, Higgins CB: Infected aortoiliofemoral grafts: Magnetic resonance imaging. *Radiology* 154: 133–136, 1985.

37. Auffermann W, Olofsson PA, Rabahie GN, Tavares NJ, Stoney RJ, Higgins CB: Incorporation versus infection of retroperitoneal aortic grafts: MR imaging features. *Radiology* 172: 359–362, 1989.

38. Hricak H, Amparo E, Fisher MR, Crooks L, Higgins CB: Abdominal venous system: Assessment using MR. *Radiology* 156: 415–422, 1985.

39. Colletti PM, Oide CT, Terk MR, Boswell WD Jr: Magnetic resonance of the inferior vena cava. *Magn Reson Imaging* 10: 177–185, 1992.

40. Cory DA, Ellis JH, Bies JR, Olson EW: Retroaortic left renal vein demonstrated by nuclear magnetic resonance imaging. *J Comput Assist Tomogr* 8: 339–340, 1984.

41. Schultz CL, Morrison S, Bryan PJ: Azygos continuation of the inferior vena cava: Demonstration by NMR imaging. *J Comput Assist Tomogr* 8: 774–776, 1984.

42. Fisher MR, Hricak H, Higgins CB: Magnetic resonance imaging of developmental venous anomalies. *Am J Roentgenol* 145: 705–709, 1985.

43. Semelka RC, Shoenut JP, Kroeker MA: The retroperitoneum and the abdominal wall. In Semelka RC, Shoenut JP (eds.), *MRI of the Abdomen with CT Correlation*. New York: Raven Press, p. 13–41, 1993.

44. Silverman SG, Hillstrom MM, Doyle CJ, Tempany CM, Sica GT: Thrombophlebitic retroperitoneal collateral veins mimicking lymphadenopathy: MR and CT appearance. *Abdom Imaging* 20: 474–476, 1995.

45. Erdman WA, Weinreb JC, Cohen JM, Buja LM, Chaney C, Peshock RM: Venous thrombosis: Clinical and experimental MR imaging. *Radiology* 161: 233–238, 1986.

46. Higgins CB, Goldberg H, Hricak H, Crooks LE, Kaufman L, Brasch R: Nuclear magnetic resonance imaging of vasculature of abdominal viscera: Normal and pathologic features. *Am J Roentgenol* 140: 1217–1225, 1983.

47. Semelka RC, Shoenut JP, Magro CM, Kroeker MA, MacMahon R, Greenberg HM: Renal cancer staging: Comparison of contrast-enhanced CT and gadolinium-enhanced fat-suppressed spin-echo and gradient-echo MR imaging. *J Magn Reson Imaging* 3: 597–602, 1993.

48. Roubidoux MA, Dunnick NR, Sostman HD, Leder RA: Renal carcinoma: Detection of venous extension with gradient-echo MR imaging. *Radiology* 182: 269–272, 1992.

49. Wendel RG, Crawford ED, Hehman KN: The "nutcracker" phenomenon: An unusual cause for renal varicosities with hematuria. *J Urol* 123: 761–763, 1980.

50. Hartman DS, Hayes WS, Choyke PL, Tibbetts GP: From the archives of the AFIP. Leiomyosarcoma of the retroperitoneum and inferior vena cava: Radiologic-pathologic correlation. *Radiographics* 12: 1203–1220, 1992.

51. Cyran KM, Kenney PJ: Leiomyosarcoma of abdominal veins: Value of MRI with gadolinium DTPA. *Abdom Imaging* 19: 335–338, 1994.

52. Kelekis NL, Semelka RC, Hill ML, Meyers DC, Molina PL: Malignant fibrous histiocytoma of the inferior vena cava: Appearances on contrast-enhanced spiral CT and MRI. *Abdom Imaging* 21: 461–463, 1996.

53. Lipton M, Sprayregen S, Kutcher R, Frost A: Venous invasion in renal vein leiomyosarcoma: Case report and review of the literature. *Abdom Imaging* 20: 64–67, 1995.

54. Arrive L, Hricak H, Tavares NJ, Miller TR: Malignant versus nonmalignant retroperitoneal fibrosis: Differentiation with MR imaging. *Radiology* 172: 139–143, 1989.

55. Comings DE, Skubi KB, Van Eyes J, Motulsky AG: Familial multifocal fibrosclerosis. Findings suggesting that retroperitoneal fibrosis, mediastinal fibrosis, sclerosing cholangitis, Riedel's thyroiditis, and pseudotumor of the orbit may be different manifestations of a single disease. *Ann Intern Med* 66: 884–892, 1967.

56. Van Hoe L, Oyen R, Gryspeerdt S, Baert AL, Bobbaers H, Baert L: Case report: Pseudotumoral pelvic retroperitoneal fibrosis associated with orbital fibrosis. *Br J Radiol* 68: 421–423, 1995.

57. Dent RG, Godden DJ, Stovin PG, Stark JE: Pulmonary hyalinising granuloma in association with retroperitoneal fibrosis. *Thorax* 38: 955–956, 1983.

58. Connolly J, Eisner D, Goldman S, Stutzman R, Steiner M: Benign retroperitoneal fibrosis and renal cell carcinoma. *J Urol* 149: 1535–1537, 1993.

59. Rhee RY, Gloviczki P, Luthra HS, Stanson AW, Bower TC, Cherry KJ Jr: Iliocaval complications of retroperitoneal fibrosis. *Am J Surg* 168: 179–183, 1994.

60. Gatanaga H, Ohnishi S, Miura H, Kita H, Matsuhashi N, Kodama T, Minami M, Okudaira T, Imawari M, Yazaki YRC: Retroperitoneal fibrosis leading to extrahepatic portal vein obstruction. *Intern Med* 33: 346–350, 1994.

61. Hricak H, Higgins CB, Williams RD: Nuclear magnetic resonance imaging in retroperitoneal fibrosis. *Am J Roentgenol* 141: 35–38, 1983.

62. Mulligan SA, Holley HC, Koehler RE, Koslin DB, Rubin E, Berland LL, Kenney PJ: CT and MR imaging in the evaluation of retroperitoneal fibrosis. *J Comput Assist Tomogr* 13: 277–281, 1989.

63. Rubenstein WA, Gray G, Auh YH, Honig CL, Thorbjarnarson B, Williams JJ, Haimes AB, Zirinsky K, Kazam E: CT of fibrous tissues and tumors with sonographic correlation. *Am J Roentgenol* 147: 1067–1074, 1986.

64. Cullenward MJ, Scanlan KA, Pozniak MA, Acher CA: Inflammatory aortic aneurysm (periaortic fibrosis): Radiologic imaging. *Radiology* 159: 75–82, 1986.

65. Ross JS, Delamarter R, Hueftle MG, Masaryk TJ, Aikawa M, Carter J, VanDyke C, Modic MT: Gadolinium-DTPA-enhanced MR imaging of the postoperative lumbar spine: Time course and mechanism of enhancement. *Am J Roentgenol* 152: 825–834, 1989.

66. Lane RH, Stephens DH, Reiman HM: Primary retroperitoneal neoplasms: CT findings in 90 cases with clinical and pathologic correlation. *Am J Roentgenol* 152: 83–89, 1989.

67. Kim SH, Choi BI, Han MC, Kim YI: Retroperitoneal neurilemoma: CT and MR findings. *Am J Roentgenol* 159: 1023–1026, 1992.

68. Bass JC, Korobkin M, Francis IR, Ellis JH, Cohan RH: Retroperitoneal plexiform neurofibromas: CT findings. *Am J Roentgenol* 163: 617–620, 1994.

69. Ros PR, Eshaghi N: Plexiform neurofibroma of the pelvis: CT and MRI findings. *Magn Reson Imaging* 9: 463–465, 1991.

70. Bequet D, Labauge P, Larroque P, Renard JL, Goasguen J: [Peripheral neurofibromatosis and involvement of lumbosacral nerves. Value of imaging]. *Rev Neurol (Paris)* 146: 757–761, 1990.

71. Burk DL, Jr., Brunberg JA, Kanal E, Latchaw RE, Wolf GL: Spinal and paraspinal neurofibromatosis: Surface coil MR imaging at 1.5 T1. *Radiology* 162: 797–801, 1987.

72. Pagliano G, Michel P, la Fay T, Duverger V: [Paraganglioma of the organ of Zuckerkandl.] *Chirurgie* 120: 128–133, 1994.

73. Kessler A, Mitchell DG, Israel HL, Goldberg BB: Hepatic and splenic sarcoidosis: Ultrasound and MR imaging. *Abdom Imaging* 18: 159–163, 1993.

74. Warshauer DM, Semelka RC, Ascher SM: Nodular sarcoidosis of the liver and spleen: Appearance on MR images. *J Magn Reson Imaging* 4: 553–557, 1994.

75. Mitchinson MJ: Retroperitoneal fibrosis revisited. *Arch Pathol Lab Med* 110: 784–786, 1986.

76. Johnson WK, Ros PR, Powers C, Stoupis C, Segel KH: Castleman disease mimicking an aggressive retroperitoneal neoplasm. *Abdom Imaging* 19: 342–344, 1994.

77. Vlahos L, Trakadas S, Gouliamos A, Plataniotis G, Papavasiliou C: Retrocrural masses of extramedullary hemopoiesis in betathalassemia. *Magn Reson Imaging* 11: 1227–1229, 1993.

78. Koep L, Zuidema GD: The clinical significance of retroperitoneal fibrosis. *Surgery* 81: 250–257, 1977.

79. Blackledge G, Best JJ, Crowther D, Isherwood I: Computed tomography (CT) in the staging of patients with Hodgkin's Disease: A report on 136 patients. *Clin Radiol* 31: 143–147, 1980.

80. Neumann CH, Robert NJ, Canellos G, Rosenthal D: Computed tomography of the abdomen and pelvis in non-Hodgkin lymphoma. *J Comput Assist Tomogr* 7: 846–850, 1983.

81. Rahmouni A, Tempany C, Jones R, Mann R, Yang A, Zerhouni E: Lymphoma: Monitoring tumor size and signal intensity with MR imaging. *Radiology* 188: 445–451, 1993.

82. Amparo EG, Hoddick WK, Hricak H, Sollitto R, Justich E, Filly RA, Higgins CB: Comparison of magnetic resonance imaging and ultrasonography in the evaluation of abdominal aortic aneurysms. *Radiology* 154: 451–456, 1985.

83. Hanna SL, Fletcher BD, Boulden TF, Hudson MM, Greenwald CA, Kun LE: MR imaging of infradiaphragmatic lymphadenopathy in children and adolescents with Hodgkin disease: Comparison with lymphography and CT. *J Magn Reson Imaging* 3: 461–470, 1993.

84. Lee JK, Heiken JP, Ling D, Glazer HS, Balfe DM, Levitt RG, Dixon WT, Murphy WA Jr: Magnetic resonance imaging of abdominal and pelvic lymphadenopathy. *Radiology* 153: 181–188, 1984.

85. Dooms GC, Hricak H, Crooks LE, Higgins CB: Magnetic resonance imaging of the lymph nodes: Comparison with CT. *Radiology* 153: 719–728, 1984.

86. Glazer HS, Lee JK, Levitt RG, Heiken JP, Ling D, Totty WG, Balfe DM, Emani B, Wasserman TH, Murphy WA: Radiation fibrosis: Differentiation from recurrent tumor by MR imaging. *Radiology* 156: 721–726, 1985.

87. Hricak H, Demas BE, Williams RD, McNamara MT, Hedgcock MW, Amparo EG, Tanagho EA: Magnetic resonance imaging in the diagnosis and staging of renal and perirenal neoplasms. *Radiology* 154: 709–715, 1985.

88. Fein AB, Lee JK, Balfe DM, Heiken JP, Ling D, Glazer HS, McClennan BL: Diagnosis and staging of renal cell carcinoma: A comparison of MR imaging and CT. *Am J Roentgenol* 148: 749–753, 1987.

89. Guimaraes R, Clement O, Bittoun J, Carnot F, Frija G: MR lymphography with superparamagnetic iron nanoparticles in rats: Pathologic basis for contrast enhancement. *Am J Roentgenol* 162: 201–207, 1994.

90. Anzai Y, Blackwell KE, Hirschowitz SL, Rogers JW, Sato Y, Yuh WT, Runge VM, Morris MR, McLachlan SJ, Lufkin RB: Initial clinical experience with dextran-coated superparamagnetic iron oxide for detection of lymph node metastases in patients with head and neck cancer [see comments]. *Radiology* 192: 709–715, 1994.

91. Williams WM, Kosovsky PA, Rafal RB, Markisz JA: Retroperitoneal germ cell neoplasm: MR and CT. *Magn Reson Imaging* 10: 325–331, 1992.

92. Ellis JH, Bies JR, Kopecky KK, Klatte EC, Rowland RG, Donohue JP: Comparison of NMR and CT imaging in the evaluation of metastatic retroperitoneal lymphadenopathy from testicular carcinoma. *J Comput Assist Tomogr* 8: 709–719, 1984.

93. Cohan RH, Baker ME, Cooper C, Moore JO, Saeed M, Dunnick NR: Computed tomography of primary retroperitoneal malignancies. *J Comput Assist Tomogr* 12: 804–810, 1988.

94. Bretan PN, Jr., Williams RD, Hricak H: Preoperative assessment of retroperitoneal pathology by magnetic resonance imaging. Primary leiomyosarcoma of inferior vena cava. *Urology* 28: 251–255, 1986.

95. Feinstein RS, Gatewood OM, Fishman EK, Goldman SM, Siegelman SS: Computed tomography of adult neuroblastoma. *J Comput Assist Tomogr* 8: 720–726, 1984.

96. Lee JK, Glazer HS: Psoas muscle disorders: MR imaging. *Radiology* 160: 683–687, 1986.

97. Weinreb JC, Cohen JM, Maravilla KR: Iliopsoas muscles: MR study of normal anatomy and disease. *Radiology* 156: 435–440, 1985.

98. Hahn PF, Saini S, Stark DD, Papanicolaou N, Ferrucci JT Jr: Intraabdominal hematoma: The concentric-ring sign in MR imaging. *Am J Roentgenol* 148: 115–119, 1987.

99. Rubin JI, Gomori JM, Grossman RI, Gefter WB, Kressel HY: Highfield MR imaging of extracranial hematomas. *Am J Roentgenol* 148: 813–817, 1987.

100. Unger EC, Glazer HS, Lee JK, Ling D: MRI of extracranial hematomas: Preliminary observations. *Am J Roentgenol* 146: 403–407, 1986.

101. Brasfield RD, Das Gupta TK: Desmoid tumors of the anterior abdominal wall. *Surgery* 65: 241–246, 1969.

102. Ichikawa T, Koyama A, Fujimoto H, Honma M, Saiga T, Matsubara N, Ozeki Y, Uchiyama G, Ohtomo K: Abdominal wall desmoid mimicking intra-abdominal mass: MR features. *Magn Reson Imaging* 12: 541–544, 1994.

103. Stover B, Laubenberger J, Hennig J, Niemeyer C, Ruckauer K, Brandis M, Langer M: Value of RARE-MRI sequences in the diagnosis of lymphangiomatosis in children. *Magn Reson Imaging* 13: 481–488, 1995.

CHAPTER 11

BLADDER

ELIZABETH DENNY BROWN, M.D., RICHARD C. SEMELKA, M.D.,
AND LARISSA L. NAGASE, M.D.

NORMAL ANATOMY

The bladder is located posterior to the symphysis, retropubic fat pad, and the space of Retzius. It is pyramidal in shape, with its apex pointing anteriorly toward the superior portion of the pubic symphysis. From the apex, the median umbilical fold passes up to the umbilicus. This is a fold peritoneum raised by the medium umbilical ligament, which is the remnant of urachus. The superior surface of the bladder is covered by peritoneum, which dips down posteriorly to form the anterior wall of the rectovesical (male) or uterovesical (female) pouch. The obturator internus muscles are located laterally, and the levator ani muscles are situated inferiorly [1, 2]. The bladder consists of four layers: an outer adventitial layer of connective tissue, a nonstriated muscle layer (the detrusor muscle, consisting of outer and inner longitudinal fibers, enclosing a middle circular layer), a lamina propria (submucosal connective tissue), and an inner layer of mucosa. The mucosa is rugose in the underdistended state, and becomes smoother as filling proceeds, with the exception of the trigone, which is always smooth [3]. When fully distended, the bladder is 2 mm thick. The ureteric orifices are placed at the angles of the trigone and are usually slitlike. The internal urethral orifice is at the apex of the trigone, the lowest part of the bladder.

The bladder receives its principal blood supply from the superior and inferior vesical arteries, which are branches of the internal iliac artery. Branches from the obturator and inferior gluteal arteries, as well as branches of the uterine and vaginal arteries in the female, also supply the bladder. Venous drainage is via an intricate plexus on the inferolateral surface, which eventually drains into the internal iliac veins. Lymphatics from the bladder drain mainly to the internal or common iliac group [3].

MRI TECHNIQUES

A variety of MRI techniques has been employed to study the bladder. As in other organ systems, it is useful to combine imaging techniques that demonstrate different tissue contrast. In the bladder, it is useful to combine sequences that demonstrate high-signal intensity urine (i.e., T2-weighted imaging and delayed postgadolinium imaging) with techniques that demonstrate low-intensity urine (noncontrast T1-weighted imaging with or without fat suppression and immediate postgadolinium dynamic SGE imaging). Images that show this contrast between urine and bladder wall are important in effectively evaluating abnormalities in the bladder wall and lumen.

Techniques that are particularly useful include T2-weighted echo-train spin-echo, pre- and postintravenous gadolinium, T1-weighted fat suppressed SGE, and dynamic immediate postgadolinium gradient-echo sequences. T1-weighted images are effective at demonstrating morphology but are not effective as the aforementioned techniques at demonstrating depth of tumor invasion. T1-weighted images performed as breath-hold SGE sequences have shown good spatial and temporal resolution. Recent implementation of breath-hold T2-weighted echo-train spin-echo sequences has been effective in examining the pelvis. One version of this, the half-Fourier single-shot turbo spin-echo (HASTE) technique has the additional advantage of being breathing independent. Multiplanar imaging capability of MRI permits image acquisition in different planes to minimize partial volume effects when evaluating depth of penetration of bladder cancer [4] (i.e., sagittal imaging for anterior and posterior wall and dome lesions and coronal imaging for lateral wall and dome lesions). If a tumor is not aligned in one of the three standard planes, volume averaging of tumor and bladder wall may occur and may lead to potential overstanding [4, 5].

The critical artifacts in MRI of the bladder include motion, degree of bladder distension, and chemical shift. Involuntary motion artifacts include motion from respiration, intestinal peristalsis, and bladder motion. Respiratory movements can be reduced by the use of a tight abdominal band. Bowel peristalsis can be minimized with administration of 1 mg of glucagon intramuscularly immediately before the exam. Glucagon should not be given to patients with history of pheochromocytoma, insulin-dependent diabetes, insulinoma, or prior hypersensitivity reaction [3]. Moderate bladder distention is important. If the bladder is not distended, the detrusor muscle is thickened, mimicking thickening from disease states and making it difficult to recognize small tumors. If the bladder is too distended, the patient becomes uncomfortable, and flat tumors can be missed secondary to overstretching of the muscle layer. It has been suggested that optimal bladder filling is achieved by asking the patient to void 2 h before the exam and not again until after the exam [6]. Chemical-shift artifact occurs at the water-fat interface and appears as a dark band along the lateral wall on one side and a bright band along the lateral wall on the opposite side [7]. This appearance can mimic or mask an invasive bladder cancer. To correct for this, chemically selective fat suppression can be performed, or the frequency-encoding gradient can be rotated to select the direction that least interferes with examination of bladder wall adjacent to tumor [7, 8].

The use of surface coils can significantly improve the image quality of the pelvic structures. Double surface coils have been shown to improve pelvic MR imaging

[8–10]. Even greater image improvements occur with the use of a phased-array multicoil.

Endorectal coils can be used to obtain high-resolution images of the bladder. However, these are usually most useful for imaging of tumors along the posterior wall of the bladder base [6].

NORMAL

On MRI images, the thickness of the normal bladder wall ranges from 2 to 8 mm. The normal wall appears as a low-signal intensity band on noncontrast T1-weighted images, with urine appearing near signal void. On T2-weighted images, the bladder wall appears as a low-signal intensity band, which represents the entire muscular layer. More recently, this band has been divided into two bands, of low signal intensity (inner) and intermediate signal intensity (outer), corresponding to the compact inner and looser outer smooth muscle layers [11].

The normal bladder wall does not enhance substantially on images acquired immediately after gadolinium-DTPA administration, which becomes important in tumor imaging. However, there is delayed enhancement of bladder wall, best seen by combining fat saturation with gadolinium-DTPA enhancement [3].

Normal Variants and Congenital Disease

Congenital anomalies of the urinary bladder include agenesis, hypoplasia, duplication, exstrophy, and diverticula. Agenesis and hypoplasia are extremely rare. Duplication of the bladder can be demonstrated with MR imaging. The septum dividing the two bladder cavities is low in signal on both T1- and T2-weighted images. The bladder wall of both cavities is of the same thickness and signal intensity. Although bladder exstrophy is a clinical diagnosis, MR imaging may contribute important information about the skeletal, muscular, and peritoneal anomalies associated with bladder exstrophy as well as the position of the sex organs [12].

Congenital bladder diverticula are herniations of bladder mucosa through areas of weakness in the detrusor muscle of the bladder. Most are seen in males, and most occur at the level of the bladder base. When they originate at the ureteral meatus, they are called Hutch diverticula. These may be associated with ureteral obstruction. On MR images, bladder diverticula are seen as outpouchings from the native bladder. The wall of the diverticulum is thin and hypointense on T2-weighted images. On T1-weighted images acquired after gadolinium administration, the diverticulum fills with contrast-enhanced urine. Diverticula may be associated with urinary stasis, leading to chronic infection, inflammation,

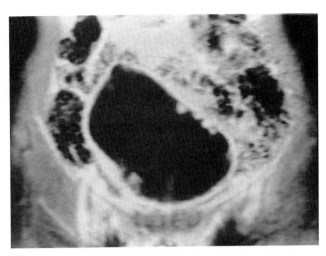

F I G . 11.1 Multiple papillary tumors. Coronal T1-weighted gadolinium-enhanced fat-suppressed spin-echo image. The enhancing papillomas are well shown as enhancing mass lesions in a background of low signal intensity of non-gadolinium-containing urine.

dysplasia, leukoplakia, and squamous metaplasia. This process may precede the development of a malignant tumor in the diverticulum. Tumors originating within diverticula are rare, occurring in 2–7% of patients with vesical diverticula. The most common cell type is transitional cell carcinoma (78%), followed by squamous cell carcinoma (17%), a combination of transitional and squamous cell types (2%), and adenocarcinoma (2%) [13].

MASS LESIONS

Benign Masses

Papilloma

Transitional cell papilloma accounts for 2–3% of all primary bladder tumors and is histologically benign but may recur or become malignant. The tumor consists of an axial fibrovascular core, which is covered by well-differentiated urothelial layers [14]. Bladder papillomas are most clearly shown on immediate postgadolinium MR images as small enhancing masses arising from lesser-enhancing wall. Dynamic postgadolinium enhanced MR images (15–45 s) may be most useful to demonstrate the superficial nature of these lesions (fig. 11.1).

Leiomyoma

Leiomyoma is the most common of the rare benign bladder tumors, affecting women 30–55 years of age. The lesion most commonly arises at the trigone but may be found on the lateral and posterior walls. Lesions may be intravesicular (60%), extravesicular (30%), or intramural (10%). Intramural and extravesicular tumors do not

cause symptoms, but intravesicle lesions may present with hematuria or dysuria. Bladder neck tumors causing bladder outlet obstruction have been reported. The lesion is intermediate in signal intensity on T1-weighted images and well shown against a background of low-signal intensity urine. On T2-weighted images, the high signal intensity of the lesion contrasts well with intermediate low-signal intensity muscle in the bladder wall, and intramural extent can be assessed. Degenerating leiomyomas can have various appearances, including medium to high signal intensity on T1-weighted images and heterogeneous mixed signal intensity on T2-weighted images. These appearances are thought to be secondary to hemorrhage, calcification, or cystic transformation [15]. Leiomyomas and leiomyosarcomas cannot be consistently distinguished on MR images [3]. However, large size, heterogeneity, and irregular margins are features suggestive of malignancy.

Pheochromocytoma

Pheochromocytomas are catecholamine-producing tumors that arise from chromaffin cells and can occur anywhere along the sympathetic nervous system from the neck to the sacrum. Ten to fifteen percent occur in an extra-adrenal location. One percent are located in the bladder and have a predilection for the trigone, followed by the region near the ureteral orifices. They are found less frequently in the dome and lateral walls of the bladder. Seven percent of bladder pheochromocytomas are malignant [14]. Males and females have an equal incidence, with a mean age of 41 years. About half of the cases present with the clinical triad of hypertension, gross intermittent hematuria, and attacks of sweating, headache and palpitations induced by micturition [16]. Characteristic MRI features help to distinguish this tumor from other tumors, including carcinoma [16, 17]. Typically, these tumors show markedly increased, homogeneous signal intensity on T2-weighted spin-echo sequences [18–20]. However, signal can be heterogeneously increased on T2-weighted images [21]. T1-weighted images demonstrate hypointense or isointense signal intensity [15].

Neurogenic tumors

Neurofibromatosis, the most common phakomatosis, is characterized by cafe au lait spots, optic gliomas, Lisch nodules, distinctive bone lesions, and neurofibromas. Genitourinary tract neurofibromas are rare but most commonly affect the bladder (fig. 11.2). Obstructive hydronephrosis, a common complication, is presumably due to neurofibromas involving the trigone. Pelvic sidewall tumors appear nodular and may extend into the obturator foramina. Neurofibromas demonstrate distinct MRI features that allow better characterization of the extent of the tumor within the bladder, pelvic sidewalls,

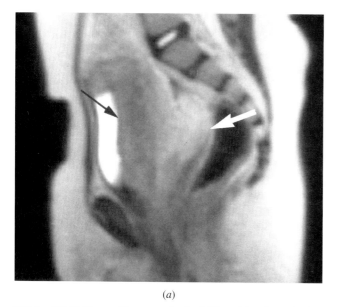

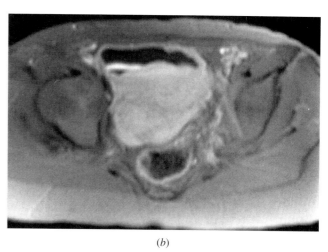

(a)

(b)

F I G . 11.2 Neurofibroma. Sagittal T2-weighted single-shot echo-train spin-echo (*a*) and T1-weighted gadolinium-enhanced fat-suppressed spin-echo (*b*) images in a patient with history of neurofibromatosis. There is a mildly heterogeneous and hypointense mass (black arrow, *a*) on the T2-weighted image that involves the posterior aspect of bladder wall and uterus (white arrow, *a*) and displaces the rectum posteriorly. After gadolinium administration, there is moderately intense and slightly heterogeneous enhancement of the tumor (*b*). Histopathology demonstrated a plexiform neurofibroma in the bladder wall.

and surrounding soft tissues than does CT imaging. The MRI appearance for Type 1 neurofibromatosis (von Recklinghausen disease) is T1-weighted signal intensity slightly greater than that of skeletal muscle and markedly increased signal intensity relative to the surrounding tissues on the T2-weighted images. Larger tumors may be inhomogeneous with markedly increased signal intensity and well-defined central areas of decreased signal intensity. Most demonstrate enhancement with gadolinium administration (fig. 11.2) [22].

Ganglioneuromas have a similar appearance; they are isointense on T1-weighted images and hyperintense on T2-weighted images and enhance substantially with gadolinium (fig. 11.3).

Hemangiomas

Hemangioma is a rare mesenchymal benign tumor of the bladder. The most common presenting symptom is gross, painless hematuria. The tumor has been reported to be low signal intensity on T1-weighted images with

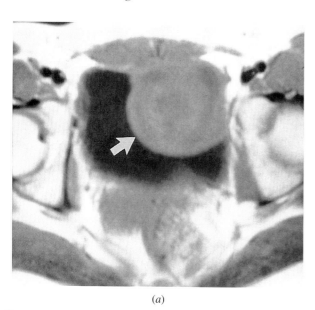

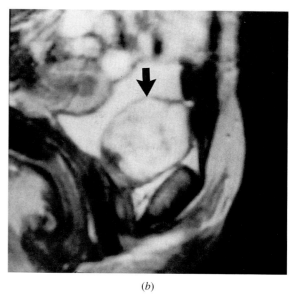

(a)

(b)

F I G . 11.3 Ganglioneuroma. T1-weighted spin-echo (*a*), sagittal T2-weighted spin-echo (*b*), and transverse (*c*) and sagittal (*d*) gadolinium-enhanced T1-weighted spin-echo images. A 4-cm ganglioneuroma arises from the anteroinferior bladder wall.

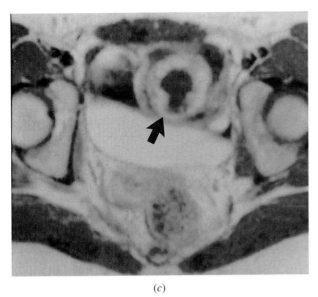

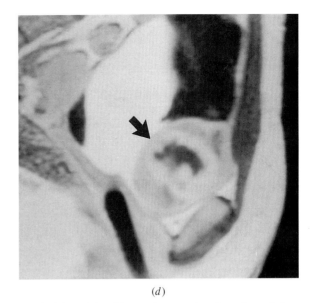

(c)

(d)

F I G . 11.3 (*Continued*) The tumor is intermediate in signal intensity on the T1-weighted image (arrow, *a*) and moderately hyperintense on the T2-weighted image (arrow, *b*) and shows substantial enhancement on interstitial-phase gadolinium-enhanced images (arrow, *c, d*) with central necrosis. (Courtesy of Hedvig Hricak, M.D., Ph.D.).

a multilocular pattern. The lesion is of very high signal intensity on T2-weighted images [23].

Calcifications

Bladder calculi may be the result of foreign body nidus, stasis, or migration of upper tract calculi, or they may be idiopathic. Foreign bodies include catheters, nonabsorbable sutures, hair, or bone fragments. Stasis may result from bladder outlet obstruction, diverticula, cystocele, or postoperative states. Bladder calculi are well shown on T2-weighted images or late postgadolinium T1-weighted images. These sequences show good contrast between high-signal intensity urine and signal-void calculi (fig. 11.4) [24].

Bilharziosis is caused by the organism *Schistosoma haematobium* in the majority of cases. Patients present with frequency urgency, dysuria, flank pain, and hematuria. The characteristic calcifications are linear and continuous along the bladder wall. These bladder wall calcifications are signal void on all MRI sequences [25].

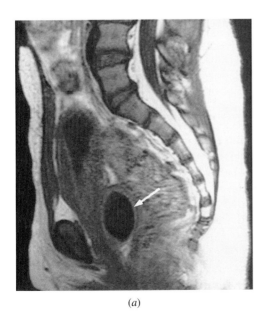

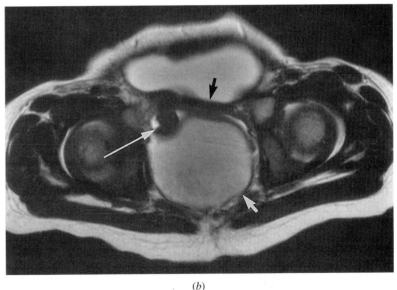

(a)

(b)

F I G . 11.4 Bladder calculus in a patient with a surgically repaired persistent cloaca. Sagittal T1-weighted spin-echo (*a*), T2-weighted fat-suppressed echo-train spin-echo (*b*), and sagittal 512-resolution T2-weighted echo-train spin-echo (*c*) images. A nearly signal-void oval structure (long white arrows, *a–c*) on the T1- and T2-weighted images represents a calculus in a bladder diverticulum.

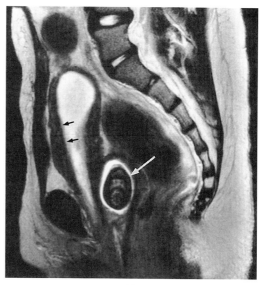

(c)

F I G . 11.4 (*Continued*) The bladder wall is thickened (black arrows, *b, c*), and the reconstructed rectum is dilated (short white arrow, *b*).

Malignant Masses

Bladder cancer is the most common cancer of the urinary tract. It accounts for 4.5% of all new malignant neoplasm and 1.9% of all cancer deaths in the United States [26]. Its incidence appears to be rising, believed to be caused by an increased exposure to multiple environmental carcinogens such as tobacco, artificial sweeteners, coffee, cyclophosphamides, and various aromatic amines. The incidence of bladder cancer increases with age and it is most commonly seen in the sixth and seventh decades. However, it is being found in an increasing number of patients less than 30 years old. Bladder cancer is three times more common in men than in women [12]. Classification of bladder tumors is based on three criteria: cell type (urothelial, squamous, or glandular), pattern of growth (papillary, nonpapillary, noninfiltrating, or infiltrating), and grading (degree of cellular differentiation). The nonpapillary urothelial tumors include invasive transitional cell carcinoma, squamous cell carcinoma, adenocarcinoma, and spindle cell carcinoma.

Primary Urothelial Neoplasm
   Transitional cell carcinoma. Transitional cell carcinoma is the most common primary bladder malignancy and accounts for 85% of all bladder malignancies. Nonpapillary or sessile urothelial tumors are typically more invasive and of a higher grade than exophytic types. Most patients have a prior history of papillary tumors, which arise from epithelial abnormalities adjacent to papillary neoplasia. Invasive urothelial cancer initially spreads radially through the wall of the bladder and then circumferentially through the muscular layer. It may then invade the perivesical fat and, depending on the location of the neoplasm, may invade the prostate, seminal vesicles, or obturator internus muscles. In women, it rarely invades the uterus or cervix. Invasion of the ureters or urethra is common when the tumor originates near one of these structures [27].

Seventy to eighty percent of bladder cancers are diagnosed as early stage, associated with a 5-year survival rate of eighty one percent. Patients with invasive tumors are at high risk of disease progression, and despite definitive therapy, the overall 5-year mortality rate is almost 50% [12]. Selection of appropriate treatment for bladder cancer depends on accurate diagnosis and staging. Superficial neoplasm can be treated with transurethral resection and instillation of chemotherapeutic agents, BCG therapy, or both. Patients with involvement of the superficial muscle layer are candidates for segmental cystectomy. Invasive neoplasm and those with limited perivesical fat involvement require radical cystectomy. Presurgical chemotherapy or palliative radiation therapy is used when extension has occurred outside of the bladder into adjacent pelvic structures [3].

The staging of bladder neoplasms is as follows:

T0	No evidence of primary tumor.
Ta	Noninvasive papillary carcinoma.
Tis	Carcinoma in situ: "flat tumor."
T1	Tumor invades subepithelial connective tissue.
T2	Tumor invades superficial muscle.
T3	Tumor invades deep muscle or perivesical fat.
T3a	Tumor invades deep muscle (outer half).
T3b	Tumor invades perivesical fat.
T4	Tumor invades any of the following: prostate, uterus, vagina, pelvic wall, or abdominal wall.
T4a	Tumor invades the prostate, uterus, or vagina.

T4b Tumor invades the pelvic or abdominal wall [19].

N0 No regional lymph node metastases.

N1 One homolateral solitary regional node (internal or external iliac).

N2–3 Contralateral or bilateral or multiple lymph node metastases.

N4 Juxtaregional (common iliac, inguinal, or aortic) lymph node metastases.

M0 No distant metastases.

M1 Distant metastases or nodes above aortic bifurcation [28].

Both T1 and T2-weighted images are useful in staging bladder cancers [29–38]. The use of T1-weighted sequences is recommended to determine invasion of the perivesical fat and surrounding organs (except the prostate) and involvement of lymph nodes and bone marrow. T2-weighted images are recommended for assessment of the extent of tumor invasion into the muscle layer of the bladder wall and prostate [7, 29–33, 36, 39].

The use of intravenous gadolinium contrast agents has improved the imaging of bladder carcinomas. Gadolinium quickly distributes in the extracellular space without passing through intact cell membranes [39] and typically provides substantial enhancement of urinary bladder carcinomas [5, 40–47]. Bladder carcinomas tend to enhance more than the surrounding bladder wall early after injection of contrast. Tumors are well seen approximately 5–15 s after arterial enhancement [43]. This early phase of enhancement also demonstrates good conspicuity of bladder tumor against gadolinium-free urine in the bladder. Fast dynamic MR imaging may also be able to differentiate between tumor and postbiopsy change, as tumor enhances earlier than postbiopsy tissue (6.5 s vs. 13.6 s) [48]. Delayed (>5 min) postcontrast T1-weighted images show high signal intensity of urine, and the intraluminal portion of a bladder tumor is usually well delineated, although small tumors may be obscured. Two- to five-minute postcontrast fat-suppressed SGE images are the most reliable to show lymph nodes and bone marrow metastases in a consistent fashion.

MRI offers several advantages over CT imaging, including higher-contrast resolution and multiplanar imaging, which permits better imaging of the bladder dome, trigone, perivesical fat, prostate, and seminal vesicles. Bladder tumors at the base or dome are better staged with MRI. Overall, accuracy of MRI in the staging of bladder carcinoma has been reported to range from 69 to 89%. Acquisition of MR images in oblique planes to demonstrate the tumor-bladder wall interface in profile has been effective for assessing depth of bladder wall invasion, with overall staging accuracy of 78% for gadolinium-enhanced T1-weighted images and 60% for T2-weighted images. Staging of small tumors, particularly, is improved with the use of immediate postgadolinium imaging [42, 44, 45, 47].

Immediate postgadolinium SGE image acquired in an oblique projection to demonstrate tumor-bladder wall interface in profile has been an effective approach, especially in the differentiation of superficial tumors and tumors with superficial muscle invasion [5].

MRI may be able to differentiate between superficial (Stage T1) (fig. 11.5) and deep invasion of the muscular layer of the bladder wall (Stage T3a) (fig. 11.6). In general, if a clearly defined dark bladder wall is visualized and appears intact on T2-weighted images, the tumor should be classified as Stage Tis, T1 or T2, whereas if the bladder wall is breached the tumor should be staged as

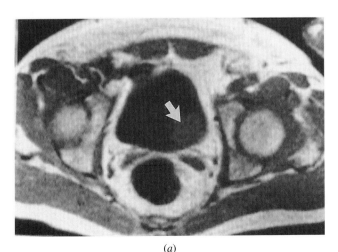

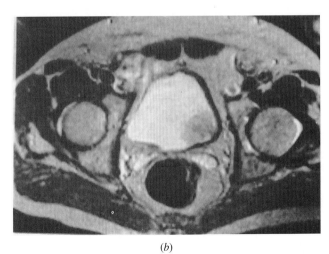

(a)   (b)

F I G . 11.5 Transitional cell cancer, superficial invasion. T1-weighted SGE (*a*), T2-weighted echo-train spin-echo (*b*), and immediate postgadolinium SGE (*c*) images in a patient with superficial T1 transitional cell bladder cancer. The tumor is intermediate in signal intensity on the T1-weighted image (arrow, *a*) and moderately high in signal intensity on the T2-weighted image (*b*).

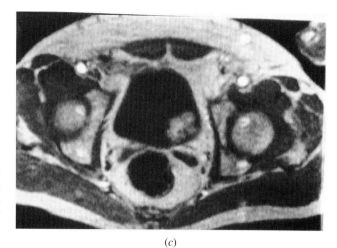

FIG. 11.5 (*Continued*) Moderately intense tumor enhancement is appreciated on the postgadolinium image (*c*), and lack of wall invasion is shown. Intact low-signal intensity muscular wall deep to the tumor is appreciated on the T2-weighted (*b*) and immediate postgadolinium SGE (*c*) images.

(*c*)

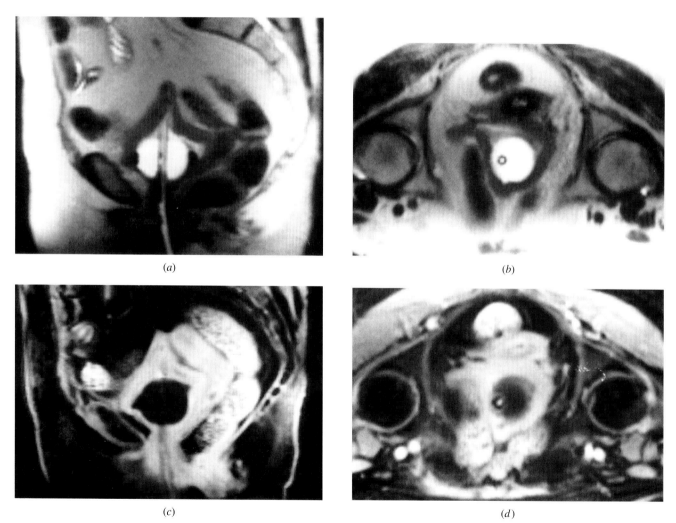

(*a*)

(*b*)

(*c*)

(*d*)

FIG. 11.6 **Invasive transitional cell carcinoma.** Sagittal (*a*) and transverse (*b*) T2-weighted single-shot echo-train spin-echo and sagittal (*c*) and transverse (*d*) T1-weighted gadolinium-enhanced fat-suppressed SGE images. Markedly diffuse thickening of the bladder wall (*a*, *b*) is present that represents diffuse tumor involvement. The tumor enhances intensely after gadolinium administration (*c*, *d*).

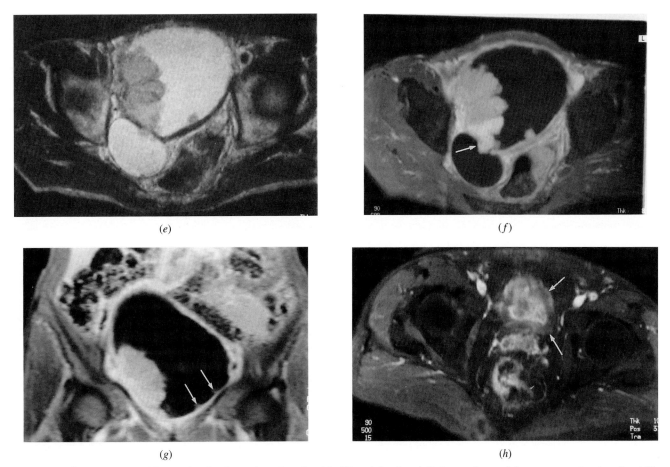

(e)

(f)

(g)

(h)

F I G . 11.6 (*Continued*) T2-weighted echo-train spin-echo (*e*), T1-weighted gadolinium-enhanced fat-suppressed spin-echo (*f*), and coronal interstitial-phase gadolinium-enhanced SGE (*g*) images in a second patient. A frondlike, T3a papillary transitional cell cancer is demonstrated arising from the right lateral wall of the bladder. Note that the lesion extends into a diverticulum (arrow, *f*). On the T2-weighted image, the low-signal intensity muscular wall is not infiltrated by tumor (*e*). Multiple small papillomas are also identified (arrows, *g*).

T1-weighted postgadolinium fat-suppressed image (*h*) in a third patient. There is diffuse, relatively symmetric thickening of the bladder wall from transitional cell cancer with heterogeneous moderate enhancement.

T3a or higher [49]. The higher-contrast resolution is most useful in the differentiation between muscular invasion (Stage T3a) and invasion into the perivesical fat (Stage T3b) [5, 29–33, 35]. For deeply infiltrative tumors (stages T3b, T4a, and T4b), MRI is generally considered the most accurate method of staging (fig. 11.7), with postgadolinium fat-suppressed images most useful. The most common cause of staging error in MRI and CT imaging studies is overstaging, and prior cystoscopic biopsy is likely a common cause of this overstaging [50]. For this reason, it is recommended that MRI studies be performed at least 3 weeks after bladder biopsy.

In the staging of lymph node metastases, MRI and CT imaging appear to be comparable. Accuracy is 83–97% for CT imaging and 73–98% for MRI. At present, distinction between enlarged hyperplastic nodes and malignant nodes cannot be made, which can result in overstaging of tumors (fig. 11.8). Additionally, because the criterion for pathologic enlargement of nodes in the pelvis is size

greater than 1 cm, small, involved nodes will not be detected. Retroperitoneal nodal involvement is not often seen in patients with bladder cancer at the time of initial diagnosis, but if present, the pelvic nodes are also usually involved [35]. After treatment with radiotherapy, relapse in retroperitoneal nodes may be seen without evidence of nodal disease in the pelvis. In treated patients, it is therefore probably prudent to examine the retroperitoneum as well as the pelvis [35]. T1-weighted images are useful for imaging lymph nodes, as their signal intensity is lower than that of the surrounding fatty tissue [51, 52]. Postgadolinium T1-weighted images with fat saturation are particularly useful for the evaluation of adenopathy, as the moderate signal intensity of enhanced nodes is conspicuous in the background of low-signal intensity fat. Three-dimensional imaging may be helpful in providing information not only about size of nodes but also about their shape [53]. MRI is superior to CT imaging in the diagnosis of bone

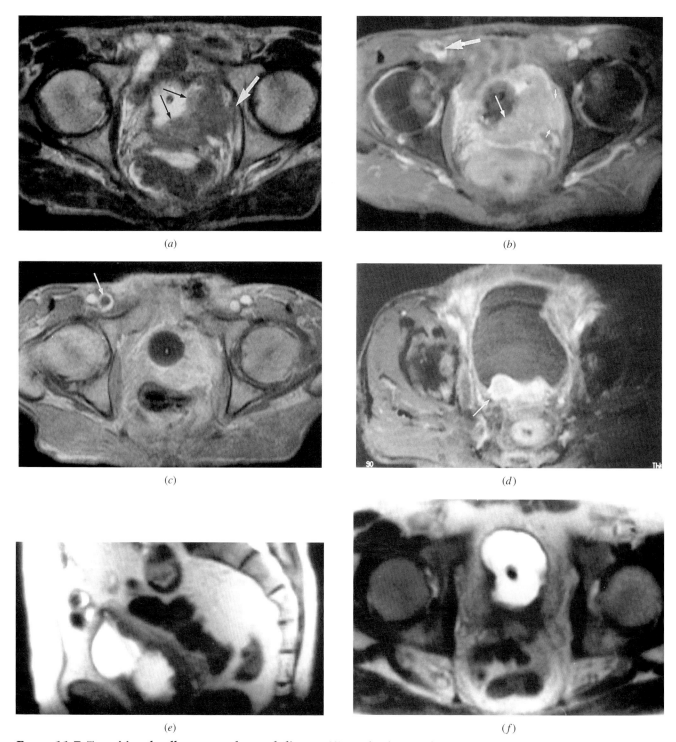

(a)

(b)

(c)

(d)

(e)

(f)

F I G . 11.7 Transitional cell cancer, advanced disease. T2-weighted spin-echo (*a*), T1-weighted gadolinium-enhanced fat-suppressed spin-echo (*b*), and T1-weighted postgadolinium SGE (*c*) images in a patient with T4bN1M0 transitional cell cancer. A large cancer arises from the left and posterior aspect of the bladder (black arrows, *a*). Invasion of the obturator internus muscle is shown (large arrow, *a*). The tumor enhances heterogeneously after gadolinium administration (large white arrow, *b*). Tumor extension into the obturator internus (small arrows, *b*) is relatively high in signal intensity compared to muscle. Thrombus in the right common iliac vein is identified (large arrow, *b* and arrow, *c*). A Foley catheter is present in the bladder (large arrow, *c*).

T1-weighted gadolinium-enhanced fat-suppressed (*d*) image in a second patient with deeply invasive transitional cell cancer. The tumor invades the posterior wall of the bladder. Deep invasion is evidenced by irregular enhancing tissue that extends through the full thickness of the bladder wall (arrow, *d*).

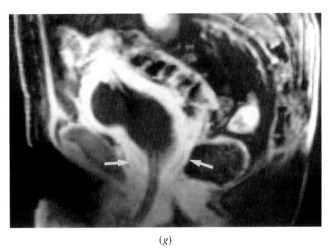
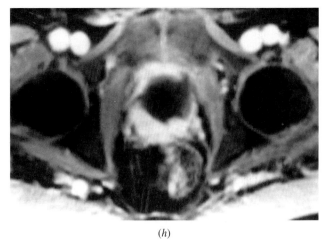

(g)   (h)

F I G . 11.7 (*Continued*) Sagittal (*e*) and transverse (*f*) T2-weighted single-shot echo-train spin-echo and sagittal (*g*) and transverse (*h*) T1-weighted gadolinium-enhanced fat-suppressed images in a second patient with high-grade invasive transitional cell carcinoma. The bladder wall is diffusely thickened and irregular (*e, f*) with moderately intense enhancement after gadolinium administration (*g, h*). The tumor extends inferiorly and invades the prostate gland (arrows, *g*). Note the Foley catheter in the bladder lumen.

marrow metastases [54]. T1-weighted images are useful in detection of bone marrow metastases, as lesions will have signal characteristics similar to those of the primary tumor (typically intermediate intensity) and will be conspicuous against the high signal intensity of fatty marrow [50]. The most accurate technique for the detection of bone marrow metastases is gadolinium-enhanced T1-weighted fat-suppressed imaging. Metastases appear as rounded or geographic regions of enhancement in a background of suppressed background fatty marrow. Unlike noncontrast T1-weighted images, which have relatively low specificity because a number of entities in

addition to metastases are low to intermediate in signal, gadolinium-enhanced fat-suppressed images have higher specificity because focal regions of enhancement are quite characteristic for metastases. Sensitivity is also higher for gadolinium-enhanced fat-suppressed images, as areas of enhancement are more conspicuous than areas of low signal.

MRI is useful in the distinction between late fibrosis and recurrence of carcinoma. One year after transurethral resection, after resolution of the acute edema, residual scar can be distinguished from recurrence of tumor using T2-weighted images [5, 36–47, 50]. Fibrosis is low in signal intensity, whereas tumor recurrence is heterogeneous and moderate in signal intensity. Before resolution of the edema, distinction between granulation tissue and recurrence is problematic [36, 42, 44, 45, 47].

MRI and clinical staging have complementary roles, and staging of urinary bladder tumors is best achieved with the use of both approaches. Because of the limitations in differentiating acute edema from tumor tissue, MRI is most helpful if performed before the clinical staging [6].

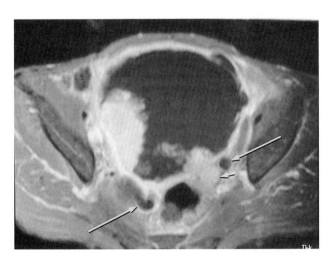

F I G . 11.8 Transitional cell cancer and hyperplasic lymph node. T1-weighted gadolinium-enhanced fat-suppressed spin-echo image. Multiple varying-sized papillary cancers are present with substantial enhancement of the mucosa after gadolinium administration. A 1.2-cm lymph node (small arrow) is shown, which was considered consistent with nodal disease. At histopathology the enlarged nodes were benign and hyperplastic. Note also the dilated ureters (long arrows).

Squamous cell carcinoma. Squamous cell carcinoma is the most common form of neoplasia in patients with chronic inflammation of the urinary bladder [12]. It is rare in western countries but is the most frequent form of bladder neoplasm (55%) in patients with schistosomiasis and is often associated with squamous metaplasia. Histologically, these tumors form squamous pearls and are graded based on the varying degrees of cellular differentiation and histologic appearance [14]. Tumors are intermediate in signal intensity on T1-weighted images and enhance with gadolinium (fig. 11.9). Their

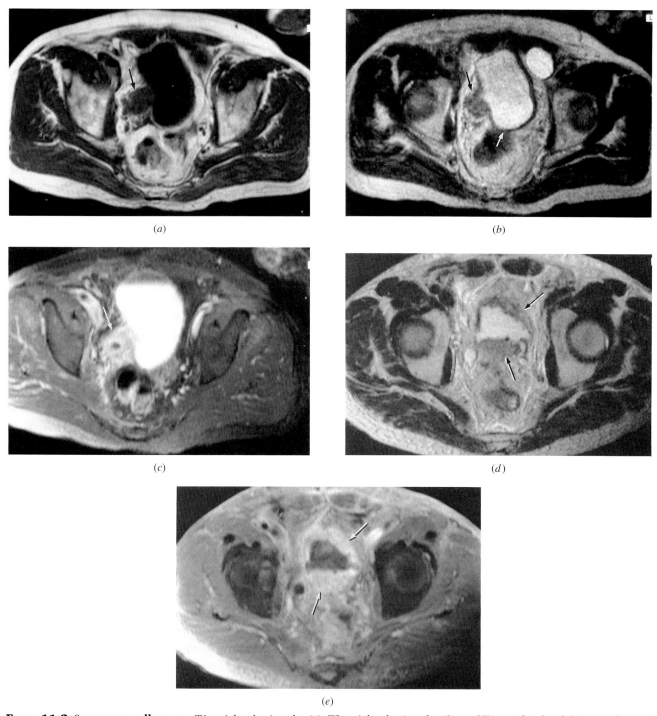

(a)   (b)

(c)   (d)

(e)

F I G . 11.9 Squamous cell cancer. T1-weighted spin-echo (*a*), T2-weighted spin-echo (*b*), and T1-weighted gadolinium-enhanced fat-suppressed spin-echo (*c*) images. Squamous cell cancer involving the distal right ureter and adjacent bladder wall is shown. The tumor is low to intermediate signal intensity on the T1-weighted image (arrow, *a*) and minimally hyperintense on the T2-weighted image (black arrow, *b*). Note that there is a transition between the involved bladder wall, which is intermediate signal intensity, and the normal wall, which is low signal intensity (white arrow, *b*). After contrast administration the tumor shows moderate, heterogeneous enhancement (arrow, *c*), and the fat planes around the tumor are ill defined with high-signal intensity reticular strands, consistent with perivesicular fat infiltration.

T2-weighted spin-echo (*d*) and T1-weighted gadolinium-enhanced fat-suppressed spin-echo (*e*) images in a second patient with squamous cell cancer of the bladder. The tumor is irregular in contour and heterogeneously and minimally hyperintense on the T2-weighted spin-echo image (arrows, *d*). After gadolinium administration there is heterogeneous enhancement of the tumor (arrows, *e*).

appearance is usually not distinguishable from that of transitional cell carcinoma.

Adenocarcinoma. Adenocarcinoma of the bladder is rare and is the most common tumor to arise at the vesicourachal remnant of the bladder dome (figs. 11.10 and 11.11). The tumor may, however, arise in any location. It is also found in patients with exstrophy of the bladder. Adenocarcinoma most commonly arises secondarily as extension from adjacent organs (see discussion below). As with squamous cell carcinoma, the prognosis is poor.

Spindle cell carcinoma. Spindle cell carcinoma, also known as carcinosarcoma, contains spindle and giant cells. The epithelial component is most often transi-

tional cell carcinoma. These tumors are bulky and invariably deeply invade the bladder wall. Prognosis is poor [14].

Malignant nonepithelial neoplasms

Malignant nonepithelial tumors include leiomyosarcoma, rhabdomyosarcoma, and lymphoma and collectively account for less than 10% of all primary bladder tumors [12]. The MRI appearance of rabdomyosarcoma has been reported as isointense on T1-weighted images and high in signal on T2-weighted images. Intravesical disease is obscured on T2-weighted images because of the similarity in signal intensity between urine and tumor. Gadolinium-enhanced T1-weighted images are helpful in some cases for detecting bladder wall involvement,

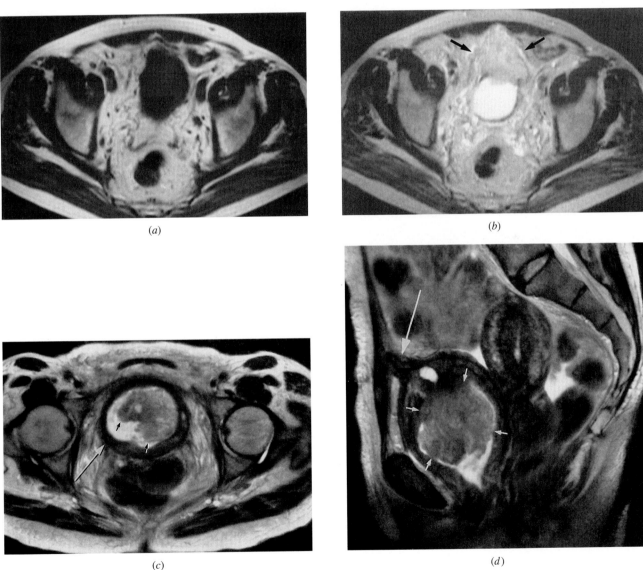

(a)

(b)

(c)

(d)

FIG. 11.10 Adenocarcinoma. T1-weighted spin-echo (*a*) and T2-weighted spin-echo (*b*) images in a patient with a patent urachus. There is a tumor arising from the bladder and extending anteriorly along the urachus, which appears low in signal intensity on the T1-weighted image (*a*) and heterogeneous and moderately high in signal intensity on the T2-weighted image (arrows, *b*).

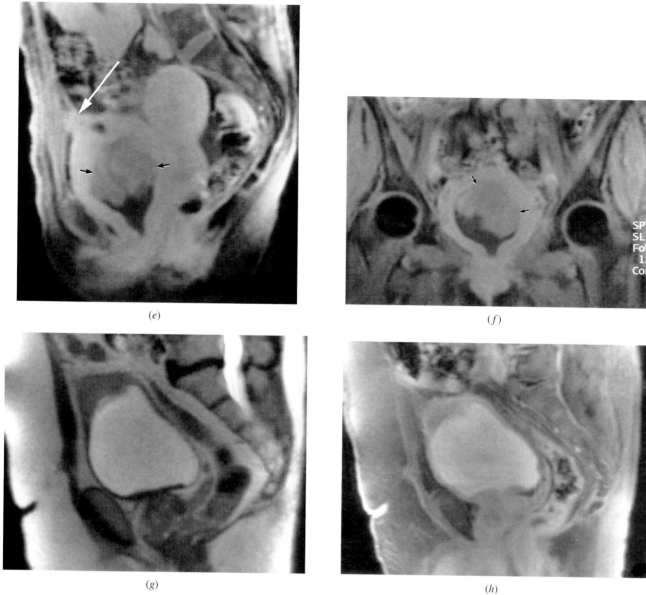

(e)

(f)

(g)

(h)

FIG. 11.10 (*Continued*) T2-weighted echo-train spin-echo (*c*), sagittal T2-weighted echo-train spin-echo (*d*) and sagittal (*e*) and coronal (*f*) T1-weighted gadolinium-enhanced fat-suppressed SGE images in a second patient. A large pedunculated adenocarcinoma (short arrows, *c–f*) arises from the dome of the bladder. Diffuse bladder wall thickening is noted (long arrow, *c*). Heterogeneous signal of the bladder wall on the T2-weighted image reflects deep bladder wall invasion. The bladder wall is more homogeneous on the postgadolinium image because it was acquired late after contrast administration. Definition of tumor invasion of the wall is not feasible on these late postcontrast images because of equilibration of contrast between wall and tumor. A urachal remnant is apparent on sagittal-plane images (long arrow, *d*, *e*).

Sagittal T2-weighted single-shot echo-train spin-echo (*g*) and sagittal T1-weighted postgadolinium fat-suppressed SGE (*h*) images in a third patient with adenocarcinoma. There is an irregular mass lesion arising from the anterosuperior aspect of the bladder wall, which is minimally hyperintense on T2 (*g*) and enhances mildly after gadolinium administration (*h*).

because with transitional cell and other epithelial tumors imaging early after gadolinium administration is important as the increased signal intensity of the urine and layering effect later postgadolinium obscures the intravesical component of the tumor [55]. As with other tumors, the multiplanar capability of MR imaging improves the ability to localize and stage tumor at diagnosis when compared to CT results [55].

Urachal Carcinoma

The urachus is a vestigial structure, representing the remnant of the embryonic allantois and cloaca. In adults, this persists as a midline musculofibrous tube that can extend from the bladder dome to the umbilicus. Neoplastic involvement is rare but can extend anywhere along the course of the urachus. Annual incidence of urachal carcinoma is estimated to be 1 in 5 million. The majority

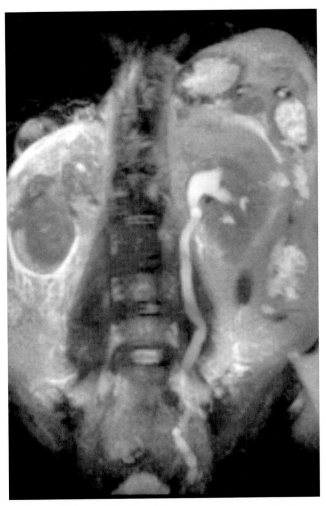

F I G . 11.11 MR urography of bladder cancer. T2-weighted thick-slab (3 cm) single-shot echo-train spin-echo image shows high-grade obstruction of the left renal collecting system to the level of the UV junction secondary to bladder carcinoma.

occur in men between the ages of 40 and 70 years [56]. At presentation, the tumor is usually advanced with a resultant poor prognosis. Overall, 5-year survival is about 10% [56].

Approximately 90% of tumors arise from the umbilical segment, and 4% arise from the umbilical end of the urachus [57]. The majority of urachals cancers are adenocarcinomas. Seventy-five percent are mucin producing and thus can be associated with calcifications on CT [56]. Demonstration of a mass in the characteristic midline supravesical location, adjacent to the anterior abdominal wall in the space of Retzius, should suggest the urachal origin of the lesion. On MR images urachal carcinoma appears as low signal on T1-weighted images and heterogeneous high signal on T2-weighted images [57], although signal characteristics vary, possibly secondary to differences in mucin content or presence of necrosis.

Metastatic Neoplasms

Direct invasion of the bladder may occur secondary to prostate (figs. 11.12 and 11.13), rectosigmoid, and uterine adenocarcinomas, and adenocarcinomas of stomach and breast may metastasize to the bladder [14]. The most common metastases to the bladder from distant sites are melanoma and gastric carcinoma. However, more commonly, metastases to the bladder arise from direct extension of pelvic neoplasms. The diagnostic accuracy of MRI in the detection of bladder mucosal invasion by pelvic tumors was reported to be 81% in one series [58]. The types of tumors studied in this series were cervical, colon, urethral, vaginal, vulvar, and lymphoid tissue. False-negative findings may arise from microscopic foci of invasion, whereas false-positive findings may stem from muscularis invasion without mucosal invasion. In this series, it was noted that postradiation changes and bullous edema are distinguishable from tumor [58].

Multiplanar imaging with precontrast T1- and T2-weighted images as well as postcontrast T1-weighted images is effective at defining tumor extension to the bladder (figs. 11.12 and 11.13). Sagittal-plane imaging is particularly effective for rectal and gynecological malignancies, and fat suppression combined with gadolinium enhancement is useful. Cervical carcinoma Stage 4a has a particular propensity to invade bladder mucosa. This invasion is well shown with the use of sagittal-plane imaging and gadolinium-enhanced T1-weighted images, which provide accurate diagnosis [59, 60].

Lymphoma

Bladder involvement is more common in non-Hodgkin lymphoma than in Hodgkin disease. Secondary bladder lymphoma, associated with more generalized disease, is more common than primary bladder lymphoma. Primary bladder lymphoma has a relatively good prognosis, with the tumor remaining localized for a long period of time [61]. Spread may eventually occur to local nodes and then become generalized. In contrast, secondary lymphoma occurs late in patients with disease; involvement of the bladder is usually by direct invasion from adjacent pelvic masses [61]. MRI appearance of bladder lymphoma appears as thickened bladder wall, with intermediate signal intensity on both T1-and T2-weighted images and mild gadolinium enhancement on early and late images. In secondary bladder lymphoma, the tumor is of similar signal intensity to involved regional lymph nodes [61].

MISCELLANEOUS

Edema

Edema of the bladder wall as a result of acute bladder disease can be distinguished from bladder wall

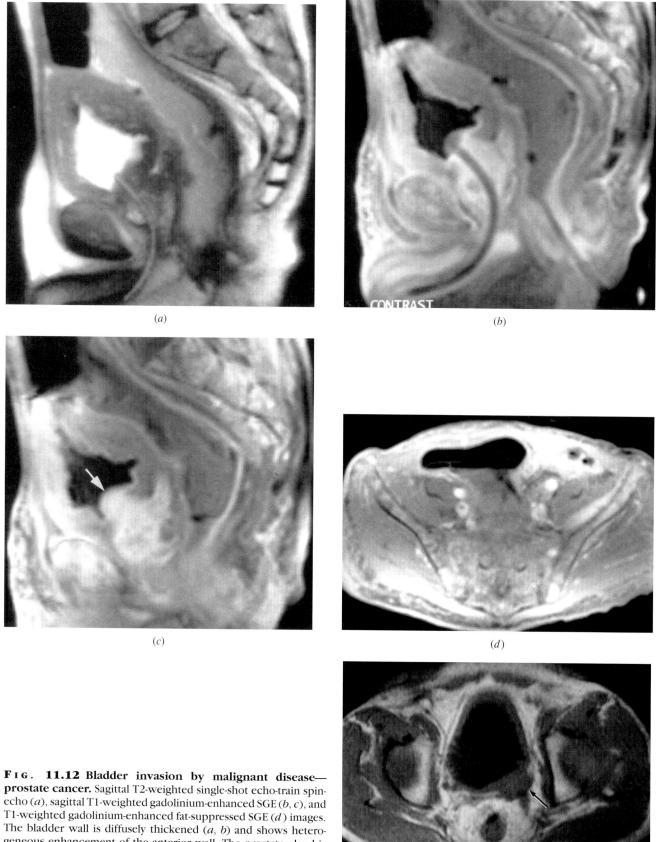

(a)

(b)

(c)

(d)

F I G .   11.12 Bladder invasion by malignant disease—prostate cancer. Sagittal T2-weighted single-shot echo-train spin-echo (*a*), sagittal T1-weighted gadolinium-enhanced SGE (*b, c*), and T1-weighted gadolinium-enhanced fat-suppressed SGE (*d*) images. The bladder wall is diffusely thickened (*a, b*) and shows heterogeneous enhancement of the anterior wall. The prostate gland is irregularly enlarged and enhances heterogeneously after contrast administration (*b, c*).

(e)

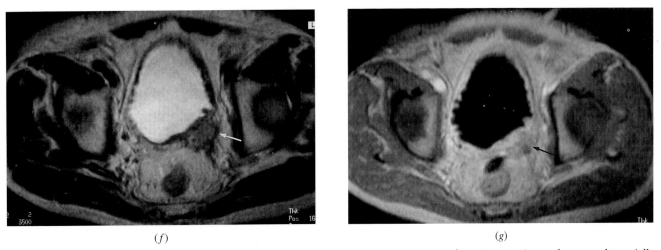

(f)   (g)

F I G . 11.12 (*Continued*) A nodule of tumor, extending superiorly from the prostate to the trigone region, enhances substantially (arrow, *c*). Note multiple bone metastases in the iliac wings that appear as high-signal enhancing foci (*d*).

T1-weighted SGE (*e*), T2-weighted single-shot echo-train spin-echo (*f*), and T1-weighted postgadolinium SGE (*g*) images in a second patient with recurrent prostate cancer invading the bladder. Tumor is intermediate in signal intensity on T1- (arrow, *e*) and T2-weighted (arrow, *f*) images and enhances minimally with gadolinium (arrow, *g*).

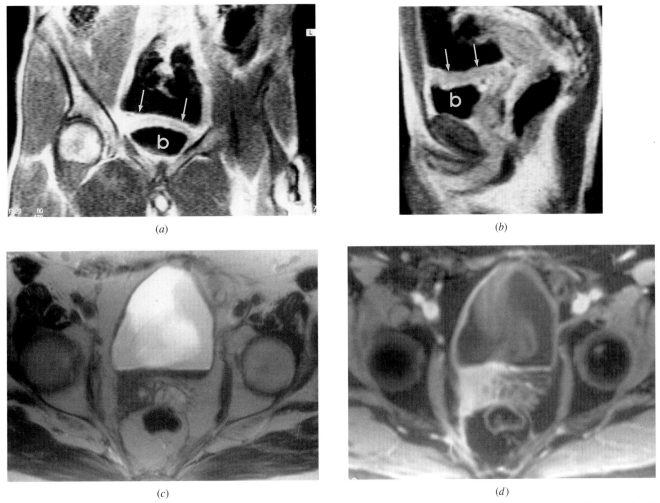

(a)   (b)

(c)   (d)

F I G . 11.13 Bladder invasion by malignant disease—rectal cancer. Coronal T1-weighted SGE (*a*) and sagittal T1-weighted immediate postgadolinium SGE (*b*) images in a patient with rectal cancer. Tumor is identified arising from the rectum and extending along the superior bladder (*b*) wall (arrows, *a*, *b*).

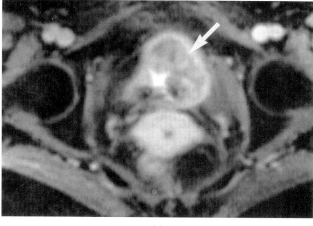

(e)

FIG. 11.13 (*Continued*) T2-weighted single-shot echo-train spin-echo (c) and T1-weighted gadolinium-enhanced fat-suppressed SGE (d) in a second patient with recurrent colorectal adenocarcinoma. The right posterior aspect of the bladder wall and the right seminal vesicle are thickened, with loss of the high signal of the seminal vesicle on the T2-weighted image (c). Tumor enhances intensely on the postgadolinium image (d), clearly defining the extent of the tumor.

T1-weighted gadolinium-enhanced fat-suppressed SGE image (e) in a third patient with rectal cancer involving the bladder. A large tumor mass is present (arrow, e), and fills much of the lumen of the bladder.

hypertrophy by its longer T2, which renders it high in signal intensity on T2-weighted images [62].

Hypertrophy

Muscular hypertrophy of the bladder wall results from bladder outlet obstruction. Underlying causes include benign prostatic enlargement (the most common cause in males), prostatic cancer, large pelvic tumors, bladder neck obstruction (functional or anatomic), and hydrocolpos.

Bladder wall hypertrophy appears as an increased thickness of the bladder wall, which is low in signal intensity on T2-weighted images and does not enhance substantially with gadolinium. Signal intensity features are similar to those of normal bladder wall (fig. 11.14). Mucosal edema related to bladder outlet obstruction is usually located around the urethral orifice and is high signal intensity on T2-weighted images.

Cystitis

Inflammation of the bladder wall may be the result of infection, foreign bodies within the bladder, peritonitis, drug toxicity, or other causes. The appearance is a thickened bladder wall that may be focal or diffuse. On T2-weighted images, four layers can be appreciated within the inflamed bladder wall. An innermost low-signal intensity and an inner high-signal intensity band represent the thickened epithelium and lamina propria, respectively. An outer low-signal intensity band and outermost intermediate-signal intensity bands represent the inner compact muscle layer and outer loose muscle layer, respectively [11]. Increased enhancement

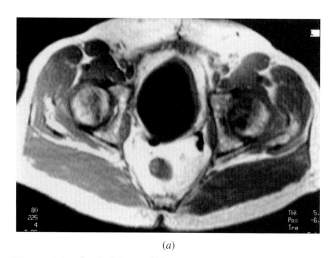

(a)

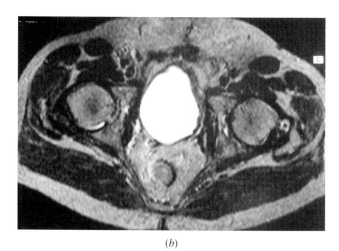

(b)

FIG. 11.14 Bladder wall hypertrophy. T1-weighted SGE (a) and transverse (b) and sagittal (c) T2-weighted echo-train spin-echo images in a patient with chronic outlet obstruction from prostate enlargement. The bladder wall is asymmetrically thickened, with low signal intensity on T1- and T2-weighted images. Note the transurethral prostatectomy defect in the bladder base on the sagittal image (arrow, c).

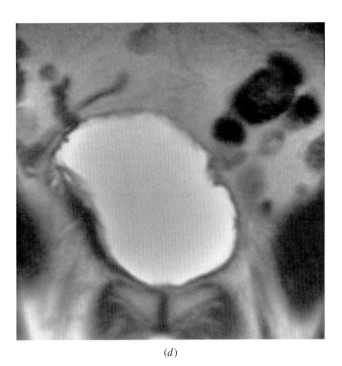

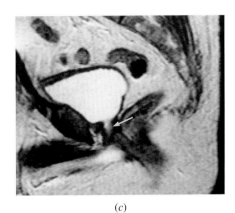

(c)

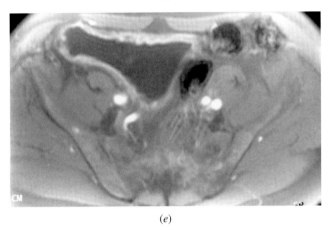

(e)

FIG. 11.14 (*Continued*) Coronal T2-weighted single-shot echo-train spin-echo (*d*) and T1-weighted gadolinium-enhanced fat-suppressed SGE (*e*) images in a second patient. The bladder is dilated with a thickened, trabeculated wall secondary to outlet obstruction from prostate enlargement. Note the moderately increased enhancement of the bladder mucosa reflecting inflammatory change (*e*). Prostate was also enlarged (image not shown), demonstrating that outlet obstruction was present.

after gadolinium administration is observed. The extent of enhancement reflects the severity of the inflammatory process (fig. 11.15).

Hemorrhagic Cystitis

Hemorrhagic cystitis is a severe form of cystitis characterized by hematuria. It may be secondary to radiation of the pelvis or infectious agents including *Escherichia coli* and viruses.

Hemorrhagic cystitis demonstrates a complex appearance on MR images based on the T1 and T2 characteristics of aging blood products. Active bleeding (oxyhemoglobin) has limited paramagnetic properties and behaves like simple fluid with a long T1 (low signal intensity on T1-weighted images) and a long T2 (high signal intensity on T2-weighted images). Acute blood (intracellular deoxyhemoglobin) has a long T1 (low signal intensity on T1-weighted images) and a short T2

(low signal intensity on T2-weighted images). Intracellular methemoglobin has a short T1 (high signal intensity on T1-weighted images) and a short T2 (low signal intensity on T2-weighted images). Extracellular methemoglobin has a short T1 (high signal intensity on T1-weighted images) and a long T2 (high signal intensity on T2-weighted images), and this appearance is most typical for subacute hemorrhage. Intracellular hemosiderin in an old hematoma has a medium T1 (intermediate signal intensity on T1-weighted images) and a short T2 (low signal intensity on T2-weighted images) [63] Thus, the appearance of hemorrhagic cystitis demonstrates not only a thickened bladder wall but also the complex signal characteristics of hemorrhage (fig. 11.16).

Cystitis Cystica

Cystitis cystica is a cystic lesion that appears in the lamina propria. The lesion may be an incidental finding at

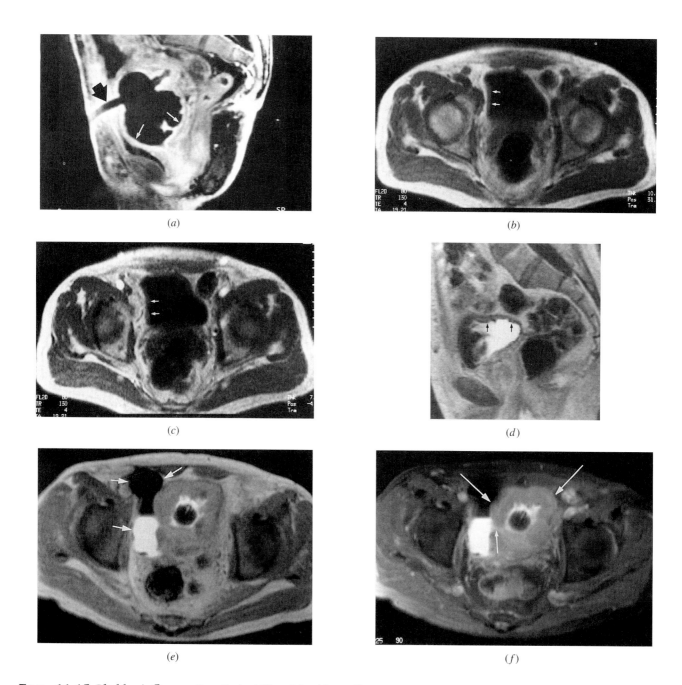

(a)

(b)

(c)

(d)

(e)

(f)

FIG. 11.15 Bladder inflammation. Sagittal T1-weighted immediate postgadolinium SGE image (*a*) in a patient with a suprapubic catheter (black arrow, *a*). Substantial enhancement of the bladder wall is demonstrated (small arrows, *a*).

T1-weighted SGE (*b*), immediate postgadolinium SGE (*c*), and sagittal 5-min postgadolinium SGE (*d*) images in a second patient with mild inflammatory cystitis. The bladder wall is irregularly thickened (arrows, *b*), with minimal enhancement after contrast admionistration (arrows, *c*, *d*).

Ninety-second postgadolinium SGE (*e*) and T1-weighted postgadolinium fat-suppressed spin-echo (*f*) images in a third patient with inflammation secondary to infection. Diffuse bladder wall thickening is present (arrows, *f*), and a large gadolinium-containing diverticulum (arrows, *e*) is identified arising from the right aspect of the bladder. A small high-signal intensity tract represents the communication between the bladder and the diverticulum (short arrow, *f*).

Ninety-second postgadolinium fat-suppressed SGE image (*g*) in a fourth patient, who had undergone intraperitoneal chemotherapy. Increased enhancement of the serosal surface of the bladder (small arrows, *g*) is present, which represents chemical peritonitis.

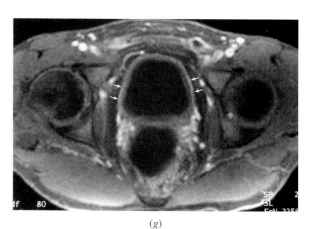

(g)

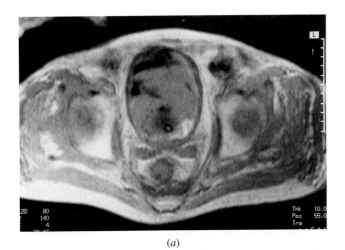

(a)

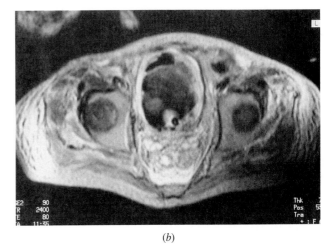

(b)

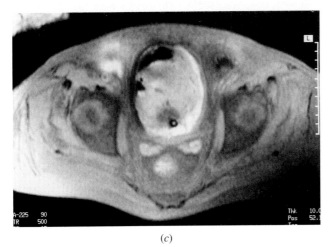

(c)

F I G. 11.16 Hemorrhagic cystitis. T1-weighted SGE (a), T2-weighted spin-echo (b), and T1-weighted fat-suppressed spin-echo (c) images in a patient with hemorrhagic cystitis. The bladder wall and intraluminal fluid show varying signal intensities, which represent the different phases of hemoglobin degradation.

biopsy but is more common in the clinical setting of chronic cystitis. Grossly, the appearance may be that of large cysts, resembling cobblestones (fig. 11.17) [64].

Granulomatous Disease

In the setting of genitourinary tuberculosis, bladder involvement is common. Patients present with dysuria and frequency. The earliest manifestations are mucosal edema and ulcerations, primarily surrounding the ureteral orifices, which can produce obstruction. Tuberculomas in the bladder wall can be large and simulate mass lesions [65]. Focal granulomatous reactions appear as intravesical lesions with high signal intensity on T2-weighted images [24]. Epithelioid granulomatous lesions, which can occur in patients undergoing immunotherapy for the treatment of malignant bladder lesions, may appear similar to malignant tumors on MRI. Although MRI accurately shows these lesions to be confined to the vesical wall, their presence can lead to false-positive findings [24].

Pelvic Lipomatosis

Pelvic lipomatosis predominantly affects black men between the ages of 25 and 55 years. Some patients present with frequency, dysuria, perineal pain, or suprapubic discomfort. Although the process is benign, the effects may be damaging, including renal failure and rectal compression [66]. The diagnosis of pelvic lipomatosis can be supported with the use of MRI. It characteristically appears as an extensive amount of fat, which appears high in signal intensity on T1-weighted images surrounding the bladder [67].

Fistulas

Pelvic fistulas may result from obstetrical procedures, surgery, trauma, radiation, infection, inflammatory bowel disease, or pelvic malignancies. Typically, patients present with urinary or fecal incontinence, pneumaturia, fecaluria, or vaginal discharge. Patients can be evaluated with cystoscopy, vaginoscopy, colonoscopy, fistulography, gastrointestinal contrast radiographic

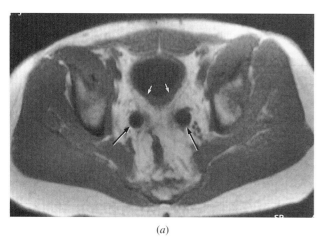 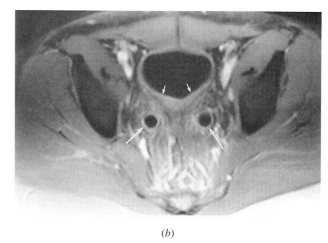

(a)   (b)

FIG. 11.17 Cystitis cystica. T1-weighted SGE (*a*) and 90-s postgadolinium fat-suppressed SGE (*b*) images. Note that the bladder wall is uniformly thickened (short arrows) and the distal ureters are thick walled and substantially dilated (long arrows).

studies, sonography, scintigraphy, computed tomography, or magnetic resonance.

The sagittal plane is particularly effective at demonstrating vesicocervical fistulas because it displays these fistulas in profile (fig. 11.18). They typically insert low in the bladder, a region less well evaluated on transverse images due to volume averaging of the pelvic floor musculature. Gadolinium-enhanced T1-weighted images best demonstrate bladder fistulas. On early postgadolinium images, the fistula wall has high signal intensity,

and the tract has low signal intensity. Late postgadolinium images may show high-signal intensity fluid within the fistula tract [68]. The addition of fat suppression increases the conspicuity of enhancing fistulous tract walls (fig. 11.19).

Postoperative Changes

Widening of the prostatic urethra occurs after all forms of prostatectomies. Immediately after prostatectomy the

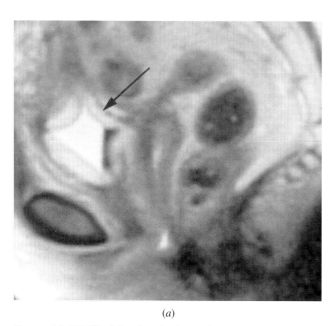 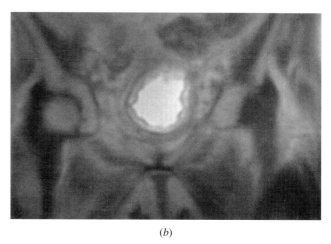

(a)   (b)

FIG. 11.18 Bladder fistula. Sagittal (*a*), coronal (*b*), and transverse (*c*) T2-weighted single-shot echo-train spin-echo and sagittal T1-weighted gadolinium-enhanced fat-suppressed SGE (*d*) images in a patient after radiation therapy for ovarian cancer. The vaginal and bladder walls are thickened, and a fistula between the bladder and vagina (arrow, *d*) is apparent. Sagittal plane, T1-weighted gadolinium-enhanced fat-suppressed images are particularly effective at demonstrating fistula between female pelvic organs and the bladder. Substantial submucosal edema of the bladder is appreciated as high signal on T2 (arrow, *a*) and lack of enhancement on postgadolinium images (*d*).

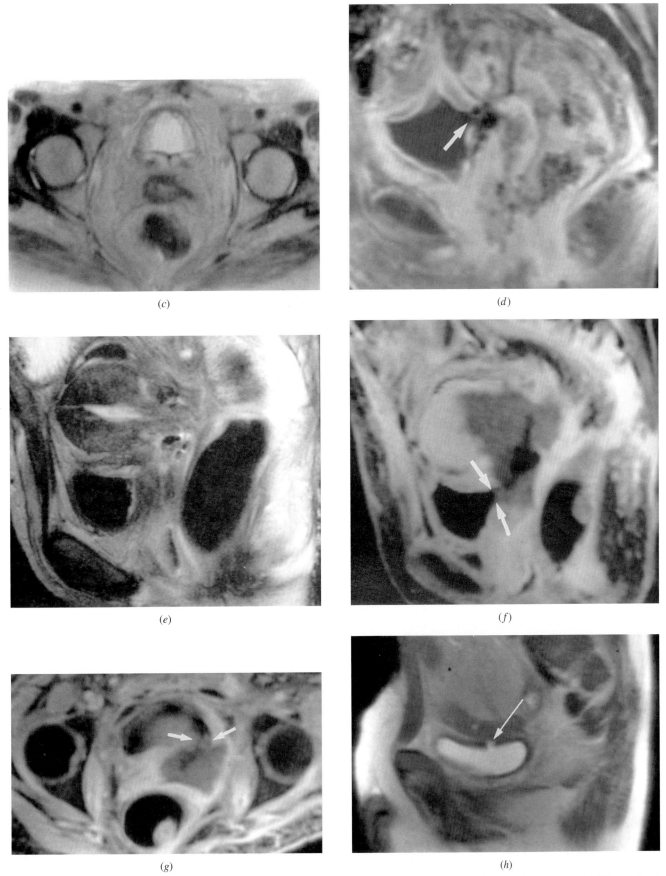

(c)

(d)

(e)

(f)

(g)

(h)

FIG. 11.18 (*Continued*) Sagittal T2-weighted single-shot echo-train spin-echo (*e*) and sagittal (*f*) and transverse (*g*) T1-weighted gadolinium-enhanced fat-suppressed SGE images in a second patient with cervical cancer after radiation therapy.

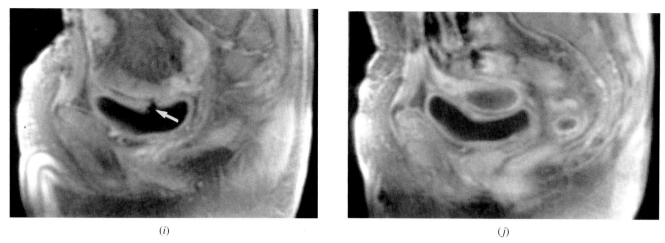

(i)　　　　　　　　　　　　　　　　　　(j)

F I G . 11.18 (*Continued*) Enlarged tissue in the region of the cervix is heterogeneous on T2- and hypointense on postgadolinium T1-weighted images (*f*, *g*), consistent with cervical necrosis. The necrotic tissue is in continuity with the posterior bladder wall, and a low-signal intensity fistulous tract is apparent on sagittal and transverse images (arrows, *f*, *g*).

Sagittal T2-weighted single-shot echo-train spin-echo (h) and sagittal T1-weighted gadolinium-enhanced fat-suppressed SGE (*i*, *j*) images in a third patient with colovesical fistula. A fistulous tract is present in the bladder dome (arrow, *h*, *i*). Adjacent sigmoid colon is thickened and demonstrates increased enhancement (*j*).

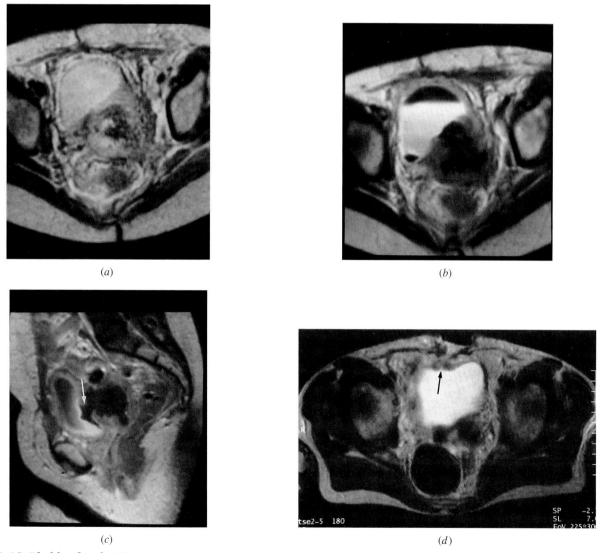

(a)　　　　　　　　　　　　　　　　　　(b)

(c)　　　　　　　　　　　　　　　　　　(d)

F I G . 11.19 Bladder fistula. T2-weighted spin-echo (*a*), transverse (*b*), and sagittal (*c*) gadolinium-enhanced T1-weighted spin-echo images. There is a cervicovesical fistula formation after radiation for cervical cancer. The fistula tract is best shown on the sagittal post-gadolinium image (arrow, *c*). (Courtesy of Hedvig Hricak, M.D., Ph.D.)

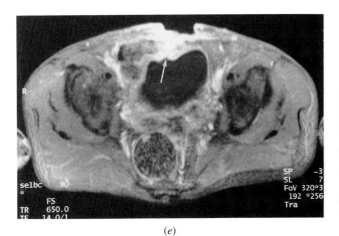

(e)

F I G . 11.19 (*Continued*) T2-weighted echo-train spin-echo (*d*) and T1-weighted gadolinium-enhanced fat-suppressed spin-echo (*e*) images in a second patient with vesicocutaneous fistula. The bladder wall shows focal irregular thickening with an overlying skin defect. A thin fistula tract is apparent and is high in signal intensity on the T2-weighted image (arrow, *d*) and low in signal intensity on the postgadolinium image (arrow, *e*). On the gadolinium-enhanced fat-suppressed image, substantial enhancement of the soft tissues surrounding the fistula and the skin is present, which is consistent with inflammatory changes.

prostatic fossa is quite wide, but it rapidly involutes to a more normal configuration over several weeks. However, a residual prostatectomy defect typically is observed for years. The configuration of the widening after cryocaustic prostate surgery is bottle shaped and different from that of transurethral resection (fig. 11.20) [69].

Bladder Reconstruction

A variety of bladder surgical procedures are performed to alter the native bladder (e.g., bladder augmentation) (fig. 11.21) or to create a neobladder (e.g., Indiana pouch) (fig. 11.22). MRI may be used to evaluate the

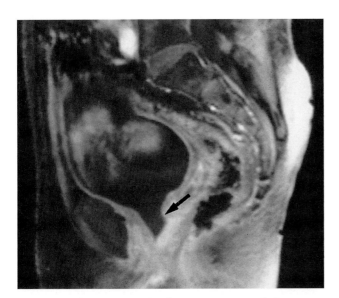

F I G . 11.20 Transurethral prostatectomy defect. Sagittal T1-weighted gadolinium-enhanced fat-suppressed SGE image showing the characteristic widening of the prostatic urethra (arrow).

reconstructed bladder to examine for surgical complications or status of the kidneys, and to detect recurrent malignant disease.

Radiation Changes

As a sequela of pelvic radiation, bullous edema may arise in the bladder and may persist for months or years. Over time, patients may develop radiation cystitis with fibrosis and a contracted bladder. Radiation changes in the bladder increase with increasing radiation dose. Radiation-induced disease is common when the dose exceeds 4,500 cGy. In one study, the incidence of bladder changes increased from 8% to 51% as the dose surpassed 4,500 cGy [70].

In patients with moderate or severe symptoms, radiation changes are detectable on MRI. However, abnormalities on MRI may be present in the absence of symptoms. Postradiation changes of the bladder have MRI appearances that correlate with the severity of histologic features. The mildest form of radiation change results in a high signal intensity of the bladder mucosa with preservation of the bladder wall thickness on T2-weighted images. The high signal intensity typically is seen at the trigone but may spread to involve the entire mucosa and could be the result of mucosal edema. With more severe injury, the wall increases in thickness (>5 mm when fully distended), and the signal characteristics are one of two patterns. The wall has either uniformly high signal intensity or low signal intensity in the inner layer with high signal intensity at the periphery. On gadolinium-enhanced studies, the bladder wall shows increased enhancement, sometimes without other morphologic changes on noncontrast images. This enhancement may occur up to 2.5 years after irradiation [71]. With extreme radiation change, formations of fistula or sinus tracts are seen. Other findings of radiation changes are commonly present (fig. 11.23).

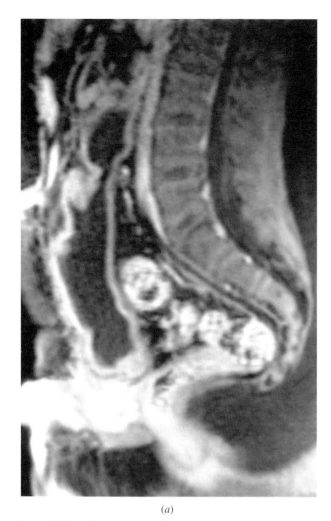

(a)

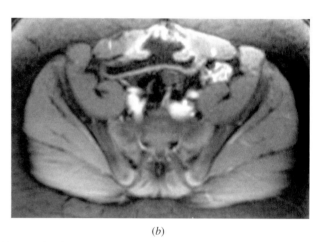

(b)

FIG. 11.21 Enterocystoplasty. Sagittal (*a*) and transverse (*b*) T1-weighted gadolinium-enhanced fat-suppressed images in a patient with enterocystoplasty using small bowel for the augmentation procedure for primary bladder exstrophy. The augmented bladder (*a*, *b*) has a large, capacious appearance with mucosal infoldings observed in bowel.

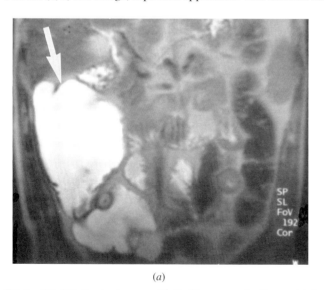

(a)

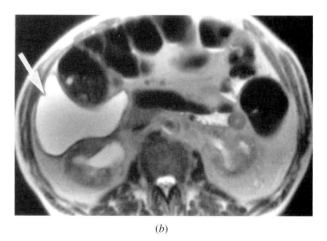

(b)

FIG. 11.22 Cystectomy with Indiana pouch. Coronal (*a*) and transverse (*b*) T2-weighted single-shot echo-train spin-echo and T1-weighted gadolinium enhanced fat-suppressed SGE (*c*) images in a patient with primary transitional cell carcinoma who underwent radical cystectomy with Indiana pouch construction. The Indiana pouch is fluid filled and located in the right anterior peritoneal cavity (arrows, *a*, *b*). Note prominent renal pelves bilaterally with atrophy of the left kidney (*b*, *c*).

Coronal (*d*) and transverse (*e*) T2-weighted single-shot echo-train spin-echo and T1-weighted gadolinium-enhanced fat-suppressed SGE (*f*) images in a second patient with an Indiana pouch. The coronal T2-weighted image provides an MRU appearance of moderately dilated ureters bilaterally (arrows, *d*).

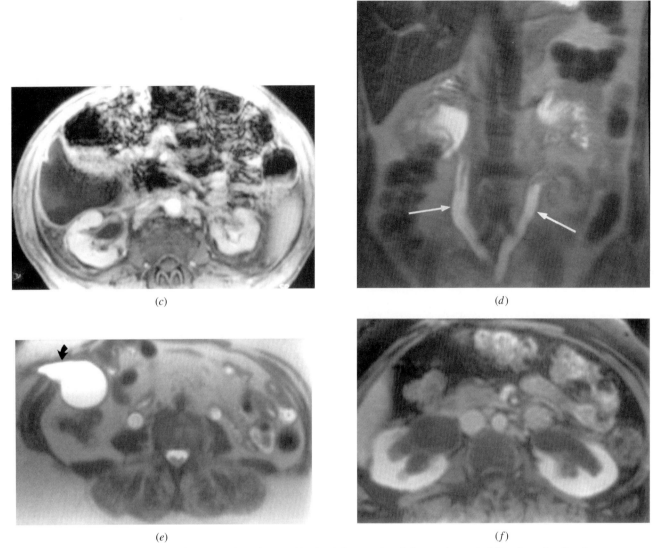

(c)

(d)

(e)

(f)

F I G. 11.22 (*Continued*) The Indiana pouch is observed in the right anterior abdomen (arrow). Dilated renal collecting systems are present on the gadolinium-enhanced image (*f*). Delayed excretion of gadolinium is evidenced by lack of visualization of gadolinium in the collecting systems by 5 min.

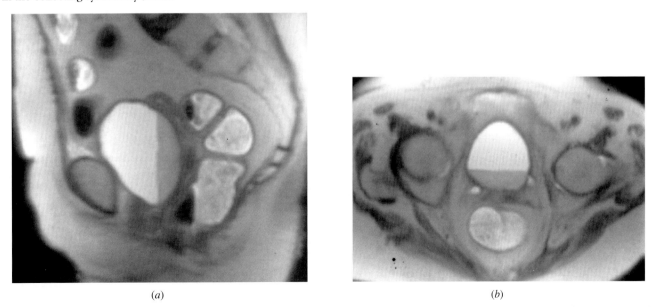

(a)

(b)

F I G. 11.23 Radiation changes. Sagittal (*a*) and transverse (*b*) T2-weighted single-shot echo-train spin-echo and sagittal (*c*) and transverse (*d*) T1-weighted gadolinium-enhanced fat-suppressed SGE images in a patient with primary cervical cancer who underwent radiation therapy.

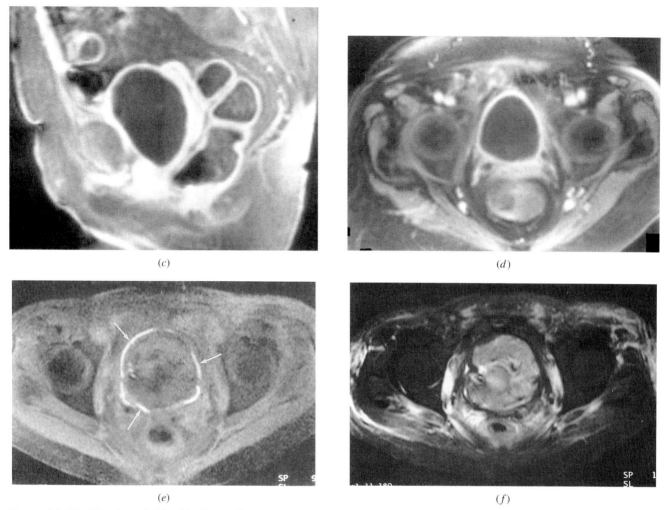

(c)

(d)

(e)

(f)

FIG. 11.23 (*Continued*) The bladder wall is diffusely thickened (*a–d*), and it enhances intensely and homogeneously after gadolinium administration (*c, d*). Note the dependently layering low-signal material in the bladder on the T2-weighted images, compatible with proteinaceous material and the clinical history of hematuria. Reticular strands in the perivesical fat and colorectal wall also enhance intensely because of inflammatory changes.

T1-weighted fat-suppressed SGE (*e*) and T2-weighted fat-suppressed spin-echo (*f*) images in a second patient. On the T2-weighted image, there is high signal intensity of the obturator internus muscles and high-signal intensity strands in the perirectal space, consistent with radiation-induced tissue damage. High signal intensity within the bladder wall on the T1-weighted fat-suppressed SGE (*e*) and low signal intensity on the T2-weighted fat-suppressed spin-echo (*f*) images are consistent with intracellular methemoglobin due to the radiation-induced hemorrhagic cystitis. The fluid in the bladder is predominantly high in signal intensity on T1- and T2-weighted images, which is consistent with extracellular metahemoglobin.

CONCLUSION

MRI is an effective technique for evaluating the full range of bladder disease. Staging of transitional cell carcinoma is the most common indication for bladder MRI investigation and is well performed with a combination of breath-hold SGE, 512-resolution T2-weighted echo-train spin-echo, and immediate and delayed postgadolinium fat-suppressed SGE techniques, with image acquisition in multiple planes and the concurrent use of a phased-array multicoil.

Future use of cine MRI may provide dynamic information regarding pattern of bladder emptying as a func-

tion of time [72]. Lymph node-specific contrast agents have been investigated that may permit differentiation of lymph-node malignant involvement versus hyperplastic enlargement. Thus the staging of bladder carcinomas may be improved [73].

REFERENCES

1. Banson ML: Normal MR anatomy and technique for imaging of the male pelvis. *MRI Clin N Am* 4: 481–496, 1996.
2. Fritzsche PJ, Wilbur MJ: The male pelvis. *Semin Ultrasound CT MR* 10: 11–28, 1989.

3. Teeger S, Sica G: MR Imaging of bladder diseases. *MRI Clin N Am* 4: 565–581, 1996.
4. Siegelman ES and Schnall MD: Contrast-enhanced MR imaging of the bladder and prostate. *MRI Clin N Am* 4: 153–169, 1996.
5. Narumi Y, Kadota T, Inoue E et al.: Bladder tumors: Staging with gadolinium-enhanced oblique MR imaging. *Radiology* 187: 145–150, 1993.
6. Barentsz JO, Ruijs SHJ, Strijk SP: The role of MR imaging in carcinoma of the urinary bladder. *Am J Roentgenol* 160: 937–947, 1993.
7. Lee JKT, Rholl KS: MRI of the bladder and prostate (review). *Am J Roentgenol* 147: 732–736, 1986.
8. Piccoli CW, Rifkin MD: Magnetic resonance imaging of the prostate and bladder. *Top Magn Reson Imaging* 2: 51–66, 1990.
9. Barentsz JO, Lemmens JAM, Ruijs SHJ, et al.: Carcinoma of the urinary bladder: MR imaging using a double surface coil. *Am J Roentgenol* 151: 107–112, 1988.
10. Reiman TH, Heiken JP, Totty WG, Lee JKT: Clinical MR imaging with a Helmholtz-type surface coil. *Radiology* 169: 564–566, 1988.
11. Narumi Y, Kadota T, Inoue E, et al.: Bladder wall morphology: In vitro MR imaging-histopathologic correlation. *Radiology* 187: 151–155, 1993.
12. Hricak H. The bladder and female urethra. In Hricak H, Carrington BM (eds.), *MRI of the Pelvis: A Text Atlas.* London: Martin Dunitz, 1991, p. 417–461.
13. Donalski M, Shite EM, Ghahremani GG et al.: Carcinoma arising in urinary diverticula: Imaging findings in six patients. *Am J Roentgenol* 161: 817–820, 1993.
14. Hahn D: Neoplasms of the urinary bladder. In Pollack HM (ed.), *Clinical Urography.* Vol. 2. Philadelphia: WB Saunders p. 1355–1377, 1990.
15. Menaham MM, Slywotzky C: Urinary bladder leiomyoma: Magnetic resonance imaging findings. *Urol Radiol* 14: 197–199, 1992.
16. Warshawsky R, Bow SN, Waldbaum RS, Cintron J: Bladder pheochromocytoma with MR correlation. *J Comput Assist Tomogr* 13: 714–716, 1989.
17. Heyman J, Cheung Y, Ghali V, Leiter E: Bladder pheochromocytoma: Evaluation with magnetic resonance imaging. *J Urol* 141: 1424–1426, 1989.
18. Fink JIJ, Reinig JW, Dwyer AJ, et al.: MR imaging of pheochromocytoma. *J Comput Assist Tomogr* 9: 454–458, 1985.
19. Falke ThM, LeStrake L, Shaff MI, et al.: MR imaging of the adrenals: Correlated with computed tomography. *J Comput Assist Tomogr* 10: 242–253, 1986.
20. Quint LE, Glazer GM, Francis IR, Shapiro B, Chenevert TL: Pheochromocytoma and paraganglioma: Comparison of MR imaging with CT and I-131 MIB6 scintigraphy. *Radiology* 165: 89–93, 1987.
21. Hencey JF, Verness M, Norman J. Urinary bladder pheochromocytoma in a patient with familial pheochromocytoma: MR and CT features. *Int Med Image Registry* 1: 123–124, 1995.
22. Shonnard KM, Jelinek JS, Benedikt RA, Kransdorf MJ: CT and MR of neurofibromatosis of the bladder. *J Comput Assist Tomgr* 16: 433–438, 1992.
23. Amano T, Kunimi K, Hisazumi H, et al.: Magnetic resonance imaging of bladder hemangioma. *Abdom Imaging* 18: 97–99, 1993.
24. Arrive L, Malbec L, Buy JN, Guinet C, Vadrot D: Male pelvis. In Vanel D, McNamara MT (eds.), *MRI of the Body.* New York: Springer, p. 242–255, 1989.
25. Bryan PJ, Butler HE, Nelson AD, Lipuma JP, Kopiwoda SY, et al.: Magnetic resonance imaging of the prostate. *Am J Roentgenol* 146: 543–548, 1986.
26. Rozanski TA, Grossman HB: Recent developments in the pathophysiology of bladder cancer. *Am J Roentgenol* 163: 789–792, 1994.
27. Heiken JP, Forman HP, Brown JJ: Neoplasm of the bladder, prostate, and testis. *Radiol Clin N Am* 32: 81–98, 1994.
28. Beahrs OH, Henson DE, Hetter RVP, eds.: *Manual for Staging of Cancer,* (4th ed.). Philadelphia: Lippincott, 1992.
29. Fisher MR, Hricak H, Tanagho EA: Urinary bladder MR imaging. Part II. Neoplasm. *Radiology* 157: 471–477, 1985.
30. Amendola MA, Glaser GM, Grossman HB, et al.: Staging of bladder carcinoma: MRI-CT-surgical correlation. *Am J Roentgenol* 146: 1179–1183, 1986.
31. Bryan PJ, Butler HE, LiPuma JP, et al.: CT and MR imaging in staging bladder neoplasms. *J Comput Assist Tomogr* 11: 96–101, 1987.
32. Rholl KS, Lee JKT, Heiken JP, et al.: Primary bladder carcinoma: Evaluation with MR imaging. *Radiology* 163: 117–123, 1987.
33. Buy JN, Moss AA, Guinet C, et al.: MR staging of bladder carcinoma: Correlation with pathologic findings. *Radiology* 169: 695–700, 1988.
34. Koebel G, Schmeidl U, Griebel J, et al.: MR imaging of urinary bladder neoplasms. *J Comput Assist Tomogr* 12: 98–103, 1988.
35. Husband JE, Oliff JF, Williams MP, Heron CW, Cherryman GR: Bladder cancer: Staging with CT and MR imaging. *Radiology* 173: 435–440, 1989.
36. Barentsz JO, Debruyne FMJ, Ruijs SHJ: *Magnetic Resonance Imaging of Carcinoma of the Urinary Bladder.* Boston: Kluwer, 1990.
37. Cheng D and Tempany CMC. Mr imaging of the prostate and bladder. *Semin Ultrasound CT MRI* 19: 67–89, 1998.
38. Piccoli CW and Rifkin MD: Magnetic resonance imaging of the prostate and bladder. *Topics Magn Reson Imaging* 2: 51–66, 1990.
39. Persad R, Kabala J, Gillatt D, Penry B, Gingell JC, Smith JB: Magnetic resonance imaging in the staging of bladder cancer. *Br J Urol* 71: 566–573, 1993.
40. Ebner F, Kressel HY, Mints MC, et al.: Tumor recurrence versus fibrosis in the female pelvis: Differentiation with MR imaging at 1.5T. *Radiology* 166: 333–340, 1988.
41. Strich G, Hagan P, Gerber KH, et al.: Tissue distribution and magnetic resonance spin lattice relaxation effects of gadolinium-DTPA. *Radiology* 154: 723–726, 1985.
42. Tachibana M, Baba S, Daguchi N, et al.: Efficacy of gadolinium-diethylene-triaminepentaacetic acid-enhanced magnetic resonance imaging for differentiation between superficial and muscle-invasive tumor of the bladder: A comparative study with computerized tomography and transurethral ultrasonography. *J Urol* 145: 1169–1173, 1991.
43. Neuerburg JM, Bohndorf K, Sohn M, et al.: Urinary bladder neoplasms: Evaluation with contrast-enhanced MR imaging. *Radiology* 172: 739–743, 1989.
44. Neuerburg JM, Bohndorf K, Sohn M, Teufl F, Gunther RW: Staging of urinary bladder neoplasms with MR imaging: Is Gd-DTPA helpful? *J Comput Assist Tomogr* 15: 780–786, 1991.
45. Sohn M, Neuerburg JM, Teufl F, Bohndorf K: Gadolinium-enhanced magnetic resonance imaging in the staging of urinary bladder neoplasms. *Urol Int* 45: 142–147, 1990.
46. Barentsz JO, van Erning LJThO, Ruijs JHJ, Bors WG, Jager G, Oosterhof G: Dynamic turbo-FLASH subtraction MR imaging: Perfusion of pelvic tumors (abstract). *Radiology* 185: 340, 1992.
47. Sparenberg A, Hamm B, Hammerer P, Samberger V, Wolf KJ: The diagnosis of bladder carcinomas by NMR tomography: Any improvement with Gd-DTPA? *Forschr Rontgenstr* 155: 117–122, 1991.
48. Barentsz JE, Jager GJ, van Vierzen PBJ, Witjes JA, Strijk SP, Peters H, Karssemeijer N, Ruijs SHJ: Staging urinary bladder cancer after transurethral biopsy: Value of fast dynamic contrast-enhanced MR imaging. *Radiology.* 201(1): 185–193, 1996.
49. Newhouse J: Clinical use of urinary tract magnetic resonance imaging. *Radiol Clin N Am* 29: 467–468, 1991.
50. Kim B, Semelka RC, Ascher SM, Chalpin D, Carroll P, Hricak H: Bladder tumor staging: Comparison of contrast enhanced CT, T1- and T2- weighted MR imaging, dynamic gadolinium-enhanced imaging, and late gadolinium-enhanced imaging. *Radiology* 193: 239–245, 1994.

51. Rarentsz JO, Witjes JA, Ruijs JH: What is new in bladder cancer imaging. *Urol Clin N Am.* 24(3): 583–602, 1997.

52. Barentsz JO, Engelbrecht M, Jager GJ, Witjes JA, de Larossete J: Fast dynamic gadolinium-enhanced MR imaging of urinary bladder and prostate cancer. *J Magn Reson Imaging.* 10(3): 295–304, 1999.

53. Barentsz JO, Jager GJ, Mugler JP 3rd, Oosterhof G, Peters H: Staging urinary bladder cancer: value of T1-weighted three-dimensional magnetization prepared-rapid gradient-echo and two-dimensional spin-echo sequences. *Am J Roentgenol.* 164(1): 109–115, 1995.

54. Algra PR, Bloem JL, Tissing H, Falke ThHM, Arndt J-W, Verboom LJ: Detection of vertebral metastases: Comparison between MR imaging and bone scintigraphy. *Radiographics* 11: 219–232, 1991.

55. Fletcher BD, Kaste SC: Magnetic resonance imaging for diagnosis and follow-up of genitourinary, pelvis and perineal rhabdomyosarcoma. *Urol Radiol* 14: 263–272, 1992.

56. Krysiewicz S: Diagnosis of urachal carcinoma by computed tomography and magnetic resonance imaging. *Clin Imaging* 14: 251–2545, 1990.

57. Rafal RB, Markisz JA: Urachal carcinoma. The role of magnetic resonance imaging. *Urol Radiol* 12: 184–187, 1991.

58. Popovich MJ, Hricak H, Sugimura Kazuro, Stern JL: The role of MR imaging in determining surgical eligibility for pelvic exenteration. *Am J Roentgenol* 160: 525–531, 1993.

59. Hricak H, Hamm B, Semelka R, Cann CE, Nauert T, Secaf E, Stern JL, Wolf K-J: Carcinoma of the uterus: Use of gadopentetate dimeglumine in MR imaging. *Radiology* 181: 95–106, 1991.

60. Janus CL, Mendelson DS, Moore S, Gendal EL, Dottino P, Brodman M: Staging of cervical carcinoma: Accuracy of magnetic resonance imaging and computed tomography. *Clin Imaging* 13: 114–116, 1989.

61. Yeoman LJ, Mason MD, Olliff JFC: Non-Hodgkin's lymphoma of the bladder—CT and MRI appearance. *Clin Radiol* 44: 39–392, 1991.

62. Rifkin MD, Piccoli CW: Male pelvis and bladder. In Stark DD, Bradley WG (eds.), *Magnetic Resonance Imaging.* Vol. 2. Baltimore: Mosby p. 2044–2057, 1992.

63. Bradley, WG Jr: Hemorrhage and brain iron. In Stark DD, Bradley WG Jr (eds.), *Magnetic Resonance Imaging.* Vol. 1. Baltimore: Mosby p. 721–728, 1992.

64. Hahn D. Neoplasms of the urinary bladder. In Pollack HM (ed.), *Clinical Urography.* Vol. 2. Philadelphia: WB Saunders, 1353–1354, 1990.

65. Elkin M. Urogenital tuberculosis. In Pollack HM (ed.), *Clinical Urography.* Vol. 1. Philadelphia: WB Saunders p. 1020–1046, 1990.

66. Saxton HM. Pelvic lipomatosis. In Pollack HM (ed.), *Clinical Urography.* Vol. 3. Philadelphia: WB Saunders p. 2458–2461, 1990.

67. Schnall MD, Connick T, Hayes CE, Lenkinski RE, Kressel HY: MR imaging of the pelvis with an endorectal-external multicoil array. *J Magn Reson Imaging* 2: 229–232, 1992.

68. Semelka RC, Hricak H, Kim B, Forstner R, Bis KG, Ascher SM, Reinhold C: Pelvic fistulas: Appearances on MR images. *Abdom Imaging* 22: 91–95, 1997.

69. Mindell HJ, Quiogue T, Lebowitz RL: Postoperative uroradiological appearances. In Pollack HM (ed.). *Clinical Urography.* Vol. 3. Philadelphia: WB Saunders, p. 2510–2531, 1990.

70. Sugimura K, Carrington, BM, Quivey JM, et al. Postirradiation changes in the pelvis: Assessment with MR imaging. *Radiology* 175: 805–813, 1990.

71. Hricak H: Magnetic resonance imaging evaluation of the irradiated female pelvis. *Semin Roentgenol* 29: 70–80, 1994.

72. Gupta RK, Kapoor R, Poptani H, Rastogi H, Gujral RB: Cine MR voiding cystourethrogram in adult normal males. *Magn Reson Imaging* 10: 881–885, 1992.

73. Guimaraes R, Clemont O, Bittoun J, Carnot F, Frija G: MR lymphadenopathy with superparamagnetic iron manoparticles in rats: Pathologic basis for contrast enhancement. *Am J Roentgenol* 162: 201–207, 1994.

chapter 12

MALE PELVIS

TARA C. NOONE, M.D., RICHARD C. SEMELKA, M.D.,
RAHEL A. KUBIK-HUCH, M.D., AND LARISSA BRAGA, M.D.

TECHNIQUE

MRI is an effective modality for the diagnosis, staging, and follow-up of a variety of diseases of the male pelvis. Our standard male pelvis imaging protocol includes 512-resolution transverse and sagittal T2-weighted echo-train spin-echo and postgadolinium transverse and sagittal fat-suppressed SGE sequences. The routine use of a phased-array multicoil results in reproducible high image quality. Several reports have emphasized the value of the high spatial resolution achieved with endorectal coil imaging [1–3]. A combination of endorectal coil and pelvis phased-array coil imaging is an alternative accepted technique. Supplemental T1-weighted imaging through the abdomen and pelvis should be performed to assess for lymphadenopathy.

PROSTATE AND POSTERIOR URETHRA

Normal Anatomy

The prostate is divided anatomically into central, transitional, and peripheral zones. The peripheral zone is most extensive within the prostatic apex, where it forms the majority of the gland, and in the midgland, where it is posterior and posterolateral in location. The central zone is periurethral in location and is situated superiorly within the base of the gland. It surrounds the verumontanum. The transitional zone surrounds the central zone and also is located predominantly within the base of the prostate. The transitional zone increases in size with patient age.

The prostate appears homogeneous and intermediate in signal intensity on T1-weighted images, and zonal anatomy is not demonstrable. The zonal anatomy of the prostate is well demonstrated on T2-weighted images (fig. 12.1). Signal intensity on T2-weighted images is directly related to the proportion of glandular elements and inversely related to the density of stromal or muscular elements. Thus there is increased signal intensity in the peripheral zone, where there is abundant glandular material, and decreased signal intensity in the central zone, where more striated muscle and stroma are present. The signal intensity of the transitional zone, where there is also a large volume of stroma, is similar to that of the central zone. Differentiation between the two cannot be made by imaging appearances but is based primarily on anatomic location.

The anterolateral prostate is cloaked by the anterior fibromuscular band, which is low in signal intensity on

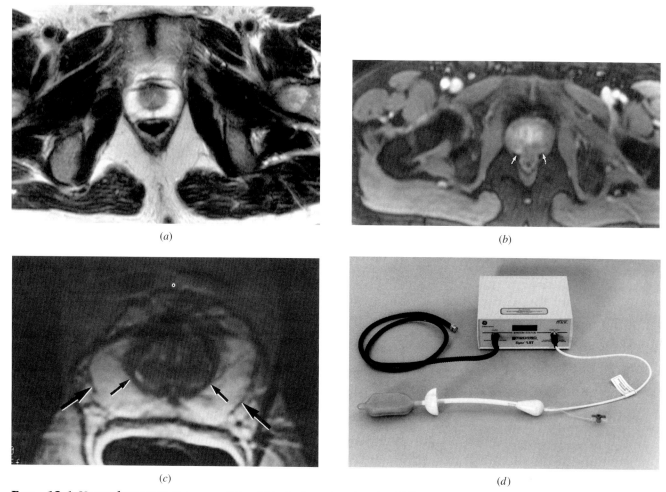

(a)

(b)

(c)

(d)

F I G. 12.1 Normal Prostate. Transverse T2-weighted echo-train spin-echo (ETSE) (*a*) image. The peripheral zone is high in signal intensity on T2-weighted images and surrounds the lower-signal intensity transitional and central zones.

Transverse immediate postgadolinium fat-suppressed SGE (*b*) image in a second patient. Note the vascular enhancement delineating the neurovascular bundles (arrows, *b*) on the postgadolinium image.

T2-weighted endorectal coil image (*c*) in a third patient with normal prostate. The zonal anatomy of the prostate is well demonstrated on T2-weighted images. The normal central zone and transitional zones are low in signal intensity (short arrows, *c*), and the normal peripheral zone is high in signal intensity (long arrows, *c*).

The endorectal coil (*d*) has a balloon tip that is inflated when the coil is placed.

both T1- and T2-weighted images. It serves as a landmark dividing the prostate from the tissues of the preprostatic space. The prostate capsule also consists of fibromuscular tissue and is low in signal intensity on T2-weighted images. The verumontanum, a central ovoid high-signal intensity structure, is located in the periurethral region at the midgland level. The neurovascular bundles are located posterolaterally at 5 and 7 o'clock within the rectoprostatic angles.

The prostatic and membranous portions of the urethra form the posterior urethra. The distal prostatic urethra is demonstrated as a low-signal intensity rounded structure within the high-signal intensity peripheral zone at the apex of the prostate (fig. 12.2). The membranous urethra extends from the prostatic apex to the

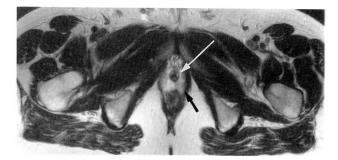

F I G. 12.2 Normal prostate level of apex. Transverse T2-weighted ETSE image. At the level of the prostatic apex the gland is comprised predominantly of the peripheral zone, which is high in signal intensity on T2-weighted images (black arrow). The muscular wall of the urethra, which is low in signal intensity on T2-weighted images, is clearly depicted (white arrow).

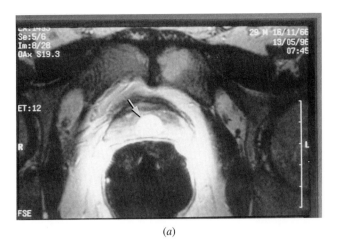

(a)

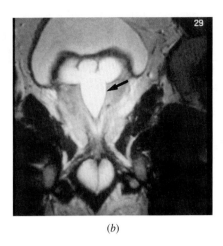

(b)

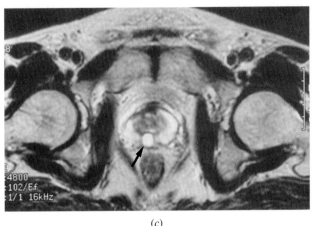

(c)

FIG. 12.3 Utricular cyst in an infertile 29-year-old male. Transverse (a) and coronal (b) T2-weighted spin-echo endorectal coil images. A rounded, central structure, which is high in signal intensity on the T2-weighted images, represents a utricular cyst (white arrow, a; black arrow, b).

Transverse T2-weighted spin-echo image (c) in a second patient. A utricular cyst located in the region of the verumontanum is high in signal intensity on this T2-weighted image (black arrow, c).

bulb of the penis. The muscular wall of the membranous urethra forms the external sphincter, and embedded within its adventitia are the paired Cowper glands.

Disease Entities

Congenital Abnormalities

Cysts are the most commonly encountered congenital anomalies of the prostate. Congenital prostatic cysts are generally high in signal intensity on T2-weighted images and of variable signal intensity on T1-weighted images, depending on the presence of infection or hemorrhage. Characterized by their location in relation to the prostate, which may be midline, paramedian, or lateral, they occur between the prostatic urethra or bladder anteriorly and the rectum posteriorly.

Midline cysts include utricular and müllerian duct cysts. Utricular cysts arise from dilatation of the prostatic utricle, originating from the verumontanum. Frequently associated with other genital anomalies, they are usually teardrop shaped and communicate with the posterior urethra (fig. 12.3) [4, 5].

In contrast, müllerian duct cysts do not communicate with the posterior urethra but are connected to the verumontanum by a stalk. Generally retrovesical in location (fig. 12.4), they are remnants of the müllerian duct

system and are rarely associated with renal agenesis. Patients may present with urinary retention, infection, and stone formation. There are associated increased incidences of both squamous cell carcinoma and adenocarcinomas [4–6].

Cysts arising from the vas deferens or ejaculatory ducts are paramedian in location. Ejaculatory duct cysts may be either congenital or postinflammatory and generally result from obstruction along the expected course of the ductal system. Cysts of the vas deferens, although extremely rare, most frequently involve the ampulla. When large, either of these paramedian cystic structures may appear identical to utricular or müllerian duct cysts. Aspirated cyst fluid contains spermatozoa, permitting differentiation from müllerian duct cysts [4, 5, 7, 8]. Cysts are high in signal intensity on high-resolution T2-weighted images and appear as signal void on postgadolinium images.

Mass Lesions

Benign Masses. Proliferation of glandular, or, less commonly, interstitial elements of the transitional zone leads to benign prostatic hyperplasia (BPH), a disease entity observed in approximately 50% of the male population older than 45 years of age [9]. When changes are focal, they may result in the formation of nodules or adenomyomata.

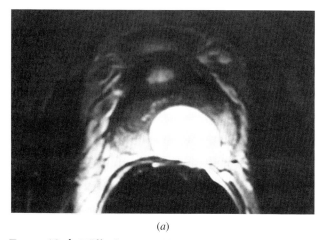
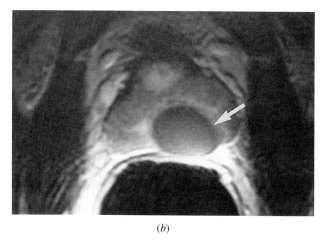

(a)   (b)

F I G . 12.4 Müllerian cyst. Transverse T2-weighted spin-echo (*a*) and immediate postgadolinium fat-suppressed T1 SGE (*b*) endorectal coil images. A large, ovoid müllerian cyst is seen in the dorsal aspect of the prostate near the midline, which is high in signal intensity on the T2-weighted image (*a*) and intermediate in signal intensity on the postgadolinium image (white arrow, *b*).

Glandular hyperplasia frequently results in enlargement of the central aspect of the prostate. BPH is low in signal intensity on T1-weighted images. On T2-weighted images BPH may be homogeneous or heterogeneous in appearance, ranging from medium to high in signal intensity [10–12]. Compression of the adjacent peripheral zone results in a low-signal intensity band referred to as the surgical pseudocapsule [12, 13]. Adenomatous changes may result in focal, nodular enlargement of the gland. Signal characteristics may be variable on T2-weighted images [10, 14]. BPH commonly occurs in conjunction with prostate cancer because both are disease processes that increase in incidence with patient age (fig. 12.5).

Distinction between interstitial hyperplasia and glandular hyperplasia has been described on MR images [11, 15]. Hyperplastic changes that predominantly involve the interstitium result in heterogeneous low signal intensity of the enlarged gland on T2-weighted images [11]. Focal alterations in signal intensity may result from infarction or cystic changes within nodules of glandular BPH [5, 15–17]. Areas of infarction may demonstrate low signal intensity on T2-weighted images [17]. Cystic ectasia, corresponding to dilatation of glandular elements, results in high signal intensity on T2-weighted images (fig. 12.6) [11, 15]. BPH may occasionally infiltrate the peripheral zone, making its distinction from carcinoma problematic [15].

Progressive enlargement of the central portion of the prostate with resultant protrusion into the bladder leads to partial bladder outlet obstruction (fig. 12.7) [11]. After the surgical removal of periurethral tissue

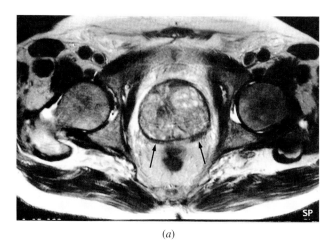
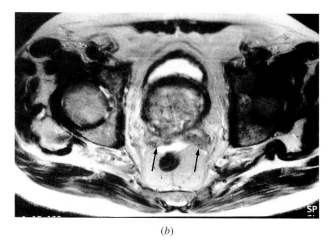

(a)   (b)

F I G . 12.5 Prostate cancer with seminal vesicle extension in the setting of massive BPH. Transverse (*a*, *b*) and sagittal (*c*) T2-weighted ETSE images. The transitional zone, which is greatly enlarged, is heterogeneous and moderately high in signal intensity. The peripheral zone of the prostate (thin arrows, *a*) is thin and diffusely low in signal intensity secondary to tumor involvement (*a*).

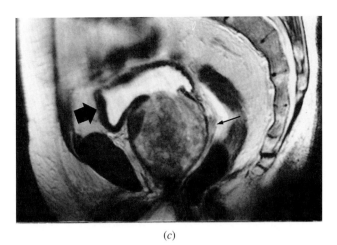

(c)

FIG. 12.5 (*Continued*) The seminal vesicles (thin arrows, *b, c*) also are low in signal intensity secondary to invasion by tumor (*b, c*). The bladder (large arrow, *c*) is elevated by the enlarged prostate and thick walled from resultant outlet obstruction.

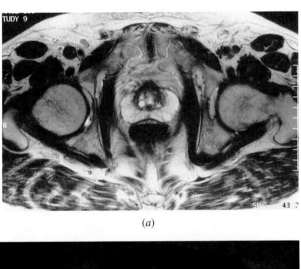

(a)

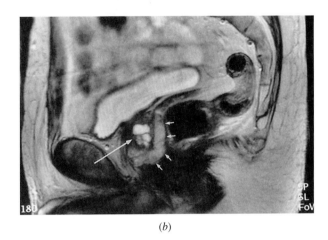

(b)

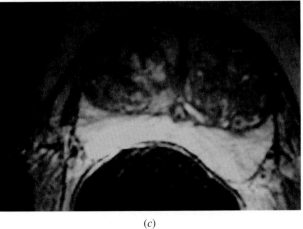

(c)

FIG. 12.6 Benign prostatic hyperplasia. Transverse (*a*) and sagittal (*b*) T2-weighted ETSE image. High-signal intensity foci are present, representing cystic elements of interstitial BPH (long arrow, *b*). Normal signal intensity is seen within the surrounding peripheral zone (short arrows, *b*).

Transverse T2-weighted ETSE endorectal coil image (*c*) in a second patient. Diffuse heterogeneous low signal intensity within an enlarged central gland is consistent with the predominately glandular subtype of BPH.

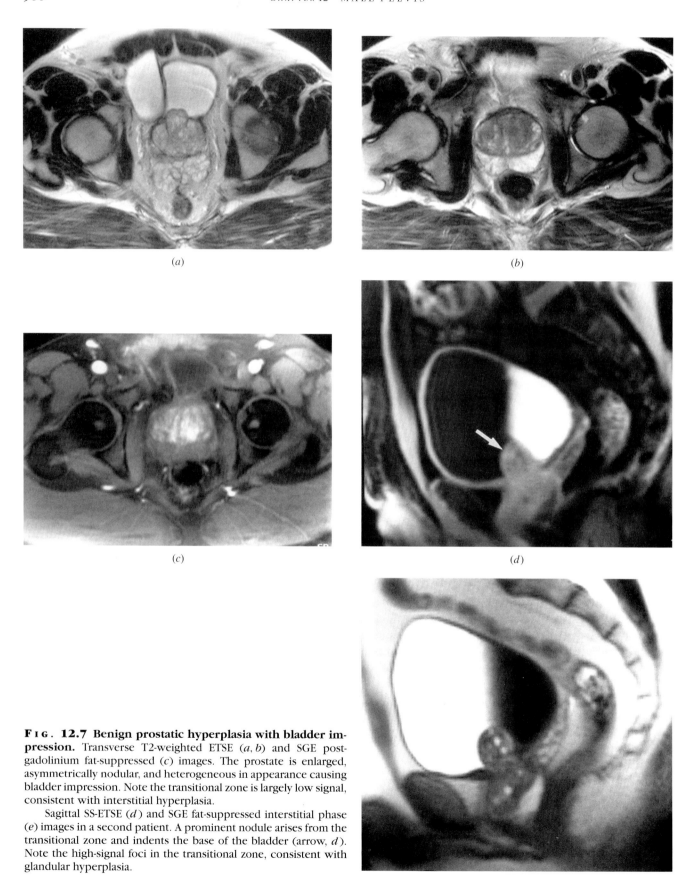

FIG. 12.7 Benign prostatic hyperplasia with bladder impression. Transverse T2-weighted ETSE (*a, b*) and SGE post-gadolinium fat-suppressed (*c*) images. The prostate is enlarged, asymmetrically nodular, and heterogeneous in appearance causing bladder impression. Note the transitional zone is largely low signal, consistent with interstitial hyperplasia.

Sagittal SS-ETSE (*d*) and SGE fat-suppressed interstitial phase (*e*) images in a second patient. A prominent nodule arises from the transitional zone and indents the base of the bladder (arrow, *d*). Note the high-signal foci in the transitional zone, consistent with glandular hyperplasia.

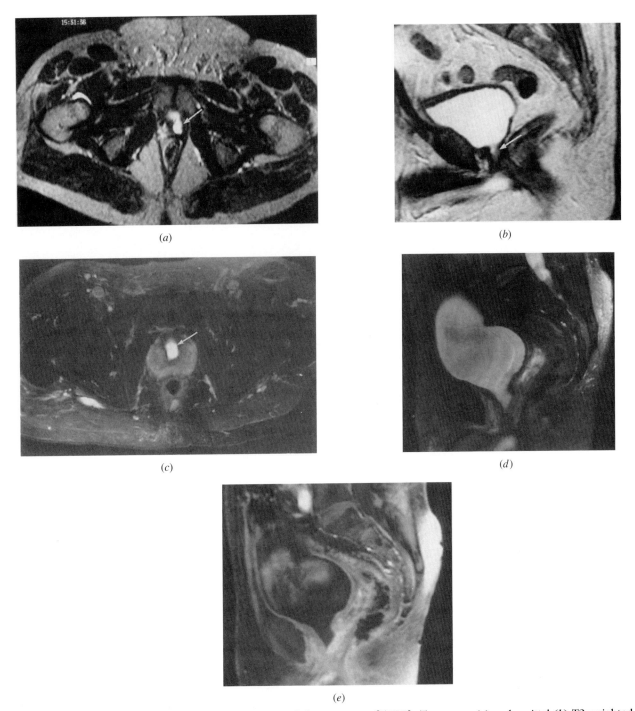

F I G . 12.8 Defect from transurethral resection of the prostate (TURP). Transverse (*a*) and sagittal (*b*) T2-weighted ETSE images. The TURP defect is seen within the base of the prostate. The posterior urethra (arrow, *a*, *b*) is dilated after the surgical removal of periurethral tissue.

Transverse T2-weighted fat-suppressed ETSE (*c*), sagittal T2-weighted fat-suppressed ETSE (*d*), and sagittal postgadolinium T1-weighted fat-suppressed SGE (*e*) images in a second patient. Dilatation of the prostatic urethra (arrow, *c*) is observed after TURP.

by transurethral, transvesical, or retropubic approaches, the adjacent prostatic urethra dilates to the level of the verumontanum. Residual hyperplastic tissue may be low to medium in signal intensity on T2-weighted images (fig. 12.8) [8]. Radical prostatectomy may result in periurethral scarring, which also is low in sig-

nal intensity on T2-weighted images (fig. 12.9). Fibrosis in the bed of the prostate and seminal vesicles after total prostatectomy is low in signal intensity on T2-weighted images and may mimic the appearance of a small, low-signal intensity prostate and seminal vesicles.

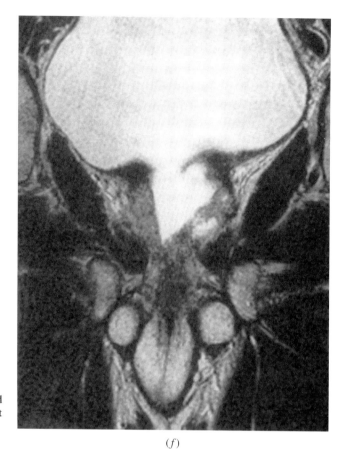

(f)

FIG. 12.8 (*Continued*) Coronal T2-weighted fat-suppressed endorectal coil image (*f*) of a third patient after TURP. Note slight irregularity of the TURP defect in the prostate.

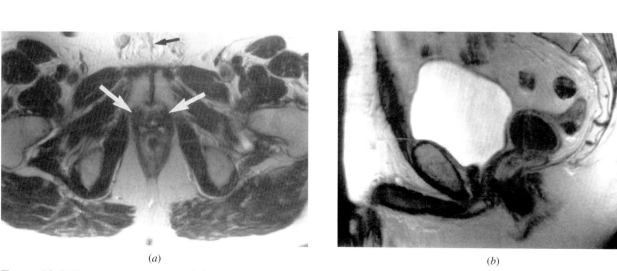

(a)   (b)

FIG. 12.9 Postprostatectomy pelvis. Transversal (*a*) and sagittal (*b*) T2-weighted ETSE images. Low-signal intensity tissue surrounds the posterior urethra within the prostatic bed (white arrows, *a*) of this patient after prostatectomy. This appearance results from fibrosis and scarring at the operative site. Note the midline scar in the subcutaneous tissue (black arrow, *a*), which is a constant observation in postprostatectomy patients.

Malignant Masses

RARE TUMORS

Squamous cell cancer, transitional cell cancer, and sarcoma are uncommon malignancies that involve the prostate and account for less than 5% of malignant tumors. In the pediatric population, prostate rhabdomyosarcoma is the most common tumor to arise from the bladder region (fig. 12.10) [8].

PROSTATE ADENOCARCINOMA

Approximately 95% of malignant prostate lesions are adenocarcinomas. Prostatic carcinoma is frequently latent. It may occur in as many as 80% of men 80 years of age or older and in as many as 50% of men 50 years of age or older [15]. Its behavior depends on histologic

grade/stage and tumor volume [19, 20]. Thus tremendous controversy regarding diagnostic and treatment options remains.

Approximately 70% of prostate cancers arise from the peripheral zone, and the remainder arise in the transitional and central zones. Detection of prostate carcinoma with MRI is limited primarily to tumors involving the peripheral zone. These tumors are generally isointense relative to surrounding peripheral zone tissue on T1-weighted images. The majority of prostate cancers are hypointense on T2-weighted images (fig. 12.11). In rare instances, tumors may be isointense or hyperintense [21–23]. These tumors frequently contain numerous mucinous elements [23, 24]. When isolated to the transition zone, adenocarcinomas may appear heterogeneous, isointense, or hypointense relative to surrounding tissue [16]. Thus these lesions may be difficult to differentiate from BPH. Tumors in the peripheral zone demonstrate increased enhancement on immediate postgadolinium fat-suppressed SGE images (fig. 12.12).

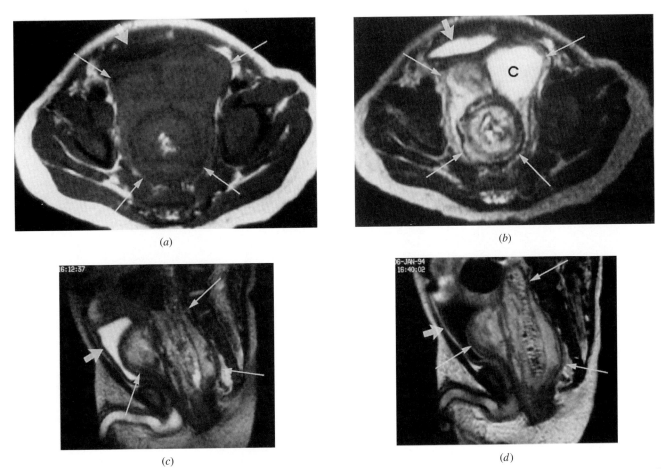

(a)   (b)   (c)   (d)

F I G . 12.10 Prostatic rhabdomyosarcoma. Transverse T1-weighted spin-echo (*a*), transverse T2-weighted spin-echo (*b*), sagittal T2-weighted spin-echo (*c*), and sagittal postgadolinium T1-weighted spin-echo (*d*) images. A complex, predominantly solid mass (long arrows, *a–c*) compresses and displaces the bladder anteriorly (arrow, *a–d*). An area of cystic ("c," *b*) change within the left aspect of the tumor is shown on the T2-weighted image (*b*).

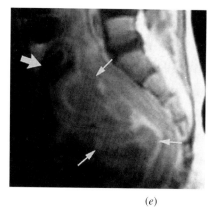

(e)

FIG. 12.10 (*Continued*) Sagittal immediate postgadolinium SGE image (*e*) in a second patient with prostatic rhabdomyosarcoma. A predominantly solid complex mass (thin arrows, *e*) impresses upon the bladder posteriorly and displaces it anteriorly. There is bladder wall thickening from outlet obstruction (large arrow, *e*).

Tumors spread first to penetrate the prostatic capsule (fig. 12.13). After capsular penetration, tumor extends to the neurovascular bundles and seminal vesicles (figs. 12.14 and 12.15). Bladder invasion occurs commonly in advanced-stage prostate cancer and may be extensive (fig. 12.16). The most common sites of metastasis are the bone marrow and lymph nodes. Infiltration of the pelvic lymphatics, particularly the obturator, external, and internal iliac chains, precedes distant metastases to the bones and retroperitoneum. Bone marrow in the iliac bones is frequently marbled in signal intensity on T1- and T2-weighted images, rendering detection of bone metastases at times problematic. On gadolinium-enhanced fat-suppressed images metastases appear as relatively well-defined focal mass lesions or diffusely enhancing extensive bony infiltration in a low-signal intensity background of fatty or fibrotic marrow (fig. 12.17).

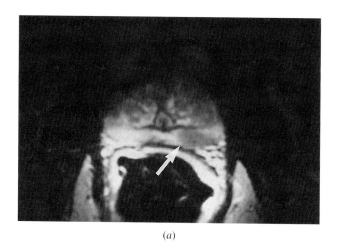

(a)

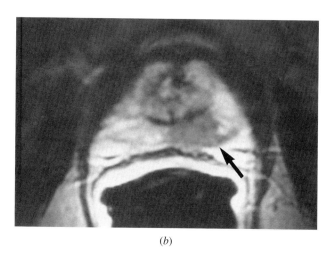

(b)

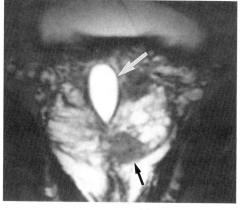

(c)

FIG. 12.11 Prostate carcinoma Stage T2. Transverse T2-weighted ETSE endorectal image (*a*). A focus of low signal intensity is seen within the peripheral zone in this patient with Stage T2 adenocarcinoma of the prostate (arrow, *a*).

Endorectal transverse T2-weighted ETSE image (*b*) in a second patient with prostate carcinoma. A hypointense tumor is seen within the peripheral zone of the prostate at the level of the apex (arrow, *b*).

Endorectal coronal T2-weighted ETSE (*c*) in a third patient with prostate carcinoma. A low-signal intensity focus within the apex of the prostate represents primary adenocarcinoma (black arrow, *c*). Note the incidental, midline utricular cyst, which is high in signal intensity on the T2-weighted image (white arrow, *c*).

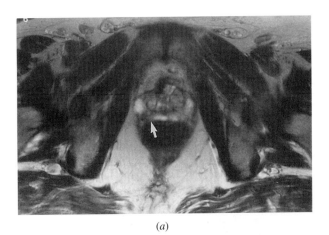

(a)

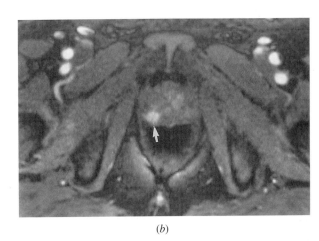

(b)

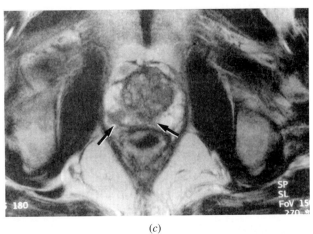

(c)

FIG. 12.12 Prostate carcinoma. Transverse T2-weighted ETSE (*a*) and transverse immediate postgadolinium fat-suppressed SGE (*b*) images. High-resolution T2-weighted image (*a*) reveals a well-defined carcinoma within the peripheral zone of the right lobe of the prostate (arrow, *a*). Smaller tumor volume is present within the left lobe (*a*). Immediate postgadolinium image demonstrates enhancement of the tumor focus within the right lobe (arrow, *b*). More ill-defined enhancement is seen within the left lobe (*b*).

Transverse T2-weighted ETSE (*c*) images in a second patient. There is a heterogeneous enlargement of the central aspect of the prostate consistent with prostatic hypertrophy. Several foci of low signal are note at the 6 and 8 o'clock positions (arrow, *c*) within the gland consistent with prostate cancer.

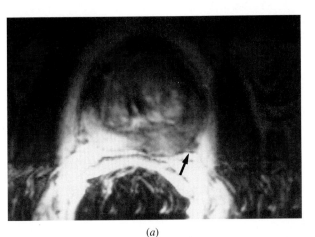

(a)

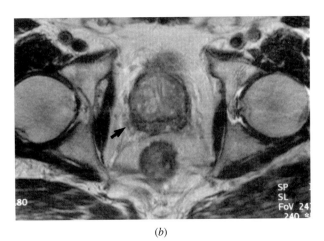

(b)

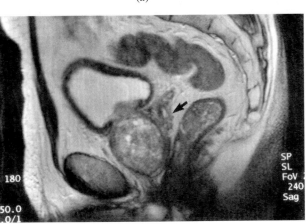

(c)

FIG. 12.13 Prostate carcinoma with capsular penetration. T2-weighted ETSE endorectal image (*a*) demonstrates low-signal intensity tumor within the peripheral zone of the prostate that extends posterolaterally (arrow, *a*), indicating capsular penetration.

Transverse (*b*) and sagittal (*c*) T2-weighted ETSE images in a second patient demonstrate diffuse low signal intensity of the peripheral zone consistent with diffuse carcinoma. Capsular penetration is observed at the 8 o'clock position (arrow, *b*). Seminal vesicle invasion is clearly shown in the sagittal projection (arrow, *c*), with involvement of the bladder base also appreciated.

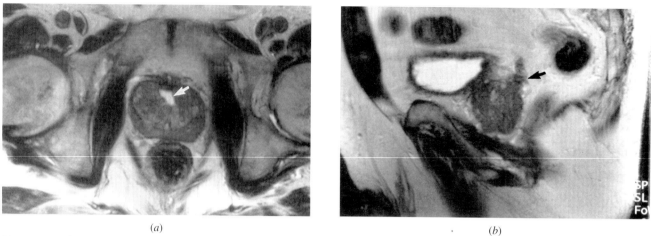

F I G . 12.14 Prostate carcinoma, diffuse involvement. Transverse (*a*) and sagittal (*b*) SS-ETSE images. The prostate is enlarged with a transurethral prostatic resection defect in the superior aspect of the gland (arrow, *a*). The peripheral zone of the prostate is diffusely low signal on T2-weighted images consistent with diffuse tumor infiltration. This is shown on both transverse and sagittal projection. Note seminal vesicle involvement on the sagittal projection (arrow, *b*).

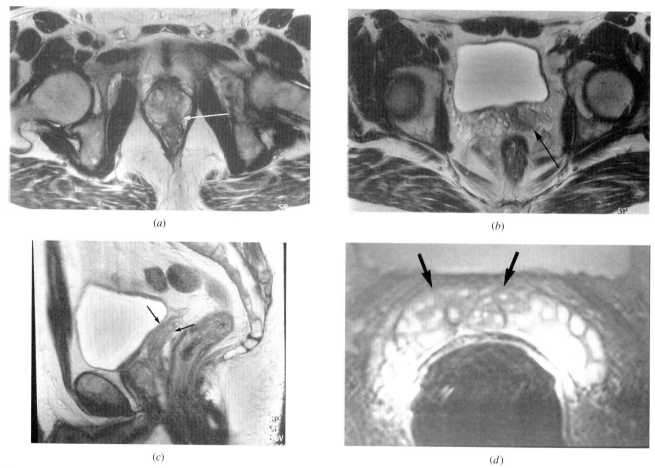

F I G . 12.15 Prostate cancer with seminal vesicle invasion. Transverse (*a, b*) and sagittal (*c*) T2-weighted ETSE images. A 1-cm tumor (white arrow, *a*) within the left aspect of the prostate at the midgland level is low in signal intensity on the T2-weighted image (*a*). The left seminal vesicle (black arrow, *b*) is diffusely low in signal intensity secondary to diffuse tumor involvement. Note the normal high-signal intensity cluster of grapes appearance of the right seminal vesicle (*b*). Loss of normal architecture and diffuse low signal intensity of the left seminal vesicle (black arrows, *c*) are confirmed on the sagittal image (*c*).

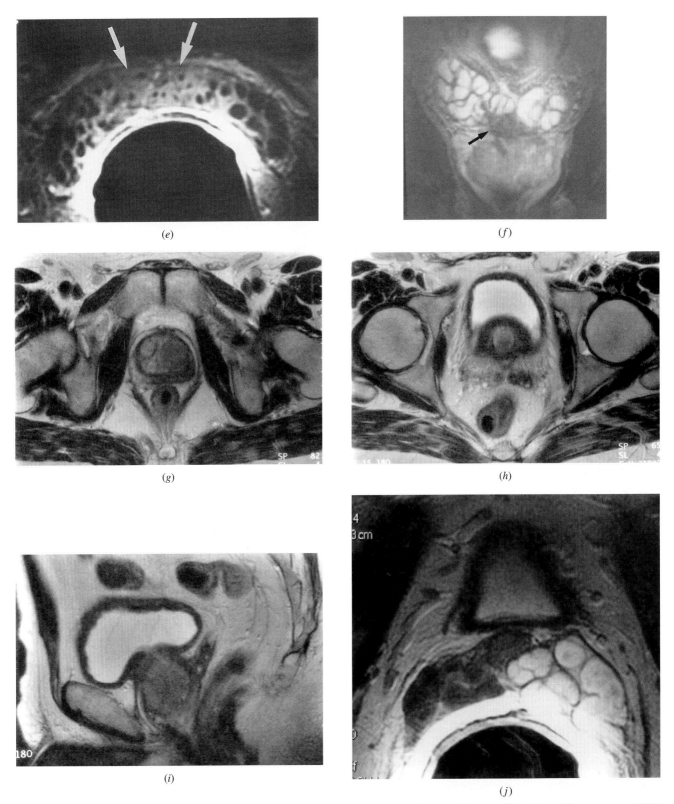

(e) *(f)*

(g) *(h)*

(i) *(j)*

FIG. 12.15 (*Continued*) Transverse T2-weighted ETSE endorectal coil (*d*) and postgadolinium T1-weighted fat-suppressed SGE endorectal coil (*e*) images in a second patient. There is ill-defined low-signal intensity tissue (arrows, *d*) within the medial aspects of the seminal vesicles on the T2-weighted image (*d*) corresponding to tumor invasion. Loss of the normal architecture of the seminal vesicles medially (arrows, *e*) indicates tumor invasion on the postgadolinium T1-weighted image (*e*).

Coronal T2-weighted ETSE endorectal coil image (*f*) in a third patient with seminal vesicle invasion. There is low signal intensity within the inferomedial aspects of the seminal vesicles (arrow, *f*) secondary to tumor invasion.

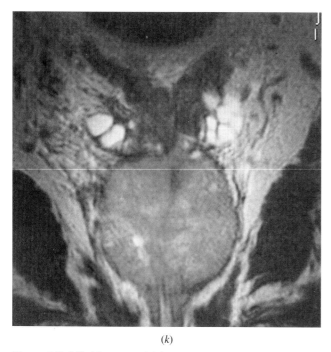

(k)

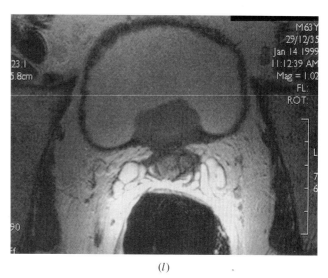

(l)

F I G . 12.15 (*Continued*) Transverse (*g*, *h*) and sagittal (*i*) T2-weighted ETSE images in a fourth patient. There is low-signal intensity tumor in the peripheral zone of the prostate at the midgland level extending from the 2:30 to 7:00 o'clock positions. Transverse and sagittal projections of the seminal vesicle demonstrate tumor involvement.

Endorectal coil T2-weighted echo-train spin-echo (*j*) image in a fifth patient demostrates involvement of the right seminal vesicle.

Endorectal T2-weighted echo-train spin-echo coronal (*k*) and transverse (*l*) images in a sixth patient demonstrates involvement of the medial portions of bilateral seminal vesicles. Imaging in two planes provides increased observer confidence of diagnosing tumor involvement.

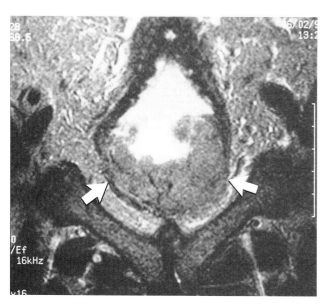

F I G . 12.16 Anaplastic prostate carcinoma. Coronal T2-weighted ETSE endorectal coil image. Lobular low-signal intensity tissue invading the urinary bladder (arrows) represents invasive prostate carcinoma in this patient with a normal prostate specific antigen level.

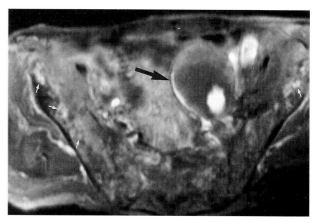

F I G . 12.17 Osseous metastases secondary to prostate carcinoma. Transverse 90-s postgadolinium fat-suppressed SGE image. Metastatic lesions are focal, well-defined enhancing lesions in a background of low-signal intensity fatty marrow on gadolinium-enhanced fat-suppressed images. Gadolinium-enhanced fat-suppressed technique enables accurate differentiation of enhancing metastatic foci (white arrows) from the frequently marbled appearance of normal bone marrow in the older patient. High-signal intensity intraluminal flow surrounded by low-signal intensity mural thrombus is seen in an incidental left internal iliac artery aneurysm (black arrow).

Table 12.1 American Joint Committee on Cancer Staging of Prostate

Carcinoma

Primary Tumor

T0	No evidence of primary tumor
T1	Clinical inapparent, not visible by imaging
T2	Tumor confined to the prostate (may involve capsule)
T3	Tumor extends beyond capsule (may involve seminal vesicles)
T4	Invasion of adjacent structures other than seminal vesicles (bladder, rectum, levator m.)

Regional Lymph Nodes

N0	No regional lymph node metastasis
N1	Metastasis in a single node, 2 cm or smaller
N2	Metastasis in single node between 2 and 5 cm in size, or in multiple nodes each 5 cm or smaller
N3	Metastasis in a single node larger than 5 cm

Distant Metastasis

M0	No distant metastasis
M1	Distant metastasis (regional nodes, bone, other sites)

Table 12.1 outlines the American Joint Committee on Cancer's TNM staging classification of prostate carcinoma [20]. The American Urological Association staging system, developed by Whitmore and Jewett, assigns alphabetical stages (A through D) to disease extent that corresponds roughly to the primary tumor staging (T1 through T4) of the TNM system [25], which is outlined briefly in Table 12.2. Histologic grading may be by degree of anaplasia, DNA ploidy (diploid, tetraploid, or anaploid), or by Gleason score, which sums the scores of the two most predominant glandular patterns of the tumor to predict aggressivity.

Currently accepted therapies for Stage A, B, and C disease include radical prostatectomy and radiation therapy, including both external beam irradiation and radioisotope implants. Radical prostatectomy is generally reserved for patients with either Stage A or Stage B disease. Stage D disease is treated palliatively with either hormonal or radiation therapies. Clinical assessment and treatment decisions are based on imaging stage, pathological grade, and prostate specific antigen levels, as well as the patient's age and general state of health. Accurate tumor staging is essential for appropriate clinical decision making.

Table 12.2 American Urological Association Staging of Prostate Carcinoma

A	Clinical inapparent
B	Tumor cofined to the prostate
C	Tumor extends beond capsule (may involve seminal vesicles)
D	Metastatic disease to pelvic or distant nodes, bones, soft tissues, or organs

Detection of extracapsular extension precludes radical prostatectomy in the younger patient. A variety of signs have been used to predict Stage C disease by MRI. These include focal contour abnormalities within the prostatic capsule, tumor volume, apical location, broad margins with the prostate capsule, and infiltration of the periprostatic fat [10, 24, 26, 27]. Seminal vesicle invasion is demonstrated by low signal intensity on T2-weighted images (fig. 12.15). Increased staging accuracy can be achieved with the use of T2-weighted endorectal coil MRI and prostate specific antigen values [28–30].

Identifying invasion of the neurovascular bundles can have important clinical implications because preservation of one or both bundles during radical prostatectomy results in a significantly decreased incidence of postoperative impotency. Identification of direct tumor extension posterolaterally into the neurovascular bundles, decreased signal intensity obliterating the rectoprostatic angle, and focal contour abnormalities within the posterolateral aspect of the gland on transverse T2-weighted images have been shown to be valuable in the prediction of neurovascular invasion [31].

Hormonal (fig. 12.18) and radiation therapies (fig. 12.19) may result in low-signal intensity within the prostate. Postbiopsy changes also may mask prostate cancer. High signal intensity in the peripheral zone (fig. 12.20) or seminal vesicles on T1- and T2-weighted images reflects postbiopsy hemorrhage, which can thereby conceal underlying tumor (fig. 12.21). Cryosurgery may result in necrosis and loss of zonal anatomy [26, 32]. Because either recent biopsy or cryosurgery may hinder differentiation from residual carcinoma, MRI should generally be delayed at least 3 weeks after intervention [26].

A variety of tumor may metastasize to the prostate. The appearance of metastases may mimic primary

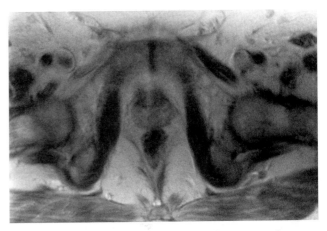

FIG. 12.18 Prostatic cancer after hormone therapy. Transverse ETSE image demonstrates a small globule-shaped heterogeneously dark prostate. This appearance, which includes decrease in prostate size and signal intensity, is typical for hormone therapy.

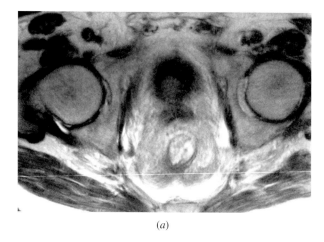

(a)

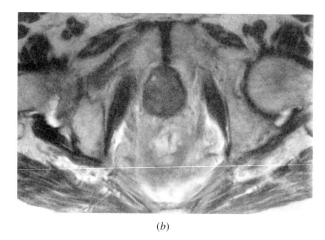

(b)

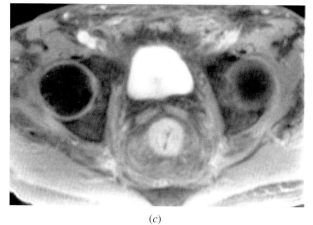

(c)

F I G . 12.19 Postradiation changes. Transverse T2-weighted ETSE (*a*, *b*), 90-s gadolinium-enhanced fat-suppressed SGE (*c*) images. The prostate is enlarged with diffuse low signal intensity of the entire gland. Radiation changes and hormonal therapy result in diffuse low-signal changes, which makes detection of persistent cancer not feasible. Substantial thickening is noted of the rectal wall (*c*) with extensive perirectal stranding (*a*, *c*) consistent with radiation changes.

tumors (fig. 12.22). The history of another primary site of malignancy is usually present.

Diffuse Disease

Prostatic Calcifications. Prostatic calcifications may be either primary or secondary in origin. Primary prostatic calcifications form within the ductal and acinar components of the gland. Acquired calcifications include those arising within the prostatic urethra or secondary to other etiologies, including infection, obstruction, necrosis, and radiation therapy [33].

Calcification appears as a signal-void focus on both T1- and T2-weighted images. Primary prostatic calcifications classically have a curvilinear configuration.

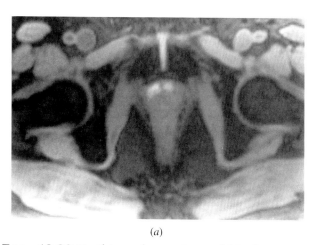

(a)

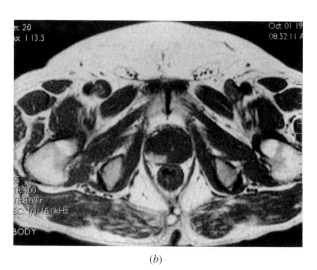

(b)

F I G . 12.20 Postbiopsy hemorrhage within the prostate. Transverse fat-suppressed SGE (*a*) image. There are two high-signal intensity foci in the anterior apex of the gland consistent with postbiopsy hemorrhage.

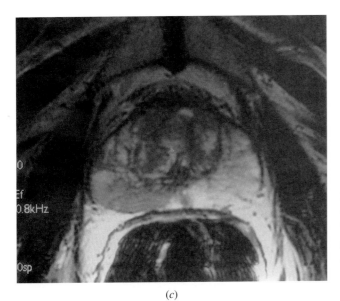

(c)

FIG. 12.20 (*Continued*) T1-weighted spin-echo (*b*) and endorectal coil T2-weighted echo-train spin-echo (*c*) images in a second patient demonstrate biopsy changes in the right aspect of the peripheral zone that appear high signal on T1 and low signal on T2. Biopsy changes may simulate or mask prostate cancer on T2-weighted images. Appreciation of high signal on T1-weighted images identifies the presence of hemorrhage.

Secondary dystrophic calculi are generally larger and more irregular in appearance [8, 13, 33].

Several age-related changes within the prostate are well recognized. The peripheral zone enlarges approximately 67%, and the central gland, which includes both the central and transitional zones, enlarges approximately 175% between the second and eighth decades [34]. Although the zonal anatomy becomes more clearly defined, the periprostatic venous plexus and anterior fibromuscular stroma are less easily distinguished in the older patient [34, 35].

Inflammation and Infection. Inflammatory processes of the prostate may be classified as either bacterial or nonbacterial in origin. Gram-negative organisms are responsible for 90–95% of infectious prostatitis cases. Approximately 80% of these result from infection with *Escherichia coli*, whereas 10–15% are the consequences of *Klebsiella, Serratia, Proteus, Pseudomonas,*

and *Enterobacter* infections. The remaining cases result from infection by Gram-positive organisms, including Enterococcus, Streptococcus, and Staphylococcus [36].

MRI of acute prostatitis frequently reveals an enlarged gland with abnormal signal intensity within the peripheral zone. Low signal intensity on T1-weighted images and higher signal intensity on T2-weighted images are often observed. Areas of inflammation demonstrate diffusely increased signal intensity after intravenous administration of gadolinium. Infiltration of the adjacent periprostatic fat and involvement of the seminal vesicles are frequent associated findings [8]. Chronic prostatitis results in lesser inflammatory changes. Focal low signal intensity within the peripheral zone may result from chronic granulomatous prostatitis, simulating the MRI appearance of prostate carcinoma (fig. 12.23) [37].

Abscesses can result in ill-defined, focal enlargement of the prostate that is appreciable on T1- and T2-weighted images. Abscesses are often very high in signal

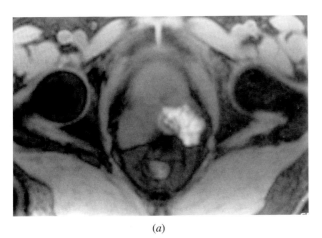

(a)

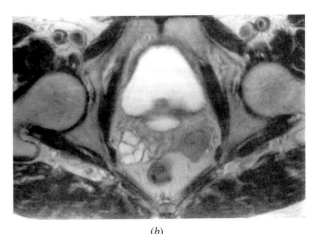

(b)

FIG. 12.21 Prostate cancer with hemorrhage in the left seminal vesicle after biopsy. Fat–suppressed SGE (*a*) and T2-weighted ETSE (*b*) images. Diffuse increased signal intensity in the left seminal vesicle on T1-weighted images (*a*) and diffuse low signal on T2-weighted images (*b*) are consistent with hemorrhage related to biopsy changes.

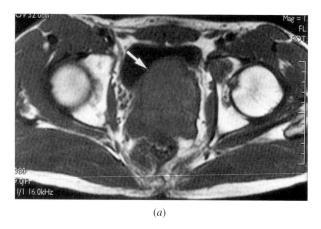

(a)

(b)

(c)

FIG. 12.22 Prostate metastasis. T1-weighted spin-echo (a), T2-weighted echo-train spin-echo (b), and endorectal coil transverse T2-weighted echo-train spin echo (c) images in a patient with colon cancer. A large metastasis is present in the prostate that is isointense on T1 (arrow, a) and heterogeneous and mildly hypointense on T2 (b, c). The left seminal vesicle is also extensively invaded (arrow, c)

intensity on T2-weighted images (fig. 12.24). There are frequently associated inflammatory changes in the periprostatic fat [13]. Enhancement of the abscess wall and inflammatory tissue surrounding a signal-void center is demonstrated on gadolinium-enhanced T1-weighted fat-suppressed images.

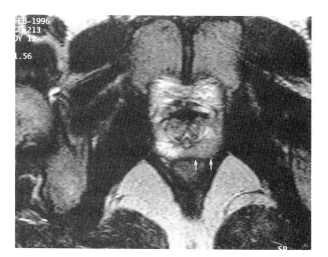

FIG. 12.23 Chronic prostatitis. Transverse T2-weighted ETSE image at the midgland level reveals low signal intensity within the peripheral zone of the prostate (arrows). This entity may mimic the appearance of carcinoma.

Trauma

Posterior urethral trauma may occur in association with crush injuries or extensive pelvic fracturing. There may be complete disruption of the prostatomembranous urethra with resultant erectile dysfunction and stricture formation. Demonstration of superior prostatic displacement on imaging studies is useful because it may alter the surgical approach [38].

Disruption of the posterior urethra is identified by urethral discontinuity and a low-signal intensity band on T2-weighted images. Stricture-associated fibrosis is shown on T1- and T2-weighted images as low-signal intensity tissue. Sagittal T2-weighted images clearly depict displacement and elevation of the prostatic apex above the pubic symphysis, which may necessitate a suprapubic approach or pubectomy [8, 38, 39].

PENIS AND ANTERIOR URETHRA

Normal Anatomy

The anterior urethra is separated into bulbous and penile portions by the suspensory ligament of the penis. It is surrounded by the corpus spongiosum, which in turn is enveloped by a thin layer of the tunica albuginea. These structures comprise the ventral compartment of

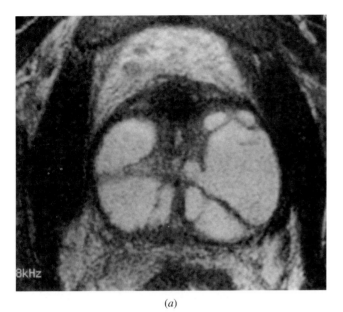

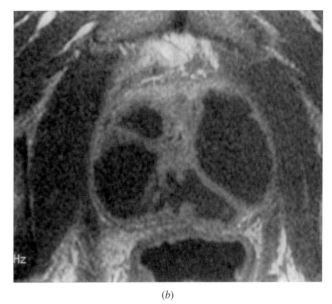

(a)   (b)

F I G . 12.24 Prostate abscess. Endorectal T2-weighted echo-train spin-echo (a) and gadolinium enhanced T1-weighted spin-echo (b) images. The prostate is enlarged and contains multiple fluid-filled spaces with intervening strands of prostate stroma. This appearance is consistent with extensive prostate abscess.

the penis. The dorsal compartment contains the paired corpora cavernosa. The two compartments are separated by Buck fascia, which encases both the thin layer of tunica albuginea surrounding the ventral compartment and a thicker layer surrounding the dorsal compartment [39].

The posterior portion of the corpus spongiosum expands to form the bulb of the penis, which is attached to the urogenital diaphragm. Immediately inferior and lateral to the bulb lies the bulbospongiosus muscle. The posterior aspects of the corpora cavernosa form the crura, which are attached to the ischiopubic ramus and are contiguous with the ischiocavernosus muscles inferomedially [40].

MRI studies should be performed with a circular surface coil or a phased-array multicoil to achieve a good signal-to-noise ratio and spatial resolution. On T1-weighted images both the corpora spongiosa and cavernosa demonstrate homogeneous, medium signal intensity. The corpus spongiosum demonstrates a homogeneous high signal intensity on T2-weighted images, whereas the corpora cavernosa may demonstrate homogeneous or heterogeneous increases in signal intensity, depending on perfusion distribution (fig. 12.25). The bulb of the penis is a useful landmark because of its high signal intensity on T2-weighted images.

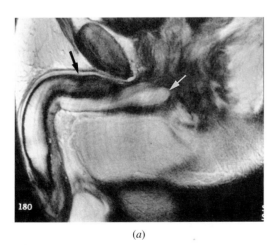

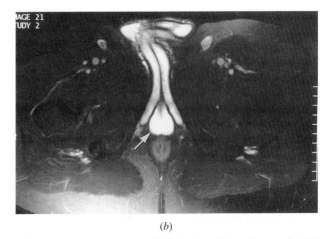

(a)   (b)

F I G . 12.25 Normal penis. Sagittal T2-weighted ETSE image (a). The corpus cavernosum is high in signal intensity on the T2-weighted image (black arrow, a). The high signal intensity of the bulb of the penis is seen posteriorly (white arrow, a).

A T2-weighted fat-suppressed ETSE image (b) in a second patient. The bulb of the penis is well defined as a high-signal intensity structure (white arrow, b).

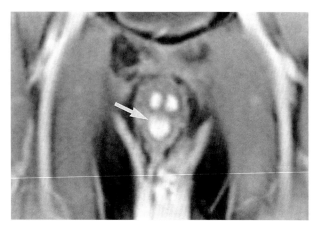

F I G . 12.26 Normal progression of enhancement of the penis. Coronal immediate postgadolinium SGE image. Enhancement of the corpus spongiosum (arrow) and corpora cavernosa commences proximally and centrally, as seen on this immediate postgadolinium image. There is subsequent progression of enhancement outward and distally within the erectile bodies.

The urethra and cavernous arteries are identified as low-signal intensity tubular structures within the centers of the corpus spongiosum and corpora cavernosa, respectively. The fascial layers demonstrate low signal intensity on both T1- and T2 weighted images. Gadolinium administration results in an increased signal intensity of both the corpus spongiosum and corpora cavernosa, enabling improved differentiation from the surrounding muscle and fascial layers (fig. 12.26). Greater delineation of anterior urethral and penile anatomy is achieved with the application of fat saturation techniques.

Disease Entities

Congenital Abnormalities

Epispadias is a rare anomaly characterized by absence of the dorsal covering of the distal urethra and ectopic placement of the proximal urethral aperture, which may be located anywhere along the length of the penis. This entity is almost always associated with bladder exstrophy and accompanying pubic diastasis.

MRI reveals separation of the corpora cavernosa and inversion of their normal relationship with the corpus spongiosum at the level of the pubic symphysis. Hence, the urethra assumes a more cephalad position. The detailed anatomic display provided by MRI enables careful surgical planning.

Hypospadias denotes a proximal, ventral location of the meatus. Perineal hypospadias is frequently associated with a ventral fibrous band, resulting in a chordee deformity. There may be foreshortening of the urethra with either epispadias or hypospadias [41].

In rare instances, partial aplasia of the corpora cavernosa may lead to erectile dysfunction. Patients frequently

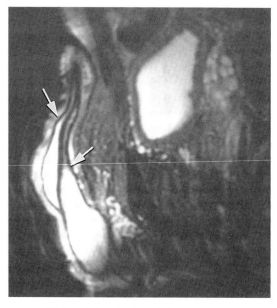

F I G . 12.27 Partial aplasia of the corpora cavernosa and spongiosum. Sagittal T2-weighted ETSE image. The distal aspects of the corpora cavernosa and spongiosa are atrophic and demonstrate a dramatic change in caliber (arrows) in this patient presenting with distal erectile dysfunction. The patient had other concomitant urogenital anomalies.

have other associated anomalies within the genitourinary tract. Irregularity of length and caliber are well shown on T2-weighted images (fig. 12.27). Diphallus is another rare anomaly resulting in partial or complete duplication of the erectile bodies and urethra. Frequently, there is associated shortening of the perineum or asymmetric development of the corpora cavernosa and ischiocavernosus muscles. Again, the detailed anatomic information provided by MRI permits accurate surgical planning. The MRI signal characteristics of the supernumerary corpora are identical to those of normally configured corpora [39, 40].

Mass Lesions

Benign Masses

■ PENILE PROSTHESES

MRI may be helpful in the postoperative evaluation of penile prostheses. These are identified as tubular structures within the central corpora cavernosa. Solid silicone prostheses appear signal void on all imaging sequences. Inflatable prostheses, however, follow the signal characteristics of the fluid they contain (fig. 12.28). Progressive decreased signal intensity on T2-weighted images within the corpora cavernosa may reflect the development of fibrosis. Other complications detected by MRI include infection and hematoma formation [39, 40].

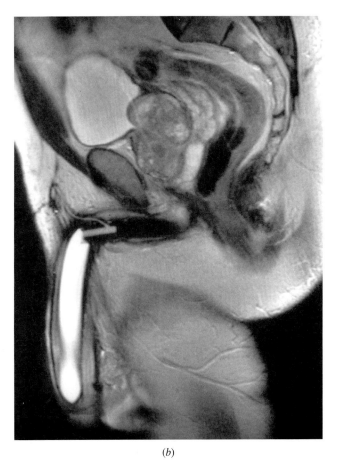

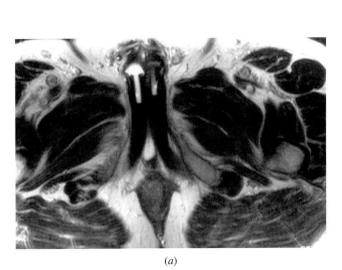

(a)　　　　　　　　　　　　　　　　　　　　(b)

F I G . 12.28 Penile prostheses. Transverse (*a*) and sagittal (*b*) T2-weighted ETSE images. An inflatable penile prostheses is present in the corpora covernosa. On the sagittal image (*b*) the prostate is enlarged, and asymmetrically nodular and protrudes into the base of the bladder.

Malignant Masses

■ PRIMARY TUMORS

Carcinomas of the urethra and penis are extremely rare, accounting for less than 1% of genitourinary cancers in males. Histologic examination reveals squamous cell carcinoma in more than 95% of cases of penile carcinoma. Approximately 78% of urethral carcinomas demonstrate this histology, whereas transitional cell carcinomas constitute approximately 15% of tumors. Adenocarcinomas account for 6% of cases and undifferentiated carcinomas the remainder [40, 42]. Metastatic penile lesions may result from contiguous spread of prostatic, testicular, bladder, and osseous neoplasms as well as from disseminated leukemia and lymphoma [39, 40].

Primary neoplasms of the urethra and penis demonstrate isointense to low signal intensity relative to the surrounding corpus spongiosum on both T1- and T2-weighted images. Metastatic lesions are also of low or intermediate signal intensity on T1-weighted images, but

they may appear hypointense, isointense, or hyperintense relative to the corpus spongiosum on T2-weighted images. Heterogeneous enhancement paralleling the appearance of the remainder of the malignant process is apparent (fig. 12.29). Regardless of the organ of origin, MRI aids in the delineation of the extent of tumor dissemination, enabling detection of invasion into the corpora cavernosa or tunica albuginea.

■ METASTASIS

Metastasis from a variety of primary tumors may involve the penis. Metastases generally have an appearance similar to primary penile tumors when they occur to the penile shaft (fig. 12.30). Direct invasion of pelvic tumors may occur to the corpora cavernosa and spongiosum, and the site of the primary tumor is usually evident.

Diffuse Disease

MRI may be employed to evaluate normal and abnormal flow phenomena within the corpora spongiosum

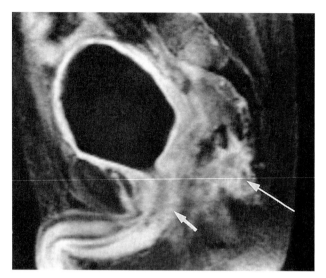

F I G . 12.29 Invasion of prostate and membranous urethra by recurrent rectal carcinoma. Sagittal 90-s post-gadolinium fat-suppressed SGE image. Heterogeneously enhancing recurrent rectal carcinoma is seen in the presacral space (long arrow). There is invasion of the prostate and membranous urethra (short arrow). Note the increased enhancement of the bladder wall secondary to radiation changes.

and cavernosa. Alteration in the normal vascular flow progression, which extends from the central cavernosal arteries outward and distally, may provide evidence for erectile dysfunction. Vascular disorders may result from impairment of the arterial supply, intracorporeal sinusoids, or venous drainage networks [43].

Amyloid may also affect the anterior urethra. Although the majority of cases represent amyloid secondary to other disease states, very rarely primary amyloid of the urethra occurs, which is identified by immunohistochemical stains. The disease may result in stricture formation and calcified plaques within the anterior urethra [44]. Focal low signal intensity on T2-weighted images may reflect amyloid deposition.

Inflammation. Peyronie disease (induratio penis plastica) is caused by focal inflammation of the tunica albuginea and corpora cavernosa. Resultant fibrosis and plaque formation lead to painful, deviated erections. Various etiologies including trauma, diabetes, gout, and hormonal dysfunction have been implicated in the development of the disease. It is most commonly observed in patients between the ages of 30 and 60 years, although occasional cases have been reported in men younger than 20 [45, 46].

On T2-weighted images heterogeneity of the corpora cavernosa may be demonstrated. In addition, low-signal intensity plaques may be visualized within the corpora cavernosa and tunica albuginea on T1- and T2-weighted images [39, 45]. Plaque detection is improved by the administration of gadolinium, with increased enhancement apparent in areas of active inflammation [45].

In rare instances fibrosis may affect Buck fascia. This entity may be observed in cases of early Peyronie disease. Alternatively, it may represent extension of fibrosis resulting from other causes including trauma, sustained priapism, and collagen vascular disease (fig. 12.31).

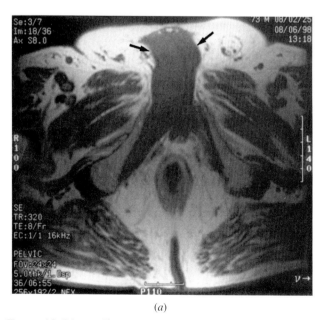

(a)

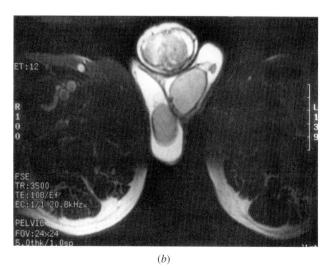

(b)

F I G . 12.30 Penile metastasis. T1-weighted spin-echo (*a*), and transverse (*b*) and sagittal (*c*) surface coil T2-weighted echo-train spin-echo images in a patient with transitional carcinoma of the urinary bladder. Enlargement of the corpora cavernosa (arrow, *a*) with loss of tissue planes by an isointense mass is appreciated on the T1-weighted image.

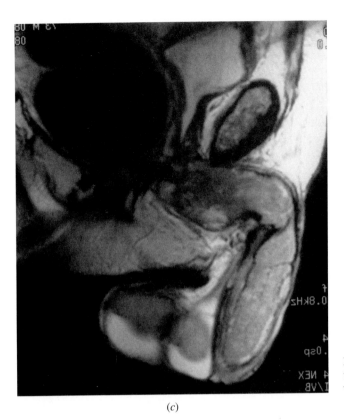

(c)

FIG. 12.30 (*Continued*) On the T2-weighted images (*b, c*), the corpora cavernosa are enlarged and heterogeneous and lack well-defined tissue planes.

Infection. Urethritis may be secondary to infection with *Neisseria gonococcus, Chlamydia trachomatis, Condylomata acuminatum,* or *Mycobacterium tuberculosis.* The periurethral glands of Littre may become distended with bacteria and leukocytes. Spread to adjacent periurethral tissues may lead to abscess formation. Aggressive infections also may result in perineal or scrotal sinus formation [47]. MRI may prove helpful in the detection of these associated complications.

Trauma

Penile trauma usually results from direct, blunt injury. The most common finding is a tear in the tunica albuginea. An adjacent hematoma is frequently visualized. There also may be fracture or avulsion of the corpora cavernosa from their ischial attachments.

MRI demonstrates discontinuity of the normal low-signal intensity ring of the tunica albuginea on

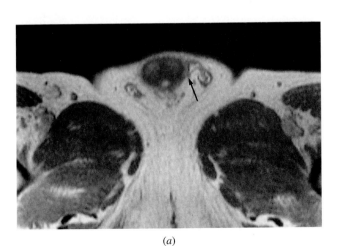

(a)

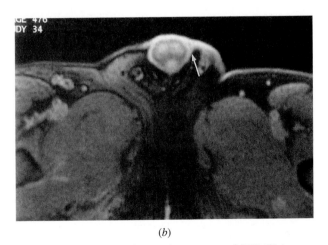

(b)

FIG. 12.31 Fibrosis of Buck fascia. Transverse T1-weighted SGE (*a*) and 90-s postgadolinium fat-suppressed SGE (*b*) images. There is increased thickness of the left aspect of Buck fascia (black arrow, *a*). Note the low-signal intensity linear markings in the adjacent fat (*a*). The thickened fascia enhances diffusely after gadolinium administration (white arrow, *b*). These changes are compatible with early Peyronie disease.

T2-weighted images after a tear. Discontinuity between the corpus cavernosum and ischium also results in focal low signal intensity on T2-weighted images. Signal characteristics of associated hematomas reflect the acuity of the traumatic event [38–40]. MRI has been shown to alter surgical planning in as many as 26% of cases [38].

SEMINAL VESICLES

Normal Anatomy

The seminal vesicles are paired accessory glands located superior to the prostate gland. Each is comprised of a single tube coiled upon itself. It is surrounded by a dense fibromuscular sheet and narrows medially, forming an excretory duct that joins with the vas deferens to form the ejaculatory duct.

Both the width and fluid content of the seminal vesicles increase after puberty, peaking within the fifth and sixth decades. On T1-weighted images the seminal vesicles demonstrate homogeneous signal intensity similar to that of muscle tissue. On T2-weighted images the signal intensity varies with the composition of fluid content. In normal men younger than 60 years of age fluid is abundant, and the seminal vesicles appear as high-signal intensity "cluster of grapes" structures (fig. 12.32). After administration of intravenous gadolinium, the convoluted walls of the vesicles enhance. The walls can be more clearly defined with concomitant application of fat

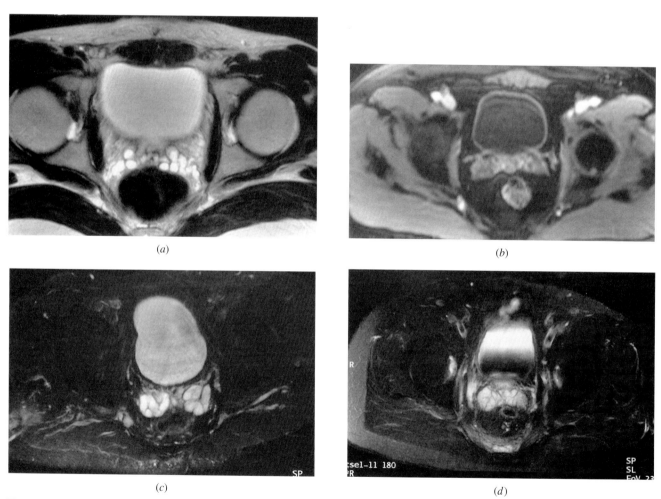

(a)

(b)

(c)

(d)

F I G . 12.32 Normal seminal vesicles. Transverse T2-weighted ETSE (*a*) image. High signal intensity is seen within the normal fluid-filled seminal vesicles on the T2-weighted image (*a*).

Immediate postgadolinium fat-suppressed SGE (*b*) image in a second patient. Note how the fat suppression increases conspicuity of the convoluted walls of the seminal vesicles, which enhance relative to the fluid that they contain (*b*).

Transverse T2-weighted fat-suppressed ETSE (*c*) in a third patient. Normal, fluid-filled seminal vesicles exhibit high signal intensity on T2-weighted images. The low signal intensity of the walls of the tubules gives the glands a cluster of grapes appearance. The external borders are clearly demarcated after the application of fat suppression.

Transverse T2-weighted fat-suppressed ETSE image (*d*) in a fourth patient. The seminal vesicles are high in signal intensity on this high-resolution T2-weighted image. Image acquisition after gadolinium administration accounts for the low signal intensity within the dependent portion of the urinary bladder.

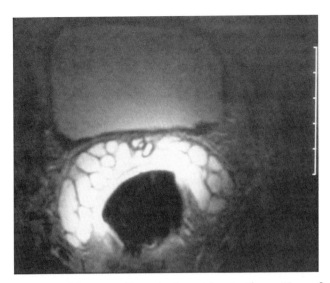

FIG. 12.33 Normal seminal vesicles in the setting of prostate carcinoma. Transverse T2-weighted fat-suppressed ETSE endorectal coil image. Normal, high signal intensity is present within the seminal vesicles in this patient with Stage T2 prostate carcinoma.

saturation techniques. The surrounding walls appear higher in signal intensity than the fluid with these techniques (see fig. 12.32). The high contrast resolution for the appearance of normally uninvolved seminal vesicles is an important feature in the staging of prostate cancer by MRI (fig. 12.33).

Beyond 60 years of age, fluid content decreases and the seminal vesicles may appear progressively lower in signal intensity. In the normal process of aging, low signal intensity is symmetric bilaterally and associated with a decrease in size.

Disease Entities

Congenital Abnormalities

Congenital abnormalities of the seminal vesicles including ectopia, hypoplasia, and agenesis are frequently associated with other anomalies of the genitourinary tract. Detection of congenital seminal vesicle abnormalities therefore warrants evaluation of the remainder of the genitourinary tract. Congenital seminal vesicle cysts are the most commonly encountered abnormalities. Approximately 80% of cases are associated with ipsilateral renal dysgenesis and approximately 8% with collecting system duplication. Seminal vesicle cysts are frequently asymptomatic but may become large enough to cause dysuria, perineal pain, increased frequency, or bladder outlet obstruction [48, 49]. Seminal vesicle cysts are easily differentiated from mullerian or utricular cysts on MRI because of their typical lack of connection to the prostate. They are of variable signal intensity on T1-weighted-images and high in signal intensity on T2-weighted images. Variable signal intensity on T1-

weighted images reflects the presence of hemorrhage or highly proteinaceous material.

Mass Lesions

Benign Masses. Vesicular tumors are rare, and among benign mass lesions leiomyomas are the most common histologic type. They generally appear well circumscribed and are of intermediate signal intensity on T1-weighted images and high signal intensity on T2-weighted images. In rare cases, lipomas, fibromas, cystadenomas, and angiomas may occur in the seminal vesicles.

Malignant Masses. Most malignant disease of the seminal vesicles results from local extension of prostatic, urinary bladder, or rectal carcinomas. Invasion by prostate carcinoma results in loss of normal architecture and decreased signal intensity on T2-weighted images (see figs. 12.5 and 12.15). Primary malignancies are rare and are usually adenocarcinomas. Leiomyosarcomas and fibrosarcomas also have been reported.

Diffuse Disease

Calcifications within the seminal vesicles are most commonly associated with diabetes mellitus. Less often, calcifications may arise secondary to infectious etiologies, which include tuberculosis and schistosomiasis [49]. Calcifications are low in signal intensity on both T1- and T2-weighted images. Abnormally low signal intensity on T2-weighted images also may be seen after prostatic biopsy [50]. This finding, if confused with tumor invasion, may prevent radical prostatectomy in eligible patients. Senile amyloidosis of the seminal vesicles is a common finding at autopsy. Appearing as low signal intensity on T2-weighted images, it also can mimic malignancy (fig. 12.34) [24, 51].

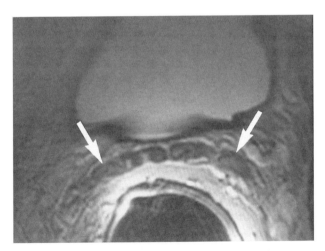

FIG. 12.34 Amyloidosis of the seminal vesicles. Transverse T2-weighted ETSE endorectal coil image. There is bilateral decreased signal intensity of the seminal vesicles secondary to amyloid deposition (arrows).

Infection. Infection of the seminal vesicles is diagnosed primarily on the basis of clinical presentation. Patients usually have associated prostatitis or epididymitis. Rare, isolated infection of the seminal vesicles classically results in hemospermia. Signal characteristics on MR images therefore reflect the presence or absence of blood products. The acutely inflamed gland also may appear enlarged and of lower signal intensity than the contralateral side. Chronic infection may result in fibrosis with concomitant loss of fluid content and a resultant decrease in signal intensity on T1- and T2-weighted images. Abscess formation may manifest as an ill-defined focus of decreased signal intensity on T1-weighted images.

TESTES, EPIDIDYMIS, AND SCROTUM

Normal Anatomy

The testes lie within the scrotum, a sac comprised of internal cremasteric and external fascial layers, dartos muscle, and skin. They are encased by the tunica albuginea, a fibrous capsule that invaginates into the testis posteriorly to form the mediastinum testis. The processus vaginalis represents an extension of peritoneum, projecting between the tunica albuginea and dartos layers. The posterior testis and mediastinum testis are not undermined by the tunica vaginalis, resulting in the bare area through which vascular structures and tubules pass. Approximately 400–600 seminiferous tubules are coiled within each testis. These converge to form the rete testis and, ultimately, the efferent ductules. The efferent ductules form the epididymal head posterior to the testis. They then unify into a single coiled duct representing the epididymal body. The narrowed tail of the epididymis ultimately leads into the vas deferens.

MRI Technique
MRI studies should be performed with a phased-array surface coil or a circular surface coil overlying the testes, which should be elevated above a folded towel placed between the thighs. The testes are clearly demarcated on both T1- and T2-weighted images by the low signal intensity of the surrounding tunica albuginea. The testes are homogeneous and isointense to muscle on T1-weighted images and higher in signal intensity on T2-weighted images. The mediastinum testis can be identified as a low-signal intensity band within the posterior testis on T2-weighted images. Low-signal intensity fibrous projections emanating from the mediastinum testis represent septulae, which divide the testis into lobules. The gubernaculum may be recognized on T2-weighted images as a low-signal intensity curvilinear rim along the inferoposterior aspect of the testis. The signal intensity of the epididymis is slightly heterogeneous and hypo- to isointense to the testis on T1-weighted images. The epididymis is more clearly differentiated from the testis on T2-weighted images because it is lower in signal intensity than the adjacent testis. Gadolinium administration results in hyperintensity of the epididymis relative to the testis [52].

Disease Entities

Congenital Abnormalities
Congenital abnormalities of the testes include unilateral or bilateral hypoplasia and agenesis as well as duplication and cryptorchidism. Congenitally duplicated testes may be classified by their location within the scrotum, inguinal canal, or retroperitoneum. Supernumerary scrotal testes are usually associated with duplication of the vas deferens and epididymis. There may be an associated ipsilateral inguinal hernia. Inguinal testes have duplicated draining systems in the majority of cases and also may have associated inguinal hernias. Retroperitoneal testes, frequently occurring near the deep inguinal ring, are always associated with ipsilateral inguinal hernias. They may or may not demonstrate separate draining structures. Polyorchia is associated with an increased incidence of testicular malignancy [53].

Cryptorchidism. MRI may be employed to localize a clinically suspected undescended testis. The testes normally descend into the scrotum during the eighth month of gestation, accounting for the increased incidence of cryptorchidism in premature births. Approximately 80% of undescended testes are located distal to the external inguinal ring [54]. A significant number of cryptorchid testes will descend spontaneously during an infant's first year of life. Fibrosis and impaired spermatogonia have been observed in undescended testes not surgically corrected by 2 years of age. Hence, as a result of subsequent increased incidences of both infertility and carcinoma, it is recommended that orchiopexy be performed between the first and second years of life [55, 56].

Undescended testes demonstrate low signal intensity on T1-weighted images and intermediate to high signal intensity on T2-weighted images. Low signal intensity on T2-weighted images may be observed in more fibrotic or atrophic testes [12, 56]. Identification of the undescended testis may be aided by identifying the mediastinum testis as a low-signal intensity structure on T2-weighted images and recognizing that undescended testes often have a larger transverse than anteroposterior (AP) diameter (fig. 12.35). In comparison, lymph nodes usually have a larger AP than transverse diameter. The low-signal intensity remnant of the gubernaculum testis on coronal T2-weighted images also serves as a helpful

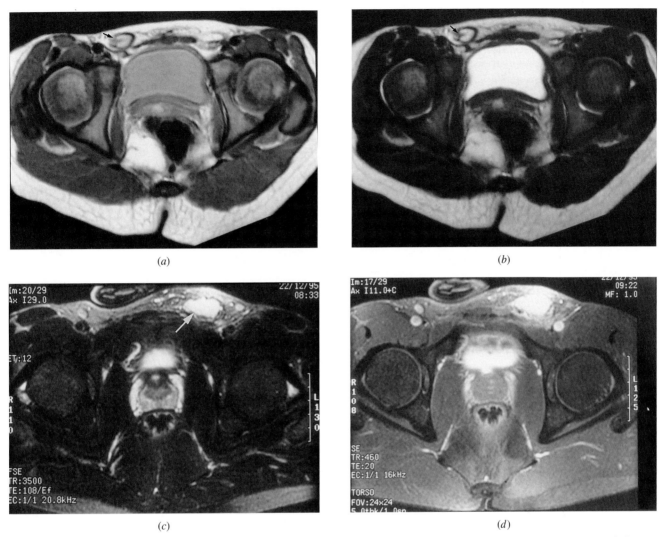

F I G . 12.35 Cryptorchidism. Transverse T1-weighted spin-echo (*a*) and T2-weighted ETSE (*b*) images. The undescended testis within the right inguinal canal is intermediate to high in signal intensity on both T1- and T2-weighted images. The mediastinum testis is shown as a low-signal intensity transverse band (arrow, *a*, *b*).

Transverse T2-weighted fat-suppressed ETSE (*c*) and transverse T1-weighted 3-min postgadolinium fat-suppressed SGE (*d*) images in a second patient. The undescended testis in the left inguinal canal (arrow, *c*) is high in signal intensity on both T2-weighted and postgadolinium T1-weighted images. Note the greater transverse than anteroposterior dimension of the ovoid testis, aiding differentiation from inguinal adenopathy.

landmark because the testis frequently lies along its medial border [56].

Mass Lesions
Benign Masses

■ TESTICULAR PROSTHESES

Testicular prostheses usually contain silicone. The older, fluid-filled silicone prostheses demonstrate low signal intensity on both T1- and T2-weighted images. Newer prostheses are composed of solid elastomers and demonstrate signal characteristics similar to those of na-

tive testes. They are of intermediate signal intensity on T1-weighted images and of high signal intensity on T2-weighted images. They are generally recognized by the presence of chemical-shift artifact and the absence of spermatic cord or other scrotal structures [57].

■ CYSTIC LESIONS

Intratesticular cysts may be solitary or multiple and may occur in up to 10% of the male population. They are characterized by distinct margins and most commonly demonstrate simple fluid signal characteristics [12].

Seminiferous tubular ectasia in the region of the rete testis may produce ovoid lesions in continuity with the edge of the testis. These cystic lesions, which contain spermatozoa, are bilateral in approximately 71% of cases and associated with an ipsilateral spermatocele in approximately 92% of cases. Centered at the mediastinum testis, they are contiguous with the adjacent spermatocele along the bare area of the testis. Seminiferous tubular ectasia is lower in signal intensity than the normal surrounding testis on T1-weighted images and nearly isointense to the surrounding testis on T2-weighted images. It has been postulated that pure intratesticular cysts originate from progressive seminiferous tubular ectasia [58]. Occasionally, cysts also may be localized to the tunica albuginea [52].

Epididymal cysts can occur along the length of the epididymis. They contain simple fluid and are low in signal intensity on T1-weighted images and high in signal intensity on T2-weighted images [12]. Spermatoceles, small cystic structures that occur most commonly in the epididymal head, may be either solitary or multiloculated. They demonstrate variable signal intensity, depending on the presence of spermatozoa, fat, lymphocytes, and cellular debris (fig. 12.36) [12, 59].

BENIGN NEOPLASMS

Only 5% of testicular neoplasms are benign. Of these, 90% are non-germ cell tumors. They may arise from Leydig cells, Sertoli cells, or connective tissue stroma [59].

The most common extratesticular neoplasm is the adenomatoid tumor. It most commonly arises in the epididymis but may be located in the spermatic cord or

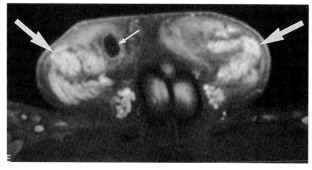

FIG. 12.36 Spermatocele and bilateral varicoceles. Transverse gadolinium-enhanced T1-weighted fat-suppressed spin-echo image demonstrates a nonenhancing ovoid structure within the right epididymal head consistent with a spermatocele (small arrow). There are also bilateral enhancing varicoceles (large arrows).

tunica. Adenomatoid tumor may be round and well defined (fig. 12.37) or occasionally, plaquelike and less well defined [60, 61]. Lipomas also may arise within the spermatic cord. They demonstrate high signal intensity on T1-weighted images and follow the signal intensity of other adipose tissues on T2-weighted images [62]. As with other fatty lesions, loss of signal intensity on fat-suppressed images is a diagnostic finding.

The paratesticular tissues also may harbor benign, fibroproliferative tumors classified as fibrous pseudotumors. They are the second most common extratesticular neoplasm after adenomatoid tumors. They may originate from the tunica albuginea or vaginalis, spermatic cord, or epididymis [63], and their etiology is uncertain [64, 65].

Patients most commonly present with painless masses. Slightly less than one-half of fibrous

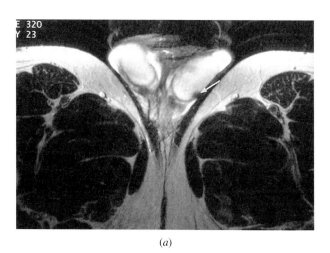

(a)

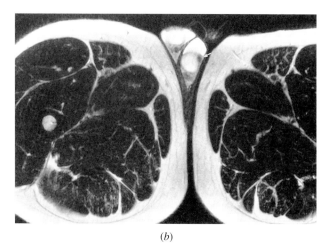

(b)

FIG. 12.37 Adenomatoid neoplasm. Transverse phased-array body coil T2-weighted ETSE (*a*), transverse circular surface coil T2-weighted ETSE (*b*), transverse phased-array body coil T1-weighted immediate postgadolinium fat-suppressed SGE (*c*), and coronal phased-array coil T1-weighted immediate post-gadolinium fat-suppressed SGE (*d*) images. The tumor is hypointense relative to the normal surrounding testis on T2-weighted imaging (arrow, *a*, *b*). After the administration of gadolinium, there is immediate increased enhancement of the tumor relative to the surrounding testis (arrow, *c*, *d*).

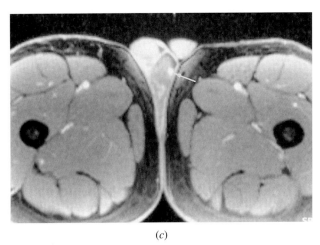

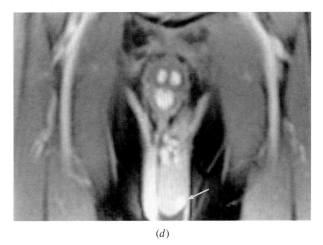

(c)

(d)

F I G . 12.37 (*Continued*) Note that the higher signal-to-noise ratio of the circular surface coil permits higher spatial resolution imaging (*b*) compared with the phased-array body coil (*a*). This is useful for imaging superficial structures such as the testicles.

pseudotumors are associated with hydroceles or hematoceles [63]. These masses are frequently lobulated, demonstrating frondlike projections, but they also may be characterized by circumferential thickening of the tunica albuginea. They are low in signal intensity on both T1- and T2-weighted images and enhance negligibly with gadolinium [62, 63].

■ OTHER BENIGN SCROTAL LESIONS

Fluid may accumulate between the parietal and visceral layers of the tunica vaginalis, producing hydroceles, pyoceles, or hematoceles. Hydroceles may occur in association with infection, tumor, or trauma. They demonstrate

signal characteristics typical of simple fluid and are low in signal intensity on T1-weighted images, high in signal intensity on T2-weighted images, and nearly signal void on postgadolinium images (fig. 12.38). Pyoceles may appear complicated with heterogeneous low signal intensity on T1-weighted images and heterogeneous high signal intensity on T2-weighted images. Hematoceles may exhibit varied signal characteristics, depending on the chronicity of the blood products they contain.

Varicoceles may occur as the result of thrombosis or extrinsic compression of the testicular venous system by organomegaly or retroperitoneal masses. They are more commonly left-sided as a result of testicular vein drainage into the left renal vein, which is lengthier and more prone to compression than the right testicular vein. MRI reveals multiple serpiginous structures in the region of the pampiniform plexus, epididymal head, and spermatic cord. Signal intensity is dependent on

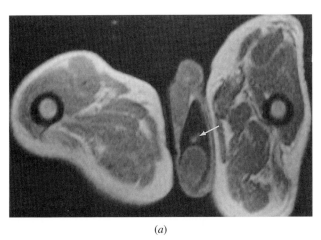

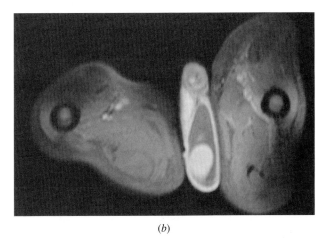

(a)

(b)

F I G . 12.38 Hydrocele. Transverse T1-weighted SGE (*a*) and transverse 1-min postgadolinium T1-weighted fat-suppressed SGE (*b*) images. A left-sided hydrocele is low in signal intensity on the T1-weighted image (*a*). A focus of high signal intensity within the fluid represents the spermatic cord (arrow, *a*). There is uniform enhancement of the testes on the postgadolinium image (*b*).

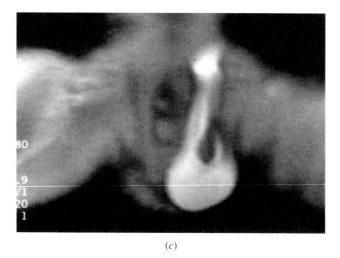

(c)

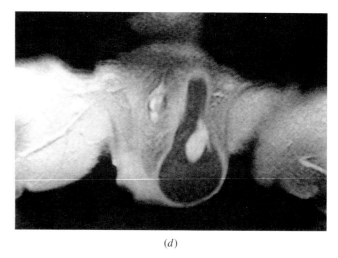

(d)

(e)

FIG. 12.38 (*Continued*) Coronal SS-ETSE (*c*) and SGE fat-suppressed (*d*) postgadolinium images in a second patient, a neonate, demonstrates a large left hydrocele. The testicle is low signal on T2 (*c*) but enhances moderately intensity on the postgadolinium image (*d*).

Surface coil T2-weighted echo-train spin-echo (*e*) in a third patient demonstrates a moderate-sized hydrocele.

flow velocity. Varicoceles often appear intermediate in signal intensity on T1-weighted images and higher in signal intensity on T2-weighted images [12, 59, 62]. On early postgadolinium gradient-echo images varicoceles are well shown as high-signal intensity tubular structures (fig. 12.39). Varicoceles often exist with hydroceles (fig. 12.39).

Scrotal hernias are most frequently diagnosed by clinical inspection. MRI evaluation may prove helpful in equivocal cases, particularly when there is marked associated pain or when physical examination is limited.

The MRI appearance of the hernia may vary with its contents. A complex mass is frequently visualized within an enlarged inguinal canal. Mesenteric fat, loops of bowel, and intraluminal air may be visualized within the scrotal sac. Imaging with single-shot echo-train spin-echo (SS-ETSE) and immediate postgadolinium fat-suppressed spoiled gradient-echo (SGE) sequence may provide helpful information regarding entrapped bowel viability.

Malignant Masses. Although testicular carcinomas comprise less than 1% of tumors in the male population, a significant number of these occur in males under the age of 40 years and approximately 95% are malignant [66, 67]. Early detection and treatment are crucial, particularly for seminomas, which are chemotherapy and radiotherapy sensitive.

Testicular carcinomas may be divided into germ cell and non-germ cell subtypes. Approximately 95% of malignant neoplasms are of germ cell origin [68]. These include seminomas (~40%) and nonseminomatous tumors. Nonseminomatous tumors may be subclassified into embryonal carcinomas (~30%), teratocarcinomas (~25%), teratoma (10%), and choriocarcinomas (1%). Another 30% of the cases are of mixed histology [69]. The remainder are comprised of Sertoli, Leydig, or mesenchymal cell carcinomas. There may also be involvement by leukemia, lymphoma, or in rare instances, metastatic disease from lung, melanoma, genitourinary, or gastrointestinal malignancies [59, 68].

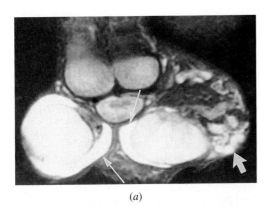

(a)

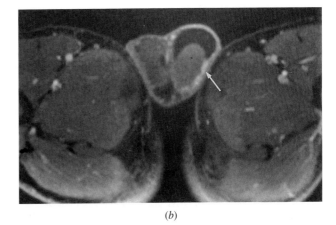

(b)

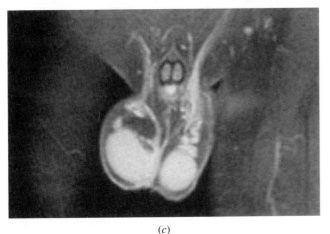

(c)

FIG. 12.39 Varicocele with bilateral hydroceles. Coronal T2-weighted ETSE image (a) demonstrates high-signal intensity serpiginous structures within the left scrotal sac representing a varicocele (thick arrow, a). There are also bilateral hydroceles (thin arrows, a).

Transverse 90-s postgadolinium fat-suppressed SGE image (b) in a second patient with a varicocele and bilateral hydroceles. High-signal intensity tubular structures represents a varicocele (arrow, b).

Coronal 3-min postgadolinium SGE (c) image in a third patient with varicocele and bilateral hydroceles with an appearance similar to the prior case.

Lymphatic drainage of the testes follows the gonadal vessels to the retroperitoneum. In the presence of epididymis or spermatic cord invasion, lymphatic drainage also extends to the pelvic nodes. Tumors are staged according to TNM criteria as outlined in Table 12.3 [70].

MRI of testicular neoplasms may reveal relative enlargement of the involved testis. Tumors are low in signal intensity on T2-weighted images, and there is degradation of normal testicular morphology. Lack of visualization of the normal septulae has been found to be a sensitive indicator of malignant infiltration [62].

Seminomas are isointense to normal tissue on T1-weighted images and hypointense to normal testicular tissue on T2-weighted images. They most commonly demonstrate homogeneous low signal intensity on T2-weighted images (fig. 12.40) [54, 62]. They may exhibit lobulation or, occasionally, central necrosis [62, 67]. Tumors enhance to a lesser degree than normal testicular tissue. Thus gadolinium administration may increase lesion conspicuity and aid detection of extension into the surrounding tunica albuginea [52, 62]. Nonseminomatous tumors appear more heterogeneous on T2-weighted images and have more ill-defined margins

Table 12.3 American Joint Committee on Cancer Staging of Testicular Carcinoma

Carcinoma

Primary Tumor	
T0	No evidence of primary tumor
T1	Tumor limited to testis, including rete testis
T2	Tumor extends beyond tunica albuginea or into epididymis
T3	Tumor invades spermatic cord
T4	Tumor invades scrotum

Lymph Nodes	
N0	No lymph node metastasis
N1	Metastasis to a single lymph node 2 cm or smaller
N2	Metastasis to a single lymph node between 2 and 5 cm in size, or to multiple nodes each 5 cm or smaller
N3	Metastasis to a single lymph node larger than 5 cm

Distant Metastases	
M0	No distant metastases
M1	Distant metastases

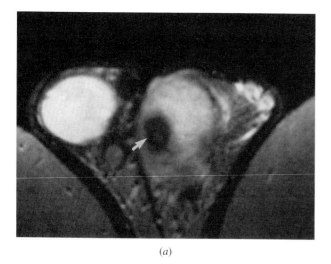

(a)

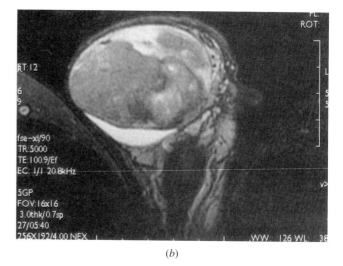

(b)

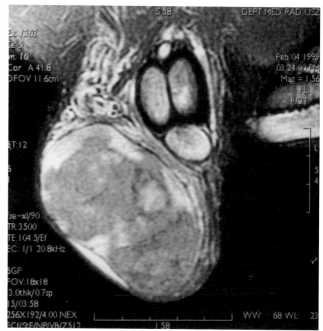

(c)

FIG. 12.40 Testicular seminoma. T2-weighted fat-suppressed ETSE (a) image using a surface coil demonstrates a well-defined, homogeneously low signal intensity 1-cm seminoma (arrow) arising in the left testicle. (Courtesy of Evan S. Siegelman, M.D., Hospital of the University of Pennsylvania).

Surface coil transverse (b) and coronal (c) T2-weighted echo-train spin-echo images demonstrate a heterogeneous low-signal intensity mass that exhibits extensive infiltration of the testicle. Remnants of uninvolved testicle appear high signal.

(fig. 12.41). Areas of increased and decreased signal intensity on T1- and T2-weighted images correspond to foci of hemorrhage and necrosis, respectively, on histologic specimens [54, 67]. These features are most marked within tumors demonstrating mixed histologies [62, 67]. Lymph nodes have a characteristic multicystic appearance.

Lymphoma may also involve the testicles. Lymphoma is typically more homogeneous than other neoplasms (fig. 12.42). Associated adenopathy is also present and is similarly homogeneous, as observed in lymphoma in general. This is different than the appearance of nonseminomatous tumors that have a more multicystic appearance.

Testicular Torsion

Acute testicular torsion arises when the bare area is not sufficiently broad to anchor the testis and its supporting structures in place, resulting in a "bell clapper" deformity. It results in irreversible ischemia in less than 30% of cases if diagnosis and surgical correction occur within 12 h of the event. The salvage rate decreases rapidly thereafter, with minimal surgical success after 24 h of ischemia [71]. Ultrasound and nuclear medicine examinations enable timely diagnosis in the acute setting. However, bilateral orchiopexy is still indicated in the subacute period, when findings may be equivocal with either of these modalities. In the setting of subacute torsion, MRI

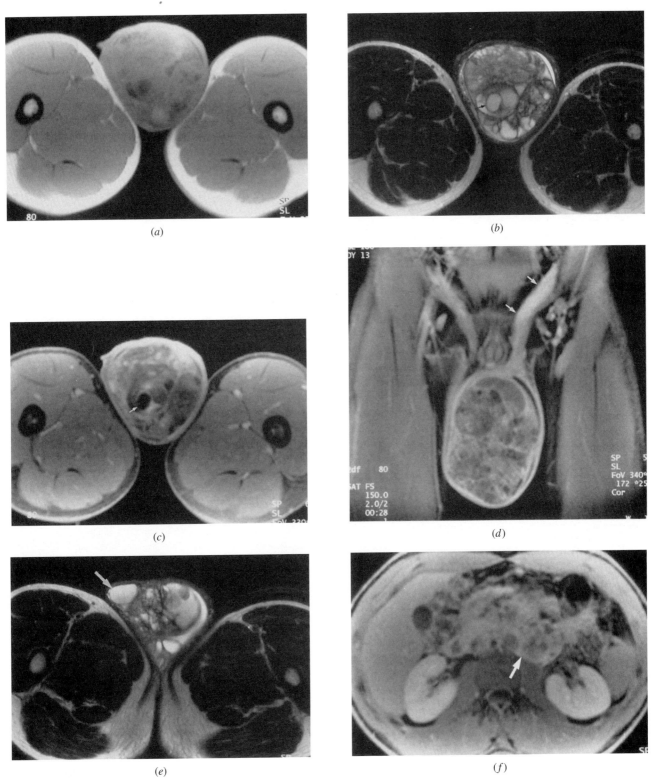

F I G . 12.41 Nonseminomatous testicular neoplasm. SGE (*a*), T2-weighted ETSE (*b*), 45-s transverse (*c*), and 90-s coronal (*d*) gadolinium-enhanced fat-suppressed SGE images. The left testicle is greatly enlarged, measuring 5 cm in diameter. Tumor replaces the testicle and is mildly heterogeneous on the T1-weighted image (*a*) and considerably heterogeneous on the T2-weighted image (*b*). The tumor contains multiple cystic spaces that are well-defined, high-signal intensity foci (arrow, *b*) on the T2-weighted image and show lack of enhancement on the postgadolinium images (arrow, *c*).

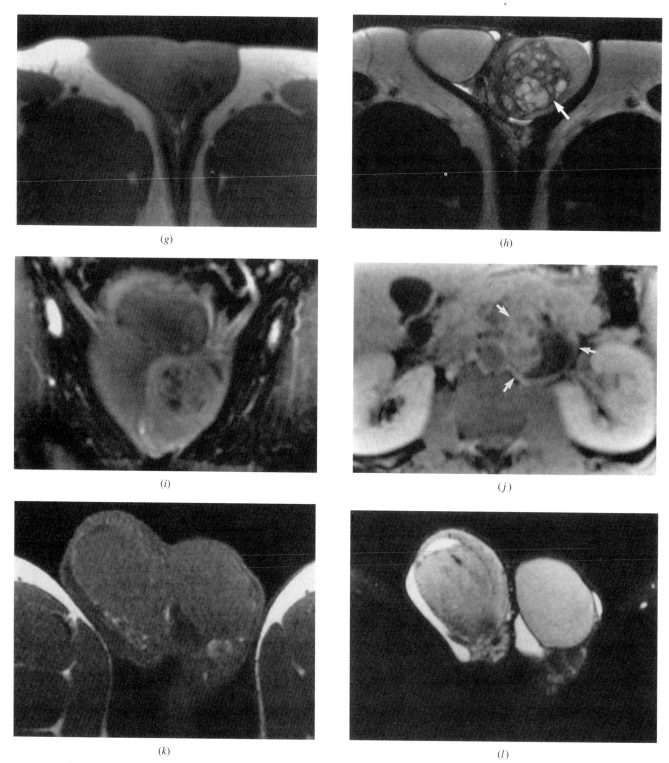

(g)

(h)

(i)

(j)

(k)

(l)

F IG . 12.41 (*Continued*) The coronal image demonstrates the vertical size of the tumor and enlargement of testicular vessels in the left inguinal canal (arrows, *d*). T2-weighted echo-train spin-echo image (*e*) from a more superior tomographic section through the scrotum demonstrates a normal high-signal intensity right testicle (arrow, *e*). On a 3-min postgadolinium fat-suppressed SGE image (*f*), a 3-cm left para-aortic lymph node (arrow, *f*) is present at the level of the left renal hilum that demonstrates a similar heterogeneous appearance to the primary tumor.

SGE (*g*), T2-weighted ETSE (*h*), and coronal interstitial phase gadolinium enhanced fat-suppressed SGE (*i*) images in a second patient. A 2.5-cm tumor is present in the left testicle (arrow, *h*). The appearance is similar to the prior case. Note in particular the well-defined high-signal intensity foci within the mass on the T2-weighted image (*h*). Heterogeneous appearance of the involved left para-aortic lymph nodes on the interstitial phase gadolinium-enhanced fat-suppressed SGE (arrows, *j*) is also comparable.

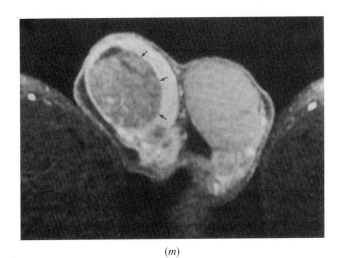

(*m*)

Fig. 12.41 (*Continued*) T1-weighted spin-echo (*k*), T2-weighted ETSE (*l*), and gadolinium-enhanced T1-weighted spin-echo (*m*) images in a third patient. The tumor in this patient is mixed embryonal carcinoma/seminoma. The tumor has a relatively homogeneous and mildly low signal intensity on the T2-weighted image (*l*). Tumor enhancement is slightly heterogeneous on post-gadolinium images (*m*) and has a relatively sharp margination (arrows, *m*) from background testicle.

may provide assistance in differentiating this entity from epididymo-orchitis.

Common findings on MRI in the subacute setting include an enlarged spermatic cord with diminished flow, diffusely decreased signal intensity of the testis, decreased testicular size, and mild to moderate thickening of the tunica albuginea and epididymis [71]. There also may be increased signal-intensity foci on T1-weighted images, reflecting hemorrhage, visualization of the pedicular attachment of the testicle in a bell-clapper deformity, or an associated hematocele. The identification of a whirling pattern within the spermatic cord and an associated low-signal intensity knot at the point of maximal torsion on T2-weighted images provides specific evidence for the diagnosis [62, 71]. Initial studies with P-31 MR spectroscopy in an animal model have revealed additional promise for the evaluation of testicular torsion in the acute setting [72].

Infection

The vast majority of acute epididymitis cases are isolated, but up to 20% may be associated with orchitis [59]. Therapy is conservative and limited to antibiotics unless there is concomitant infarction from extensive edema or abscess formation necessitating surgery [71]. With the exception of mumps orchitis, isolated acute infection of the testes is rare [36]. When pyogenic abscesses occur, they are frequently accompanied by pyoceles [59, 71].

On MRI, epididymal inflammation is most commonly manifested by generalized enlargement of the organ [52, 62]. The involved epididymis may be hyperintense on T1-weighted images and of variable signal intensity relative to the contralateral side on T2-weighted images [52, 59, 62]. There is heterogeneous enhancement after gadolinium administration [52]. Testicular inflammation also is commonly manifested by generalized

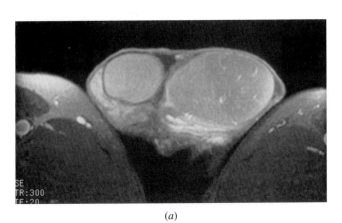

(*a*)

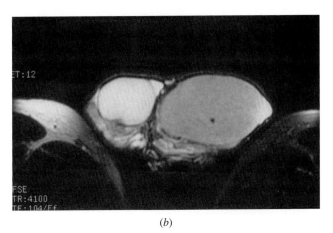

(*b*)

Fig. 12.42 Testicular lymphoma. T1-weighted SE (*a*) and T2-weighted echo-train spin-echo (*b*) images. The left testicle is enlarged and exhibits diffuse infiltration with homogeneous tumor that is isointense on T1 and mildly hypointense on T2. Lymphoma is typically more homogeneous in appearance than other neoplasms.

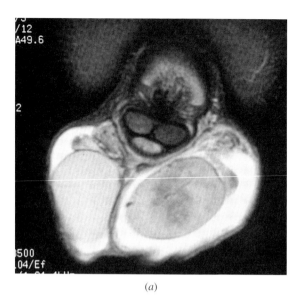

(a)

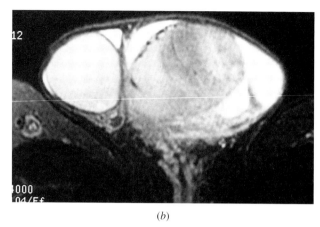

(b)

FIG. 12.43 Mumps orchitis. Coronal T2-weighted fat-suppressed echo-train spin-echo (a), transverse T2-weighted fat-suppressed ETSE (b), and T1-weighted postgadolinium fat-suppressed spin-echo (c) images. There is enlargement of the left testis relative to the contralateral side (b, c). The affected testis is heterogeneous and low in signal intensity on the T2-weighted images (a, b) and enhances slightly more than unaffected testis on the postgadolinium image (c). Note the enhancing, thickened septations within the scrotal sac (arrow, c). There are accompanying hydroceles, bilaterally.

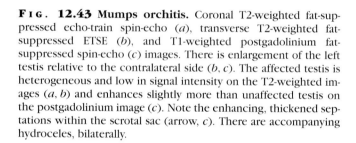

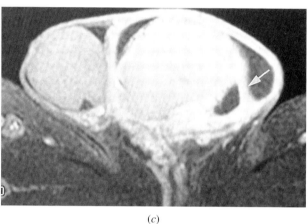

(c)

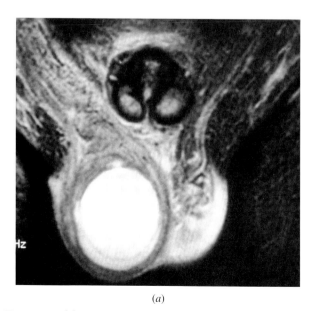

(a)

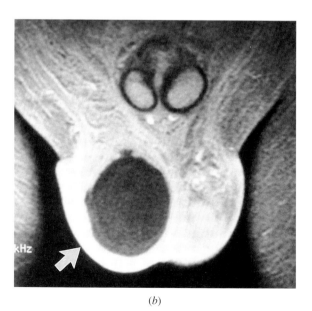

(b)

FIG. 12.44 Testicular abscess. Coronal T2-weighted ETSE (a) and gadolinium-enhanced T1-weighted spin-echo (b) images. A complex fluid collecion within the right testis is heterogeneously high in signal intensity on the T2-weighted image (a) and heterogeneously low in signal intensity on the post-gadolinium T1-weighted image, which is consistent with an abscess. There is extensive enhancement of the surrounding scrotal tissues secondary to adjacent inflammatory changes (arrow, b).

enlargement (fig. 12.39) [12, 52, 71]. There is frequently decreased signal intensity of the involved testis on T2-weighted images [52, 59, 62]. The testicular septulae remain well defined but thickened, a finding that is in contrast to the loss of normal architecture frequently observed with invasive neoplastic disease [62]. Intense enhancement of the involved testis is seen after gadolinium administration [52]. Abscesses are accompanied by pyoceles in the majority of patients [71]. Heterogeneous high signal intensity on T2-weighted images is observed both in these extratesticular fluid collections and in the infected fluid intercalating between the testicular septulae (fig. 12.44) [62].

Acute inflammation often results in enlargement and edema of the spermatic cord [52, 71]. However, in contrast to the avascularity of the cord observed in cases of torsion, there is increased vascularity of the cord in the setting of infection. On gadolinium-enhanced images, there is marked enhancement of the inflamed structure and surrounding tissues [52]. These findings serve as helpful differentiating factors in equivocal cases. Identification of the bare area of the testis also virtually excludes the possibility of a bell clapper deformity, and thus of torsion as well [71].

Trauma

MRI may provide information important for clinical management after testicular trauma. Hemorrhage is well demonstrated on T1- and T2-weighted images. Intratesticular hematomas may appear high in signal intensity on T1-weighted images and variable in signal intensity on T2-weighted images [52, 62]. They may also result in alternating bands of increased and decreased signal intensity on T1-weighted images [62]. Blood intersecting between the layers of the tunica vaginalis may result in hematoceles, which also follow the signal intensity of blood products.

Contusion in the absence of focal hemorrhage may also be detected by MRI. There is a resultant decrease in signal intensity of the involved testis on T2-weighted images as well as a relative decrease in gadolinium enhancement [52].

Careful inspection of the tunica albuginea is necessary to evaluate for the possibility of acute testicular rupture. This may be manifested by discontinuity in the normal low signal intensity of the tunica albuginea on T2-weighted images. Detection of testicular rupture often necessitates surgical intervention [62].

SPECTROSCOPY

The high signal-to-noise ratio, high spatial resolution, and lack of difficulty with localization achievable with endorectal coils for prostate disease and surface coils for

testicular disease have resulted in clinical applicability of spectroscopy for distinguishing prostate cancer from fibrosis and testicular cancer from other disease entities [72–74].

Magnetic resonance spectroscopy (MRS) may prove a particularly useful adjunct to the MR evaluation of prostate cancer. The addition of a spectroscopy sequence to routine MR evaluation of the prostate can provide direct correlation between morphologic and biochemical alterations. It may be possible to differentiate among normal tissue, BPH, postbiopsy hemorrhage and carcinoma [75]. Recent studies have revealed increased levels of choline, creatinine, *myo*-inositol, and mobile lipids relative to that of citrate in the prostate cancer patient [76–78]. An increase in overall accuracy and specificity has been reported in the detection of tumor within the postbiopsy prostate [79]. MRS also may prove helpful in the evaluation of recurrent disease, as well as the far lateral peripheral zone and prostatic apex, which are less amenable to traditional biopsy [80–81].

The emergency of managed care and fiscal constraint has led to the search for comprehensive imaging evaluation of the oncology patient with a single modality. In addition to the promise of a combined approach, employing contrast MRI and MRS, a survey examination for osseous metastatic disease may be merited for patients at higher risk. These examinations could include a limited number of sequences for the assessment of those anatomic areas most likely to harbor metastases, the spine, pelvis, and femurs [82]. The most consistent results for the detection of bone marrow metastases is gadolinium-enhanced fat-suppressed SGE.

CONCLUSIONS

MRI is an effective modality for detecting the full range of disease entities involving the male pelvis because of high intrinsic soft tissue contrast resolution, high spatial resolution, and multiplanar imaging. Although MRI is excellent at evaluating testicular disease, the lower cost and acceptable accuracy of other imaging approaches has relegated MRI to a problem-solving modality. The greatest role for MRI has been in the staging of prostate cancer. The variety of diagnostic options and uncertainty in patient outcome after therapeutic intervention has limited the widespread use of MRI in this setting. Continued refinement of MR spectroscopy techniques may ultimately permit comprehensive imaging evaluation of the cancer patient.

REFERENCES

1. Mirowitz SA, Heiken JP, Brown JJ: Evaluation of fat saturation technique for T2-weighted endorectal coil MRI of the prostate. *Magn Reson Imaging* 12: 743–747, 1994.

2. Nunes LW, Scheibler MS, Rauschning W, Schnall MD, Tomaszewski JE, Pollack H, Kressel H: The normal prostate and periprostatic structures: Correlation between MR images made with an endorectal coil and cadaveric microtome sections. *Am J Roentgenol* 164: 923–927, 1995.

3. Hricak H, White S, Vigneron D, et al.: Carcinoma of the prostate gland: MR imaging with pelvic phased-array coils versus integrated endorectal-pelvic phased-array coils. *Radiology* 193: 703–709, 1994.

4. McDermott VG, Meakem III TJ, Stolpen AH, Schnall MD: Prostatic and periprostatic cysts: Findings on MR imaging. *Am J Roentgenol* 164: 123–127, 1995.

5. Nghiem HT, Kellman GM, Sandberg SA, Craig BM: Cystic lesions of the prostate. *Radiographics* 10: 635–650, 1990.

6. Thurnher S, Hricak H, Tanagho EA: Mullerian duct cyst: Diagnosis with MR imaging. *Radiology* 168: 25–28, 1988.

7. Gevenois PA, Van Sinoy ML, Sintzoff SA Jr, Stallenberg B, Salmon I, Regemorter GV, Struyven J: Cysts of the prostate and seminal vesicles: MR findings in 11 cases. *Am J Roentgenol* 155: 1021–1024, 1990.

8. Hricak H: The prostate gland. In Hricak H, Carrington BM (eds.), *MRI of the Pelvis*. Norwalk, CT: Appleton & Lange, p. 249–312, 1991.

9. Keetch DW, Andriole GL: Medical therapy for benign prostatic hyperplasia. *Am J Roentgenol* 164: 11–15, 1995.

10. Kahn T, Burrig K, Schmitz-Drager B, Lewin JS, Furst G, Modder U: Prostatic carcinoma and benign prostatic hyperplasia: MR imaging with histopathologic correlation. *Radiology* 173: 847–851, 1989.

11. Schiebler ML, Tomaszewski JE, Bezzi M, Pollack HM, Kressel HY, Cohen EK, Altman HG: Prostatic carcinoma and benign prostatic hyperplasia: Correlation of high resolution MR and histopathologic findings. *Radiology* 172: 131–137, 1989.

12. Fritzsche PJ, Wilbur MJ: The male pelvis. *Semin Ultrasound CT MR* 10: 11–28, 1989.

13. Chang Y, Hricak H: Magnetic resonance imaging of the prostate gland. *Semin Ultrasound CT MR* 9: 343–351, 1988.

14. Way WG, Brown JJ, Lee JKT, Gutierrez E, Andriole GL: MR imaging of benign prostatic hypertrophy using a Helmholtz-type surface coil. *Magn Reson Imaging* 10: 341–349, 1992.

15. Lovett K, Rifkin MD, McCue PA, Choi H: MR imaging characteristics of noncancerous lesions of the prostate. *J Magn Reson Imaging* 2: 35–39, 1992.

16. Sommer FG, Nghiem HV, Herfkens R, McNeal J: Gadolinium-enhanced MRI of the abnormal prostate. *Magn Reson Imaging* 11: 941–948, 1993.

17. Phillips M, Kressel H, Spritzer C, et al.: Prostatic disorders: MR imaging at 1.5 T. *Radiology* 164: 386–392, 1987.

18. Hricak H, Thoeni R: Neoplasms of the prostate gland. In Pollack H (ed.), *Clinical Urography*. Philadelphia: WB Saunders, p. 1382–1383, 1990.

19. Hricak H: Imaging prostatic carcinoma. *Radiology* 169: 569–571, 1988.

20. American Joint Committee on Cancer: Prostate. In *Manual for Staging Cancer* (4th ed.). Philadelphia: Lippincott, p. 181–183, 1992.

21. Schnall M, Imai Y, Tomaszewski J, Pollack H, Lenkinski R, Kressel H: Prostate cancer: Local staging with endorectal surface coil MR imaging. *Radiology* 178: 797–802, 1991.

22. Carter H, Brem R, Tempany C, Yang A, Epstein J, Walsh P, Zerhouni E: Nonpalpable prostate cancer: Detection with MR imaging. *Radiology* 178: 523–525, 1991.

23. Outwater E, Schiebler M, Tomaszewski J, Schnall M, Kressell H: Mucinous carcinomas involving the prostate: Atypical findings at MRI. *J Magn Reson Imaging* 2: 597–600, 1992.

24. Schiebler M, Schnall M, Pollack H, Lenkinski R, Tomaszewski J, Wein A, Whittington R: Current role of MR imaging in the staging of adenocarcinoma of the prostate. *Radiology* 189: 339–352, 1993.

25. Steinfeld A: Questions regarding the treatment of localized prostate cancer. *Radiology* 184: 593–598, 1992.

26. Quinn S, Franzini D, Demlow T, Rosencrantz D, Kim J, Hanna R, Szumowski J: MR imaging of prostate cancer with an endorectal surface coil technique: Correlation with whole mount specimens. *Radiology* 190: 323–327, 1994.

27. Harris R, Schned A, Heaney J: Staging of prostate cancer with endorectal MR imaging: Lessons from a learning curve. *Radiographics* 15: 813–829, 1995.

28. Huch Boni R, Boner J, Debatin J, Trinkler F, Knonagel H, Von Hochstetter A, Helfenstein U, Krestin G: Optimization of prostate carcinoma staging: Comparison of imaging and clinical methods. *Clin Radiol* 50: 593–600, 1995.

29. Huch Boni R, Boner J, Lutolf U, Trinkler F, Pestalozzi D, Krestin G: Contrast-enhanced endorectal coil MRI in local staging of prostate carcinoma. *J Comput Assist Tomogr* 19(2): 232–237, 1995.

30. Huch Boni R, Meyenberger C, Pok Lundquist J, Trinkler F, Lutolf U, Krestin G: Value of endorectal coil versus body coil MRI for diagnosis of recurrent pelvic malignancies. *Abdom Imaging* 21: 345–352, 1996.

31. Tempany C, Rahmouni A, Epstein J, Walsh P, Zerhouni E: Invasion of the neurovascular bundle by prostate cancer: Evaluation with MR imaging. *Radiology* 181: 107–112, 1991.

32. Kalbhen CL, Hricak H, Shinohara K, et al.: Prostate carcinoma: MR imaging findings after cryosurgery. *Radiology* 198: 807–811, 1996.

33. McCollum RW, Banner MP: Calculous disease of the urinary tract. In Pollack H (ed.), *Clinical Urography*. Philadelphia: WB Saunders, p. 1908–1912, 1990.

34. Allen KS, Kressel HY, Arger PH, Pollack HM: Age-related changes of the prostate. *Am J Roentgenol* 152: 77–81, 1989.

35. Hricak H, Dooms GC, Jeffrey RB, et al.: Prostatic carcinoma: Staging by clinical assessment, CT, and MR imaging. *Radiology* 162: 331–336, 1987.

36. Rifkin M: Inflammation of the lower genitourinary tract: The prostate, seminal vesicles and scrotum. In Pollack H (ed.), *Clinical Urography*. Philadelphia: WB Saunders, p. 940–960, 1990.

37. Gevenois PA, Stallenberg B, Sintzoff SA, Salmon I, Van Regemorter G, Struyven J: Granulomatous prostatitis: A pitfall in MR imaging of prostatic carcinoma. *Eur Radiol* 2: 365–367, 1992.

38. Narumi Y, Hricak H, Armenakas NA, Dixon CM, McAninch JW: MR imaging of traumatic posterior urethral injury. *Radiology* 188: 439–443, 1993.

39. Hricak H, Marotti M, Gilbert TJ, Lue TF, Wetzel LH, McAninch JW, Tanagho EA: Normal penile anatomy and abnormal penile conditions: Evaluation with MR imaging. *Radiology* 169: 683–690, 1988.

40. Hricak H: The penis and male urethra. In Hricak H, Carrington BM (eds.), *MRI of the Pelvis*. Norwalk, CT: Appleton & Lange, p. 383–416, 1991.

41. Amis ES, Newhouse JH: *Essentials of Uroradiology*. Boston: Little, Brown, p. 69, 1991.

42. McCollum RW: Urethral neoplasms. In Pollack HM (ed.), *Clinical Urography*. Philadelphia: WB Saunders, p. 1406–1409, 1990.

43. Kaneko K, De Mouy EH, Lee BE: Sequential contrast-enhanced MR imaging of the penis. *Radiology* 191: 75–77, 1994.

44. Noone T, Clark R: Primary, isolated urethral amyloidosis. *Abdom Imag*. In press.

45. Helweg G, Judmaier W, Buchberger W, Wicke K, Oberhauser H, Knapp R, Ennemoser O, Zur Nedden D: Peyronie's disease: MR findings in 28 patients. *Am J Roentgenol* 158: 1261–1264, 1992.

46. Schneider HJ, Rufendorff EW, Rohrborn C: Pathogenesis, diagnosis, and therapy of induratio penis plastica. *Int Urol Nephrol* 17: 235–244, 1985.

47. Di Santis D: Urethral inflammation. In Pollack H (ed.), *Clinical Urography*. Philadelphia: WB Saunders, p. 925–939, 1990.

48. King BF, Hattery RR, Lieber MM, Berquist TH, Williamson B Jr, Hartman GW: Congenital cystic disease of the seminal vesicle. *Radiology* 178: 207–211, 1991.

49. King BF, Hattery RR, Lieber MM, Williamson B Jr, Hartman GW, Berquist TH: Seminal vesicle imaging. *Radiographics* 9: 653–676, 1989.

50. Mirowitz S: Seminal vesicles: Biopsy-related hemorrhage simulating tumor invasion at MR imaging. *Radiology* 185: 373–376, 1992.

51. Ramchandani P, Schnall MD, LiVolsi VA, Tomaszewski JE, Pollack HM: Senile amyloidosis of the seminal vesicles mimicking metastatic spread of prostatic carcinoma on MR images. *Am J Roentgenol* 161: 99–100, 1993.

52. Muller-Leisse C, Bohndorf K, Stargardt A, et al.: Gadolinium-enhanced T1-weighted imaging of scrotal disorders: Is there an indication for MR imaging? *J Magn Reson Imaging* 4: 389–395, 1994.

53. Hancock RA, Hodgins TE: Polyorchidism. *Urology* 24: 303–307, 1984.

54. Johnson JO, Mattrey RF, Philipson J: Differentiation of seminomatous from nonseminomatous testicular tumors with MR imaging. *Am J Roentgenol* 154: 539–543, 1990.

55. Giwercman A, Grindsted J, Hansen B, et al.: Testicular cancer risk in boys with maldescended testis: A cohort study. *J Urol* 138: 1214–1216, 1987.

56. Kier R, McCarthy S, Rosenfield AT, Rosenfield NS, Rapoport S, Weiss RM: Nonpalpable testes in young boys: Evaluation with MR imaging. *Radiology* 169: 429–433, 1988.

57. Semelka R, Anderson M, Hricak H: Prosthetic testicle: Appearance at MR imaging. *Radiology* 173: 561–562, 1989.

58. Tartar VM, Trambert MA, Balsara ZN, Mattrey RF: Tubular ectasia of the testicle. *Am J Roentgenol* 160: 539–542, 1993.

59. Hricak H: The testis. In Hricak H, Carrington BM (eds.). *MRI of the Pelvis.* Norwalk. CT: Appleton & Lange, p. 343–382, 1991.

60. Faysal MH, Strefling A, Kosek JC: Epididymal neoplasms: A case report and review. *J Urol* 129: 843–844, 1983.

61. Pavone-Macaluso M, Smith PH, Bagshaw MA: *Testicular Cancer and Other Tumors of the Genitourinary Tract.* New York: Plenum, 1985.

62. Cramer BM, Schiegel E, Thuroff J: MR imaging in the differential diagnosis of scrotal and testicular disease. *Radiographics* 11: 9–21, 1991.

63. Grebenc ML, Gorman JD, Sumida FK: Fibrous pseudotumor of the tunica vaginalis testis: Imaging appearance. *Abdom Imaging* 20: 379–380, 1995.

64. Sajjad SM, Azizi MR, Llamas L: Fibrous pseudotumor of the testicular tunic. *Urology* 19: 86–88, 1982.

65. Parveen T, Fleischmann, J, Petrelli M: Benign fibrous tumor of the tunica vaginalis testis. *Arch Pathol Lab Med* 116: 277–280, 1992.

66. Parker SL, Tong T, Bolden S, Wingo PA: Cancer statistics, 1996. *CA Cancer J Clin* 65: 5–27, 1996.

67. Reinges MHT, Kaiser WA, Miersch WD, Vogel J, Reiser M: Dynamic MRI of benign and malignant testicular lesions: Preliminary observations. *Eur Radiol* 5: 615–622, 1995.

68. Richie JP: Detection and treatment of testicular cancer. *CA Cancer J Clin* 43: 151–175, 1993.

69. Mostofi FK: Proceedings: Testicular tumors: Epidemiologic, etiologic, and pathologic features. *Cancer* 32: 1186–1201, 1973.

70. American Joint Committee on Cancer: Testis. In *Manual for Staging Cancer* (4th ed.). Philadelphia: Lippincott, p. 187–189, 1992.

71. Trambert MA, Mattrey RF, Levine D, Berthoty DP: Subacute scrotal pain: Evaluation of torsion versus epididymitis with MR imaging. *Radiology* 175: 53–56, 1990.

72. Tzika AA, Vigneron DB, Hricak H, Moseley ME, James TL, Kogan BA: P-31 MR spectroscopy in assessing testicular torsion: Rat model. *Radiology* 172: 753–757, 1989.

73. Chew W, Hricak H: P-31 MRS of human testicular function and viability. *Invest Radiol* 24: 997–1000, 1989.

74. Cornel E, Smits G, Oosterhof G, Karthaus H, Deburyne F, Schalken J, Heerschap A: Characterization of human prostate cancer, benign prostatic hyperplasia and normal prostate by in vitro ^{1}H and ^{31}P magnetic resonance spectroscopy. *Urology* 150: 2019–2024, 1993.

75. Yu KK, Hricak H: Imaging prostate cancer. *Radiol Clin N Am* 38: 59–85, 2000.

76. Garcia-Segura JM, Sanchez-Chapado M, Ibarburen C, Viano J, Angulo JC, Gonzalez J, Rodriguez-Vallejo JM: In vivo proton magnetic resonance spectroscopy of diseased prostate: Spectroscopic features of malignant versus benign pathology. *Magn Reson Imaging* 17(5): 755–65, 1999.

77. Van der Graaf M, van den Boogert HJ, Jager GJ, Barentsz JO, Heerschap A: Human prostate: Multisection proton MR spectroscopic imaging with a single spin-echo sequence-preliminary experience. *Radiology* 213(3): 919–925, 1999.

78. Heerschap A, Jager GJ, van der Graaf M, Barentsz JO, de la Rosette JJ, Oosterhof GON, Ruijter ETG, Ruijs SHJ: In vivo proton MR spectroscopy reveals altered metabolite content in malignant prostate tissue. *Anticancer Res* 17: 1455–1460, 1997.

79. Kaji Y, Kurhanewicz J, Hricak H, Sokolov DL, Huang LR, Nelson SJ, Vigneron DB: Localizing prostate cancer in the presence of post-biopsy changes on MR images: Role of proton MR spectroscopic imaging. *Radiology* 206(3): 785–90, 1998.

80. Bahnson RR: Editorial: Improving prostate cancer detection. *J Urology* 164(2): 405, 2000.

81. Parivar F, Hricak H, Shinohara K, Kurhanewicz J, Vigneron DB, Nelson SJ, Carroll PR: Detection of locally recurrent prostate cancer after cryosurgery: Evaluation by transrectal ultrasound, magnetic resonance imaging, and three-dimensional proton magnetic resonance spectroscopy. *Urology* 48(4): 594–599, 1996.

82. Freedman GM, Negenank WG, Hudes GR, Shaer AH, Hanks GE: Preliminary results of a bone marrow magnetic resonance imaging protocol for patients with high-risk prostate cancer. *Urology* 54(1): 118–23, 1999.

FEMALE URETHRA AND VAGINA

LARA B. EISENBERG, M.D., RICHARD C. SEMELKA, M.D.,
MONICA S. PEDRO M.D., AND EVAN S. SIEGELMAN, M.D.

FEMALE URETHRA

Introduction

Evaluation and diagnosis of pathology involving the female urethra has been challenging and difficult because of the poor specificity of clinical symptoms and the lack of a suitable imaging modality. Because of its multiplanar imaging capability and superior soft tissue contrast, MRI has proven to be the most sensitive modality for the detection and staging of benign and malignant urethral pathology.

Normal Anatomy

The female urethra originates at the trigone of the bladder and terminates anterior to the opening of the vagina. It is a thin-walled muscular channel and measures approximately 4 cm in length. The lower two-thirds of the urethra is lined by stratified squamous epithelium, whereas the proximal one-third, like the urinary bladder, has a transitional cell epithelial lining. The urethra has a three-layered zonal anatomy, which consists of the inner mucosal layer, the highly vascular submucosal layer, and the outer muscular layer. The muscular layer consists of an inner longitudinal smooth muscle layer and an outer striated circular muscle layer. Extensions of the endopelvic fascia, the urethropelvic and pubourethral ligaments, help to stabilize the urethra in addition to contributing to urinary continence. The submucosal and striated muscle fibers of the urethra aid in urinary continence as well. The paraurethral and periurethral submucosal glands are not typically seen [1–3].

MRI Technique

Routine imaging for urethral pathology should include transverse, high-resolution, small field-of-view T1-weighted images before and after intravenous contrast administration, particularly in cases of suspected tumor. The addition of fat suppression may increase conspicuity of disease. Orthogonal transverse and sagittal high-resolution T2-weighted images are also routinely obtained [1, 4].

Coronal high-resolution T2-weighted images may be helpful in select cases. Endorectal and endovaginal coil imaging provides superior anatomic resolution and can help to better delineate the zonal anatomy of the urethra as well as define extent of disease processes. [4–6]

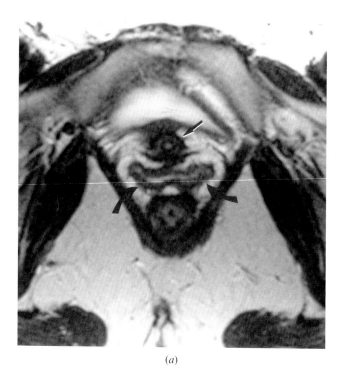

(a)

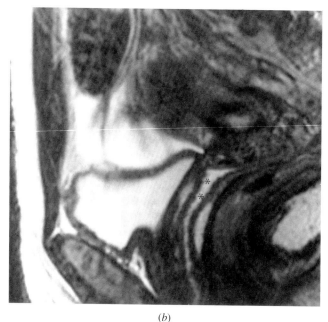

(b)

FIG. 13.1 Normal anatomy of the female urethra and vagina. Transverse (a) and sagittal (b) ETSE images show the normal urethral zonal anatomy (from central to peripheral): high-signal intensity (SI) central spot, low-SI mucosa, moderately high-SI submucosa and low-SI muscularis (arrow, a). The vagina is located posteriorly and reveals (from central to peripheral): high-signal mucosa/secretions, low-SI muscular wall (curved arrow, a) and high-SI perivaginal venous plexus. The normal rugae of the vaginal wall are well depicted (**, b).

T2-weighted ETSE image (c) in a second patient demonstrates the central low-SI mucosal layer, higher-SI surrounding submucosal layer, and low-SI outer ring representing the muscular layer of the urethra.

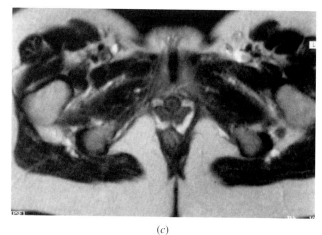

(c)

Normal

On transverse T2- and enhanced T1-weighted images the female urethra demonstrates a "target" appearance with a low-signal intensity outer ring, a high-signal intensity middle ring, and a low signal intensity central dot (fig. 13.1) [1, 4]. The dark outer ring corresponds to both the outer striated and inner longitudinal and circular smooth muscle layers [4, 7–10]. The middle high-signal intensity ring represents the vascular submucosal layer, whereas the dark central dot represents the mucosal layer. This target appearance is seen more commonly in the middle urethra than in the proximal or distal urethra. The low-signal intensity outer layer thins toward the distal urethra. Occasionally, a tiny dot of high signal intensity is seen in the center of the urethra on high-resolution T2-weighted images and is thought to be caused by urine or mucus in the lumen [10, 11]. With endovaginal coil imaging, the separate muscle layers of the urethra can be discerned [12]. The zonal anatomy of the urethra is not always apparent in postmenopausal women, and decreased zonal definition should not be assumed to be abnormal. On enhanced T1-weighted images, the most common pattern seen is marked enhancement in the middle submucosal layer with little to no enhancement of the remaining urethra [1, 10].

Normal Variants and Congenital Disease

Duplication. Urethral duplication is cause by delayed fusion of the urogenital sinus and müllerian ducts. It may occur alone or in concert with bladder duplication or other abnormalities of the genitalia. It is typically discovered in infants, but affected adults may present with a double urinary stream, incontinence, or recurrent urinary infections [13, 14]. The accessory urethra usually drains into the clitoris. Surface coil imaging and postgadolinium T1-weighted fat-suppressed gradient-echo techniques may be useful in the evaluation of suspected urethral duplication.

Ectopic Ureterocele. A cause of urinary incontinence, ectopic ureteroceles can drain into the urethrovaginal septum or into the posterior urethral wall [15–17].

Mass Lesions

Benign Masses

Urethral Leiomyoma. Urethral leiomyomas are unusual benign tumors, which arise from the smooth muscle layer of the urethra [18]. Presenting clinical symptoms of dysuria or a palpable mass may be mistaken for a urethral diverticulum [19, 20]. Like uterine fibroids, these masses may grow during pregnancy. Urethral leiomyomas are usually of low to intermediate signal intensity on T1- and T2-weighted images secondary to their smooth muscle content [4, 21, 22]. Malignant degeneration has not been reported. Symptomatic tumors can be removed by transurethral resection [18].

Malignant Masses

Primary Urethral Carcinomas. Primary urethral carcinoma is an uncommon entity that occurs in middle-aged or older women. Most urethral carcinomas are of squamous cell origin and arise from the distal (anterior) urethra. Transitional cell carcinomas and adenocarcinomas most commonly originate from the proximal (posterior) urethra [23, 24]. A TNM staging approach is used for urethral carcinomas (Table 13.1). Urethral carcinoma spreads contiguously to adjacent sites and then lymphatically to distant sites. Regional nodal involvement relates to the initial location of the tumor. Anterior urethral lesions usually involve the inguinal nodes, with subsequent spread to pelvic nodal groups. Posterior urethral lesions drain to iliac, obturator, and para-aortic lymph nodes [1, 23, 25]. Patients often present with advanced disease because of nonspecific symptomatology combined with difficulty in detecting lesions clinically. Treatment for advanced lesions includes anterior pelvic exenteration, radiation, or chemotherapy [25, 26]. Lesions that are Stage Ta-2N0M0 or less may be treated with surgery alone.

Table 13.1 TNM Staging for Female Urethral Carcinoma

Primary Tumor

Tx	Primary tumor cannot be assessed
T0	No evidence of primary tumor
Tis	Carcinoma in situ
T1	Tumor invades subepithelial, connective tissue
T2	Tumor invades periurethral muscle
T3	Tumor invades the bladder neck or anterior vaginal wall
T4	Tumor invades other adjacent organs

Regional Lymph Nodes

Nx	Regional lymph nodes cannot be assessed
N0	No regional lymph node metastasis
N1	Metastasis in one lymph node is 2 cm or smaller
N2	Metastasis on one node in between 2 and 5 cm in size
N3	Metastasis in one node is larger than 5 cm

Metastases

Mx	Distant metastases cannot be assessed
M1	No distant metastases
M2	Distant metastases

The combination of T2- and T1-weighted images before and after contrast administration provides complementary information (figs. 13.2 and 13.3). Transverse and sagittal T2-weighted images are useful for depicting tumor invasion of the muscular wall of the bladder, vagina and pelvic floor. T1-weighted images, on the other hand, demonstrate extension into periurethral fat [8]. Although proven to be a sensitive modality for this entity, MRI is limited by difficulty in differentiating tumor from secondary inflammatory change, which can lead to overestimation of disease extent [1, 10].

Secondary Urethral Malignancies. Secondary urethral malignancies include metastases from renal cell carcinoma or melanoma, and contiguous spread from carcinomas of the bladder, uterus, cervix, and vagina (fig. 13.4). MRI is useful in demonstrating the extent of involvement in these cases and thereby influencing staging and treatment [27].

Miscellaneous

Urethral Diverticulum

Urethral diverticula are saccular outpouchings from the urethra, which are thought to result from recurrent infection and obstruction of the periurethral glands [28–30]. The dilated glands then rupture and drain into the urethral lumen. They are often asymptomatic but can become infected, form stones or, less often, cause dyspareunia, dribbling, or a palpable mass [31]. These lesions often are difficult to diagnose because of nonspecific symptomatology [32]. Traditional evaluation for

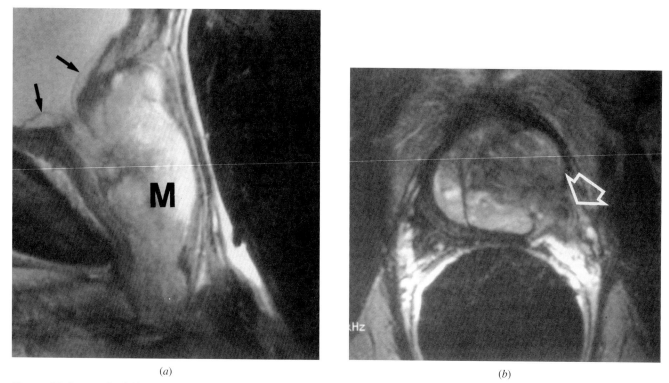

(a)   (b)

F I G . 13.2 Poorly differentiated adenocarcinoma of the urethra with vaginal invasion. Sagittal (*a*) and tranverse (*b*) ETSE endorectal coil images in a 50-year-old woman with palpable urethral mass. Sagittal image (*a*) shows a heterogeneous high-SI mass (M) whose center is in the posterior urethra. The mass extends from the widened bladder neck to the meatus. Normal collapsed high-SI vaginal mucosa (arrows, *a*) can be seen posterior to the mass. Transverse image (*b*) at the level of the proximal urethra shows a tumor-filled widened bladder neck, as well as thinning and poor definition of the left posterior urethral muscularis and anterior vaginal wall, with gross tumor involvement of the left paravaginal/paraurethral venous plexus (hollow arrow, *b*) representing contiguous spread of tumor.

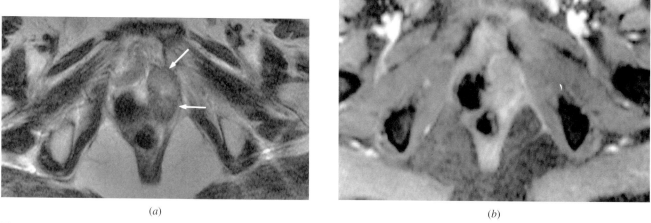

(a)   (b)

F I G . 13.3 Recurrent urethral cancer. Transverse T2-weighted ETSE (*a*) and gadolinium-enhanced fat-suppressed SGE (*b*) images in a patient who underwent anterior pelvic exenteration for urethral cancer show an irregular left-sided mass (arrows, *a*) with heterogeneous enhancement (*b*) consistent with local recurrence.

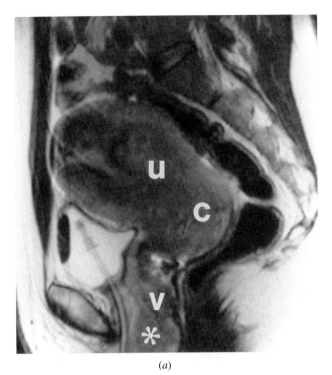

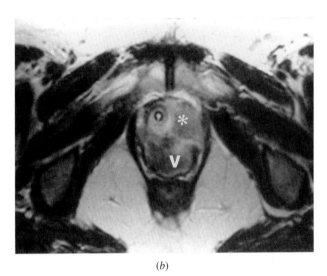

(a)   *(b)*

F I G . 13.4 Poorly differentiated cervical carcinoma with vaginal and urethral invasion. Sagittal (*a*) and transverse (*b*) ETSE images show an aggressive mass centered within the cervix (C) with proximal extension into the uterus (U) and distal spread inferiorly through the cervix into the anterior vagina (V) and periurethral soft tissues (*). A Foley catheter reveals the urethral lumen.

urethral diverticula has been done with voiding cystourethrography, double-balloon urethrography, and/or urethroscopy. These modalities are not always successful [1, 33]. Ultrasound has been advocated by some as an economical way to evaluate this condition, but ultrasound may not be able to distinguish a diverticulum from a paravaginal cyst, nor can it often localize the ostium of the diverticulum [34, 35].

MRI is an excellent imaging modality for evaluation of symptomatic urethral diverticula. Its accuracy and sensitivity exceed both urethrography and urethroscopy,

and MRI has the added advantages of visualizing the surrounding anatomy and being a noninvasive test [35]. MRI findings include an enlarged urethra with a focal area of low signal intensity on T1-weighted images and high signal intensity on T2-weighted images corresponding to the diverticulum. Multiplanar T2-weighted images are useful for the accurate localization of diverticula (figs. 13.5 and 13.6). Gadolinium-enhanced T1-weighted fat-suppressed images have proven useful in demonstrating the cystic nature of diverticula. Contrast-enhanced images may also detect the presence of granulation tissue

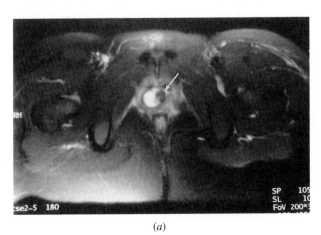

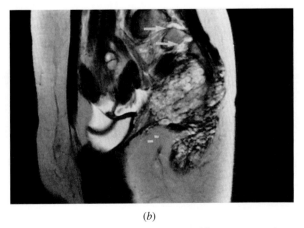

(a)   *(b)*

F I G . 13.5 Urethral diverticulum. Transverse (*a*) and sagittal (*b*) T2-weighted fat-suppressed ETSE images. The transverse image (*a*) shows the high-signal intensity diverticulum surrounding the lower-signal intensity urethra (arrow, *a*), which is displaced laterally. The sagittal image (*b*) demonstrates the high-signal intensity diverticulum (arrow, *b*), which projects posteriorly and causes mass effect on the adjacent vagina.

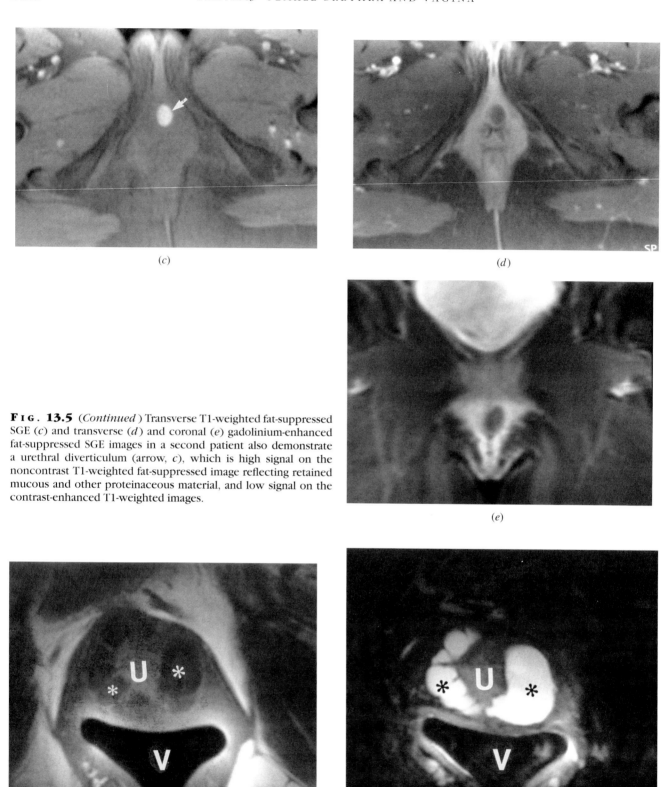

(c)

(d)

F I G . 13.5 (*Continued*) Transverse T1-weighted fat-suppressed SGE (*c*) and transverse (*d*) and coronal (*e*) gadolinium-enhanced fat-suppressed SGE images in a second patient also demonstrate a urethral diverticulum (arrow, *c*), which is high signal on the noncontrast T1-weighted fat-suppressed image reflecting retained mucous and other proteinaceous material, and low signal on the contrast-enhanced T1-weighted images.

(e)

(a)

(b)

F I G . 13.6 Endovaginal coil demonstration of a saddlebag urethral diverticulum. Transverse T1-weighted (*a*), transverse (*b*) and sagittal (*c*) T2-weighted ETSE endovaginal coil images show a multiloculated diverticulum (*) that almost entirely surrounds the circumference of the urethra. The vaginal coil (V) is positioned posterior to the urethra.

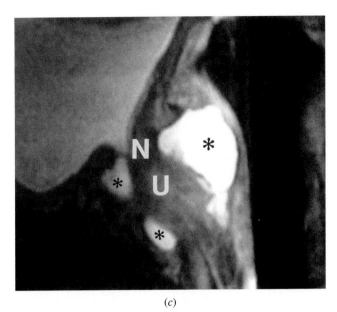

(c)

FIG. 13.6 (*Continued*) Sagittal T2-weighted image (*c*) reveals the superior extent of the diverticulum relative to the bladder neck ("N," *c*) and also shows the portions of the diverticulum located anterior to the urethra ("U," *c*).

or carcinoma [35, 36]. Carcinomas arising within diverticula are very rare and most often adenocarcinomas, reflecting the ductal origin of the diverticula [37]. The ability of MRI to clearly delineate the anatomy of the diverticulum and its relationship to the bladder neck significantly aids in planning the surgical repair of these lesions [30, 33, 35, 37–39].

Caruncle

Urethral caruncles are small, benign, often asymptomatic inflammatory masses that typically occur in older postmenopausal women and arise on or near the external meatus. Occasionally, these lesions can cause pain or hematuria [28]. Histologically, caruncles demonstrate hyperplastic squamous epithelium with underlying submucosal vascularity, fibrosis, and inflammation [40]. This entity has become uncommon with the widespread use of estrogen replacement in the postmenopausal population. MR imaging is useful in localizing the lesion to the urethral meatus and in excluding adenopathy that would suggest a malignant neoplasm [4, 41].

Urethral Trauma and Strictures

MRI is useful in the evaluation of urethral trauma in males by demonstrating in detail the anatomy of the urethral and periurethral tissues. For the same reasons, MR imaging has been useful in preoperative evaluation of posttraumatic and postinfectious strictures in men [42–44]. Urethral trauma and strictures are very rare in women, and the MR appearance has not yet been described [24].

Stress Incontinence

Single-shot echo-train spin echo and fast gradient-echo imaging has been used to evaluate women with pelvic floor relaxation and secondary stress incontinence [45–48]. Sagittal images are typically obtained at rest and during straining. Urethral hypermobility is depicted at MR imaging by a change in the normal vertical orientation of the urethra to a horizontal orientation during straining [47]. Urethral hypermobility can be treated with surgical urethral suspension, collagen injection, or mechanical sphincters. Periurethral collagen is well shown on T2-weighted images and appears high in signal intensity (fig. 13.7) [49–52]. Complications of mechanical sphincters such as fistula formation, periurethral abscess, and erosion can also be depicted [53]. Sagittal single-shot echo-train spin-echo technique is also valuable for demonstrating enteroceles and cystoceles that are also associated with pelvic floor relaxation [47, 54, 55].

Urethral Fistula

Urethrovaginal fistulas occur most often as a complication of urethral diverticulectomy or vaginal surgery [56]. Crohn and Behçet disease are uncommon causes, whereas traumatic childbirth is a common cause in developing countries [57–59]. Rectourethral fistulas are usually developmental abnormalities and are usually associated with complex anorectal abnormalities [60]. Spinal cord injury patients with decubitus ulcers are at risk for developing urethroperineal fistulas [61]. Infection with gonorrhea or tuberculosis can cause periurethral abscesses that can rupture through the skin and form urethroperineal fistulas as well. Transverse and sagittal T2-weighted images demonstrate these abnormalities as high-signal intensity tracts, whereas postgadolinium T1-weighted fat-saturated images can demonstrate the enhancing sinus tract walls.

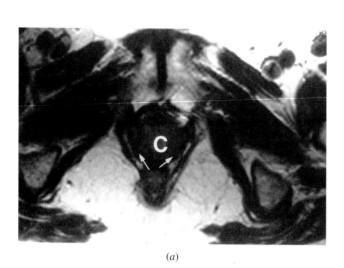

(a)

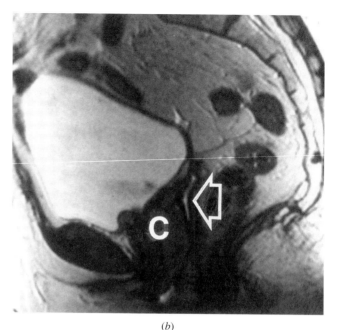

(b)

FIG. 13.7 Periurethral collagen injection for urinary incontinence. Transverse (*a*) and sagittal (*b*) ETSE images in a 72-year-old woman show an intermediate-signal intensity mass that is centered around the urethra (arrows, *a*). The collapsed vagina is present posterior to the mass (arrow, *b*). Without a history of prior collagen injections, it would be difficult to differentiate this mass from a urethral carcinoma.

Transverse T2-weighted spin-echo image (*c*) in a second patient demonstrates high-signal intensity collagen (large arrow) surrounding the low-signal intensity urethra (small arrow).

(c)

Conclusion

MRI is the ideal imaging modality for the evaluation of urethral abnormalities because of to its superior contrast resolution, lack of ionizing radiation, multiplanar capability, and nonnephrotoxic contrast material. Most common indications include evaluation of incontinence and pelvic floor relaxation and evaluation for diverticula in patients with recurrent infection. MRI is also excellent for evaluation of the more uncommon conditions of malignancy and congenital abnormalities.

THE VAGINA

The high contrast resolution, the ability to achieve both small and large fields of view, and multiplanar capability render MRI superior to CT imaging and ultrasound

for evaluation of many benign and malignant conditions of the vagina. In addition, the lack of invasiveness and added extraluminal anatomic detail make MRI preferable to vaginography for the evaluation of congenital anomalies [62].

Normal Anatomy

The vagina is a 7 to 9-cm-long fibromuscular tube lying between the bladder and rectum. The upper one-third is derived from müllerian duct fusion, whereas the lower two-thirds originates from the urogenital sinus [63]. The layers of the vagina consist of the inner mucosal layer, middle submucosal and muscular layer, and an outer adventitial layer that contains the vaginal venous plexus [10, 64]. The anterior, posterior, and lateral fornices of the vagina surround the cervix and are best seen on sagittal and transverse images. For descriptive purposes, it is useful to divide the vagina into thirds. The upper third is considered to be at the level of the lateral fornices, the middle third at the level of the base of the bladder, and the lower third at the level of the urethra.

MRI Technique

As in the evaluation of the pelvis in general, T2-weighted images are critical because they differentiate the layers of the vaginal wall to the best advantage. T1-weighted images are complementary, particularly combining fat suppression with gadolinium administration. Fat suppression is required to differentiate fat from proteinaceous or hemorrhagic contents [65] and for detection of peritoneal enhancement or tumor [66]. The transverse plane is ideal for the evaluation of pathology with respect to the vaginal wall, and sagittal plane imaging demonstrates the relationship to the bladder and rectum. Coronal images can demonstrate levator ani muscle involvement. Thin (≤5 mm) sections are preferable. Patients should be asked to remove tampons before imaging to avoid obscuring detail. Routine use of torso or pelvic phased-array coils is ideal to allow acquisition of high-resolution, small field-of-view images [67, 68].

When even smaller field-of-view and higher resolution images are needed, endovaginal or endorectal coils may be employed [5].

Normal

The mucosal layer and any intraluminal fluid and mucus appear as a central area of low signal intensity on T1-weighted images and high signal intensity on T2-weighted images (fig. 13.8) [64]. The thickness of the endoluminal mucus has been shown to correlate with estrogen levels and becomes more prominent during the late proliferative and early secretory phases of the menstrual cycle. Pregnant patients often have medium to high signal intensity of the mucus layer, vaginal wall, and surrounding tissues. In contrast, premenarchal females and postmenopausal females have a low-signal intensity wall and a very thin high-signal intensity mucus layer. The middle layer of the vagina is low in signal intensity on both T1- and T2-weighted images and consists of the submucosa and muscularis layers. The muscularis consists of inner longitudinal and outer circular smooth muscle layers. The vaginal venous plexus in the adventitial layer is high in signal intensity on T2-weighted images because of slow venous flow. After gadolinium administration, the vaginal wall enhances, and occasionally, a

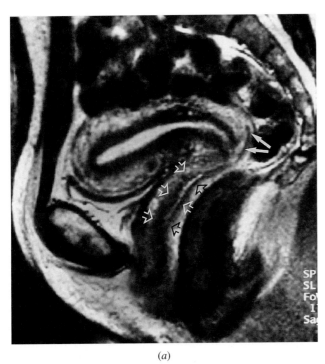

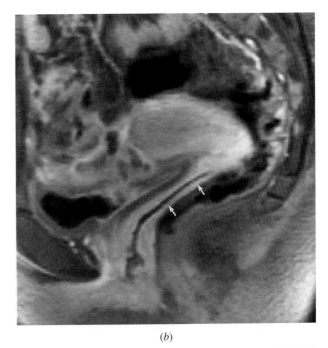

(a)   (b)

F I G . 13.8 Normal vagina. Sagittal T2-weighted echo-train spin-echo (*a*) and immediate postgadolinium fat-suppressed SGE (*b*) images. On the T2-weighted images the low-signal intensity muscular wall and the central higher-signal intensity mucosal layer of the vagina are apparent. The sagittal T2-weighted image (*a*) shows vagina (open arrows, *a*) as well as the posterior vaginal fornix (closed arrows, *a*). Relationship with uterus and cervix is well seen. On the immediate postgadolinium fat-suppressed image (*b*), intense enhancement of vaginal mucosa (arrows, *b*) is present. (Courtesy of Susan M. Asher, M.D., Dept. of Radiology, Georgetown University Medical Center, Washington, D.C.)

low-signal intensity line is present centrally, which may represent the lumen or inner epithelial layer [10].

Normal Variants and Congenital Disease

Congenital and developmental anomalies of the vagina can be divided into four categories: absence and partial absence, duplication and partial duplication, abnormalities of gonadal differentiation, and ambiguous genitalia. MRI provides a noninvasive method of determining the presence of the uterus, cervix, vagina, gonads, and penile bulb and thus is ideally suited for evaluation of these abnormalities [69–74].

Vaginal Agenesis and Partial Agenesis

Vaginal agenesis and partial agenesis are rare conditions that are classified under the larger category of müllerian duct anomalies. The incidence of all müllerian duct anomalies in women has been reported to be 1–15%. One in 4000–5000 women is estimated to have vaginal agenesis [71, 75]. These patients typically have normal ovaries and external genitalia but can have associated abnormalities of the uterus, cervix, upper urinary tract, and skeleton (fig. 13.9). If no functioning endometrium is present, these patients will often present with primary amenorrhea. If functioning endometrium is present, however, patients present after menarche with pain and mass effect from hematometra.

The surgical management of these patients is determined by the presence of functioning endometrium and a cervix. Complete vaginal agenesis with no functioning endometrium and only a small uterine bulb is treated

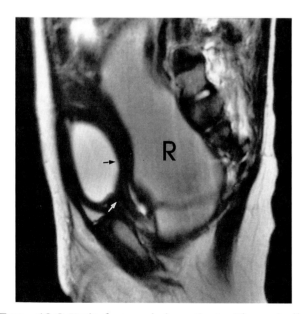

F I G . 13.9 Vaginal agenesis in patient with surgically repaired persistent cloaca. Sagittal SS-ETSE image. No vagina is seen. The urethra (white arrow) is elongated and superiorly positioned. The bladder has a thickened wall (black arrow). The reconstructed rectum (R) is dilated.

with vaginoplasty. If the uterine bulb contains functioning endometrium, vaginoplasty along with open surgery to remove the uterine remnant are required to prevent endometriosis. When a uterus with endometrium but no cervix accompanies complete agenesis, hysterectomy and vaginoplasty are required. If patients have a partial vaginal agenesis with a normal uterus and cervix, creation of an external vaginal opening alone is required, and pregnancy is possible [75].

Mayer-Rokitansky-Küster-Hauser syndrome is the name given to the müllerian duct anomaly with vaginal and uterine agenesis, normal tubes and ovaries, and variable urinary tract anomalies (fig. 13.10). This disorder occurs in approximately 1 in 5000 female births, with most patients having a normal karyotype [76]. Uterine and/or vaginal rudiments may be present, and documentation of their presence is also important for planning of the surgical approach [70]. Vaginal agenesis, partial agenesis, and cloacal abnormalities are best imaged using MRI. Thin-section T2-weighted transverse images accurately demonstrate agenesis, and in cases of partial agenesis, combined transverse and sagittal images delineate vaginal length, which is important in surgical planning [70, 73, 77, 78]. MRI also shows the presence or absence of the uterus, cervix, and kidneys. Exquisite sensitivity in evaluating blood makes MRI ideal for identifying functioning endometrium.

Duplication and Partial Duplication

Duplication and partial duplication of the vagina are typically seen in association with the didelphic anomaly of the uterus. This anomaly is well seen on transverse T2-weighted images. Vaginal duplication can result in a longitudinal vaginal septum that can be a cause of dyspareunia [79]. T2-weighted images demonstrate the low-signal intensity septum contrasted by the high signal intensity of the adjacent vaginal secretions and mucosal layer. Vaginal and uterine duplication can also be complicated by a transverse vaginal septum causing obstruction of the affected hemivagina and its associated uterine cavity [80]. Patients begin menses at a normal age at puberty, because of the presence of the nonobstructed uterine horn, but can present with a palpable mass. Untreated cases can result in the development of endometriosis [79, 81]. This abnormality is also associated with ipsilateral renal agenesis.

A transverse vaginal septum is the result of failure of fusion of the down-growing müllerian duct with the up-growing urogenital sinus. Like patients with imperforate hymen, these patients present at puberty with amenorrhea and cyclical abdominal pain (fig. 13.11). Treatment of transverse vaginal septum includes resection of the septum and vaginal reconstruction. In more severe cases, agenesis of the cervix is also found and hysterectomy with vaginoplasty is required [79, 82, 83].

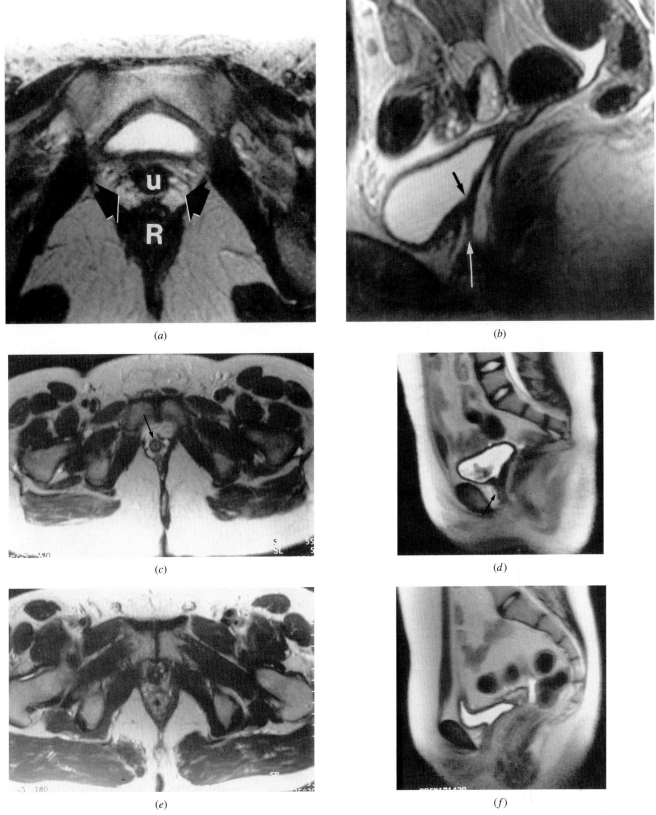

FIG. 13.10 Mayer-Rokitansky-Küster-Hauser syndrome. Transverse (*a*) and sagittal (*b*) T2-weighted ETSE images in a 17-year-old female with primary amenorrhea show a normal urethra ("U," *a*), rectum (R) and vaginal venous plexus (arrows, *a*). No normal vaginal wall is present. On the sagittal image (*b*) the absence of the uterus, cervix, and vagina is well demonstrated.

Transverse (*c*) and sagittal (*d*) SS-ETSE images in a second patient. The vagina and uterus are absent, and the urethra (arrow, *c*, *d*) is more posteriorly positioned than normal. Partial absence of the sacrum with abnormal elevation of the pelvic floor is present.

Transverse 512-resolution echo-train spin-echo (*e*) and sagittal SS-ETSE (*f*) images in a third patient demonstrate similar findings of absent vagina and uterus with posterior positioned urethra.

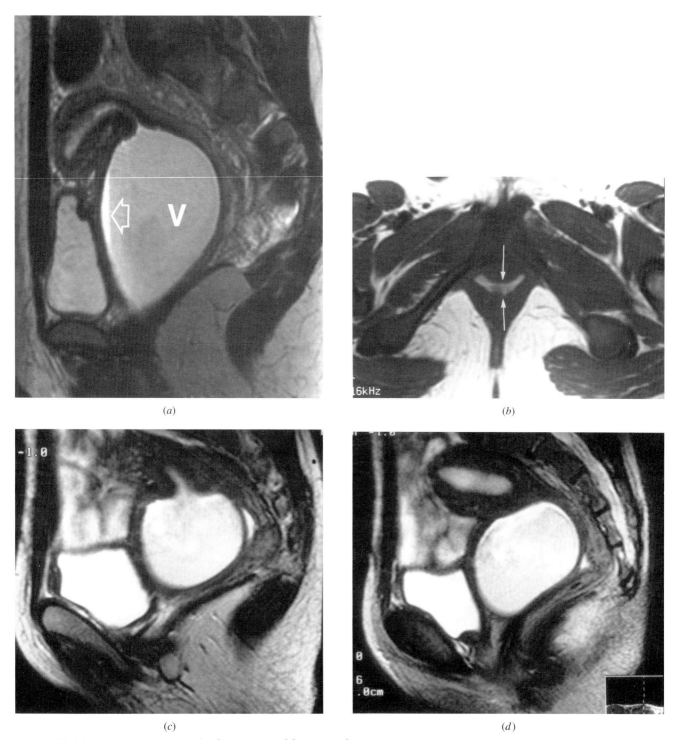

(a)

(b)

(c)

(d)

F I G . 13.11 Low transverse vaginal septum and hematocolpos. Sagittal T2-weighted ETSE (*a*) and transverse T1-weighted (*b*) images in a 12-year-old girl with pelvic pain show a distended vaginal canal that is filled with complex fluid with a fluid-fluid level (arrow, *a*). T1-weighted image (*b*) obtained through the lower vagina shows that the distended vaginal canal contains high-signal intensity representing the T1-shortening effects of protein and/or methemoglobin within subacute blood. A low transverse septum may have a similar appearance to an imperforate hymen on MR imaging. The treatment of the two conditions, however, is similar.

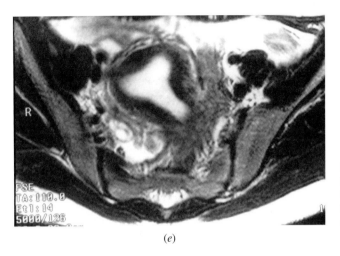

(*e*)

F I G . 13.11 (*Continued*) Sagittal (*c*, *d*) and transverse (*e*) T2-weighted ETSE images in a second patient, who has a transverse vaginal septum, demonstrate marked distension of the vagina and uterine cavity consistent with hematocolpometra. (Courtesy of Andrea Oliveira, MD, Brasilia, Brazil.)

Abnormalities of Gonadal Differentiation

Abnormalities of gonadal differentiation include true hermaphroditism and gonadal dysgenesis. True hermaphrodites have both ovarian and testicular tissues, which can exist together as an ovotestis or in separate discrete gonads [84, 85]. Although the internal genitalia are variable, most patients have a uterus. Ovatestes and testes are often intra-abdominal or cryptorchid, whereas ovaries are typically intra-abdominal [85]. Most (80%) have XX karyotype, with the remaining 20% evenly divided between XY and mosaic karyotypes [69, 70]. Development of the internal ducts usually corresponds with the gonad on that side. Sex assignment of true hermaphrodites is usually made by the external genitalia, which are variable in appearance. MRI evaluation can be helpful in demonstrating the internal anatomy. Presence of the vagina or prostate is well established with transverse imaging, and sagittal views display the uterus, penile bulb, and prostate well [64, 69, 73, 85]. The gonads in these patients are at increased risk of neoplasms.

The term "pure gonadal dysgenesis" refers to the presence of bilateral streak gonads, which are fibrous in nature and contain no germ cells [85]. The basic underlying defect is typically an abnormal second sex chromosome. The majority of these patients are of the XO phenotype known as Turner syndrome. These patients have infantile external genitalia, a uterus and vagina, as well as bilateral streak ovaries. They often have other abnormalities such as a webbed neck and short stature. Other karyotypes occur with gonadal dysgenesis and include mixed gonadal dysgenesis in which the patients have a mosaic karyotype (XO/XY, XO/XYY). These patients have one testis and one streak gonad [85]. A 46 XY combination also exists with abnormal testicular development. This entity differs from testicular feminization in that female internal ducts are usually present as well as external female genitalia. The feminization may be incomplete if the testes are able to produce some testosterone or müllerian regression factor [85]. In patients with gonadal dysgenesis, Y chromosome-containing gonads are at increased risk for malignant transformation and should be removed. Although karyotype analysis is the most critical in the evaluation of these patients, MRI can be helpful in demonstrating the degree of differentiation of internal organs as well as identifying streak gonads, seen as low signal intensity on T2-weighted images.

Ambiguous Genitalia.

Patients with normal genotype but ambiguous genitalia are classified as pseudohermaphrodites. Male pseudohermaphrodites have testes but possess ambiguous internal and/or external genitalia [85]. The most common etiology is testicular feminization (fig. 13.12), which is an X-linked recessive disorder in which there is an absence of cytoplasmic testosterone receptors. These patients are phenotypically female but have a blind-ended vagina with no uterus or fallopian tubes because the testes make normal müllerian regression factor [84]. T2-weighted MR imaging is helpful in preoperative location of the testes, which are removed because of increased risk of malignancy [85].

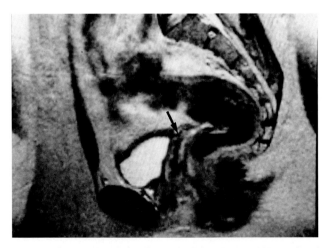

F I G . 13.12 Testicular feminization. Sagittal T2-weighted echo-train spin-echo image. Note absence of the uterus and the blind-ended vagina (arrow).

Other forms of male pseudohermaphroditism include incomplete testicular feminization with partially masculinized genitalia, inability of tissues to convert testosterone to dihydrotestosterone, congenital errors of testosterone synthesis, and inability of the testes to respond to hypothalamic gonadotropin [69].

Female pseudohermaphrodites have normal 46 XX karyotypes and normal ovaries but have virilized external genitalia because of androgen exposure in utero [64, 85]. The most common etiology is 21-hydroxylase deficiency, which is one form of congenital adrenal hyperplasia. This deficiency leads to an excess of androgenic sex steroids, which leads in turn to ambiguous genitalia if exposure occurs before the 12th week of gestation and to clitoromegaly if exposure occurs later. Development of male internal genitalia does not occur because this requires local androgen exposure rather than systemic exposure. Other more rare causes of female pseudohermaphroditism include androgen-producing ovarian or adrenal tumors or maternal ingestion of androgen-containing drugs during the first trimester. With surgical and/or hormonal treatment,

these females can have normal fertility and near-normal female phenotype. MRI is important in identifying uterus, ovaries, vagina, and penile bulb, if present.

Mass Lesions

Benign Masses

Bartholin Cyst. Bartholin glands are mucus-secreting glands that open into the posterolateral aspect of the vaginal vestibule. Trauma or chronic inflammation in this region is thought to lead to retention of secretion in these glands and cyst formation. Unless these cysts become infected, they usually do not incite symptoms. *Neisseria gonorrhoeae* is the most common infecting organism. In addition to antibiotic therapy, aspiration, incision and drainage, laser vaporization, and marsupialization can be employed [86, 87]. These cysts are seen on MR images as small fluid-filled structures in the lower third of the vagina. They are high in signal intensity on T2-weighted images and medium to high in signal intensity on T1-weighted images, depending on the protein content of the fluid (fig. 13.13) [62, 88]. Rim

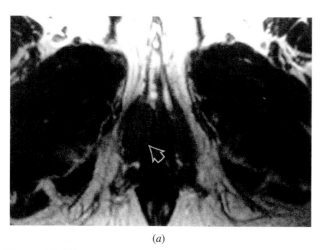

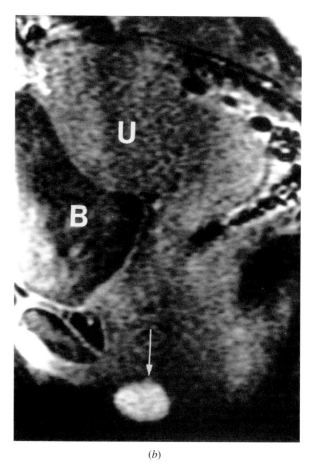

F I G . 13.13 Asymptomatic Bartholin gland cyst. Transverse T2-weighted ETSE (*a*) and sagittal T1-weighted fat-suppressed SGE (*b*) images show a low-signal intensity mass on the T2-weighted image (arrow, *a*) within the lateral aspect of the distal vagina near the introitus.

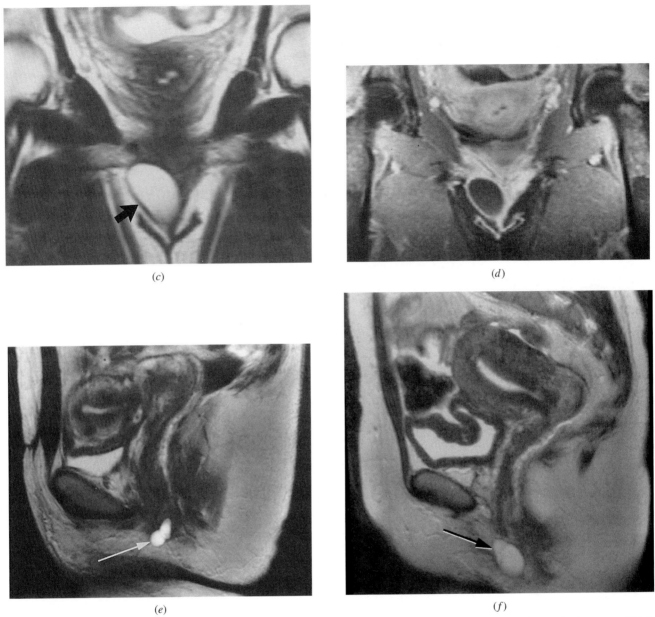

(c)

(d)

(e)

(f)

FIG. 13.13 (*Continued*) On the sagittal T1-weighted fat-suppressed image this mass appears high signal intensity because of high protein content (arrow, *b*). Bladder (B); uterus (U).

Coronal T2-weighted ETSE (*c*) and coronal gadolinium-enhanced fat-suppressed SGE (*d*) images in a second patient. The cyst is high in signal intensity on the T2-weighted image (arrow, *c*) and demonstrates an enhancing cyst wall with low-signal intensity cyst contents on the postgadolinium image (*d*).

Sagittal 512-resolution T2-weighted ETSE (*e*, *f*) images in 2 other patients show Bartholin duct cysts (arrow, *e*, *f*).

enhancement after gadolinium administration suggests infection of the cyst.

Gartner Duct Cyst. Gartner duct cysts are formed from mesonephric duct or wolffian duct remnants and represent the most common benign vulvovaginal lesion in children. Usually asymptomatic, these lesions are found incidentally in 1–2% of female pelvic MRI examinations [62]. Occasionally larger lesions are seen

and may cause dyspareunia or difficult vaginal delivery. Gartner duct cysts arise from the anterolateral wall of the proximal vagina. These lesions have signal characteristics typical for cysts that are low in signal intensity on T1-weighted images and high in signal intensity on T2-weighted images. These cysts can exhibit high signal intensity on T1-weighted images when the contents are proteinaceous or hemorrhagic (fig. 13.14) [89]. Rim enhancement is not a typical feature. Gartner duct cysts

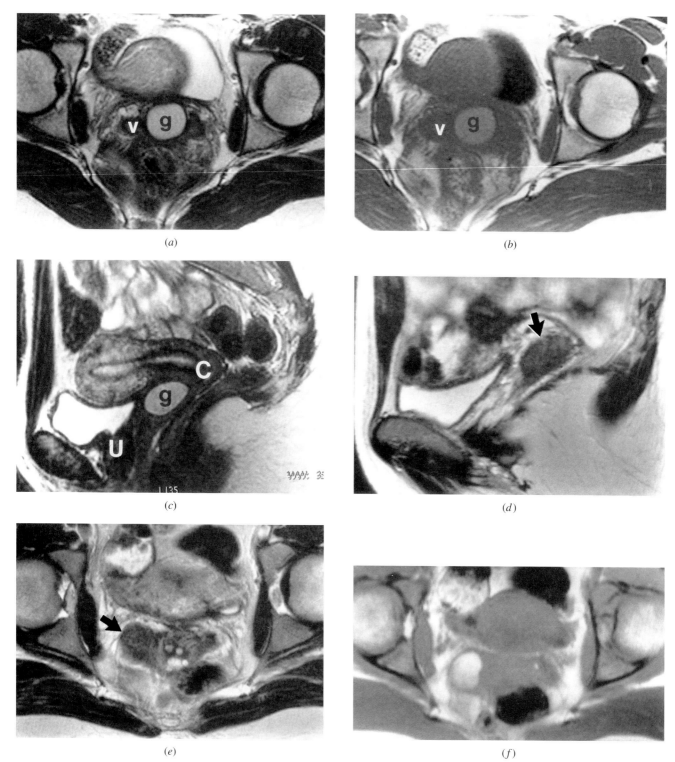

FIG. 13.14 Gartner duct cyst. Transverse T2-weighed ESTE (*a*), transverse T1-weighted ETSE (*b*), and sagittal T2-weighted ETSE (*c*) images in a 22-year-old woman with an asymptomatic palpable paracervical mass. There is a well-circumscribed mass representing a Gartner duct cyst ("g," *a–c*), with high signal intensity on T1- and T2-weighted images, centered within the left side of the proximal vagina ("v," *a, b*). The high signal on T1 reflects intracystic protein. Sagittal T2-weighted image (*c*) reveals that the mass is located above the urethra ("U," *c*) and below the cervix ("C," *c*) within the proximal vagina. The normal zonal anatomy of the uterus is present.

Sagittal (*d*) and transverse (*e*) T2-weighted ETSE and transverse SGE (*f*) images in a second patient. There is a round, well-defined lesion in the upper vagina in the right lateral fornix (arrow, *d, e*). The cyst is high signal on the T1-weighted image (*f*) and low signal on T2-weighted images (*d, e*) consistent with intracystic protein in a Gartner duct cyst.

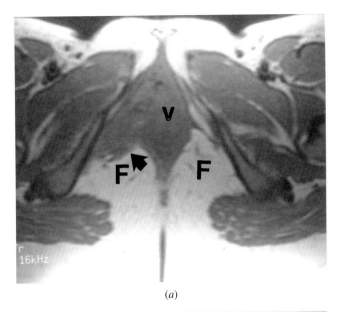

(a)

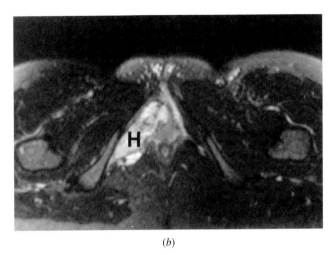

(b)

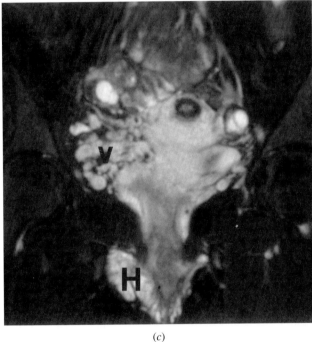

(c)

Fig. 13.15 Recurrent perivulvar cavernous hemangioma. Tranverse T1-weighted (*a*) and transverse (*b*) and coronal (*c*) T2-weighted fat suppressed ETSE images in a 26-year-old woman who underwent resection of perivulvar hemangioma 12 years before imaging. The T1-weighted image (*a*) at the level of the perineum shows effacement (arrow, *a*) of the anterior ischiorectal fat ("F," *a*) adjacent to the right side of the vagina. On T2-weighted images (*b, c*) this area is ill defined and shows high signal intensity ("H," *b*), representing the patient's known vascular malformation. Coronal image (*c*) shows the longitudinal extent of the lobular malformation ("H," *c*). Note the asymmetry of the more central pelvic veins ("V," *c*) because of the increased venous outflow of the malformation.

can be associated with genitourinary abnormalities such as Herlyn-Werner-Wunderlich syndrome where it is associated with ipsilateral renal agenesis [90]. Communication of an ectopic ureter with a Gartner duct cyst has been reported and is a cause of incontinence [91].

Cavernous Hemangioma. Cavernous hemangiomas of the vulva or vagina are most common in infants and tend to stabilize or regress during childhood and adolescence. Symptoms are unusual but can include

bleeding, ulceration, or hemorrhage during vaginal delivery [92–94]. STIR and fat-suppressed T2-weighted images demonstrate high signal intensity in the serpiginous vascular lakes that make up the neoplasm (fig. 13.15) [95].

Malignant Masses
Primary Vaginal Malignancies. Relatively rare lesions, vaginal carcinomas account for less than 3% of all gynecological malignancies. Up to 95% of primary

Table 13.2 TNM Staging for Vaginal Carcinoma

Primary Tumor
Tx   Primary tumor cannot be assessed
T0   No evidence of primary tumor
Tis   Carcinoma in situ
T1   Tumor confined to the vagina
T2   Tumor invades paravaginal tissues but dose not extend to the pelvic
T3   Tumor extends to the pelvic wall
T4   Tumor invades mucosa of bladder or rectum and/or extends beyond

Regional Lymph Nodes
Nx   Regional lymph nodes cannot be assessed
N0   No regional lymph node metastasis
                Upper two-thirds of vagina
N1   Regional lymph node metastasis
                Lower third of vagina
N2   Regional lymph node metastasis
      Bilateral inguinal lymph node metastasis

Metastases
M1   Distant metastases

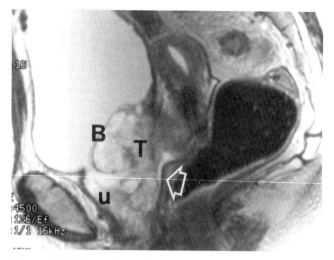

FIG. 13.16 Invasive clear cell adenocarcinoma of the vagina. Sagittal T2-weighted ETSE image in a 68-year-old woman unrelated to DES exposure shows a large heterogeneous intermediate- to high-signal intensity mass (T) in the anterior wall of the proximal vagina with gross invasion of the posterior bladder wall ("B") and the posterior urethra ("U"). The posterior vaginal wall is preserved (white arrow).

vaginal malignancies are of squamous cell histology, and they are usually well differentiated [96, 97]. This entity affects older patients, with a peak age incidence of 60–70 years. Infection with human papilloma virus has been shown to be a risk factor for these tumors [98]. Patients are often asymptomatic but can present with increased vaginal discharge or spotting. Either TNM or FIGO classification schemes can be used for staging (Table 13.2). These lesions typically arise from the upper posterior vagina and then spread through the wall to invade adjacent pelvic structures. Lesions in the upper third of the vagina spread to the iliac nodes, whereas tumors in the lower two-thirds initially involve the inguinal nodes.

Clearcell adenocarcinomas make up 3% of primary vaginal malignancies and occur in less than 0.14% of women who have suffered in utero diethylstilbestrol (DES) exposure [99–101]. Most of these patients were born between 1951 and 1953. These tumors most often arise from the anterior aspect of the upper third of the vagina (fig. 13.16). There is an 80% 5-year survival rate for women presenting with vaginally confined disease and only a 20% 5-year survival for women with locally advanced or metastatic tumors [98].

The contrast resolution of MRI has made it the modality of choice in the evaluation of vaginal tumors. It can be used to assess the extent of disease at initial presentation, and it can be used to detect tumor recurrence [102]. Differentiation of inflammatory changes from primary or metastatic lesions may be problematic, but

one group of investigators has shown MRI to be 92% accurate in demonstrating metastatic disease and 82% accurate in depicting recurrence [103]. Vaginal tumors are of intermediate signal intensity on T1-weighted images and may be occult when small. However, these lesions are well-seen on T2-weighted images and demonstrate moderately high signal intensity [102, 104]. Vaginal neoplasms show variable enhancement after gadolinium administration (figs. 13.17, 13.18).

Detection of tumor recurrence after hysterectomy may be an important role for MRI. The vaginal cuff can have a very irregular appearance because of postoperative fibrosis and granulation tissue. Tumor is generally irregular in contour and usually high in signal intensity on T2-weighted images, whereas fibrosis and granulation tissue are low in signal intensity on T2-weighted images [103, 105]. Recurrent tumor frequently enhances in a heterogeneous intense fashion on gadolinium-enhanced fat-suppressed images. Inflammatory changes within 9 months to 1 year after radiation therapy result in increased signal intensity on T2-weighted images and may mimic tumor recurrence [106]. Close follow-up with MRI may be useful in selected cases.

Other rare primary vaginal malignancies include leiomyosarcomas in adults, endodermal sinus tumors in infants, and lymphoma and melanoma [102, 107–109]. Leiomyosarcoma and endodermal sinus tumors are highly malignant with poor prognosis. Melanoma may be high in signal intensity on T1-weighted images [94]. The high signal intensity within melanin can be

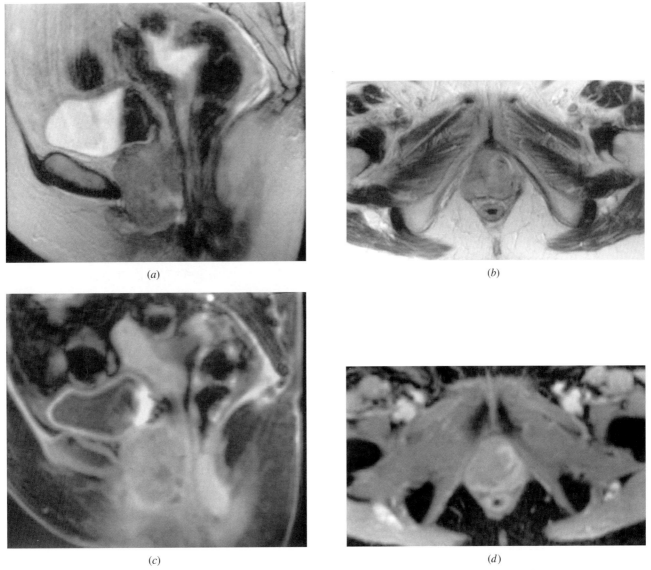

FIG. 13.17 Vaginal carcinoma. Sagittal (*a*) and tranverse (*b*) T2-weighted ETSE and sagittal (*c*) and transverse (*d*) interstitial-phase gadolinium-enhanced fat-suppressed SGE images. There is a large, irregular soft tissue mass arrising from the vagina and involving the urethra. The uterus is small and low signal secondary to prior radiation therapy.

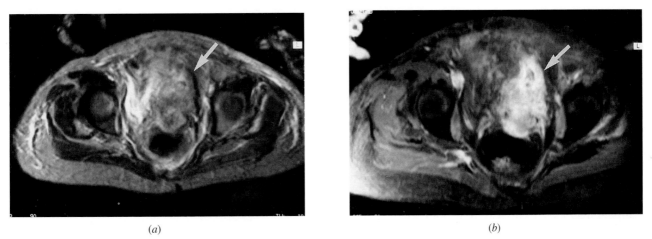

FIG. 13.18 Vaginal carcinoma with bladder and rectum invasion. Transverse T2-weighted spin-echo (*a*) and transverse gadolinium-enhanced T1-weighted fat-suppressed spin-echo (*b*) images. A large heterogeneous vaginal cancer is identified on the T2-weighted image (arrow, *a*) arising from the anterior vaginal wall. Postradiation changes in the pelvis are also heterogeneous in signal intensity, and the margins of the tumor are not well defined. The tumor enhances heterogeneously and intensely after gadolinium administration (arrow, *b*), and invasion of the bladder is clearly shown.

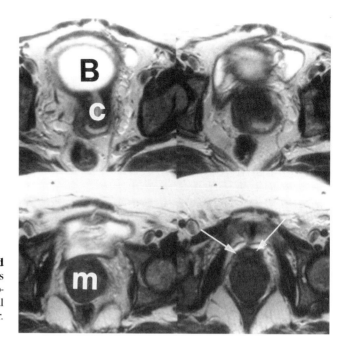

F I G . 13.19 Primary vaginal leiomyoma in a 40-year-old woman. Four consecutive transverse T2-weighted ETSE images show a homogeneous low-signal intensity mass ("m") that is separate from the cervix ("c") and urethra (arrows). The low signal intensity on T2 reflects the smooth muscle content of the tumor. B = bladder.

secondary to either intratumoral hemorrhage or from the T1-shortening effects of paramagnetic metals such as iron that are associated with melanin [110]. Primary vaginal leiomyomas have a similar appearance as uterine fibroids. Tumors that are not degenerated reveal homogenous low signal intensity on T2-weighted images secondary to the smooth muscle content of the tumor (fig. 13.19) [22, 111].

Vaginal Metastases. Secondary vaginal malignancies make up 80% of all vaginal tumors [85]. Local spread from cervical and endometrial carcinoma comprises the majority of reported cases (figs. 13.20 and 13.21) [112].

Sagittal- and transverse-plane images are useful for the demonstration of tumor extension to the vagina. Both T2-weighted fast spin-echo images and gadolinium-enhanced T1-weighted fat-suppressed images define tumor involvement.

Vulvar and Perineal Carcinomas. Vulvar carcinomas are uncommon lesions that occur in older patients and are typically of squamous cell origin. Most of the patients have vulvar pruritus, although pain, bleeding, and palpable mass are often typical symptoms. A TNM system is used for staging (Table 13.3). Modern treatment includes local resection with inguinal lymphadenectomy. Postoperative adjuvant radiation therapy has replaced pelvic lymphadenectomy [113, 114]. MRI is a sensitive modality for the evaluation of both primary and recurrent vulvar carcinoma (figs. 13.22 and 13.23).

Other more rare malignancies involving the vulva include Bartholin gland carcinoma, Paget disease, melanoma, basal cell carcinoma, rhabdomyosarcoma, and aggressive angiomyxoma [62, 109, 115].

Bartholin Gland Carcinoma. Bartholin gland carcinomas are very rare, with fewer than 50 reported cases in the literature [116]. Most are adenoid cystic carcinomas and grow slowly with local spread preceding metastatic disease. Treatment includes radical vulvectomy with regional nodal dissection and adjuvant radiation if complete resection is not obtained [117]. At least in part because of the slow rate of growth of this neoplasm, greater than 80% 5-year survival is usually seen.

Table 13.3 TNM Staging for Carcinoma of the Vulva

Primary Tumor

T1	Tumor 2 cm or smaller confined to the vulva
T2	Tumor larger than 2 cm confined to the vulva
T3	Tumor of any size with adjacent spread to the urethra and/or perineum
T4	Tumor of any size infiltrating the bladder mucosa and/or the rectum

Regional Lymph Nodes

N0	No nodes palpable
N1	Noes palpable in either groin, not enlarged, mobile
N2	Nodes palpable in either one or both groins, enlarged, firm, and mobile
N3	Fixed or ulcerated nodes

Metastases

M0	No clinical metastases
M1	Palpable deep pelvic lymph nodes
M2	Other distant metastases

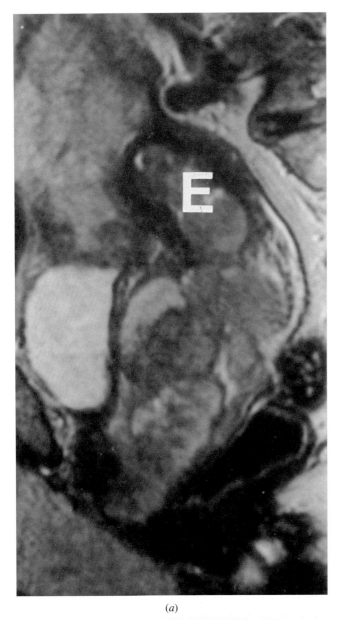

(a)

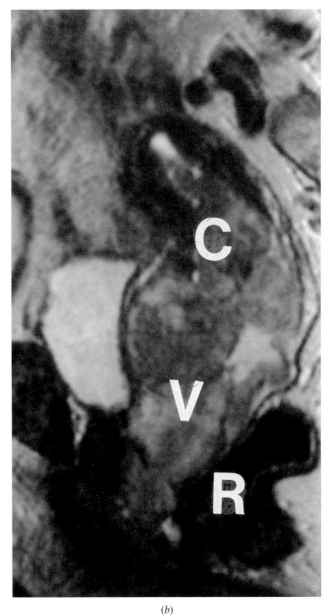

(b)

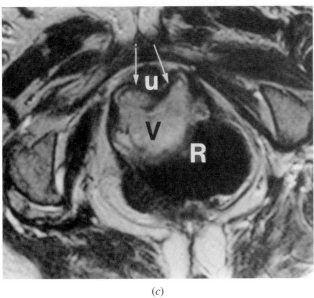

(c)

F I G . 13.20 Vaginal invasion. Sagittal (*a*, *b*) and transverse (*c*) T2-weighted ETSE images, in a 78-year-old woman who has endometrial carcinoma and presents with an introital mass, show distended endometrial (E), cervical (C), and vaginal (V) canals that are filled with solid tumor. Transverse image (*c*) demonstrates that the anterior vaginal wall is intact (white arrows) and the urethra (u) spared. However, the posterior vaginal wall and rectovaginal septum are indistinct, indicating invasive adenocarcinoma.

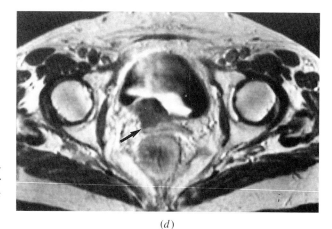

(d)

FIG. 13.20 (*Continued*) Transverse T2-weighted spin-echo image (*d*) in a second patient, who has bladder cancer. The bladder cancer (arrow, *d*) arises from the posterior wall and invades the anterior wall of the vagina.

Miscellaneous

Radiation Change. The appearance of radiation changes of the vagina varies depending on the time interval between therapy and imaging. Acute radiation changes of less than 1 year reflect histologic changes of interstitial edema and capillary leakage. The vaginal wall shows generalized thickening and is high in signal intensity on T2-weighted and gadolinium-enhanced T1-weighted images (fig. 13.24). Chronic changes after more than 1 year result in fibrosis, diminished interstitial fluid, and diminished vascularity. The vaginal wall may become atrophic, has low signal intensity on T2-weighted images, and demonstrates diminished enhancement after gadolinium administration. Necrosis of the vaginal wall with secondary fistula formation can also occur [106, 118, 119].

Fistulas

Fistulas to the vagina occur most commonly in the setting of gynecological malignancy after radiation therapy, hysterectomy, inflammatory bowel disease, or a combination of these. Imaging in the sagittal and transverse planes with T2-weighted and postgadolinium T1-weighted images is important to maximize detection (fig. 13.25). The addition of fat suppression to the T1-weighted images increases the conspicuity of the enhancing sinus tract walls. Vaginal fistulas can be diagnosed with vaginography, contrast enema, and retrograde cystography, but MR imaging has the added advantage of being able to evaluate the surrounding soft tissue structures, which can often determine whether the fistula is caused by benign or malignant disease [120–122].

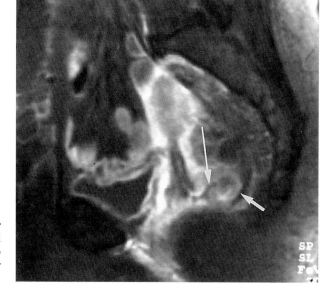

FIG. 13.21 Rectal carcinoma with spread to posterior vaginal fornix. Sagittal immediate postgadolinium fat-suppressed SGE image. A lobulated intermediate-signal intensity mass (arrow) extends from the lower rectum anteriorly to involve the posterior vaginal fornix (long arrow), which appears expanded.

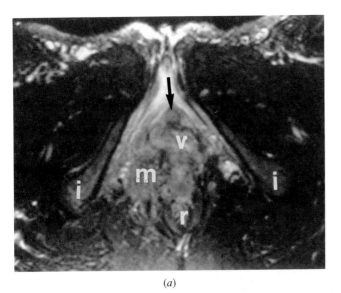

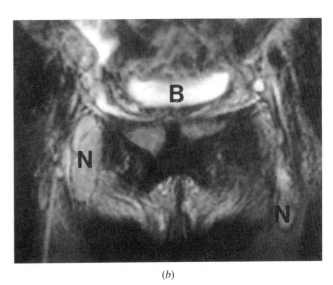

(a)   *(b)*

F I G . 13.22 Invasive squamous cell carcinoma of the vulva. Transverse (*a*) and coronal (*b*) T2-weighted fat-suppressed ETSE images in a 37-year-old woman with history of human papilloma virus infection and condylomata accuminata. There is a heterogeneous mass ("m," *a*) of intermediate to high signal intensity in the perineum with obliteration of the expected location of the normal low-signal intensity anterior rectal wall ("r," *a*) and posterior vaginal wall ("v," *a*). The distal urethra is not involved (arrow, *a*). Coronal image (*b*) shows bilateral inguinal adenopathy ("N," *b*). This image alone is not specific for metastatic adenopathy. The presence of central necrosis within lymph nodes on postcontrast MR and CT images is very specific for malignancy in the setting of squamous cell carcinomas of the pelvis. i = Ischial tuberosities, B = bladder.

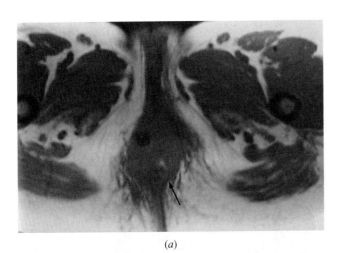

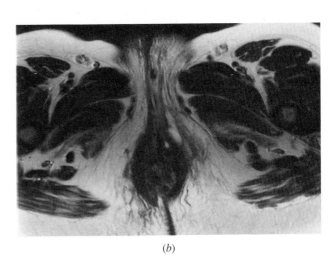

(a)   *(b)*

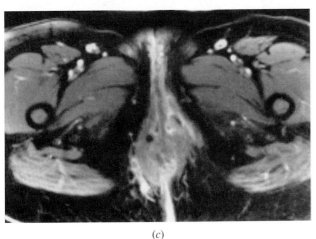

F I G . 13.23 Vulvar carcinoma. Transverse SGE (*a*), 512-resolution T2-weighted echo-train spin-echo (*b*), and 90-s post-gadolinium fat-suppressed SGE (*c*) images. The T1-weighted image (*a*) shows an irregular low-signal intensity mass arising from the vulva with posterior extension to involve the anus (arrow). On the T2-weighted image (*b*), the mass is intermediate in signal intensity. In part, this reflects the high signal intensity of fat on echo-train spin-echo sequences. Heterogeneous enhancement of tumor is seen on postgadolinium imaging (*c*).

(c)

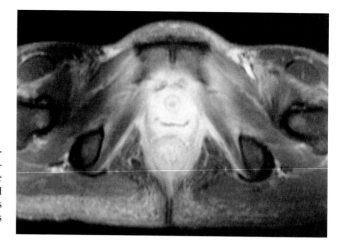

FIG. 13.24 Radiation changes after treatment for vaginal carcinoma. Transverse gadolinium-enhanced T1-weighted fat-suppressed spin-echo image. Enhancing tissue is seen involving the urethra, vagina, and anal canal. Diffuse thickening of the vaginal wall is appreciated. Enhancement from acute radiation changes cannot be easily distinguished from tumor, but symmetric changes favor benign disease.

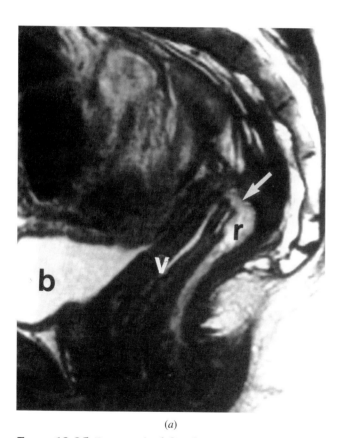

(a)

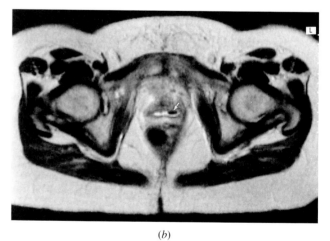

(b)

FIG. 13.25 Rectovaginal fistula. Sagittal T2-weighted ETSE image (*a*) in a 36-year-old woman with history of inflammatory bowel disease and prior subtotal colectomy reveals high-signal intensity content of the fistula (arrow, *a*) that is continuous with the remaining rectal segment ("r," *a*) and the vagina ("v," *a*), b = bladder.

Transverse 512-resolution T2-weighted echo-train spin-echo (*b*), sagittal 512-resolution T2-weighted echo-train spin-echo (*c*), and sagittal 45-s postgadolinium SGE (*d*) images in a second patient who is status posthysterectomy for cervical cancer. A signal-void focus of air is present in the vagina on T2-weighted images (small arrow, *b*, *c*) consistent with a fistulous communication with bowel. The superior aspect of the vagina expands into an abscess cavity (long arrow, *c*), which is well shown on sagittal plane images.

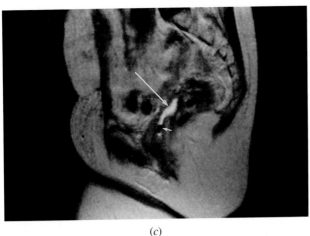

(c)

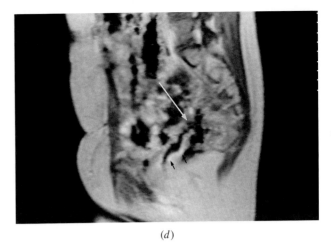

(d)

F i g. 13.25 (*Continued*) The gadolinium-enhanced image shows increased enhancement and thickness of the vaginal wall, which is consistent with inflammatory changes (short arrows, *d*). A fistulous tract is apparent on this sagittal image (long arrow, *d*) in continuity with adjacent bowel.

Conclusion

MRI is the modality of choice for evaluation of vaginal pathology. The noninvasive nature of the test, the lack of ionizing radiation, and its ability to demonstrate the surrounding soft tissue structures make it superior to vaginography for evaluation of congenital abnormalities. Multiplanar capability, high soft tissue contrast, and nonnephrotoxic contrast media make it the examination of choice for evaluation of benign or malignant masses.

REFERENCES

1. Hricak H, Secaf E, Buckley DW, Brown JJ, Tanagho EA, McAninch JW: Female urethra: MR imaging. *Radiology* 1991; 178: 527–535.
2. Moore K: *Clinically Oriented Anatomy.* (2nd ed.) Baltimore: Williams and Wilkens, 1985.
3. Countouris N: [The mucosal zones of the female urethra]. *Urologe A* 1992; 31: 81–84.
4. Siegelman ES, Banner MP, Ramchandani P, Schnall MD: Multicoil MR Imaging of symptomatic female urethral and periurethral disease. *Radiographics* 1997; 17: 349–365.
5. Tan IL, Stoker J, Lameris JS: Magnetic resonance imaging of the female pelvic floor and urethra: Body coil versus endovaginal coil. *Magma* 1997; 5: 59–63.
6. Nurenberg P, Zimmern PE: Role of MR imaging with transrectal coil in the evaluation of complex urethral abnormalities. *Am J Roentgenol* 1997; 169: 1335–1338.
7. Strohbehn K, Quint LE, Prince MR, Wojno KJ, Delancey JO: Magnetic resonance imaging anatomy of the female urethra: A direct histologic comparison. *Obstet Gynecol* 1996; 88: 750–756.
8. Klutke CG, Siegel CL: Functional female pelvic anatomy. *Urol Clin N Am* 1995; 22: 487–498.
9. Sugimura K, Yoshikawa K, Okizuka H, Kaji Y, Ishida T: [Normal female urethra and paraurethral structure—evaluation with MR imaging]. *Nippon Igaku Hoshasen Gakkai Zasshi* 1991; 51: 901–905.
10. Lipson SA, Hricak H: The urinary bladder and female urethra. In: Higgins CB, Hricak H, Helms CA (eds.), *Magnetic Resonance Imaging of the Body.* (3rd ed.) New York: Lippincott-Raven, 1997, p. 929–956.
11. Tempany CMC: Normal magnetic resonance imaging anatomy. In: Tempany CMC (ed.), *MR and Imaging of the Female Pelvis.* Philadelphia: Mosby, 1995, p. 35–54.
12. Yang A, Mostwin J, Genadry R, Saunders R: High resolution magnetic resonance imaging of urethral and periurethral structures using intravaginal surface coil and quadrature phased array surface coil. *Neurourol Urodyn* 1993; 12: 329–330.
13. Bellinger MF, Duckett JW: Accessory phallic urethra in the female patient. *J Urol* 1982; 127: 1159–1164.
14. Ramon J, Mekras JA, Webster GD: Accessory phallic urethra in adult female. *Urology* 1990; 36: 280–282.
15. Nino-Murcia M, Friedland GW, DeVries PA: Congenital anomalies of the papillae, calyces, renal pelvis, ureter, and ureteral orifice. In: Pollack HM, McClennan BL (eds.), *Clinical Urography.* (2nd ed.). Philadelphia: WB Saunders, 2000, vol 1, p. 764–825.
16. Hochhauser L, Alton DJ: Prolapse of an ectopic ureterocele into both urethra and ipsilateral orthotopic ureter. *Pediatr Radiol* 1986; 16: 167–168.
17. Leese T, Osborn DE: Ectopic ureterocele in an adult with prolapse through the urethra. *J Urol* 1985; 133: 269–270.
18. Cornella JL, Larson TR, Lee RA, Magrina JF, Kammerer-Doak D: Leiomyoma of the female urethra and bladder: Report of twenty-three patients and review of the literature. *Am J Obstet Gynecol* 1997; 176: 1278–1285.
19. Leidinger RJ, Das S: Leiomyoma of the female urethra. A report of two cases. *J Reprod Med* 1995; 40: 229–231.
20. Cheng C, Mac-Moune Lai F, Chan PS: Leiomyoma of the female urethra: A case report and review. *J Urol* 1992; 148: 1526–1527.
21. Siegelman SS, Khouri NF, Scott WW Jr., et al.: Pulmonary hamartoma: CT findings. *Radiology* 1986; 160: 313–317.
22. Siegelman ES, Outwater EK: Tissue characterization in the female pelvis by means of MR imaging. *Radiology* 1999; 212: 5–18.
23. Benson RC, Tunca JC, Buchler DA, Uehling DT: Primary carcinoma of the female urethra. *Gynecol Oncol* 1982; 14: 313–318.
24. Hayes WS: The urethra. In: Davidson AJ, Hartman DS (eds.), *Radiology of the kidney and urinary tract.* Philadlephia: W.B. Saunders, 1994, p. 649–667.
25. Narayan P, Konety B: Surgical treatment of female urethral carcinoma. *Urol Clin N Am* 1992; 19: 373–382.

26. Gheiler EL, Tefilli MV, Tiguert R, de Oliveira JG, Pontes JE, Wood DP: Management of primary urethral cancer. *Urology* 1998; 52: 487–493.

27. De Paepe ME, Andre R, Mahadevia P: Urethral involvement in female patients with bladder cancer. A study of 22 cystectomy specimens. *Cancer* 1990; 65: 1237–1241.

28. Dmochowski RR, Ganabathi K, Zimmern PE, Leach GE: Benign female periurethral masses. *J Urol* 1994; 152: 1943–1951.

29. Lee RA: Diverticulum of the urethra: Clinical presentation, diagnosis, and management. *Clin Obstet Gynecol* 1984; 27: 490–498.

30. Khati NJ, Javitt MC, Schwartz AM, Berger BM: MR imaging diagnosis of a urethral diverticulum. *Radiographics* 1998; 18: 517–522.

31. DiSantis SJ: Inflammatory conditons of the urethra. In: Pollack HM, McClennan BL (eds.), *Clinical Urography.* (2nd ed.) Philadelphia: W. B. Saunders, 2000, p. vol 1, 1041–1057.

32. Romanzi LJ, Groutz A, Blaivas JG: Urethral diverticulum in women: Diverse presentations resulting in diagnostic delay and mismanagement. *J Urol* 2000; 164: 428–433.

33. Neitlich JD, Foster HE, Glickman MG, Smith RC: Detection of urethral diverticula in women: Comparison of a high resolution fast spin echo technique with double balloon urethrography. *J Urol* 1998; 159: 408–410.

34. Keefe B, Warshauer DM, Tucker MS, Mittelstaedt CA: Diverticula of the female urethra: Diagnosis by endovaginal and transperineal sonography. *Am J Roentgenol* 1991; 156: 1195–1197.

35. Kim B, Hricak H, Tanagho EA: Diagnosis of urethral diverticula in women: Value of MR imaging. *Am J Roentgenol* 1993; 161: 809–815.

36. Hickey N, Murphy J, Herschorn S: Carcinoma in a urethral diverticulum: Magnetic resonance imaging and sonographic appearance. *Urology* 2000; 55: 588–589.

37. Thomas RB, Maguire B: Adenocarcinoma in a female urethral diverticulum. *Aust NZ J Surg* 1991; 61: 869–871.

38. Blander DS, Broderick GA, Rovner ES: Images in clinical urology. Magnetic resonance imaging of a "saddle bag" urethral diverticulum. *Urology* 1999; 53: 818–819.

39. Daneshgari F, Zimmern PE, Jacomides L: Magnetic resonance imaging detection of symptomatic noncommunicating intraurethral wall diverticula in women. *J Urol* 1999; 161: 1259–1261.

40. Marshall PC, Uson AC, Melicow MM: Neoplasms and caruncles of the female urethra. *Surg Gynecol Obstet* 1960; 110: 723–733.

41. Khatib RA, Khalil AM, Tawil AN, Shamseddine AI, Kaspar HG, Suidan FJ: Non-Hodgkin's lymphoma presenting as a urethral caruncle. *Gynecol Oncol* 1993; 50: 389–393.

42. Narumi Y, Hricak H, Armenakas NA, Dixon CM, McAninch JW: MR imaging of traumatic posterior urethral injury. *Radiology* 1993; 188: 439–443.

43. Dixon CM, Hricak H, McAninch JW: Magnetic resonance imaging of traumatic posterior urethral defects and pelvic crush injuries. *J Urol* 1992; 148: 1162–1165.

44. Maubon AJ, Roux JO, Faix A, Segui B, Ferru JM, Rouanet JP: Penile fracture: MRI demonstration of a urethral tear associated with a rupture of the corpus cavernosum. *Eur Radiol* 1998; 8: 469–470.

45. Comiter CV, Vasavada SP, Barbaric ZL, Gousse AE, Raz S: Grading pelvic prolapse and pelvic floor relaxation using dynamic magnetic resonance imaging. *Urology* 1999; 54: 454–457.

46. Mostwin JL, Yang A, Sanders R, Genadry R: Radiography, sonography, and magnetic resonance imaging for stress incontinence. *Urol Clin N Am* 1995; 22: 539–549.

47. Pannu HK, Kaufman HS, Cundiff GW, Genadry R, Bluemke DA, Fishman EK: Dynamic MR imaging of pelvic organ prolapse: Spectrum of abnormalities. *Radiographics* 2000; 20: 1567–1582.

48. Yang A, Mostwin JL, Rosenshein NB, Zerhouni EA: Pelvic floor descent in women: Dynamic evaluation with fast MR imaging and cinematic display. *Radiology* 1991; 179: 25–33.

49. McGuire EJ, English SF: Periurethral collagen injection for male and female sphincteric incontinence: Indications, techniques, and result. *World J Urol* 1997; 15: 306–309.

50. Maki DD, Banner MP, Ramchandani P, Stolpen A, Rovner ES, Wein AJ: Injected periurethral collagen for postprostatectomy urinary incontinence: MR and CT appearance. *Abdom Imaging* 2000; 25: 658–662.

51. Carr LK, Herschorn S, Leonhardt C: Magnetic resonance imaging after intraurethral collagen injected for stress urinary incontinence. *J Urol* 1996; 155: 1253–1255.

52. Corcos J, Fournier C: Periurethral collagen injection for the treatment of female stress urinary incontinence: 4-year follow-up results. *Urology* 1999; 54: 815–818.

53. Martins FE, Boyd SD: Post-operative risk factors associated with artificial urinary sphincter infection-erosion. *Br J Urol* 1995; 75: 354–358.

54. Kirschner-Hermanns R, Wein B, Niehaus S, Schaefer W, Jakse G: The contribution of magnetic resonance imaging of the pelvic floor to the understanding of urinary incontinence. *Br J Urol* 1993; 72: 715–718.

55. Fielding JR, Griffiths DJ, Versi E, Mulkern RV, Lee ML, Jolesz FA: MR imaging of pelvic floor continence mechanisms in the supine and sitting positions. *Am J Roentgenol* 1998; 171: 1607–1610.

56. Lee RA, Symmonds RE, Williams TJ: Current status of genitourinary fistula. *Obstet Gynecol* 1988; 72: 313–319.

57. Jafri SZH, Roberts JL, Berger BD: Fistulas of the genitourinary tract. In: Pollack HM, McClennan BL (eds.), *Clinical Urography* (2nd ed.) Philadelphia: WB Saunders, 2000, vol 3, p. 2992–3012.

58. Gerber GS, Schoenberg HW: Female urinary tract fistulas [see comments]. *J Urol* 1993; 149: 229–236.

59. Waidelich RM, Brunschweiger SM, Schmeller NT: [Urethrovaginal fistula in Behcet disease.] *Urologe A* 1994; 33: 163–166.

60. Takamatsu H, Noguchi H, Tahara H, et al.: Ano-urethral fistula, a special type of anomaly: Report of two cases. *Surg Today* 1993; 23: 1116–1118.

61. Rousson B, Verzeaux E, Leriche A, Monnet F: [Urethroplasty using polyglactin mesh in urethral fistula caused by decubitus ulcer of the perineum in spinal cord injuries. Apropos of 7 cases.] *Ann Chir Plast Esthet* 1994; 39: 10–14.

62. Siegelman ES, Outwater EK, Banner MP, Ramchandani P, Anderson TL, Schnall MD: High-resolution MR imaging of the vagina. *Radiographics* 1997; 17: 1183–1203.

63. Hopkins KL, Nino-Murcia M, Friedland GW, DeVries PA: Miscellaneous congential anomalies of the genitourinary tract. In: Pollack HM, McClennon BL (eds.), *Clinical Urography.* (2nd ed.) Philadelphia: W. B. Saunders, 2000, vol 1, p. 892–911.

64. Hricak H, Chang YC, Thurnher S: Vagina: Evaluation with MR imaging. Part I. Normal anatomy and congenital anomalies. *Radiology* 1988; 169: 169–174.

65. Gougoutas CA, Siegelman ES, Hunt J, Outwater EK: Pelvic endometriosis: Various manifestations and MR imaging findings. *Am J Roentgenol* 2000; 175: 353–358.

66. Low RN, Barone RM, Lacey C, Sigeti JS, Alzate GD, Sebrechts CP: Peritoneal tumor: MR imaging with dilute oral barium and intravenous gadolinium-containing contrast agents compared with unenhanced MR imaging and CT. *Radiology* 1997; 204: 513–520.

67. Outwater EK, Mitchell DG: Magnetic resonance imaging techniques in the pelvis. *MRI Clin N Am* 1994; 2: 481–488.

68. Smith RC: Magnetic resonance imaging of the female pelvis: Technical considerations. *Top Magn Reson Imaging* 1995; 7: 3–25.

69. Secaf E, Hricak H, Gooding CA, et al.: Role of MRI in the evaluation of ambiguous genitalia. *Pediatr Radiol* 1994; 24: 231–235.

70. Fedele L, Dorta M, Brioschi D, Giudici MN, Candiani GB: Magnetic resonance imaging in Mayer-Rokitansky-Kuster-Hauser syndrome. *Obstet Gynecol* 1990; 76: 593–596.

71. Togashi K, Nishimura K, Itoh K, et al.: Vaginal agenesis: Classification by MR imaging. *Radiology* 1987; 162: 675–677.

72. Carrington BM, Hricak H, Nuruddin RN, Secaf E, Laros RK, Jr., Hill EC: Mullerian duct anomalies: MR imaging evaluation. *Radiology* 1990; 176: 715–720.

73. Reinhold C, Hricak H, Forstner R, et al.: Primary amenorrhea: Evaluation with MR imaging. *Radiology* 1997; 203: 383–390.

74. Fielding FR: MR imaging of Mullerian anomalies: Impact on therapy. *Am J Roentgenol* 1996; 167: 1491–1495.

75. Capraro VJ, Gallego MB: Vaginal agenesis. *Am J Obstet Gynecol* 1976; 124: 98–107.

76. Strubbe EH, Willemsen WN, Lemmens JA, Thijn CJ, Rolland R: Mayer-Rokitansky-Kuster-Hauser syndrome: Distinction between two forms based on excretory urographic, sonographic, and laparoscopic findings. *Am J Roentgenol* 1993; 160: 331–334.

77. Letterie GS: Combined congenital absence of the vagina and cervix. Diagnosis with magnetic resonance imaging and surgical management. *Gynecol Obstet Invest* 1998; 46: 65–67.

78. Lang IM, Babyn P, Oliver GD: MR imaging of paediatric uterovaginal anomalies. *Pediatr Radiol* 1999; 29: 163–170.

79. Rock JA: Anomalous development of the vagina. *Semin Reprod Endocrinol* 1986; 4: 13–31.

80. Tanaka YO, Kurosaki Y, Kobayashi T, et al.: Uterus didelphys associated with obstructed hemivagina and ipsilateral renal agenesis: MR findings in seven cases. *Abdom Imaging* 1998; 23: 437–441.

81. Lin CC, Chen AC, Chen TY: Double uterus with an obstructed hemivagina and ipsilateral renal agenesis: Report of 5 cases and a review of the literature. *J Formos Med Assoc* 1991; 90: 195–201.

82. Niver DH, Barrette G, Jewelewicz R: Congenital atresia of the uterine cervix and vagina: Three cases. *Fertil Steril* 1980; 33: 25–29.

83. Neal MR, Angtuaco TL, Shah HR: Vaginal agenesis. *J Ultrasound Med* 1994; 13: 333–334.

84. Saenger P: Abnormal sex differentiation. *J Pediatr* 1984; 104: 1–17.

85. Gambino J, Caldwell B, Dietrich R, Walot I, Kangarloo H: Congenital disorders of sexual differentiation: MR findings. *Am J Roentgenol* 1992; 158: 363–367.

86. Cheetham DR: Bartholin's cyst: Marsupialization or aspiration? *Am J Obstet Gynecol* 1985; 152: 569–570.

87. Andersen PG, Christensen S, Detlefsen GU, Kern-Hansen P: Treatment of Bartholin's abscess. Marsupialization versus incision, curettage and suture under antibiotic cover. A randomized study with 6 months' follow-up. *Acta Obstet Gynecol Scand* 1992; 71: 59–62.

88. Kier R: Nonovarian gynecologic cysts: MR imaging findings. *Am J Roentgenol* 1992; 158: 1265–1269.

89. Moulopoulos LA, Varma DG, Charnsangavej C, Wallace S: Magnetic resonance imaging and computed tomography appearance of asymptomatic paravaginal cysts. *Clin Imaging* 1993; 17: 126–132.

90. Lee MJ, Yoder IC, Papanicolaou N, Tung GA: Large Gartner duct cyst associated with a solitary crossed ectopic kidney: Imaging features. *J Comput Assist Tomogr* 1991; 15: 149–151.

91. Rosenfeld DL, Lis E: Gartner's duct cyst with a single vaginal ectopic ureter and associated renal dysplasia or agenesis. *J Ultrasound Med* 1993; 12: 775–778.

92. Haley JC, Mirowski GW, Hood AF: Benign vulvar tumors. *Semin Cutan Med Surg* 1998; 17: 196–204.

93. Lazarou G, Goldberg MI: Vulvar arteriovenous hemangioma. A case report. *J Reprod Med* 2000; 45: 439–441.

94. O'Neal MF, Amparo EG: MR demonstration of extensive pelvic involvement in vulvar hemangiomas. *J Comput Assist Tomogr* 1988; 12: 219–221.

95. Saks AM, Paterson FC, Irvine AT, Ayers BA, Burnand KG: Improved MR venography: use of fast short inversion time inversion-recovery technique in evaluation of venous angiomas. *Radiology* 1995; 194: 908–911.

96. Dixit S, Singhal S, Baboo HA: Squamous cell carcinoma of the vagina: A review of 70 cases. *Gynecol Oncol* 1993; 48: 80–87.

97. Piura B, Rabinovich A, Cohen Y, Glezerman M: Primary squamous cell carcinoma of the vagina: Report of four cases and review of the literature. *Eur J Gynaecol Oncol* 1998; 19: 60–63.

98. Merino MJ: Vaginal cancer: The role of infectious and environmental factors. *Am J Obstet Gynecol* 1991; 165: 1255–1262.

99. Herbst AL, Anderson D: Clear cell adenocarcinoma of the vagina and cervix secondary to intrauterine exposure to diethylstilbestrol. *Semin Surg Oncol* 1990; 6: 343–346.

100. Herbst AL, Anderson D: Clear cell adenocarcinoma of cervix and vagina and DES-related abnormalities. In: Coppleson M (ed.), *Gynecologic Oncology*. New York: Churchill Livingstone, 1992, vol 1, p. 523–540.

101. Mittendorf R: Teratogen update: Carcinogenesis and teratogenesis associated with exposure to diethylstilbestrol (DES) in utero. *Teratology* 1995; 51: 435–445.

102. Tsuda K, Murakami T, Kurachi H, et al.: MR imaging of non-squamous vaginal tumors. *Eur Radiol* 1999; 9: 1214–1218.

103. Chang YC, Hricak H, Thurnher S, Lacey CG: Vagina: Evaluation with MR imaging. Part II. Neoplasms. *Radiology* 1988; 169: 175–179.

104. Gilles R, Michel G, Chancelier MD, Vanel D, Masselot J: Case report: clear cell adenocarcinoma of the vagina: MR features. *Br J Radiol* 1993; 66: 168–170.

105. Brown JJ, Gutierrez ED, Lee JK: MR appearance of the normal and abnormal vagina after hysterectomy. *Am J Roentgenol* 1992; 158: 95–99.

106. Blomlie V, Rofstad EK, Tvera K, Lien HH: Noncritical soft tissues of the female pelvis: Serial MR imaging before, during, and after radiation therapy. *Radiology* 1996; 199: 461–468.

107. McNicholas MM, Fennelly JJ, MacErlaine DP: Imaging of primary vaginal lymphoma. *Clin Radiol* 1994; 49: 130–132.

108. Moon WK, Kim SH, Han MC: MR findings of malignant melanoma of the vagina. *Clin Radiol* 1993; 48: 326–328.

109. Piura B, Rabinovich A, Dgani R: Malignant melanoma of the vulva: Report of six cases and review of the literature. *Eur J Gynaecol Oncol* 1999; 20: 182–186.

110. Enochs WS, Petherick P, Bogdanova A, Mohr U, Weissleder R: Paramagnetic metal scavenging by melanin: MR imaging. *Radiology* 1997; 204: 417–423.

111. Murase E, Siegelman ES, Outwater EK, Perez-Jaffe LA, Tureck RW: Uterine leiomyomas: Histopathologic features, MR imaging findings, differential diagnosis, and treatment. *Radiographics* 1999; 19: 1179–1197.

112. Outwater EK: CT and MRI of neoplasms metastatic to the genital tract. In: Andersen JC (ed.), *Gynecologic Imaging*. London: Churchill LIvingstone, 1999, p. 519–534.

113. Morgan MA, Mikuta JJ: Surgical management of vulvar cancer. *Semin Surg Oncol* 1999; 17: 168–172.

114. Hacker NF: Radical resection of vulvar malignancies: A paradigm shift in surgical approaches. *Curr Opin Obstet Gynecol* 1999; 11: 61–64.

115. Outwater EK, Marchetto BE, Wagner BJ, Siegelman ES: Aggressive angiomyxoma: Findings on CT and MR imaging. *Am J Roentgenol* 1999; 172: 435–538.

116. DePasquale SE, McGuinness TB, Mangan CE, Husson M, Woodland MB: Adenoid cystic carcinoma of Bartholin's gland:

A review of the literature and report of a patient. *Gynecol Oncol* 1996; 61: 122–125.

117. Duun S: Adenoid cystic carcinoma of Bartholin's gland—a review of the literature and report of a patient. *Acta Obstet Gynecol Scand* 1995; 74: 78–80.

118. Blomlie V, Rofstad EK, Trope C, Lien HH: Critical soft tissues of the female pelvis: Serial MR imaging before, during, and after radiation therapy. *Radiology* 1997; 203: 391–397.

119. Grigsby PW, Russell A, Bruner D, et al.: Late injury of cancer therapy on the female reproductive tract. *Int J Radiat Oncol Biol Phys* 1995; 31: 1281–1299.

120. Healy JC, Phillips RR, Reznek RH, Crawford RA, Armstrong P, Shepherd JH: The MR appearance of vaginal fistulas. *Am J Roentgenol* 1996; 167: 1487–1489.

121. Outwater E, Schiebler ML: Pelvic fistulas: findings on MR images. *Am J Roentgenol* 1993; 160: 327–330.

122. Semelka RC, Hricak H, Kim B, et al.: Pelvic fistula: appearances on MR images. *Abdom Imaging* 1997; 22: 91–95.

123. Yang WT, Lam WW, Yu MY, Cheung TH, Metreweli C: Comparison of dynamic helical CT and dynamic MR imaging in the evaluation of pelvic lymph nodes in cervical carcinoma. *Am J Roentgenol* 2000; 175: 759–766.

CHAPTER 14

UTERUS AND CERVIX

RAHEL A. KUBIK-HUCH, M.D., CAROLINE REINHOLD, M.D.,
RICHARD C. SEMELKA, M.D., SVEN C. A. MICHEL, M.D.,
AND MONICA S. PEDRO, M.D.

INTRODUCTION

Because of recent technical developments including the advent of fast pulse sequences and phased-array multicoil technology, magnetic resonance imaging (MRI) is gaining increasing importance for the imaging of the cervix and uterus. In benign conditions, for example, congenital müllerian duct anomalies or leiomyoma, endovaginal ultrasound remains the primary imaging modality. The role of MRI is limited to that of a problem-solving tool in patients for whom the ultrasound examination is not feasible, inconclusive, or technically suboptimal. However, MRI has been shown to be the modality of choice for preoperative characterization and staging of gynecologic tumors, especially for the preoperative assessment of endometrial and cervical carcinoma.

MRI does not employ ionizing radiation, and there is no evidence of teratogenic or other adverse fetal effects [1–5]. The technique is thus well suited for imaging women of reproductive age and especially for pregnant women, for example, for MR pelvimetry, assessment of maternal complications during pregnancy, and, because of technical advances in ultrafast imaging techniques, more recently for fetal imaging.

MRI TECHNIQUE

Patient Preparation

For imaging the cervix and uterus no special patient preparation is required. A tampon should not be routinely applied by the patient. On occasion, the presence of tampon may aid tumor staging and diagnosis of recurrent disease because of improved delineation of the vaginal lumen (fig. 14.1).

Immediately before the examination, the patient should be asked to void. This minimizes "ghosting" in the phase-encoding direction, namely, artifacts of the distended urinary bladder induced by motion of the patient. Furthermore, in the setting of an overly distended urinary bladder, the fundus of the uterus will be displaced superiorly. Not only does this frequently bring it into close contact with small bowel, resulting in artifacts from intestinal peristalsis, but uterine compression may alter the appearance of normal and pathological structures and the normally visible fat plane between the uterus and urinary bladder—an important criteria to exclude tumor invasion of the bladder wall in gynecologic tumor staging—might be obliterated.

The usual contraindications to MRI also apply to examinations of the uterus. The presence of orthopedic

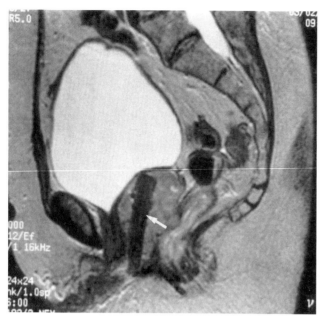

FIG. 14.1 Patient preparation: Tampon. T2-weighted ETSE image. A tampon (arrow) was applied in this patient with a history of hysterectomy and recurrent cervical carcinoma to improve delineation of the vaginal lumen to define the perivaginal tumor extension.

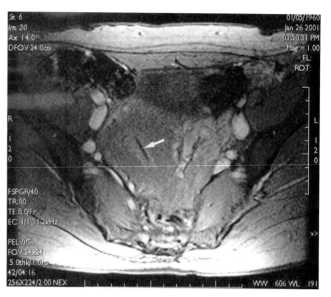

FIG. 14.2 Intrauterine contraceptive device. T1-weighted SGE image. A correctly positioned IUD is shown as a low-signal intensity linear structure within the endometrial cavity (arrow), which could not be delineated on spin-echo images (not shown). Patients with IUD are safely imaged by MRI. Most IUDs, as in this case, do not cause sufficient signal loss to render the examination of the uterus nondiagnostic.

devices, although not hazardous to the patient, can impair image quality. Extensive signal loss is usually present at the site of a metallic device. In patients with a hip prosthesis, the signal loss may extend as far across as the midpelvis. To minimize magnetic susceptibility artifacts, spin-echo sequences should be favored over gradient-echo sequences in these cases. In particular, the single-shot echo-train spin-echo (SS-ETSE) sequence is very resistent to magnetic susceptibility artifacts from hip protheses, rendering it the optimal MR or CT approach for evaluating the pelvis in patients with these devices.

Patients with intrauterine contraceptive devices (IUD) are safely imaged. The device usually demonstrates a signal void on T1- and T2-weighted sequences, which is most prominent on gradient-echo imaging (fig. 14.2). Most IUDs do not cause signal loss sufficient to render the examination of the uterus nondiagnostic. No deflection, turning motion, or temperature change has been observed when exposing a copper IUD to a magnetic field, and according to the literature there appears to be no reason to exclude women with IUDs from MR imaging [6].

In selected cases, gastrointestinal motion may cause significant imaging degradation in the pelvis by obscuring the tissue planes of the urinary bladder, rectum, and female genital organs. Although this problem has currently been largely overcome with the advent of faster sequences and compensation techniques, artifacts from peristalsis can be further diminished by the prescan

administration of glucagon, if needed. A routine 5- to 6-hour fast before scanning is usually sufficient to minimize artifacts from peristalsis.

Surface Coils

Examinations are usually performed in the supine position. To obtain high-quality images, a pelvic phased-array coil should be used routinely if available. In obese or pregnant patients, better results are usually achieved without the use of a phased-array coil, as signal loss in the center of the patient may create excessive signal variation across the image.

Multicoil ("phased array") arrangements use multiple separate receiver coils simultaneously acquiring and subsequently combining data. This means that the signal from each receiver is separately transformed and generates separate data sets being reconstructed into a single composite image. This technique allows for the inclusion of a larger area, but with the same signal-to-noise ratio of a smaller-diameter coil [7, 8].

Endoluminal surface coils further increase the signal-to-noise ratio. Whereas endorectal coils have been shown to be useful in imaging the prostate, neither endorectal nor endovaginal coils are routinely used for imaging of the uterus [9–13]. They would also add significant cost to the MRI examination. Furthermore, it has been shown in one prior report that accuracy of overall staging in patients with cervical carcinoma was not improved with their use [14].

Imaging Protocol

Pulse Sequences and Imaging Planes

T1- and T2-weighted sequences are standard techniques for evaluating the uterine corpus and cervix. Transverse and sagittal T2-weighted echo-train spin-echo images are most important for the assessment of normal MR anatomy, for example, the uterine zonal anatomy, as well as the depiction of pathology.

Sagittal sections image the uterus in its long axis. In addition, the cervix, including the pars vaginalis and the posterior vaginal fornix, is well demonstrated in this plane on T2-weighted sequences. On sagittal images, the bladder, rectum, and pouch of Douglas are all visualized in a single plane of section. Fat suppression may not be of value for sagittal T2-weighted sequences, because the hyperintense fat planes between urinary bladder and uterus and uterus and rectum are removed. The visualization of these fat planes is an important criterion for staging of gynecologic tumors and for localizing masses to their organ of origin. Fat suppression may at times be used on transverse T2-weighted sequences. Transverse sections demonstrate the uterus and cervix, as well as the parametrium. They are also most commonly used to detect the presence of lymphadenopathy. Coronal sections, although very helpful for the depiction of ovarian pathologies, are not routinely used for imaging of the uterus.

In specific instances, off-axis imaging planes may be helpful; for example, an oblique transverse section parallel to the endometrium results in a long-axis view, which is ideal for imaging the fundal contour in congenital uterine anomalies (fig. 14.3). An oblique section obtained perpendicular to the cervical canal results in a short-axis view and allows accurate assessment of cervical zonal anatomy, such as cervical carcinoma staging [15].

T1-weighted sequences maximize the image contrast between muscle and fat and are helpful for the detection of enlarged pelvic lymph nodes. In addition, the demonstration of hemorrhage or fat within a lesion benefits from acquiring T1-weighted images.

Gadolinium-enhanced T1-weighted sequences (fig. 14.4) are recommended for evaluating the endometrium and staging endometrial carcinoma, being most useful in evaluating the depth of endometrial tumor invasion. They are not needed for most benign uterine conditions and are not routinely performed in cervical carcinoma [16–20]. For detailed fetal imaging, evaluation is best performed with fast T2-weighted imaging, such as T2-weighted single-shot echo-train spin-echo, half-Fourier single-shot echo-train spin-echo, and 0.5-signal acquired single-shot echo-train spin-echo sequences [21]. Images are acquired according to maternal or fetal position in the transverse, coronal,

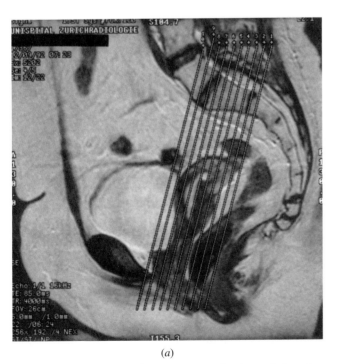

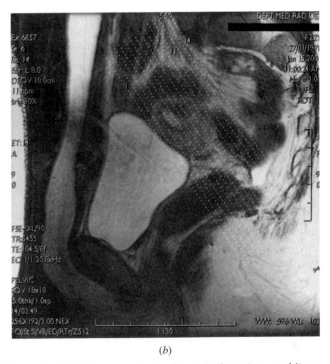

(a)　　　　　　　　　　　　　　　　　　(b)

F I G . 14.3 Imaging planes: Long-axis view of the uterus. T2-weighted ETSE image (*a*). On the sagittal section an oblique imaging plane parallel to the endometrium is prescribed graphically in this patient with a retroverted uterus.

T2-weighted ETSE (*b, c*) in a second patient. On the sagittal section an oblique imaging plane parallel to the endometrium is prescribed graphically in this patient with an anteverted uterus and suspected congenital uterine malformation.

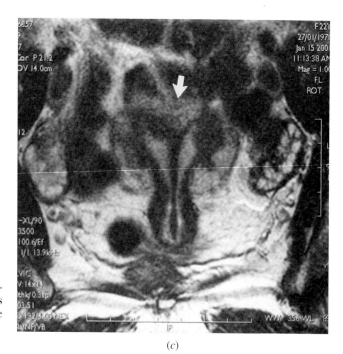

(c)

FIG. 14.3 (*Continued*) The resultant image (*c*) shows the outward convexity of the fundal contour (arrow, *c*) as well as a fibrous septum extending the full length of the uterine cavity into the cervix in this patient with a septate uterus.

and sagittal planes. Image acquisition is sequential with acquisition time for each individual image being under 1 s, yielding excellent image quality devoid of motion artifacts [21–27]. If needed, T1-weighted imaging can be obtained with conventional spin-echo or breath-hold spoiled gradient-echo sequences. These sequences are, however, slower and thus more susceptible to motion

artifacts [21]. Patients are imaged in the supine position. To alleviate patient discomfort, MRI during the late third trimester might also be performed in an oblique or decubitus position. Depending on the age of gestation at the time of MRI, and thus maternal abdominal circumference, a pelvic phased array, a torso coil or—in the third trimester—even the body coil will be used.

NORMAL ANATOMY AND CHANGES WITH MENSTRUAL CYCLE/ MENOPAUSE

Uterine Corpus

The uterus is divided into three major segments, 1) the fundus, 2) the body or corpus, and 3) the cervix. In women of reproductive age the entire uterus measures 6–9 cm in length with the uterine corpus measuring 4–6 cm and the cervix 2.5–3.2 cm. The uterus measures approximately 4 cm in thickness and 6 cm in its maximal transverse dimension [28, 29]. Histologically, the uterine corpus is divided into three tissue layers, 1) the serosa, which consists of the peritoneum, 2) the myometrium, consisting of smooth muscle, and 3) the endometrium.

On MRI, the uterus is best depicted on T2-weighted sagittal images. On T1-weighted images, the zonal anatomy of the uterine corpus is usually not apparent. On T2-weighted imaging three distinct zones can be recognized in women of reproductive age: 1) A high-signal intensity central stripe representing the normal

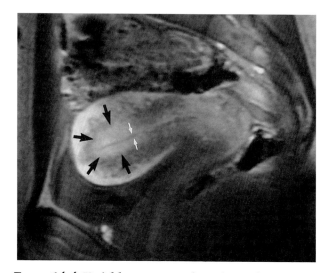

FIG. 14.4 Variable patterns of uterine enhancement. Sagittal gadolinium-enhanced fat-suppressed SGE image. Early enhancement of the inner myometrium may be observed during the menstrual phase. The endometrial stripe is thin and hypointense (small arrows). There is early enhancement of the junctional zone (arrows) relative to the outer myometrium.

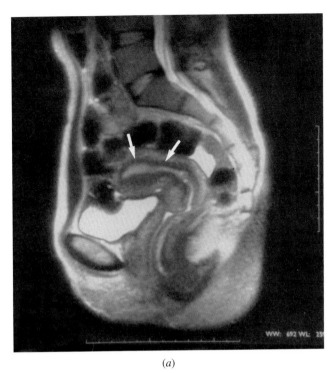

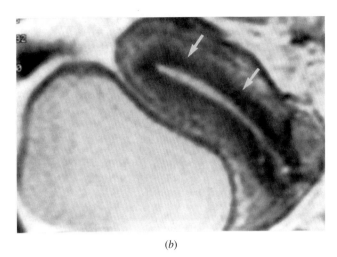

(*a*)   (*b*)

F I G . 14.5 Zonal anatomy of the uterine corpus. Sagittal T2-weighted ETSE images (*a*, *b*) in 2 different patients. The central, high-signal intensity stripe represents the endometrium. The band of low signal intensity subjacent to the endometrial stripe represents the inner myometrium, termed junctional zone (JZ) (arrows, *a*, *b*). The outer layer of the myometrium is of intermediate signal intensity.

endometrium and secretions within the endometrial cavity; 2) the junctional zone, a band of low-signal intensity tissue, histologically corresponding to the innermost layer of the myometrium, and 3) the outer layer of the myometrium of intermediate signal intensity [28–30] (figs. 14.5 and 14.6).

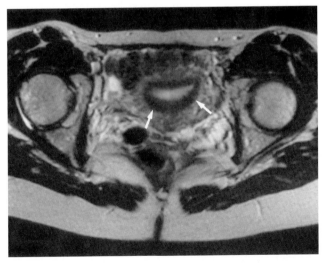

F I G . 14.6 Short-axis view of the uterus. T2-weighted ETSE image. The zonal anatomy is well depicted: hyperintense endometrium; junctional zone (arrows), representing the innermost part of the myometrium, of low signal intensity; and the myometrium of intermediate signal intensity.

The endometrium occupies the central portion of the uterus. Endometrial thickness varies with the menstrual cycle, being thinnest at time of menstruation. The endometrium increases in width rapidly during the follicular or proliferative phase and continues to increase during the secretory phase, although at a slower rate [31]. The thickness of the endometrial stripe is reported to vary widely with averages of 3–6 mm in the follicular phase and 5–13 mm during the secretory phase (figs. 14.7 and 14.8) [29, 32–34]. The low-signal intensity junctional zone is seen immediately subjacent to the endometrial stripe (figs. 14.5 and 14.6). This zone has no actual anatomic correlate but has been shown to represent the innermost layer of the myometrium [35–37]. The histologic basis for the low signal intensity of the junctional zone has not yet been definitely established, but a number of factors are likely to contribute to this imaging appearance. McCarthy et al. [35] found that the water content of the junctional zone was significantly lower than that of the endometrium and outer myometrium. Brown et al. [37] hypothesized that the compact smooth muscle bundles, as well as the orientation of the fibers within the junctional zone, may contribute to the low signal on T2-weighted images. The group of Scoutt et al. [38] found a threefold increase in percentage of nuclear area in the junctional zone in comparison with the outer myometrium, reflecting an increase in both size and number of nuclei. Considerable variation in

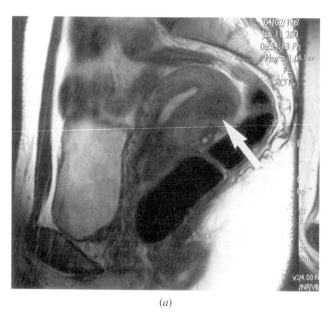

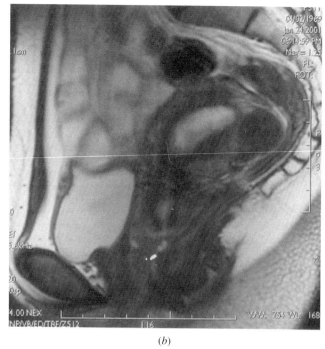

(a)   (b)

FIG. 14.7 Physiological changes during menstrual cycle in a 32-year-old woman. Sagittal T2-weighted ETSE (*a, b*) images at different phases of the menstrual cycle. Retroverted uterus with a small hypointense intramural leiomyoma (large arrow, *a*) is apparent. During the follicular phase (day 5) (*a*), the high-signal intensity endometrial stripe is thin. During the secretory phase (day 18) (*b*), the endometrial stripe widens considerably and the endometrial complex and myometrium show increased signal intensity.

the normal thickness of the junctional zone has been reported, with a mean thickness ranging from 2 to 8 mm [28, 37]. During the menstrual phase, intense early enhancement of the junctional zone may be observed at dynamic gadolinium-enhanced SGE imaging [39].

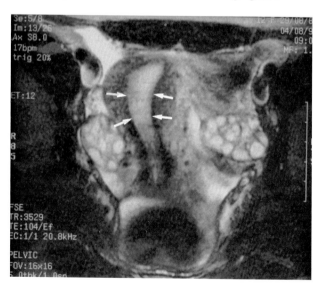

FIG. 14.8 Hormonal overstimulation syndrome in 14-year-old female patient presenting with primary amenorrhea. Transverse T2-weighted fat-suppressed ETSE image. A wide endometrial stripe is seen (arrows). The junctional zone can be well delineated. There are also multiple cysts of similar size in both ovaries as well as fluid in the pouch of Douglas.

The outer layer of the myometrium is of intermediate signal intensity on T2-weighted images and increases in signal intensity in the midsecretory phase. During the menstrual cycle, the thickness of the myometrium increases slightly and is greatest during the secretory phase [31].

On precontrast and gadolinium-enhanced T1-weighted images, the difference in contrast between the various uterine layers is considerably less apparent than on T2-weighted sequences, and frequently the uterine zonal anatomy is completely obscured [40]. On gadolinium-enhanced images, the appreciation of the zonal anatomy can be observed within 1 min after injection however.

In postmenopausal women, the uterus is small and the zonal anatomy is indistinct. The signal intensity of the myometrium on T2-weighted sequences is decreased compared to the uteri of premenopausal females, and the junctional zone is not consistently visualized.

On T2-weighted sequences the endometrial stripe can be identified as a thin, hyperintense structure. The use of exogenous hormones does result in preservation of zonal anatomy in postmenopausal women. A maximal endometrial thickness of 3 mm in women not receiving exogenous hormones and a thickness of 4–6 mm in women receiving hormonal replacement therapy has been reported on MRI [30, 32, 41].

Cervix

The cervix is separated from the corpus of the uterus by the internal os, which corresponds to a slight constriction visible externally and at which level the uterine vessels enter the uterus. On high-resolution T2-weighted sequences the cervix demonstrates three to four distinct zones. Centrally, in many cases, a hyperintense zone representing the mucus within the endocervical canal can be seen. This is followed by an inner area of high signal intensity representing the endocervix, which is composed of columnar epithelium as well as central mucus. The combined thickness of the endocervical canal and mucosa on conventional T2-weighted spin-echo images ranges from 2 to 3 mm. Surrounding the endocervix is the hypointense fibrous stroma of the cervix of 3–8 mm thickness, which has a high concentration of elastic fibrous tissue. Smooth muscle strands predominate toward the periphery of the cervix. This layer is continuous with the outer myometrium of the uterine corpus and appears of medium signal (fig. 14.9). In contrast to the zonal anatomy of the uterus, the MRI appearance of the cervical zonal anatomy does not appear to vary with the hormonal status of women. The signal intensity of the cervical fibrous stroma does alter late in the third trimester of pregnancy, changing from low signal to high signal, as described below. On T1-weighted precontrast images the zonal anatomy of the cervix usually is not apparent. After gadolinium administration, the endocervical mucosa enhances rapidly, whereas the stroma shows more gradual enhancement. The fibrous stroma enhances at a slower rate relative to the outer zone of smooth muscle [9, 42].

Parametrium

The parametrium is located between the layers of the broad ligament adjacent to the lateral margins of the uterine corpus and cervix. It may serve as pathways for local spread of disease, for example, tumor extension of cervical carcinoma. The parametrium is composed largely of loose connective tissue and contains a high number of blood and lymphatic vessels. It is usually of intermediate signal intensity on T1-weighted sequences and iso- or hyperintense to fat on T2-weighted sequences. On postgadolinium images, intense enhancement of the parametrium is noted [43].

Exogenous Hormone Therapy

In addition to reproductive status and age, the MR appearance of the uterus is affected by exogenous hormones. With prolonged use of oral contraceptives a decrease in uterine size may be seen; the endometrial thickness averages 2 mm, and negligible variation with

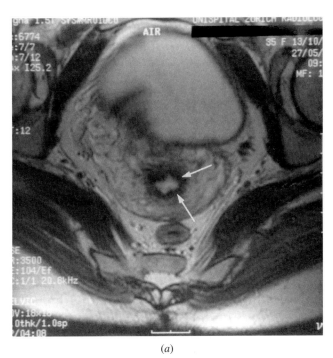
(a)

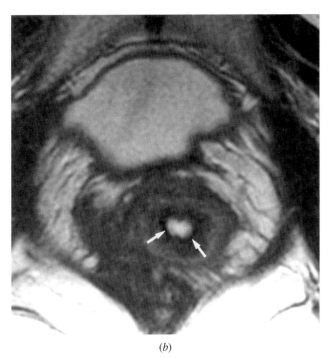
(b)

F I G . 14.9 Zonal anatomy of the cervix. Transverse-oblique T2-weighted ETSE images (a, b) in 2 patients. A thin hypointense fibrous cervical stroma (arrows a, b) is seen surrounding a high-signal intensity central area representing the cervical mucosa and some cervical mucus.

the course of the menstrual cycle is seen. The junctional zone is less prominent, and the signal intensity of the myometrium on T2-weighted images is increased, compared with women who do not use oral contraceptives [29, 32].

Tamoxifen is an orally administered nonsteroidal antiestrogen that is widely used as an adjuvant therapy in women with breast carcinoma. In addition to its antiestrogen effects on breast tissue, tamoxifen acts as a weak estrogen agonist on the postmenopausal endometrium of the uterus and may thus cause adverse effects at the uterine level. A spectrum of endometrial abnormalities has been reported in patients receiving tamoxifen therapy, including proliferative changes, hyperplasia, polyps, and carcinoma [44–46]. Currently, no definitive screening guidelines for monitoring patients on tamoxifen therapy have been established, but a combination of endovaginal ultrasound and endometrial sampling is most frequently used [47]. The role of MRI in evaluating this group of patients is under development. At MR imaging, two different imaging patterns have been described: 1) homogenously hyper-intense endometrium on T2-weighted images with a mean thickness of 0.5 mm, combined with enhancement of the endometrial-myometrial interface and signal-void endometrial cavity on gadolinium-enhanced images, and 2) heterogeneous, widened endometrium (mean thickness 1.8 cm) on T2-weighted images combined with enhancement of the endometrial-myometrial interface and a latticelike enhancement, circumscribing well-defined cystic spaces on gadolinium-enhanced images. (fig. 14.10)

CONGENITAL UTERINE ANOMALIES

Müllerian Duct Anomalies

The incidence of congenital müllerian duct anomalies (MDA) among women of reproductive age is estimated to be up to 0.5%. Congenital uterine anomalies result from either nondevelopment, or partial or complete nonfusion of the müllerian ducts. Failure of the paired müllerian ducts to develop results in various degrees

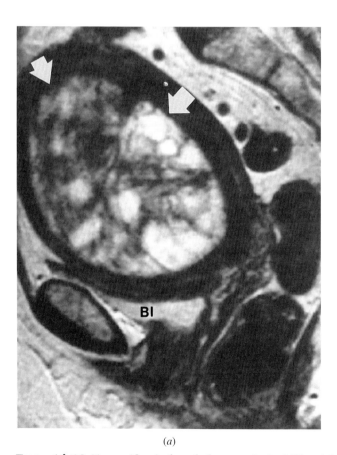

(a)

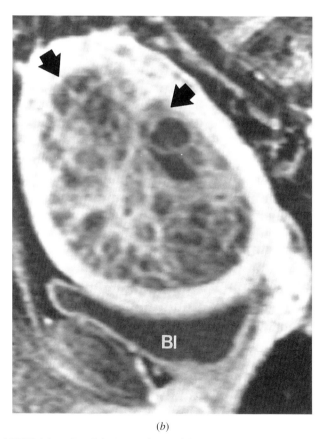

(b)

F I G . 14.10 Tamoxifen-induced changes. Sagittal T2-weighted ETSE (*a*) and gadolinium-enhanced fat-suppressed SGE (*b*) images. The endometrial complex is markedly enlarged (arrows, *a, b*) and shows heterogeneous signal intensity. A latticelike pattern of enhancement is present. A benign polyp was found at histopathology. Bl, bladder.

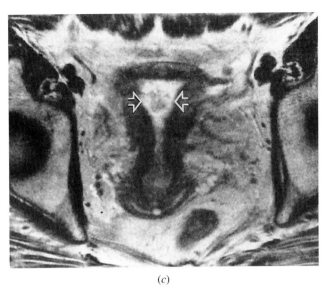

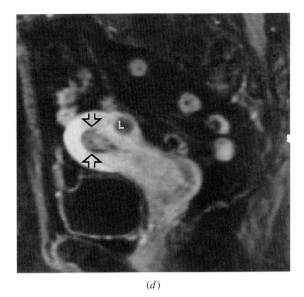

(c)   (d)

F I G. 14.10 (*Continued*) Transverse T2-weighted ETSE (*c*) and sagittal gadolinium-enhanced fat-suppressed SGE (*d*) images in a second patient show heterogeneous signal intensity of the endometrial complex (open arrows, *c*). Gadolinium-enhanced fat-suppressed image demonstrates a latticelike pattern of enhancement traversing the endometrial canal, which is consistent with a polyp (open arrows). L, leiomyoma.

of uterine, cervical, and vaginal agenesis. Didelphic or bicornuate uteri result from absent or incomplete fusion of the uterine horns, respectively. Finally, if fusion does occur but is followed by absent or incomplete resorption of the septum between müllerian duct components, a septate uterus will result. Because of the proximity of the müllerian and wolffian systems embryologically, MDAs are frequently associated with urinary tract anomalies, particularly renal agenesis or ectopia [48].

Many of these uterine anomalies are entirely asymptomatic, but they can be associated with primary amenorrhea, menstrual disorders, impaired fertility, and problems during pregnancy, including recurrent miscarriage, premature labor, or intrauterine growth retardation.

Transvaginal ultrasound, hysterosalpingography (HSG), and laparoscopy are the mainstays for diagnosis of these malformations. HSG, however, has several limitations in classifying patients with uterine anomalies. First, only horns that communicate with the main endometrial cavity are opacified. Second, the external contour of the uterus cannot be evaluated, thereby limiting accurate differentiation between bicornuate and septate uteri. MRI is currently used as a problem-solving modality in cases inconclusive at US and HSG, in teenage girls in whom transvaginal ultrasound is not desirable or in patients with multiple and complex abnormalities. In patients undergoing MRI for suspected MDA, it is advisable to perform a screening coronal T1-weighted sequence (e.g., SGE) to evaluate for renal agenesis or ectopia [49, 50]. MR hysterosalpingogra-

phy is at present still in an experimental state but might become a promising technique as an adjunct to conventional MR pelvic imaging in the future [51].

The treatment options for different uterine anomalies vary considerably, and accurate preoperative diagnosis is essential for appropriate patient management. The classification proposed by Buttram and Gibbons, which divides anomalies into classes with similar clinical features, prognoses, and treatment options, is widely used (fig. 14.11). Five different classes can be distinguished: **Class I: segmental agenesis or hypoplasia** (vaginal, cervical, fundal, tubal, or combined), **class II: unicornuate uterus** (with or without rudimentary horn), **class III: uterus didelphys, class IV: bicornuate uterus** (complete division down to internal os, partial division, arcuate uterus), and **class V: septate uterus** (complete or incomplete) [52]. It should, however, be emphasized that congenital anomalies represent a spectrum of disorders rather than discrete entities, and thus not all malformations can be classified into one particular class.

MR appearance of MDAs

Class I: Uterine agenesis or hypoplasia is the result of non-development or rudimentary development of the müllerian ducts. It may occur as part of a congenital syndrome or as a result of chromosomal defects (figs. 14.12 and 14.13). Sagittal T2-weighted sequences are best suited for documenting the absence or hypoplasia of the uterus [50].

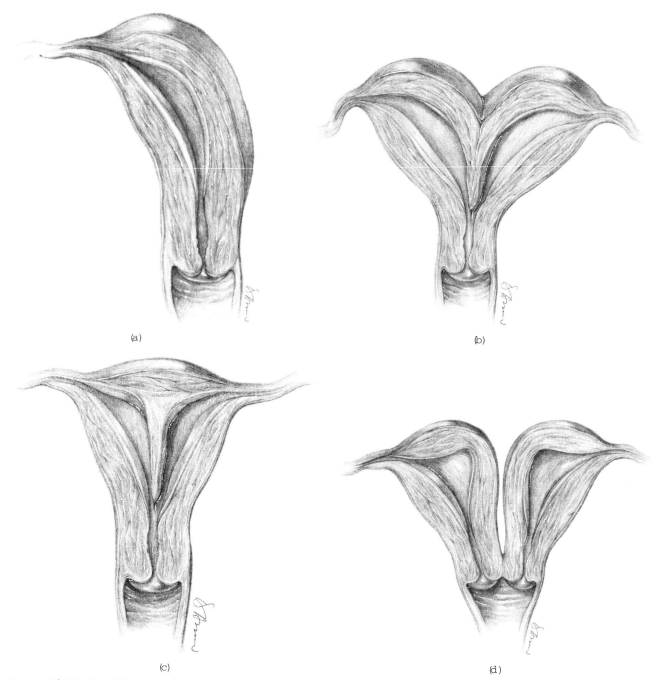

(a)

(b)

(c)

(d)

FIG. 14.11 Classification of uterine anomalies. (*a*) unicornuate uterus (*b*) bicornuate uterus (*c*) septate uterus (*d*) uterus didelphys.

The most common type of class I MDA is the combined form, as seen in patients with Mayer-Rokitansky-Küster-Hauser syndrome. In patients with this syndrome, the presence of vaginal agenesis or hypoplasia with intact ovaries and fallopian tubes is accompanied by variable anomalies of the uterus, urinary tract, and skeletal system. Primary amenorrhea is the presenting symptom in these patients (fig. 14.14) [53, 54].

Class II: An unicornuate uterus is characterized on MRI by its elongated, curved, banana-shaped configuration as the result of non-development or rudimentary development of one müllerian duct. The unicornuate uterus demonstrates normal zonal anatomy on T2-weighted images, but the overall uterine volume is reduced (fig. 14.15). When there is incomplete development of the second müllerian duct, a rudimentary horn

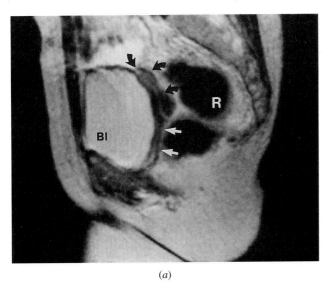

(a)

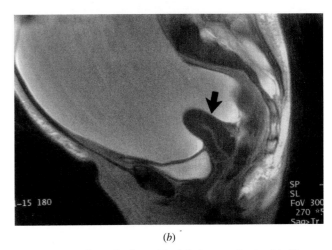

(b)

FIG. 14.12 Gonadal dysgenesis. Sagittal T2-weighted spin-echo image (*a*) through the midpelvis in a patient with Turner syndrome. There is uterine hypoplasia (curved arrows) with a uterus-to-cervix ratio of 1 to 1. Vaginal hypoplasia (arrows) is also noted. Ovaries were not identified. Bl, bladder; R, rectum. (Reprinted with permission from Reinhold C, Hricak H, Forstner R, et al.: Primary amenorrhea: Evaluation with MR imaging. *Radiology* 203(2): 383–390,1997.)

Sagittal T2-weighted ETSE (*b*) image in a second patient, who has Noonan syndrome, demonstrates uterine hypoplasia (arrow, *b*). Note also the large-volume ascites secondary to cirrhosis.

is seen that may or may not contain endometrium. T2-weighted short- and long-axis views, as well as parasagittal sections, are used to image the rudimentary horn. The presence or absence of the hyperintense endometrial stripe, and its continuity with the main uterine cavity, can be accurately determined with MRI [49, 50, 55].

Class III: Uterus didelphys is diagnosed at MRI when two separate normal-sized uteri and cervices are seen. Although a septate vagina may be seen with any of the MDAs, it is most commonly associated with uterus didelphys (fig. 14.16). When transverse, the septum can obstruct the outflow of blood from the vagina and result in hematocolpometra (fig. 14.17). In these cases, MRI demonstrates a distended vagina and uterine horn

whose contents follow the signal characteristics of blood on T1- and T2-weighted sequences [49, 50].

Class IV: The diagnosis of bicornuate uterus on MRI requires two criteria: 1) divergent uterine horns with an intercornual distance exceeding 4 cm divided by a septum that consist of low-signal intensity fibrous tissue in addition to intermediate-signal intensity myometrium on T2-weighted images and 2) an identation of the fundal contour or external fundal cleft measuring more than 1 cm in depth (figs. 14.18–14.20). In addition to standard MRI planes, a long-axis view of the uterus should be obtained. The septum of a bicornuate uterus may terminate at the level of the internal os (uterus bicornuate unicollis) or extend down to the external os (uterus bicornuate bicollis). At times it may be difficult to

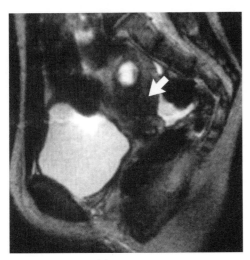

(a)

FIG. 14.13 Cervical atresia. Sagittal (*a*) and transverse (*b, c*) T2-weighted ETSE images.

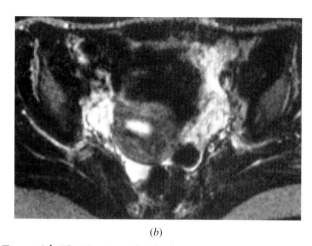

(b)

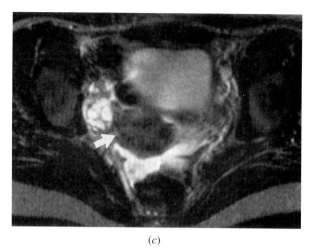

(c)

F I G . 14.13 *(Continued)* The lower uterine and cervical canals are atretic as evidenced by lack of central high signal intensity on sagittal (arrow, *a*) and transverse (arrow, *c*) images. The upper endometrial canal is expanded and fluid filled secondary to the obstruction (*b*).

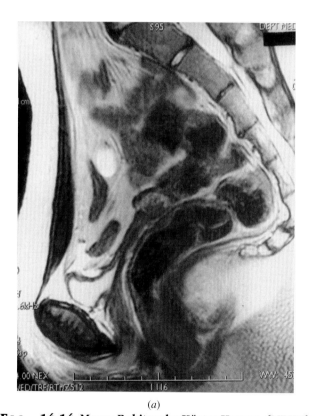

(a)

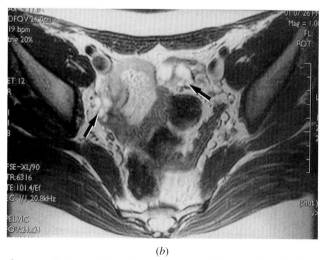

(b)

F I G . 14.14 Mayer-Rokitansky-Küster-Hauser (MRKH) syndrome. Sagittal (*a*) and transverse (*b*) T2-weighted ETSE, coronal T2-weighted fat-suppressed ETSE (*c*, *d*) and T1-weighted SGE (*e*) images in a 16-year-old patient presenting with primary amenorrhea.

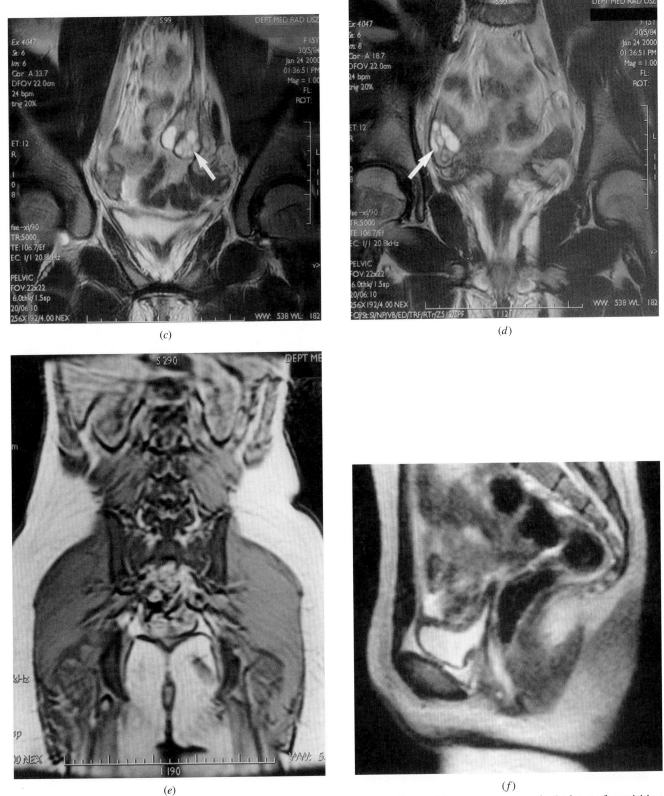

(c)

(d)

(e)

(f)

FIG. 14.14 (*Continued*) There is vaginal and uterine agenesis, with no evidence of these structures on the 3 planes of acquisition (*a–d*). Coronal and transverse sections through the midpelvis show both ovaries with small hyperintense follicular cysts (arrows, *b–d*). Both kidneys are delineated (*e*).

Sagittal (*f*) and transverse, at superior (*g*) and inferior (*h*) levels, T2-weighted ETSE images in a second patient demonstrate the absence of the uterus and vagina. No muscular wall of vagina is appreciated posterior to the urethra on sagittal (*f*) and transverse (*h*) images.

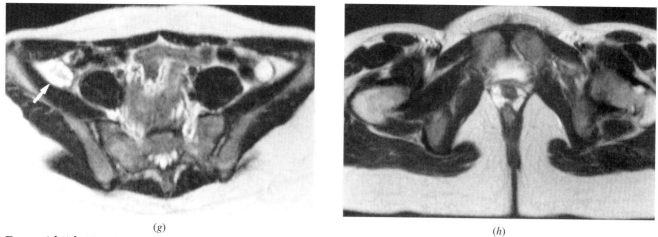

(g)

(h)

FIG. 14.14 (*Continued*) Note the normal ovaries bilaterally with follicles well shown in the right ovary (arrow, *g*) at this tomographic level (*g*).

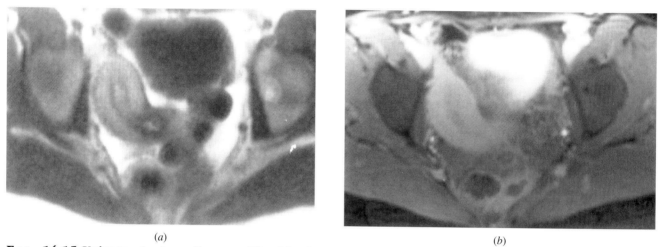

(a)

(b)

FIG. 14.15 Unicornuate uterus. Transverse T2-weighted SS-ETSE (*a*) and interstitial-phase gadolinium-enhanced fat-suppressed SGE (*b*) images demonstrate a curved and elongated uterus that represents a unicornuate uterus. No rudimentary horn on the left is identified. Note that the zonal anatomy is normal.

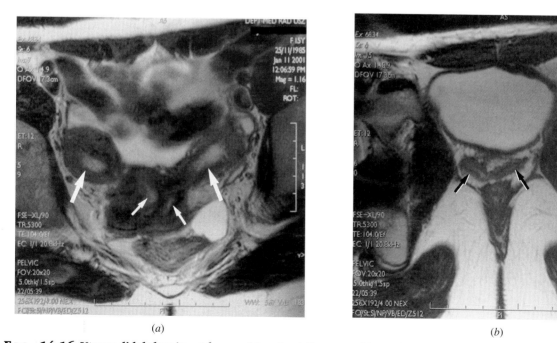

(a)

(b)

FIG. 14.16 Uterus didelphys in a 16-year-old patient. Transverse T2-weighted ETSE images at the level of the uterine corpus (*a*) and vagina (*b*) and T1-weighted spin-echo image of the upper abdomen (*c*).

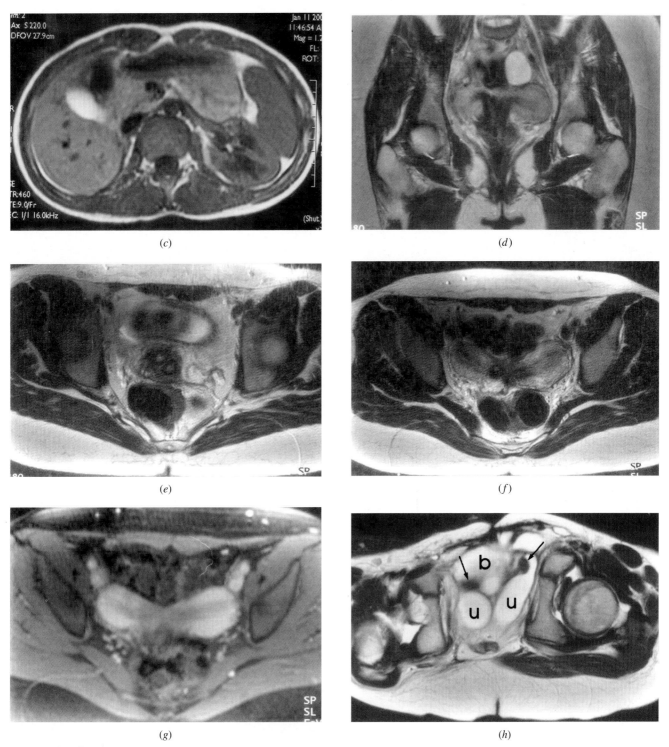

(c)

(d)

(e)

(f)

(g)

(h)

FIG. 14.16 Complete uterine duplication with 2 separate, normal-sized corpora (arrows, *a*) is present, and 2 cervices are seen, with 2 hyperintense endocervical canals (small arrows, *a*). Two separate vaginas (black arrows, *b*) are present. The patient has associated right renal agenesis (*c*).

Coronal (*d*) and transverse (*e*, *f*) T2-weighted ETSE and tranverse interstitial-phase gadolinium-enhanced SGE (*g*) images in a second patient. Two normal-sized uteri and cervices are identified. Note that normal zonal anatomy of the uteri is present.

Transverse T2-weighted ETSE image (*h*) in a third patient who is 2 years of age and has a surgically repaired common cloaca. A didelphys uterus is present, and the two uterine horns (arrows, *h*) are low signal intensity on T2-weighted image (*h*). Ureters ("u") are dilated because of bladder ("b") outlet obstruction.

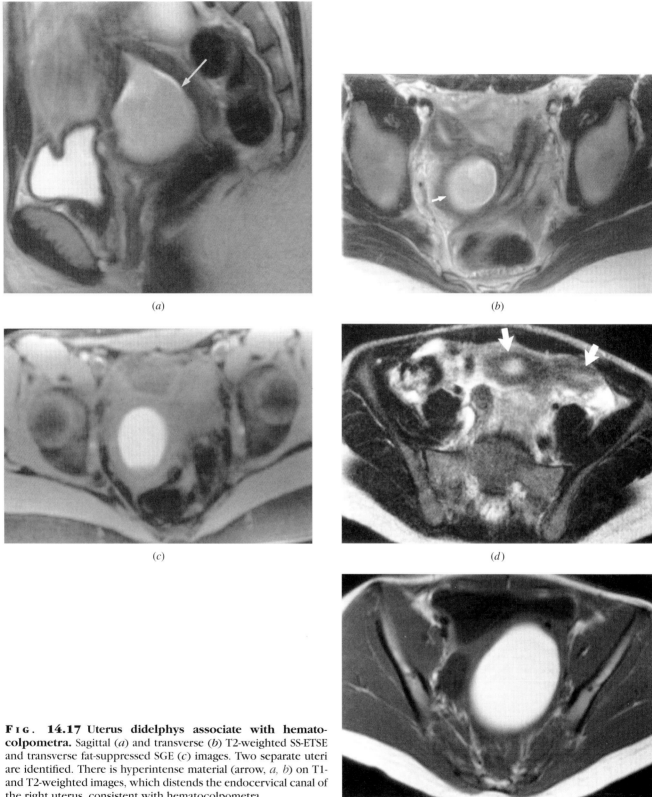

(a)

(b)

(c)

(d)

FIG. 14.17 Uterus didelphys associate with hemato-colpometra. Sagittal (*a*) and transverse (*b*) T2-weighted SS-ETSE and transverse fat-suppressed SGE (*c*) images. Two separate uteri are identified. There is hyperintense material (arrow, *a, b*) on T1- and T2-weighted images, which distends the endocervical canal of the right uterus, consistent with hematocolpometra.

(e)

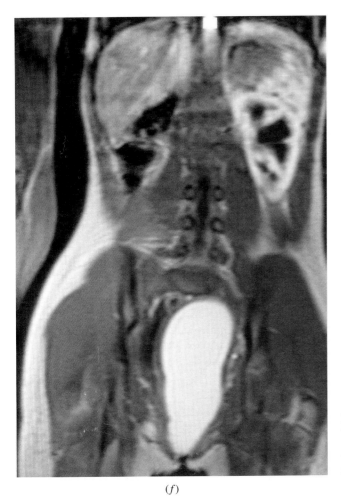

(*f*)

F I G . 14.17 (*Continued*) Transverse T2-weighted ETSE (*d*) and transverse (*e*) and coronal (*f*) SGE images in a second patient show 2 separate uteri (arrows, *d*) with distension of the right endometrial cavity and vagina by a hyperintense material consistent with hematocolpometra.

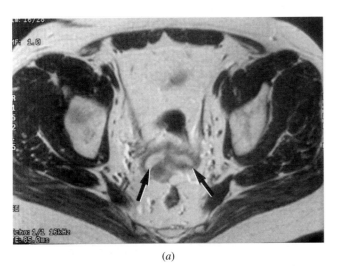

(*a*)

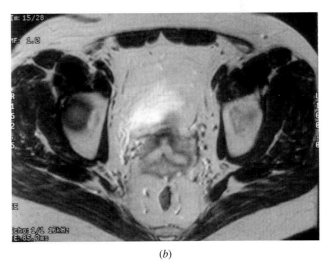

(*b*)

F I G . 14.18 Bicornuate retroverted uterus. Transverse T2-weighted ETSE images (*a, b, c*) from superior to inferior.

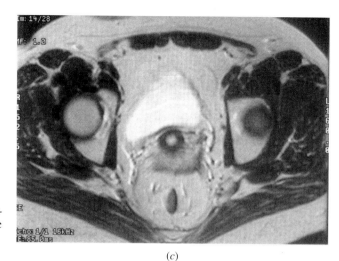

FIG. 14.18 (*Continued*) Widely divergent uterine horns (arrows, *a*) are present with a large intercornual distance. A single cervix is present (uterus bicornuate unicollis).

(c)

differentiate a double cervix from a cervical septation at MRI. Although a bicornuate uterus infrequently requires surgery, a transabdominal approach is used to fuse the uterine horns in symptomatic patients [49, 50].

Class V: Failure of resorption of the final fibrous septum between the two müllerian ducts results in a septate uterus The external contour of the uterine fundus is the main differentiating feature between a septate and bicornuate uterus (fig. 14.21). Laparoscopy was at one time the only reliable method of differentiating these entities. Several studies have demonstrated the high accuracy of MRI in diagnosing septate and bicornuate uteri [49, 50, 56]. Septate uteri have a convex, flat, or minimally indented fundal contour, whereas bicornuate uteri have a large fundal cleft [49]. In addition, septate uteri

maintain a normal intercornual distance (range 2–4 cm) [50]. Accurate distinction between septate and bicornuate uteri is important for proper patient management. Septate uteri are associated with a higher rate of reproductive failure, with two-thirds of pregnancies terminating in abortion (fig. 14.22). In contrast to bicornuate uteri, septate uteri are successfully treated with hysteroscopic excision of the septum and do not require abdominal surgery.

Diethylstilbesterol Exposure

Diethylstilbesterol (DES), a synthetic estrogen agent, was used from approximately 1950 to 1970 in pregnant women with vaginal bleeding in an attempt to prevent

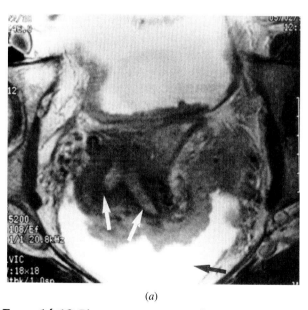

(a)

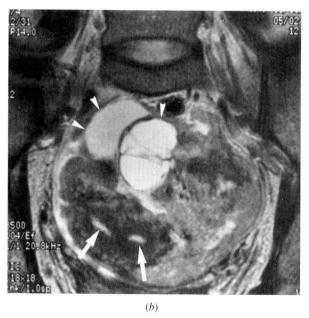

(b)

FIG. 14.19 Bicornuate retroverted uterus as a incidental finding in a patient with stage IV ovarian carcinoma. Transverse (*a*) and coronal (*b*) T2-weighted ETSE images. Widely divergent uterine horns (arrows, *a*, *b*) are present, with a large intercornual distance. A cystic-solid ovarian lesion (arrowheads, *b*) and ascites (black arrow, *a*) are also seen. Ovarian cancer invades along the surface of the uterus (*a*).

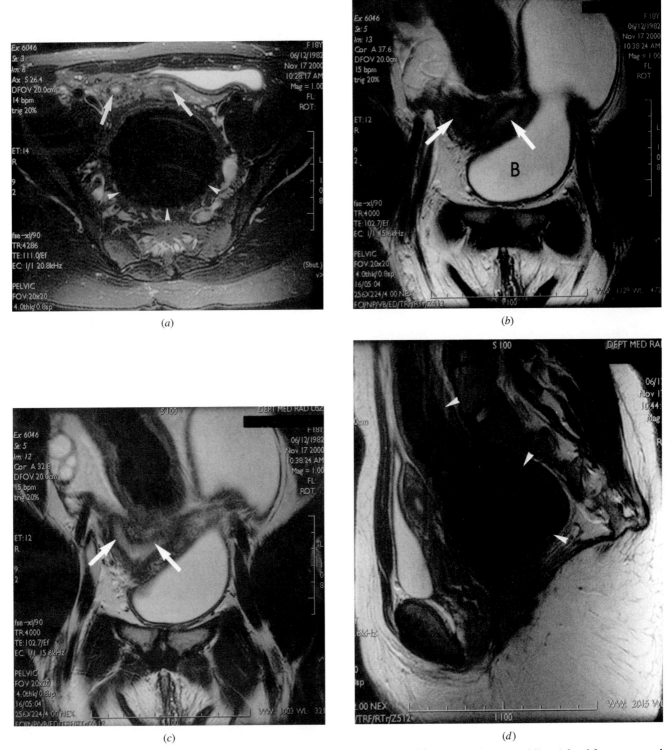

F I G . 14.20 Bicornuate uterus and repaired anal atresia in an 18-year-old patient. Transverse T2-weighted fat-suppressed ETSE (*a*) and coronal (*b, c*) and sagittal T2-weighted ETSE (*d*) images demonstrate widely divergent uterine horns (arrows, *a–c*), with a large intercornual distance. An irregularly shaped urinary bladder ("B," *b*) is present, and there is a large volume of stool (arrowheads, *a, d*) in the rectum reflecting postsurgical anal stenosis.

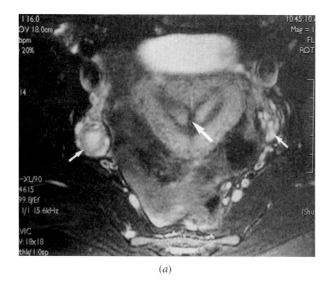

(a)

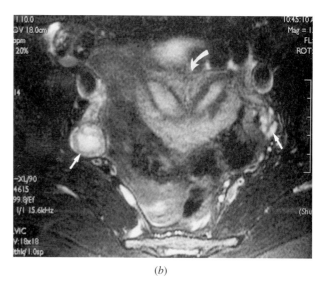

(b)

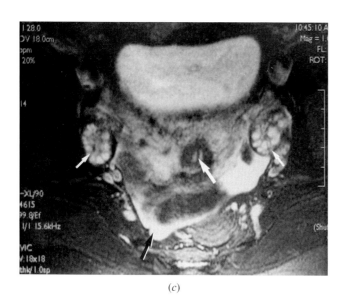

(c)

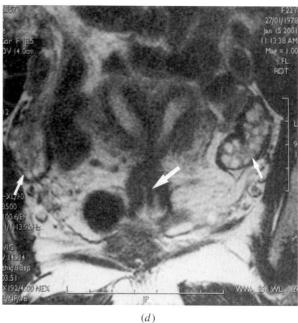

(d)

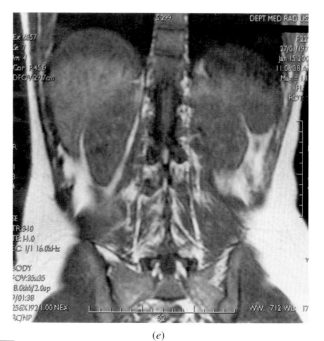

(e)

FIG. 14.21 Septate uterus. Transverse T2-weighted fat-suppressed ETSE images at the level of the uterine corpus (*a, b*) and cervix (*c*), transverse-oblique T2-weighted ETSE (*d*), and coronal T1-weighted spin-echo (*e*) images. A uterine septum is identified (large arrow, *a*). The long-axis (oblique transverse) view demonstrates a flat surface along the fundus of the uterus consistent with a septate uterus (curved arrow, *b*). The septum extends through the cervix (arrow, *c, d*). The ovaries are well shown because of the visualization of hyperintense cysts (small arrows, *a–d*). Fluid is seen in the pouch of Douglas (black arrow, *c*). Both kidneys are present (*e*).

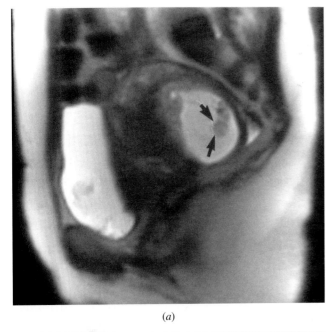

(a)

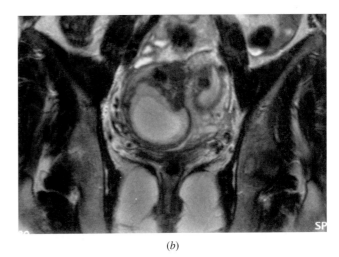

(b)

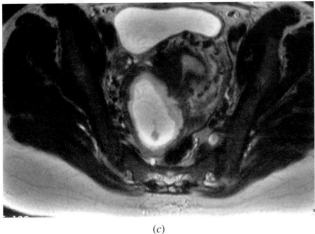

(c)

F I G . 14.22 Septate uterus with pregnancy in 1 horn. Sagittal T2-weighted SS-ETSE (*a*) and coronal (*b*) and transverse (*c*) ETSE images in a patient with a septate uterus and first-trimester pregnancy. A gestational sac is identified in the right horn of the uterus. The fetus is well shown (arrows, *a*). Incidental note is made of multiple small leiomiomas (*b*).

miscarriage. The female offspring of these patients exposed to DES in utero have an almost 50% incidence of congenital uterine anomalies including hypoplasia, T shape, constrictions, polypoid defects, synechiae, and marginal irregularities of the uterine cavity and are at risk for developing clear cell carcinoma of the vagina. On MRI, long-axis views have been shown to be well suited to demonstrate the anomalies of the endometrial cavity. At the site of uterine cavity constriction, localized thickening of the junctional zone has been described on T2-weighted images. Hypoplasia of the cervix and uterine cavity is seen, whereas normal zonal uterine anatomy is preserved. No increased incidence of urinary tract anomalies has been reported in patients with DES exposure. [57, 58].

Congenital Disorders of Sexual Differentiation

Congenital disorders of sexual differentiation are divided into four categories: male and female pseudohermaphroditism, mixed gonadal dysgenesis, and true hermaphroditism. A multidisciplinary approach is usually required in these patients, including hormonal studies, karyotyping, and anatomic information for accurate diagnosis and treatment. The excellent soft tissue differentiation and multiplanar imaging capability of MRI make it a useful noninvasive tool to determine the presence or absence of a uterus and vagina as well as to preoperatively identify the position of undescended testes (fig. 14.23) [59]. This topic is further described in Chapter 13, *Female Urethra and Vagina*.

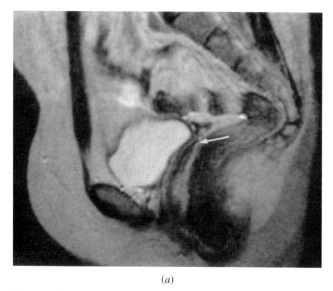

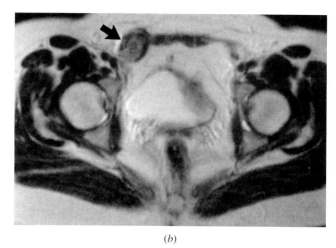

(a)   (b)

FIG. 14.23 Testicular feminization. Sagittal (*a*) and transverse (*b*) T2-weighted ETSE images in a patient with complete androgen insensivity (testicular feminization). There is a blind-ending vagina (arrow, *a*), and the uterus is absent (a). Note the rounded structure (arrow, *b*) in the right inguinal canal, consistent with a testes, evident by the lack of follicles.

BENIGN DISEASES OF THE UTERINE CORPUS

Endometrial Hyperplasia and Endometrial Polyps

Endovaginal sonography is the imaging modality of choice to assess the endometrium in symptomatic patients, for example, for the evaluation of the endometrium in abnormal postmenopausal bleeding [60]. Sonographic studies of endometrial thickness in postmenopausal women have suggested an upper limit of 5 mm in patients without hormone replacement and 8 mm for patients receiving hormonal therapy [60–63].

The presence of endometrial thickening on ultrasonography is, however, a nonspecific finding and may be due to endometrial hyperplasia, polyps, or carcinoma. The final diagnosis will usually be established by endometrial sampling [60]. Currently, MRI has no established role in screening for endometrial pathology.

Endometrial hyperplasia usually presents as diffuse thickening of the endometrial stripe on T2-weighted images. The signal intensity of the endometrial stripe is isointense or slightly hypointense compared to normal endometrium. These imaging characteristics, however, are nonspecific and are also seen with endometrial carcinoma [41].

Polyps of the endometrium are seen in about 10% of all uteri, typically in postmenopausal patients. In many cases, they are asymptomatic but may cause irregular or persistent bleeding. Malignant transformation into endometrial cancer is seen in less than 1% of cases [20].

On T2-weighted images, endometrial polyps most frequently appear as isointense or slightly hypointense masses relative to normal endometrium. At times, however, they may be entirely isointense and appear as diffuse or focal thickening of the endometrial stripe. Large polyps result in distension of the endometrial cavity. Polyps show pronounced enhancement on gadolinium-enhanced T1-weighted sequences. On the basis of signal intensity and gadolinium enhancement, they are distinguishable from submucosal leiomyomas; the latter appear hypointense on T2-weighted sequences with usually only slight contrast enhancement (figs. 14.24 and 14.25) [20, 64].

Although MRI can help to distinguish most polyps from endometrial carcinoma on the basis of morphologic features, accuracy is not sufficient to obviate biopsy, partly because carcinomas and polyps frequently coexist [65].

Leiomyomas

Leiomyomas (also termed fibroids, fibroleiomyoma) are benign neoplasms of smooth muscle cell origin and are the most common uterine tumor. Leiomyomas are usually classified according to location: submucosal, intramural, subserosal, or cervical (fig. 14.26). Five to ten percent of leiomyomas arise submucosally or protrude into the uterine cavity. Subserosal leiomyomas may occasionally mimic a solid ovarian mass. Uncommonly, a leiomyoma may be situated in the broad ligament or be entirely detached from the uterus, parasitizing the blood supply from other vascular beds, usually the omentum [66]. As

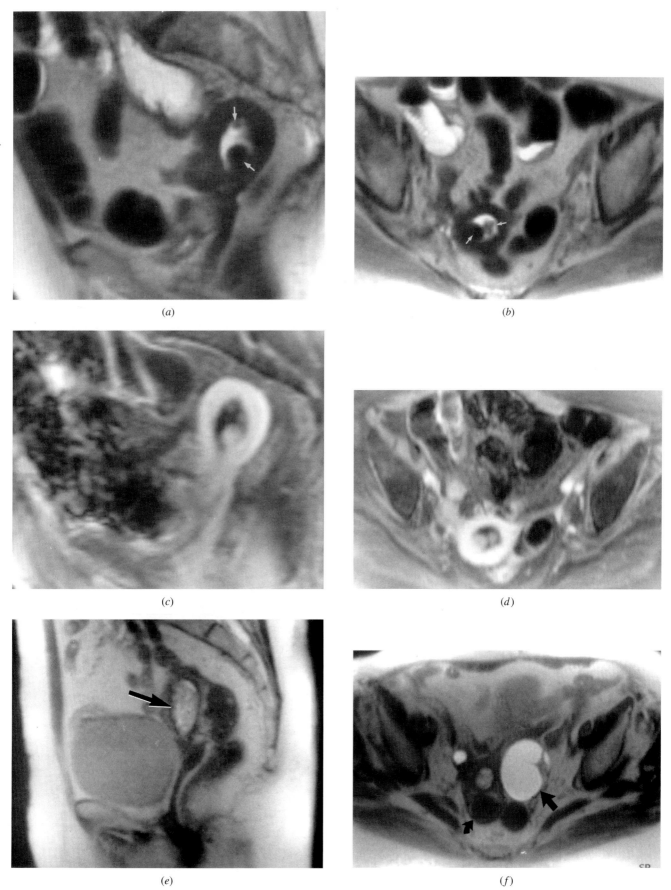

(a)

(b)

(c)

(d)

(e)

(f)

F I G . 14.24 Endometrial polyp. Sagittal (*a*) and transverse (*b*) T2-weighted SS-ETSE and sagittal (*c*) and transverse (*d*) interstitial-phase gadolinium-enhanced fat-suppressed SGE images.

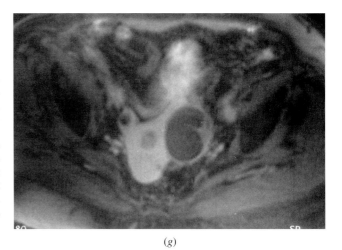

(g)

FIG. 14.24 (*Continued*) The uterine cavity is mildly distended and contains multiple polypoid lesions (arrows, *a, b*), consistent with polyps. Note that the polyps are isointense with myometrium on the T2-weighted images (*a, b*) and enhance comparable to the myometrium on the postgadolinium images (*c, d*).

Sagittal (*e*) and transverse (*f*) SS-ETSE and transverse interstitial-phase gadolinium-enhanced fat-suppressed SGE (*g*) images in a second patient with an endometrial polyp (arrow, *e*) that distends the uterine cavity. The polyp enhances with contrast, distinguishing it from blood products (*g*). Note also the presence of a left adnexa mass (arrow, *f*), consistent with ovarian cancer, and a leiomyoma (curved arrow, *f*) in the posterior aspect of the uterus.

leiomyomas enlarge, they may outgrow their blood supply. Especially when tumors exceed 8 cm in diameter, they are likely to undergo some degree of degeneration, which contributes to the variable appearance of these large tumors on imaging. In addition, leiomyomas frequently calcify, particularly in older women.

Although the majority of leiomyomas are asymptomatic, presenting as incidental findings, they may be associated with a variety of symptoms. The most common is bleeding disorder, but pressure effects, infertility, second-trimester abortions, dystocia or palpable abdominopelvic mass also are observed. Torsion, infection, and sarcomatous degeneration are rare complications. Pain is usually the result of acute degeneration, including hemorrhagic infarction of a leiomyoma

during pregnancy, torsion of pedunculated subserosal leiomyoma, or prolapse of a submucosal leiomyoma. [20, 67–69].

The role of imaging in evaluating patients with suspected leiomyomas includes lesion detection, characterization, and localization. Ultrasound remains the primary imaging modality for clinically suspected leiomyomas, and in the vast majority of routine clinical presentations no additional investigation is needed. In patients scheduled for uterine-sparing surgery, however, accurate preoperative localization of leiomyomas is not always possible sonographically. This is of great importance in planning myomectomy, because submucosal leiomyomas may be resected hysteroscopically, whereas laparoscopic or transabdominal myomectomy is required

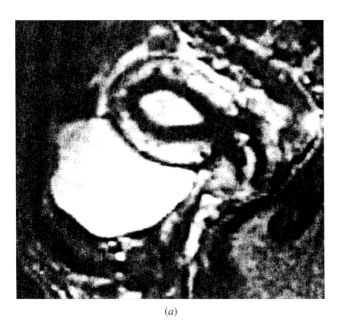

(a)

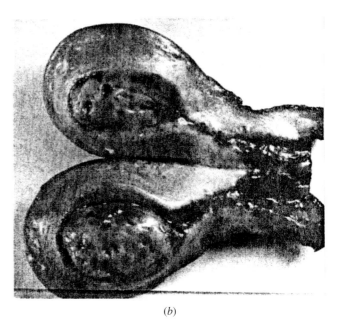

(b)

FIG. 14.25 Endometrial polyp. Sagittal T2-weighted spin echo image (*a*) and gross specimen (*b*). The endometrial polyp is of slightly lower signal intensity than adjacent endometrium. The junctional zone is intact. (Reprinted with permission from Hamm B, Kubik-Huch RA, Fleige B: MR imaging and CT of the female pelvis: Radiologic-pathologic correlation. *Eur Radiol* 1999; 9: 13–15.)

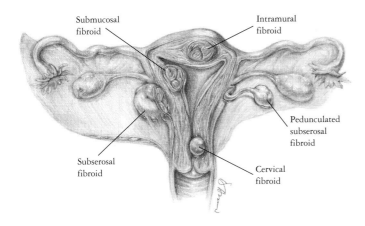

F I G . 14.26 Classification of uterine leiomyomas.

for intramural or subserosal leiomyomas. Similarly, visualization of the endometrium or ovaries may be obscured in patients with large or multiple leiomyomas. The distinction between a pedunculated leiomyoma and a solid ovarian mass may not always be possible on ultrasound [70, 71].

MRI can thus be recommended in selected cases as a problem-solving modality, for example, to distinguish between a pedunculated leiomyoma and a solid ovarian mass, to demonstrate the exact size and location of the lesion (i.e., subserosal, intramural or submucosal origin) before uterine-sparing surgery, or to distinguish leiomyomas from adenomyosis. Several studies have demonstrated MRI to be superior to ultrasound for the detection and localization of uterine leiomyomas and to be

an useful adjunct to differentiate leiomyomas from other pathological conditions [70–76].

Leiomyomas of the uterus have a typical appearance on MRI. They are depicted as sharply marginated lesions of low signal intensity on both T1- and T2-weighted sequences. Dark signal on T2-weighted images permits differentiation from malignant tumors which are almost never low signal (figs. 14.27–14.32). The lesions are surrounded by a pseudocapsule of compressed neighboring tissue. A small hyperintense rim due to dilated lymphatic clefts, dilated veins, and minimal edema surrounding the leiomyoma may be seen on T2-weighted imaging (fig. 14.28). These histologic findings have been shown to correspond to perilesional rim enhancement on gadolinium-enhanced images [64].

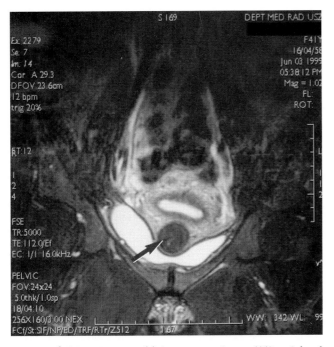

F I G . 14.27 Intramural leiomyoma. Coronal T2-weighted fat-suppressed ETSE image demonstrates a small sharply marginated, hypointense intramural leiomyoma (arrow).

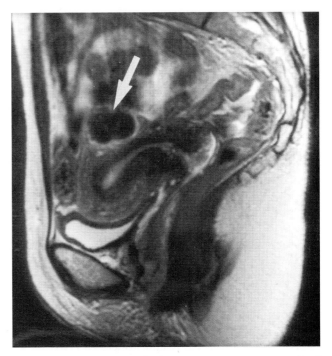

F I G . 14.28 Subserosal leiomyoma. Sagittal T2-weighted ETSE demonstrates a subserosal, sharply marginated hypointense mass with a hyperintense rim (arrow).

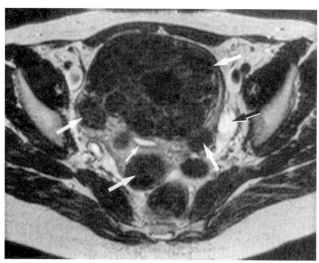

F I G . 14.29 Multiple uterine leiomyomas. Transverse T2-weighted fat-suppressed ETSE image. Multiple leiomyomas of different size are shown as sharply marginated low-signal intensity masses (white arrows). The relationship of the fibroids to the endometrial cavity (small arrow) is shown. (Black arrow = left ovary).

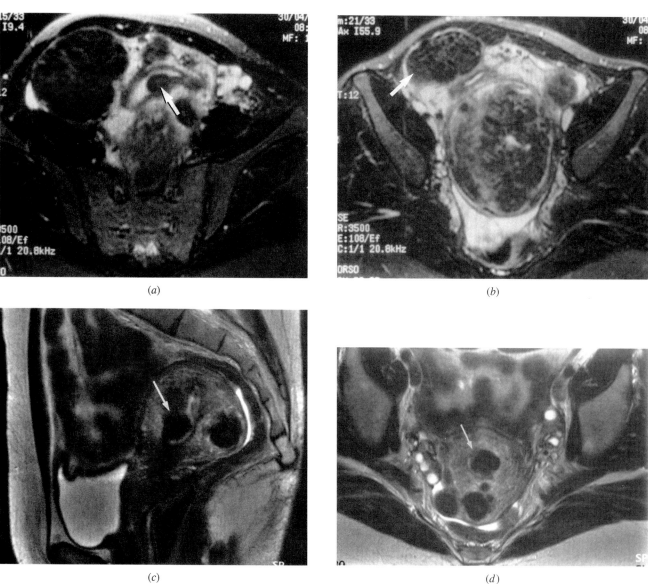

(a)

(b)

(c)

(d)

F I G . 14.30 Multiple uterine leiomyomas. Transverse T2-weighted fat-suppressed ETSE image (*a*). Multiple leiomyomas of different size are shown as sharply marginated masses of low signal intensity on T2-weighted images. One lesion (arrow, *a*) is submucosal in origin and results in widening of the endometrial cavity. The lesion's hypointense signal distinguishes it from an endometrial polyp or carcinoma.

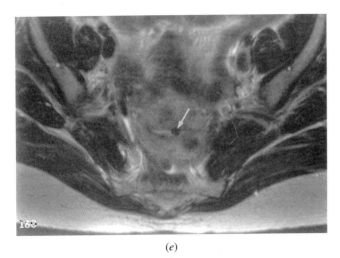

(*e*)

FIG. 14.30 Transverse fat-suppressed T2-weighted ETSE image (*b*) in a second patient. Multiple leiomyomas are present as sharply marginated masses of low signal intensity. The subserosal lesion on the right (arrow, *b*) was mistaken for a solid ovarian lesion on ultrasound, which prompted the MRI study.

Sagittal (*c*) and transverse (*d, e*) T2-weighted ETSE images in a third patient demonstrate several hypointense masses within the uterus. Note the presence of both large (arrow, *c, d*) and small (arrow, *e*) submucosal leiomyomas.

In addition to standard sagittal and transverse views, coronal or oblique views may be indicated for accurate localization and for establishing the myometrial origin of a lesion. The absence of a fat plane between the mass and the uterus on T1-weighted sequences may aid in differentiating a pedunculated leiomyoma from a solid ovarian mass. Gadolinium-enhanced T1-weighted images are not usually helpful in the detection or characterization of uterine leiomyomas. The majority of leiomyomas enhance to a lesser degree than the surrounding myometrium and remain well marginated. Moderately intense enhancement of fibroids on immediate postgadolinium images correlates with a greater likelihood of good response to therapeutic intervention, either embolization or pharmacologic intervention.

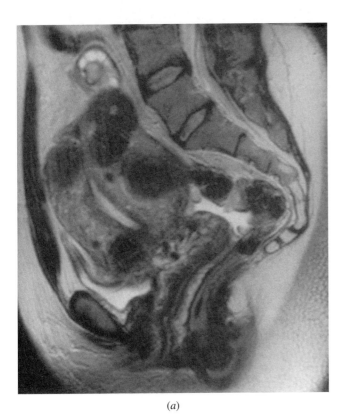

(*a*)

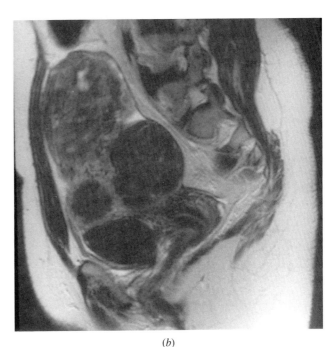

(*b*)

FIG. 14.31 Multiple uterine leiomyomas with gadolinium enhancement.

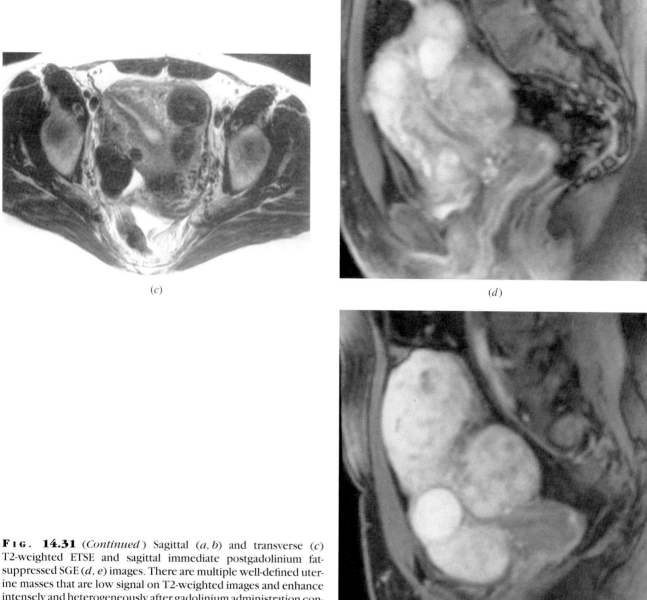

(c)

(d)

(e)

FIG. 14.31 (*Continued*) Sagittal (*a, b*) and transverse (*c*) T2-weighted ETSE and sagittal immediate postgadolinium fat-suppressed SGE (*d, e*) images. There are multiple well-defined uterine masses that are low signal on T2-weighted images and enhance intensely and heterogeneously after gadolinium administration consistent with multiple leiomyomas. The intense early enhancement of the leiomyomas reflects extensive vascularity. Well-vascularized leiomyomas will generally respond well to therapeutic intervention.

Leiomyomas may undergo degenerative changes resulting in varying MR signal intensity, which most often appear as inhomogeneous high signal intensity on T2-weighted sequences and lack of enhancement on gadolinium-enhanced T1-weighted sequences (fig. 14.33). In leiomyomas undergoing hemorrhagic degeneration (so called red degeneration), which occurs most often during pregnancy, hyperintense areas on T1-weighted images are typically seen [69].

Secondary calcification occurs in about 4% of leiomyomas [77]. Demonstration of these characteristic calcifications, which are well shown on computed tomography or plain films, is difficult by MRI, because signal-void calcification is nearly imperceptible within a

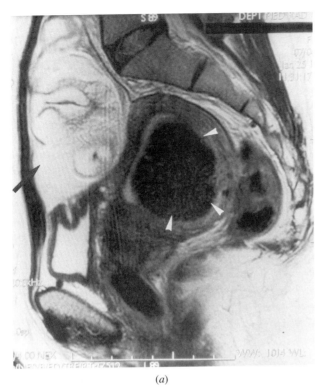

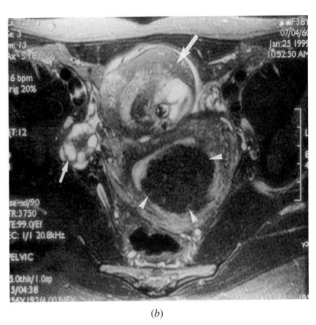

(a) (b)

F I G . 14.32 Leiomyoma in a patient with mature teratoma of the left ovary. Sagittal T2-weighted ETSE (*a*) and transverse T2-weighted fat-suppressed ETSE (*b*) images. A large sharply marginated, hypointense leiomyoma (arrowheads, *a, b*) is observed in this patient referred for investigation of an ovarian mass. The ovarian lesion is hyperintense on T1- (not shown) and T2-weighted images (black arrow, *a*) with signal loss after fat suppression (large arrow, *b*), diagnostic for a mature teratoma, which was histologically confirmed. Normal right ovary (small arrow, *b*).

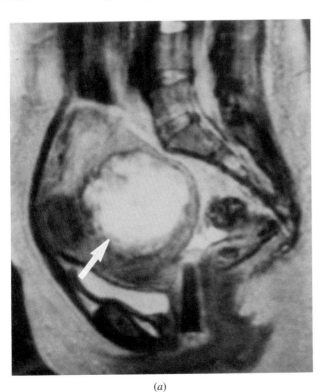

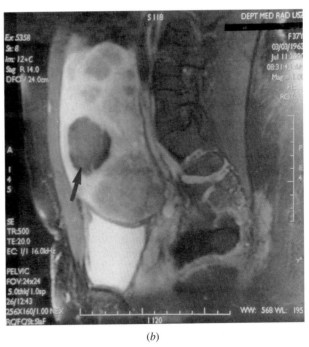

(a) (b)

F I G . 14.33 Degenerated uterine leiomyomas. Sagittal T2-weighted ETSE (*a*) image. There is a small hypointense leiomyoma and a sharply demarcated large leiomyoma (arrows, *a*) along the posterior aspect of the uterus, with increased signal intensity corresponding to areas of degeneration.

T1-weighted interstitial-phase gadolinium-enhanced fat-suppressed SE image (*b*) in a second patient demonstrates a degenerated leiomyoma (arrow, *b*) that does not enhance, in comparison to the other leiomyomas, which show enhancement.

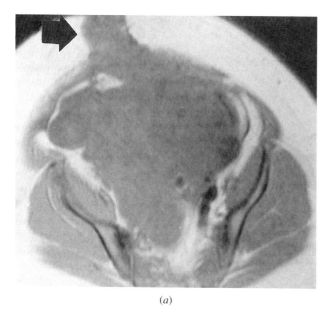

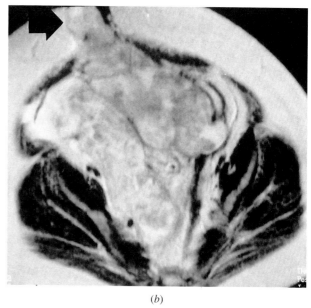

(a)

(b)

F ı g . 14.34 Benign metastasizing leiomyoma (low-grade leiomyosarcoma). T1-weighted SGE (*a*), transverse (*b*) and sagittal (*c*) T2-weighted ETSE, and 1-min postgadolinium SGE (*d*) images. A massive uterine tumor is present involving the entire uterus. The tumor extends through the peritoneum at the level of the umbilicus into subcutaneous tissue (arrows, *a*, *b*). The tumor is moderately low in signal intensity, comparable to skeletal muscle on the T1-weighted image (*a*), and heterogeneous and moderately high in signal intensity on the T2-weighted images (*b*, *c*).

hypointense mass. This, however, is not problematic because the correct diagnosis is readily established by the characteristic appearance of leiomyomas as described above [20, 67, 68].

MRI can be useful in differentiating leiomyomas from other solid pelvic masses [71]. Establishing the myometrial origin of a mass by demonstrating splaying of the uterine serosa or myometrium usually allows a confident diagnosis of leiomyoma to be made. Signal characteristics will give additional information. If a mass is well defined and predominantly of low signal intensity relative to myometrium on T2-weighted images, the diagnosis of leiomyoma is virtually certain. Although the signal characteristics of leiomyomas may be indistinguishable from those of ovarian fibroma and Brenner tumors of the ovary, the consequence of a misdiagnosis is probably not significant because these latter tumors are also rarely malignant [71, 78].

Submucosal leiomyomas may be differentiated from an endometrial pathology, namely, endometrial polyps, hyperplasia or endometrial carcinoma, by confirming their myometrial origin and by their typical low signal intensity on T2-weighted images (figs. 14.29 and 14.30). However, leiomyomas may exhibit variable signal intensities, and overlap in signal characteristics between leiomyomas and endometrial pathologies has been described [41].

Lipoleiomyoma is a rare, specific type of leiomyoma that contains a substantial amount of fat, which on MRI has a signal intensity similar to that of subcutaneous fat on all pulse sequences [77].

Malignant degeneration of a leiomyoma is uncommon but is suspected if a leiomyoma enlarges suddenly, especially after menopause, or if indistinct borders or irregular contours are noted, particularly in massive tumors. MRI signal characteristics are not reliable in differentiating leiomyomas from leimyosarcomas. Often it is the appreciation of metastatic disease, such as lung metastases, that permits the diagnosis of malignancy.

Benign metastasizing leiomyoma, actually a low-grade leiomyosarcoma, is an unusual variant that consists of smooth muscle cell tumors in the lungs, lymph nodes, or abdomen that appear to have originated from a benign uterine leiomyoma, which may have been removed years earlier (fig. 14.34) [77].

For patients with symptomatic leiomyomas, either medical, namely, administration of gondatotropin-releasing hormone (GnRH) analogs, or surgical treatment, namely, hysterectomy or myomectomy, may be indicated. More recently, uterine artery embolization has been advocated as a promising new method to treat symptomatic leiomyomas. As a percutaneous interventional technique, this procedure offers the advantages of avoidance of surgical risks, potential preservation of fertiliy, and shorter hospitalization [69].

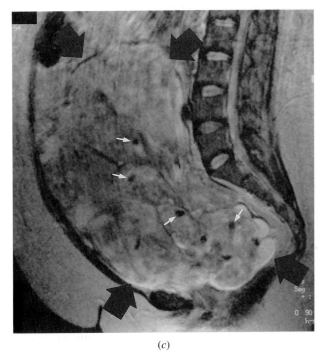

(c)

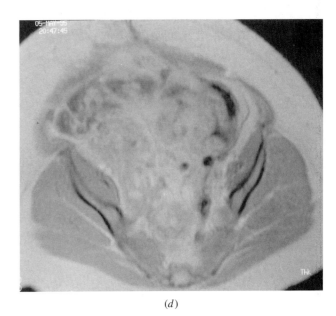

(d)

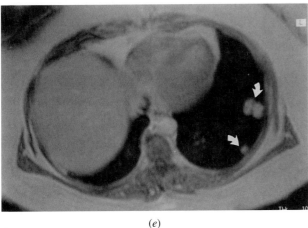

(e)

FIG. 14.34 (*Continued*) The sagittal-plane image clearly defines the longitudinal extent of tumor (arrows, *c*). Multiple signal-void calcific foci are present in the mass (small arrows, *c*). Relatively intense diffuse heterogeneous enhancement is present on the early postgadolinium image (*d*). A 3-min postgadolinium SGE image (*e*) through the lung bases in this patient demonstrates several enhancing metastases in the left lung base (curved arrows).

MRI enables quantitative monitoring of GnRH analog therapy documenting the change in size of individual leiomyomas. It can also demonstrate postprocedural complications such as hematoma, abscess, uterine rupture, and peritoneal inclusion cyst. In women undergoing myomectomy, the surgical bed may be seen as an area of moderately high signal intensity on both T1- and T2-weighted sequences. These signal characteristics suggest the presence of a subacute hematoma within the myometrium at the myomectomy site (fig. 14.35) [69].

More recently, MRI has been shown to be useful in monitoring the result of embolization by demonstrating the degree of shrinkage and loss of enhancement of the leiomyomas. Furthermore, it has been shown that in patients undergoing uterine arterial embolization, MR imaging characteristics of leiomyomas before embolization can help predict the success of the procedure with more vascular tumors having a greater response [69, 79, 80].

Adenomyosis

Uterine adenomyosis is a common disease that affects women during their menstrual life. Histologically it is demonstrated in up to 24% of all hysterectomy specimens. Clinical manifestations include dysmenorrhea and menorrhagia and are similar to those of uterine leiomyoma. Adenomyosis is defined as the presence of aberrant endometrial stroma and glands within the myometrium. Because the ectopic endometrium in adenomyosis consists almost exclusively of tissue derived from the basal layer, it is not affected by hormonal stimulation and will not contain hemorrhage. This is in contrast to endometriosis, which is characterized by the aberrant

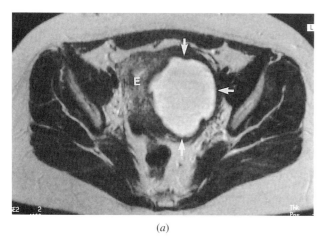
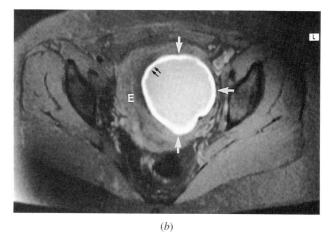

(a) *(b)*

FIG. 14.35 Postmyomectomy hematoma. T2-weighted ETSE (*a*) and T1-weighted fat-suppressed SGE (*b*) images. A well-delineated mass of moderately high signal intensity (arrows, *a, b*) consistent with a hematoma is present in the surgical bed. Note the peripheral rim of higher signal intensity on the T1-weighted image (small arrows, *b*), which is typical of a subacute hematoma. E, endometrium.

occurrence of functional endometrial tissue. Adenomyosis is commonly associated with leiomyomas. Adenomyosis may be microscopic, focal, or diffuse. The term adenomyoma is reserved for the focal, nodular form of adenomyosis [20, 64, 81–83].

Adenomyosis may be entirely asymptomatic or present with symptoms of pelvic pain, hypermenorrhea, and uterine enlargement. Symptoms typically manifest in the fourth to fifth decade with a higher incidence in multiparous women. These symptoms and signs, however, are nonspecific and can be seen in other common gynecological disorders such as dysfunctional uterine bleeding, leiomyomas, and endometriosis. Physical examination demonstrates an enlarged uterus, which is of softer consistency than a myomatous uterus. Establishing the correct diagnosis preoperatively is essential because uterine-conserving therapy is possible with leiomyomas, whereas hysterectomy is the definitive treatment for debilitating adenomyosis [20].

The findings of adenomyosis on endovaginal ultrasound may be subtle, but correct diagnosis can be established when the exam is performed meticulously and in real time by an experienced operator. Several studies have demonstrated MRI to be as, or more, accurate in diagnosing adenomyosis, with a sensitivity and specificity ranging from 86 to 100% [64, 73, 81, 84, 85].

On MRI, adenomyosis is diagnosed on T2-weighted sequences. Thickening of the hypointense junctional zone of 12 mm or more is suggestive of the diagnosis, with irregularly marginated thickening increasing the likelihood of diagnosis. Thickening of the junctional zone of more than 5 mm is not recommended as a threshold value for diagnosing adenomyosis, as this is within the normal range. On T2-weighted images, multiple spots of hyperintensity are frequently observed,

which most likely represent islands of ectopic endometrium, cystically dilated endometrial glands, or hemorrhagic fluid [84, 85].

Bright foci on T1-weighted images are seen much less frequently and correspond to areas of hemorrhage. The exact mechanism of hemorrhage is unclear because adenomyosis involves only the basal, nonfunctional layer of the endometrium. When the degree of hemorrhage is extensive, cystic adenomyosis can result, appearing on MR images as well-circumscribed, cystic myometrial lesions with hemorrhage in different stages of organization [83].

The diffuse form of adenomyosis affects the entire uterus (figs. 14.36 and 14.37), and often results in uterine enlargement. The focal form, the so-called adenomyoma, appears as either a region of thickening of the junctional zone, which exhibits blurring of its myometrial border, or as a low-signal intensity myometrial mass with ill-defined borders (fig. 14.38).

Gadolinium-enhanced sequences have not been shown to provide additional information for the diagnostic assessment of adenomyosis or for its differentiation from leiomyomas [20, 64].

The differential diagnosis of adenomyosis includes transient myometrial contractions, postpartum changes, and leiomyoma. Although MRI is shown to be highly accurate in differentiating adenomyosis from leiomyomas, the imaging characteristics may overlap, particularly in the case of adenomyoma. Features favoring the diagnosis of adenomyosis include a lesion with poorly defined borders, a lesion with an elliptical shape extending along the endometrium, minimal mass effect on the endometrium relative to the size of the lesion, linear striations radiating from the endometrium into the myometrium, and small, high-signal foci [73, 85].

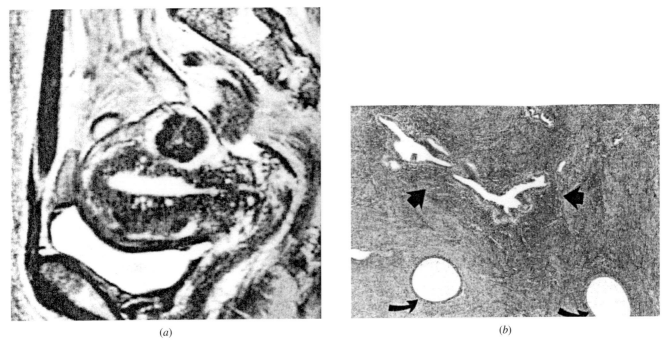

(a)   (b)

F I G . 14.36 Diffuse adenomyosis and leiomyomas. Sagittal T2-weighted ETSE image (*a*) and histologic specimen (hematoxylin & eosin staining) (*b*). Generalized thickening of the junctional zone with multiple small hyperintense foci is observed. A leiomyoma arising in the posterior uterine wall is also present surrounded by a narrow, hyperintense rim of dilated lymphatic clefts and veins. Histology confirms adenomyosis with ectopic endometrial tissue in the myometrium with glandular (arrows, *b*) and cystic portions (curved arrows, *b*). The cystic portions correlate with the hyperintense foci on T2-weighted images. (Reprinted with permission from Hamm B, Kubik-Huch RA, Fleige B: MR imaging and CT of the female pelvis: Radiologic-pathologic correlation. *Eur Radiol* 1999; 9: 13–15.)

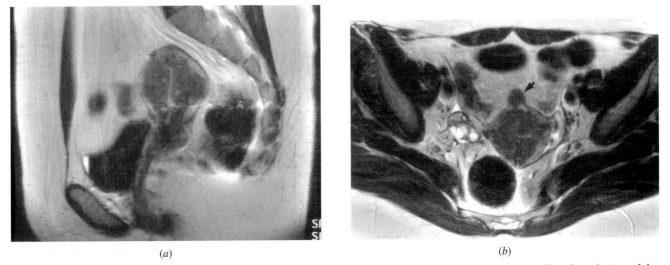

(a)   (b)

F I G . 14.37 Diffuse adenomyosis. Sagittal (*a*) and transverse (*b*) T2-weighted ETSE images. There is diffuse broadening of the junctional zone of the uterine body consistent with diffuse adenomyosis. Note also a small subserosal leiomyoma (arrow, *b*) located anteriorly.

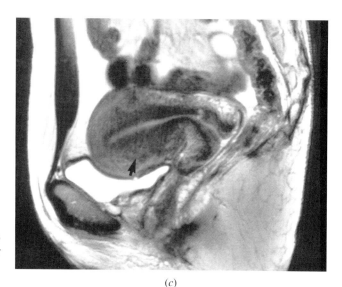

(c)

FIG. 14.37 (*Continued*) Sagittal T2-weighted ETSE image (*c*) in a second patient with diffuse adenomyosis demonstrates a lesser degree of broadening of the junctional zone.

BENIGN DISEASE OF THE CERVIX

Nabothian Cysts

Nabothian cysts result from mucous distention of endocervical glands or clefts. They can be the result of an inflammatory process or squamous metaplasia. The cysts are common and only rarely present with symptoms, and therefore they usually do not require treatment.

They may, however, reach up to 4 cm in diameter and, when multiple, may result in marked enlargement of the cervix.

On MRI, nabothian cysts are well depicted on T2-weighted sagittal and transverse images. Nabothian cysts are generally intermediate signal intensity on T1-weighted images and hyperintense on T2-weighted images (fig. 14.39). They show no enhancement after gadolinium administration. Nabothian cysts are

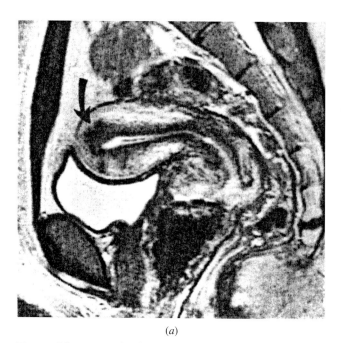

(a)

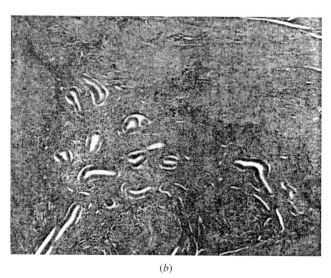

(b)

FIG. 14.38 Focal adenomyosis of the uterine fundus in a patient with cervical carcinoma. Sagittal T2-weighted ETSE image (*a*) and histologic specimen (hematoxylin & eosin staining) (*b*). Focal thickening (arrow, *a*) of the junctional zone of the uterine fundus is present on the T2-weighted image. Histology confirmed ectopic endometrial tissue in the myometrium (*b*). A large cervical carcinoma, that appears hyperintense is present, extending into the upper vagina. (Reprinted with permission from Hamm B, Kubik-Huch RA, Fleige B: MR imaging and CT of the female pelvis: Radiologic-pathologic correlation. *Eur Radiol* 1999; 9: 13–15.)

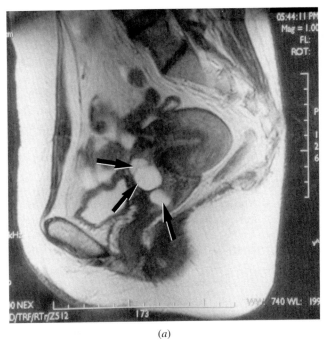

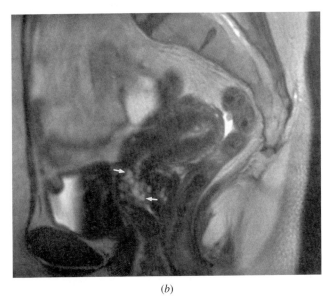

(a)   (b)

FIG. 14.39 Nabothian cysts. Sagittal T2-weighted ETSE image demontrates several 1-cm, well-defined, hyperintense nabothian cysts (arrows) in the cervix. The uterus is retroverted.

Sagittal T2-weighted SS-ETSE images in a second patient shows multiple small, <5 mm, cystic lesions in the cervix, consistent with nabothian cysts.

differentiated from cervical carcinoma by their well-defined margins, generally small (<1 cm) size, and very high signal intensity on T2-weighted images.

MALIGNANT DISEASE OF THE UTERINE CORPUS AND CERVIX

Endometrial Carcinoma

Endometrial carcinoma is the most common malignancy of the female genital tract, primarily occurring in postmenopausal women. Approximately 2–5% of cases occur in women below the age of 40 years. Postmenopausal bleeding is the most common, and often the only, symptom in these patients. Adenocarcinomas account for 80–90% of all endometrial carcinomas. Currently, the diagnosis is established by fractional abrasion. Fractionation is employed to exclude or confirm involvement of the endocervix, corresponding to FIGO stage II disease [20, 86].

Endometrial carcinoma invades the myometrium but rarely extends through the serosa into the abdominal cavity. In about 10% of cases, the cervix will be involved at the time of diagnosis. Lymphatic and hematogenous spread of endometrial carcinoma occurs later than in cervical carcinoma, with a close correlation between the depth of myometrial invasion and lymphatic spread. The FIGO classification is used for tumor staging (Table 14.1) [87].

Whereas superficial myometrial invasion (FIGO stage IB) is associated with lymph node metastases in 3% of cases, metastatic nodes will be seen in 40% of patients with deep (FIGO stage IC) myometrial involvement. The extent of myometrial invasion is, therefore, next to the histologic grade of the tumor, an important prognostic factor. Depth of invasion may be the factor most responsible for the extreme variation in the 5-year survival of patients with stage I disease: from 40 to 60% in the most invasive cases to 90 to 100% in cases with little or no myometrial involvement [88–91].

Nodal involvement most often extends from pelvic lymph nodes superiorly in a contiguous fashion. Para-aortic lymphadenopathy may occur without involvement of pelvic lymph nodes if the tumor spreads via lymphatics accompanying the ovarian vessels. Hematogenous metastases occur in patients with disseminated disease and most frequently involve the lungs [20, 86, 89, 92].

MRI may be the imaging modality of choice for preoperative staging of endometrial carcinoma. Prior studies have shown that gadolinium-enhanced MR imaging is significantly superior to endovaginal ultrasonography for staging, using fractional abrasion correlation [93–95].

A cost analysis of the use of preoperative MR imaging in the management of endometrial carcinoma has shown that staging with MRI has lesser costs and

Table 14.1   Revised FIGO Staging of Endometrial Carcinoma with Corresponding MRI Findings

Revised FIGO Staging[1]

Stage 0		Carcinoma in situ
Stage I		Tumor confined to corpus
	IA	Tumor limited to endometrium
	IB	Invasion <50% of myometrium
	IC	Invasion >50% of myometrium
Stage II		Tumor invades cervix but does not extend beyond uterus
	IIA	Invasion of endocervix
	IIB	Cervical stromal invasion
Stage III		Tumor extends beyond uterus but not outside true pelvis
	IIIA	Invasion of serosa, adnexa, or positive peritoneal cytology
	IIIB	Invasion of vagina
	IIIC	Pelvic and/or para-aortic lymphadenopathy
Stage IV		Tumor extends outside of true pelvis of invades bladder or rectal mucosa
	IVA	Invasion of bladder or rectal mcosa
	IVB	Distant metastases (includes intra-abdominal or inguinal lymphadenopathy)

Corresponding MR Findings[2]

Stage 0		Normal or thickened endometrial stripe
Stage I	IA	Thickened endometrial stripe with diffuse or focal abnormal signal intensity. Endometrial stripe may be normal. Intact junctional zone with smooth endometrial-myometrial interface[3]
	IB	Signal intensity of tumor extends into myometrium <50% Partial or full-thickness disruption of junctional zone with irregular endometrial-myometrial interface
	IC	Signal intensity of tumor extends into myometrium >50% Full-thickness disruption of junctional zone[3] Intact stripe of normal outer myometrium
Stage II	IIA	Internal os and endocervical canal are widened Low signal intensity of fibrous stroma remains intact
	IIB	Disruption of fibrous stroma
Stage III	IIIA	Disruption of continuity of outer myometrium Irregular uterine configuration
	IIIB	Segmental loss of hypointense vaginal wall
	IIIC	Regional lymph nodes >1.0 cm in diameter
Stage IV	IVA	Tumor signal disrupts normal tissue planes with loss of low signal intensity of bladder or rectal wall
	IVB	Tumor masses in distant organs or anatomic sites

[1]All stages are further subdivided into three tumor grades (not shown).
[2]MRI findings seen on T2-weighted or contrast-enhanced T1-weighted images.
[3]For patients with adenomyosis, criteria may not apply.

equivalent accuracy to that of conventional surgical staging with intraoperative nodal dissection. Furthermore, the results of this study demonstrate that the number of unnecessary lymph node dissections might decrease with the use of MRI [96].

MRI is indicated for patients in whom advanced disease is suspected on clinical grounds and for patients with histologic subtypes that signify a worse prognosis. In addition, MRI can be performed in cases in which endovaginal US is technically limited or indeterminate and in patients with coexisting myometrial pathology such as leiomyomas. The decision to evaluate patients with MRI will depend to a large extent on cost, availability of equipment, local expertise, and the potential impact on patient management. It is useful to assess the depth of myometrial invasion with a reported accuracy of approximately 80% and to identify invasion of the cervix and/or extrauterine spread (figs. 14.40–14.43) [94, 97].

On MRI, T2-weighted sequences are used to identify and stage endometrial carcinoma because they provide optimal depiction of the uterine zonal anatomy. In addition to standard sagittal and transverse imaging planes, short-axis views of the uterine corpus are helpful for assessing myometrial invasion. Signal intensities of small endometrial tumors are similar to that of normal endometrium on T2-weighted sequences, limiting the ability of tumor delineation, whereas larger tumors result in widening of the endometrial cavity. A disruption of the junctional zone by hyperintense tumor is indicative of myometrial invasion. A problem, however, is that the junctional zone is not always visualized in postmenopausal women rendering correct image interpretation difficult in these cases. Deep myometrial invasion is suggested by the presence of hyperintense tumor in the outer half of the myometrium. Intravenous administration of gadolinium agents is helpful for MR staging of endometrial carcinoma, with the cancer demonstrating less pronounced contrast enhancement than surrounding uterine tissue. Most studies report that contrast-enhanced sequences are a useful addition as they improve assessment of myometrial invasion and differentiation of vital tumor from necrosis, debris or fluid-accumulation, namely, hematometra (fig. 14.41) [20, 94, 98, 99].

The MR appearance of noninvasive endometrial carcinoma (FIGO stage IA) is nonspecific. The uterus may appear entirely normal, or the endometrial carcinoma may appear as a widening of the endometrial stripe in postmenopausal women. In some cases, a heterogeneous mass with areas of high and low signal intensity distending the endometrial cavity may be noted [41]. Because these changes are also seen in endometrial hyperplasia, endometrial polyps, or coagulated blood, MRI has no role as a screening modality and histologic sampling is required to establish the diagnosis [41]. After

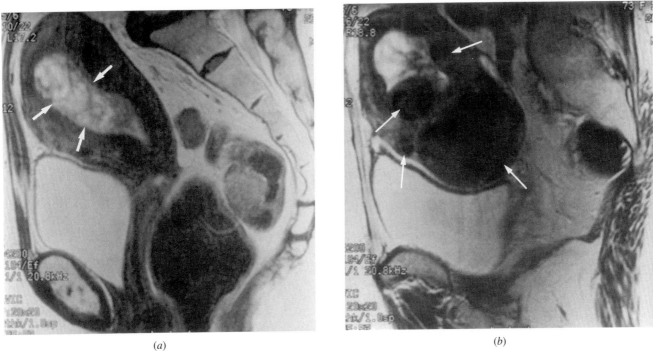

(a)   *(b)*

F I G . 14.40 Endometrial carcinoma stage IA, multiple leiomyomas. Sagittal T2-weighted ETSE images (*a*, *b*).The patient was referred to MRI for staging of endometrial carcinoma, detected by D&C, which was suspected as clinically advanced. MRI shows widening of the endometrial cavity due to inhomogeneously hyperintense tumor. The tumor (arrows, *a*) is well defined and the junctional zone is intact, consistent with stage IA. The large uterus found at clinical examination, and considered suspicious of advanced tumor stage, reflected the presence of multiple sharply delineated, hypointense leiomyomas (arrows, *b*).

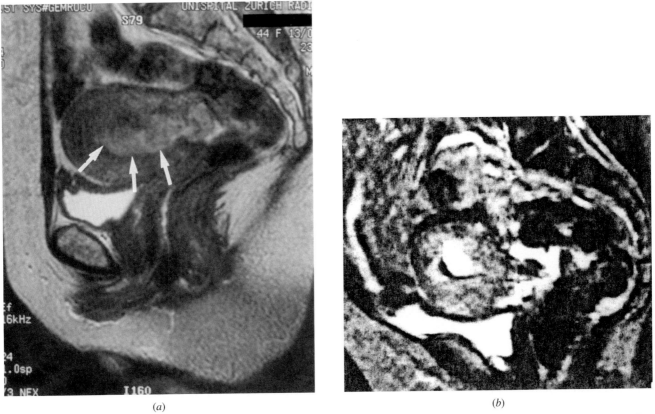

(a)   *(b)*

F I G . 14.41 Endometrial carcinoma stage IC. Sagittal T2-weighted ETSE image (*a*). An endometrial carcinoma is present that is isointense with endometrium and causes asymmetric widening of the endometrium. The junctional zone (arrows, *a*) is intact anteriorly, but tumor invasion is appreciated of the inner myometrium along the posterior aspect.

1085

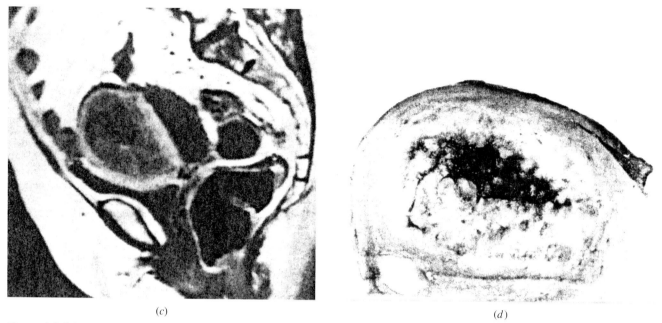

(c)

(d)

FIG. 14.41 (*Continued*) Sagittal T2-weighted spin-echo (*b*) and T1-weighted gadolinium-enhanced spin-echo (*c*) images and gross specimen (*d*) in a second patient. On the T2-weighted image (*b*), an increased volume of fluid is seen within the uterine cavity. The endometrial carcinoma is not well delineated on T2. On the gadolinium-enhanced image (*c*), substantially better demarcation of the carcinoma relative to the myometrium is observed. The tumor extent shows good correlation to the gross specimen. (Reprinted with permission from Hamm B, Kubik-Huch RA, Fleige B: MR imaging and CT of the female pelvis: Radiologic-pathologic correlation. *Eur Radiol* 1999; 9: 13–15.)

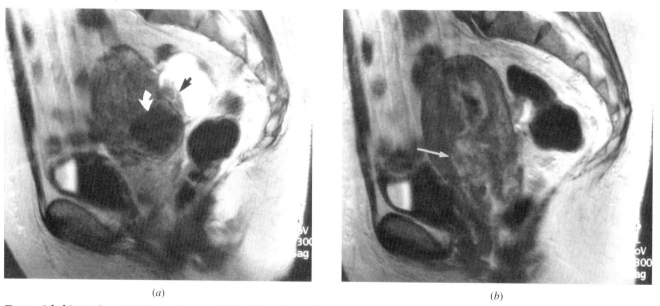

(a)

(b)

FIG. 14.42 Endometrial carcinoma with right adnexal metastasis. Sagittal (*a, b*) and transverse (*c*) T2-weighted ETSE and transverse interstitial-phase gadolinium-enhanced SGE (*d*) images. There is marked irregularity of endometrial tissue that shows heterogeneous enhancement after gadolinium administration. Deep invasion is shown in the anterior inferior uterine body (arrow, *b*). The zonal anatomy of the uterus body is lost. A cystic mass with an anterior solid nodule (arrow, *a, c, d*) is seen within the right adnexa, consistent with metastatic disease.

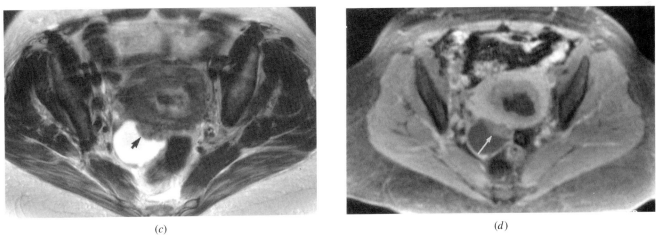

FIG. 14.42 (*Continued*) A leiomyoma (curved arrow, *a*) is present in the posteroinferior aspect of the uterus body. The post-gadolinium image (*d*) distinguishes between endometrial cancer and nonenhancing fluid in the endometrial canal.

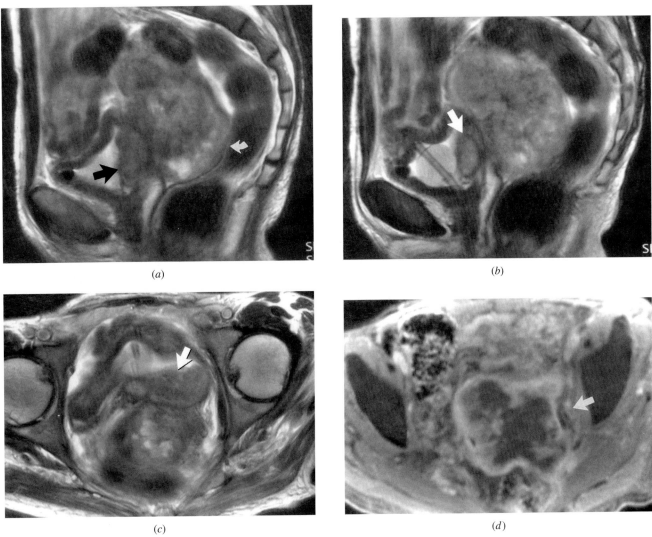

FIG. 14.43 Endometrial carcinoma, extensive disease. Sagittal (*a*, *b*) and transverse (*c*) T2-weighted ETSE and gadolinium-enhanced fat-suppressed SGE (*d*) images. A large necrotic endometrial mass is seen with invasion of the posterior wall of the urinary bladder (arrow, *a*–*c*) as well as extension to the left pelvic sidewall (arrow, *d*). This mass extends to the sigmoid colon and rectum (curved arrow, *a*). Liver metastases (not shown) were also identified.

gadolinium administration, endometrial carcinoma typically enhances to a lesser extent than the adjacent myometrium. In patients with FIGO stage IA disease, the junctional zone will remain intact (fig. 14.40), whereas in patients with myometrial invasion (stages FIGO IB and IC), segmental or complete disruption of the junctional zone by the tumor can be seen on T2-weighted sequences (Table 14.1; fig. 14.41). The accuracy of MRI in differentiating noninvasive from invasive endometrial carcinoma has been reported to range from 69 to 88% [41, 94, 95, 97, 99–101].

Superficial extension of endometrial carcinoma to the cervical mucosa (FIGO stage IIA) is best demonstrated on sagittal T2-weighted images by the observation that tumor widens the endocervical canal. Invasion of the cervical fibrous stroma (FIGO stage IIB) is diagnosed when hypointense cervical stroma is disrupted by the hyperintense tumor mass.

The ovaries may be involved by contiguous spread or by metastatic extension. Secondary involvement of the ovaries is suggested when a mass with heterogeneous signal characteristics is noted within the ovary [41].

FIGO stage III and FIGO stage IV, characterized by tumor extension beyond the uterus, can likewise be assessed by MRI. Ascites may be present in advanced disease.

Lymph nodes are well shown on noncontrast T1-weighted images or gadolinium-enhanced T1-weighted fat-suppressed images because of the good soft tissue contrast between low- to moderate-signal intensity nodes and the high-signal intensity surrounding fat or enhancing nodes and low signal fat, respectively. Assessment of metastatic lymphadenopathy in patients with endometrial and cervical carcinoma on MRI is based on lymph node size. Nodes with a size exceeding 1.0 cm in short-axis diameter are considered pathologic [41, 102]. In general, signal intensity characteristics have not been useful in differentiating metastatic from hyperplastic lymphadenopathy in the pelvis. A recent study by Yang et al. [103], however, showed that central necrosis of a lymph node, as shown on gadolinium-enhanced images, is an accurate criterion to diagnose metastasis in a pelvic node. Necrosis is not, however, commonly observed in malignant lymph nodes. The administration of lymph node specific contrast agents (USPIO: ultrasmall superparamagnetic iron oxide) might be a promising new approach to improve MR accuracy in lymph node staging in the near future [104].

Uterine Sarcoma

Uterine sarcomas are rare, constituting only 2–3% of all uterine malignancies. They encompass four histologic subtypes, malignant mixed mesodermal tumors,

leiomyosarcomas, and, rarely, endometrial stromal sarcomas and adenosarcomas [86].

For uterine sarcomas, no specific staging system exists. Uterine sarcomas invade blood vessels, lymphatics, and contiguous pelvic structures once they have extended beyond the uterus. The lung is the most common site of distant metastases. MRI signal characteristics are not reliable in differentiating sarcomas from other benign or malignant uterine neoplasms, but the presence of a large, heterogeneous mass with indistinct borders or irregular contours should raise concern (figs. 14.44 and 14.45) [105, 106]. Often the finding that establishes the diagnosis of malignancy is the demonstration of metastases.

Cervical Carcinoma

Invasive cervical carcinoma is the third most common malignancy of the female genital tract and is typically seen in younger women. The average age at diagnosis of patients with cervical carcinoma is 45 years. Early cytological detection of cervical intraepithelial neoplasia (CIN), a precursor lesion of cervical carcinoma, with routine cervical Papanicolaou (Pap) smears has led to a significant reduction in mortality. Intermenstrual bleeding is the most common symptom of invasive cervical carcinoma [86].

Up to 90% of all cervical carcinomas are squamous cell carcinomas. The remaining histologic types consist of adenocarcinomas, adenosquamous carcinomas, and undifferentiated carcinomas. Adenocarcinomas tend to have a worse prognosis. Other indicators of a poor prognosis include young age, lymphadenopathy, tumor diameter larger than 4 cm, depth of stromal invasion greater than 5 mm, and advanced stage at presentation [86, 98].

Cervical carcinoma advances predominately via direct extension and local spread. External iliac lymph nodes are most frequently involved, followed by obturator and common iliac and internal iliac nodes. Para-aortic lymph nodes are involved in approximately 45% of patients with tumor extension to the pelvic side wall or lower vagina. With tumor extension to the lower vagina, metastases may occur to inguinal lymph nodes. Hematogenous spread is rare and occurs only in the presence of advanced disease. The liver and lung are the most common sites of hematogenous metastases [86].

Cervical carcinoma is staged clinically according to the FIGO staging system (Table 14.2) [87]. Correct preoperative assessment of stage of disease is important, because it not only influences prognosis but also defines the choice of treatment. Patients with FIGO stage Ia are usually treated with simple hysterectomy or even fertility-preserving surgery, namely, trachelectomy [107], whereas patients with invasive carcinoma (FIGO

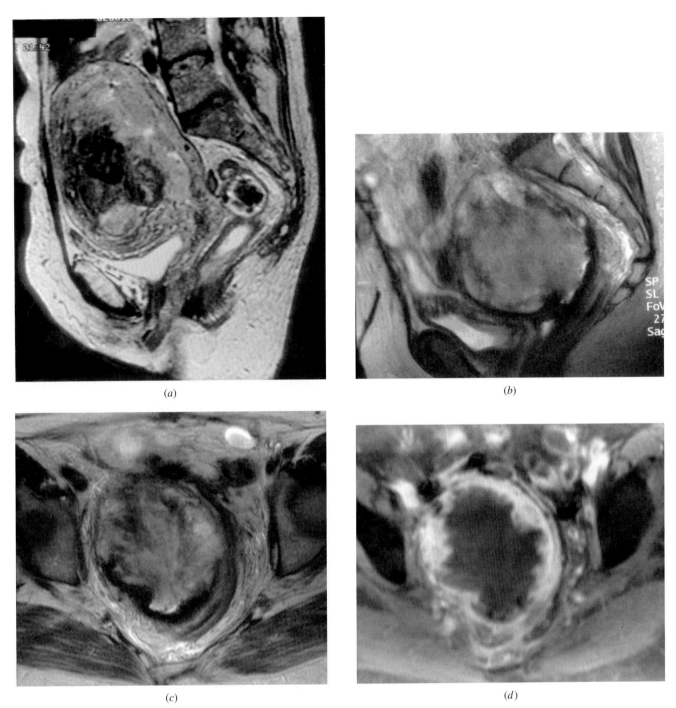

(a)

(b)

(c)

(d)

F I G . 14.44 Endometrial sarcoma. Sagittal T2-weighted ETSE image (*a*). A large, heterogeneous uterine mass with indistinct borders is demonstrated.

Sagittal (*b*) and transverse (*c*) T2-weighted ETSE and transverse gadolinium-enhanced SGE (*d*) images in a second patient with uterine sarcoma also demonstrate an ill-defined, large, heterogeneous mass, with central necrosis and peripheral enhancement.

stage Ib) or tumor extending to the upper vagina (FIGO stage IIa) are generally treated with radical hysterectomy and pelvic lymph node dissection. Patients with more advanced disease (Stage IIB or beyond) are treated with radiation therapy in many institutions.

Despite well-known limitations of the FIGO staging system, clinical staging remains the standard of reference by which treatment protocols are instituted in patients with invasive cervical carcinoma [108]. Staging errors of clinical staging ranging from 17 to 32% for Stage IB

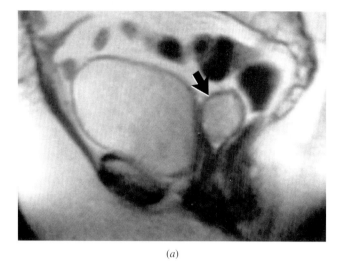

(a)

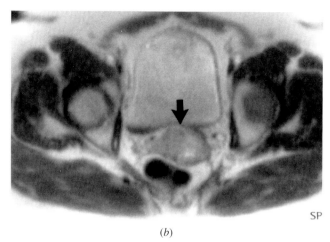

(b)

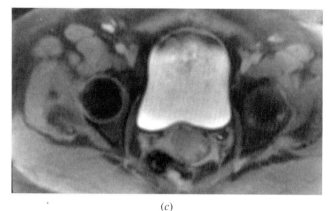

(c)

FIG. 14.45 Recurrent uterine carcinosarcoma. Sagittal (a) and transverse (b) T2-weighted SS-ETSE and transverse interstitial-phase gadolinium-enhanced fat-suppressed SGE (c) images in a patient who had previously undergone hysterectomy for uterine carcinosarcoma. There is a soft tissue mass (arrow, a, b) in the superior aspect of the vagina consistent with tumor recurrence.

disease and from 39 to 64% for Stage II disease have been reported [109–111]. Furthermore, although the presence of lymphadenopathy, large tumor volume, and tumor extension to the uterine corpus may have important prognostic and therapeutic implications, these factors are not evaluated in the FIGO staging system.

In recent years, however, the role of imaging in preoperative assessment of cervical carcinoma has steadily increased. Imaging is not used for detection of carcinoma but for staging of disease extent. Transvaginal ultrasound is usually the first imaging modality employed. Additional cross-sectional imaging is useful if the tumor volume is large. MRI has been shown to be superior to CT in the local staging of cervical carcinoma [112]. A recent cost-effectiveness study demonstrated significant cost savings when comparing MRI to the traditional evaluation including tests such as cystoscopy, barium enema, and intravenous pyelography [108].

MRI surpasses CT imaging and clinical staging in assessing the depth of stromal invasion, with reported accuracies ranging from 77 to 85%, and assessing parametrial invasion, with accuracy rates ranging from 80 to 94% [16, 85, 112–115].

Currently MRI may not be indicated in all patients with cervical carcinoma. Patients with tumors larger than

2 cm in size or with tumors located entirely within the endocervical canal have been shown to benefit most from undergoing MRI evaluation [108]. Furthermore, MRI is particularly useful in patients with concomitant pelvic masses and is currently the best imaging procedure for evaluating pregnant patients with cervical carcinoma (fig.14.46).

On MRI, the T2-weighted sequence is the most important sequence for the staging of cervical cancer, providing optimal contrast between tumor and residual cervix. Transverse and sagittal sequences are routinely performed. One study reported that additional oblique images, perpendicular to the cervical canal, can further improve staging accuracy [15]. Cervical cancer appears high signal intensity compared to the hypointense cervical stroma (figs. 14.47–14.54). Stage FIGO IB carcinoma is restricted to the cervix and demonstrates a fully preserved hypointense rim of normal cervical stroma surrounding the tumor on T2-weighted images (figs. 14.47 and 14.48).

Tumor is classified as Stage IIA when it invades the upper two-thirds of the vagina (see Table 14.2). On MRI, this is best established on sagittal T2-weighted images. Disruption of the low signal intensity of the vaginal wall or the presence of a thickened hyperintense vagina

Table 14.2 FIGO Staging of Cervical Carcinoma with Corresponding MRI Findings

FIGO Staging[1]

Stage 0		Carcinoma in situ
Stage I		Tumor confined to cervix (extension to corpus should be disregarded)
	IA	Microinvasion
	IB	Clinically invasive. Invasive component >5 mm in depth and >7 mm in horizontal spread
Stage II		Tumor extends beyond cervix but not to pelvic side wall or lower third of vagina
	IIA	Vaginal invasion (no parametrial invasion)
	IIB	Parametrial invasion
Stage III		Tumor extends to lower third of vagina or pelvic side wall; ureter obstruction
	IIIA	Invasion of lower third of vagina (no pelvic side-wall extension)
	IIIB	Pelvic side wall extension or ureteral obstruction
Stage IV		Tumor extends outside true pelvis of invades bladder or rectal mucosa
	IVA	Invasion of bladder or rectal mucosa
	IVB	Distant metastases

Corresponding MRI findings[2]

Stage 0		No tumor mass present
Stage I	IA	No tumor mass or localized widening of the endocervical canal with a small tumor mass. Fibrous stroma intact and symmetric
	IB	Partial or complete disruption of low-signal-intensity fibrous stroma. Rim of intact cervical tissue surrounding tumor
Stage II	IIA	Segmental disruption of hypointense vaginal wall (upper two-thirds)
	IIB	Complete disruption of low signal intensity fibrous stroma with tumor signal extending into parametrium
Stage III	IIIA	Segmental disruption of hypointense vaginal wall (lower third)
	IIIB	Same findings as IIB with tumor signal, most frequently extending to involve obturator internus, piriformis, or levator ani muscles. Dilated ureter
Stage IV	IVA	Tumor signal disrupts normal tissue planes with loss of low signal intensity of bladder or rectal wall
	IVB	Tumor masses in distant organs or anatomic sites

[1]The presence of metastatic lymph nodes is not included in the FIGO classification.
[2]MRI findings seen on T2-weighted or contrast-enhanced T1-weighted images.

indicate tumor invasion. A more important criterion that influences therapeutic decisionmaking, is the presence or absence of parametrial invasion, namely, FIGO stage IIb. Parametrial extension is diagnosed with MRI when there is complete disruption of the cervical stroma often associated with irregularity or stranding within the parametrial fat. Studies have shown that a completely intact ring of low-signal intensity cervical stroma is highly accurate in excluding parametrial invasion (fig. 14.51) [85, 112, 114].

In FIGO stage IIIa disease, the tumor mass extends to involve the lower third of the vagina. This is best evaluated on sagittal T2-weighted images (fig. 14.52). Because the distal portion of the vagina drains to the lymph nodes in the groin, the groin region should be examined in cases of extensive tumor growth.

Invasion of the pelvic side wall or obstruction of one or both ureters corresponds to stage IIIb disease. A dilated ureter can be well delineated along the psoas muscle by a variety of MR sequences including T2-weighted fat-suppressed and interstitial-phase gadolinium-enhanced T1-weighted fat-suppressed sequence, both of which show excellent contrast between tumor, surrounding tissue and ureter. Pelvic side wall invasion is shown when the normal low signal intensity of the levator ani, pyriformis, or obturator internus muscle is disrupted on T2-weighted images. Invasion of the urinary bladder or rectal wall (stage Iva) is demonstrated, when the normally present fat planes between organs is obliterated combined with a hyperintense disruption of the otherwise hypointense urinary bladder or rectal wall on T2-weighted images. Nodular wall thickening or intraluminal masses may be present (figs. 14.53 and 14.54) [20]. Transverse and sagittal T1-weighted sequences, T2-weighted fat-suppressed sequences and/or interstitial-phase gadolinium-enhanced T1-weighted fat-suppressed sequences are used to detect the presence of lymphadenopathy as with other malignancies.

Gadolinium-enhanced images are not routinely used for the staging of cervical carcinoma, because prior studies have shown that, in distinction to staging of endometrial carcinoma, they provide little additional information in patients with cervical carcinoma. Gadolinium enhancement is useful in cases of suspected invasion of the bladder or rectum, large tumor volume, necrotic areas, or suspected fistulas, particularly in the setting of postradiation treatment (fig. 14.55) [16–20].

Cervical carcinoma may result in cervical outlet obstruction, and thus when the obstruction of the cervix is high grade, hematometra or pyometra. On MRI, the uterine cavity is distended by material of variable signal intensity, depending on its composition, for example, retained secretions, blood, or tumor. Other cause of cervical stenosis include postradiation, congenital, inflammatory, neoplastic, or iatrogenic origins as well as the presence of endometrial carcinoma [116].

Recurrent Cervical Carcinoma

After treatment of cervical carcinoma, either by surgery or radiation therapy, recurrent disease may develop at

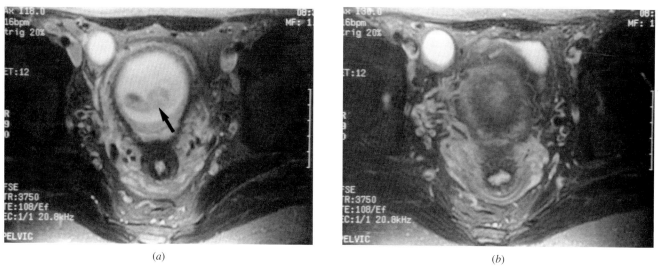

FIG. 14.46 FIGO stage I cervical carcinoma in a pregnant patient at 11 weeks gestation. Transverse T2-weighted ETSE images (*a, b*) at superior (*a*) and inferior (*b*) levels. The cervical carcinoma is not clearly visualized, reflecting small tumor size. The MR image shows that the hypointense cervical stroma is not disrupted: thus parametrial invasion could be excluded. Trachelectomy was performed and definitive treatment delayed until after delivery (black arrow = fetus, *a*).

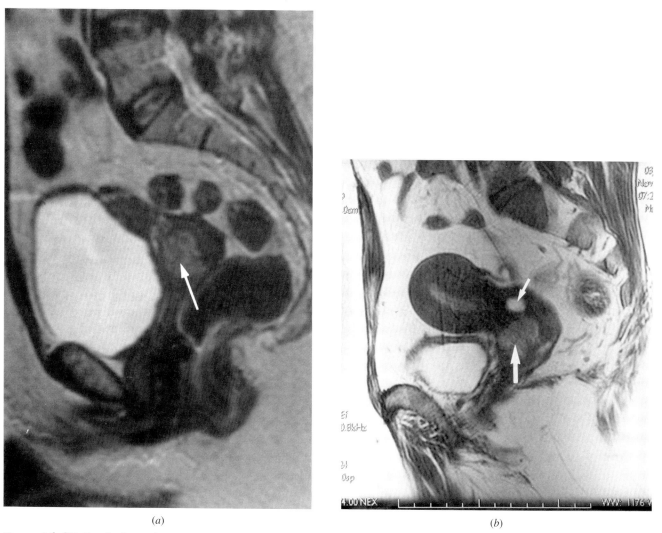

FIG. 14.47 Cervical carcinoma stage IB. Sagittal T2-weighted ETSE image (*a*). A tumor (arrow, *a*) of intermediate signal is shown within the cervix. The uterus in this postmenopausal patient is atrophic.

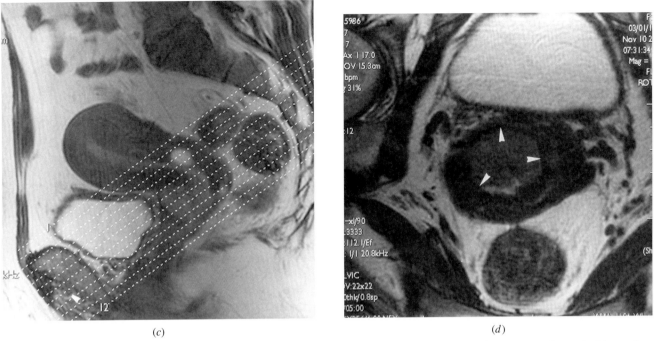

(c)   (d)

F I G . 14.47 (*Continued*) Sagittal T2-weighted ETSE (*b*, *c*) and transverse (*d*) images in a second patient. On the sagittal image in *c* an oblique imaging plane perpendicular to the cervical canal is prescribed graphically. The resulting transverse-oblique T2-weighted fast spin-echo image is shown in *d*. A tumor (arrow, *b*) of intermediate signal is shown within the cervix. The tumor is surrounded by normal hypointense cervical stroma along its entire circumference (arrowheads, *d*), excluding parametrial invasion. Incidental nabothian cysts (small arrow, *b*) are seen within the cervix.

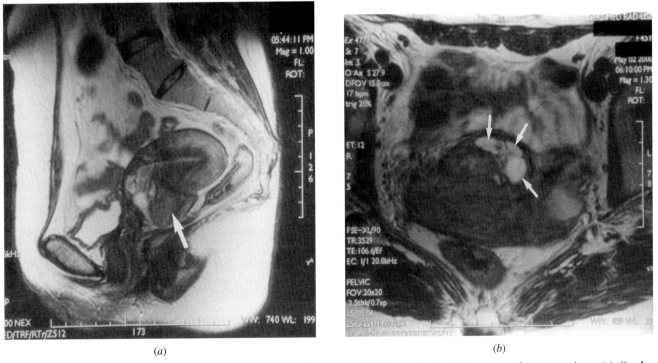

(a)   (b)

F I G . 14.48 Cervical carcinoma stage IB. Sagittal (*a*) and transverse (*b*) T2-weighted ETSE images and gross specimen (*c*). On the sagittal image a tumor (arrow, *a*) of intermediate signal is shown within the posterior aspect of the cervix. The tumor is surrounded by a thin stripe of normal hypointense cervical stroma.

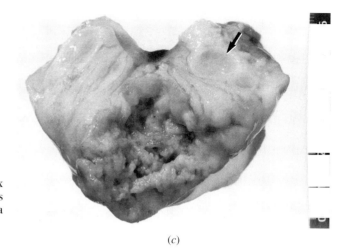

(c)

FIG. 14.48 (*Continued*) The fat plane between the cervix and the rectal wall is well delineated. Incidentally, nabothian cysts (small arrows, *b*) are seen within the cervix. A stage IB carcinoma was histologically confirmed (arrow, *c*: nabothian cyst).

multiple sites. Typical manifestations include a recurrent pelvic mass and lymphadenopathy; less common sites of recurrence are solid organs, including liver or bones, and peritoneal carcinomatosis [117]. Approximately 30% of women with invasive cervical carcinoma will die as a result of recurrent or persistent disease [118]. Recurrent disease may come to clinical attention of the basis of follow-up imaging studies, or symptoms resulting from swelling of lower extremities due to lymphatic obstruction, pain due to nerve compression or invasion, or tumor obstruction of the ureters. MRI and computed tomography perform comparably to detect distant recurrence, whereas MRI likely performs better at detecting local recurrence in the pelvis (fig. 14.56).

Irradiation of the uterus in premenopausal patients results in a decrease in the size of the uterus, thinning of the endometrium, decreased signal intensity of the myometrium, and loss of uterine zonal anatomy on T2-weighted sequences, resembling the appearance of

a nonirradiated postmenopausal uterus. These changes likely reflect a combination of direct radiation effects on the uterus and loss of hormonal stimulation from ovarian function suppression. The appearance of the uterus in postmenopausal women does not significantly change after radiation therapy.

Patients who have undergone radiation therapy present a diagnostic challenge because differentiation between radiation changes and residual or recurrent disease is frequently difficult. MRI has been shown to be of value in evaluation of patients who have undergone radiation therapy and is superior to CT [119–123].

In patients with recurrent tumor, who are more than 12 months out from radiation therapy, areas of tumor tissue appear hyperintense relative to adjacent muscle and fat on T2-weighted imaging, whereas radiation fibrosis appears hypointense. One cautionary note is that on long echo-train sequences fat has a relatively high signal that may be higher than tumor recurrence. Therefore,

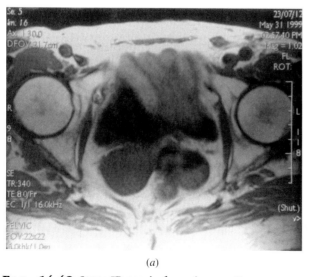

(a)

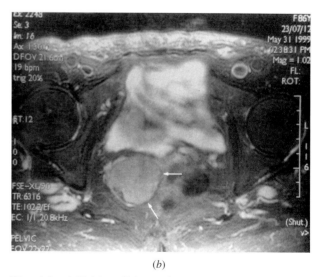

(b)

FIG. 14.49 Stage IB cervical carcinoma. Transverse precontrast T1-weighted SE (*a*) and T2-weighted fat-suppressed ETSE (*b*) images. The cervical tumor is of large volume, however, on the T2-weighted images a thin hypointense stripe of cervical stroma (arrows, *b*) is seen surrounding the entire circumference of the cancer, and parametrial invasion was thus excluded. This finding was confirmed by histology.

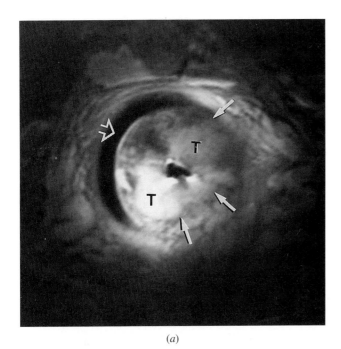
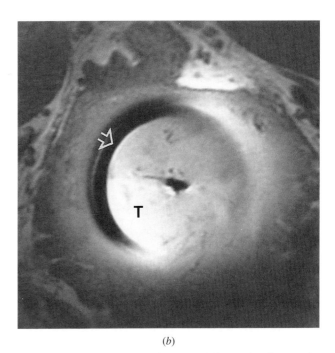

(a)   *(b)*

F IG. 14.50 Stage IB cervical carcinoma, endovaginal coil. Transverse T2-weighted spin-echo (*a*) and T1-weighted spin-echo (*b*) images using a solenoid geometry ring endovaginal coil (open arrow, *a, b*). A susceptibility artifact is present centrally within the cervix from a recent biopsy (*a, b*). An intermediate-signal intensity tumor (T) is expanding the cervix (*a, b*), but an intact stripe of residual cervical stroma is seen around the periphery (arrows, *a*). (Courtesy of Dr. Naudita De Souza, MRI Unit, Hammersmith Hospital, London, UK. Reprinted with permission from De Souza NM, Scoones D, Krausz T, Gilderale DJ, Soutter WP: High-resolution MR imaging of Stage I cervical neoplasia with a dedicated transvaginal coil: MR features and correlation of imaging and pathological findings. *AM J Roentgenol* 166: 553–559, 1996.)

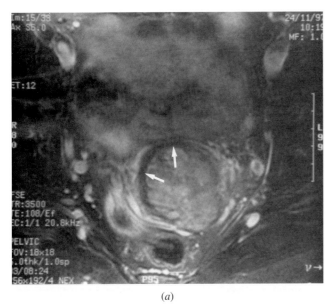
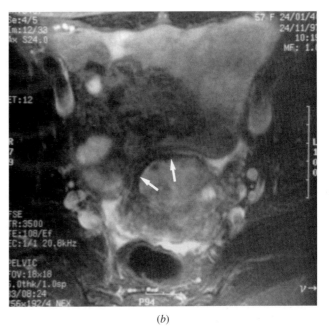

(a)   *(b)*

F IG. 14.51 Cervical carcinoma stage IIB. Transverse T2-weighted fat-suppressed ETSE images (*a, b*). A large heterogeneous hyperintense cervical tumor is seen. Normal hypointense cervical stroma can be delineated along the anterior aspect (arrows, *a, b*), but it is disrupted posteriorly. The diagnosis of parametrial invasion was histologically confirmed.

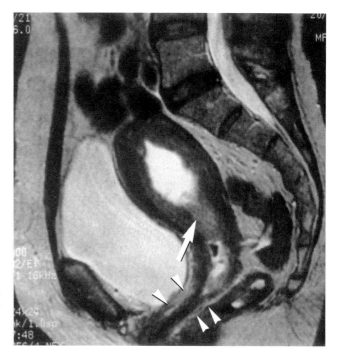

FIG. 14.52 Cervical carcinoma with vaginal extension. Sagittal T2-weighted ETSE image. Hyperintense cervical carcinoma (arrow) is present with extension into the vagina. The tumor results in cervical obstruction with fluid retention within the uterine cavity. Note that the fat planes between the cervix and urinary bladder and cervix and rectal wall are preserved (arrowheads), excluding bladder or rectal wall invasion.

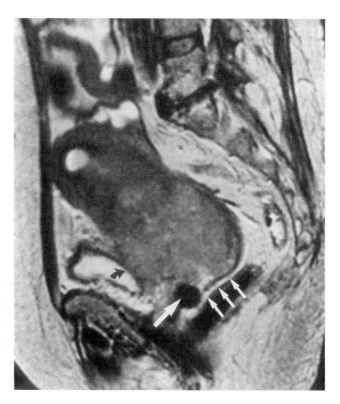

FIG. 14.53 Cervical carcinoma with urinary bladder invasion (FIGO IV). Sagittal T2-weighted ETSE image. Cervical carcinoma is present, which is hyperintense and shows extension into the vagina (large arrow = tampon) and urinary bladder. The inner aspect of the bladder wall (curved arrow) is not invaded as shown by the preservation of low signal intensity. Note that the fat plane between the cervix and rectal wall is preserved (small arrows), excluding rectal wall invasion.

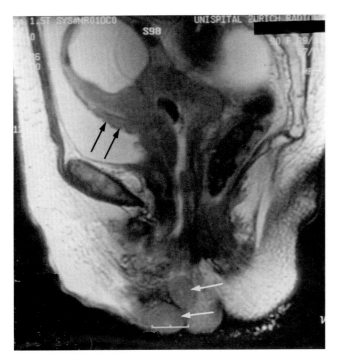

FIG. 14.54 Cervical carcinoma, extensive disease. Sagittal T2-weighted ETSE image. A large cervical carcinoma is present, which appears hyperintense and shows extension to the vagina, the labia majora (white arrows), and the urinary bladder (black arrows). Fluid retention in the uterine cavity reflects obstruction of the cervical canal.

when these sequences are employed more emphasis must be placed on morphology of tissue (i.e., masslike favors recurrence) and less emphasis on the signal of tissue relative to fat. During the initial 6–12 months after treatment, areas of radiation fibrosis may appear increased signal intensity on T2-weighted sequences due to acute inflammation, edema, and increased capillary vascularity. Both tumor recurrence and radiation fibrosis are low signal intensity on T1-weighted sequences. In the early posttreatment period, the presence of an identifiable mass lesion favors recurrence [119, 121, 122]. The

extent of gadolinium enhancement of the cervix is relatively nonspecific and may be observed not only in recurrent tumor but also in postirradiation fibrosis, inflammation or radiation necrosis [119], particularly within 12 months of treatment. In our experience, increased enhancement of radiation fibrosis may last up to 2 years, whereas increased signal on T2 usually lasts for a shorter time period, generally up to 12 months. If superimposed infection has occurred, then both increased enhancement and increased signal on T2 will be apparent for an ever longer period of time. Gadolinium-enhanced

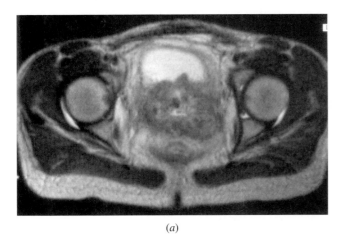

(*a*)

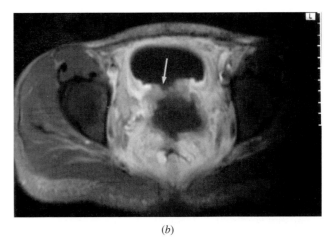

(*b*)

FIG. 14.55 Large cervical cancer after radiation therapy with necrosis and bladder fistula. Transverse T2-weighted ETSE (*a*) and transverse interstitial-phase gadolinium-enhanced fat-suppressed SGE (*b*) images. The T2-weighted image (*a*) demonstrates a large mass in the cervix. After gadolinium enhancement (*b*), extensive necrosis secondary to radiation therapy is identified. A fistula to the bladder (arrow, *b*) is well seen. Bladder fistula are usually best shown on postgadolinium images as a low-signal linear structure reflecting lack of enhancement of the tract, often associated with increased enhancement of the tract wall.

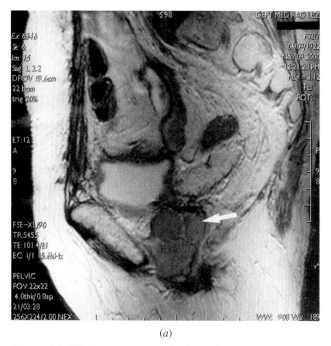
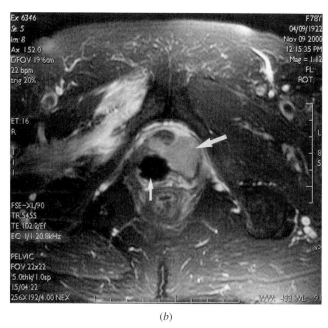

(a)   *(b)*

F I G . 14.56 Recurrent cervical carcinoma. Sagittal T2-weighted ETSE (*a*) and transverse T2-weighted fat-suppressed ETSE (*b*) images. There is a large tumor recurrence (arrows, *a, b*) involving the entire vagina, which appears intermediate signal intensity. The patient has a history of hysterectomy for cervical carcinoma. A tampon is present (small arrow, *b*).

imaging has, however, been shown to be helpful in demonstrating parametrial and pelvic side wall recurrence [121]. As a rule, radiation changes tend to be small volume, with symmetric involvement of tissue and organs, and confined to the expected radiation portal, whereas tumor recurrence tends to be of larger volume, with nodular or irregular involvement of tissue and organs, and of asymmetric distribution, including outside the expected radiation portal. Of course, changes of radiation injury and recurrence commonly coexist, making accurate diagnosis very challenging.

MRI AND PREGNANCY

General Considerations

The choice of imaging techniques in pregnant patients is limited by the potential risks to the fetus. Because low-dose irradiation of the fetus may increase the likelihood of childhood cancer, the use of ionizing radiation during pregnancy should be avoided whenever possible. Ultrasonography (US) is routinely used in the evaluation of the fetus and pregnant women because it is safe, inexpensive, and widely available. In experienced hands, US is highly accurate in the diagnosis of most complications associated with pregnancy. In recent years, several studies have reported the results of MRI in the evaluation of fetal and maternal disorders. Although US remains the imaging technique of choice for prenatal

assessment of fetal (mal)development, the advent of ultrafast MR sequences has currently increased the clinical indications for fetal MRI. Fast MR imaging techniques provide excellent resolution for imaging of fetal and maternal anatomies without the need for sedation [23, 24, 27, 124–127].

Safety Issues

MRI is considered safe for the pregnant patient and developing fetus. At present, there is no clinical or experimental evidence of teratogenic or other adverse fetal effects from MR imaging in pregnancy [1, 3, 4, 128–130], although a few studies have demonstrated that prolonged or high-level exposure to electromagnetic radiation might result in disorders of embryogenesis and teratogenicity in laboratory animals [130, 131]. In a survey of female MR workers, no substantial increase in adverse pregnancy outcome was found [132].

A statement from the National Institute of Health Consensus Development Conferences on MRI indicated that "MRI should be used during the first trimester of pregnancy only when there are clear medical indications and when it offers a definite advantage over other tests" [87]. Thus prudence currently dictates that MRI should be avoided during the first trimester not only because of biosafety aspects, because this is the time when rapid organogenesis is taking place, but also because of the limited results of the benefits fetal imaging studies at this gestational age.

Extracellular MRI contrast agents, such as gadopentetate dimeglumine, have been demonstrated to cross the placental barrier when injected into primates. These agents are then excreted by the fetal urinary tract into the amniotic cavity and subsequently swallowed by the fetus [133]. Although a study performed in pregnant mice, with gadopentetate dimeglumine injected into the peritoneal cavity, failed to demonstrate any adverse effects [134], gadolinium contrast media should in general be avoided during pregnancy, because no controlled studies have been performed in humans. Gadolinium contrast should only be used if not using the agent has the potential to seriously impact in a negative fashion on the medical management of the woman or fetus in the investigation of major medical illness.

The Fetus

At present, ultrasonography, as an inexpensive and widely available real-time investigation, remains the imaging technique of choice for prenatal assessment of the fetus. With the advent of motion-insensitive T2-weighted sequences over the last few years, the role of fetal MRI is increasing in the routine clinical setting (figs. 14.57–14.72).

Although ultrasonography is not limited by motion artifacts (still not completely obviated in fetal MRI) and can additionally provide Doppler blood flow information, there are some advantages inherent to the MR technique: the investigation is not as operator dependent, the complete study can be easily stored for subsequent analysis or transmission to another facility (this may be especially useful in difficult cases and at isolated or small institutions), the field of view obtained with MRI is larger than that obtained with ultrasound, which facilitates anatomic orientation and allows for a global evaluation of the fetus and maternal pelvis, and image quality is not adversely affected by the presence of air or bony structures or by maternal obesity. MR imaging might develop an important role in those situations where the sonographic examination is impaired, for example, by maternal obesity, oligohydramnios, or fetal head engagement in late pregnancy.

With the advent of fetal MR imaging, knowledge of normal fetal anatomy is essential to detect maldevelopment in utero. MR imaging can demonstrate fetal anatomy in detail. Major developmental structures of the fetus, particularly the CNS, lungs, and major abdominal viscera, can be adequately evaluated by MRI as early as the beginning of the second trimester. Because of its small size and cardiac motion artifacts, MRI of the heart is still limited at present.

The majority of clinically indicated obstetric MR studies involve either evaluation of the fetal brain or the assessment of complex malformation syndromes, because it has been shown that MRI performs very well in the evaluation of fetal cerebral pathologies. Its diagnostic accuracy is superior to sonography in selected

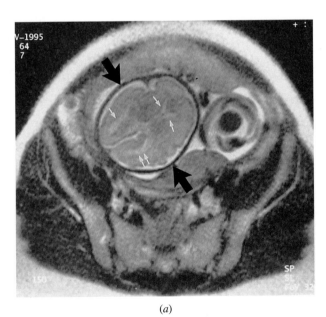

(a)

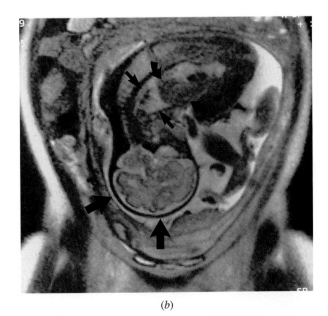

(b)

FIG. 14.57 Normal fetus. Central nervous system (CNS) third trimester. Transverse (*a*) and coronal SS-ETSE (*b*) sequences through the maternal pelvis. The contour of the fetal head (large arrows, *a, b*) and the cerebral hemispheres are well delineated. Cerebral ventricles (small arrows, *a*) are hyperintense relative to brain tissue. Fetal lungs (arrows, *b*) are of high signal intensity because of their water content. The liver (curved arrows, *b*) is of intermediate signal intensity and occupies most of the abdominal cavity. The lung-liver interface outlines the diaphragm.

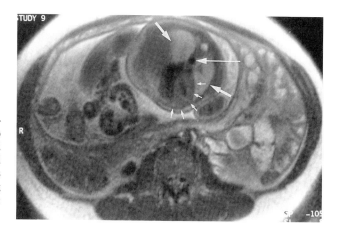

FIG. 14.58 Normal fetus. Heart and vessels. Transverse SS-ETSE sequence through the maternal pelvis. Fetal lungs (arrows) are depicted on either side of the thorax. The heart is visible, and the contrast between the signal-void left ventricule chamber and the intermediate-signal intensity myocardium (small arrows) allows assessment of ventricule wall thickness. The thoracic aorta (long thin arrow) is depicted as a signal-void structure anterior to the thoracic spine.

cases of cerebral malformations, because of the high soft tissue contrast resolution, and in complex fetal disorders [27, 124, 135].

Changes in fetal brain maturation proceed through different stages in an predictable fashion that can be reliably evaluated with fast T2-weighted imaging. At 12–23 weeks of gestation, the brain demonstrates a smooth surface, except for the interhemispheric fissure. Two to three layers in the cerebral cortex can be delineated at this time. At 24–26 weeks, a few shallow groves will be seen in the central sulcus, and the three different layers, the immature cortex, the intermediate zone, and the germinal matrix, can be differentiated. Sulcus

formation is observed in various regions of the brain parenchyma between 27 and 29 weeks and sulcation in the whole cerebal cortex is seen from 30 weeks on, whereas infolding of the cortex and opercular formation will not be seen before 33 weeks. At 23 weeks, cerebral ventricles are large, corresponding to normal fetal hydrocephalus, gradually becoming smaller thereafter. The subarachnoid space overlying the cortical convexities is slightly dilated at all gestational ages, most markedly at 21–26 weeks of gestation [126, 136].

In the thorax, the lung, and the tracheobronchial tree, both filled with amniotic fluid, appear hyperintense on T2-weighted images. Sagittal, coronal, and transverse

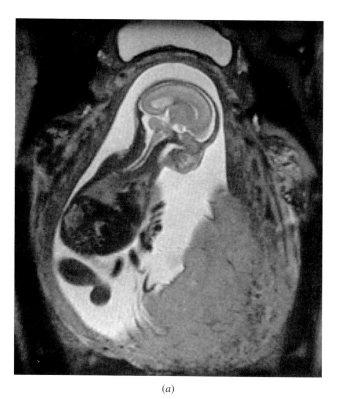
(a)

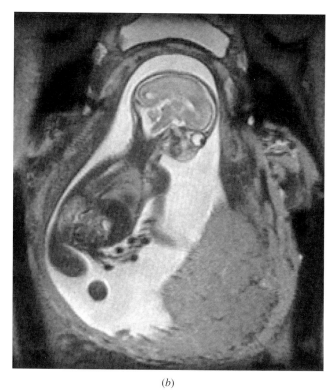
(b)

FIG. 14.59 Normal pregnancy at 22 weeks of gestation. Sagittal T2-weighted SS-ETSE (*a, b, c*) images of the fetus; 3D reconstruction of the 2D MR data set of the fetus and placenta (*d, e, f, g*).

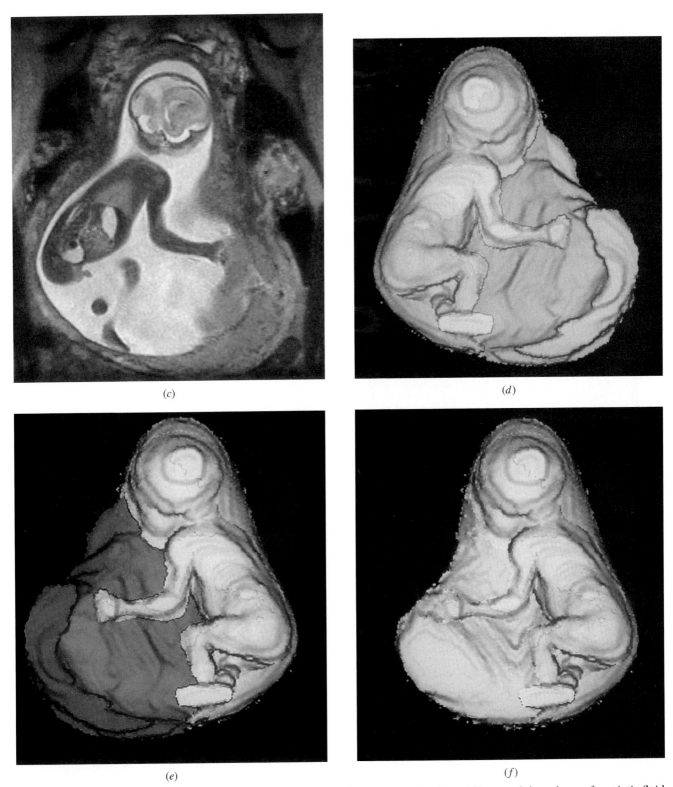

(c)   *(d)*

(e)   *(f)*

F I G. 14.59 (*Continued*) Fetal volume was determined to be 349 cc, placental volume 390 cc, and the volume of amniotic fluid 486 cc. (Reprinted with permission from Kubik-Huch RA, Wildermuth S, Cettuzzi L, Rake A, Seifert B, Chaoui R, Marincek B: Ultrafast magnetic resonance imaging of the fetus and utero-placental unit: 3-Dimensional reconstruction and volumetry. *Radiology.* In press.)

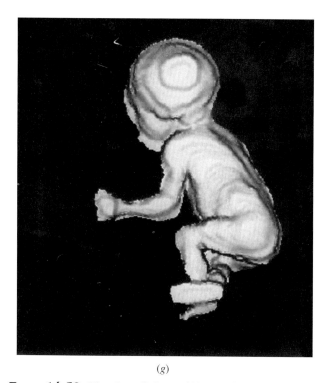

(g)

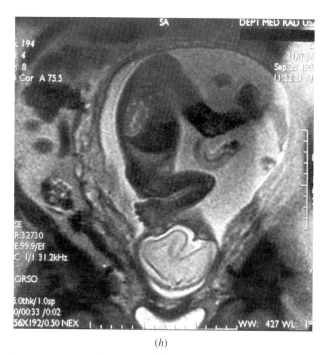

(h)

FIG. 14.59 (*Continued*) Sagittal T2-weighted SS-ETSE (*b*) image demonstrates another normal fetus in the second trimester of pregnancy.

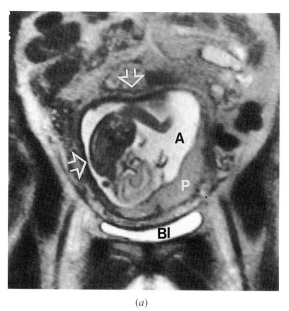

(a)

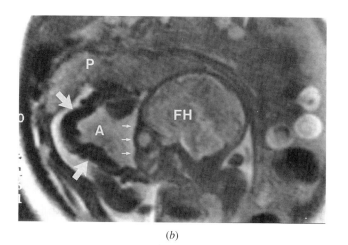

(b)

FIG. 14.60 Normal fetus. Coronal SS-ETSE sequence through the maternal pelvis (*a*). Because of short acquisition times, the gestational sac (open arrows) and fetal contours are clearly depicted, without motion-related artifacts. A, amniotic fluid; P, placenta; Bl, maternal bladder.

Coronal SS-ETSE sequence through the maternal pelvis (*b*) in a second patient shows the fetal face (small arrows) and a segment of the umbilical cord (arrows) in the amniotic fluid (A). FH, fetal head; P, placenta.

Coronal SS-ETSE sequence through the maternal pelvis (*c*) in a third patient shows the fetal face (small arrows) and upper extremity (arrows). FH, fetal head; P, placenta.

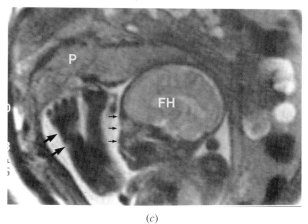

(c)

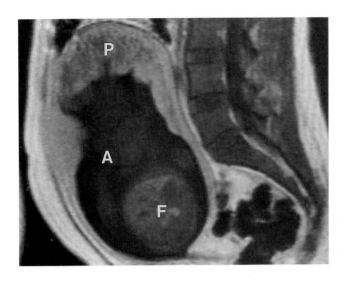

FIG. 14.61 Normal fetus. Sagittal SGE sequence through the maternal pelvis shows a gravid uterus with amniotic fluid (A), fetal parts (F), and a placenta (P). The low signal intensity of the amniotic fluid serves as a native contrast to outline the inner contour of the placenta.

images of the fetus clearly permit distinction between structures of the thorax and abdomen and can be used to assess diaphragmatic integrity [21]. Diagnosis of maldevelopment, for example, congenital diaphragmatic hernia, adenomatoid-cystic pulmonary malformation (fig. 14.70) or bronchopulmonary sequestration may be established by MRI. Accurate assessment of lung volume can be determined that may have potentially important

clinical applications in the assessment of pulmonary hypoplasia in the future [127, 137].

The heart, pulmonary vasculature, and great vessels of the thorax appear as hypointense structures. At present, the value of fetal MRI for assessment of the heart is limited because of the small size of the organ, the lack of flow information, and the fact that the fetal heart rate commonly exceeds 140 beats per

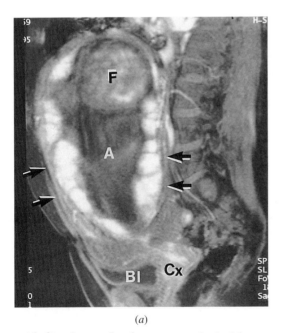

(a)

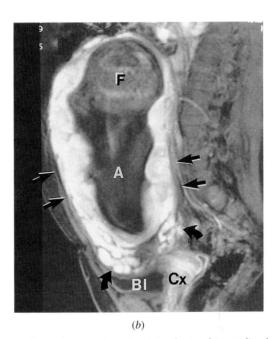

(b)

FIG. 14.62 Placental enhancement. Sagittal fat-suppressed SGE images through the maternal pelvis obtained immediately (*a*) and at 1 min (*b*) after gadolinium administration in the third trimester. The placenta (arrows, *a*, *b*) shows rapid, intense enhancement. The placenta exhibits a cotyledon pattern of enhancement on the immediate postgadolinium image (*a*) which becomes more homogeneous at 1 min (*b*), consistent with the appearance of a third trimester placenta. In contrast, second trimester placentas show uniform enhancement and thickness. Note enlarged uterine vessels (curved arrows, *b*) around the lower uterine segment. A, amniotic fluid; F, fetal parts; Bl, maternal bladder; Cx, cervix.

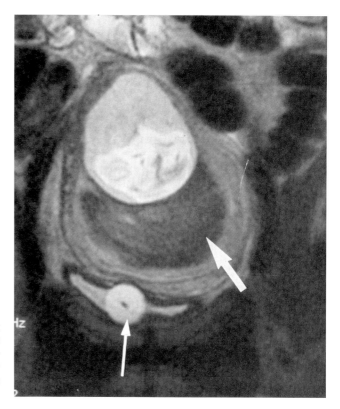

FIG. 14.63 Uterine hematoma in a cornual pregnancy at 12 weeks of gestation. Coronal SS-ETSE sequence through the maternal pelvis shows a hypointense uterine hematoma (large arrow). Intrauterine growth retardation was also present secondary to cornual implantation. A Foley catheter can be delineated in the maternal urinary bladder (small arrow).

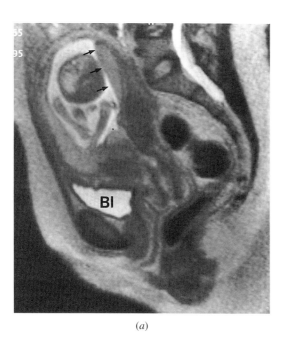

(a)

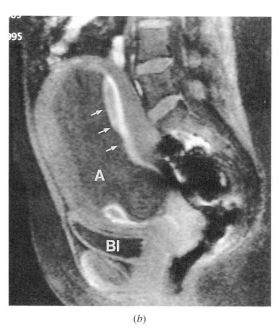

(b)

FIG. 14.64 Subchorionic hematoma. Sagittal SS-ETSE (*a*) and fat-suppressed SGE (*b*) images through the maternal pelvis. A lenticular area of decreased signal intensity on the T2-weighted image (arrows, *a*) and moderately high signal on the SGE image (arrows, *b*) is consistent with a subchorionic hematoma. Note the peripheral rim of higher signal intensity on the SGE sequence indicating subacute hemorrhage. A, amniotic fluid; Bl, maternal bladder.

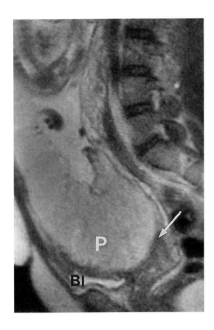

F I G . 14.65 Complete placenta previa. Sagittal SS-ETSE image through the maternal pelvis shows that the placenta (P) completely covers the internal cervical os (arrow). Bl, maternal bladder.

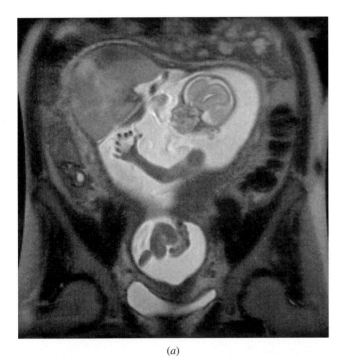

(a)

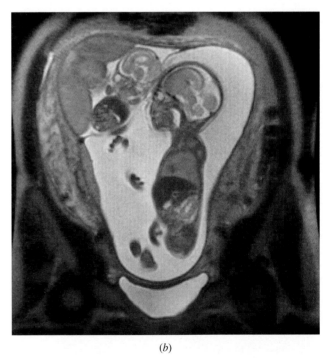

(b)

F I G . 14.66 Twin pregnancy at 21 weeks of gestation. Intrauterine growth retardation of 1 fetus caused by hemo-dynamic impairment. Coronal T2-weighted SS-ETSE images (*a, b*) demonstrate a smaller size of 1 of the twins, reflecting growth retardation. The placenta of this twin is also small in size and of compact architecture. (Reprinted with permission from Kubik-Huch RA, Wildermuth S, Cettuzzi L, Rake A, Seifert B, Chaoui R, Marincek B: Ultrafast magnetic resonance imaging of the fetus and utero-placental unit: 3-Dimensional reconstruction and volumetry. *Radiology.* In press.)

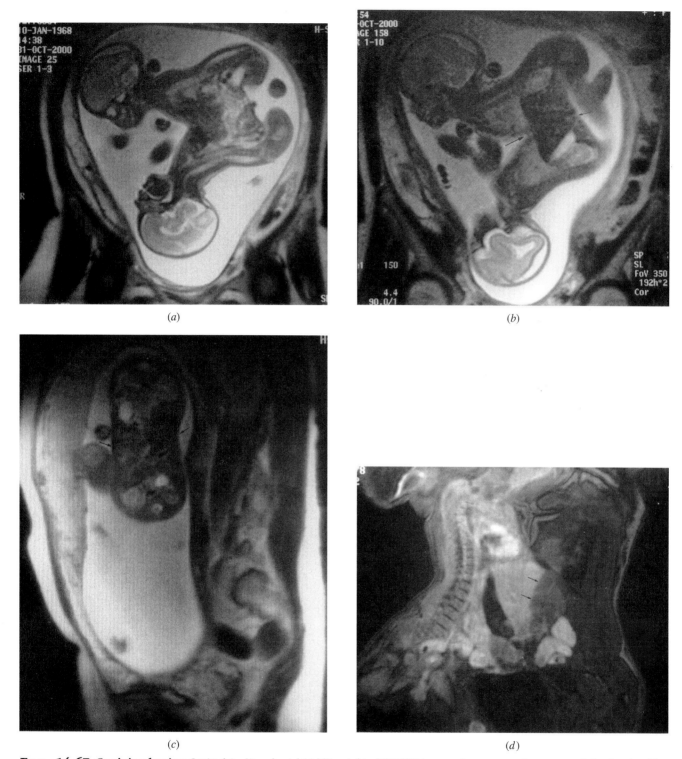

(a)

(b)

(c)

(d)

F I G . 14.67 Conjoined twins. Sagittal (*a, b*) and axial (*c*) T2-weighted SS-ETSE images demonstrate in utero conjoined twins. The peritoneal cavities of the conjoined twins are in continuity, and the livers are attached (arrows, *b, c*).

Interstitial-phase gadolinium-enhanced fat-suppressed SGE (*d*). Gadolinium administered to 1 of the 2 neonates 1 day after birth demonstrates sharp demarcation of enhancing and nonenhancing livers (arrows, *d*), signifying that the hepatic vasculatures of the twins are separate.

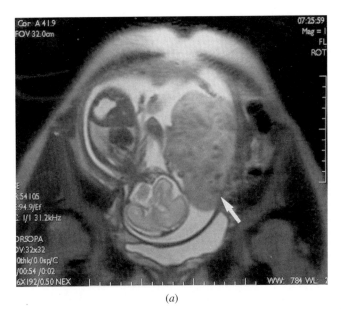

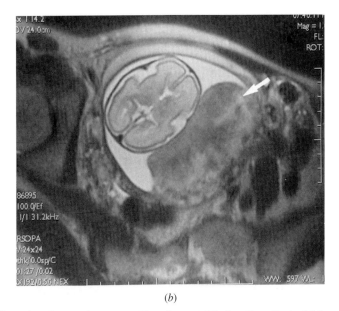

(a)   (b)

FIG. 14.68 Intrauterine growth retardation of a fetus at 26 weeks of gestation caused by placental infarction. Sagittal (*a*) and transverse (*b*) T2-weighted SS-ETSE images of a fetus. The placenta shows an atypical compact shape as well as an inhomogeneous signal intensity (arrows, *a, b*). Intrauterine growth retardation of the fetus is present. Placental infarction was diagnosed at time of delivery.

minute, resulting in slight blurring of the cardiac chambers [21].

Although the fine detail of the internal structures of the abdomen and pelvis is not well demonstrated with fast T2-weighted sequences, delineation of the visceral organs is possible. Because of their fluid content, stomach, esophagus, intestine, urinary collecting system, and

bladder appear high signal intensity. The liver, spleen, and kidneys appear low to intermediate in signal. Because of the pattern of distribution of the fetal circulation, both lobes of the liver are similar in size [21]. On T1-weighted images, the intestinal loops appear relatively high signal intensity because the presence of meconium [138].

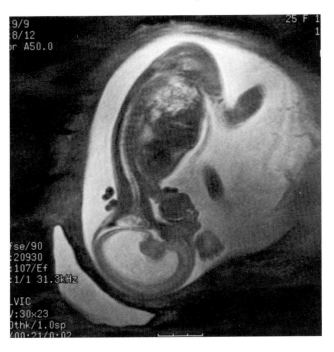

FIG. 14.69 Hydrocephalus in a fetus at 22 weeks of gestation. Sagittal T2-weighted SS-ETSE image shows marked dilatation of lateral ventricles.

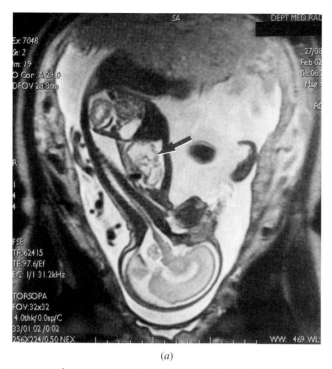

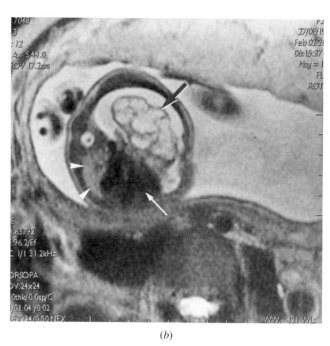

(*a*)   (*b*)

F I G . 14.70 Fetus with adenomatoid cystic malformation at 28 weeks of gestation. Sagittal (*a*) and transverse (*b*) T2-weighted SS-ETSE images of the fetus. A predominantly cystic, hyperintense lesion is seen within the left hemithorax (black arrows, *a*, *b*). The heart (white arrow, *b*) is pushed to the contralateral side. Displacement into the right hemithorax of mediastinal structures has resulted in hypoplasia of the right lung (arrowheads, *b*). Associated polyhydramnios is present.

The extremities are easily recognized on T2-weighted images as low-signal intensity structures within the high-signal intensity amniotic fluid. MRI can provide accurate assessment of their dimensions. A disadvantage compared to ultrasonography, however, is the lack of real-time information, namely, the prenatal assessment of function, which is important, for example, in cases of myelomeningocele [21, 27].

Accurate assessment of fetal weight during and at the end of pregnancy is useful for the management of

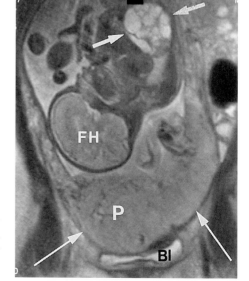

F I G . 14.71 Multicystic dysplastic kidney disease. Coronal SS-ETSE sequence through the maternal pelvis. The fetal kidney (arrows) shows multiple high-signal intensity cysts, which is consistent with multicystic dysplastic renal disease. In addition, a complete placenta previa is demonstrated (long thin arrows). FH, fetal head; P, placenta; Bl, maternal bladder.

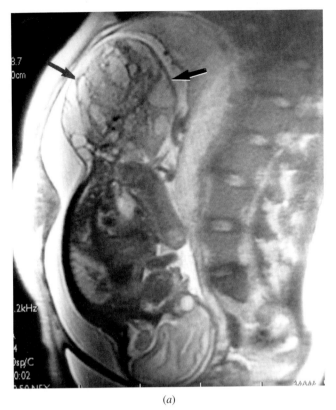
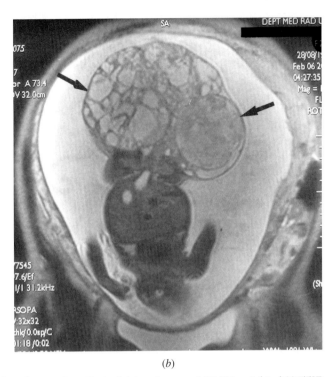

(a)

(b)

F I G . 14.72 Fetus with sacrococcygeal teratoma at 28 weeks of gestation. Sagittal (*a*) and coronal (*b*) T2-weighted SS-ETSE images of the fetus. A large, predominantly cystic, hyperintense lesion is delineated in the sacral region (arrows, *a*, *b*) consistent with a sacrococcygeal teratoma. Associated polyhydramnios is present.

labor and the perinatal period, because both intrauterine growth retardation and fetal macrosomia increase the risks of perinatal morbidity and mortality. MRI was recently shown to be of value for the intrauterine assessment of growth retardation. Baker et al. [139] demonstrated that a single measurement of fetal liver volume with echoplanar imaging could accurately identify fetuses with a birth weight below the 10th percentile. Furthermore, it was shown that measurements of total fetal volume obtained with MRI (fig. 14.59) correlate as well or even better with actual birth weight than those obtained with ultrasonography, because US at present only measures fetal weight indirectly from anatomic measurements, for example, fetal head circumference, abdominal circumference, and femur length [130, 140].

Normal amniotic fluid, similar to other simple biologic fluids, is hypointense on T1-weighted sequences and hyperintense on T2-weighted sequences. Volume measurements of amniotic fluid can be performed with MRI, which allows detection of oligohydramnios and polyhydramnios (fig. 14.59) [140]. Ex vivo studies performed on amniotic fluid have shown promising results in quantifying the concentration of meconium in the amniotic fluid during the third trimester [141], but this tech-

nique is not yet used in the clinical investigation of fetal distress.

MRI, because of its multiplanar capabilities, allows exact assessment of the placental position size and volume. The normal placenta appears of homogeneous intermediate signal intensity. Because of its ability to image the long axis of the entire uterine cavity and cervical canal, MRI has been shown to be highly accurate in the diagnosis of placenta previa (see fig. 14.65) and is an important adjunct to US in inconclusive cases [142, 143]. Placenta previa is diagnosed when the placenta covers a portion (marginal placenta) or all of the internal cervical os. Short duration sequences such as T2-weighted single-shot echo-train spin-echo or T1-weighted SGE acquired in the sagittal plane are effective at defining the relationship between the placenta and internal cervical os, with the occasional need of orthogonal planes of image acquisition. Clinically, placenta previa usually presents as painless vaginal bleeding during the course of the third trimester.

MRI can also visualize the umbilical cord and its insertion. Furthermore, MRI clearly demonstrates the lie of the fetus and can thus be useful to demonstrate breech and cephalic presentations [21, 140]. It has been observed on immediate postgadolinium SGE images that the normal placenta alters from a relatively homogeneous structure in the second trimester to a cotyledonous structure in the third trimester (fig. 14.62), as also observed on sonographic examination [144].

Gestational Trophoblastic Disease

The term gestational trophoblastic disease includes a variety of disease entities, including complete or partial hydatidiform mole, invasive mole, and choriocarcinoma. Clinically, a molar pregnancy is suspected in a patient with hyperemesis gravidarum, severe preeclampsia before 24 weeks of gestation, a large-for-date uterus, or first-trimester bleeding. Laboratory findings are diagnostic with markedly elevated levels of human chorionic gonadotropin (β-HCG). The most common form is a complete hydatidiform mole, characterized by trophoblastic proliferation without the development of an embryo. A partial hydatidiform mole is a distinct entity, and both mole and fetus exhibit a triploid karyotype. Whereas patients with partial hydatidiform mole rarely develop an invasive mole or choriocarcinoma, invasive moles are seen in approximately 10% of patients treated for complete hydatidiform mole and are characterized by myometrial invasion. Approximately 50% of chorio-

carcinomas arise from a preexisting molar pregnancy, whereas the other 50% will develop after any gestational event including abortion and ectopic or term pregnancy. Choriocarcinomas metastasize most frequently to the maternal lung.

The role of imaging in this patient population is limited, because the diagnosis and follow-up of patients with GTD is primarily based on β-HCG testing [145]. Computed tomography is the imaging procedure employed most often for the detection of extrapelvic metastases. The consistent results with the detection of small lung metastases with CT may support this approach currently. However, MRI is superior at the detection of small hypervascular liver metastases, as is observed with choriocarcinoma, and gadolinium-enhanced 3D imaging is effective at detecting 3-mm lung nodules (see Chapter 1). MRI is, however, effective at evaluating the primary uterine disease, for example, the degree of myometrial invasion in patients with invasive moles or choriocarcinomas (figs. 14.73 and 14. 74). In complete hydatidiform moles, MRI demonstrates a heterogeneous mass with multiple cystic spaces distending the endometrial cavity. A rim of hypointense myometrium may be visible at the periphery of a molar pregnancy. The uterine zones are distorted or obliterated, and an irregular boundary between tumor and myometrium is seen. On T1-weighted

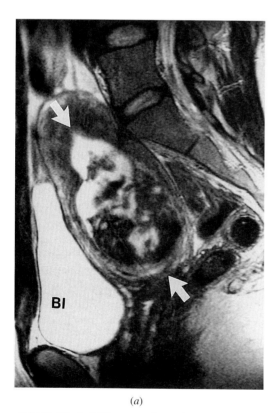

(a)

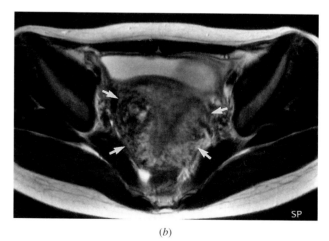

(b)

F I G . 14.73 Hydatidiform mole and invasive mole. Sagittal T2-weighted ETSE image (*a*) in a patient with a partial hydatidiform mole. A large heterogeneous mass is seen within the endometrial cavity (arrows) in a patient with elevated serum β-HCG levels. Note that there is no definite evidence of myometrial invasion.

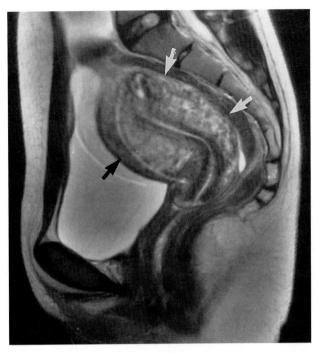

FIG. 14.73 (*Continued*) Transverse (*b*) and sagittal (*c*) T2-weighted ETSE images in a second patient who has an invasive mole. Note that in distinction from the patient with the hydatid mole there is diffuse heterogeneous high signal intensity of the myometrium consistent with invasion (arrows *b, c*). Bl, bladder.

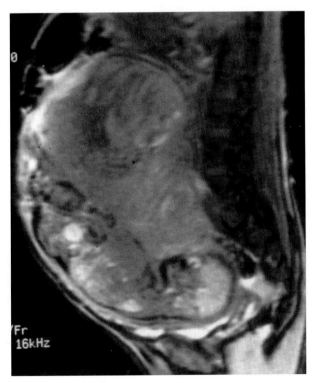

FIG. 14.74 Hydatidiform mole in a twin pregnancy. Sagittal T2-weighted ETSE image demonstrates a large heterogeneous mass within the endometrial cavity (arrows) in a patient with elevated serum β-HCG levels.

sequences, foci of high signal intensity corresponding to areas of hemorrhage may be seen. The mole is hypervascular and thus enhances intensely after gadolinium administration [146–148].

Pelvimetry

Pelvimetry is performed in patients who desire a trial of labor and have complicating factors including fetus in breech presentation, a history of secondary cesarean section due to dystocia, or maternal pelvic deformity.

The use of X-ray pelvimetry has decreased steadily in the last two decades. MRI offers the benefit of accurate measurements of the bony structures of the pelvis without exposure to ionizing radiation (fig. 14.75). Furthermore, MRI can clearly delineate the soft tissues of the maternal pelvis. The use of gradient-echo sequences has been advocated for MR pelvimetry, because acquisition times are shorter compared to T1-weighted spin-echo sequences and they are characterized by a relatively low specific absorption rate [25, 149–152]. Single-shot T2-weighted images perform also well.

Maternal Imaging

MRI has been shown to be useful in the diagnosis of maternal complications during pregnancy, both pregnancy- and non-pregnancy-related. Physical examination in pregnancy is impaired by the presence of the gravid uterus, making assessment of abdominal or pelvic pathology difficult. Because of the potential harmful effects of exposure of the fetus to ionizing radiation, radiologic assessment using computed tomography or plain film imaging is often not desirable. Ultrasonography remains the primary imaging modality; however, its value is restricted because of the enlarged uterus as well as lack of tissue specificity. MRI has thus been shown to be useful in the detection and characterization of abdominal and pelvic disease in pregnant women [153].

The diagnosis of an adnexal mass during pregnancy poses a diagnostic challenge. The most common adnexal mass in a pregnant patient is a corpus luteal cyst. It usually measures less than 6 cm in size and does not enlarge during pregnancy. The criteria to differentiate benign and malignant ovarian lesion are described in Chapter 15, *Adnexa*. MRI permits differentiation between simple cysts and more complex lesions, and the relationship between the mass and the pregnant uterus can be established. Because of the increased pressure in the pelvic cavity, adnexal masses may become symptomatic during pregnancy as a result of extrinsic compression, hemorrhage, or torsion (figs. 14.76 and 14.77) [154].

Uterine leiomyomas demonstrate the same imaging characteristics during pregnancy as in the nongravid uterus; however, they have a propensity to undergo degeneration in pregnancy. The most common pattern is hemorrhagic infarction and necrosis, termed red degeneration. The leiomyoma will contain peripheral or diffuse high signal intensity on T1-weighted images and variable signal intensities, with or without low-signal intensity rim, on T2-weighted images [67, 69, 155].

Precise mapping of all leiomyomas should be performed with ultrasound early during pregnancy because evaluation becomes more difficult during the second and third trimesters. When the gestational contents preclude accurate assessment with ultrasound, MRI is indicated. MRI is useful to identify whether degenerated leiomyomas are the cause of a suspected adnexal mass or pelvic pain. When multiple or large leiomyomas are present, their location, for example in the lower uterine segment, may influence the decision about route of delivery, that is, vaginal delivery versus cesarean section (fig. 14.78).

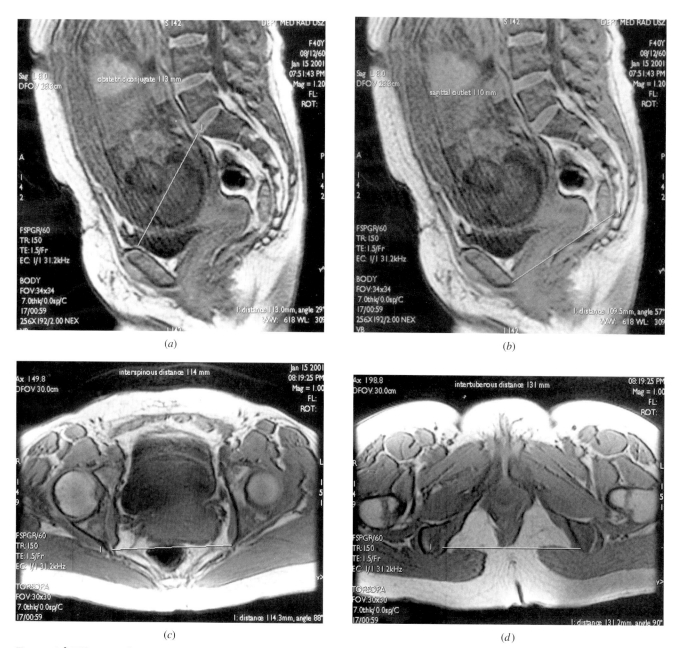

(a)

(b)

(c)

(d)

F I G . 14.75 MR pelvimetry performed in a pregnant patient. T1-weighted SGE images (*a–f*). Obstetric conjugate (*a*) and sagittal outlet (*b*) are measured on a midsagittal plane, interspinous distance (*c*) and intertuberous distance (*d*) on transverse planes.

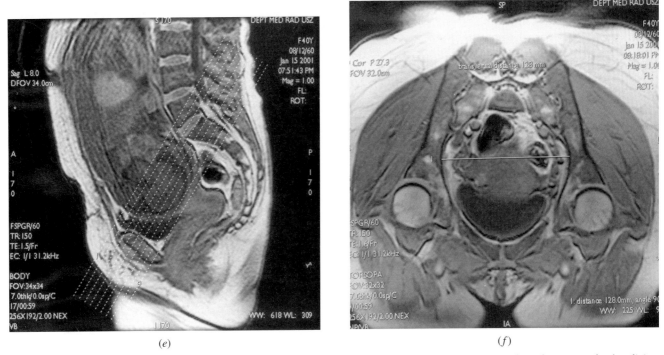

(e)   (f)

F I G . 14.75 (*Continued*) The transversal distance (*f*) is measured on an oblique plane acquired as shown on the localizing image (*e*).

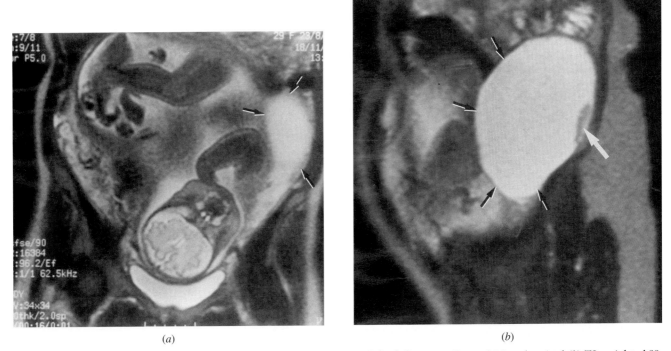

(a)   (b)

F I G . 14.76 Pregnant women with borderline ovarian tumor of the left ovary. Coronal (*a*) and sagittal (*b*) T2-weighted SS-ETSE images through the maternal pelvis. A 12-cm cystic ovarian lesion (black arrows, *a, b*) with a solitary nodule along the posterior wall (white arrow, *b*) is present in a pregnant patient. The pregnancy was carried to term. Surgery was performed, and histology showed a borderline ovarian tumor.

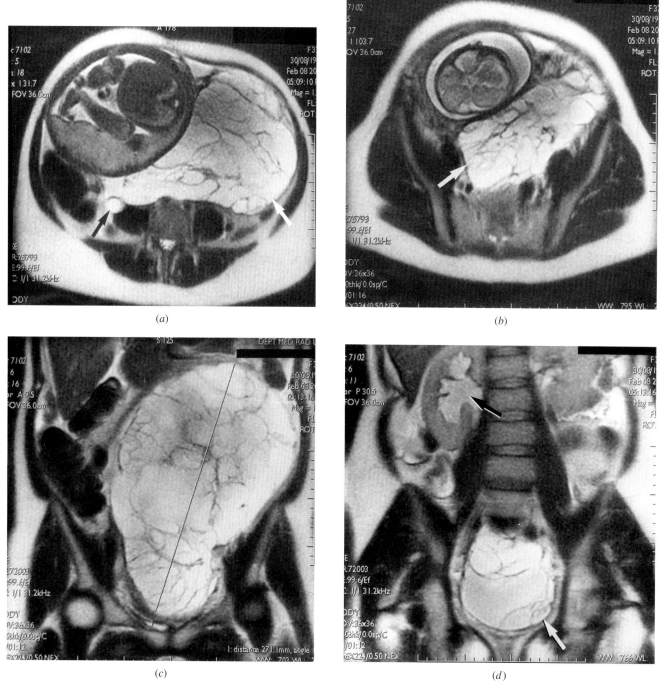

(a)

(b)

(c)

(d)

F I G . 14.77 Ovarian carcinoma in a pregnant patient at 28 weeks of gestation. Transverse (*a*, superior; *b*, inferior) and coronal (*c*, anterior; *d*, posterior) T2-weighted SS-ETSE images of the maternal lower abdomen and transverse T2-weighted fat-suppressed ETSE image of the upper abdomen. A large predominantly cystic lesion with a maximal diameter of 27 cm is seen (white arrows, *a*, *b*, *d*) consistent with ovarian carcinoma. The pregnant uterus is displaced to the right.

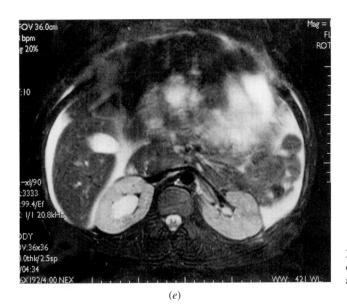

(e)

FIG. 14.77 (*Continued*) Ascites is present (*e*). Right-sided hydronephrosis (black arrow, *d*) and dilated ureter (black arrow, *a*) are observed.

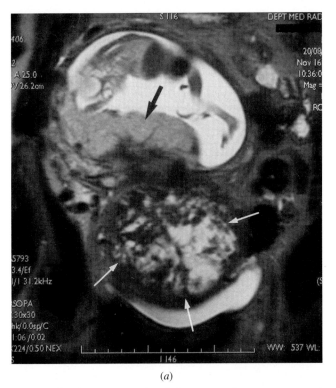

(a)

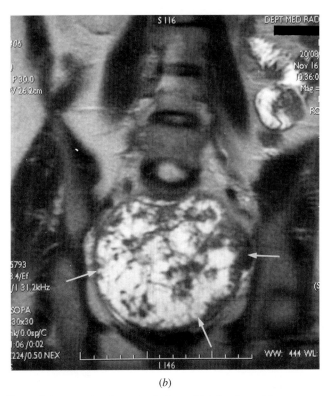

(b)

FIG. 14.78 Large uterine leiomyoma in pregnant patient. Coronal (*a*, anterior; *b*, posterior), sagittal (*c, d*), and transverse (*e*) T2-weighted SS-ETSE images. The large uterine leiomyoma (arrows, *a, b*) shows multiple foci of increased signal intensity corresponding to areas of degeneration. Note also the normal pregnancy and placenta (black arrow, *a*).

Coronal SS-ETSE (*e*) and coronal interstitial-phase gadolinium-enhanced fat-suppressed SGE (*f*) images. An 8-cm leiomyoma arises from the right superolateral aspect of the uterus. The leiomyoma is low in signal intensity and well defined on the SS-ETSE image (arrows, *e*), which is the typical appearance for a leiomyoma. Ill-defined subtle high signal intensity (long white arrow, *e*) is appreciated on the T2-weighted image (*e*), which corresponds to a region of lack of gadolinium enhancement on the gadolinium-enhanced fat-suppressed SGE image (*f*), reflecting degeneration. Clear definition of the uterine origin of the mass was appreciated on images obtained in multiple planes.

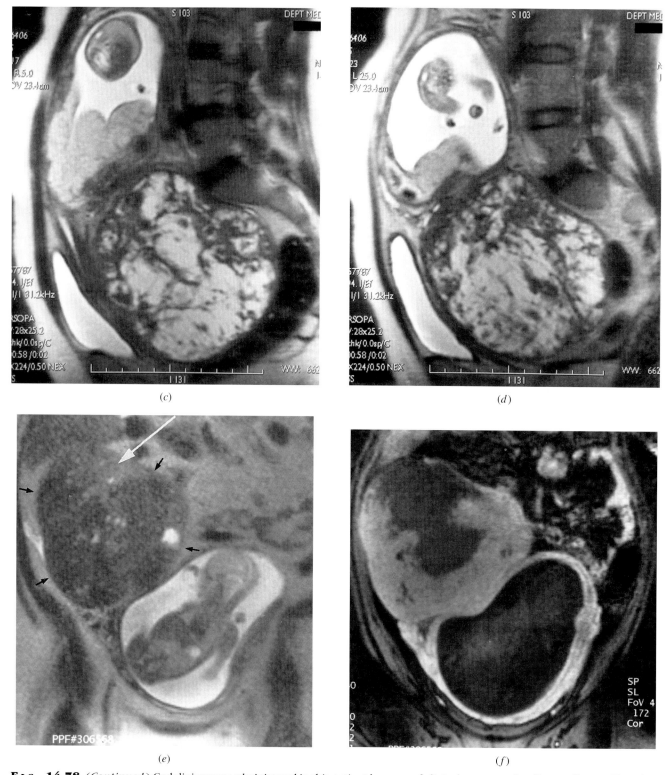

(c)

(d)

(e)

(f)

FIG. 14.78 (*Continued*) Gadolinium was administered in this patient because of clinical concern of malignant disease. Note that even though data acquisition is 20 s using the breath-hold SGE sequence (*f*), fetal motion blurs out definition of the fetus. In contrast, the 1-s data acquisition of SS-ETSE freezes fetal motion, rendering the fetus clearly defined.

Cervical carcinoma in association with pregnancy is rare, with an incidence of approximately 1 per 1200–10,000 pregnancies. The association of cervical carcinoma with pregnancy, however, raises difficult management issues. MRI is currently the best imaging modality for evaluating pregnant patients with cervical carcinoma (fig. 14.46). (See the earlier subsection, Cervical Carcinoma, in the section on Malignant Disease of the Uterine Corpus and Cervix for a more complete discussion on the role of MRI in the staging of cervical carcinoma). With close surveillance, deliberate delay of therapy to achieve fetal maturity is a reasonable option for patients with early stage cancer, because tumor growth and maternal survival may not be adversely effected by pregnancy [156].

Another promising application of MRI in pregnant women is urography. Dilatation of the urinary tract, usu-ally more prominent on the right side, is a physiologic finding during pregnancy, with the dilated ureter extending to the sacral promontory, at which level it tapers in caliber to normal for the lower third of the ureter. MRI can be helpful in distinguishing physiologic hydronephrosis (fig. 14.77) from other causes of urinary tract dilatation, including the presence of calculi [25, 157].

Postpartum Uterus

The greatest reduction in size of the uterine corpus and cervix occurs within 1 week after delivery. The uterus has returned to its normal size by 6 months (fig. 14.79). The presence of acute or subacute blood in the endometrial cavity is a common occurrence in the immediate postpartum period and resolves usually within 1 week.

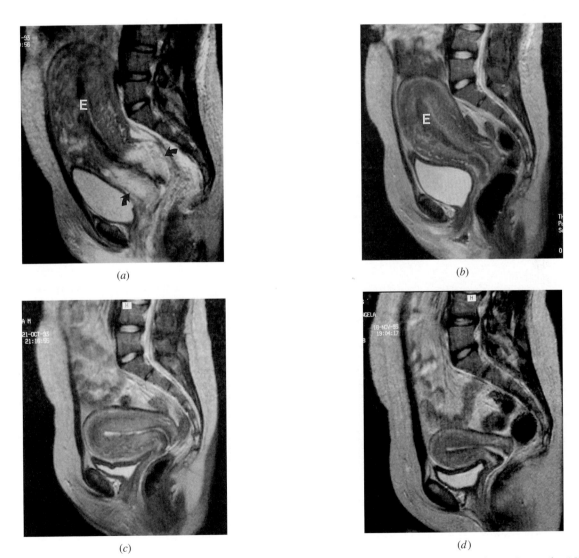

(a) (b)

(c) (d)

F I G . 14.79 Postpartum uterus. Sagittal T2-weighted ETSE images at 24 h (*a*), 1 week (*b*), 1 month (*c*), 2 months (*d*), and 6 months (*e*) after delivery. Acute and/or subacute blood is shown within the endometrial cavity (E) in the first week postpartum (*a*, *b*). The outer cervical stroma or smooth muscle layer is hyperintense (curved arrows, *a*) in the first 30 h after delivery.

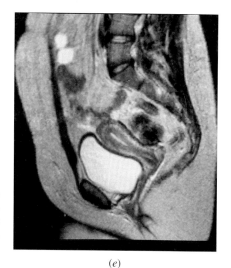

(e)

FIG. 14.79 (*Continued*) The inner fibrous stroma, however, remains hypointense throughout the postpartum period (*a-e*). The myometrium is of intermediate and heterogeneous signal intensity during the early postpartum period (*a-c*). By 6 months, complete reconstitution of the junctional zone (JZ) is evident (*e*). Note the gradual decreases in size of the uterus from *a* to *e*.

The junctional zone will start to be visualized again 2 weeks after delivery, with complete reconstitution after 6 months. A small amount of free pelvic fluid is a normal finding in the postpartum patient [158, 159].

In women undergoing cesarean section, the incision is typically seen as an area of moderately high signal intensity within 1 month of the procedure on both T1- and T2-weighted sequences consistent with subacute hematoma within the myometrium, although the signal intensity may be variable (fig. 14.80) [158].

Ovarian vein thrombosis is a relatively rare complication often associated with postpartum endometritis. It occurs most commonly in the right ovarian vein. The diagnosis of ovarian vein thrombosis is frequently difficult with ultrasound, and MRI or computed tomography are indicated to establish the correct diagnosis [158, 160].

Conclusions

MRI has an established role in the investigation of the uterus and cervix. Detection and characterization of benign disease, such as leiomyoma and adenomyosis, is routinely performed at many centers. MRI is excellent at staging malignant disease, although the clinical impact has not been great in the majority of institutions, as clinical staging is still the routine. Fetal imaging is an emerging area of interest with clinical applications still in evolution.

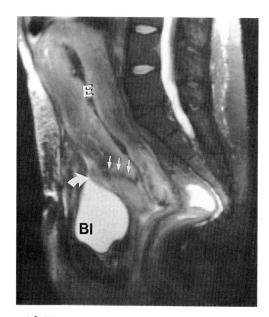

FIG. 14.80 Postcesarean section uterus. Sagittal T2-weighted fat-suppressed ETSE image in a patient 5 days after cesarean section. A hypointense scar is visible in the lower uterine segment (small arrows), as well as a bladder flap (curved arrow). The low signal intensity of the endometrial cavity (E), due to the presence of acute and/or subacute blood, and the lack of zonal differentiation of the myometrium are normal findings in the early postpartum period. Bl = bladder.

REFERENCES

1. Budinger TF: Nuclear magnetic resonance (NMR) in vivo studies: known thresholds for health effects. *J Comp Assist Tomogr* 5: 800–811, 1981.

2. Reid A, Smith FW, et al.: (1982). Nuclear magnetic resonance imaging and its safety implications: Follow-up of 181 patients. *Br J Radiol* 55: 784–786.

3. McRobbie D, Foster MA: Pulsed magnetic field exposure during pregnancy and implications for NMR foetal imaging: A study with mice. *Magn Reson Imaging* 3: 231–234, 1985.

4. Heinrichs WL, Fong P, et al.: Midgestational exposure of pregnant BALB/c mice to magnetic resonance imaging conditions. *Magn Reson Imaging* 6: 305–313, 1988.

5. Baker PN, Johnson IR, et al.: Fetal weight estimation by echo-planar magnetic resonance imaging. *Lancet* 343: 644–645, 1994.

6. Pasquale SA, Russer TJ, et al.: Lack of interaction between magnetic resonance imaging and the copper-T380A IUD. *Contraception* 55: 169–173, 1997.

7. Roemer PB, Edelstein WA, et al.: The NMR phased array. *Magn Reson Med* 16: 192–225, 1990.

8. Hayes CE, Hattes N, et al.: Volume imaging with MR phased arrays. *Magn Reson Med* 18: 309–319, 1991.

9. DeSouza NM, Hawley IC, et al.: The uterine cervix on in vitro and in vivo MR images: A study of zonal anatomy and vascularity using an enveloping cervical coil. *Am J Roentgenol* 163: 607–612, 1994.

10. Huch Boni RA, Boner JA, et al.: Optimization of prostate carcinoma staging: comparison of imaging and clinical methods. *Clin Radiol* 50: 593–600, 1995.

11. Huch Boni RA, Boner JA, et al.: Contrast-enhanced endorectal coil MRI in local staging of prostate carcinoma. *J Comput Assist Tomogr* 19: 232–237, 1995.

12. Huch Boni RA, Meyenberger C, et al.: Value of endorectal coil versus body coil MRI for diagnosis of recurrent pelvic malignancies. *Abdom Imaging* 21: 345–352, 1996.

13. Kubik Huch RA, Hailemariam S, et al.: CT and MRI of the male genital tract: Radiologic-pathologic correlation. *Eur Radiol* 9: 16–28, 1999.

14. Kim MJ, Chung JJ, et al.: Comparison of the use of the transrectal surface coil and the pelvic phased-array coil in MR imaging for preoperative evaluation of uterine cervical carcinoma. *AJR Am J Roentgenol* 168: 1215–1221, 1997.

15. Shiraiwa M, Joja I, et al.: Cervical carcinoma: Efficacy of thin-section oblique axial T2-weighted images for evaluating parametrial invasion. *Abdom Imaging* 24: 514–519, 1999.

16. Sironi S, De Cobelli F, et al.: Carcinoma of the cervix: Value of plain and gadolinium-enhanced MR imaging in assessing degree of invasiveness. *Radiology* 188: 780–797, 1993.

17. Hawighorst H, Knapstein PG, et al.: Cervical carcinoma: Comparison of standard and pharmacokinetic MR imaging. *Radiology* 201: 531–539, 1996.

18. Semelka RC, Hricak H, et al.: Pelvic fistulas: appearances on MR images. *Abdom Imaging* 22: 91–95, 1997.

19. Scheidler J, Heuck AF, et al.: Parametrial invasion in cervical carcinoma: Evaluation of detection at MR imaging with fat suppression. *Radiology* 206: 125–129, 1998.

20. Hamm B, Kubik Huch RA, et al.: MR imaging and CT of the female pelvis: Radiologic-pathologic correlation. *Eur Radiol* 9: 3–15, 1999.

21. Amin RS, Nikolaidis P, et al.: Normal anatomy of the fetus at MR imaging. *Radiographics* 19: 201–214, 1999.

22. Levine D, Edelman RR: Fast MRI and its application in obstetrics. *Abdom Imaging* 22: 589–596, 1997.

23. Levine D, Barnes PD, et al.: Fetal fast MR imaging: Reproducibility, technical quality, and conspicuity of anatomy. *Radiology* 206: 549–554, 1998.

24. Kubik Huch RA, Wisser J, et al.: Prenatal diagnosis of fetal malformations by ultrafast magnetic resonance imaging. *Prenat Diagn* 18: 1205–1208, 1998.

25. Levine D, Barnes PD, et al.: Obstetric MR imaging. *Radiology* 211: 609–617, 1999.

26. Levine D, Barnes PD, et al.: Fetal CNS anomalies revealed on ultrafast MR imaging. *AJR Am J Roentgenol* 172: 813–828, 1999.

27. Kubik Huch RA, Huisman TA, et al.: Ultrafast MR imaging of the fetus. *Am J Roentgenol* 174: 1599–1606, 2000.

28. Lee JK, Gersell DJ, et al.: The uterus: In vitro MR-anatomic correlation of normal and abnormal specimens. *Radiology* 157: 175–189, 1985.

29. McCarthy S, Tauber C, et al.: Female pelvic anatomy: MR assessment of variations during the menstrual cycle and with use of oral contraceptives. *Radiology* 160: 119–123, 1986.

30. Hricak H, Alpers C, et al.: Magnetic resonance imaging of the female pelvis: Initial experience. *Am J Roentgenol* 141: 1119–1128, 1983.

31. Haynor DR, Mack LA, et al.: Changing appearance of the normal uterus during the menstrual cycle: MR studies. *Radiology* 161: 459–462, 1986.

32. Demas BE, Hricak H, et al.: Uterine MR imaging: Effects of hormonal stimulation. *Radiology* 159: 123–136, 1986.

33. Wiczyk HP, Janus CL, et al.: Comparison of magnetic resonance imaging and ultrasound in evaluating follicular and endometrial development throughout the normal cycle. *Fertil Steril* 49: 969–972, 1988.

34. Janus CL, Bateman B, et al.: Evaluation of the stimulated menstrual cycle by magnetic resonance imaging. *Fertil Steril* 54: 1017–1020, 1990.

35. McCarthy S, Scott G, et al.: Uterine junctional zone: MR study of water content and relaxation properties. *Radiology* 171: 241–253, 1989.

36. Mitchell DG, Schonholz L, et al.: Zones of the uterus: Discrepancy between US and MR images. *Radiology* 174: 827–831, 1990.

37. Brown HK, Stoll BS, et al.: Uterine junctional zone: Correlation between histologic findings and MR imaging. *Radiology* 179: 409–413, 1991.

38. Scoutt LM, Flynn SD, et al.: Junctional zone of the uterus: Correlation of MR imaging and histologic examination of hysterectomy specimens. *Radiology* 179: 403–407, 1991.

39. Yamashita Y, Harada M, et al.: Normal uterus and FIGO stage I endometrial carcinoma: Dynamic gadolinium-enhanced MR imaging. *Radiology* 186: 495–501, 1993.

40. Hricak H, Kim B: Contrast-enhanced MR imaging of the female pelvis. *J Magn Reson Imaging* 3: 297–306, 1993.

41. Hricak H, Stern JL, et al.: Endometrial carcinoma staging by MR imaging. *Radiology* 162: 297–305, 1987.

42. Scoutt LM, McCauley TR, et al.: Zonal anatomy of the cervix: Correlation of MR imaging and histologic examination of hysterectomy specimens. *Radiology* 186: 159–162, 1993.

43. Togashi K, Nishimura K, et al.: Uterine cervical cancer: Assessment with high-field MR imaging. *Radiology* 160: 431–435, 1986.

44. Fornander T, Rutqvist LE, et al.: Adjuvant tamoxifen in early breast cancer: Occurrence of new primary cancers. *Lancet* 1: 117–120, 1989.

45. De Muylder X, Neven P, et al.: Endometrial lesions in patients undergoing tamoxifen therapy. *Int J Gynaecol Obstet* 36: 127–130, 1991.

46. Ascher SM, Johnson JC, et al.: MR imaging appearance of the uterus in postmenopausal women receiving tamoxifen therapy for breast cancer: Histopathologic correlation. *Radiology* 200: 105–110, 1996.

47. Cohen I, Rosen DJ, et al.: Ultrasonographic evaluation of the endometrium and correlation with endometrial sampling in postmenopausal patients treated with tamoxifen. *J Ultrasound Med* 12: 275–280, 1993.

48. Buttram VC, Jr: Mullerian anomalies and their management. *Fertil Steril* 40: 159–163, 1983.

49. Pellerito JS, McCarthy SM, et al.: Diagnosis of uterine anomalies: Relative accuracy of MR imaging, endovaginal sonography, and hysterosalpingography. *Radiology* 183: 795–800, 1992.

50. Carrington BM, Hricak H, et al.: Mullerian duct anomalies: MR imaging evaluation. *Radiology* 176: 715–720, 1990.

51. Frye RE, Ascher SM, et al.: MR hysterosalpingography: Protocol development and refinement for simulating normal and abnormal fallopian tube patency—feasibility study with a phantom. *Radiology* 214: 107–112, 2000.

52. Buttram VC Jr, Gibbons WE: Mullerian anomalies: A proposed classification. (An analysis of 144 cases). *Fertil Steril* 32: 40–46, 1979.

53. Reinhold C, Hricak H, et al.: Primary amenorrhea: Evaluation with MR imaging. *Radiology* 203: 383–390, 1997.

54. Wiesner W, Kubik Huch RA, et al.: [Mayer-(von)Rokitansky-Kuster syndrome] Original title: Mayer-(von)Rokitansky-Kuster-Syndrom. *Schweiz Rundsch Med Prax* 87: 1257–1259, 1998.

55. Fedele L, Dorta M, et al.: Magnetic resonance imaging of unicornuate uterus. *Acta Obstet Gynecol Scand* 69: 511–513, 1990.

56. Woodward PJ, Wagner BJ, et al.: MR imaging in the evaluation of female infertility. *Radiographics* 13: 293–310, 1993.

57. Kaufman RH, Binder GL, et al.: Upper genital tract changes associated with exposure in utero to diethylstilbestrol. *Obstet Gynecol Surv* 32: 611–613,1977.

58. Van Gils AP, Tham RT, et al.: Abnormalities of the uterus and cervix after diethylstilbestrol exposure: Correlation of findings on MR and hysterosalpingography. *Am J Roentgenol* 153: 1235–1238, 1989.

59. Gambino J, Caldwell B, et al.: Congenital disorders of sexual differentiation: MR findings. *Am J Roentgenol* 158: 363–367, 1992.

60. Atri M, Nazarnia S, et al.: Transvaginal US appearance of endometrial abnormalities. *Radiographics* 14: 483–492, 1994.

61. Lin MC, Gosink BB, et al.: Endometrial thickness after menopause: Effect of hormone replacement. *Radiology* 180: 427–432, 1991.

62. Varner RE, Sparks JM, et al.: Transvaginal sonography of the endometrium in postmenopausal women. *Obstet Gynecol* 78: 195–199, 1991.

63. Sheth S, Hamper UM, et al.: Thickened endometrium in the postmenopausal woman: Sonographic-pathologic correlation. *Radiology* 187: 135–139, 1993.

64. Hricak H, Finck S, et al.: MR imaging in the evaluation of benign uterine masses: Value of gadopentetate dimeglumine-enhanced T1-weighted images. *Am J Roentgenol* 158: 1043–1050, 1992.

65. Grasel RP, Outwater EK, et al.: Endometrial polyps: MR imaging features and distinction from endometrial carcinoma. *Radiology* 214: 47–52, 2000.

66. Rader JS, Binette SP, et al.: Ileal hemorrhage caused by a parasitic uterine leiomyoma. *Obstet Gynecol* 76: 531–534, 1990.

67. Boni RA, Hebisch G, et al.: Multiple necrotic uterine leiomyomas causing severe puerperal fever: Ultrasound, CT, MR, and histological findings. *J Comput Assist Tomogr* 18: 828–831, 1994.

68. Kubik Huch RA: Female pelvis. *Eur Radiol* 9: 1715–1721, 1999.

69. Murase E, Siegelman ES, et al.: Uterine leiomyomas: Histopathologic features, MR imaging findings, differential diagnosis, and treatment. *Radiographics* 19: 1179–1197, 1999.

70. Zawin M, McCarthy S, et al.: High-field MRI and US evaluation of the pelvis in women with leiomyomas. *Magn Reson Imaging* 8: 371–376, 1990.

71. Weinreb JC, Barkoff ND, et al.: The value of MR imaging in distinguishing leiomyomas from other solid pelvic masses when sonography is indeterminate. *Am J Roentgenol* 154: 295–299, 1990.

72. Hricak H, Tscholakoff D, et al.: Uterine leiomyomas: Correlation of MR, histopathologic findings, and symptoms. *Radiology* 158: 385–391, 1986.

73. Mark AS, Hricak H, et al.: Adenomyosis and leiomyoma: Differential diagnosis with MR imaging. *Radiology* 163: 527–529, 1987.

74. Dudiak CM, Turner DA, et al.: Uterine leiomyomas in the infertile patient: Preoperative localization with MR imaging versus US and hysterosalpingography. *Radiology* 167: 627–630, 1988.

75. Togashi K, Ozasa H, et al.: Enlarged uterus: Differentiation between adenomyosis and leiomyoma with MR imaging. *Radiology* 171: 531–534, 1989.

76. Panageas E, Kier R, et al.: Submucosal uterine leiomyomas: Diagnosis of prolapse into the cervix and vagina based on MR imaging. *Am J Roentgenol* 159: 555–558, 1992.

77. Ueda H, Togashi K, et al.: Unusual appearances of uterine leiomyomas: MR imaging findings and their histopathologic backgrounds. *Radiographics* 19: 131–145, 1999.

78. Hamlin DJ, Fitzsimmons JR, et al.: Magnetic resonance imaging of the pelvis: Evaluation of ovarian masses at 0.15 T. *Am J Roentgenol* 145: 585–590, 1985.

79. Burn PR, McCall JM, et al.: Uterine fibroleiomyoma: MR imaging appearances before and after embolization of uterine arteries. *Radiology* 214: 729–734, 2000.

80. Jha RC, Ascher SM, et al.: Symptomatic fibroleiomyomata: MR imaging of the uterus before and after uterine arterial embolization. *Radiology* 217: 228–235, 2000.

81. Reinhold C, Atri M, et al.: Diffuse uterine adenomyosis: Morphologic criteria and diagnostic accuracy of endovaginal sonography. *Radiology* 197: 609–614, 1995.

82. Byun JY, Kim SE, et al.: Diffuse and focal adenomyosis: MR imaging findings. *Radiographics* 19: 161–170, 1999.

83. Reinhold C, Tafazoli F, et al.: Uterine adenomyosis: Endovaginal US and MR imaging features with histopathologic correlation. *Radiographics* 19: 147–160, 1999.

84. Togashi K, Nishimura K, et al.: Adenomyosis: Diagnosis with MR imaging. *Radiology* 166: 111–114, 1988.

85. Togashi K, Nishimura K, et al.: Carcinoma of the cervix: Staging with MR imaging. *Radiology* 171: 245–251, 1989.

86. Goodman A: Premalignant & malignant disorders of the uterine coprus. *Current Obstetric & Gynecologic Diagnosis & Treatment*, Nordwalk, CT: Appelton & Lange vol. 8, p. 937–953, 1994.

87. American Joint Committee on Cancer: *Manual for Staging of Cancer* (3rd ed.). Philadelphia: Lippincott, p. 151–153, 1988.

88. Nolan JF, Huen A: Prognosis in endometrial cancer. *Gynecol Oncol* 4: 384–390, 1976.

89. Chen SS, Lee L: Retroperitoneal lymph node metastases in Stage I carcinoma of the endometrium: Correlation with risk factors. *Gynecol Oncol* 16: 319–325, 1983.

90. Figge DC, Otto PM, et al.: Treatment variables in the management of endometrial cancer. *Am J Obstet Gynecol* 146: 495–500, 1983.

91. DiSaia PJ, Creasman WT, et al.: Risk factors and recurrent patterns in Stage I endometrial cancer. *Am J Obstet Gynecol* 151: 1009–1015, 1985.

92. Piver MS, Lele SB, et al.: Paraaortic lymph node evaluation in stage I endometrial carcinoma. *Obstet Gynecol* 59: 97–100, 1982.

93. Gordon AN, Fleischer AC, et al.: Preoperative assessment of myometrial invasion of endometrial adenocarcinoma by sonography (US) and magnetic resonance imaging (MRI). *Gynecol Oncol* 34: 175–179, 1989.

94. Yamashita Y, Mizutani H, et al.: Assessment of myometrial invasion by endometrial carcinoma: Transvaginal sonography vs contrast-enhanced MR imaging. *Am J Roentgenol* 161: 595–599, 1993.

95. DelMaschio A, Vanzulli A, et al.: Estimating the depth of myometrial involvement by endometrial carcinoma: Efficacy of transvaginal sonography vs MR imaging. *Am J Roentgenol* 160: 533–538, 1993.

96. Hardesty LA, Sumkin JH, et al.: Use of preoperative MR imaging in the management of endometrial carcinoma: Cost analysis. *Radiology* 215: 45–49, 2000.

97. Hricak H, Hamm B, et al.: Carcinoma of the uterus: Use of gadopentetate dimeglumine in MR imaging. *Radiology* 181: 95–106, 1991.

98. Hricak H, Rubinstein LV, et al.: MR imaging evaluation of endometrial carcinoma: Results of an NCI cooperative study. *Radiology* 179: 829–832, 1991.

99. Sironi S, Colombo E, et al.: Myometrial invasion by endometrial carcinoma: Assessment with plain and gadolinium-enhanced MR imaging. *Radiology* 185: 207–212, 1992.

100. Olson MC, Posniak HV, et al.: MR imaging of the female pelvic region. *Radiographics* 12: 445–465, 1992.

101. Frei KA, Kinkel K, et al.: Prediction of deep myometrial invasion in patients with endometrial cancer: Clinical utility of contrast-

enhanced MR imaging—a meta-analysis and Bayesian analysis. *Radiology* 216: 444–449, 2000.

102. Popovich MJ, Hricak H, et al.: The role of MR imaging in determining surgical eligibility for pelvic exenteration. *Am J Roentgenol* 160: 525–531, 1993.

103. Yang WT, Lam WW, et al.: Comparison of dynamic helical CT and dynamic MR imaging in the evaluation of pelvic lymph nodes in cervical carcinoma. *Am J Roentgenol* 175: 759–766, 2000.

104. Harisinghani MG, Saini S, et al.: MR lymphangiography using ultrasmall superparamagnetic iron oxide in patients with primary abdominal and pelvic malignancies: Radiographic-pathologic correlation. *Am J Roentgenol* 172: 1347–1351, 1999.

105. Shapeero LG, Hricak H: Mixed mullerian sarcoma of the uterus: MR imaging findings. *Am J Roentgenol* 153: 317–319, 1989.

106. Pattani SJ, Kier R, et al.: MRI of uterine leiomyosarcoma. *Magn Reson Imaging* 13: 331–333, 1995.

107. Peppercorn PD, Jeyarajah AR, et al.: Role of MR imaging in the selection of patients with early cervical carcinoma for fertility-preserving surgery: Initial experience. *Radiology* 212: 395–399, 1999.

108. Hricak H, Powell CB, et al.: Invasive cervical carcinoma: Role of MR imaging in pretreatment work-up—cost minimization and diagnostic efficacy analysis. *Radiology* 198: 403–409, 1996.

109. Van Nagell JR Jr, Roddick JW Jr, et al.: The staging of cervical cancer: Inevitable discrepancies between clinical staging and pathologic findings. *Am J Obstet Gynecol* 110: 973–978, 1971.

110. Averette HE, Dudan RC, et al.: Exploratory celiotomy for surgical staging of cervical cancer. *Am J Obstet Gynecol* 113: 1090–1096, 1972.

111. Lagasse LD, Creasman WT, et al.: Results and complications of operative staging in cervical cancer: Experience of the Gynecologic Oncology Group. *Gynecol Oncol* 9: 90–98, 1980.

112. Kim SH, Choi BI, et al.: Uterine cervical carcinoma: Comparison of CT and MR findings. *Radiology* 175: 45–51, 1990.

113. Rubens D, Thornbury JR, et al.: Stage IB cervical carcinoma: Comparison of clinical, MR, and pathologic staging. *Am J Roentgenol* 150: 135–138, 1988.

114. Sironi S, Belloni C, et al.: Carcinoma of the cervix: Value of MR imaging in detecting parametrial involvement. *Am J Roentgenol* 156: 753–756, 1991.

115. Subak LL, Hricak H, et al.: Cervical carcinoma: Computed tomography and magnetic resonance imaging for preoperative staging. *Obstet Gynecol* 86: 43–50, 1995.

116. Hill EC, Pernoll ML: Benign disorders of the uterine cervix. In DeCherney AH. Pernoll ML (eds.), *Current Obstetrics & Gynecologic* vol. 8, p. 713–730, 1994.

117. Fulcher AS, O'Sullivan SG, et al.: Recurrent cervical carcinoma: Typical and atypical manifestations. *Radiographics* 19: 103–116, 1999.

118. Cannistra SA, Niloff JM: Cancer of the uterine cervix. *N Engl J Med* 334: 1030–1038, 1996.

119. Ebner F, Kressel HY, et al.: Tumor recurrence versus fibrosis in the female pelvis: Differentiation with MR imaging at 1.5 T. *Radiology* 166: 333–340, 1988.

120. Flueckiger F, Ebner F, et al.: Cervical cancer: Serial MR imaging before and after primary radiation therapy—a 2-year follow-up study. *Radiology* 184: 89–93, 1992.

121. Hricak H, Swift PS, et al.: Irradiation of the cervix uteri: Value of unenhanced and contrast-enhanced MR imaging. *Radiology* 189: 381–388, 1993.

122. Weber TM, Sostman HD, et al.: Cervical carcinoma: Determination of recurrent tumor extent versus radiation changes with MR imaging. *Radiology* 194: 135–139, 1995.

123. Yamashita Y, Harada M, et al.: Dynamic MR imaging of recurrent postoperative cervical cancer. *J Magn Reson Imaging* 6: 167–171, 1996.

124. Levine D, Barnes PD, et al.: Fetal central nervous system anomalies: MR imaging augments sonographic diagnosis. *Radiology* 204: 635–642, 1997.

125. Yamashita Y, Namimoto T, et al.: MR imaging of the fetus by a HASTE sequence. *Am J Roentgenol* 168: 513–519, 1997.

126. Levine D, Barnes PD: Cortical maturation in normal and abnormal fetuses as assessed with prenatal MR imaging. *Radiology* 210: 751–758, 1999.

127. Hubbard AM, Adzick NS, et al.: Congenital chest lesions: Diagnosis and characterization with prenatal MR imaging. *Radiology* 212: 43–48, 1999.

128. Schwartz JL, Crooks LE: NMR imaging produces no observable mutations or cytotoxicity in mammalian cells. *Am J Roentgenol* 139: 583–585, 1982.

129. Kay HH, Herfkens RJ, et al.: Effect of magnetic resonance imaging on *Xenopus laevis* embryogenesis. *Magn Reson Imaging* 6: 501–506, 1988.

130. Baker PN, Johnson IR, et al.: A three-year follow-up of children imaged in utero with echo-planar magnetic resonance. *Am J Obstet Gynecol* 170: 32–33, 1994.

131. Tyndall DA, and Sulik KK: Effects of magnetic resonance imaging on eye development in the C57BL/6J mouse. *Teratology* 43: 263–275, 1991.

132. Kanal E, Gillen J, et al.: Survey of reproductive health among female MR workers. *Radiology* 187: 395–399, 1993.

133. Panigel M, Wolf G, et al.: Magnetic resonance imaging of the placenta in rhesus monkeys, *Macaca mulatta*. *J Med Primatol* 17: 3–18, 1998.

134. Rofsky NM, Pizzarello DJ, et al.: Effect on fetal mouse development of exposure to MR imaging and gadopentetate dimeglumine. *J Magn Reson Imaging* 4: 805–807, 1994.

135. Coakley FV, Hricak H, et al.: Complex fetal disorders: effect of MR imaging on management—preliminary clinical experience. *Radiology* 213: 691–696, 1999.

136. Lan LM, Yamashita Y, et al.: Normal fetal brain development: MR imaging with a half-Fourier rapid acquisition with relaxation enhancement sequence. *Radiology* 215: 205–210, 2000.

137. Duncan KR, Gowland PA, et al.: Assessment of fetal lung growth in utero with echo-planar MR imaging. *Radiology* 210: 197–200, 1999.

138. Benson RC, Colletti PM, et al.: MR imaging of fetal anomalies. *Am J Roentgenol* 156: 1205–1207, 1991.

139. Baker PN, Johnson IR, et al.: Measurement of fetal liver, brain and placental volumes with echo-planar magnetic resonance imaging. *Br J Obstet Gynaecol* 102: 35–39, 1995.

140. Kubik-Huch RA, Wildermuth S, et al.: Fetus and utero-placental unit: Foot MR imaging with three-Dimensional reconstruction and volumetry-feasibility study. *Radiology* 219: 567–573, 2001.

141. Borcard B, Hiltbrand E, et al.: Estimating meconium (fetal feces) concentration in human amniotic fluid by nuclear magnetic resonance. *Physiol Chem Phys* 14: 189–192, 1982.

142. Powell MC, Buckley J, et al.: Magnetic resonance imaging and placenta previa. *Am J Obstet Gynecol* 154: 565–569, 1986.

143. Kay HH, Spritzer CE: Preliminary experience with magnetic resonance imaging in patients with third-trimester bleeding. *Obstet Gynecol* 78: 424–429, 1991.

144. Marcos HB, Semelka RC, Worawattanakul S: Normal placenta: Gadolinium-enhanced, dynamic MR imaging. *Radiology* 205: 493–496, 1997.

145. Wagner BJ, Woodward PJ, et al.: From the archives of the AFIP. Gestational trophoblastic disease: Radiologic-pathologic correlation. *Radiographics* 16: 131–148, 1996.

146. Hricak H, Demas BE, et al.: Gestational trophoblastic neoplasm of the uterus: MR assessment. *Radiology* 161: 11–16, 1986.

147. Powell MC, Buckley J, et al.: Magnetic resonance imaging and hydatidiform mole. *Br J Radiol* 59: 561–564, 1986.

148. Barton JW, McCarthy SM, et al.: Pelvic MR imaging findings in gestational trophoblastic disease, incomplete abortion, and ectopic pregnancy: Are they specific? *Radiology* 186: 163–168, 1993.

149. Stark DD, McCarthy SM, et al.: Pelvimetry by magnetic resonance imaging. *Am J Roentgenol* 144: 947–950, 1985.

150. Weinreb JC, Lowe TW, et al.: Magnetic resonance imaging in obstetric diagnosis. *Radiology* 154: 157–161, 1985.

151. Pfammatter T, Marincek B, et al.: MR-pelvimetrische Referenzwerte. *Rofo Fortschr Geb Rontgenstr Neuen Bildgeb Verfahr* 153: 706–710, 1990.

152. Sigmund G, Bauer M, et al.: [A technic of magnetic resonance tomographic pelvimetry in obstetrics] Original title: Technik der kernspintomographischen Beckenmessung in der Geburtshilfe. *Rofo Fortschr Geb Rontgenstr Neuen Bildgeb Verfahr* 154: 370–374, 1991.

153. Weinreb JC, Brown CE, et al.: Pelvic masses in pregnant patients: MR and US imaging. *Radiology* 159: 717–724, 1986.

154. Curtis M, Hopkins MP, et al.: Magnetic resonance imaging to avoid laparotomy in pregnancy. *Obstet Gynecol* 82: 833–836, 1993.

155. Kawakami S, Togashi K, et al.: Red degeneration of uterine leiomyoma: MR appearance. *J Comput Assist Tomogr* 18: 925–928, 1994.

156. Nguyen C, Montz FJ, et al.: Management of Stage I cervical cancer during pregnancy. *Gynecol Surv* 55: 633–643, 2000.

157. Roy C, Saussine C, et al.: Fast imaging MR assessment of ureterohydronephrosis during pregnancy. *Magn Reson Imaging* 13: 767–772, 1995.

158. Woo GM, Twickler DM, et al.: The pelvis after cesarean section and vaginal delivery: Normal MR findings. *Am J Roentgenol* 161: 1249–1252, 1993.

159. Willms AB, Brown ED, et al.: Anatomic changes in the pelvis after uncomplicated vaginal delivery: Evaluation with serial MR imaging. *Radiology* 195: 91–94, 1995.

160. Kubik Huch RA, Hebisch G, et al.: Role of duplex color Doppler ultrasound, computed tomography, and MR angiography in the diagnosis of septic puerperal ovarian vein thrombosis. *Abdom Imaging* 24: 85–91, 1999.

CHAPTER 15

ADNEXA

DEBORAH. A. BAUMGARTEN, M.D., SUSAN M. ASCHER, M.D.,
RICHARD C. SEMELKA, TOMOFUMI MOTOHARA, M.D.,
LARISSA L. NAGASE, M.D., AND ERIC K. OUTWATER, M.D.

MRI has many advantages over other imaging modalities with respect to imaging the adnexa. Inherent high soft tissue contrast, multiplanar capabilities, and lack of ionizing radiation are but a few. This chapter outlines the current use of MRI in imaging a variety of benign and malignant processes involving the adnexa.

OVARY

Normal Anatomy

The position and appearance of the ovary are dependent on age and hormonal milieu. During the first year of life, the ovaries migrate into the true pelvis to lie within the ovarian fossa, a depression within the pelvic sidewall. The ovarian fossa is defined by the external iliac vessels anteriorly and the ureter and internal iliac vessels posteriorly. Although this is the typical location of the ovaries, there is some variability based on multiparity, the size of the bladder and uterus, and prior surgery. The ovaries are held in position by the ovarian suspensory ligament (or infundibulopelvic ligament) superiorly and medially, by the broad ligament (proper ovarian ligament)

inferiorly and anteriorly, and by the mesovarium anteriorly. In general, the ovaries are lateral to the uterus and inferior to the fallopian tubes.

The blood supply of the ovaries is derived from the ovarian artery, a branch of the aorta below the renal artery, as well as the ovarian branch of the uterine artery (which is a branch of the internal iliac artery). These anastomose to form an arcade of approximately 10 arterial branches that penetrate the ovary. The ovarian artery and vein pass through the ovarian suspensory ligament. The venous drainage of the ovaries differs slightly between left and right, with the left ovarian vein draining into the left renal vein and the right ovarian vein draining directly into the IVC near the right renal vein. The lymphatic drainage of the ovaries follows the venous drainage into para-aortic nodes.

Ovarian size varies with age; in the neonate, ovaries measure approximately $1.5 \times 2.5 \times 3$ mm [1]. In the premenopausal female, ovarian volume is 5–8 g with increases during ovulation and pregnancy. A decrease in size begins at age 30, and after menopause ovarian atrophy is more pronounced [2]. The use of hormonal replacement therapy may affect the rate of atrophy.

Histologically, the ovary is divided into medullary (central) and cortical (peripheral) regions. The medulla contains the stromal cells, lymphatics, blood vessels, and nerves. The cortex is composed of follicles differing in their stage of maturation; the number of follicles is greatest at birth and progressively declines, disappearing after menopause [1]. During the reproductive years, one graafian follicle matures each month, releasing an ovum and becoming a corpus luteum. In the absence of pregnancy, the corpus luteum degenerates into a corpus albicans and eventually completely involutes. Oral contraceptive tablets interfere with this process, suppressing graafian follicle maturation and ovum release.

MRI Technique

Bowel peristalsis can cause significant degradation of images in the pelvis. To reduce this artifact, patients can fast for 4–6 h before scanning or an antiperistaltic drug such as glucagon can be employed (1 mg given intramuscularly 15-30 min before the scan). Respiratory motion is not as much of a problem as in the abdomen but if needed, respiratory gating or compensation or compression belts can be utilized. To reduce the presence of flow-related artifacts, saturation pulses can be placed above and below the volume of interest. In addition, having the patient void before imaging improves comfort and decreases motion artifact.

MRI may be particularly useful in the pregnant patient for characterization of symptomatic or incidentally discovered adnexal masses. The advantages of superior tissue characterization over ultrasound and the lack of ionizing radiation make it an ideal modality, limiting surgical intervention and directing appropriate management [3, 4]. Most studies have failed to show any harmful effects of MRI on the human fetus [5].

Use of the phased-array torso coil has improved MR imaging in the pelvis, increasing the signal-to-noise ratio in the center of the body compared with the conventional body coil [6, 7]. However, the surface coil cannot be used in every patient. Large body habitus either from obesity or a large amount of ascites precludes placement of the coil, and penetration may not be adequate even if placement is possible. Postsurgical patients with recent incisions or ostomies or those women with significant pelvic discomfort may not tolerate coil placement [8]. Other considerations include artifact caused by the coils near field sensitivity. Fat beneath the coil is bright in signal intensity and motion-related ghost artifact might be a problem [9]. A variety of techniques have been described to moderate this effect [10, 11].

Standard sequences used for the adnexa include transverse T1-weighted spoiled gradient-echo (SGE), transverse T1-weighted SGE with fat suppression, transverse fast spin-echo (SE) T2-weighted, sagittal or coronal breath-hold or single-shot fast SE, and postgadolinium SGE with fat suppression.

Normal ovary

In a recent study of the histologic and anatomic basis of MR imaging features of the ovary [12], two patterns of ovarian anatomy were seen with T2-weighted images. The first is a lower-signal intensity cortex and stroma with higher signal in the medulla; this pattern is more prevalent in premenopausal subjects (figs. 15.1 and 15.2). The second pattern is a more homogeneous low signal of the cortex and medulla. This pattern is more common in postmenopausal women. On T1-weighted images the ovaries have signal intensity homogeneously isointense to the myometrium. After the administration of gadolinium, the ovarian enhancement differs with hormonal status. In premenopausal women ovarian enhancement tends to be less than the enhancement of the myometrium, whereas in postmenopausal women, enhancement is equivalent [13]. Transposed ovaries have imaging patterns similar to normal ovaries. (fig. 15.3)

Functional cysts have very high signal on T2-weighted images and are of low to intermediate signal on T1-weighted images. These include follicular, corpus luteal, and corpus albicans cysts. Cysts are common in ovaries regardless of age and hormonal status. In one series of asymptomatic postmenopausal women, 17% had at least one cyst [14]. Cyst walls are generally of decreased signal intensity on T2-weighted images; wall enhancement after gadolinium is variable (fig. 15.4). Corpus luteal cysts tend to have more thickened and irregular walls and show intense wall enhancement after contrast [15]. Because these features can also be seen with malignancy, follow-up may be necessary to distinguish the two. Furthermore, corpus luteal cysts may also hemorrhage, altering their T1- and T2-weighted signal characteristics (fig. 15.5). When hemorrhagic, their signal intensity is intermediate to high on both sequences and they can be confused with endometriomas [16]. Follow-up can be helpful in this situation as well.

Congenital abnormalities

These entities are discussed more fully in the chapters: female urethra and vagina and the uterus and cervix (Chapters 13 and 14, respectively) and include complete and mixed gonadal dysgenesis and true and pseudo-hermaphroditism. MRI is very important in demonstrating the internal reproductive organs and can identify the presence of normal ovaries, streak gonads, or ovotestes [17, 18]. Gonadoblastoma, a neoplasm occurring in up to one-third of patients with mixed gonadal dysgenesis can also be detected [17, 19].

Mass Lesions

Benign Masses

Functional Cysts. The imaging characteristics were discussed in the section on normal anatomy. When

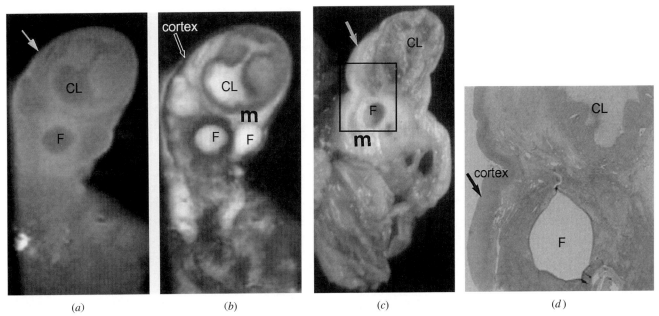

(a)   *(b)*   *(c)*   *(d)*

F I G . 15.1 High resolution specimen images of the normal ovary. T1-weighted (*a*) and T2-weighted ETSE (*b*) images, gross specimen photograph (*c*), and specimen photomicrograph (*d*) of a normal ovary in a woman of reproductive age. T2-weighted images highlight ovarian zonal anatomy: an outer rim of low signal intensity circumscribing an inner region of high signal intensity. These areas correspond to the cortex (arrows, *a–d*) and medulla ("m," *b, c*), respectively, on the gross specimen photograph and photomicrograph. Follicles (F, *a–d*) are also seen. On the T2-weighted image, they possess a uniform and thin low-signal intensity rim versus the high signal intensity of their contents. In contrast, an involuting corpus luteum ("CL," *a–d*) possesses an uneven and focally thickened intermediate-signal intensity periphery. This is typical of the luteinized cell lining of involuting corpus lutea. (Parts *a, b,* and *c* are reprinted with permission from Outwater EK, Schiebler ML: Magnetic resonance imaging of the ovary. *Radiol Clin N Am* 2: 245–274, 1994.)

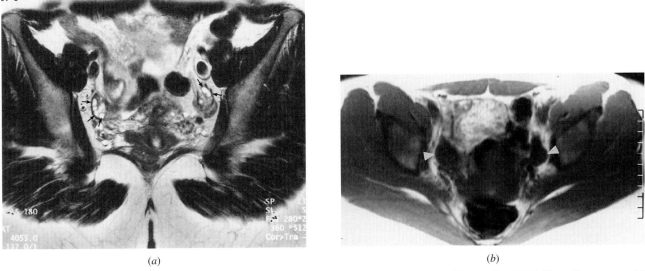

(a)   *(b)*

F I G . 15.2 Normal ovaries. Paracoronal 512-resolution T2-weighted ETSE (*a*), transverse T1-weighted SGE (*b*), and transverse (*c*) and sagittal (*d*) gadolinium-enhanced T1-weighted fat-suppressed SGE images of a woman with normal ovaries. The ovaries reside in the ovarian fossa and are intermediate in signal intensity on the unenhanced T1-weighted image (arrowheads, *b*). On the T2-weighted image (*a*), follicles are identified as high-signal intensity structures (arrows, *a*). After contrast the ovarian parenchyma enhances, whereas the follicles (arrows, *c, d*) are signal-void foci. The enhanced images show some of the anatomic boundaries of the ovarian fossa: the bifurcation of the common iliac vessels superiorly (open arrow, *d*), obliterated umbilical artery anteriorly (open arrow, *c*), and the internal iliac vessels posteriorly (curved arrow, *d*).

T2-weighted ETSE image (*e*) of a normal ovaries in a second patient. Ovaries are readily visualized because of the presence of follicles, which appear as high-signal intensity, small, rounded foci (arrows, *e*).

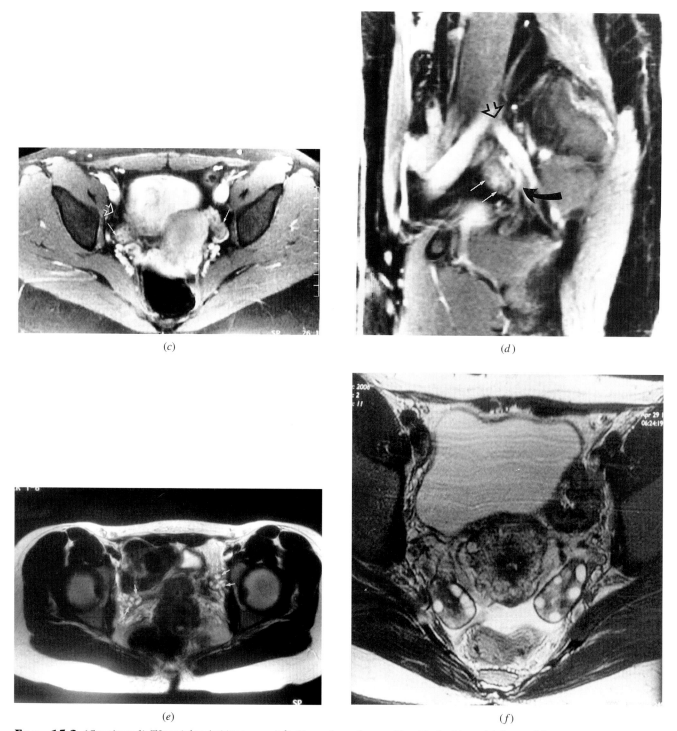

(c)

(d)

(e)

(f)

FIG. 15.2 (*Continued*) T2-weighted ETSE image (*f*). Normal ovaries are identified with multiple small hyperintense follicles. A small volume of fluid is present in the pouch of Douglas. (Courtesy of Rahel Kubik-Huch MD, Department of Radiology, University Hospital of Zurich, Zurich, Switzerland.)

uncomplicated, functional cysts are not a diagnostic dilemma. However, when complicated (generally by hemorrhage) differentiation from endometriomas and neoplasm may be difficult. Follow-up showing resolution of the cyst easily classifies it as functional; however, on any single study there are features that can aid in this differentiation. Papillary projections are an important differential feature of neoplastic cysts (fig. 15.6) and are not present in functional cysts (fig. 15.7) [20] and are more fully discussed in the section on neoplastic cysts.

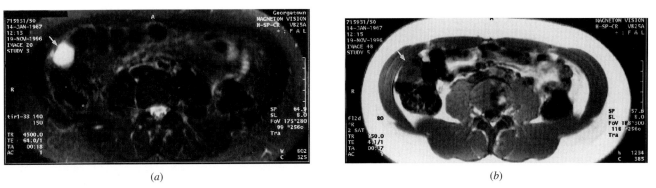

(a)   (b)

F I G . 15.3 Transposed right ovary. T2-weighted ETSE (*a*) and T1-weighted SGE (*b*) of a transposed normal right ovary (arrow, *a, b*) in a woman with cervical cancer treated with radiation therapy.

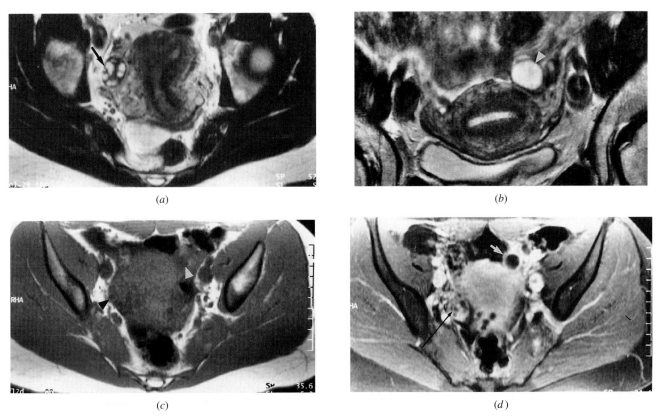

(a)   (b)

(c)   (d)

F I G . 15.4 Normal ovary with a functional cyst. Transverse (*a*) and coronal (*b*) 512-resolution T2-weighted ETSE, T1-weighted SGE (*c*), and transverse (*d*) and sagittal (*e*) gadolinium-enhanced T1-weighted fat-suppressed SGE images in a woman with normal ovaries. On the unenhanced T1-weighted image (*a*), the ovarian stroma is isointense to the uterus with the follicles and functional cyst being lower in signal intensity (arrowheads, *c*). The high-resolution T2-weighted images (*a, b*) show the follicle-laden right ovary (arrow, *a*) and a cyst-containing left ovary (arrowhead, *b*). The cortex containing the follicles is lower in signal intensity than the medulla. After contrast, the ovarian parenchyma enhances, including the rims of the follicles (long arrow, *d, e*) and cyst (short arrow, *d, e*). The remainder of the left ovary is draped around the functional cyst. Simple functional cysts are low to intermediate in signal intensity on T1-weighted images and high in signal intensity on T2-weighted images, and have variable thin mural enhancement after contrast administration.

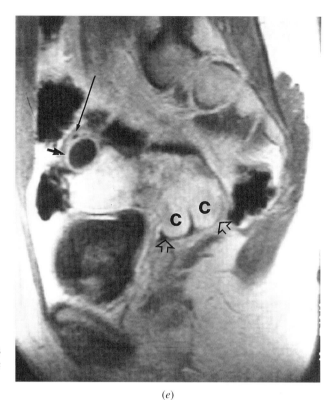

FIG. 15.4 (*Continued*) Note that the cervix ("c," *e*) protrudes into the vaginal fornices (open arrows, *e*) and is well seen with the contrast-enhanced fat-suppressed SGE technique.

(*e*)

Endometriomas generally have profound T1 shortening, rendering them high signal, and T2 shortening, rendering them low signal [16].

Mature Cystic Teratoma. The most common ovarian neoplasm is the mature cystic teratoma or dermoid cyst, comprising between 26 and 44% of ovarian neoplasms, depending upon the series [2]. The peak incidence is during the midreproductive years, although they can be detected at any age. Approximately 85% are detected between 20 and 50 years of age. Roughly 90% are unilateral [2] and many are incidentally discovered in an asymptomatic woman. These are slow-growing tumors, and symptoms, when present, are related to the size of the tumor (mass effect causing pressure or pain) or to torsion, infection or rupture, which are much

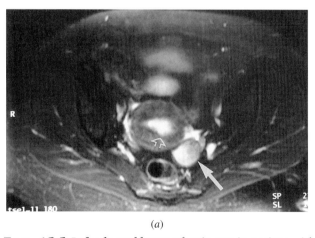

(*a*)

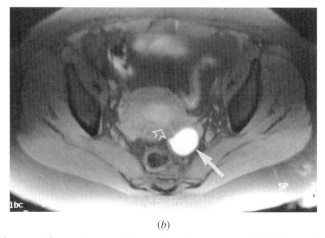

(*b*)

FIG. 15.5 **Left adnexal hemorrhagic cyst in patient with endometrial carcinoma.** T2-weighted fat-suppressed ETSE (*a*) and T1-weighted fat-suppressed SGE (*b*) images. Hemorrhagic cysts can mimic endometriomas with high signal intensity on T1-weighted images (arrow, *b*) and heterogeneous high signal intensity on T2-weighted images (arrow, *a*). Note the focus of endometrial carcinoma that thins the junctional zone (open arrow, *a*, *b*).

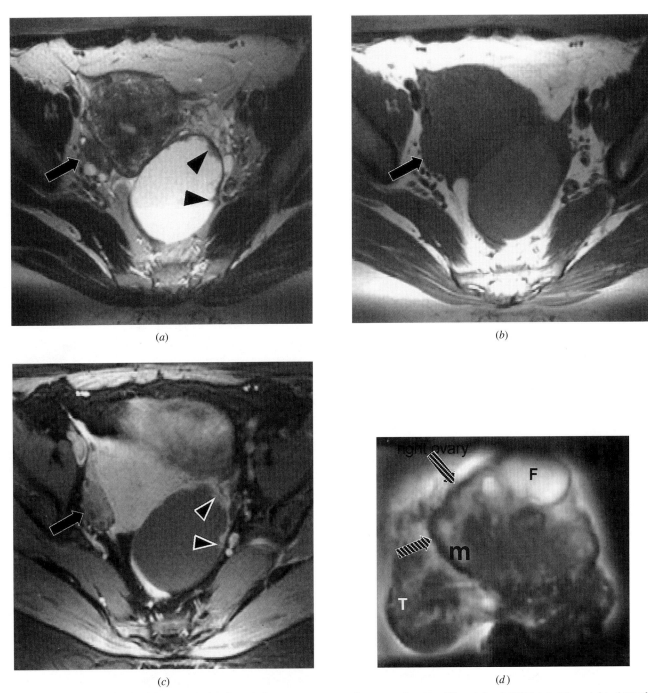

FIG. 15.6 Normal right ovary and left ovarian serous cystadenocarcinoma. T2-weighted ETSE (*a*), T1-weighted SE (*b*), gadolinium-enhanced T1-weighted fat-suppressed SGE (*c*) images, and specimen T2-weighted SE (*d*) and T1-weighted SE (*e*) images in a 40-year-old woman with a left adnexal mass. The normal right ovary (arrow, *a–c*) contains several follicles that have enhancing rims after contrast. Note that the ovarian stroma enhances less than adjacent myometrium. The specimen right ovary image accentuates the difference in signal intensity between the ovarian cortex (hatched arrow, *d*) low signal intensity, and the ovarian medulla ("m," *d*) high signal intensity. Note the adjacent normal coiled fallopian tube ("T," *d,e*). In contrast, the left ovary has been replaced by a primarily cystic mass.

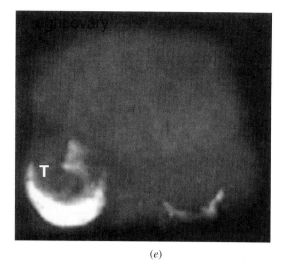

F I G . 15.6 (*Continued*) Apparent thickening of the wall of the cyst (arrowheads, *a*) is confirmed on the postgadolinium image, which demonstrates enhancing papillary projections (arrowheads, *c*). F, follicle (Parts *a*, *c*, *d*, and *e* are reprinted with permission from Outwater EK, Mitchell DG: Normal ovaries and functional cysts: MR appearance. *Radiology* 198: 397–402, 1996.)

(e)

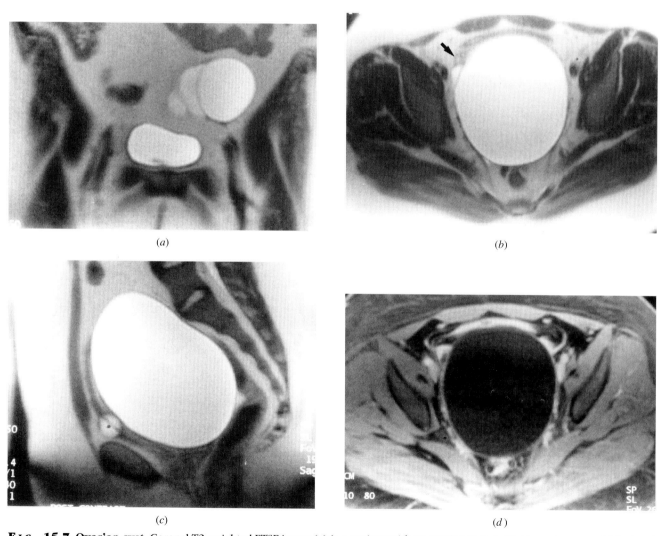

(a)

(b)

(c)

(d)

F I G . 15.7 Ovarian cyst. Coronal T2-weighted ETSE image (*a*) in a patient with an ovarian cyst. A simple cyst appears high signal intensity on the T2-weighted image without mural thickening or nodularity. Adnexal cyst shown on transverse (*b*) and sagittal (*c*) T2-weighted SS-ETSE and transverse (*d*) and sagittal (*e*) interstital phase images in a second patient.

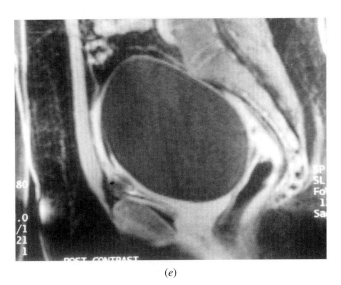

(e)

FIG. 15.7 (*Continued*) A large well-defined cyst with simple fluid content and no mural irregularity is apparent arising from the right ovary (arrow, *b*).

rarer complications. In 1–3% of cases, malignant transformation can occur [2] and is more frequent in postmenopausal women.

Histopathologically, these tumors are composed of varying amounts of endodermal, mesodermal, and ectodermal elements giving rise to the bone, teeth, hair, cartilage, skin, muscle, fat, bronchus, salivary gland, thyroid, pancreas, neural tissue, and retina that have been found within them [2]. In most cases, they are unilocular, with an ectodermal lining, and contain keratin and sebum, secreted by sebaceous glands. Septations may also be present, giving a multilocular appearance. These are managed by conservative surgery, either cystectomy, ovarirectomy or salgingo-oophorectomy depending on the size and location of the tumor and the patient's desire for future fertility. When malignant transformation does occur, the neoplasm is similar to other adult neoplasms, with squamous cell carcinoma accounting for the majority; other cell types include adenocarcinoma, sarcoma,

transitional cell carcinoma, and melanoma [2, 21, 22]. The prognosis after malignant transformation is poor, with most patients surviving less than 1 year [2].

The MR features of cystic teratomas have been extensively described. Characteristic features include fat within the lesion, fat-fluid or fluid-fluid levels, layering debris, low-signal intensity calcification (usually teeth), and Rokitansky nodules (dermoid plugs attached to the cyst wall) [24–26]. The fat within the lesion follows fat signal on all sequences. Interfaces between the fat and water and/or soft tissue in the lesion also causes chemical shift artifact, present in about 60% of cases [27]. Standard T1- and T2-weighted imaging sequences can support the diagnosis of a teratoma; however, fat saturated or out-of-phase T1-weighted images will improve diagnostic confidence (fig. 15.8) [27–29]. Accuracies up to 96% have been reported using these techniques [27]. It is possible that out-of-phase imaging may have an advantage in lesions with only small amounts of lipid [30].

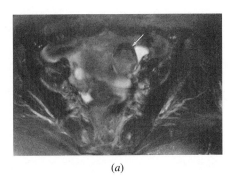

(a)

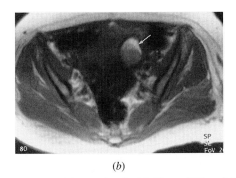

(b)

FIG. 15.8 Dermoid. Transverse 512-resolution T2-weighted fat-suppressed ETSE (*a*), T1-weighted SGE (*b*), and T1-weighted fat-suppressed SGE (*c*) images in a woman with a left adnexal mass. On the nonsuppressed image, a high-signal intensity component, similar to the pelvic and subcutaneous fat, is noted in the nondependent portion of the mass (arrow, *b*). Although this is suggestive of a lipid-containing mass, methemoglobin may appear similarly. On the fat-suppressed sequences (*a, c*) this area diminishes in signal intensity (arrow, *a, c*), comparable to the pelvic, marrow, and subcutaneous fat, confirming the diagnosis of a dermoid cyst.

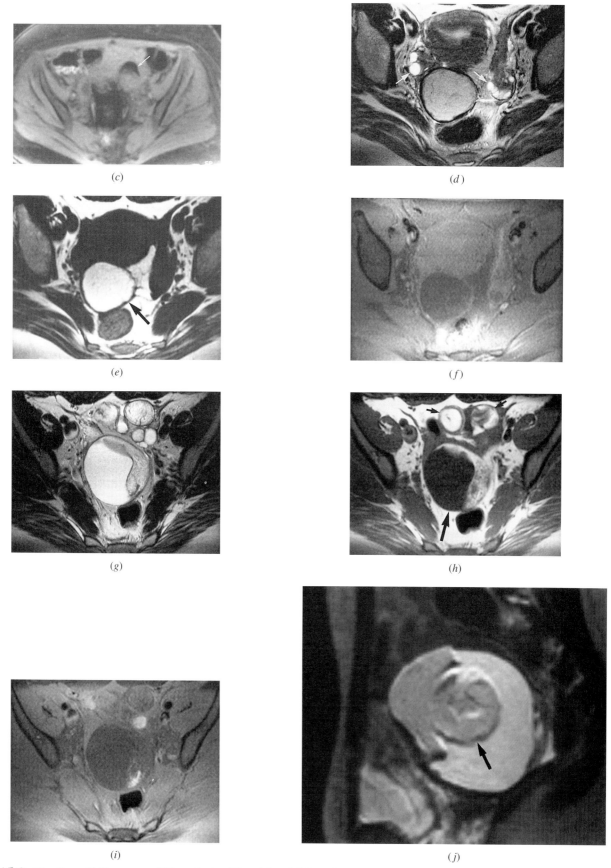

(c)

(d)

(e)

(f)

(g)

(h)

(i)

(j)

F I G . 15.8 (*Continued*) Transverse 512-resolution T2-weighted ETSE (*d*), T1-weighted SE (*e*), and T1-weighted fat-suppressed SE (*f*) images in a second patient. An exophytic right ovarian dermoid is present that is uniformly high in signal intensity on the T1-weighted image (arrow, *e*) and suppresses uniformly on the fat-suppressed image (*f*).

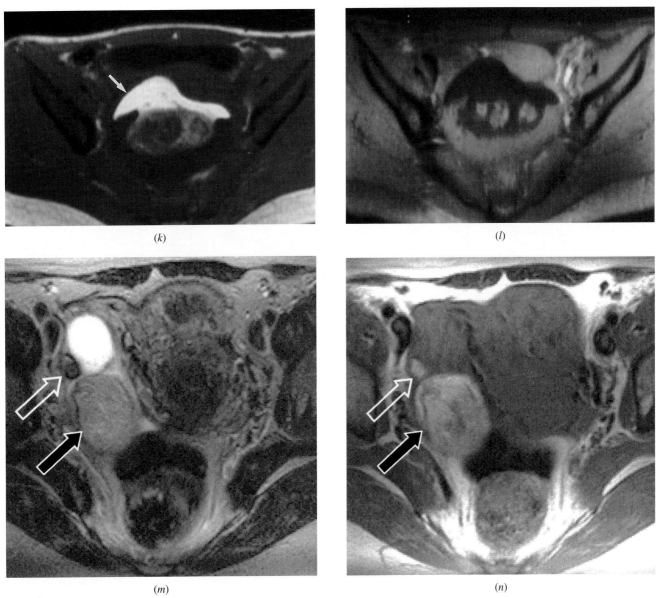

(k)   *(l)*

(m)   *(n)*

FIG. 15.8 *(Continued)* Follicles are well shown in both ovaries (arrows, *d*) on the high-resolution image, and the exophytic nature of the dermoid is clearly demonstrated.

Transverse 512-resolution T2-weighted ETSE (*g*), T1-weighted SE (*h*), and T1-weighted fat-suppressed SE (*i*) images in a third patient with bilateral dermoids. A large right (large arrow, *h*) and two smaller left (small arrows, *h*) ovarian dermoids are present. The signal intensities of the dermoids are complex on T1- (*h*) and T2-weighted (*g*) images because of a mixture of substances they contain. The fat components suppress on the fat-suppressed image (*i*).

Sagittal T2-weighted ETSE (*j*), T1-weighted SGE (*k*), and T1-weighted fat-suppressed SE (*l*) images in a fourth patient. A 5-cm dermoid is present that contains fat and hair. A layer of fatty material is present in the top portion of the dermoid that is high in signal intensity (arrow, *k*) on the T1-weighted image (*k*) and suppresses on the fat-suppressed image (*l*). A ball of hair is suspended in the midportion of the dermoid (arrow, *j*). (Courtesy of Ann B. Willms MD).

Transverse T2-weighted echo-train spin-echo (*m*), T1-weighted spin-echo (*n*), and T1-weighted fat-suppressed SGE (*o*) images in a fifth patient with mature cystic teratoma and endometriosis. T2-weighted image shows heterogenous internal signal intensity of the larger mass (black arrows, *m*), with punctate high signal. The smaller mass (open arrows, *m*) shows low signal intensity "shading" typical of endometrioma. T1-weighted spin-echo image shows 2 high-signal intensity masses of the right ovary (arrows, *n*). T1-weighted fat-suppressed SGE image shows saturation of the larger cyst contents (black arrow, *n*), whereas the hemorrhagic endometriosis (open arrow, *n*) remains high signal intensity.

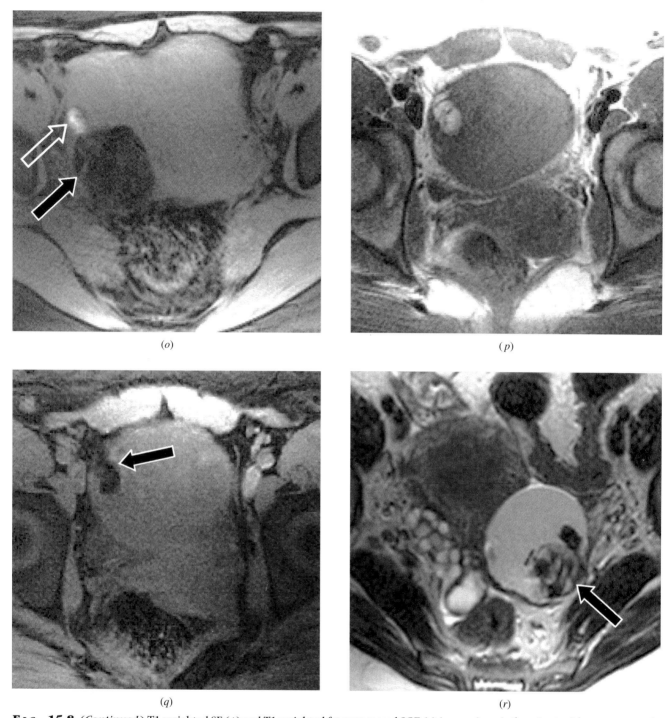

(o)

(p)

(q)

(r)

F I G . 15.8 (*Continued*) T1-weighted SE (*p*) and T1-weighted fat-suppressed SGE (*q*) images in a sixth patient with a mature cystic teratoma. T1-weighted image (*p*) shows a high-signal intensity nodule in the wall of the mass. T1-weighted fat-suppressed image shows saturation of the fatty nodule (arrow, *q*). The majority of the lesion is nonfatty.

T2-weighted ETSE (*r*), T1-weighted SE (*s*), and T1-weighted fat-suppressed SGE (*t*) images in a seventh patient with mature cystic teratoma. T2-weighted image shows a high-signal intensity mature cystic teratoma (arrow, *r*) in the left ovary. The Rokitansky nodule contains areas that are high signal intensity, representing fat, and signal voids representing teeth.

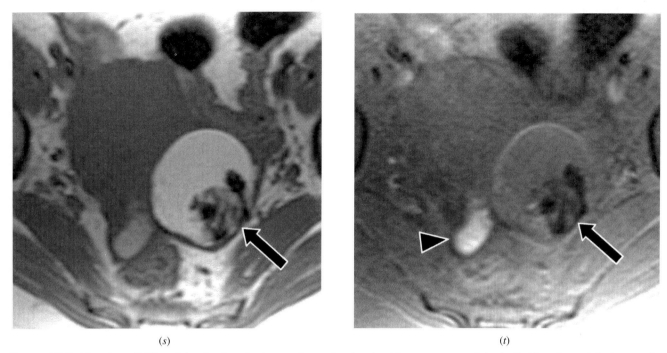

(s)   (t)

F I G . 15.8 (*Continued*) T1-weighted spin-echo image shows the signal voids represent teeth in the Rokitansky nodule (arrow, *s*). T1-weighted fat-suppressed SGE image (*t*) shows osseous signal intensity both within the cyst contents and and within the Rokitansky nodule itself. The high signal intensity hematosalpinx (arrowhead, *t*) does not suppress.

There is a subset of teratomas composed entirely or almost entirely of thyroid tissue; these are referred to as struma ovarii. Most reports in the literature describe these tumors as complex multilocular masses with solid components [31–34]. The different locules may have vari-able signal intensity due to the differences in viscosity within the fluid; the signal is often low to intermediate on T1- and very low on T2-weighted images [35]. The solid components demonstrate significant enhancement after gadolinium and correspond to thyroid tissue (fig. 15.9)

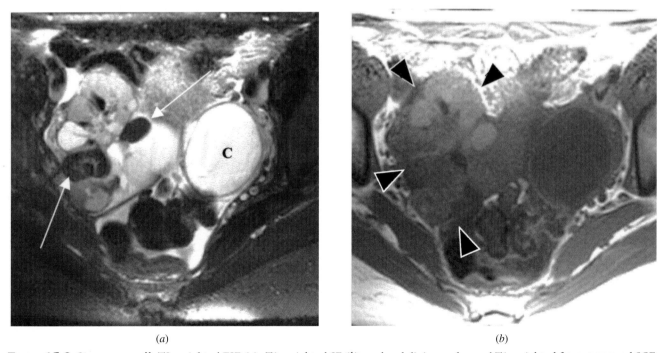

(a)   (b)

F I G . 15.9 Struma ovarii. T2-weighted FSE (*a*), T1-weighted SE (*b*), and gadolinium-enhanced T1-weighted fat- suppressed SGE (*c*) images in a patient with struma ovarii.

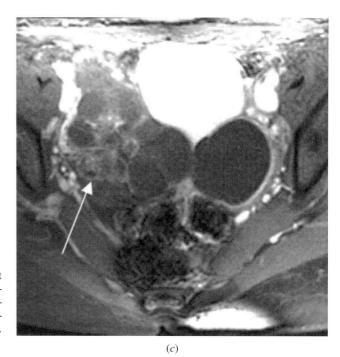

(c)

FIG. 15.9 *(Continued)* Note a multiloculated mass in the right ovary (arrowheads, *b*), which shows lacelike enhancement on post-gadolinium images (arrows, *c*). Some cysts show low signal intensity on T2-weighted images (arrows, *a*). Struma ovarii is a monodermal teratoma in which the tumor may produce thyroid hormones.

[35]. An additional recent article reports three cases lacking this solid component [36]. However, the same signal pattern within the locules was noted in the multilocular cases.

Cystadenomas. Serous cystadenomas are common epithelial neoplasms, accounting for about 20% of benign ovarian neoplasms [2]. Whereas the malignant counterpart of this lesion tends to occur in older women, benign cystadenomas develop in women between 20 and 50 years of age; about 20% are bilateral, also in distinction to the malignant version, which is more frequently bilateral [37]. The most common presentation is of a thin-walled unilocular cyst; however, there have been descriptions of papillary projections [38]. These projections are very important to recognize as they are the hallmark of epithelial neoplasms and may be a predictor of malignancy [20]. Benign epithelial tumors have fewer and smaller projections than borderline or frankly malignant lesions [20]. When benign, these lesions can be treated by simple resection or unilateral ovarirectomy and do not recur or spread.

On MRI, these lesions follow water on all imaging sequences: dark on T1 and bright on T2-weighted sequences, if uncomplicated (fig. 15.10). When complicated by hemorrhage, both the T1 and T2 signal

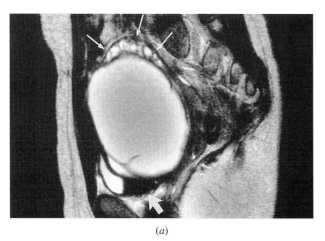

(a)

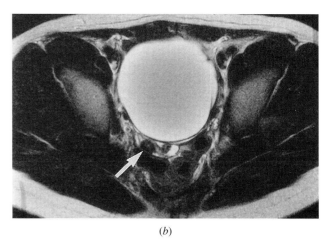

(b)

FIG. 15.10 Serous cystadenoma. Sagittal (*a*) and transverse (*b*) 512-resolution T2-weighted ETSE images in a 10-year-old girl with precocious puberty. A large septate mass occupies the pelvis. Note the pubertal-sized, follicle-containing ovary draped over the mass (long arrows, *a*).

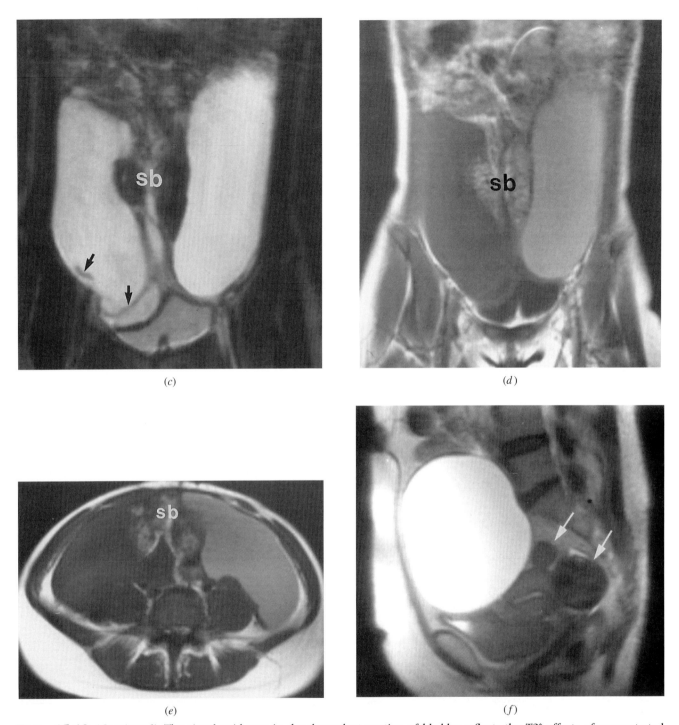

(c)

(d)

(e)

(f)

FIG. 15.10 (*Continued*) The signal void area in the dependent portion of bladder reflects the T2* effects of concentrated gadolinium (short arrow, *a*). The ovarian mass displaces the uterine corpus and cervix (arrow, *b*) posteriorly. At surgery a benign serous cystadenoma was resected.

Coronal T2-weighted ETSE (*c*), coronal (*d*) and transverse (*e*) T1-weighted SE images in a second young girl who presented with an enlarging abdomen. Bilateral cystic masses originate in the pelvis and extend into the abdomen. The right-sided mass has signal characteristics suggesting simple fluid, whereas the left-sided mass has signal characteristics of proteinaceous or hemorrhagic fluid. Septations are more conspicuous on the T2-weighted image (arrows, *c*). At surgery, bilateral serous cystadenomas were found: the left-sided one was complicated by hemorrhage, accounting for its imaging features. Note that the small bowel ("sb," *c, d, e*) is compressed between the two masses.

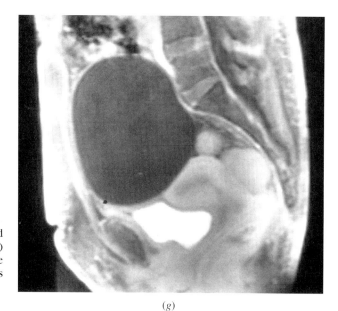

FIG. **15.10** (*Continued*) Sagittal T2-weighted ETSE (*f*) and sagittal gadolinium-enhanced T1-weighted fat-suppressed SGE (*g*) in a third patient with an ovarian serous cystadenoma. A large simple cystic mass is present. Note exophytic subserosal fibroids (arrows, *f*).

(*g*)

characteristics are altered because of shortening of relaxation times (fig. 15.10). When unilocular and thin walled, these lesions can be mistaken for simple functional cysts. When multilocular, they may be mistaken for malignant tumors or fallopian tube pathology such as hydrosalpinx. The presence of papillary projections should be carefully sought; the use of IV gadolinium may aid in their detection.

Mucinous cystadenomas are also of epithelial origin and account for another 20% of benign ovarian neo-

plasms. They are less frequently bilateral (about 5%) and are more common after age 40 [2]. These lesions tend to be multilocular, another feature that may help to distinguish them from the serous type, although treatment is the same.

On MRI, these lesions demonstrate multiple locules with varying signal intensity on T1- and T2-weighted images because of their protein content [39]. Hemorrhage may also be seen in one or more locules, also causing variation in the T1 and T2 signals (fig. 15.11) [38]. Like

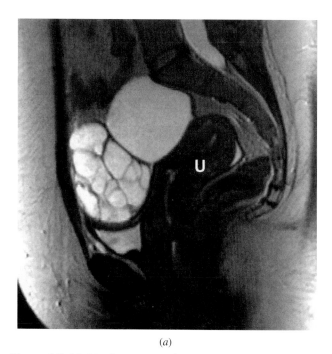

(*a*)

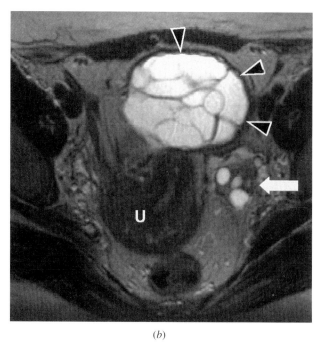

(*b*)

FIG. **15.11 Mucinous cystadenoma.** Sagittal (*a*) and transverse (*b*) T2-weighted ETSE and transverse T1-weighted SE (*c*) images. Multiple internal cysts and septations are typical findings in mucinous cystadenoma. The low-signal intensity fibrotic wall of the mass (arrowheads, *b*) and the adjacent normal left ovary (arrow, *b*) are noted.

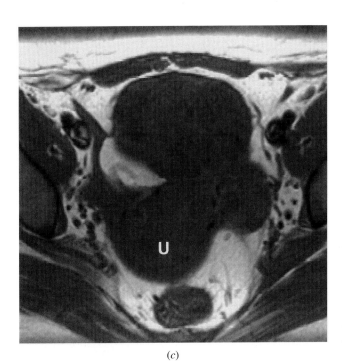

(c)

FIG. 15.11 (*Continued*) The sagittal image (*a*) demonstrates displacement of the uterus (uterus = u, *a–c*) posteriorly by the mass.

serous cystadenomas, papillary projections are suggestive of malignancy.

Endometriosis. Endometriosis is a generally benign entity affecting women in their reproductive years. It may be an incidental finding or can present with pain or infertility. Although very rare (occurring in <1%), malignant transformation can occur, with the most common tumor types being endometrioid carcinoma, clear cell carcinoma and carcinosarcoma [2, 40]. Enlargement of an endometrioma during pregnancy can be the result of changes in the hormonal milieu and does not necessarily mean malignant transformation [41]. By strict pathologic criteria, ectopic endometrial glands with surrounding endometrial stroma must be found; however, repeated hemorrhage often causes obliteration of the endometrial lining [42, 43]. In order of decreasing incidence, the most common sites of involvement are the ovaries, cul de sac and posterior uterine wall, uterosacral ligaments, anterior uterine wall, and bladder dome [43–45]. Other sites of involvement are the sigmoid colon, the fallopian tubes, and the distal ureters. Involvement in any of these sites may be by endometrial implants; the term endometrioma is generally reserved for ovarian involvement.

Numerous theories have been postulated as to the histogenesis of endometriosis. The major theories are 1) reflux of endometrial cells through the fallopian tubes with direct implantation onto pelvic structures, 2) coelomic metaplasia in which totipotential cells are transformed by repeated exposure to hormonal stimuli, and 3) vascular dissemination in which endometrial cells are transported by the blood vessels or lymphatics [46].

Thick-walled cysts with extensive surrounding fibrosis and adhesions to adjacent structures characterize endometriomas. It is the endometrioma that is most often diagnosed by imaging; endometrial implants are not as easily detected. On T1-weighted images, endometriomas are of high signal intensity; this signal intensity is more conspicuous on fat-suppressed images because of the removal of the high signal of adjacent fat. Several groups of investigators have shown that the detection of endometriomas on MR is improved, including those less than 1 cm in size, with this technique [47–49]. On T2-weighted images, endometriomas demonstrate a gradient of low signal intensity (shading) presumably caused by repeated bleeding and the build-up of blood products that shorten T2 (figs. 15.12–15.14). This profound T2 shortening is uncommon in functional or hemorrhagic cysts [15]. When using all of these signal characteristics, the sensitivity of MR for detecting endometriomas ranges from 90–92%, whereas the specificity ranges from 91 to 98% [47, 50, 51]. Variable mural enhancement is also evident with endometriomas and may cause confusion with other processes such as tubo-ovarian abscess or hemorrhagic cysts if all of the sequences are not considered [50, 52, 53]. Currently, the use of gadolinium to detect endometriomas is not considered useful [54].

As noted, the diagnosis of endometrial implants is more elusive. High-resolution MR imaging may detect implants as high-signal lesions on T1-weighted sequences, especially those with fat suppression [47, 48]. Some implants also exhibit enhancement after gadolinium

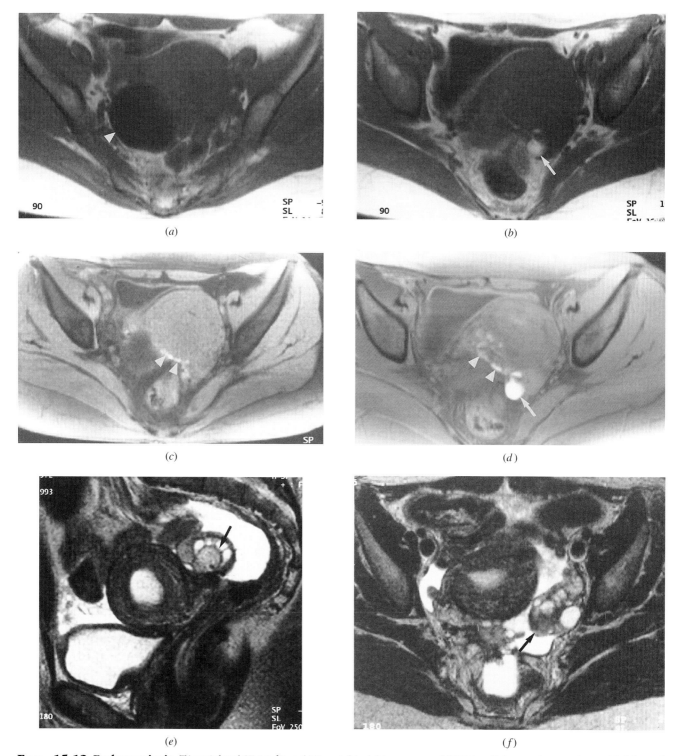

FIG. 15.12 Endometriosis. T1-weighted SE (*a, b*) and T1-weighted fat-suppressed SGE (*c, d*) images in a patient with bilateral adnexal masses, previously shown on transvaginal ultrasound. The right adnexal mass is low in signal intensity on the unenhanced image (arrowhead, *a*). There is also a high-signal intensity mass applied to the left ovary on the T1-weighted image (arrow, *b*), which is more conspicuous on the fat-suppressed image (arrow, *d*). Note that the small endometrial implants applied to the uterine serosa are well seen with fat-suppression technique (arrowheads, *c, d*).

Sagittal (*e*) and transverse (*f*) T2-weighted ETSE, sagittal (*g*) and transverse (*h*) T1-weighted SE, T1-weighted fat-suppressed SE (*i*), and sagittal (*j*) and transverse (*k*) gadolinium-enhanced T1-weighted fat-suppressed SE images in an adolescent girl with amenorrhea and pelvic pain. High-signal intensity endometriomas on the conventional T1-weighted images demonstrate characteristic shading on the T2-weighted images (arrows, *e, f*). With the addition of fat suppression, small endometriosis implants that were indistinguishable from pelvic fat on non- suppressed images become more conspicuous (arrows, *i*).

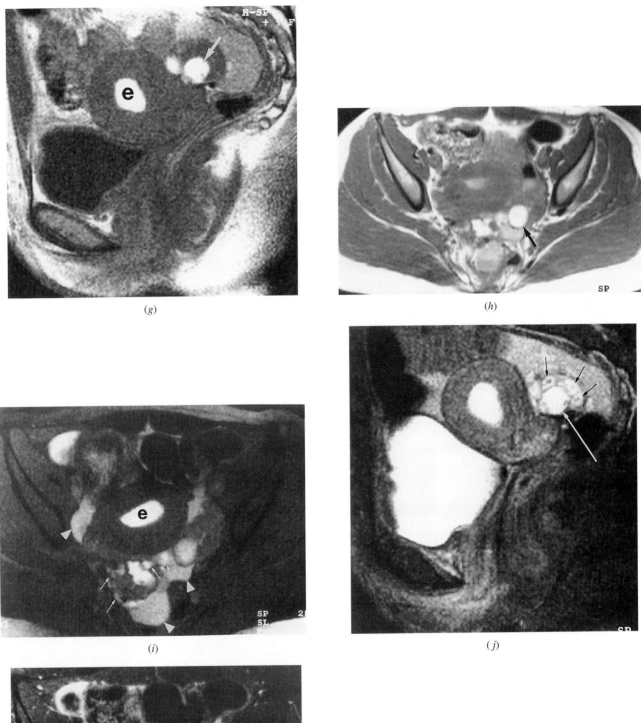

(g)

(h)

(i)

(j)

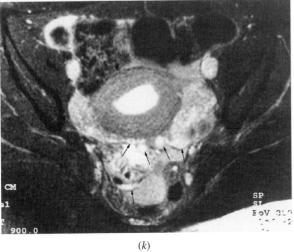

(k)

FIG. 15.12 (*Continued*) Note that the endometrial canal ("e," *g*, *i*) and free fluid (arrowheads, *i*) in the pelvis are higher in signal intensity than usual, which is consistent with hematometra and hemoperitoneum, respectively. The endometriomas and endometriosis implants have variable enhancement after contrast administration (arrows, *k*). Note the enhancing follicle rims (short arrows, *j*) surrounding the endometrioma (long arrow, *j*). This patient had cervical atresia and retrograde menses, which presumably account for her endometriosis. Surgery confirmed endometriosis and hemorrhagic free pelvic fluid; the hysterectomy specimen revealed cervical agenesis.

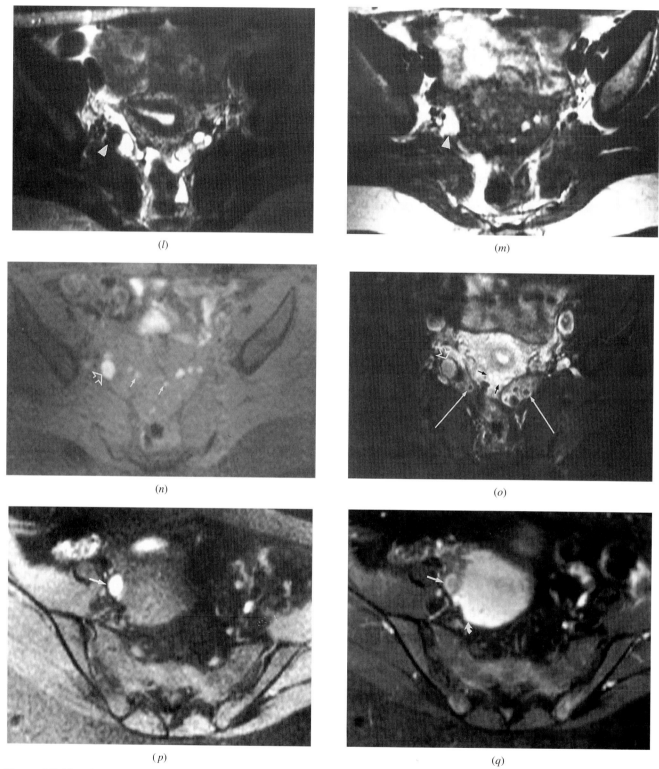

FIG. 15.12 (*Continued*) T2-weighted ETSE (*l*), T1-weighted SE (*m*) T1-weighted fat-suppressed SE (*n*), and gadolinium-enhanced T1-weighted fat-suppressed SE (*o*) images in a 39-year-old woman with pelvic pain. Endometriosis was not prospectively suggested on the nonsuppressed conventional SE images. Fat suppression highlights the endometriomas (open arrow, *n*) and endometrial implants (solid arrows, *n*) applied to the serosa of the posterior uterus. After contrast, the ovarian parenchyma and right endometrioma rim (open arrow, *o*) and follicle rims (long solid arrows, *o*) enhance. The endometrial implants remain high in signal intensity after gadolinium (short solid arrows, *o*). Retrospectively, the right endometrioma (arrowhead, *l*, *m*) and serosal implants can be identified. (Reprinted with permission from Ascher SM, Agrawal R, Bis KG, et al: Endometriosis: Appearance and detection with conventional and contrast-enhanced fat-suppressed SE techniques. *J Magn Reson Imaging* 5: 251–257, 1995.)

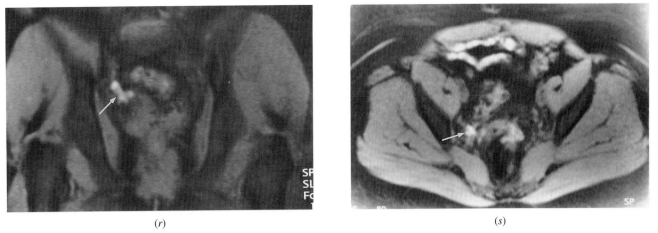

(r)

(s)

FIG. 15.12 (*Continued*) T1-weighted fat-suppressed SE (*p*) and gadolinium-enhanced T1 fat-suppressed SE (*q*) images in a fourth patient who is a 35-year-old woman with increasing pelvic pain. A right adnexal mass has high-signal intensity on the unenhanced image, which is consistent with blood (arrow, *p*). After contrast the rim enhances (arrow, *q*). This finding has been observed in both endometriomas and hemorrhagic cysts. Note the intense enhancement along the posterior uterine serosa (curved arrow, *q*). At surgery this region was studded with endometriosis implants. Ill-defined enhancement may be useful as an ancillary sign of endometriosis, although it may not be a sensitive or specific finding.

Coronal (*r*) and transverse (*s*) T1-weighted fat-suppressed SGE images in a fifth patient with right sciatic pain. An irregular, 1.5-cm high-signal intensity focus (arrow, *r*, *s*) of endometrial implant is in the right pelvis immediately adjacent to the sciatic nerve. Note the linear radiation of fibrotic tissue that extends from the mass and presumably tethers the sciatic nerve.

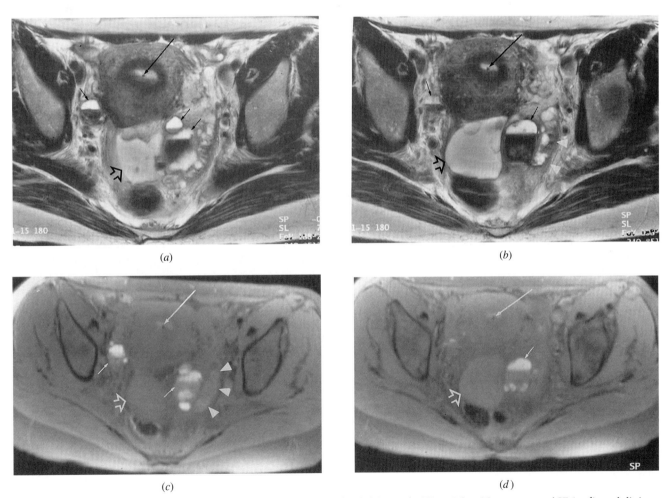

(a)

(b)

(c)

(d)

FIG. 15.13 Endometriosis. Transverse 512-resolution T2-weighted ETSE (*a*, *b*), T1-weighted fat-suppressed SE (*c*, *d*), gadolinium-enhanced T1-weighted fat-suppressed SE (*e*, *f*), sagittal T2-weighted ETSE (*g*), and coronal gadolinium-enhanced T1-weighted fat-suppressed SE (*h*) images in a 42-year-old woman with a 2-month history of pelvic pain, elevated CA-125, and complex adnexal masses on transvaginal sonography.

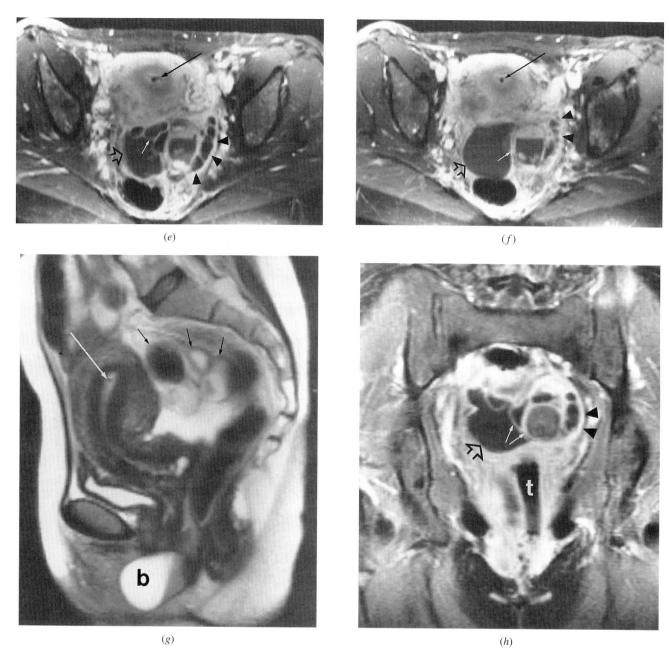

(e)

(f)

(g)

(h)

FIG. 15.13 (*Continued*) Bilateral adnexal masses have high-signal intensity components on T1-weighted images, which demonstrate shading with fluid-fluid levels on T2-weighted images consistent with endometriomas (short solid arrows, *a–d*). Note the serpentine left hydro/hematosalpinx (arrowheads, *b, c, e, f, h*). Posterior to the uterus is a polygonal fluid collection (open arrow, *a–f, h*). After contrast, both the rims and septations of the masses (short solid arrows, *e–h*) enhance, as do the walls of the dilated left fallopian tube (arrowheads, *e, f, h*). The polygonal fluid collection has similar enhancement characteristics. Orthogonal views confirm the findings. Note the IUD within the endometrium (long solid arrow, *a–g*), Bartholin duct cyst ("b," *g*) and tampon ("t," *h*). At laparoscopy, bilateral endometriomas, endometriosis implants, left hydro/hematosalpinx, adhesions, and a peritoneal pseudocyst behind the uterus were found. MRI can add specificity to the finding of an elevated CA-125.

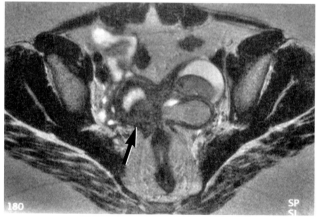

(i)

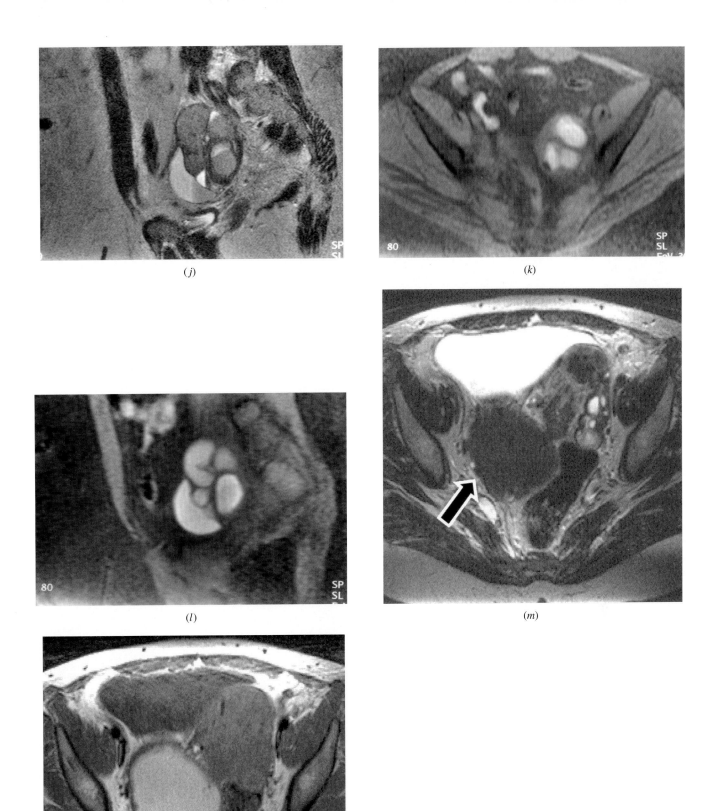

(j)

(k)

(l)

(m)

(n)

FIG. 15.13 (*Continued*) Transverse (*i*) and sagittal (*j*) T2-weighted ETSE and transverse (*k*) and sagittal (*l*) T1-weighted fat-suppressed SGE in a second patient with a complex left ovarian endometrioma. Adenomyosis is also present (arrow, *i*)

T2-weighted echo-train spin-echo (*m*) and T1-weighted spin-echo (*n*) images in a third patient. T2-weighted image (*m*) shows very low signal intensity to the mass, also termed "shading." T1-weighted image (*n*) shows the high-signal intensity mass in the right ovary, with a discrete wall. These findings are typical for endometrioma.

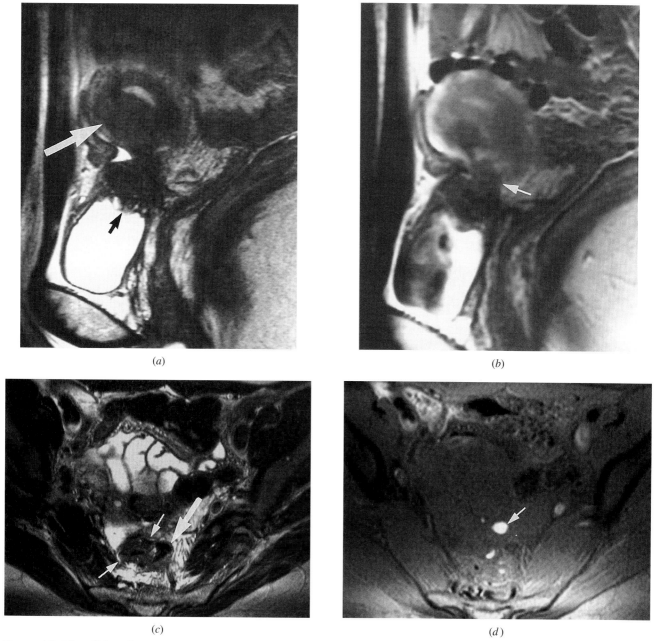

(a)

(b)

(c)

(d)

FIG. 15.14 Solid endometrioma. Sagittal 512-resolution T2-weighted ETSE (*a*) and sagittal gadolinium-enhanced T1-weighted SE (*b*) images. A 4-cm ill-defined mass is present that invades the dome of the bladder (arrow, *a*) and the anterior myometrium (arrow, *b*). The mass is low in signal intensity on T1-weighted (not shown), T2-weighted (*a*), and gadolinium-enhanced T1-weighted (*b*) images. Diffuse adenomyosis of the uterus is noted (large arrow, *a*). Cystoscopic biopsy had suspected the diagnosis of sarcoma. The correct diagnosis was made on the MRI study and confirmed at surgery. (Courtesy of Caroline Reinhold MD, Dept. of Radiology, McGill University.)

Transverse 512-resolution T2-weighted ETSE (*c*) and T1-weighted fat-suppressed SE (*d*) images in a second patient with a solid endometrioma. A low-signal intensity mass is demonstrated (arrows, *c*) invading the outer wall of the upper rectum (large arrow, *c*). On T1- fat suppressed image a 1-cm endometrioma is demonstrated as a high-signal intensity focus (arrow, *d*).

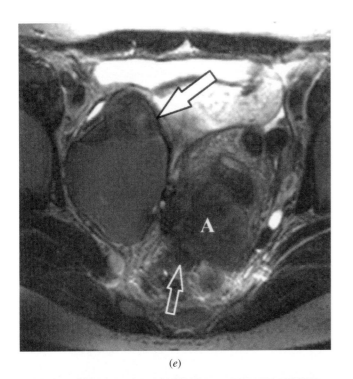

(e)

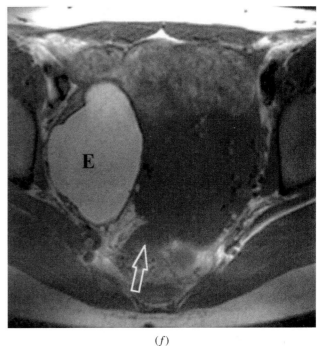

(f)

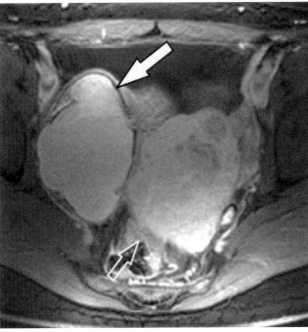

(g)

FIG. 15.14 (*Continued*) T2-weighted echo-train spin-echo (*e*), T1-weighted spin-echo (*f*), and gadolinium-enhanced T1-weighted fat-suppressed SGE (*g*) images in a third patient with right endometrioma and cul de sac endometrial implants. The T2-weighted image (*e*) shows the endometrioma (E = endometrioma, *f*) with low signal intensity (shading) (arrow, *e*) A fibrotic cul de sac solid endometrioma implant (open arrow, *e, f, g*) infiltrates the perirectal fat. (A = adenomyosis, *e*) Gadolinium-enhanced T1-weighted fat-suppressed SGE image (*g*) shows a layered appearance to the endometriomal (arrows, *g*) with a high-signal intensity superior layer (arrow, *g*), corresponding to the low-signal layer on T2, reflecting paramagnetic effects of blood products.

[50]. High-signal lesions on T2-weighted images have also been described, presumed due to detection of actual endometrial glands [51]. Most of the time, however, the implants are low-signal intensity masses on T2-weighted images due to surrounding fibrosis; foci of hemorrhage may also be detected [56]. Laparoscopic or surgical diagnosis, staging, and treatment are still often necessary. Ancillary findings such as adhesions and fibrosis are also difficult to detect with MR imaging.

Polycystic Ovary Disease. Polycystic ovary disease is a hormonally mediated disorder, seen in association with Stein-Leventhal syndrome in a minority of cases (hirsutism, amenorrhea, and anovulation leading to infertility). The most common cause is a hormone imbalance leading to stimulation of the ovaries without maturation of a dominant follicle. As a result, the ovaries are left with numerous follicles of nearly the same size, generally at the periphery of the ovary. When present,

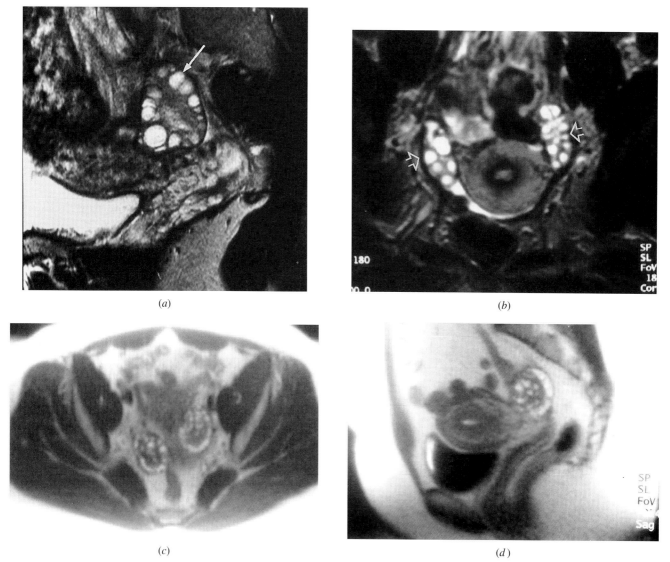

(a)

(b)

(c)

(d)

F I G . 15.15 Polycystic ovary disease. Sagittal 512-resolution T2-weighted ETSE image (a) demonstrates a mildly enlarged ovary that contains multiple, similar-sized cysts (arrow, a). Central ovarian tissue is low in signal intensity, reflecting increased medullary cellular stroma.

Paracoronal T2-weighted ETSE image (b) in a second patient shows enlargement of the ovaries bilaterally (open arrows, b) with multiple similar-sized peripheral cysts.

Transverse (c) and sagittal (d) T2-weighted SS-ETSE images in a third patient with polycystic ovary disease. Similar findings are appreciated.

ovarian enlargement is due to an increase in the stromal tissues; capsular hypertrophy is also present [2, 57]. The disease always affects both ovaries.

With MR imaging, the ovaries have a distinctive pattern of multiple small follicles of nearly the same size just below the ovarian capsule (fig. 15.15). As hemorrhagic complication has not been reported, the signal intensity of the cysts on T2-weighted images is universally high. With high-resolution imaging, a thickened fibrotic capsule may be evident [58]. The central stroma of the ovary is hypointense on T2-weighted images [59]. These ovaries differ in appearance from the normal ovary with

multiple functional cysts in that in the normal ovary the cysts vary in size and may be complicated by hemorrhage resulting in nonuniformity of signal intensity [58].

Theca-Lutein Cysts. Elevated circulating levels of human chorionic gonadotropin (β-hCG), usually seen in women with gestational trophoblastic disease, cause gross enlargement of the ovaries due to the presence of multiple theca-lutein cysts. Of women with gestational trophoblastic disease, 26–46% are found to have theca-lutein cysts depending on whether physical examination or ultrasound is used for detection [60]. In these cases,

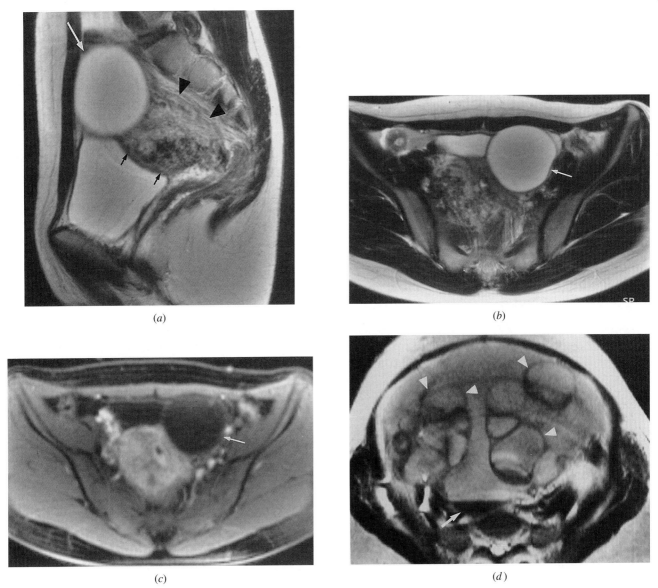

(a)

(b)

(c)

(d)

F I G . 15.16 Theca-lutein cysts. Sagittal (*a*) and transverse (*b*) 512-resolution T2-weighted ETSE and gadolinium-enhanced fat-suppressed T1-weighted SGE (*c*) in a woman with an invasive mole. The combination of an infiltrating endometrial mass and enlarged and cystic ovaries (long arrow, *a–c*) should suggest the diagnosis of gestational trophoblastic disease. Note the high signal of myometrium in the area of marked molar invasion (arrowheads, *a*) versus the area where it is relatively spared (short arrows, *a*). Whereas theca-lutein cysts are present in up to one-third of women with gestational trophoblastic disease, they also occur in other conditions associated with elevated human chorionic gonadotropin (β-hCG) levels.

the ovaries become congested and edematous. Numerous cysts, often multilocular and measuring up to 4 cm are noted. Overall the ovaries are generally between 6 and 12 cm but can enlarge to upwards of 20 cm [60]. Although usually asymptomatic, women may present with pain if there is cyst rupture or hemorrhage or if the ovary torses. Women undergoing ovulation induction for infertility can have a similar ovarian response if hyperstimulated (ovarian hyperstimulation syndrome).

On MR, theca-lutein cysts have a variable appearance with low to high signal on T1- and high signal on T2-weighted sequences [61, 62]. If there is also an associated hypervascular endometrial mass, a diagnosis of gestational trophoblastic disease is likely (fig. 15.16). Accompanying simple or hemorrhagic ascites may indicate ovarian hyperstimulation syndrome given the appropriate clinical scenario. In these cases, an intrauterine or ectopic gestation may also be evident.

Paraovarian and Peritoneal Cysts. Almost any sort of benign or malignant ovarian cyst can arise adjacent to the ovary within the broad ligament or

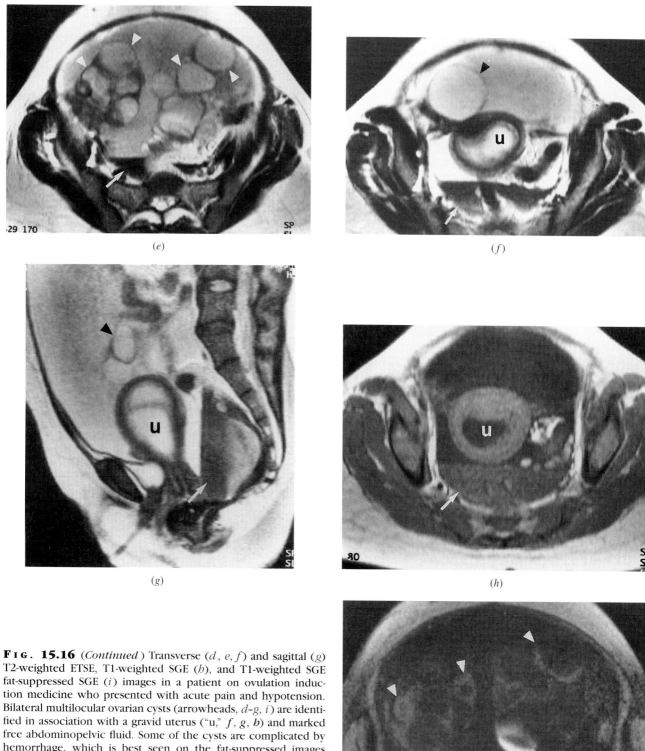

(e)

(f)

(g)

(h)

(i)

FIG. 15.16 *(Continued)* Transverse (*d*, *e*, *f*) and sagittal (*g*) T2-weighted ETSE, T1-weighted SGE (*h*), and T1-weighted SGE fat-suppressed SGE (*i*) images in a patient on ovulation induction medicine who presented with acute pain and hypotension. Bilateral multilocular ovarian cysts (arrowheads, *d–g, i*) are identified in association with a gravid uterus ("u," *f, g, h*) and marked free abdominopelvic fluid. Some of the cysts are complicated by hemorrhage, which is best seen on the fat-suppressed images (curved arrow, *i*). There is also evidence of hemoperitoneum. Note that the dependent fluid is intermediate in signal intensity on the T1-weighted images and is decreased in signal intensity on T2-weighted images, which is consistent with intracellular methemoglobin (arrow, *d–i*). The hyperstimulation syndrome is a well-recognized, life-threatening complication of ovulation induction therapy for infertility.

parovarium, and collectively these cysts are termed paraovarian cysts [2]. They may account for 10–20% of adnexal masses, based on surgical reports [63]. A common subset of these cysts is hydatid cysts of Morgagni that arise from müllerian duct remnants. These occur at the fimbriated end of the fallopian tube and are generally asymptomatic unless they are complicated by torsion. Multiplicity and bilaterality have been reported. The cysts are round or ovoid and may be indistinguishable from ovarian cysts unless a normal ipsilateral ovary is identified separate from the cystic lesion. These lesions are low signal intensity on T1-weighted images and high signal on T2-weighted images.

Peritoneal inclusion cysts or peritoneal pseudocysts require two conditions for formation: an ipsilateral functioning ovary and adhesions. These are, therefore, most often seen in women with prior abdominal or pelvic surgery or endometriosis. These pseudocysts do not have true walls; rather, because they are ascitic fluid collections contained by mesothelial lined adhesions, they conform to the surrounding structures and can be irregular in shape. This distinguishing feature is well shown by MRI; in one series, MRI was more useful than CT or US in their diagnosis [64]. Inclusion cysts can also mimic other adnexal cysts [65].

Benign Solid Tumors. The most common benign solid ovarian tumors arise from the stromal elements of the ovary and are composed of fibrous cells, thecal cells, or a combination of the two. If purely one or the other, they are termed fibromas or thecomas; because the histologic appearance can overlap, the term fibrothecoma may be more appropriate in many cases. Pure thecomas arise most often in menopausal or perimenopausal women; 15% have concomitant endometrial hyperplasia, whereas 29% have frank endometrial carcinoma [2]. Given the associated endometrial disease, many of these tumors are discovered during a work-up for abnormal bleeding. Other symptoms are nonspecific and include pelvic pain or discomfort. Pure fibromas are diagnosed more frequently in younger women (under 50) and are usually asymptomatic. Rarely patients can present with ascites; if a right pleural effusion is also present, this is termed Meigs syndrome, a rare presentation of fibroma [2]. These tumors are treated by surgical excision.

The MR characteristics of fibromas, thecomas, and fibrothecomas are similar: hypointensity on both T1- and T2-weighted images (fig. 15.17). Because of these signal characteristics, these tumors can be difficult to distinguish from nondegenerative subserosal or pedunculated leiomyomata [66]. The multiplanar capability of MR aids in the differentiation of masses of adnexal versus uterine origin. An exophytic leiomyoma will often exhibit what has been coined the "bridging vascular sign" in which curvilinear tortuous vascular structures will be seen crossing and/or between the uterus and the pelvic mass [67]. The detection of compressed ovarian tissue surrounding the ovarian tumor can also be of use. After the administration of gadolinium, these tumors have variable enhancement with reports of both negligible

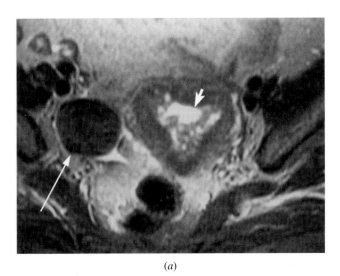

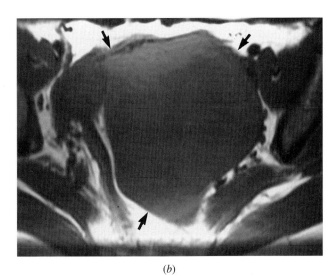

(a)   (b)

F I G . 15.17 Fibroma/thecoma. T2-weighted ETSE image (*a*) demonstrates a 3-cm right ovarian fibroma (long arrow, *a*) that is well defined and very low in signal intensity. Changes in the uterus (arrow, *a*) are due to adenomyosis and recent dilation and curettage for endometrial hyperplasia.

T1-weighted SE (*b*), sagittal 512-resolution T2-weighted ETSE (*c*), and gadolinium-enhanced T1-weighted SE (*d*) images in a second patient with ovarian fibroma. A 12-cm mass is present in the pelvis that is homogeneous in signal intensity on the T1-weighted image (arrows, *b*) and heterogeneous on the T2-weighted image (*c*), and enhances in a mild and heterogeneous fashion with cystic areas (arrow, *d*).

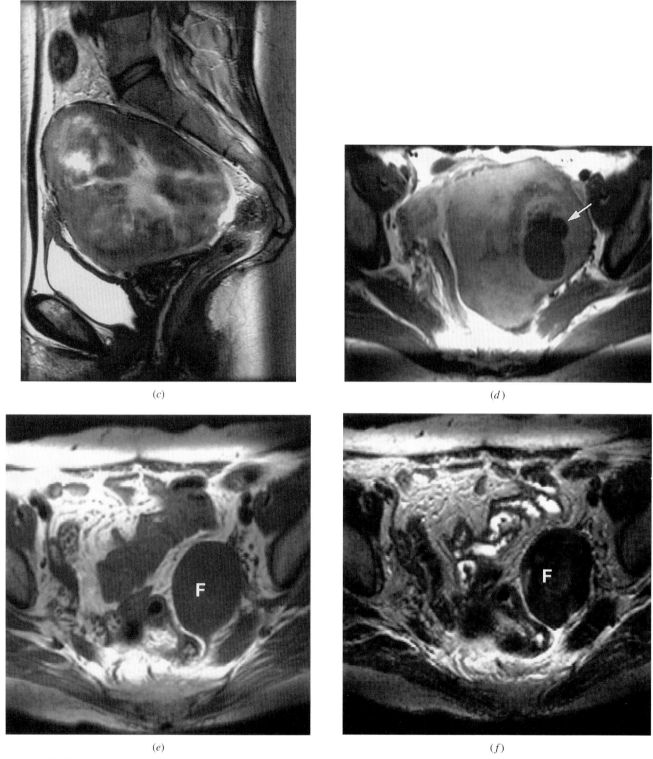

(c)

(d)

(e)

(f)

F I G . 15.17 (*Continued*) T1-weighted SE (*e*) and transverse (*f*) and sagittal (*g*) T2-weighted ETSE images in a third patient with a left ovarian fibroma ("F", *e–g*). The tumor is well defined and low in signal intensity on T1-weighted (*e*) and T2-weighted (*f*, *g*) images. A small volume of pelvic fluid (arrowheads, *g*) is noted posterior and adjacent to the mass.

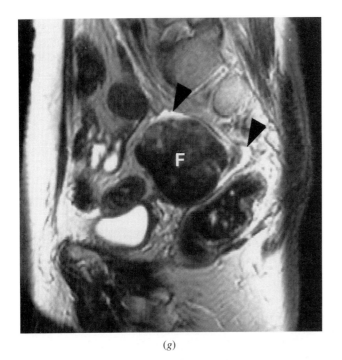

(g)

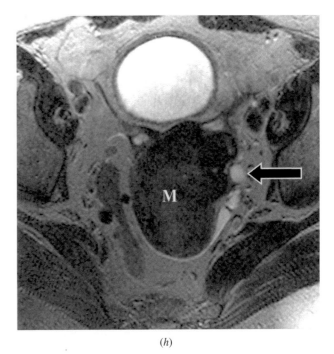

(h)

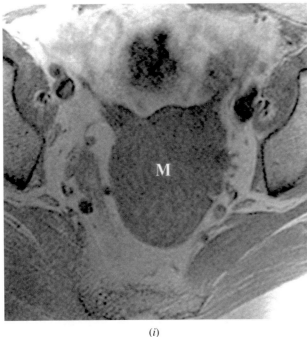

(i)

F I G. 15.17 (*Continued*) T2-weighted echo-train spin-echo (*h*) and T1-weighted spin-echo (*i*) images in a fourth patient with prior hysterectomy and an ovarian fibroma. T2-weighted image (*h*) shows very low signal intensity of the mass, similar to muscle, characteristic of an ovarian fibroma. Small ovarian cysts (arrows, *h*) at the margin of the mass identify the mass as ovarian. T1-weighted image (*i*) shows the mass as comparable signal to muscle.

and significant enhancement [68–71]. There has been one report of a fibroma exhibiting atypical high T2 signal due to pronounced microscopic myxomatous change [72]. In another series all but the very smallest tumor had associated ascites [73].

A less common solid neoplasm is the Brenner tumor arising from the surface epithelium of the ovary [74]. These account for 2–3% of all ovarian neoplasms; the majority of these are benign with few reports of borderline or malignant counterparts. The benign Brenner tumor has signal characteristics on MR more similar to

the fibroma than to other nonfibrous ovarian masses; these tumors are of decreased homogeneous signal on T2-weighted images [75]. Larger tumors may show cystic areas [74]. Brenner tumors are frequently associated with other ovarian tumors; this occurs in about 30% of cases, usually in the ipsilateral ovary.

Ovarian Torsion. Torsion of the ovary occurs most frequently in prepubertal girls and during pregnancy [76]. The presence of an underlying ovarian mass predisposes the ovary to torsion. Although most patients present with acute onset of pelvic pain, some patients present with episodic pain presumably related to intermittent ovarian torsion. The pathologic and imaging changes reflect the degree of vascular compromise and are related to whether there is venous or both venous and arterial compromise. In the earliest stages, only the venous flow is restricted; this causes enlargement of the ovary from congestion, edema, and interstitial hemorrhage. As arterial flow is restricted, necrosis of the ovary and any associated mass will commence. In cases of chronic intermittent torsion, massive ovarian edema may occur.

Three MR findings have been described that are considered diagnostic of acute ovarian torsion: 1) an adnexal protrusion continuous with the uterus or to which engorged blood vessels converge, 2) thick, straight vessels draping around the lesion, and 3) complete absence of enhancement [77]. The first sign, the adnexal protrusion, is felt to represent the pedicle connecting the ovary and/or lesion to the uterus or vascular supply. This torsion knot is generally of low signal intensity on T1- and T2-weighted images (fig. 15.18), but areas of high-signal may be seen reflecting the presence of hemorrhage or congestion [58, 77]. The second sign, the draping vessels,

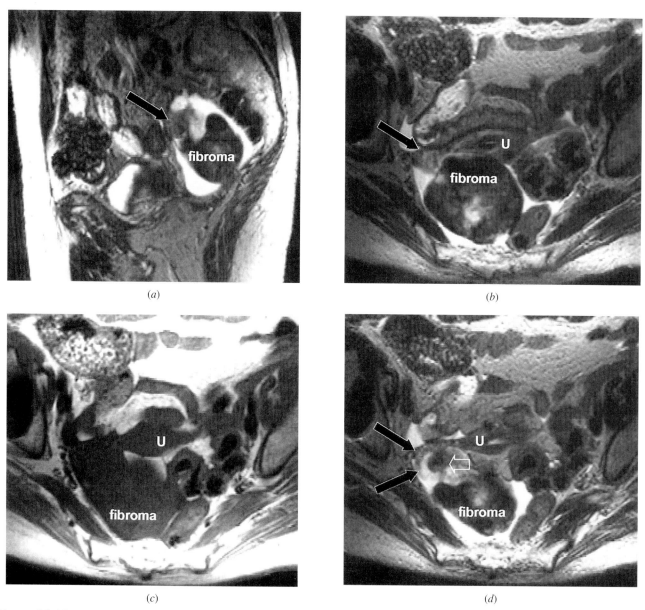

(a)

(b)

(c)

(d)

F I G . 15.18 Ovarian torsion. Sagittal (*a*) and transverse (*b*) T2-weighted ETSE, T1-weighted SE (*c*), T2-weighted ETSE (*d*), and gadolinium-enhanced T1-weighted fat-suppressed SGE (*e*) images in a patient with pelvic pain. T1- and T2-weighted images show a primarily low-signal intensity mass, that represents a fibroma in the cul de sac. The right fallopian tube is enlarged, edematous, and applied to the uterus; this appearance has been termed "protrusion" and is suggestive of torsion (arrow, *a*, *b*, *d*, *e*). Within the convoluted tube is the low-signal intensity torsion knot (open arrow, *d*). After contrast, the tube wall (anterior arrow, *e*), torsion knot (posterior arrow, *e*), and fibroma enhance, excluding complete arterial compromise. *u*, Uterus.

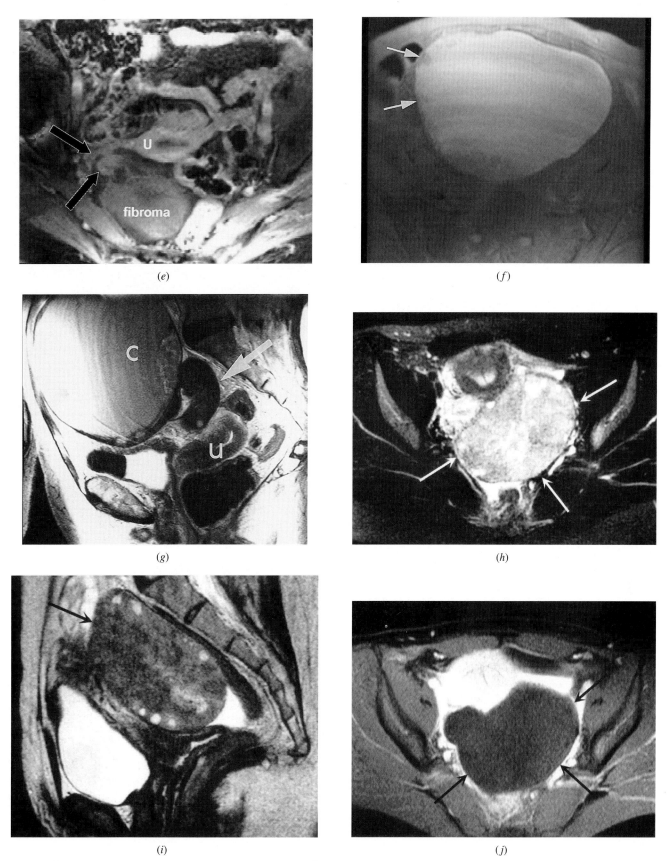

(e)   *(f)*

(g)   *(h)*

(i)   *(j)*

F I G . 15.18 (*Continued*) T1-weighted fat-suppressed SE (*f*) and sagittal 512-resolution T2-weighted ETSE (*g*) images in a second patient with ovarian torsion. A large hemorrhagic cyst is shown on the T1-weighted fat-suppressed image that contains small peripheral excrescences (arrows, *f*). The sagittal plane image demonstrates a dilated blood-filled fallopian tube (large arrow, *g*). The low signal intensity of the blood is consistent with deoxyhemoglobin or intracellular methemoglobin reflecting acute blood. A gradation of signal intensity in the large hemorrhagic ovarian cyst is seen, representing layering of blood products. *u*, Uterus, c, cyst.

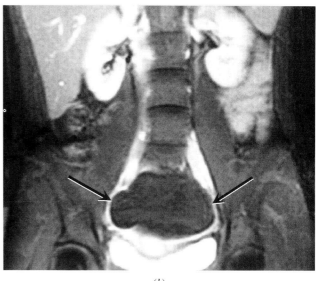

(*k*)

F I G . 15.18 (*Continued*) Transverse (*h*) and sagittal (*i*) T2-weighted ETSE and transverse (*j*) and coronal (*k*) gadolinium- enhanced T1-weighted SGE in a third patient, who presented with pelvic pain, low-grade fever, and mild leukocytosis. T2-weighted images (*h*, *i*) show a large, solid pelvic mass posterior to the uterus. Peripheral follicles are noted on the sagittal image indicating that the mass is a markedly enlarged ovary. Gadolinium-enhanced T1-weighted images (*j*, *k*) show no enhancement of the pelvic mass consistent with infarction. Surgery confirmed ovarian torsion with an infarcted ovary. Histopathologic evaluation showed an infarcted ovary with hemorrhagic necrosis. (Courtesy of Russell N. Low M.D., Sharp Clinic, San Diego.)

are vessels on the surface of the ovary and/or lesion distal to the torsion. The third sign, lack of enhancement, indicates significant arterial compromise; when the torsion involves only the vein or incompletely involves the artery, some enhancement will still be detected. This enhancement may be better seen with the use of MR subtraction imaging [78]. Occasionally, a high signal intensity rim surrounds the adnexal mass on T1-weighted images. This reflects the presence of hemorrhage within the lesion but is a nonspecific finding seen in any subacute hematoma [79].

The MR findings of chronic intermittent torsion (massive ovarian edema) have also been described. The most common finding is marked enlargement of the ovary with increased T2 signal [80–82]. In one report, the process was confused for an ovarian cyst [83].

Malignant Masses

Primary Ovarian Carcinoma. Ovarian cancer comprises 4% of all cancers in women. In the year 2000, 23,100 women were diagnosed with ovarian cancer, the second most common gynecological malignancy, and 14,000 succumbed to this illness, the number one cause of death from reproductive tract malignancies. There does, however, appear to be a decrease in tumor incidence. According to information available on the American Cancer Society website, during the period between 1992 and 1996, the rate of new diagnosis of ovarian cancer declined [www.cancer.org]. Ovarian cancer is primarily a diagnosis of middle-aged and older women, with the incidence increasing with age. The median age at diagnosis is 61 years. Risk factors associated with ovarian cancer include early menarche, low parity, older age at first pregnancy, infertility, late menopause, and family history. In contrast, oral contraceptives appear to confer a protective effect presumably due to the decrease in

the number of times a woman ovulates during her lifetime. There have also been suggestions of environmental risk factors, but none have been conclusively proven [84]. Survival depends on the stage at diagnosis; because most women present with advanced disease, the overall 5-year survival is very poor (46%). If women present with localized disease, the 5-year survival is 93%; with disease spread beyond the pelvis, this figure drops to 25% [85]. Ovarian carcinoma derives most often from the epithelium of the ovary but can also arise from the ovarian stroma/sex cords or germ cells.

The main strength of MR in the diagnosis of women with pelvic masses is its ability to accurately determine the origin of a pelvic mass and, if ovarian, to determine whether it is likely neoplastic, and if neoplastic, benign or malignant. Studies have reported very high accuracy rates for these determinations [27, 50, 86–89]. One series reported five criteria of malignancy: 1) size >4 cm; 2) solid mass or a large solid component; 3) wall thickness of >3 mm; 4) septa thickness >3 mm or the presence of nodularity or vegetations; and (5) necrosis. Four additional findings were also indicative of malignancy: 1) involvement of adjacent organs or the pelvic sidewall; 2) peritoneal, mesenteric, or omental disease; 3) ascites; and 4) adenopathy. When gadolinium was used in this series, an accuracy rate of 95% was achieved in the diagnosis of malignancy when at least one of the primary criteria and one additional finding are present [90]. A more recent series reported similar findings and described the following significant predictors of malignancy in univariate analysis: predominantly solid mass or wall thickness >3 mm; heterogeneous internal architecture, necrosis, massive ascites, and bilaterality. In the logistic regression, massive ascites was the most significant predictor of malignancy [88]. The usefulness of gadolinium has been confirmed in other series [91].

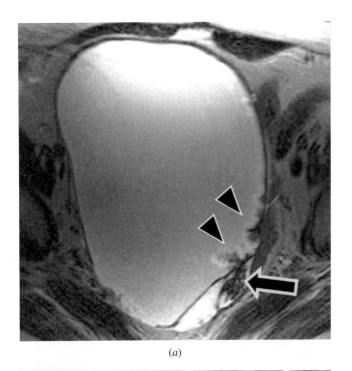

(a)

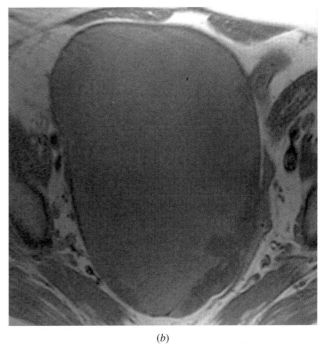

(b)

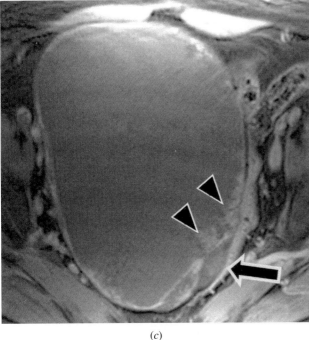

(c)

F I G . 15.19 Cystadenofibroma with borderline futures.
T2-weighted echo-train spin-echo (*a*), T1-weighted spin-echo (*b*), and gadolinium-enhanced T1-weighted fat-suppressed SGE (*c*) images in a patient with cystadenofibroma with borderline features. T2-weighted image (*a*) shows papillary projections (arrowheads, *a*) consisting of low-signal intensity fibrous core and barely visible edematous stroma. A prominent very low-signal intensity fibrous component (arrow, *a*) is seen in the wall. Gadolinium-enhanced T1-weighted fat-suppressed SGE image (*c*) shows enhancement of the papillary projections (arrowheads, *c*) but less enhancement of the fibrous component (arrow, *c*).

Epithelial Origin. There are four major cell types of ovarian epithelium: mucinous, serous, clear cell, and endometrioid. Masses arising from these cell types account for 60% of all ovarian neoplasms and 85% of malignant neoplasms [92]. The benign lesions arising from these cell types have been previously discussed (serous and mucinous cystadenomas). A second category of masses is those with borderline (fig. 15.19) or low malignancy potential. These tumors have an excellent prognosis despite sharing histologic features of

frankly malignant masses; what they lack is destructive growth (invasion) [84]. The final category is those that are overtly malignant.

Cancers arising from the serous cell type account for about half of all ovarian malignancies [93]. In 50% of these patients, the disease is bilateral. These tumors are predominantly unilocular cysts (figs. 15.20 and 15.21); as the degree of cellular differentiation decreases, the incidence of hemorrhage, solid elements, and necrosis increases. Papillary projections, both macro- and

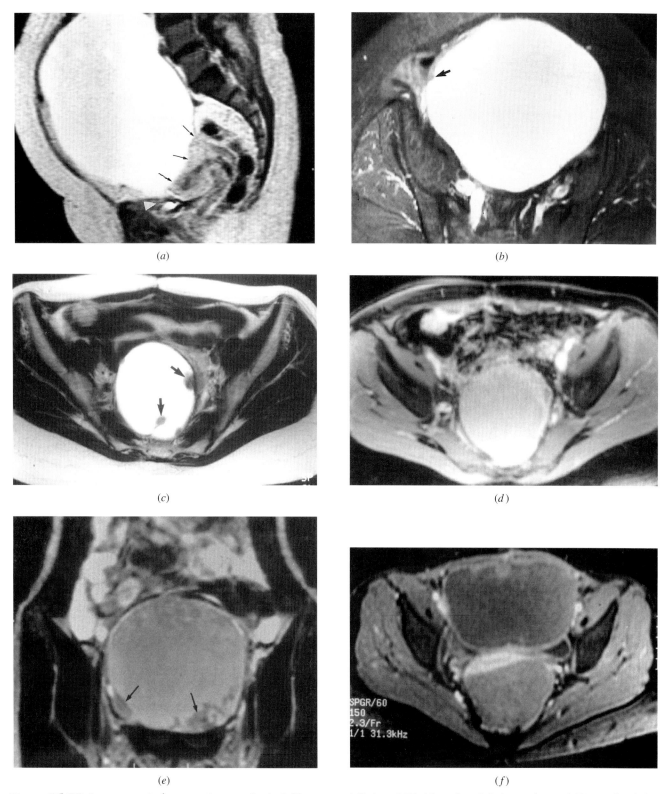

FIG. 15.20 Serous cystadenocarcinoma. Sagittal 90-s postgadolinium SGE (*a*) and gadolinium-enhanced T1-weighted fat-suppressed SE (*b*) images. A high-signal intensity lesion on both nonsuppressed (*a*) and fat-suppressed (*b*) images accurately characterizes it as hemorrhagic. The sagittal plane delineates the relationship of the mass to the uterus (arrows, *a*) and bladder (arrowhead, *a*). Multiplanar MR images are superior to other cross-sectional studies in defining the origin of a pelvic mass and its relationship to adjacent structures. Note the mural nodule along the sidewall (arrow, *b*). (Reprinted with permission from Semelka RC, Lawrence PH, Shoenut JP, et al.: Primary ovarian cancer: Prospective comparison of contrast-enhanced CT and pre- and postcontrast, fat-suppressed MR imaging with histologic correlation. *J Magn Reson Imaging* 3: 99–106, 1993.)

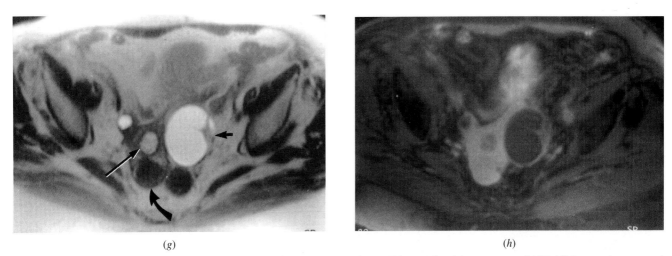

(g)   *(h)*

F I G . 15.20 *(Continued)* T2-weighted ETSE (*c*) and gadolinium-enhanced T1-weighted fat-suppressed SGE (*d*) images in a second patient demonstrate a large cystic mass with mural nodules (arrows, *c*).

Coronal T2-weighted (*e*) and transverse gadolinium-enhanced T1-weighted fat-suppressed SGE (*f*) images in a third patient demonstrate a large cystic mass with mural nodularity. (Courtesy of Rahel A. Kubik-Huch MD, Dept. of Radiology, University of Zurich, Zurich, Switzerland.)

T2-weighted ETSE (*g*) and gadolinium-enhanced T1-weighted fat-suppressed SGE (*h*) images in a fourth patient demonstrate a left ovarian mass that is largely cystic with left mural nodular irregularity (arrow, *g*). Histology revealed a moderately differentiated serous cystadenocarcinoma. A fibroid is present in the posterior uterus (curved arrow, *g*) and an endometrial polyp (long arrow, *g*) is identified.

Serous cystadenocarcinomas are usually solitary cystic lesions with mural nodularity, as these cases illlustrate.

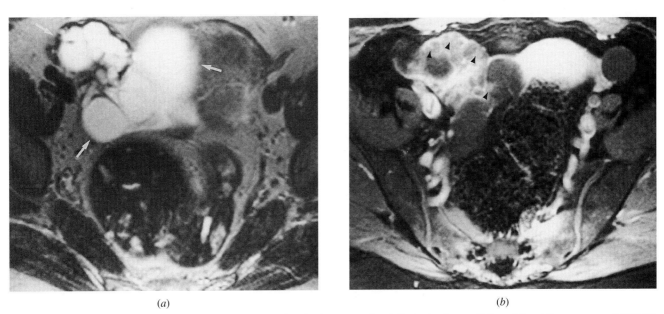

(a)   *(b)*

F I G . 15.21 Serous cystadenocarcinoma. T2-weighted ETSE (*a*) and gadolinium-enhanced T1-weighted fat-suppressed SGE (*b*) images in a woman with a right adnexal mass. A lobulated mass replaces the right ovary (arrows, *a*). After contrast, small internal papillary projections (arrowheads, *b*) enhance.

Coronal (*c*) and transverse (*d*) T2-weighted ETSE, T1-weighted SGE (*e*), and gadolinium-enhanced T1-weighted (*f*) SE images in a second patient, a 19-year-old woman with a low malignant potential serous tumor. Complex bilateral adnexal masses are noted. The T2-weighted images demonstrate papillary projections ("p," *c, d*). After gadolinium administration, the papillary projections show marked enhancement ("p," *f*). Contrast administration helps to differentiate between vascularized solid elements and debris within cystic masses.

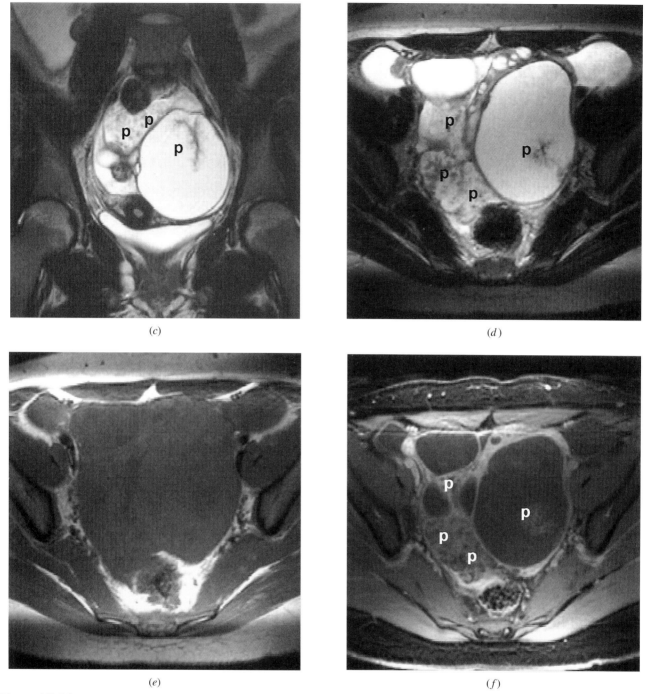

(c)

(d)

(e)

(f)

FIG. 15.21 (*Continued*) Sagittal T2-weighted ETSE (*g*) and sagittal gadolinium-enhanced T1-weighted SE images (*h*) in a third patient with stage II serous cystadenocarcinoma. A complex mass ("m," *g*, *h*) is anterior to, but also indents, the uterus (arrows, *g*). After contrast, the solid elements, including the masses scalloping the uterus (arrows, *h*), enhance. There is a moderate amount of ascites. Serous adenocarcinoma is usually unilocular, but solid elements, hemorrhage, and necrosis occur with increasing frequency with higher-grade tumors. Incidental note is made of adenomyosis ("a," *g*, *h*) affecting the posterior uterine corpus.

T2-weighted ETSE (*i*) and gadolinium-enhanced T1-weighted fat-suppressed SGE (*j*) images in a fourth patient, who has recurrent serous ovarian carcinoma FIGO grade II. Bilateral peritoneal masses are present (arrows, *i*, *j*).

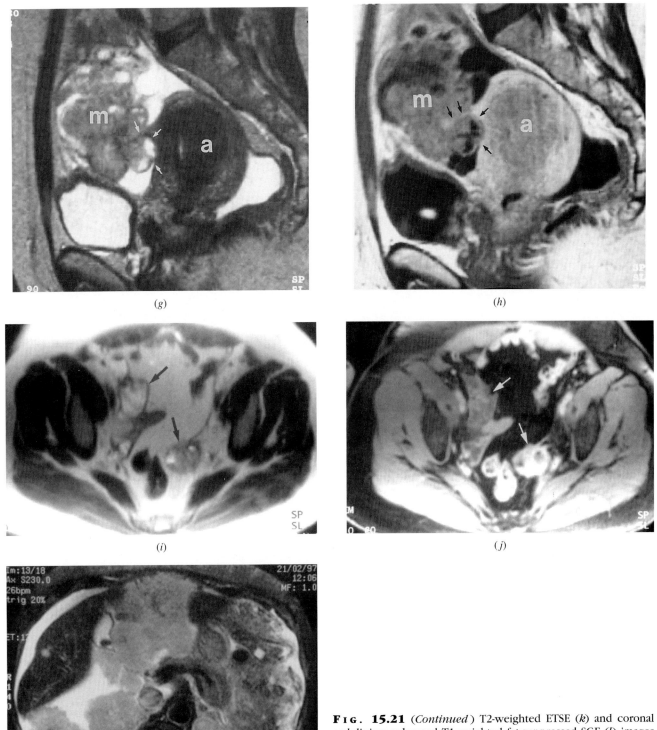

(g)

(h)

(i)

(j)

(k)

FIG. 15.21 (*Continued*) T2-weighted ETSE (*k*) and coronal gadolinium-enhanced T1-weighted fat-suppressed SGE (*l*) images in a fifth patient, with serous ovarian carcinoma FIGO grade IV and peritoneal carcinomatosis and liver metastases. Large peritoneal tumor masses are apparent (*k, l*). (Courtesy of Rahel A. Kubik-Huch MD, Dept. of Radiology, University Hospital of Zurich, Zurich, Switzerland.)

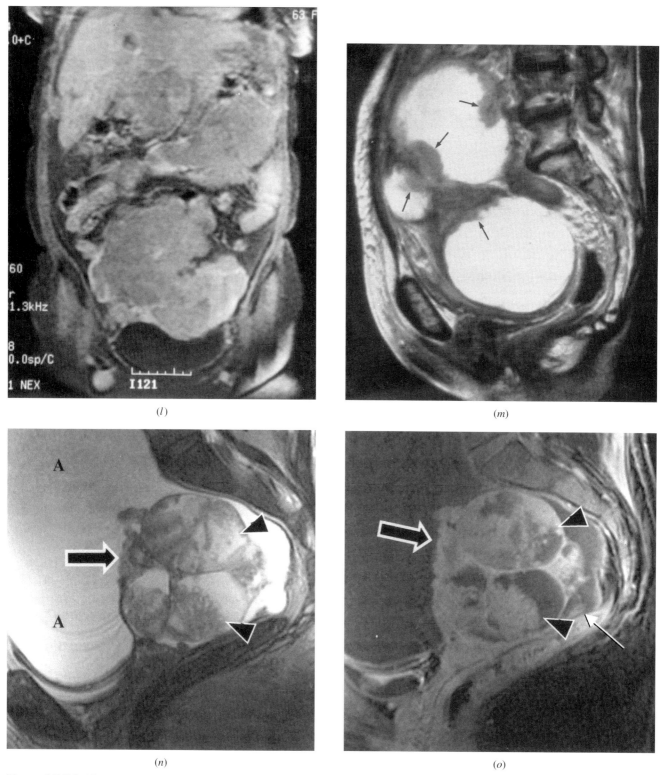

(l)

(m)

(n)

(o)

F I G .   15.21 (*Continued*) Sagittal T2-weighted ETSE image (*m*) in a sixth patient with serous ovarian cancer. A large cystic/solid mass is present, with dominant cysts with mural nodularity (arrows, *m*).

Sagittal T2-weighted ETSE image (*n*) and sagittal T1-weighted fat-suppressed SGE (*o*) images in a seventh patient. The T2-weighted image shows a right ovarian mass with irregular solid components (arrow, *n, o*) and florid intracystic papillary projections (arrowheads, *n, o*). Ascites is present with implants in the cul de sac. Gadolinium-enhanced T1-weighted fat-suppressed SGE image shows enhancement of the papillary projections (arrowheads) and solid components (arrow) and implants (thin arrow).

microscopic are characteristic and 30% contain psammoma bodies [94].

Cancers arising from the mucinous cell type are more aggressive than those of serous origin, more frequently having spread beyond the ovary at initial presentation. These tumors are generally very large and at higher stages are more frequently bilateral. Unlike serous tumors, these tumors are multilocular and the septations are variable in thickness. Areas of hemorrhage, necrosis and solid elements may all be seen (fig. 15.22).

Cancers arising from the endometrioid cell type are invariably invasive and account for 15% of ovarian cancers. They can arise either de novo within the ovary or from foci of endometriosis. These tumors are associated with endometrial hyperplasia or frank endometrial carcinoma in up to one-third of cases. Despite this association, they are felt to represent separate tumors and not foci of metastatic disease. They are less commonly bilateral serous or mucinous tumors (25%) and are generally composed of a mixture of cystic and solid elements.

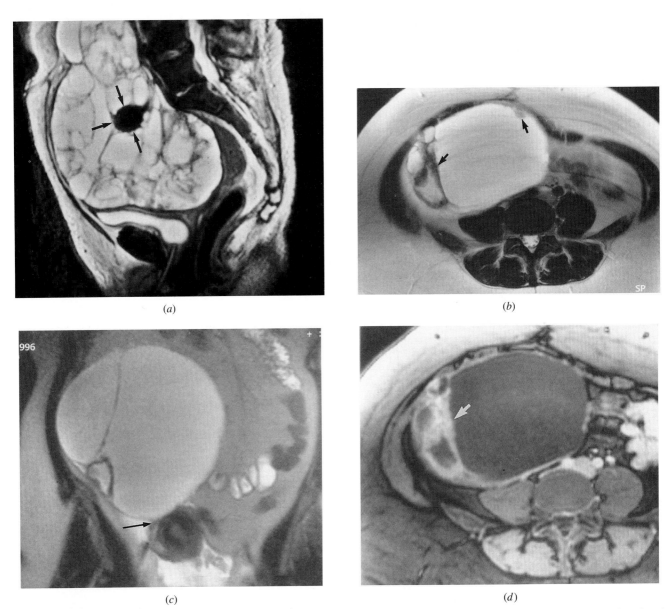

(a)

(b)

(c)

(d)

F I G . 15.22 Mucinous cystadenocarcinoma. Sagittal T2-weighted ETSE image (*a*) in a patient with a large multiloculated mucinous cystadenocarcinoma. One of the locules is complicated by hemorrhage; intracellular methemoglobin is low in signal intensity on T2-weighted images (arrows, *a*). Hemorrhage into a tumor locule is common with mucinous neoplasms.

Transverse 512-resolution T2-weighted ETSE (*b*), coronal T2-weighted SS-ETSE (*c*), and transverse gadolinium-enhanced T1-weighted fat-suppressed SGE (*d*) images in a second patient, with advanced mucinous ovarian cancer. A large cystic mass with septations and nodules (arrows, *b*) abuts the uterus (arrow, *c*). After contrast, the enhancing tumor excrescences are well shown (arrow, *d*).

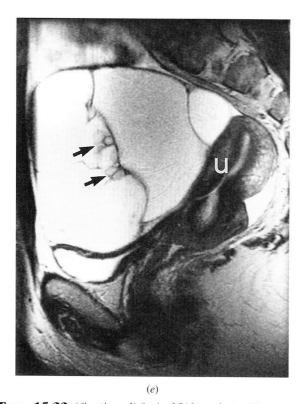

(e)

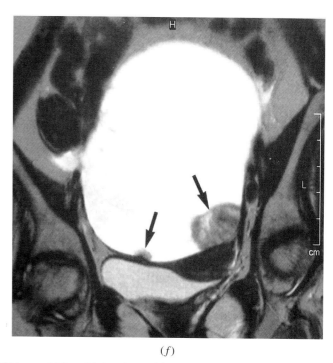

(f)

FIG. 15.22 (*Continued*) Sagittal 512-resolution T2-weighted ETSE image (*e*) in a third patient with mucinous cystadenocarcinoma demonstrates a large cystic mass in the anterior cul de sac that displaces the uterus ("u," *e*) posteriorly. Multiple irregularly thickened internal septations (arrows, *e*) are present.

Coronal T2-weighted ETSE image (*f*) in a fourth patient with a large low-grade malignant mucinous ovarian cancer. A large cystic mass that contains mural nodules (arrows, *f*) is present superior to the uterus.

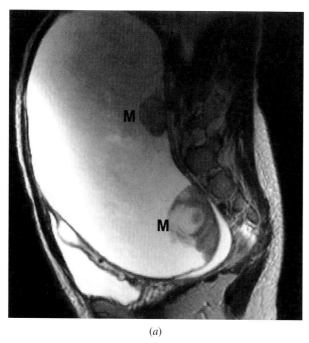

(a)

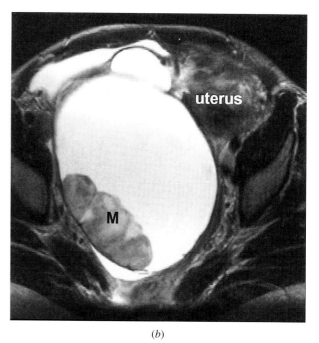

(b)

FIG. 15.23 Clear cell carcinoma. Sagittal (*a*) and transverse (*b*) T2-weighted ETSE, T1-weighted SE (*c*) and gadolinium-enhanced T1-weighted fat-suppressed SGE (*d*) images in a 51-year-old woman with an ovarian mass.

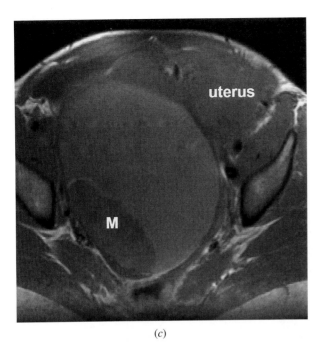

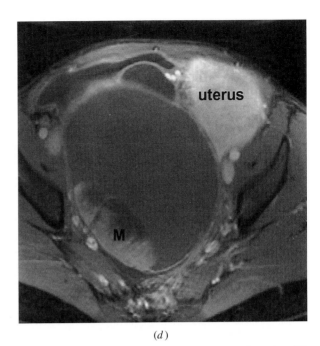

(c)   (d)

F i g . 15.23 (*Continued*) A large primarily unilocular cystic lesion with peripheral masses ("M," *a–c*) arises from the pelvis. The masses enhance after contrast ("M," *d*). This appearance is typical of clear cell carcinoma.

Rarely lesions are purely solid; papillary projections are very uncommon.

Cancers arising from the clear cell type are less common, comprising only 5% of ovarian cancers. Like endometrioid types, these are also invariably invasive but unlike the other cell types, they generally present more often with local disease and therefore carry a better overall prognosis. These are generally unilocular tumors with mural nodules and can mimic the appearance of serous tumors. Clear cell cancers are less frequently bilateral than the other types (13%) (figs. 15.23 and 15.24).

A final classification is the undifferentiated epithelial neoplasm. They do not fit into any category based on one of the four cell types of origin. These carry the poorest prognosis with widespread disease generally present at diagnosis (fig. 15.25).

Approximately 75–85% of patients with epithelial neoplasms present with peritoneal disease (fig. 15.26); even women with apparently localized disease may have metastases detected in peritoneal washings or biopsy of the omentum or diaphragm [84]. Another method of spread is via the lymphatics to the para-aortic lymph nodes. Lymphatic channels also facilitate spread along the broad ligament to pelvic lymph nodes (internal and external iliac and obturator chains). Most patients present with nonspecific symptoms, as abdominal discomfort or pain, and abdominal distension. The latter is attributable to malignant ascites or a large primary mass. Traditionally, complete staging requires surgical removal of the uterus, ovaries, and fallopian tubes, sampling of the para-aortic and retroperitoneal lymph nodes, excision of the omentum, biopsies of the peritoneum and

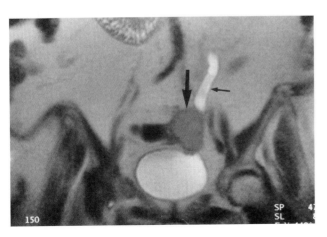

F i g . 15.24 Mixed clear cell and endometrial carcinoma. Coronal T2-weighted echo-train spin-echo image in a second patient with recurrent mixed clear cell and endometrioid adenocarcinoma. A solid mass (arrow) is present that obstructs the left ureter (short arrow).

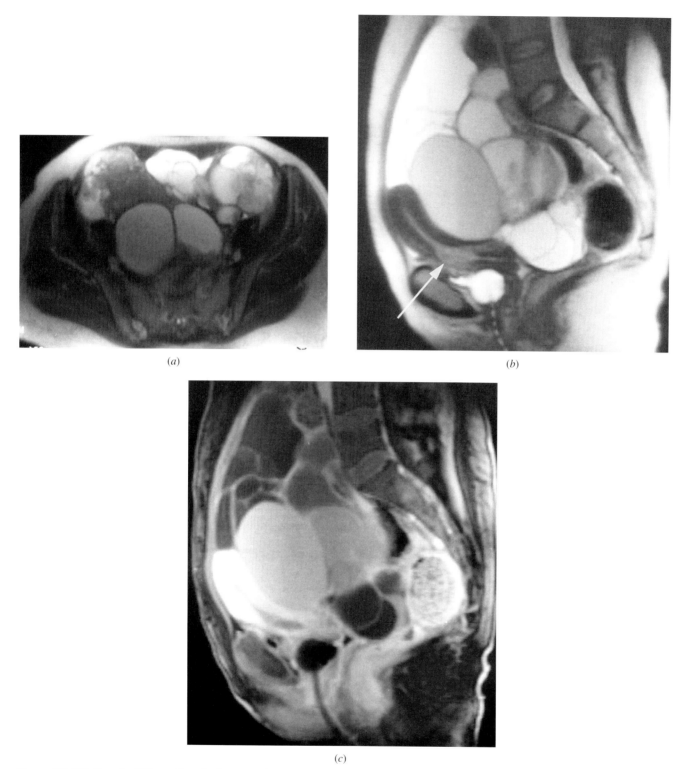

(a)

(b)

(c)

FIG. 15.25 Poorly differentiated adenocarcinoma. Transverse (*a*) and sagittal (*b*) T2-weighted ETSE and sagittal (*c*) gadolinium-enhanced T1-weighted fat-suppressed SGE images in a patient with poorly differentiated ovarian adenocarcinoma and endometrial cancer. A large cystic/solid mass is present in the pelvis representing poorly differentiated ovarian adenocarcinoma. A separate high-signal tumor (arrow, *b*) is appreciated in the lower endometrial canal, consistent with endometrial carcinoma.

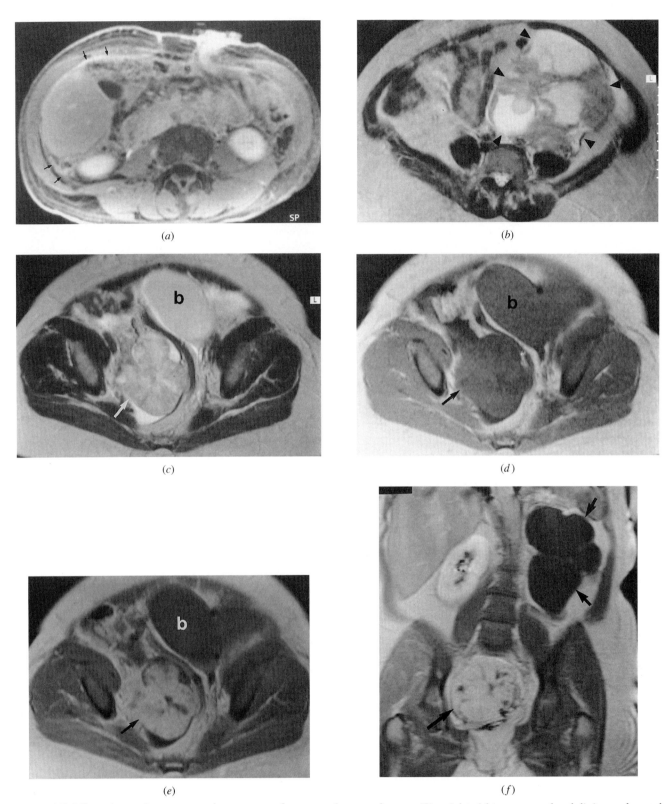

(a)

(b)

(c)

(d)

(e)

(f)

F I G . 15.26 Peritoneal metastases/recurrence from ovarian carcinoma. T1-weighted fat-suppressed gadolinium-enhanced SGE image (*a*) demonstrates extensive peritoneal metastases (arrows, *a*) along the liver capsule and adjacent peritoneum in a patient with peritoneal metastases from recurrent ovarian cancer.

Transverse 512-resolution T2-weighted ETSE (*b, c*), T1-weighted SGE (*d*), transverse (*e*) and coronal (*f*) gadolinium-enhanced T1-weighted SGE images, and MIP MR urogram (*g*) in a second patient with ovarian cancer. A primarily solid mass is seen in the pelvis (arrow, *c, d*), whereas a more cystic mass (arrowheads, *b*) is noted in the left lower abdomen. Gadolinium enhancement improves identification of the solid components (arrow, *e, f*). The pelvic mass displaces the urinary bladder ("b", *c–e*) anteriorly and superiorly, whereas the lower abdominal mass compresses the ureter.

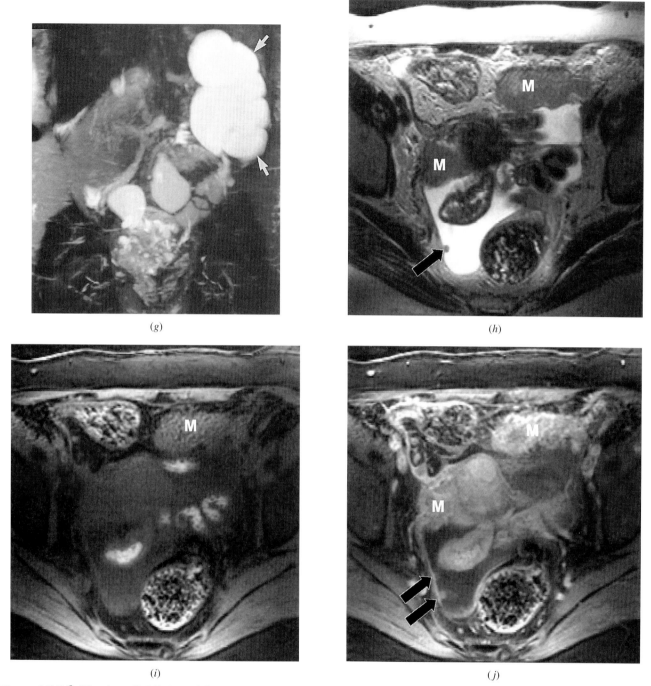

(g)

(h)

(i)

(j)

F I G . 15.26 (*Continued*) Dilation of the intrarenal collection system is well shown on the postcontrast coronal SGE image and the MIP reconstruction (short arrows, *f, g*).

T2-weighted ETSE (*h*), T1-weighted fat-suppressed (*i*), and gadolinium-enhanced T1-weighted fat suppressed (*j*) SE images in a third patient, a 69-year-old woman with advanced ovarian carcinoma, stage III. The peritoneum is diffusely thickened and has superimposed nodules. Peritoneal metastases (arrow, *h*) are most conspicuous on T2-weighted images in the setting of ascites and are consistently well seen after gadolinium administration on T1-weighted fat-suppressed images (arrows, *j*). Note the larger metastatic masses distributed in the pelvis ("M," *h–j*). Contrast-enhanced T1-weighted fat-suppressed technique increases staging accuracy of ovarian carcinomas.

Gadolinium-enhanced T1-weighted fat-suppressed SGE (*k*) image in a fourth woman with ovarian cancer metastatic to the peritoneum. The involved peritoneum enhances and is thickened (short arrows, *k*). A larger discrete peritoneal-based mass is also identified (long arrow, *k*).

T2-weighted fat-suppressed ETSE (*l*) and gadolinium-enhanced T1-weighted fat-suppressed SGE (*m*) images in a fifth patient with diffuse peritoneal disease. Note the metastatic thickening of the peritoneum surrounding the liver (short arrows, *l*). Tumor nodules indent and scallop the posterior aspect of the right lobe of the liver (arrowheads, *l*). After contrast, peritoneal disease in the pelvis enhances (arrows, *m*). The combination of fat suppression and gadolinium is the most sensitive technique for assessing peritoneum-based metastases.

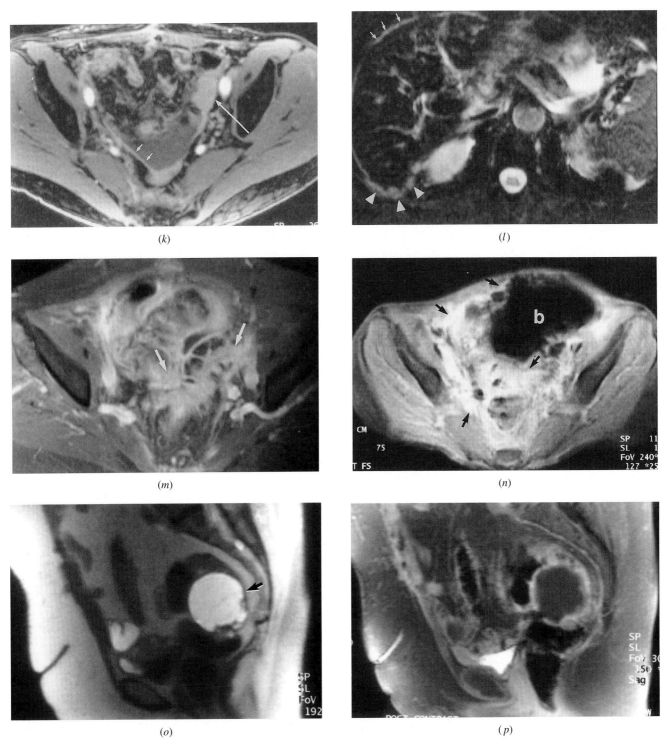

(k)

(l)

(m)

(n)

(o)

(p)

FIG. 15.26 (*Continued*) Gadolinium-enhanced T1-weighted fat-suppressed SGE image (*n*) in a sixth patient, who has a history of ovarian carcinoma status post transabdominal hysterectomy, bilateral ovarirectomy, omentectomy, lymphadenectomy, peritoneal sampling, and adjuvant chemotherapy. The patient presented with complaints of bowel obstruction. Diffuse liver metastases and dilated loops of bowel ("b" = bowel, *n*) are identified. Enhancing recurrent ovarian cancer of the peritoneum and serosa encases the colon (arrows, *n*) and causes distal large bowel obstruction. MRI is useful for identifying which patients may benefit from second-look surgery. No therapeutic benefit for patients with recurrent disease greater than 2 cm has been demonstrated, although debulking surgery may provide symptomatic relief.

Sagittal T2-weighted echo-train spin-echo (*o*) and sagittal gadolinium-enhanced T1-weighted fat-suppressed SGE (*p*) image in a seventh patient, with recurrent ovarian cancer. A 3-cm cystic mass (arrow, *o*) with a thickened irregular wall is present in the presacral space.

diaphragm, and evaluation of peritoneal washings; stages are assigned using the International Federation of Gynecology and Obstetrics (FIGO) schema. Many investigators have attempted to prove the worth of noninvasive methods for staging. A major initiative of the Radiological Diagnostic Oncology Group (RDOG) is to examine the diagnostic accuracy of Doppler US, CT, and MR in the diagnosis and staging of ovarian cancer. Their primary analysis showed no difference for the three modalities with an area under the receiver-operator characteristic curve (ROC) of 0.91 [95]. A subsequent study of advanced stage disease (stages III and IV) showed an advantage of using either MR or CT over US in these patients [96]. Prognosis depends on tumor stage, residual disease after initial surgery, and tumor grade. Beyond surgery, many patients are treated with chemotherapy and/or radiation therapy. In up to 80%, the CA-125 level will be elevated at presentation; this level can be followed to assess for response to treatment. However, there are limitations to this blood test, as a normal value does not exclude the presence of tumor [97]. In one series of 69 patients, MRI accurately determined the presence of residual or recurrent subclinical disease in 20 of 23 patients [97].

The MR appearance of primary epithelial neoplasms is variable, a combination of cystic and solid components. Gadolinium administration is useful for the detection of solid and necrotic components as well as intraperitoneal implants. There is considerable overlap in the appearance of tumors of the various cell types, but some features are more characteristic of a particular cell type. Papillae are suggestive of tumors of serous origin; these are seen at MR as intermediate-signal intensity projections within a cystic lesion. These projections enhance after gadolinium administration.

Mucinous tumors are generally multiloculated and have been termed "stained glass" by one group because of the differences in signal intensity in the different locules; these signal differences are due to differences in content of the locules [98]. Septae between the locules enhance with gadolinium.

Clear cell carcinomas tend to be large unilocular masses with solid mural elements.

Sex Cord Stromal Origin. Masses arising from the specialized gonadal stroma account for 5% of all ovarian neoplasms [99]. These are further classified according to the differentiation of the tumor toward ovarian follicles, testicular tubules, Leydig cells, or adrenal cortical cells [99]. Granulosa cell tumors are the most common of this category. About 50% are seen in postmenopausal women; about 5% are seen in prepubertal girls. Both types are associated with excretion of estrogen. This can cause precocious puberty in the child and uterine bleeding in adults. There is also an association with endometrial hyperplasia/polyps/cancer. The adult form has a variety of histologic patterns; in turn, the gross appearance is also variable ranging from predominantly solid to unilocular to multicystic [100].

The MR appearance of tumors of sex cord stromal origin is likewise variable. Granulosa cell tumors are generally solid with variable amounts of cystic change and intratumoral hemorrhage (fig. 15.27); on T1-weighted images the tumors are of intermediate signal intensity, whereas on T2-weighted images the tumors are of heterogeneous high signal. After gadolinium, the solid areas will enhance whereas the areas of cystic change or hemorrhage will not. Local invasion, especially into the sacrum, is well seen with sagittal imaging. Associated uterine changes due to hormone elaboration are

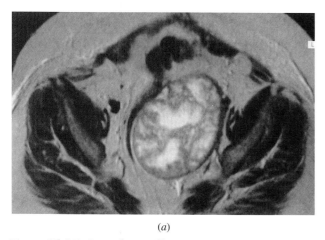

(a)

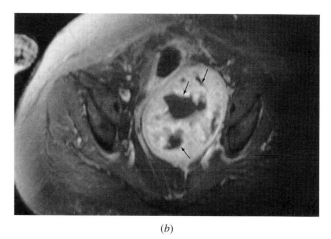

(b)

F I G . 15.27 Granulosa cell tumor. T2-weighted ETSE (*a*), and gadolinium-enhanced T1-weighted fat-suppressed SGE (*b*) images in a woman with a granulosa cell ovarian tumor. The tumor is heterogeneous on the T2-weighted image, and after contrast the solid elements enhance. Necrotic foci interspersed in an otherwise solid mass is a common feature of granulosa-cell tumors (arrows, *b*).

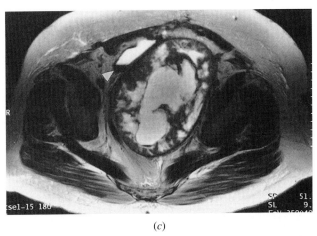

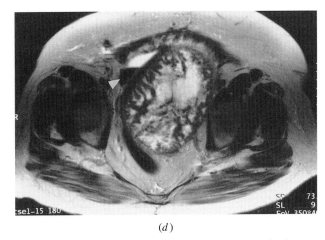

(c) (d)

FIG. 15.27 *(Continued)* Transverse 512-resolution T2-weighted ETSE (*c, d*) images 9 months later show interval growth of tumor and increasing necrosis. Note that the bladder is displaced anterolaterally by the mass. Low-signal intensity in the dependent portion of the bladder reflects excreted concentrated gadolinium (arrowhead, *c, d*).

seen in most patients and include uterine enlargement and thickening of the endometrium [101]. These features are also well demonstrated on sagittal images.

Germ Cell Origin. Dysgerminomas are the most common germ cell neoplasms, occurring predominantly in adolescents and young women. Diagnosis after age 35 is virtually unheard of. The disease is bilateral in up to 15%, even with stage I disease [99]. Unlike other ovarian malignancies, lymphatic spread is more common than peritoneal seeding and the tumors are very radiosensitive. These tumors are generally solid (fig. 15.28).

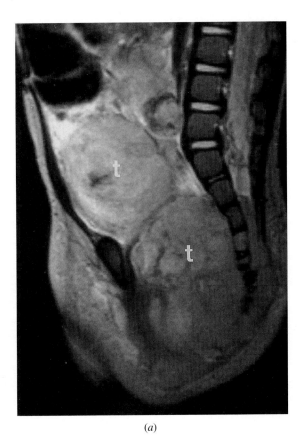

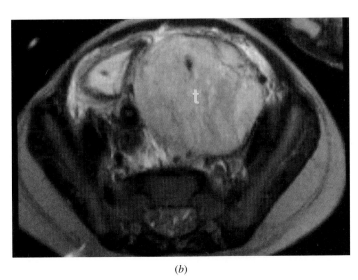

(a) (b)

FIG. 15.28 Germ cell carcinomas. Sagittal (*a*) and transverse (*b*) T2-weighted ETSE images in a young girl with an endodermal sinus tumor. A large tumor originated in the ovary but has spread contiguously into the abdomen and spine (*a, b*). These tumors tend to be solid and are very aggressive, with rapid growth and a poor prognosis.

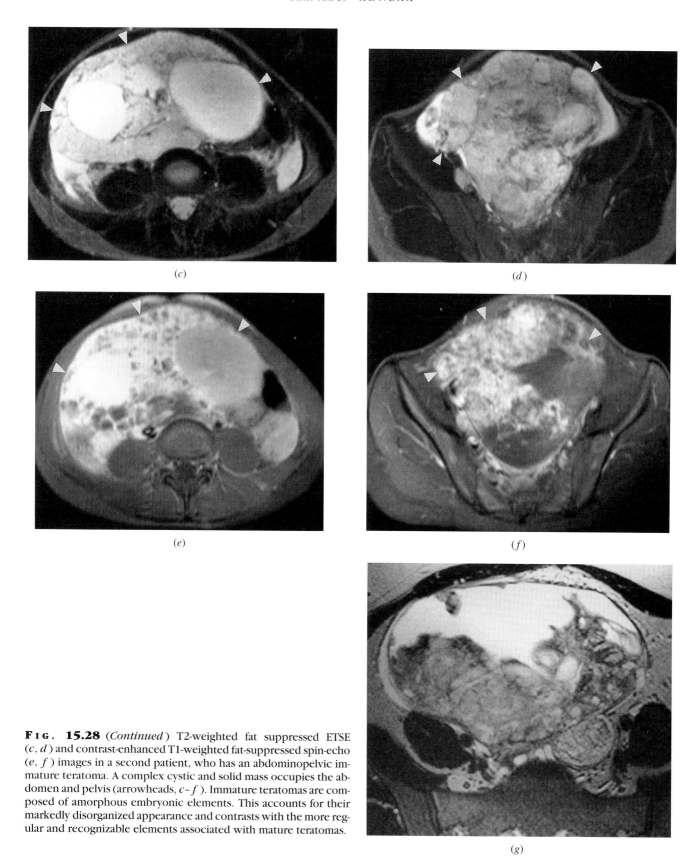

FIG. 15.28 (*Continued*) T2-weighted fat suppressed ETSE (*c, d*) and contrast-enhanced T1-weighted fat-suppressed spin-echo (*e, f*) images in a second patient, who has an abdominopelvic immature teratoma. A complex cystic and solid mass occupies the abdomen and pelvis (arrowheads, *c–f*). Immature teratomas are composed of amorphous embryonic elements. This accounts for their markedly disorganized appearance and contrasts with the more regular and recognizable elements associated with mature teratomas.

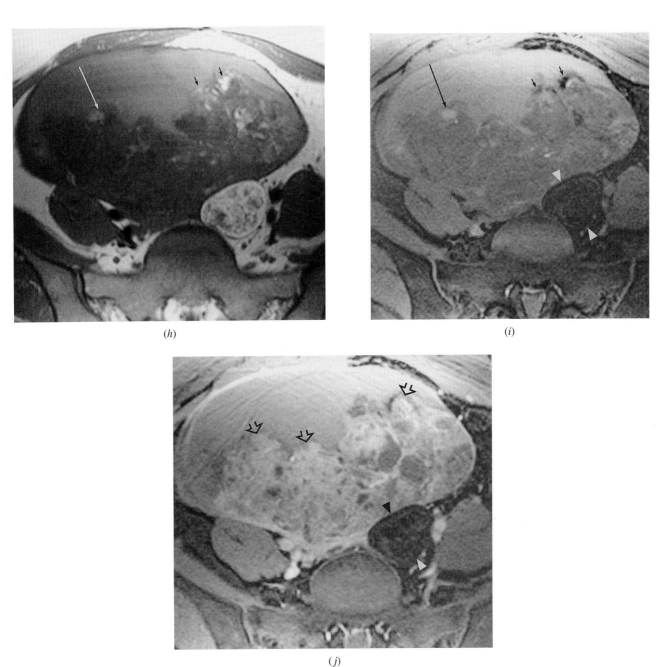

(h)

(i)

(j)

F IG. 15.28 *(Continued)* T2-weighted ETSE (*g*), T1-weighted SE (*h*), T1-weighted fat-suppressed SGE (*i*), and gadolinium-enhanced T1-weighted fat-suppressed SGE (*j*) images in third patient who has complex right adnexal masses. The two masses have variable amounts of fatty elements, which are high in signal intensity on the conventional T1-weighted SE image and suppress on the fat-suppressed images (short arrows, *g, i*). Note that some of the high-signal intensity foci in the larger mass retain their high signal intensity on the fat-suppressed images, which is consistent with coexisting hemorrhage (long arrow, *g, i*). The smaller posterior mass shows nearly complete suppression on the fat-suppressed image (arrowheads, *i*). After contrast, there is a profusion of solid tissue enhancing in the larger mass (open arrows, *j*). The smaller mass does not enhance appreciably, which is consistent with a cystic structure (arrowheads, *j*). Extensive solid elements in a fat-containing mass are atypical of a dermoid cyst and should raise the suspicion of an immature teratoma. This was proven at surgery, whereas the posterolateral mass represented a mature teratoma (dermoid cyst). (*g–j* reprinted with permission from Outwater EK, Dunton CJ: Imaging of the ovary and adnexa: Clinical issues and applications of MR imaging. *Radiology* 194: 1–18, 1992.)

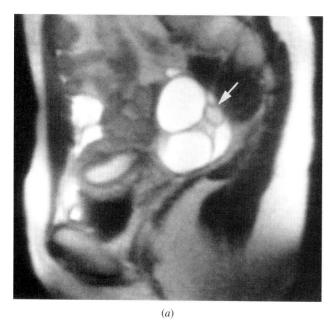
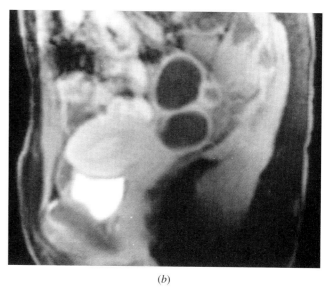

F I G . 15.29 Endodermal sinus tumor. Sagittal T2-weighted echo-train spin-echo (*a*) and sagittal gadolinium-enhanced T1-weighted fat-suppressed SGE (*b*) images in a patient with an endodermal sinus tumor. A cystic tumor (arrow, *a*) with irregular thickened septations is present.

Endodermal sinus tumors have a similar age distribution to the other germ cell tumors and are the second most common of this category. These tumors are some of the most malignant arising in the ovary (fig. 15.29), but most cases are confined to one ovary. Rupture and ascites are not uncommon [99]. The prognosis with this cell type is poor without surgery and aggressive chemotherapy regimens [102].

Immature teratomas comprise about 20% of germ cell tumors and also occur in children and young adults. Histologically, these tumors are comprised of tissues normally seen in the human embryo. They are usually large at presentation, averaging 18 cm, but are usually unilateral [2]. They tend to spread by seeding the peritoneum; the peritoneal implants may show spontaneous maturation into benign tissues, generally glial [99].

The MR appearance of tumors of germ cell origin is also nonspecific. These tumors may be quite large at presentation; immature teratomas may contain foci of fat; these foci will follow fat signal on all sequences and may be best proven with fat-suppression techniques.

Other Primary Tumors. Almost all types of soft tissue tumors have been reported to arise within the ovary; these tumors are similar in appearance to their counterparts elsewhere within the body. Of the mesenchymal tumors, those of smooth muscle origin are the most common, with most being benign leiomyomas. The MR appearance of malignant transformation of a benign leiomyoma has been reported [103]. Leiomyosarcomas are rare [2]. Also reported are lipoleiomyoma,

hemangioma, myxoma, fibrosarcoma, rhabdomyosarcoma, schwannoma, osteosarcoma, chondrosarcoma, fibrosarcoma, and endometrial stromal sarcoma [2].

Lymphoma. Rare cases of primary ovarian lymphoma have also been reported in women in whom treatment restricted to ovariectomy has proven curative [2]. Generally, ovarian involvement with lymphoma is part of a disseminated disease presentation (fig. 15.30). The most common forms of lymphoma to involve the ovary are non-Hodgkin, which affects children and younger women, and large cell, which is more common in adults. The diagnosis of lymphoma may be suspected when bilateral masses with homogeneous hypointensity on T1-weighted images and homogeneous slight hyperintensity on T2-weighted images are present. Contrast enhancement is mild to moderate and is more evident with fat suppression techniques [104]. Physiologic follicles may be retained [105].

Metastases. Metastases account for 10% of tumors seen in surgical series, but the percentage presenting as a primary ovarian mass is smaller [2]. The most common sites of origin are the intestines, stomach, breast, and hematopoietic tissues [106]. The functioning, more highly vascularized ovaries of premenopausal women are more receptive to metastatic deposits than the ovaries of older women. For the common primary sites, women with ovarian involvement are on average significantly younger than women without ovarian involvement [106]. The mode of spread of metastatic

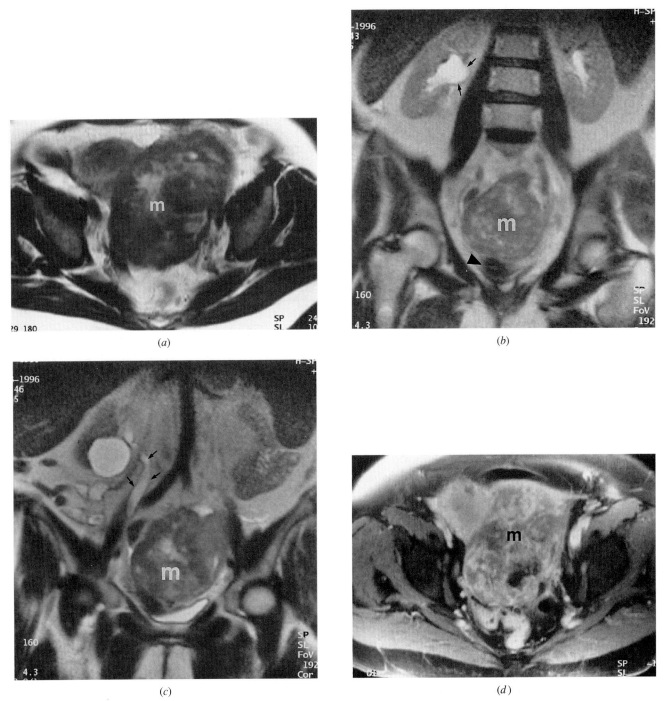

F I G . 15.30 Disseminated lymphoma. Transverse 512-resolution T2-weighted spin-echo (*a*), coronal T2-weighted SS-ETSE (*b, c*), and transverse gadolinium-enhanced fat-suppressed T1-weighted SGE (*d*) images in a woman with disseminated lymphoma. Primary lymphoma of the ovary is rare, and ovarian involvement usually is seen in the setting of diffuse disease. A large mass ("m," *a–d*) occupies the pelvis and obstructs the right distal ureter. Contiguous coronal SS-ETSE images highlight the pelvocaliectasis and proximal ureterectasis (arrows, *b, c*). After contrast, the lymphomatous mass enhances in a mildly intense and heterogenous fashion. The uterus is displaced inferiorly (arrowhead, *b*). Discrete ovaries were not identified on any of the imaging sequences. At surgery, disseminated non-Hodgkin lymphoma with invasion of the adnexa was found. This pattern of enhancement is typical of lymphoma with mild enhancement and slight heterogeneity, with usually negligible necrosis despite large tumor size (compare to cystic ovarian cancers).

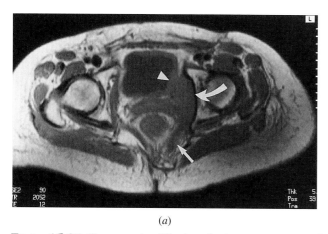 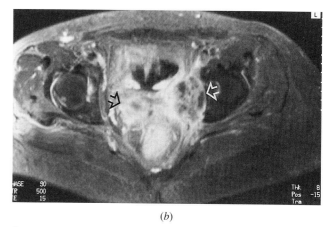

(a)   (b)

FIG. 15.31 Recurrent müllerian duct cancer metastatic to the ovaries. Proton density (*a*) and gadolinium-enhanced T1-weighted fat-suppressed SE (*b*) images in a woman with recurrent müllerian duct cancer. Note the left pelvic mass, which invades the obturator externus muscle (curved arrow, *a*). Associated thickening of the left bladder wall (arrowhead, *a*) and levator ani muscle (straight arrow, *a*) suggests that the imaging findings may be related to previous radiotherapy. However, at a slightly higher level after contrast, bilateral adnexal masses are present that demonstrate heterogeneous enhancement, consistent with metastases to the ovaries (open arrows, *b*). Uterine carcinoma is one of the more common primary tumors to metastasize to the ovaries.

disease can be by one of several routes: direct extension from adjacent organs, via the bloodstream or lymphatics, or by serosal implantation of cells shed into the peritoneal cavity. The term "Krukenberg tumor" specifically refers to tumors in which malignant mucin-filled signet ring cells are found within the abundant and hypercellular ovarian stroma [2]. Although this term is classically associated with tumors of gastric origin, tumors arising from the breast, colon, and appendix can also give rise to these histologic features. Tumors from the gallbladder, pancreas, biliary tract, urinary bladder, and cervix are more rare sources of this tumor type [106]. Almost all patients die within a year of diagnosis of Krukenberg tumors.

The gross appearance of metastatic disease to the ovaries varies with the primary carcinoma and route of spread. The ovary may retain its shape but be enlarged, may be replaced by a multicystic mass with solid components, or may exhibit tumor nodules on its surface. Ovaries can also be of normal size but have widespread lymphatic involvement. The MR appearance of metastatic disease to the ovary is likewise variable (fig. 15.31). Although rare, metastatic melanoma in the ovary may be differentiated from other masses in a patient with the appropriate history if melanin is present; in these cases, peripheral high T1 signal may be noted within the mass [107]. Kruckenberg tumors generally have both cystic and solid components (fig. 15.32). The cystic components will be variable in signal on T1-weighted images, largely reflecting the content of mucin and or blood, both of which will appear high signal. Cystic regions are generally high signal on T2, but may be variable for the same reasons as T1, and the cystic component will shown lack of enhancement on postgadolinium images. The solid components may be hypointense

on T1-and T2-weighted images; this corresponds to areas of dense collagenous stroma. The solid components may show intense enhancement after gadolinium [108–110].

Inflammation

Pelvic Inflammatory Disease/Tubo-Ovarian Abscess

Pelvic inflammatory disease (PID) is a condition of women of reproductive age and refers to a variety of pelvic infections. The route of spread of the infection is ascending; women who have undergone hysterectomy are not at risk for this condition. A variety of microorganisms have been implicated including *Chlamydia trachomatis*, *Neisseria gonorrhoeae*, *Bacteroides* species, and a variety of other Gram-negative and positive aerobic and anaerobic bacteria. Mixed infections are also common. A subset of women is at particular risk for PID, those with an intrauterine device (IUD). Actinomyces is especially common in these women [111]. Women with PID present with fever and abdominal and pelvic pain; cervical motion tenderness and a discharge may be detected during the physical examination. An associated palpable adnexal mass suggests a concurrent tubo-ovarian abscess (TOA) or pyosalpinx. Uncomplicated PID (myometritis, endometritis, and oophoritis) can generally be managed conservatively with antibiotics. TOA or pyosalpinx may require percutaneous or surgical drainage for cure. Long-term sequelae of PID include infertility, chronic pelvic pain, and an increased risk of ectopic pregnancy.

Most cases of PID/TOA are suspected and confirmed on the basis of the clinical picture and physical examination and with the aid of transabdominal or transvaginal ultrasound. In one series of highly selected patients

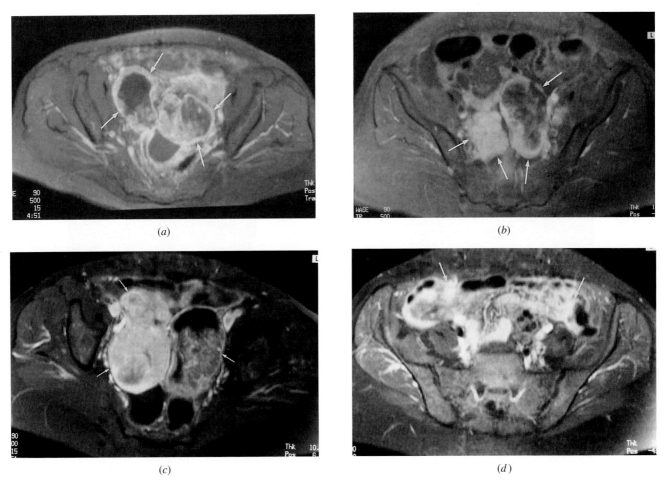

FIG. 15.32 Krukenberg tumors. Gadolinium-enhanced T1-weighted fat-suppressed SE (*a–d*) images in 3 patients with malignant signet cell metastases to the ovaries termed, Krukenberg tumors. The most common malignancies to cause Krukenberg tumors are gastric, pancreas (*a*), breast, colon (*b, c,* and *d*) and gallbladder carcinomas. Involvement is often bilateral; the ovaries are enlarged but retain an ovoid morphology (arrows, *a–c*). The metastases are primarily solid, although cystic regions are common. Gadolinium-enhanced T1-weighted fat-suppressed technique demonstrates the ovarian involvement and coexisting peritoneal disease (arrows, *d*).

admitted to the hospital for suspicion of PID, MR proved more accurate in the diagnosis of PID than transvaginal US [112]. MR was also helpful in detecting other causes for the patients' presenting symptoms. MR can define the extent of inflammation as ill-defined hyperintense areas on fat-suppressed T2-weighted images that enhance markedly on postgadolinium fat suppressed T1-weighted images (fig. 15.33) [111]. These areas are also seen as curvilinear and hypointense on routine T1-weighted imaging. A TOA has a variable MR appearance but is generally seen as round or tubular thick-walled, fluid-filled mass in the adnexal region (fig. 15.34). In one series, the abscesses were generally hypointense on T1-weighted images and hyperintense or heterogeneous on T2-weighted images [113]. Within the innermost portion of the abscess wall, a thin rim was observed; this rim was hyperintense or of intermediate signal on T1-weighted images and hypointense on T2-weighted images in almost every case. Dense enhancement was observed after gadolinium administration. This rim corresponds

histologically with a layer of granulation tissue, heavily infiltrated by inflammatory cells and containing fresh hemorrhage. The differential diagnosis of a TOA includes endometrioma, ovarian neoplasm, infected ovarian cyst, and an abscess from another source such as Crohn disease, appendicitis, or diverticulitis. Chronic PID/TOA results in similar but less severe changes. MR findings related to the fallopian tubes are discussed below.

FALLOPIAN TUBES

Normal Anatomy

The fallopian tubes form from the unfused proximal portions of the müllerian ducts during the third phase of müllerian development [114]. They are encased within the superior portion of the broad ligament and assume a relatively horizontal orientation during the migration of the ovaries. The normal tube is approximately 10 cm in

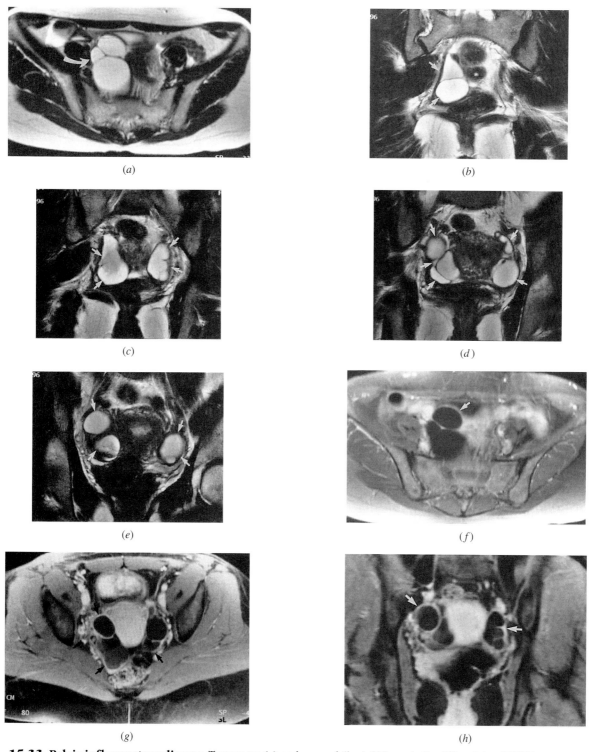

F I G . 15.33 Pelvic inflammatory disease. Transverse (*a*) and coronal (*b–e*) 512-resolution T2-weighted ETSE, transverse (*f, g*) and coronal (*h*) gadolinium-enhanced T1-weighted fat-suppressed SGE images in a patient with acute pelvic pain and fever. A complex cystic right adnexal mass is seen (curved arrow, *a*). On a lower section (not shown) a similar mass was seen on the left. Coronal images demonstrate that the masses are not ovarian cysts but the inflamed dilated fallopian tubes, folded upon themselves (arrows, *b–e*), which flank the uterus. After contrast the tube walls enhance and further demonstrate that the masses are not adjacent discrete cysts but rather continuous structures (arrows, *f –h*).

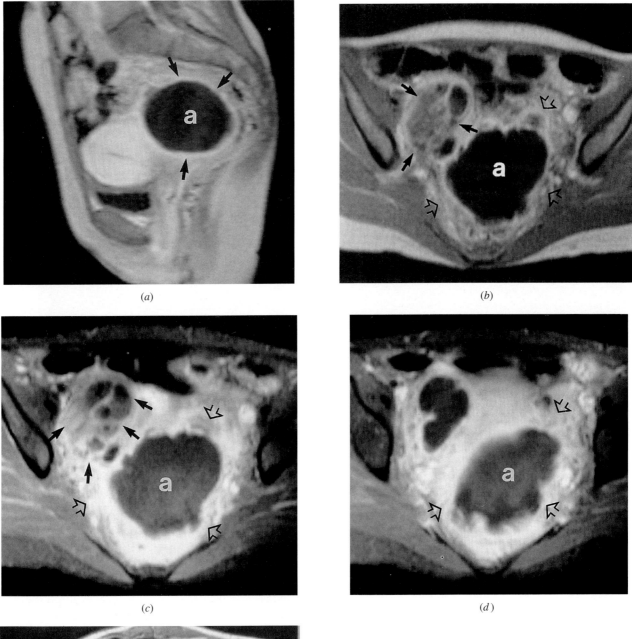

F I G . 15.34 Tubo-ovarian abscess. Sagittal (*a*) and transverse (*b*) gadolinium-enhanced T1-weighted SGE and gadolinium- enhanced T1-weighted fat-suppressed SE (*c, d*) images in a woman with fever and a fluctuant adnexal mass on bimanual exam. A large loculated abscess occupies the posterior pelvis ("a," *a–d*). The right ovary is enlarged and is invested with an abscess (solid arrows, *b, c*). The well-formed abscess capsule (arrows, *a*) and septations enhance markedly, as does the inflammation in the surrounding fat (open arrows, *b–d*). The associated inflammatory changes are more conspicuous on the fat-suppressed images. Tubo-ovarian abscess is a well-recognized complication of PID, and whereas most cases of PID can be managed conservatively, the presence of an abscess usually necessitates surgical intervention.

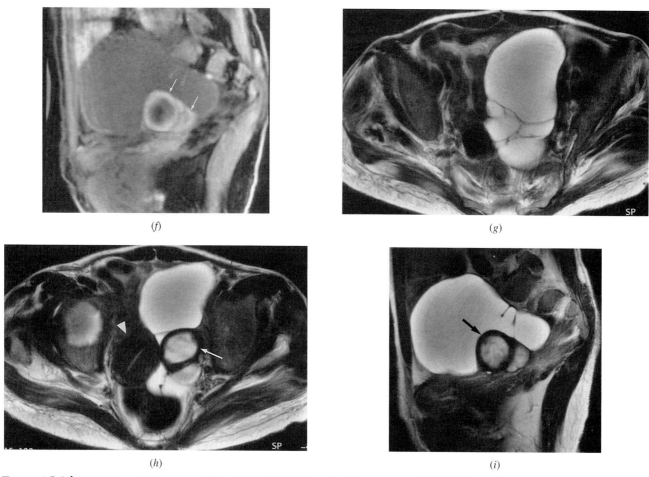

(f)

(g)

(h)

(i)

FIG. 15.34 (*Continued*) Transverse T1-weighted SGE (*e*), sagittal fat-suppressed SGE (*f*), and transverse (*g, h*) and sagittal (*i*) 512-resolution T2-weighted ETSE images in a second young woman, with chronic low-grade fever, pelvic pain, and a pelvic mass. A complex cystic adnexal mass displaces the uterus to the right. The dilated fallopian tube resembles septations coursing through the posterior aspect of the mass. The hydrosalpinx contains hemorrhage that has high-signal intensity rims on T1-weighted images (arrows, *e, f*) that are low in signal intensity on T2-weighted images (arrow, *h, i*). This is consistent with intracellular methemoglobin. (uterus = arrowhead, *h*).

length and has a 1- to 4-mm luminal diameter [115]. Four segments are recognized (medial to lateral): interstitial portion, isthmus, ampulla, and infundibulum or fimbriated end. The wall of the fallopian tube is somewhat complex, consisting of longitudinal folds and mucosal rugae whose size and number increase from medial to lateral. The mucosal surface contains ciliated cells that aid in the passage of the ovum to the uterine cavity.

MRI Technique

The techniques outlined for optimal imaging of the ovaries are also applicable to the fallopian tubes. In addition, there has been a report of the use of gadolinium-DPTA for proving tubal patency [116]. In this case, MR imaging was obtained 30 min after the injection of gadolinium into the uterine cavity using a balloon catheter. Fat-suppressed T1-weighted transverse

and sagittal images were examined for the presence of contrast material in the peritoneal cavity implying that at least one tube is patent.

Normal Fallopian Tubes
The normal fallopian tube is not routinely seen with MR imaging.

Congenital Abnormalities
The Buttram classification of müllerian duct defects groups disorders based on their similar embryonic and anatomic features [115]. Included among the class 1 anomalies is fallopian tube agenesis, a bilateral condition. Among the class 2 anomalies is a unicornuate uterus in which one tube can be aplastic. Class 6 anomalies are diethylstilbestrol related and include shortened, convoluted tubes with abnormal, withered fimbria and very narrowed fimbrial openings and bandlike constrictions in the intramural portions of the tube [117].

Mass Lesions

Benign Masses

Benign diseases that affect the ovaries and/or uterus can also affect the fallopian tubes, including endometriosis, leiomyomata, adenomatoid tumors, and teratoma. Endometriosis of the fallopian tubes generally affects the surface of the tube, with the endometrial glands and stroma confined to the subserosal layer of the tube [118]. Leiomyomata of the tubes are exceedingly rare and generally asymptomatic, discovered incidentally [119]. The MR characteristics of this and other benign diseases are the same as those described above for the ovary.

Hydrosalpinx. Occlusion of the fimbriated end of the tube uncomplicated by hemorrhage or infection produces tubal dilation resulting in a hydrosalpinx. If complicated by hemorrhage the term hematosalpinx may be applied; if complicated by infection, the term pyosalpinx is used. The causes of tubal obstruction include PID, endometriosis, adjacent tumors, and adhesions from prior surgery. On MRI, the dilated fallopian tube appears as a tubular fluid-filled structure folded on itself to form an S or C shape (fig. 15.35) [120]. The multiplanar capability of MR is especially useful in proving that a multicystic structure is actually a dilated tube. The signal intensity of the fluid on T1- and T2-weighted images may provide a clue as to the cause of the obstruction. Fluid that is of increased signal on T1-weighted images is associated with endometriosis.

Ectopic Pregnancy. The most common sites for an extrauterine gestation are the fallopian tubes and ovaries. Because of the increased use of ovulation-stimulating drugs as well as other treatments for infertility, the incidence of ectopic pregnancy is on the

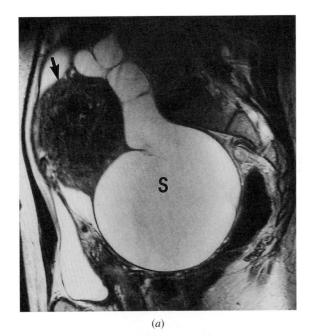

(a)

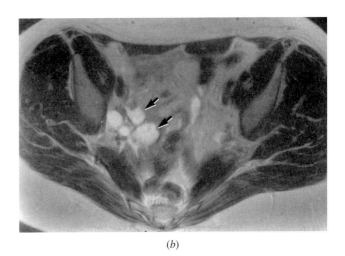

(b)

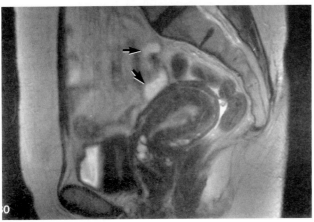

(c)

F I G . 15.35 Hydrosalpinx. Sagittal 512-resolution T2-weighted ETSE image (*a*) demonstrates a large hydrosalpinx (S). Adenomyosis of the uterus (arrow) is also present.

Transverse (*b*) and sagittal (*c*) T2-weighted ETSE images in a second patient demonstrate a fluid-filled structure that on the transverse image appears to represent cysts (arrows, *b*), whereas on the sagittal image (*c*) the tubular shape of the hydrosalpinx (arrows, *c*) is shown.

rise. Because most ectopic pregnancies are confirmed with transvaginal ultrasound, few reports of the MR features have been published [121–123]. Features described include a fallopian tube hematoma, enhancement of the fallopian tube wall, a gestational saclike structure, bloody ascites, and a heterogeneous adnexal mass. The hematoma is of intermediate to high signal on T1-weighted images [123], and the ascites is of increased signal intensity on fat-suppressed T1-weighted images. An enhancing treelike region within the heterogeneous mass has been reported to represent villous-containing fibrin strands in the fetoplacental tissue [121].

Malignant Masses

Primary Fallopian Tube Carcinoma. Primary fallopian tube carcinoma is a rare disease entity, with a reported incidence in the United States of 3.6 cases per million women per year [124]. It comprises only 0.5% of all gynecologic tumors. The most common histology is adenocarcinoma; sarcomas (leiomyosarcoma, carcinosarcomas and mixed müllerian tumors) and choriocarcinoma are even more rare. The typical patient is older (average age 55 years) and presents with such nonspecific symptoms as abdominal pain, abnormal vaginal bleeding, and vaginal discharge [125]. The poor prognosis of fallopian tube malignancies relates to the late stage at diagnosis rather than to a particular aggressiveness of the tumor; the average 5-year survival is less than 50% [v]. At presentation most women have widespread disease; the tumor can spread directly through the fimbriated end of the tube, through the wall of the tube, or via the lymphatics to the para-aortic, iliac and lumbar nodes as well as to the ovaries, other pelvic organs, or more distant sites. The prognosis is dependent on disease burden

at diagnosis. Both FIGO staging and an alternative similar to the Duke classification for colon cancer have been advocated [124]. Treatment is primarily surgical; adjuvant chemotherapy is also used. Radiation therapy at present does not appear to confer additional benefit.

The MR appearance of fallopian tube carcinoma has been described. Typically, the tumor is a small adnexal mass with low T1 signal and high T2 signal. Enhancement is seen after the administration of gadolinium (fig. 15.36). Associated findings include hydrosalpinx, peritumoral ascites, and intrauterine fluid [125].

Metastases. Metastatic disease involving the fallopian tube is more common than primary carcinoma and is generally the result of direct extension from the ovary, endometrium, or cervix. Tumors arising outside of the genital system that can metastasize to the tubes include breast and gastrointestinal cancers. Lymphatic spread accounts for the majority of this involvement. The appearance of metastatic disease to the fallopian tubes has not been described in series. Anecdotal reports suggest that the appearance is similar to that of ovarian metastatic disease (fig. 15.37).

Inflammation

Salpingitis

The epidemiological and clinical features of PID/TOA as well as findings related to the ovary are described above. The findings of salpingitis include tubal enlargement due to obstruction of the fimbriated end of the tube. On MR, this is seen as a serpentine adnexal lesion; the central signal varies with the tube contents. Purulent material is of variable signal on T1- and T2-weighted images but

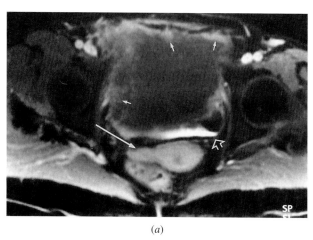

(a)

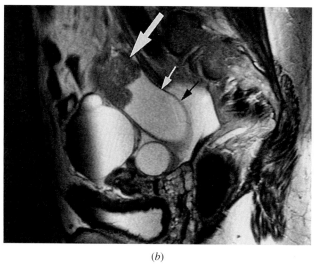

(b)

F I G . 15.36 Fallopian tube adenocarcinoma. Gadolinium-enhanced T1-weighted fat-suppressed SGE image (*a*) demonstrates a solid right fallopian tube cancer (long arrow, *a*) and multiple peritoneal metastases (short arrows, *a*). The bladder (open arrow, *a*) contains high-signal intensity gadolinium.

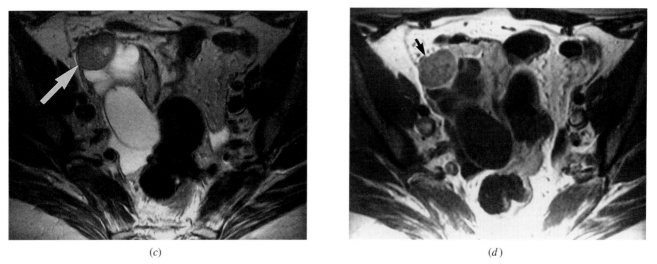

(c)   *(d)*

F I G . 15.36 *(Continued)* Sagittal (*b*) and transverse (*c*) 512-resolution T2-weighted ETSE and gadolinium-enhanced T1-weighted SE (*d*) images in a second patient. The fallopian tube is shown as a dilated tubular structure (arrows, *b*) that contains solid tumor components (large arrow, *b, c*). Heterogeneous enhancement of the tumor nodules is present (arrow, *d*) after gadolinium administration.

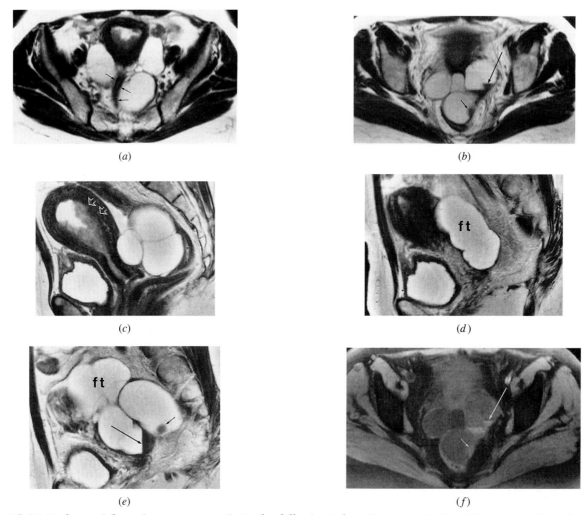

(a)   *(b)*

(c)   *(d)*

(e)   *(f)*

F I G . 15.37 Endometrial carcinoma metastatic to the fallopian tubes. Transverse (*a, b*), midline sagittal (*c*), right sagittal (*d*), and left sagittal (*e*) high-resolution T2-weighted ETSE, T1-weighted fat-suppressed SGE (f), and transverse (*g, h*) and sagittal (*i, j*) gadolinium-enhanced T1-weighted fat-suppressed SGE images in a woman with metastatic mixed papillary serous and clear cell endometrial carcinoma complaining of a change in bowel habits.

1183

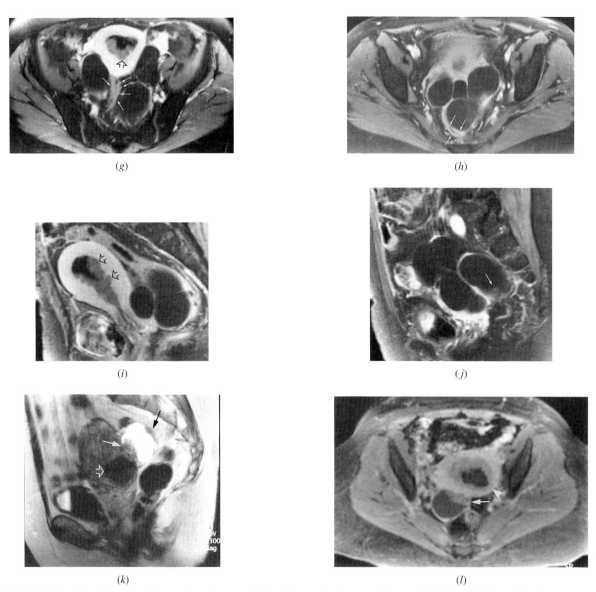

(g)

(h)

(i)

(j)

(k)

(l)

F IG . 15.37 (*Continued*) The endometrium is expanded and contains intermediate- and high-signal intensity elements on the T2-weighted image (*c*). The junctional zone is effaced posteriorly (open arrow, *c*). Bilateral adnexal cystic masses compress and surround the sigmoid colon (arrows, *a*). On the right parasagittal image the adnexal cysts appear in continuity with a dilated fallopian tube ("ft," *d*), a hydrosalpinx. Similar findings are noted on the left. In addition, the contents of the left tube appear complex; there is blood dependently (hematosalpinx) (long arrow, *b, e, f*) and nodularity of the tube wall (short arrow, *b, e, f*). The ovaries (not shown) were displaced anteriorly and superiorly by the diseased tubes. After contrast, the viable endometrial tumor enhances and scallops the posterior myometrium (open arrows, *g, i*). The compressed wall of the sigmoid colon is tethered to, and adherent, to the dilated fallopian tubes (solid arrows, *g, h*). Note an enhancing metastatic nodule in the fallopian tube (arrow, *j*).

Sagittal 512-resolution gadolinium-enhanced T2-weighted ETSE (*k*) and transverse gadolinium-enhanced T1-weighted fat-suppressed SGE (*l*) images in second patient who has invasive endometrial carcinoma metastatic to the right fallopian tube. There is a complex fallopian tube metastasis. The solid components are intermediate in signal intensity on the T2-weighted image (solid arrows, *k*). After contrast, the endometrial carcinoma enhances less than adjacent normal myometrium (arrowhead, *l*). Intravenous gadolinium administration is mandatory to accurately assess myometrial invasion. The solid portions of the fallopian tube metastasis also enhance (solid arrow, *l*). Incidental note is made of an intramural fibroid (open arrow, *k*).

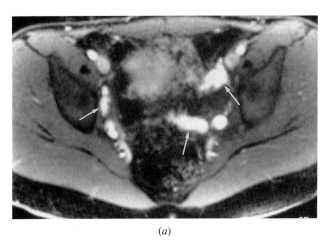

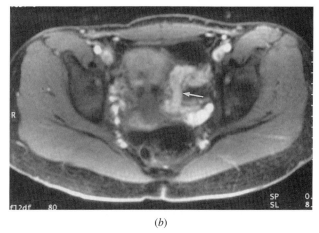

(a)   *(b)*

F i g . 15.38 Pelvic varices. Transverse 45-s postgadolinium fat-suppressed SGE images (*a, b*) in a patient with chronic pelvic pain. Pelvic varices, left greater than right, show marked enhancement after intravenous gadolinium administration (arrows, *a, b*). The concurrent use of fat suppression increases the conspicuity of the dilated vessels by removing the competing high-signal intensity of fat. Pelvic varices are a common, though rarely recognized, cause of chronic pelvic pain. In imaging a patient with pelvic pain of unknown etiology, the presence or absence of varices should be noted.

may show a fluid-debris level. After the administration of gadolinium, the tube wall enhances, a finding highlighted with fat suppression techniques (fig. 15.34).

Pelvic Varices

Primary pelvic varices are associated with the pelvic pain syndrome, chronic pelvic pain without obvious cause. In one series, women undergoing laparoscopy for pelvic pain had dilated veins within the broad ligament and surrounding the ovary as their sole finding [126]. This is an entity generally affecting multiparous women of reproductive age; patients complain of a deep, dull pelvic ache made worse by activity or actions that increase intra-abdominal pressure [127]. In contrast, secondary pelvic varices are not generally associated with pain but do signal a potentially serious underlying abnormality such as inferior vena caval obstruction, portal hypertension, increased pelvic blood flow, or vascular malformations [127]. MR is not the first line in diagnosis of this entity, however; pelvic varices can be detected as part of a work-up or may be noted incidentally [128]. On T1-and T2-weighted images, serpentine parauterine and paraovarian structures are noted. These enhance to a significant degree after gadolinium administration, especially if an appropriate delay is employed (2 min) (fig. 15.38).

Future Directions

Work continues on the development of an MR equivalent of hysterosalpingography. In a recent paper, a phantom model of the normal uterus and fallopian tubes as well as unilateral and bilateral hydrosalpinx was studied [129]. Work included optimizing the imaging sequences and determining the correct agent to demonstrate fallopian tube patency. Further in vivo investigation is required

before the technique can gain widespread acceptance in the work-up of infertility.

CONCLUSION

MRI offers distinct advantages over other modalities in the characterization of adnexal lesions, not only with regard to their organ of origin but also with regard to their pathology. Dermoids, teratomas, endometriomas, simple and hemorrhagic cysts, fibromas, and hydrosalpinges can be diagnosed with a high degree of confidence. MRI may also be the most sensitive technique for the detection of peritoneal spread of ovarian carcinoma. In women of childbearing age and in women who are pregnant, the lack of ionizing radiation and safety of gadolinium are of paramount importance. Several studies have attempted to address the possible cost savings of MRI in the management of women with a variety of gynecological disorders [130–132]. Further work is needed in this era of rising health care costs to determine the best utilization of this technique.

REFERENCES

1. Haller JO, Freidman AP, Schaffer R, et al.: The normal and abnormal ovary in childhood and adolescence. *Semin Ultrasound* 4: 206–214, 1983.
2. Zaloudek C. The ovary. In Gompel C and Silverberg SG (eds.), *Pathology in Gynecology and Obstetrics*, Philadelphia: Lippincott, p. 313–413, 1994.
3. Curtis M, Hopkins MP, Zarlingo T, et al.: Magnetic resonance imaging to avoid laparotomy in pregnancy. *Obstet Gynecol* 82: 833–836, 1993.

4. Kier R, McCarthy SM, Scoutt LM, et al.: Pelvic masses in pregnancy: MR imaging. *Radiology* 176: 709–713, 1990.

5. Colleti P, Sylvestre PB: Magnetic resonance imaging in pregnancy. *Magn Reson Imaging Clin N Am* 2: 291–307, 1994.

6. Smith RC, Reinhold C, McCauley TR, et al.: Multicoil high resolution fast spin-echo MR imaging of the female pelvis. *Radiology* 184: 671–675, 1992.

7. Hayes CE, Dietz MJ, King BF, et al.: Pelvic imaging with phased-array coils: Quantitative assessment of signal-to-noise ratio improvement. *J Magn Res Imaging* 2: 321–326, 1992.

8. Hricak H: Current trends in MR imaging of the female pelvis. *Radiographics* 13: 913–919, 1993.

9. McCauley TR, McCarthy S, Lange R: Pelvic phased-array coil: Image quality assessment for spin-echo MR imaging. *Magn Reson Imaging* 10: 513–522, 1992.

10. Outwater EK, Mitchell DG: Magnetic resonance imaging techniques in the pelvis. *Magn Reson Imaging Clin N Am* 2: 161–188, 1994.

11. Tempany MC, Fielding JR: Female pelvis. In Edelman RR, Hasselink JR, Zlatkin MB (eds.), *Clinical Magnetic Resonance Imaging.* Philadelphia: WB Saunders, p. 1432–1465, 1996.

12. Outwater EK, Talerman A, Dunton C: Normal adnexa uteri specimens: anatomic basis of MR imaging features. *Radiology* 201: 751–755, 1996.

13. Outwater EK, Mitchell DG: Normal ovaries and functional cysts: MR appearance. *Radiology* 198: 397–402, 1996.

14. Levine D, Gosink B, Wolf SL, et al.: Simple adnexal cysts: The natural history in postmenopausal women. *Radiology* 184: 653–659, 1992.

15. Outwater EK, Dunton CJ: Imaging of the ovary and adnexa: clinical issues and applications of MR imaging. *Radiology* 194: 1–18, 1995.

16. Outwater EK, Schiebler ML, Owens RS, et al.: MRI characterization of hemorrhagic adnexal masses: A blinded reader study. *Radiology* 186: 489–494, 1993.

17. Gambino J, Caldwell B, Dietrich R, et al.: Congenital disorders of sexual differentiation: MR findings. *AM J Roentgenol* 158: 363–367, 1992.

18. Choi HK, Cho KS, Lee HW, Kim KS: MR Imaging of intersexuality. *Radiographics* 18: 83–96, 1998.

19. Secaf E, Hricak H, Gooding CA, et al.: Role of MRI in the evaluation of ambiguous genitalia. *Pediatr Radiol* 24: 231–235, 1994.

20. Outwater EK, Huang AB, Dunton CJ, et al.: Papillary projections in ovarian neoplasms: Appearance on MRI. *J Magn Reson Imaging* 7: 689–695, 1997.

21. Koonings PP, Campbell K, Mishell DR Jr, Grimes DA: Relative frequency of primary ovarian neoplasms: A 10-year review. *Obstet Gynecol* 74: 921–926, 1989.

22. Isoda H, Setoh H, Oka A, et al.: Squamous cell carcinoma arising in a mature teratoma with metastasis to the urinary bladder. *Comput Med Imaging Graphics* 23: 223–225, 1999.

23. Dooms BC, Hricak H, Tscholakoff D: Adnexal structures: MR imaging. *Radiology* 158: 639–646, 1986.

24. Kido A, Togashi K, Konishi I, et al.: Dermoid cyst of the ovary with malignant transformation: MR appearance. *Am J Roentgenol* 172: 445–449, 1999.

25. Togashi K, Nishimura K, Itoh K, et al.: Ovarian cystic teratomas: MR imaging. *Radiology* 162: 669–673, 1987.

26. Mitchell DG, Mintz MC, Spritzer CE, et al.: Adnexal masses: MR imaging observations at 1.5 T with US and CT correlation. *Radiology* 162: 319–324, 1987.

27. Stevens SK, Hricak H, Campos Z: Teratomas versus cystic hemorrhagic adnexal lesions: Differentiation with proton-selection fat saturation MR imaging. *Radiology* 186: 481–488, 1993.

28. Kier R, Smith RC, McCarthy SM: Value of lipid- and water-suppression MR images in distinguishing between blood and lipid within ovarian masses. *AM J Roentgenol* 158: 321–325, 1992.

29. Yamashita Y, Toraxhima M, Hatanaka Y, et al.: Value of phase-shift gradient-echo MR imaging in the differentiation of pelvic lesions with high signal intensity at T1-weighted imaging. *Radiology* 191: 759–764, 1994.

30. Mitchell DG: Chemical shift magnetic resonance imaging: Applications in the abdomen and pelvis. *Top Magn Res Imaging* 4: 46–63, 1992.

31. Matsumoto F, Yoshioka H, Hamada T, et al.: Struma ovarii: CT and MR findings. *J Comput Assist Tomagr* 14: 310–312, 1990.

32. Dohke M, Watanabe Y, Takahashi A, et al.: Struma ovarii: MR findings. *J Comput Assist Tomagr* 21: 265–267, 1997.

33. Yamashita Y, Hatanaka Y, Takahashi M, et al.: Struma ovarii: MR appearances. *Abdom Imaging* 22: 100–102, 1997.

34. Joja I, Asakawa T, Shirakawa M: Uterus and ovary. *Jpn J Diag Imaging* 18: 291–299, 1998.

35. Matsuki M, Kaji Y, Matsuo M, Kobashi Y: Struma ovarii: MRI findings. *Br J Radiol* 73: 87–90, 2000.

36. Ojada S, Ohaki Y, Kawamura T, et al.: Cystic struma ovarii: imaging findings. *J Comput Assist Tomagr* 24: 413–415, 2000.

37. Morrow CP, Curran JP: Tumors of the ovary: classification; the adnexal mass. In Morrow CP, Curran JP (eds.), *Synopsis of Gynecological Oncology.* New York: Churchill Livingstone, p. 215–232, 1998.

38. Ghossain MA, Buy JN, Ligneres C, et al.: Epithelial tumors of the ovary: Comparison of MR and CT findings. *Radiology* 181: 863–870; 1991.

39. Kinoshita T, Ishii K, Naganuma H, et al.: MR findings of ovarian tumors with cystic components. *Br J Radiol* 73: 333–339, 2000.

40. Gompel C, Silverberg SG: Endometriosis. In Gompel S, Silverberg SG (eds.), *Pathology in Gynecology and Obstetrics* (4th ed.). Philadelphia: Lippincott, p. 425–431, 1994.

41. Miyakoshi K, Tanaka M, Gabionza D, et al.: Decidualized ovarian endometriosis mimicking malignancy. *Am J Roentgenol* 171: 1625–1626, 1998.

42. Nezhat F, Nezhat C, Allan CJ, et al.: Clinical and histological classification of endometriomas: Implication for a mechanism of pathogenesis. *J Reprod Med* 37: 771–776; 1992.

43. Clement PB: Pathology of endometriosis. In: Rosen PP, Fechner RE (eds.), *Pathology Annual* Vol 25. Norwalk, CT: Appleton and Lange, p. 245–295, 1990.

44. Gerbie AB, Merrill JA: Pathology of endometriosis. *Clin Obstet Gynecol.* 31: 779–786, 1988.

45. Weitzman GA, Buttram VCl: Classification of endometriosis. *Obstet Gynecol Clin N Am* 16: 61–77, 1989.

46. Hesla JS, Rock JA: Endometriosis. In Rock JA, Thompson JD (eds.), *TeLinde's Operative Gynecology.* Philadelphia: Lippincott-Raven, p. 585–595, 1997.

47. Sugimura K, Okizuka H, Iamaoka I, et al.: Pelvic endometriosis: detection and diagnosis with chemical shift MR imaging. *Radiology* 188: 435–438, 1993.

48. Ha HK, Lim YT, Kim HS, et al.: Diagnosis of pelvic endometriosis: Fat suppressed T1-weighted vs. conventional MR images. *Am J Roentgenol* 163: 127–131, 1994.

49. Ascher SM, Agrawal R Bis KG, et al.: Endometriosis: Appearance and detection with conventional and contrast-enhanced fat-suppressed spin-echo technique. *J Magn Reson Imaging* 5: 251–257, 1995.

50. Togashi K, Nishimura K, Kimura I, et al.: Endometrial cyst: Diagnosis with MR imaging. *Radiology* 180: 73–78, 1991.

51. Scoutt LM, McCarthy SM, Lange R, et al.: MR evaluation of clinically suspected adnexal masses. *J Comput Assist Tomagr* 18: 609–618, 1994.

52. Thurnher S, Hudler J, Baer S, et al.: Gadolinium DOTA-enhanced MR imaging of adnexal tumors. *J Comput Assist Tomagr* 14: 939–949, 1990.

53. Thurnher SM: MR imaging of pelvic masses in women: Contrast-enhanced vs. unenhanced images. *Am J Roentgenol* 159: 1243–1250, 1992.

54. Woodward PJ, Sohaey R, Mettetti TP: Endometriosis: Radiologic-pathologic correlation. *Radiographics* 21: 193–216, 2001.

55. Arrive L, Hricak H, Martin MC: Pelvic endometriosis: MR imaging. *Radiology* 171: 687–692, 1989.

56. Siegelman ES, Outwater EK, Wang T, et al.: Solid pelvic masses caused by endometriosis: MR imaging features. *Am J Roentgenol* 163: 357–361, 1994.

57. Franks S: Polycystic ovary syndrome. *N Engl J Med* 333: 853–861, 1995.

58. Outwater EK, Schiebler ML: Magnetic resonance imaging of the ovary. *Radiol Clin N Am* 2: 245–274, 1994.

59. Kimura I, Togashi K, Kawakami S, et al.: Polycystic ovaries: implications of diagnosis with MR imaging. *Radiology* 201: 549–552, 1996.

60. Berkowitz RS, Goldstein DP: Gestational trophoblastic disease. In Hoskins WJ, Perez CA, Young RC (eds.), *Principles and Practice of Gynecologic Oncology*. Philadelphia: Lippincott, p. 1117–1138, 2000.

61. Hricak H, Demas BE, Braga CA, et al.: Gestational trophoblastic neoplasm of the uterus: MR assessment. *Radiology* 161: 11–16, 1986.

62. Barton JW, McCarthy SM, Kohorn EL, et al.: Pelvic MR imaging findings in gestational trophoblastic disease, incomplete abortion, and ectopic pregnancy: Are they specific? *Radiology* 186: 163–168, 1993.

63. Kier R: Nonovarian gynecologic cysts: MR imaging findings. *Am J Roentgenol* 158: 1265–1269, 1992.

64. Kurachi H, Murakami T, Nakamura H, et al.: Imaging of peritoneal pseudocysts: Value of MR imaging compared with sonography and CT. *Am J Roentgenol* 160: 589–591, 1993.

65. Jain KA: Imaging of peritoneal inclusion cysts. *Am J Roentgenol* 174: 1559–1563, 2000.

66. Murase E, Siegelman ES, Outwater EK, et al.: Uterine leiomyomas: histopathologic features, MR imaging findings, differential diagnosis, and treatment. *Radiographics* 19: 1179–1197, 1999.

67. Kim JC, Kim SS, Park YJ: "Bridging vascular sign" in the MR diagnosis of exophytic uterine leiomyoma. *J Comput Assist Tomagr* 24: 57–60, 2000.

68. Thurnher S, Hodler J, Baer S, et al.: Gadolinium-DOTA enhanced MR imaging of adnexal tumors. *J Comput Assist Tomagr* 14: 939–949, 1990.

69. Stevens SK, Hricak H, Stern JL: Ovarian lesions: detection and characterization with gadolinium-enhanced MR imaging at 1.5 T. *Radiology* 181: 481–488, 1991.

70. Schwartz RK, Levine D, Hatabu H, Edelman RR: Ovarian fibroma: Findings by contrast-enhanced MRI. *Abdom Imaging* 22: 535–537, 1997.

71. Outwater EK, Siegelman ES, Talerman A, Dunton C: Ovarian fibromas and cystadenofibromas: MRI of the fibrous component. *JMRI* 7: 465–471, 1997.

72. Ueda J, Furukawa T, Higashino K, et al.: Ovarian fibroma of high signal intensity on T2-weighted MR image. *Abdom Imaging* 23: 657–658, 1998.

73. Troiano RN, Lazzarini KM, Scoutt LM, et al.: Fibroma and fibrothecoma of the ovary: MR imaging findings. *Radiology* 204: 795–798, 1997.

74. Moon WJ, Koh BH, Kim SK, et al.: Brenner tumor of the ovary: CT and MR findings. *J Comput Assist Tomagr* 24: 72–76, 2000.

75. Outwater EK, Siegelman ES, Kim B, et al.: Ovarian Brenner tumors: MR imaging characteristics. *Magn Reson Imaging* 16: 1147–1153, 1998.

76. Jain KA: Magnetic resonance imaging findings in ovarian torsion. *Magn Reson Imaging* 13: 111–113, 1995.

77. Kimura I, Togashi K, Kawakami S, et al.: Ovarian torsion: CT and MR imaging appearances. *Radiology* 190: 337–341, 1994.

78. Dohke M, Watanabe Y, Okumura A, et al.: Comprehensive MR imaging of acute gynecologic diseases. *Radiographics* 20: 1551–1556, 2000.

79. Kawakami K, Murata K, Kawaguchi N, et al.: Hemorrhagic infarction of the diseased ovary: a common MR finding in two cases. *Magn Reson Imaging* 11: 595–597, 1993.

80. Lee AR, Kim KH, Lee BH, et al.: Massive edema of the ovary: Imaging findings. *Am J Roentgenol* 161: 343–344, 1993.

81. Umesaki N, Tanaka T, Miyana M, et al.: Successful preoperative diagnosis of massive ovarian edema aided by comparative imaging study using magnetic resonance and ultrasound. *Eur J Obstet Gynecol Repro Biol* 89: 97–99, 2000.

82. Kramer LA, Lalani T, Kawashima A: Massive edema of the ovary: High resolution MR findings using a phased-array pelvic coil. *J Magn Reson Imaging* 7: 758–760, 1997.

83. Hall B, Printz D, Rith J: Massive ovarian edema: Ultrasound and MR characteristics. *J Comput Assist Tomagr* 17: 477–479, 1993.

84. Ozols RF, Rubin SC, Thomas GM, Robboy S: Epithelial ovarian cancer. In Hoskins WJ, Perez CA, Young RC (eds.), *Principles and Practice of Gynecologic Oncology*. Philadelphia: Lippincott, p. 981–1058, 2000.

85. American Cancer Society: *Cancer Facts and Figures: 1998*. Atlanta, GA: American Cancer Society, 1998, p. 13.

86. Yamashita Y, Torashima M, Hatanaka Y, et al.: Adnexal masses: Accuracy of characterization with transvaginal US and precontrast and postcontrast MR imaging. *Radiology* 194: 557–565, 1995.

87. Komatsu T, Konishi I, Mondai M, et al.: Adnexal masses: Transvaginal US and gadolinium-enhanced MR imaging assessment of intratumoral structure. *Radiology* 198: 109–115, 1996.

88. Yamashita Y, Hatanaka Y, Torashima M, et al.: Characterization of sonographically indeterminate ovarian tumors with MR imaging—a logistic regression analysis. *Acta Radiol* 38: 572–577, 1997.

89. Jain KA, Friedman DL, Pettinger TW, et al.: Adnexal masses: Comparison of the specificity of endovaginal US and pelvic MR imaging. *Radiology* 186: 697–704, 1993.

90. Stevens SK, Hricak H, Stern JL: Ovarian lesions: Detection and characterization with gadolinium-enhanced MR imaging at 1.5T. *Radiology* 181: 481–488.

91. Semelka RC, Lawrence PH, Shoenut JP, et al.: Primary ovarian cancer: Prospective comparison of contrast-enhanced CT and pre- and postcontrast fat-suppressed MR imaging with histologic correlation. *J Magn Imaging* 3: 99–106, 1993.

92. Jeong YY, Outwater EK, Kang HK: Imaging of ovarian masses. *Radiographics* 20: 1445–1470, 2000.

93. Sutton CL, McKinney CD, Jones JE, Gay SB: Ovarian masses revisited: Radiologic and pathologic correlation. *Radiographics* 12: 853–877, 1992.

94. Wagner BJ, Buck JL, Seidman JD, McCabe KM: Ovarian epithelial neoplasms: Radiologic-pathologic correlation. *Radiographics* 14: 1351–1274, 1994.

95. Kurtz AB, Tsimikas JV, Tempany CMC, et al.: The comparative values of Doppler and conventional US, CT and MR imaging correlated with surgery and histopathologic analysis: report of the Radiologic Diagnostic Oncology Group. *Radiology* 212: 19–27, 1999.

96. Tempany CMC, Zou KH, Silverman SG, et al.: Staging of advanced ovarian cancer: comparison of imaging modalities—report of the

Radiologolic Diagnostic Oncology Group. *Radiology* 215: 761–767, 2000.

97. Low RN, Saleh F, Song SYT, et al.: Treated ovarian cancer: Comparison of MR Imaging with serum CA-125 level and physical examination—a longitudinal study. *Radiology* 211: 519–528, 1999.

98. Tanaka YO, Nishida M, Kurosaki Y, et al.: Differential diagnosis of gynaecological "stained glass" tumors on MRI. *Br J Radiol* 72: 414–420, 1999.

99. Morrow CP, Curtin JP: Tumors of the ovary: Sex cord stromal tumors and germ cell tumors. In Morrow CP, Curtin JP (eds.): *Synopsis of Gynecologic Oncology*. New York: Churchill Livingstone, p. 281–306, 1998.

100. Ko SF, Wan YL, Ng SH, et al.: Adult granulosa cell tumors: Spectrum of sonographic and CT findings with pathologic correlation. *AmJ Roentgenol* 172: 1227–1233, 1999.

101. Morikawa K, Hatabu H, Togashi K, et al.: Granulosa cell tumor of the ovary: MT findings. *J Comput Assist Tomagr* 21: 1001–1004, 1997.

102. Levitan A, Haller KD, Cohen HL, et al.: Endodermal sinus tumor of the ovary: imaging evaluation. *AmJ Roentgenol* 167: 791–793, 1996.

103. Kohno A, Yoshikawa W, Yunoki M, et al.: MR findings in degenerated ovarian leiomyoma. *Br J Radiol* 72: 1213–1215, 1999.

104. Ferrozzi F, Tognini G, Bova D, Zuccoli G: Non-Hodgkin lymphomas of the ovaries: MR findings. *J Comput Assist Tomagr* 24: 416–420, 2000.

105. Mitsumori A, Joja I: MRI appearance of Non-Hodgkin's lymphoma of the ovary. *AmJ Roentgenol* 173: 245, 1999.

106. Young RH, Scully RE: Metastatic tumors in the ovary. In Blaustein A (ed.), *Pathology of the Female Genital Tract*. New York: Springer p. 939–974, 1994.

107. Moselhi M, Spencer J, Lane G: Malignant melanoma metastatic to the ovary: Presentation and radiological characteristics. *Gynecol Oncol* 69: 165–168, 1998.

108. Kim SH, Kim WH, Park KJ, et al.: CT and MR findings of Kruenberg tumors. Comparison with primary ovarian tumors. *J Comput Assist Tomagr* 20: 393–398, 1996.

109. Cho JY, Seong CK, Kim SH: Krukenberg tumor findings at color and power Doppler US: Correlation with findings at CT, MR, and pathology. *Acta Radiol* 39: 327–329, 1998.

110. Ha HK, Baek SY, Kim SH, et al.: Krukenberg's tumor of the ovary: MR imaging features. *AmJ Roentgenol* 164: 1435–1439, 1995.

111. Dohke M, Watanabe Y, Okumura A, et al.: Comprehensive MR imaging of acute gynecologic diseases. *Radiographics* 20: 1551–1566, 2000.

112. Tukeva TA, Aronen NJ, Karjalainen PT, et al.: MR imaging in pelvic inflammatory disease: Comparison with laparoscopy and US. *Radiology* 210: 209–216, 1999.

113. Ha HK, Lim GY, Cha ES, et al.: MR imaging of tubo-ovarian abscess. *Acta Radiol* 36: 510–514, 1995.

114. O'Neill MJ, Yoder IC, Connolly SA, Mueller PR: Imaging evaluation and classification of developmental anomalies of the female reproductive system with emphasis on MR imaging. *AmJ Roentgenol* 173: 407–416, 1999.

115. Rowling SE, Ramchandani P: Imaging of the fallopian tubes. *Semin Roentgenol* 31: 299–311, 1996.

116. Furuhashi M, Miyabi Y, Katsumata Y, et al.: Magnetic resonance imaging with gadolinium diethylenetriamine pentaacetic acid is useful in the assessment of tubal patency in a patient with iodine-induced hypothyrodisim. *Magn Reson Imaging* 16: 339–341, 1998.

117. DeCherney AH, Cholst I, Naftolin F: Structure and function of the fallopian tubes following exposure to diethylstilbestrol DES during gestation. *Fertil Steril* 36: 741–745, 1981.

118. Bis KG, Vrachliotics TG, Agrawal R, et al.: Pelvic endometriosis: MR imaging spectrum with laparoscopic correlation and diagnostic pitfalls. *Radiographics* 17: 639–655, 1997.

119. Misao R, Niwa K, Shimokawa K, Tamaya T: Leiomyoma of the fallopian tube. *Gynecol Obstet Invest* 49: 279–280, 2000.

120. Outwater EK, Siegelman ES, Chiowanich P, et al.: Dilated fallopian tubes: MR imaging characteristics. *Radiology* 208: 463–469, 1998.

121. Ha HK, Jung JK, Kang SK, et al.: MR imaging in the diagnosis of rare forms of ectopic pregnancy. *AmJ Roentgenol* 160: 1229–1232, 1993.

122. Outwater EK: Magnetic resonance imaging of acute and chronic pelvic pain disorders. In Fleischer AC, Javitt MC, Jefffrey RB, Jones HW (eds.), *Clinical Gynecologic Imaging*. Philadelphia, Lippincott-Raven, p.263–271, 1997.

123. Kataoka ML, Togashi K, Kobayashi H, et al.: Evaluation of ectopic pregnancy by magnetic resonance imaging. Human Reproduction 14: 2644–2650, 1999.

124. Gompel C, Silverberg SG: The fallopian tube. In Gompel C, Silverberg SG (eds.), *Pathology in Gynecology and Obstetrics*. Philadelphia, Lippincott, p. 284–311, 1994.

125. Kawakami S, Togashi K, Kimura I, et al.: Primary malignant tumor of the fallopian tube: Appearance at CT and MR imaging. *Radiology* 186: 503–508, 1993.

126. Gupta A, McCarthy S: Pelvic varices as a cause for pelvic pain: MRI appearance. *Magn Reson Imaging* 12: 679–681, 1994.

127. Coakley FV, Varghese SL, Hricak H: CT and MRI of pelvic varices in women. *J Comput Assist Tomagr* 23: 429–434, 1999.

128. Gullo G, Russ PD: Pelvic varices diagnosed with endorectal surface coil magnetic resonance imaging: Case report. *Can Assoc Radiol J* 51: 23–27, 2000.

129. Frye RE, Ascher SM, Thomasson D: MR hysterosalpingography: protocol development and refinement for simulating a normal and abnormal fallopian tube patency—feasibility study with a phantom. *Radiology* 214: 107–112, 2000.

130. Schwartz LB, Panageas E, Lange R, et al.: Female pelvis: Impact of MR imaging on treatment decisions and net cost analysis. *Radiology* 192: 55–60, 1994.

131. Yu KK, Hricak H: Can MRI of the pelvis be cost effective? *Abdom Imaging* 22: 587–601, 1997.

132. Hardesty LA, Sumkin JH, Nath ME, et al.: Use of preoperative MR imaging in the management of endometrial carcinoma: Cost analysis. *Radiology* 215: 45–9, 2000.

Figure Credits

The following figures were first published in *MRI of the Abdomen and Pelvis: A Text-Atlas* (1997). Richard C. Semelka, Susan M. Ascher, and Caroline Reinhold. Wiley-Liss, Inc., New York.

Figure 4.1e	Figure 4.26a	Figure 4.51a	Figure 4.83c
Figure 4.1f	Figure 4.26b	Figure 4.51b	Figure 4.86a
Figure 4.1g	Figure 4.26c	Figure 4.51c	Figure 4.86b
Figure 4.1h	Figure 4.26d	Figure 4.51d	Figure 4.86c
Figure 4.1i	Figure 4.26e	Figure 4.51e	Figure 4.86d
Figure 4.1j	Figure 4.26f	Figure 4.52	Figure 4.88a
Figure 4.1k	Figure 4.27a	Figure 4.54a	Figure 4.88b
Figure 4.1l	Figure 4.27b	Figure 4.54b	Figure 4.88c
Figure 4.1m	Figure 4.27c	Figure 4.54c	Figure 4.88d
Figure 4.1n	Figure 4.30j	Figure 4.54d	Figure 4.89a
Figure 4.1o	Figure 4.30k	Figure 4.57a	Figure 4.89b
Figure 4.2b	Figure 4.35a	Figure 4.57b	Figure 4.89c
Figure 4.3c	Figure 4.35b	Figure 4.57c	Figure 4.89d
Figure 4.2d	Figure 4.35c	Figure 4.57d	Figure 5.1a
Figure 4.2e	Figure 4.35d	Figure 4.58a	Figure 5.1b
Figure 4.2f	Figure 4.35e	Figure 4.59a	Figure 5.2a
Figure 4.2g	Figure 4.37a	Figure 4.59b	Figure 5.2b
Figure 4.2h	Figure 4.37b	Figure 4.59c	Figure 5.3
Figure 4.3a	Figure 4.37c	Figure 4.59d	Figure 5.4
Figure 4.3b	Figure 4.37d	Figure 4.59e	Figure 5.5
Figure 4.4a	Figure 4.37e	Figure 4.59f	Figure 5.6a
Figure 4.4b	Figure 4.38a	Figure 4.62	Figure 5.6b
Figure 4.4c	Figure 4.38b	Figure 4.67a	Figure 5.6c
Figure 4.6a	Figure 4.38c	Figure 4.67b	Figure 5.10a
Figure 4.6b	Figure 4.38d	Figure 4.67c	Figure 5.10b
Figure 4.8d	Figure 4.38e	Figure 4.68a	Figure 5.11
Figure 4.8e	Figure 4.38f	Figure 4.68b	Figure 5.12a
Figure 4.8f	Figure 4.38g	Figure 4.68c	Figure 5.12b
Figure 4.8g	Figure 4.39a	Figure 4.68d	Figure 5.12c
Figure 4.8h	Figure 4.39b	Figure 4.68e	Figure 5.13a
Figure 4.8i	Figure 4.39c	Figure 4.68f	Figure 5.13b
Figure 4.8j	Figure 4.40	Figure 4.69a	Figure 5.13c
Figure 4.8k	Figure 4.41a	Figure 4.69b	Figure 5.13d
Figure 4.9a	Figure 4.41b	Figure 4.69c	Figure 5.15a
Figure 4.9b	Figure 4.41c	Figure 4.69d	Figure 5.15b
Figure 4.10a	Figure 4.42f	Figure 4.69e	Figure 5.15c
Figure 4.10b	Figure 4.43a	Figure 4.70a	Figure 5.15d
Figure 4.13a	Figure 4.43b	Figure 4.70b	Figure 5.15e
Figure 4.13b	Figure 4.44a	Figure 4.70c	Figure 5.15f
Figure 4.13c	Figure 4.44b	Figure 4.72a	Figure 5.15g
Figure 4.13d	Figure 4.44c	Figure 4.72b	Figure 5.15h
Figure 4.13e	Figure 4.44d	Figure 4.72c	Figure 5.15i
Figure 4.13f	Figure 4.44e	Figure 4.72d	Figure 5.15j
Figure 4.13g	Figure 4.45a	Figure 4.72e	Figure 5.16a
Figure 4.13h	Figure 4.45b	Figure 4.72f	Figure 5.16b
Figure 4.13i	Figure 4.45c	Figure 4.72g	Figure 5.17a
Figure 4.13j	Figure 4.47a	Figure 4.72h	Figure 5.17b
Figure 4.15a	Figure 4.47b	Figure 4.72i	Figure 5.17c
Figure 4.15b	Figure 4.47c	Figure 4.73a	Figure 5.17d
Figure 4.17a	Figure 4.47d	Figure 4.73b	Figure 5.17e
Figure 4.17b	Figure 4.48a	Figure 4.73c	Figure 5.17f
Figure 4.17c	Figure 4.48b	Figure 4.73d	Figure 5.18
Figure 4.17d	Figure 4.48c	Figure 4.73e	Figure 5.19a
Figure 4.17l	Figure 4.48d	Figure 4.73f	Figure 5.19b
Figure 4.17m	Figure 4.49a	Figure 4.73g	Figure 5.19c
Figure 4.17n	Figure 4.49b	Figure 4.76a	Figure 5.20
Figure 4.22a	Figure 4.49c	Figure 4.76b	Figure 5.21a
Figure 4.22b	Figure 4.49d	Figure 4.76c	Figure 5.21b
Figure 4.22c	Figure 4.50a	Figure 4.83a	Figure 5.21c
Figure 4.22d	Figure 4.50b	Figure 4.83b	Figure 5.23a

Figure 12.10d
Figure 12.10e
Figure 12.11a
Figure 12.11b
Figure 12.11c
Figure 12.12a
Figure 12.12b
Figure 12.13a
Figure 12.15a
Figure 12.15b
Figure 12.15c
Figure 12.15d
Figure 12.15e
Figure 12.15f
Figure 12.16a
Figure 12.17
Figure 12.23
Figure 12.25a
Figure 12.25b
Figure 12.26
Figure 12.27
Figure 12.29
Figure 12.31a
Figure 12.31b
Figure 12.32b
Figure 12.32c
Figure 12.32d
Figure 12.33
Figure 12.34a
Figure 12.35a
Figure 12.35b
Figure 12.35c
Figure 12.35d
Figure 12.36
Figure 12.37a
Figure 12.37b
Figure 12.37c
Figure 12.37d
Figure 12.38a
Figure 12.38b
Figure 12.39a
Figure 12.39b
Figure 12.40a
Figure 12.41a
Figure 12.41b
Figure 12.41c
Figure 12.41d
Figure 12.41e
Figure 12.41f
Figure 12.41g
Figure 12.41h
Figure 12.41i
Figure 12.41j
Figure 12.41k
Figure 12.41l
Figure 12.41m
Figure 12.43a
Figure 12.43b
Figure 12.43c
Figure 12.44a
Figure 12.44b
Figure 13.1c
Figure 13.5a
Figure 13.5b
Figure 13.7c
Figure 13.8a

Figure 13.8b
Figure 13.9
Figure 13.10c
Figure 13.10d
Figure 13.10e
Figure 13.10f
Figure 13.12
Figure 13.13c
Figure 13.13d
Figure 13.13e
Figure 13.18a
Figure 13.18b
Figure 13.20d
Figure 13.21
Figure 13.23a
Figure 13.23b
Figure 13.23c
Figure 13.24
Figure 13.25b
Figure 13.25c
Figure 13.25d
Figure 14.4
Figure 14.10a
Figure 14.10b
Figure 14.10c
Figure 14.10d
Figure 14.12a
Figure 14.34a
Figure 14.34b
Figure 14.34c
Figure 14.34d
Figure 14.34e
Figure 14.35a
Figure 14.35b
Figure 14.50a
Figure 14.50b
Figure 14.57a
Figure 14.57b
Figure 14.58
Figure 14.60a
Figure 14.60b
Figure 14.60c
Figure 14.61
Figure 14.62a
Figure 14.62b
Figure 14.64a
Figure 14.64b
Figure 14.65
Figure 14.71
Figure 14.73a
Figure 14.73b
Figure 14.73c
Figure 14.78e
Figure 14.78f
Figure 14.79a
Figure 14.79b
Figure 14.79c
Figure 14.79d
Figure 14.79e
Figure 14.80
Figure 15.1a
Figure 15.1b
Figure 15.1c
Figure 15.1d
Figure 15.2a
Figure 15.2b

Figure 15.2c
Figure 15.2d
Figure 15.3a
Figure 15.3b
Figure 15.4a
Figure 15.4b
Figure 15.4c
Figure 15.4d
Figure 15.4e
Figure 15.5a
Figure 15.5b
Figure 15.6a
Figure 15.6b
Figure 15.6c
Figure 15.6d
Figure 15.6e
Figure 15.8a
Figure 15.8b
Figure 15.8c
Figure 15.8d
Figure 15.8e
Figure 15.8f
Figure 15.8g
Figure 15.8h
Figure 15.8i
Figure 15.8j
Figure 15.8k
Figure 15.8l
Figure 15.10a
Figure 15.10b
Figure 15.10c
Figure 15.10d
Figure 15.10e
Figure 15.11a
Figure 15.11b
Figure 15.11c
Figure 15.12a
Figure 15.12b
Figure 15.12c
Figure 15.12d
Figure 15.12e
Figure 15.12f
Figure 15.12g
Figure 15.12h
Figure 15.12i
Figure 15.12j
Figure 15.12k
Figure 15.12l
Figure 15.12m
Figure 15.12n
Figure 15.12o
Figure 15.12p
Figure 15.12q
Figure 15.12r
Figure 15.12s
Figure 15.13a
Figure 15.13b
Figure 15.13c
Figure 15.13d
Figure 15.13e
Figure 15.13f
Figure 15.13g
Figure 15.13h
Figure 15.14a
Figure 15.14b
Figure 15.14c

Figure 15.14d
Figure 15.15a
Figure 15.15b
Figure 15.16a
Figure 15.16b
Figure 15.16c
Figure 15.16d
Figure 15.16e
Figure 15.16f
Figure 15.16g
Figure 15.16h
Figure 15.16i
Figure 15.17a
Figure 15.17b
Figure 15.17c
Figure 15.17d
Figure 15.17e
Figure 15.17f
Figure 15.17g
Figure 15.18a
Figure 15.18b
Figure 15.18c
Figure 15.18d
Figure 15.18e
Figure 15.18f
Figure 15.18g
Figure 15.20a
Figure 15.20b
Figure 15.21a
Figure 15.21b
Figure 15.21c
Figure 15.21d
Figure 15.21e
Figure 15.21f
Figure 15.21g
Figure 15.21h
Figure 15.22a
Figure 15.22b
Figure 15.22c
Figure 15.22d
Figure 15.22e
Figure 15.23a
Figure 15.23b
Figure 15.23c
Figure 15.23d
Figure 15.26a
Figure 15.26b
Figure 15.26c
Figure 15.26d
Figure 15.26e
Figure 15.26f
Figure 15.26g
Figure 15.26h
Figure 15.26i
Figure 15.26j
Figure 15.26k
Figure 15.26l
Figure 15.26m
Figure 15.26n
Figure 15.27a
Figure 15.27b
Figure 15.27c
Figure 15.27d
Figure 15.28a
Figure 15.28b
Figure 15.28c

INDEX